The Little Black Book of Neu

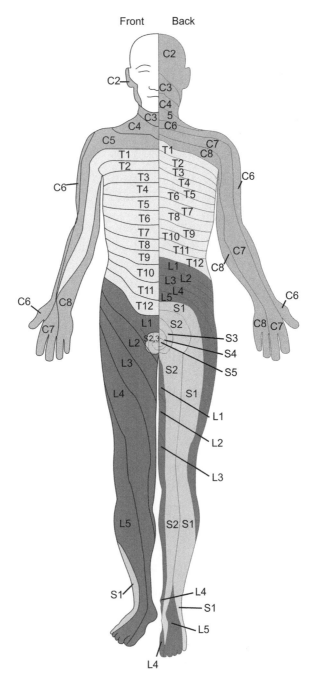

Anterior and Posterior Views of the Human Dermatomes

Mike R. Schoenberg · James G. Scott
Editors

The Little Black Book
of Neuropsychology

A Syndrome-Based Approach

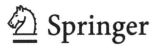 Springer

Editors

Mike R. Schoenberg
University of South Florida
College of Medicine
Departments of Psychiatry and
Neurosciences, Neurology, and
Neurosurgery
Tampa, Florida
USA
mschoenb@health.usf.edu

James G. Scott
University of Oklahoma
Health Sciences Center
College of Medicine
Departments of Psychiatry and
Behavioral Sciences
Oklahoma City, Oklahoma
USA
jim-scott@ouhsc.edu

ISBN 978-0-387-70703-7   e-ISBN 978-0-387-76978-3
DOI 10.1007/978-0-387-76978-3
Springer New York Dordrecht Heidelberg London

Printed on acid-free paper

Springer is part of Springer Science+Business Media (www.springer.com)

Acknowledgments

This book would not have been possible without the encouragement of Mariann Suarez. The assistance, wisdom and guidance of Jim Scott, my co-editor, allowed me to laugh when things seemed darkest, and the book would not have been finished without his friendship and support. I would also like to thank the contributing authors to this book. The breadth and depth of knowledge and expertise brought to this volume frankly astounds me. A special thanks to Grant Iverson who contributed to several substantive areas. A note of gratitude to the many colleagues who have shaped my thinking about neuropsychology, including Russell Adams, Lyle Baade, Darwin Dorr, Kevin Duff, Philip Fastenau, Herman Jones, Jim Scott, Mary Ann Werz, and David (DJ) Williamson. A dedication to Bob Maciunas, a true friend, pinnacle of professional integrity, and perhaps the smartest and most genuine individual I have ever known. Continue to conquer the world, my friend! A nod of appreciation to Patrick Marsh, friend and an expert in handling professional and personal life challenges. Finally, I would like to thank Janice Stern for her unending support, advice, encouragement and nudges to complete the work.

Mike R. Schoenberg

Thanks first to my spouse (Vickie) and children (Remi and Logan) who made as many sacrifices in this effort as I did. Also, a big thanks to my co-editor who sowed the seed for the book, weeded, fertilized, and made gardening fun. A big thank you to all our contributors not only for your excellent contributions but for your indulgence of Mike and I as we asked for additions, deletions and re-writes. I also want to thank those behind the scene who were my mentors, including F. William Black, Oscar Parsons, Russell Adams, and Herman Jones. While I have benefited from being taught by many in neuropsychology, your teaching continues to give me inspiration. I would be remiss if I didn't thank all the neuropsychology interns and postdoctoral fellows with whom it has been my pleasure to work over the years (many of whom are represented on the title pages of this volume). You have all reinforced my belief that learning really is a two-way street.

Jim Scott

The editors thank Elena DuPont, Cleveland, OH, USA and Tina Pavlatos of Visual Anatomy Limited, Springfield, OH, USA for the original artwork appearing in this volume. Elena provided some initial artwork and encouraged us to contact Tina as the project increased in scope. Tina was responsible for the majority of artwork in this volume and provided indispensable recommendations for illustrating various neuropsychological concepts.

Preface

Neuropsychology is the study of brain–behavior relationships. This book attempts to provide a general review of the science and clinical practice of neuropsychology. The book was designed to offer those interested in neuropsychology a reference guide in the tradition of pocket references in medicine subspecialities. As such, information is presented to aide in the development of, and maintenance of, evidenced-based clinical neuropsychology practice (Chelune 2010).

Neuropsychology practice and science has exhibited an exponential growth to assist in the diagnosis and treatment of known or suspected dysfunction of the central nervous system. The clinical application of neuropsychological evaluation has increased in a variety of settings, including primary care offices, acute care (e.g., emergency departments, intensive care centers, acute trauma centers) as well as a multitude of tertiary care and rehabilitation centers. Furthermore, the research application of neuropsychology has expanded, with increased emphasis in measures of cognitive, behavioral and emotional functions (attention/executive, memory, language, visuoperceptual, and/or mood/affect) as important end points in a variety of treatment and research areas. Assessment of neuropsychological functions among individuals with diseases that are known or suspected to affect the central nervous system has become increasingly integrated in the management of patient health care. Furthermore, neuropsychological evaluation has become increasingly important in studies evaluating the effectiveness of pharmacologic and surgical therapies. Measurement of cognitive functions is also being used to assess for neuropsychological processes that may be early signs of disease or a marker for a disease course or outcome. In addition to scientific application of neuropsychological assessment to better understand brain processes, markers of disease, evaluate treatment course, or predict outcome, these data guide the emergence of evidenced-based clinical neuropsychology practice, and are being increasingly applied to clinical and forensic applications. Over the past decade, neuropsychological evaluations have become important in legal proceedings to assist in understanding the cause and ramifications of known or suspected central nervous system dysfunction on behavior, emotion and cognition, including decision-making and judgment.

Neuropsychological science has expanded at a breakneck pace, with an ever-increasing understanding of the processes underlying traditionally held models of neuropsychological functioning, such that new models for learning and memory, visuoperceptual, and executive functions have emerged (e.g., Lezak et al. 2004; Heilman et al. 2007; Strauss et al. 2006). There has also been an evolution in task engagement or effort on testing, with a sea change in the appreciation of the impact of task engagement on neuropsychological evaluations, changing theories of dissimulation, somatization, and test taking effort, and in the development of measures to assess test taking effort (e.g., see Lezak et al. 2004; Strauss et al. 2006 for review). Finally, neuropsychology has seen the increasing emphasis on evidenced-based neuropsychology practice (Chelune 2010). With these advancements come increasing complexity. Neuropsychological practice has emerged as a true psychological subspecialty, requiring unique training and qualifications (e.g., Hannay et al. 1998; Reports of the INS-Division 40 task force on education, accreditation, and credentialing 1987). However, the practice of neuropsychology is not limited to clinical psychologists. The assessment of neuropsychological functions is routinely evaluated by various physician specialties including neurologists, neurological surgeons, and psychiatrists. This book aims to address the needs of licensed practitioners and to provide an overview of neuropsychology practice and science to medical and healthcare specialties having an interest in neuropsychology assessment. To meet these goals, the first three chapters provide an overview for understanding referrals from healthcare providers, how to read the medical chart when conducting a neuropsychological evaluation, and a primer to the clinical neuropsychologist for understanding the common short-hand and little notations made by physicians and nurses so often seen in the medical chart. For physicians in training (medical students, residents, and fellows), we include a special section in Chap. 1 about how to understand and interpret a neuropsychological evaluation report, what the qualitative descriptors mean to neuropsychologists, and the basic premises and theories underlying clinical neurpsychological practice. Chapter 3 provides a review of functional neuroanatomy.

A unique aspect of this book is neuropsychology science and practice is approached from two different perspectives. The first section of this book approaches neuropsychological evaluations from a presenting symptoms perspective. We believe the first section is particularly well suited to clinicians faced with common clinical practices. There is a patient referred for a clinical neuropsychological evaluation, and the diagnosis is unknown. What assessment procedures should be implemented and based on the history, behavioral observations, and obtained neuropsychological data, what might the clinician determine? Thus, the clinician may review chapters about attention problems (see Chaps. 4, 5, and 6) and/or forgetfulness (Chaps. 8 and 10) to obtain helpful assessment procedures which is then followed by diseases or neuroanatomical correlates of observed behavior and test scores. This provides a neuropsychological method to systematically assess cognitive and behavioral signs and symptoms in order to formulate hypothesis about lesion lateralization, localization, and diagnosis within a brief, consultative assessment framework. This, we believe, is complementary to the great tradition of neurology in which the question of where is the lesion leads to differential diagnoses of the etiology for the lesion.

The next section is a more traditional approach to neuropsychology principals and science, in which the diagnosis is specified (e.g., epilepsy, dementia, or stroke), and the neuropsychological evaluations attempts to answer questions based on this diagnosis. Thus, these chapters provide an overview of the disease states and how these may present clinically. Special emphasis is given to neuropsychological features of diseases, giving recommendations for assessment procedures and data to assist interpretation. Each chapter is designed with comprehensive neuropsychological evaluations in mind, with the authors providing their clinical pearls, recommendations of the neuropsychological, neurological, and psychological domains to assess as well as helpful clinical information such as Reliable Change Indices (RCI's, Jacobson and Truax 1991; Chelune et al. 1993) when these are available as of January 2009.

The book includes another section for the neuropsychologist, which is also likely to be of interest to consumers of neuropsychological evaluations (e.g., physicians, nurses, social workers, and our patients). A section includes a practical review of psychometrics including a clinically focused overview of measurement of change in cognitive functioning over time, RCIs, and issues about validity and common errors in interpreting neuropsychological data. Increasing sophistication in the measurement of neuropsychological processes and associated psychometrics along with better appreciation for the natural variation in neuropsychological function among healthy individuals has led to an evolution for the interpretation of neuropsychological data to identify disease. Chapters explicitly review methods to interpret neuropsychological data founded in psychometric principles and neuropathologic science, and subsequently to integrate data to improve the diagnostic accuracy of making diagnoses of neuropsychological impairment (i.e., cognitive disorders). In addition, this text provides a brief review of emerging technologies in the application of neuropsychological evaluation in rehabilitation and how an empirically validated intervention for changing a variety of health behaviors, termed Motivational Interviewing (Miller and Rollnick 2002, 2009), may be applied to neuropsychology practice. Collectively, we strongly believe the material provided this book provides a foundation for the clinician in evidence-based clinical neuropsychological practice.

References

American Board of Clinical Neuropsychology (2007). American Academy of Clinical Neuropsychology (AACN) practice guidelines for neuropsychological assessment and consultation. *The Clinical Neuropsychologist, 21*, 209–231.

Bush, S. S., Ruff, R. M., Troster, A. I., Barth, J. T., Koffler, S. P., Pliskin, N. H., Reynolds, C. R., & Silver, C. H. (2005). Symptom validity assessment: Practice issues and medical necessity. NAN Polocy and Planning Committee. *Archives of Clinical Neuropsychology, 20*, 419–426.

Chelune, G. J. (2003). Assessing reliable neuropsychological change. In R. D. Franklin (Ed.), *Prediction in forensic and neuropsychology: Sound statistical practices* (pp. 65–88). Mahwah, NJ: Lawrence Erlbaum Associates.

Chelune, G. J. (2010). Evidenced-based research and practice in clinical neuropsychology. *The Clinical Neuropsychologist*, *24*, 454–467.

Hannay, H. J., Bieliauskas, L. A., Crosson, B. A., Hammeke, T. A., Hamsher, K. DeS., & Koffler, S. P. (1998). Policy statement. Proceedings of the Houston conference on specialty education and training in clinical neuropsychology. *Archives of Clinical Neuropsychology*, *13*, 160–166.

Heilman, K. M., & Valenstein, E. (2007). *Clinical neuropsychology* (4th ed.). New York: Oxford University Press.

Jacobson, N. S., & Truax, P. (1991). Clinical significance: A statistical approach to defining meaningful change in psychotherapy research. *Journal of Consulting and Clinical Psychology*, *59*(1), 12–19.

Lezak, M. D., Howieson, D. B., & Loring, D. W. (2004). *Neuropsychological assessment* (4th ed.). New York: Oxford University Press.

Miller, W. R., & Rollnick, S. R. (2002). *Motivational interviewing: Preparing people for change* (2nd ed.). New York: Guilford Press.

Miller, W. R., & Rollnick, S. R. (2009). Ten things that motivational Interviewing is not. *Behavioural and Cognitive Psychotherapy*, *37*, 129–140.

Reports of the INS-Division 40 task force on education, accreditation, and credentialing (1987). *The Clinical Neuropsychologist*, *1*, 29–34.

Strauss, E., Sherman, E. M. S., & Spreen, O. (2006). *A compendium of neuropsychological tests: Administration, norms, and commentary* (3rd ed.). New York: Oxford University Press.

Contents

1 The Neuropsychology Referral and Answering the Referral Question 1
Mike R. Schoenberg and James G. Scott

2 Deconstructing the Medical Chart 39
Alan J. Lerner and Mike R. Schoenberg

3 Neuroanatomy Primer: Structure and Function of the Human Nervous System 59
Mike R. Schoenberg, Patrick J. Marsh, and Alan J. Lerner

4 Components of the Neuropsychological Evaluation 127
James G. Scott

5 Arousal: The Disoriented, Stuporous, Agitated or Somnolent Patient 139
James G. Scott

6 Attention/Concentration: The Distractible Patient 149
James G. Scott

7 Language Problems and Assessment: The Aphasic Patient 159
James G. Scott and Mike R. Schoenberg

8 Memory and Learning: The Forgetful Patient 179
James G. Scott and Mike R. Schoenberg

9 Deficits in Visuospatial/Visuoconstructional Skills and Motor Praxis 201
James G. Scott and Mike R. Schoenberg

10   Frontal Lobe/Executive Functioning... 219
James G. Scott and Mike R. Schoenberg

11   Affect, Emotions and Mood 249
James G. Scott and Mike R. Schoenberg

12   Aphasia Syndromes... 267
Mike R. Schoenberg and James G. Scott

13   Cerebrovascular Disease and Stroke... 293
Cathy Sila and Mike R. Schoenberg

14   Dementias and Mild Cognitive Impairment in Adults 357
Mike R. Schoenberg and Kevin Duff

15   Episodic Neurologic Symptoms 405
Heber Varela and Selim R. Benbadis

16   Epilepsy and Seizures 423
Mike R. Schoenberg, Mary Ann Werz, and Daniel L. Drane

17   Neuropsychology of Psychogenic Nonepileptic Seizures 521
Daniel L. Drane, Erica L. Coady, David J. Williamson,
John W. Miller, and Selim Benbadis

**18   Somatoform Disorders, Factitious Disorder,
and Malingering**.. 551
Kyle Boone

19   Parkinson's Disease and Other Movement Disorders 567
Steven A. Gunzler, Mike R. Schoenberg, David E. Riley,
Benjamin Walter, and Robert J. Maciunas

20   Multiple Sclerosis and Other Demyelinating Disorders..................... 647
Julie A. Bobholz and Shelley Gremley

21   Moderate and Severe Traumatic Brain Injury 663
Grant L. Iverson and Rael T. Lange

22   Mild Traumatic Brain Injury.. 697
Grant L. Iverson and Rael T. Lange

23   Sport-Related Concussion 721
Grant L. Iverson

24 Post-Concussion Syndrome.. 745
Grant L. Iverson and Rael T. Lange

25 Pediatric Traumatic Brain Injury (TBI): Overview........................... 765
Cathy Catroppa and Vicki A. Anderson

26 Brain Tumors.. 787
Kyle E. Ferguson, Grant L. Iverson, and Mike R. Schoenberg

27 Neurotoxicity in Neuropsychology.. 813
Raymond Singer

28 Cognitive Decline in Childhood or Young Adulthood........................ 839
Mike R. Schoenberg and James G. Scott

**29 Application of Motivational Interviewing
    to Neuropsychology Practice: A New Frontier
    for Evaluations and Rehabilitation**... 863
Mariann Suarez

30 Reliability and Validity in Neuropsychology....................................... 873
Elisabeth M.S. Sherman, Brian L. Brooks, Grant L. Iverson,
Daniel J. Slick, and Esther Strauss

**31 Psychometric Foundations for the Interpretation
    of Neuropsychological Test Results**.. 893
Brian L. Brooks, Elisabeth M.S. Sherman, Grant L. Iverson,
Daniel J. Slick, and Esther Strauss

32 Improving Accuracy for Identifying Cognitive Impairment.............. 923
Grant L. Iverson and Brian L. Brooks

Index.. 951

Contributors

Vicki A. Anderson
Department of Psychology, Australian Centre for Child Neuropsychology Studies, Murdoch Children's Research Institute, Royal Children's Hospital, University of Melbourne, Parkville, Melbourne, Australia
Vicki.anderson@rch.org.au

Selim R. Benbadis
Department of Neurology, University of South Florida College of Medicine and Tampa General Hospital, Tampa, FL, USA
sbenbadi@health.usf.edu

Julie A. Bobholz
Department of Neurology, Medical College of Wisconsin, Milwaukee, WI, USA
and
Alexian Neurosciences Institute, Elk Grove Village, IL, USA
jbobholz@mcw.edu

Kyle Boone
Center for Forensic Studies, Alliant International University, Alhambra, CA, USA
kboone@alliant.edu

Brian L. Brooks
Alberta Children's Hospital, University of Calgary, Calgary, AB, Canada
brian.brooks@albertahealthservices.ca

Cathy Catroppa
Department of Psychology, Australian Centre for Child Neuropsychology Studies, Murdoch Children's Research Institute, Royal Children's Hospital, University of Melbourne, Parkville, Melbourne, Australia
cathy.catroppa@mcri.edu.au

Erica L. Coady
MINCEP Epilepsy Care, Minneapolis, MN, USA
coadye@gmail.com

Daniel L. Drane
Assistant Professor, Department of Neurology, Emory University
School of Medicine, Atlanta, GA, USA
and
Adjunct Professor, Department of Neurology,
University Washington School of Medicine, Seattle, WA, USA
ddrane@emory.edu

Kevin Duff
Department of Neurology, University of Utah School of Medicine,
Salt Lake City, UT, USA
Kevin.Duff@hsc.utah.edu

Kyle E. Ferguson
British Columbia Mental Health & Addiction Services & University of Nevada,
Reno, NV, USA
KFerguson@bcmha.bc.ca

Shelley Gremley
Alexian Neurosciences Institute, Elk Grove Village, IL, USA
gremleys@alexian.net

Steven A. Gunzler
Department of Neurology, The Neurological Institute, University Hospitals Case
Medical Center and Case Western Reserve University School of Medicine,
Cleveland, OH, USA
Steven.Gunzler@UHhospitals.org

Grant L. Iverson
University of British Columbia, Vancouver, BC, Canada
and
British Columbia Mental Health and Addiction Services, Coquitlam, BC, Canada
giverson@interchange.ubc.ca

Rael T. Lange
British Columbia Mental Health and Addiction Services, Coquitlam, BC, Canada
rlange@dvbic.org

Alan J. Lerner
Department of Neurology, The Neurological Institute, University Hospitals Case
Medical Center and Case Western Reserve Unviersity School of Medicine,
Cleveland, OH, USA
Alan.Lerner@UHhospitals.org

Robert J. Maciunas
Department of Neurological Surgery, The Neurological Institute, University
Hospitals Case Medical Center and Case Western Reserve University School of
Medicine, Cleveland, OH, USA
Robert.Maciunas@UHhospials.org

Patrick J. Marsh
Department of Psychiatry and Neurosciences, University of South Florida
College of Medicine, Tampa, FL, USA
pmarsh@health.usf.edu

John W. Miller
Department of Neurology, University of Washington School of Medicine,
Seattle, WA, USA
millerjw@u.washington.edu

David E. Riley
Department of Neurology, The Neurological Institute, University Hospitals Case
Medical Center and Case Western Reserve Unviersity School of Medicine,
Cleveland, OH, USA
David.Riley@UHhospitals.org

Mike R. Schoenberg
Departments of Psychiatry and Neurosciences, Neurology, and Neurosurgery,
University of South Florida College of Medicine, Tampa, FL, USA
mschoenb@health.usf.edu

James G. Scott
Department of Psychiatry and Behavioral Sciences, University of Oklahoma
Health Sciences Center College of Medicine, Oklahoma City, Oklahoma, USA
jim-scott@ouhsc.edu

Elisabeth M.S. Sherman
Alberta Children's Hospital, University of Calgary, Calgary, AB, Canada
elisabeth.sherman@albertahealthservices.ca

Cathy Sila
Department of Neurology, The Neurological Institute, University Hospitals Case
Medical Center and Case Western Reserve University School of Medicine,
Cleveland, OH, USA
Cathy.Sila@UHhospitals.org

Raymond Singer
Sante Fe, New Mexico, USA
ray.singer@gmail.com

Daniel J. Slick
Alberta Children's Hospital, University of Calgary, Calgary, AB, Canada
daniel.slick@albertahealthservices.ca

Esther Strauss
Department of Psychology, University of Victoria, Victoria, BC, Canada
estrauss@uvic.ca

Mariann Suarez
Department of Psychiatry and Neurosciences, University of South Florida College
of Medicine, Tampa, FL, USA
msuarez1@health.usf.edu

Heber Varela
Department of Neurology, University of South Florida College of Medicine
and James A. Haley Veterans Affairs Medical Center, Tampa, FL, USA
heberluis@yahoo.com

Benjamin Walter
Department of Neurology, The Neurological Institute, University Hospitals Case
Medical Center and Case Western Reserve University School of Medicine,
Cleveland, OH, USA
Benjamin.Walter@UHhospitals.org

Mary Ann Werz
Department of Neurology, University of Iowa Carver School of Medicine,
Iowa City, IA, USA
mary-werz@uiowa.edu

David J. Williamson
Ortho-McNeil Janssen Scientific Affairs, LLC, Mobile, AL, USA
dj.williamson@alumni.duke.edu

Chapter 1
The Neuropsychology Referral and Answering the Referral Question

Mike R. Schoenberg and James G. Scott

Abstract Neuropsychological evaluations provide a wealth of information to the referring clinician and patient, offering a host of answers to important diagnostic and treatment-related questions. The range of questions a neuropsychological evaluation can answer are broad, but generally fall under six broad categories (e.g., Lezak et al., Neuropsychological assessment, 4th edn. Oxford University Press, New York, 2004):

1. Diagnoses: Identifying the existence of brain dysfunction [and differentiating brain dysfunction from non-lesional psychiatric diagnosis or otherwise reversible causes of cognitive dysfunction (e.g., depression)].
   - *Example*: Distinguishing dementia from depression or identifying the presence of mild cognitive impairment (MCI).
2. Describing neuropsychological status: Detailing how a disease or lesion(s) is expressed from cognitive, behavioral and affective perspectives.
   - *Example*: Describing how a traumatic brain injury (TBI) has affected a patient's cognitive and emotional functioning, including the severity and extent of neuropsychological deficits.
3. Treatment planning, treatment facility placement or evaluating for resource utilization.
   - *Example*: Identifying if a patient meets inclusion/exclusion criteria for placement in a rehabilitation facility. An increasing emphasis within neuropsychology is predicting neuropsychological outcome from proposed medical treatment (e.g., temporal lobectomy for intractable epilepsy or DBS for Parkinson's disease).
4. Identifying the effects of treatment (often includes measuring change in function over time).
   - *Example*: Evaluation of effects of a speech/language therapy program for a patient.
5. Research evaluation tool: Identifying basic and central nervous system processes and/or the effects of other agents on the central nervous system.
   - *Example*: Evaluating the neuropsychological effects of a medication to treat epilepsy in a randomized controlled trial.

M.R. Schoenberg (✉)
University of South Florida College of Medicine, Tampa, FL, USA
e-mail: mschoenb@health.usf.edu

M.R. Schoenberg and J.G. Scott (eds.), *The Little Black Book of Neuropsychology: A Syndrome-Based Approach*, DOI 10.1007/978-0-387-76978-3_1,
© Springer Science+Business Media, LLC 2011

6. Forensic applications: Neuropsychological evaluations are increasingly being used to assist fact-finding bodies to determine if, or the extent to which, an alleged event resulted in damage to the CNS. Another use is to assist courts in evaluating if a defendant is capable of managing his/her affairs independently. Also used forensically to evaluate mental state/competence/decision making capacity of individuals, particularly those alleged to be involved in criminal activities

---

Key Points and Chapter Summary

- Neuropsychology is the study of brain–behavior relationships
- Neuropsychology evaluations provide unique information about a person's cognitive and behavioral functioning that is quantified and medically necessary, and can be essential for (1) diagnosis (e.g., Mild Cognitive Impairment), (2) describing neuropsychological status, (3) treatment planning/program placement, (4) monitoring effect of treatment(s), (5) the identification of underlying processes for cognition and/or effects of treatments/other agents, and (6) forensic applications.
- Referring health providers for neuropsychological consult should clearly identify the purpose of the referral (i.e., identify the referral question(s) the neuropsychological study is to answer).
- Neuropsychological report should clearly specify if the neuropsychological study is abnormal (vs normal), recommendations based on referral question(s), and in most cases, diagnosis.
- Neuropsychological consult reports will typically: (1) characterize cognitive and behavioral deficits and strengths, (2) relate deficits to functional neuroanatomy, (3) provide diagnostic considerations, and (4) offer etiology for neuropsychological deficits.
- Interpretation of the neuropsychological study and study results should be communicated to the patient in most cases.
- Conclusions as to presence or absence of neuropsychological deficits are based upon deficit measurement which requires that a comparison standard be established. The comparison standard is used as a benchmark against which current performance is compared to determine the presence or absence of neuropsychological deficits.
- Comparison standard may be of two broad types: (1) normative comparison standards (i.e., population average or species wide expectations) or (2) individual comparison standards (i.e., using individual factors such as education, occupation, and/or previous indicators of cognitive ability).
- Neuropsychological studies are increasingly part of medico-legal proceedings, including questions of competence and functional capacity, and evaluation is used to quantify functioning across cognitive, behavioral and emotional domains as they relate to forensic issues.

Evidenced Based Neuropsychological Practice

The unique information provided by neuropsychological evaluations identified above has been demonstrated to impact the management of patients (and claimants in medico-legal contexts) and improve patient outcomes, an essential component for evidence-based medicine and evidence-based clinical neuropsychology practice (Chelune 2010). Evidence-based neuropsychological practice (EBNP) (we prefer not using "clinical" as a descriptor, and think evidence-based neuropsychology is sufficient) is emerging to provide guidelines for neuropsychologists to integrate outcomes research, clinical expertise, the unique aspects of the patient, referral questions, and available costs and resources to the provision of neuropsychology services.

As a new diagnostic tool, the neuropsychological examination can contribute essential information of cognitive and/or behavioral dysfunction that is required to make a diagnosis [e.g., dementia and/or mild cognitive impairment (MCI), learning disorders, intellectual disability, HIV-associated mild neurocognitive disorder, mild traumatic brain injury, and toxic encephalopathies]. The description of the type and extent of neuropsychological dysfunction can provide indispensable information to health providers for patient management and/or clinical research. For example, even when the lesion and its etiology are known, the neuropsychological evaluation offers *unique* information as to the type and severity of cognitive or behavioral problems the individual exhibits, and how the patient's functioning may affect his/her ability for self-care, follow medical recommendations, and/or complete activities of daily living (ADLs). Because of individual variability in functional neuroanatomy and disease characteristics, the expression of similar left hemisphere strokes involving the middle cerebral artery can vary substantially from patient to patient (see Heilman and Valenstein 2003; Lezak et al. 2004; Mesulam 2000; Ropper and Samuels 2009, for reviews). Thus, while it may be known a patient has disease (e.g., Parkinson's disease, epilepsy, or a traumatic brain injury), the impact of the disease or lesion on the patient's cognitive functioning and behavior may *only* be objectively quantified through neuropsychological assessment.

Finally, the neuropsychological evaluation can provide predictive information with respect to outcome from a suspected or known condition. As an example, neuropsychological variables are predictive of a variety of functional outcomes (return to work, school, living independently, etc.) following traumatic brain injury (Ponsford et al. 2008; Ross et al. 1997; Sherer et al. 2002). Likewise, neuropsychological evaluations can predict cognitive outcome from temporal lobectomy (e.g., Chelune 1995; Chelune and Najm 2001; Davies et al. 1998; Hermann et al. 1999; Lineweaver et al. 2006), contribute unique variance to identifying laterality of seizure focus (Busch et al. 2005; Drane et al. 2006) and to predicting the likelihood a patient will be seizure free following temporal lobectomy (e.g., Sawrie et al. 1999). Similarly, neuropsychological data adds unique predictive value to distinguish patients with relapsing remitting multiple sclerosis (MS) from patients with secondarily progressive MS (Chelune and Stone 2005; Chelune 2010). Indeed, neuropsychological results have provided predictive value beyond other neuroimaging and clinical variables to identify those individuals at increased risk for cognitive decline over time (and disease progression) across a variety of medical conditions, such as epilepsy (e.g., Hermann et al. 2007; Seidenberg et al. 2007), multiple sclerosis (e.g., Achiron et al. 2005), Parkinson's disease (e.g., Dujardin et al. 2004), and mild cognitive impairment (e.g., Fleisher et al. 2008) to name a few. Clearly, there is a body of emerging literature supporting evidence-based neuropsychology in a variety of diseases and clinical practice areas.

Description of Neuropsychological Functioning

Neuropsychological evaluations describe an individual's brain–behavior function. However, the neuropsychological evaluation should generally *not* be limited to describing the neuropsychological scores a patient obtained, or simply a patient's cognitive strengths and weaknesses. Rather, the clinical neuropsychologist should state whether (or not) there is evidence for brain dysfunction, the degree of impairment, and relate this description to the patient's functioning (i.e., the individual's level of adjustment, and/or how the individual's needs for care and/or treatment/rehabilitation/educational programming may be affected). Indeed, we argue that providing a detailed description of the patient's neuropsychological functioning, in and of itself, is often the least important aspect of a neuropsychological evaluation. The most important is to relate how the patient's cognitive and emotional functioning is likely to affect their ability to adhere to their treatment, interact within their physical and/or social environment, affect their treatment plan, and/or affect their ability to make decisions, etc. In other words, the neuropsychologist's report answers the consulting clinician's questions by the interpretation, and not just description, of a patient's neuropsychological functions. We also advocate that neuropsychologists follow recommendations of Chelune (2010) for EBNP, and consider base rates for neuropsychological performances such that the frequency of discrepancy among scores and the subsequent interpretation of the pattern of scores is transparent (see also Chap. 32, this volume, by G. Iverson and colleagues, for a systematic, empirically guided approach for diagnosing mild neurocognitive disorder).

Often, a referral question will entail providing an opinion regarding a patient's treatment, ability for self care, and/or challenges to successfully live independently, work, learn, and/or complete activities of daily living. Exceptions to this exist, as in neuropsychological assessments for research purposes or other selected uses, and a brief description of cognitive performances may be sufficient. In general, EBNP dictates that it is essential to identify the explicit referral question(s) that necessitated the assessment procedures, and that the interpretation and recommendations logically flow from the questions in order to form the neuropsychological basis for improving patient care.

Structure and Organization of the Evaluation

At a basic level, the neuropsychological evaluation should provide a written document in which the referral question(s) are clearly answered. We strongly advocate answers to referral questions be clearly specified in a section of the report, often identified as "conclusions" or "diagnostic impressions" (see below). Subsequent recommendations for the patient's care should be clearly specified (see below). In general, the report should identify the following information of service provision:

1. Date and time (when the patient was seen and the report was prepared). The chart should specify the time when the patient was seen and who provided the service
2. What information was used (patient report, report of family member, medical records, etc.)
3. Where information was obtained (from patient, medical records, etc.)
4. Procedures used for the evaluation (tests, interview, sensory-perceputal exam, etc.)
5. Results/conclusions drawn from the assessment data.
6. Whether or not the results were discussed with the patient (and/or caregiver) and to whom the results were provided.
7. Recommendations, which in most circumstances, should be provided to consulting clinician and patient. We also believe it is best practice to obtain consent to provide the consult report to the patient's primary care physician

The neuropsychological evaluation report need not be lengthy. In some cases, a single page report is sufficient. While we do not wish to dictate report formats (as these will be guided by the individual needs of the patient, the providers, and institutional/cultural variables), we provide a sample report format of a routine inpatient consultation in Appendix 1 and a more detailed outpatient evaluation in Appendix 2 to illustrate the headings and organization of reports outlined above. Regardless of the report format one wishes to use, the neuropsychological report should always include answers to the referral questions. These should be clearly labeled. In most cases, the neuropsychologist should first identify the neuropsychological study as normal or abnormal, and the reason why the study was abnormal (a study may also be equivocal, see detailed review below). This will generally involve describing which cognitive or functional domains were impaired. However, this statement should be limited to one or two concise sentences (e.g., "The neuropsychological study was abnormal due to mild impairment in memory and visuoconstructional skills."). The etiology and expected course should be identified along with a statement regarding the confidence of these opinions. This information should then be related to functional capacities specific to the referral source such as medication management, safety to live independently, driving, returning to work/school, and any accommodations/rehabilitation which may be helpful to the patient.

Rule of thumb: Structure of neuropsychological evaluation

- Current complaints and history
- Past medical and psychiatric history
- Psychosocial history
- Medications
- Procedures
- Results
- Conclusions/Interpretation of the data incorporating referral question, patient complaints, and past medical, psychiatric, and psychosocial history
- Diagnosis
- Recommendations, which must answer referral question(s) and incorporate interpretation of data in light of the patient's unique history

How to Answer the Referral Question(s)

To answer the referral question(s), the neuropsychologist must have referral questions to answer. All too often, the referral question is something akin to "evaluate for organicity" or "poor school performance." Often what the referring provider seeks to know is "Are this patient's complaints (or the complaints from others) due to a brain disease or due to psychiatric/psychological/drug problems?" For children, the referral is often "evaluate for learning disorder" or "school problems." A more detailed interpretation of this referral is "Something is wrong with this child as he/she is unable to learn or behave appropriately in school and/or home. Is the problem(s) psychiatric or neurological, and please provide recommendations to identify how to improve the child's academics or decrease undesirable behaviors?" Ideally, the referral question(s) will be more specific, such as "The patient is a surgical candidate for left temporal lobectomy, please determine cognitive functioning and risks to surgery" or "The patient has memory complaints and history of cardiac arrest. Can the patient live alone?" Regardless of the specificity in the referral provided, the neuropsychologist should endeavor to clarify what information is being requested by the referring provider (or entity). In addition, the neuropsychologist should identify how the evaluation can be of assistance to the patient.

It is therefore incumbent upon the neuropsychologist to identify the question(s) of the referral source. In addition, the patient (and/or patient's family) may also have questions they would like answered. We believe it is best to inquire if the patient has any questions the evaluation may assist in answering. In the case of the children and adolescents, it is best to endeavor to answer questions the patient's family may have. We also encourage the neuropsychologist to interpret performance in reference to potential problems and/or recommendations for the child's academic, social, and vocational development. It is typically *not* adequate for the neuropsychological report to describe scores and provide no further interpretation and/or recommendations. The neuropsychologist should always endeavor to interpret the neuropsychological data in the setting of the patient's medical, psychiatric, and social circumstances/history/background and equate these findings to specifically answer the referral question(s). If a neuropsychologist does not believe the evaluation or rehabilitative service is able to answer the referral question(s), the clinical neuropsychologist should discuss this with the referring health care provider.

Responding to Referrals: Timelines as an Important Variable in the Neuropsychological Referral

There are at least two temporal issues in the neuropsychological referral, each impacting the type of referral questions a clinical neuropsychologist can answer. The first aspect of time reflects when a referral is first made for a patient with known or suspected disease onset (i.e., Is the referral made within days to weeks of onset or after months to years of onset?). The second time issue refers to the duration during which symptoms presented (e.g., did symptoms present slowly over months to years, or did the symptoms present over a period of seconds? Did symptom onset appear to wax and wane?). Both aspects of time have broad implications for the clinical neuropsychologist. As an example, referral for evaluation shortly (within hours, days, or in some cases weeks) after the onset of symptoms that presented over several minutes (e.g., embolic stroke) is likely to have different questions and a different assessment approach than the evaluation of a patient having slowly progressive symptoms over several years. The clinical neuropsychologist should carefully consider the likely etiology and course of the condition, designing an assessment appropriately. As an example, a patient sustaining a moderate to severe traumatic brain injury may be assessed with a brief bedside screening to evaluate for post-traumatic amnesia and when declarative memory functions return. Likewise, a referral for neuropsychological evaluation acutely after stroke may be used to guide treatment planning (rehabilitation programming). However, changes in neuropsychological functioning over days, weeks, and even hours should be anticipated, and in most cases, the neuropsychologist will be unable to answer questions about stability of deficits with certainty. Alternatively, patients with mild TBI may be administered a more comprehensive assessment within weeks of the injury, as most individuals neuropsychological functioning have returned to baseline within this time frame. Timing of symptom onset is an important variable, as symptoms occurring insidiously over months to years may lead to a different assessment procedure, and certainly different hypothesis regarding etiology, compared to a patient having symptoms presenting rapidly over the course of minutes, days, or weeks.

Rule of thumb: Answering referral question(s)

- Neuropsychological evaluations must endeavor to answer referral question(s)
- Answers to referral question(s) should be clearly specified
- Time is an important aspect of neuropsychological evaluations in terms of establishing the assessment procedures and the referral question(s) that may be answered by a neuropsychological study
  - Assessment results within days to weeks of acute insult is likely dynamic
  - Assessment results of patient(s) with subacute or chronic loss of function is more stable

The timeline for responding to referrals are often dictated by institutional rules and/or policies. Commonly, inpatient consultations should be responded to within 24–48 hours. Neuropsychological reports for outpatient studies are typically completed within 5–10 working days, but certainly can be more rapid. More detailed evaluations and medico-legal evaluations may be completed over the period of weeks or even months as data are collected from multiple sources.

Providing Results and Recommendations

We recommend the neuropsychological report/evaluation includes a specific section entitled "Conclusions" or "Results" or "Diagnosis." A section entitled "Recommendations" is also encouraged. Often "Conclusions and Recommendations" may be combined, and an example is provided in Appendix 1. Having sections highlighted, particularly the conclusions (and recommendations if separate) will assist the reader quickly identify this crucial information. It is often the only part of the report the referral source will read prior to seeing the patient in follow up, so its importance cannot be overstated. In pediatric cases, reports should be tailored for the referral source which may be the parent or school and must be detailed enough to answer the questions that initiated the referral (i.e. Diagnosis, Educational implications, Behavioral management, etc.).

The "Conclusions (and Recommendations)" section should be short and concise. The neuropsychologist should clearly state his/her interpretation of the obtained data. We advocate a summary sentence specifying if the neuropsychological study was interpreted as "normal," "equivocal" or "abnormal." While this section may include a brief discussion of the neuropsychological scores, this is secondary to interpreting these scores for the intended recipient of the report.

The Conclusions (and Recommendations if combined) section should also include the patient's diagnosis(es). Because neuropsychological evaluations may be completed for either neurological/medical conditions or, in some cases, psychiatric/learning disorder cases, the neuropsychologist needs to assure diagnoses follow logically from the conclusions drawn from the data, and the referral question(s). For example, a neurological diagnosis should be provided when the patient has a neurological disorder, while a psychiatric diagnosis is given when the condition is psychiatric in nature. The clinical neuropsychologist should conform to regional and local practices for reporting diagnostic codes.

The "Recommendations" section, whether incorporated with the Conclusions section or not, should be *concise* and *unambiguous*. We recommend providing recommendations in a point by point fashion. Regardless, recommendations should provide the neuropsychologist's opinions as to what interventions may be of benefit to the patient. The neuropsychological recommendations should integrate ongoing medical and/or psychiatric care. Recommendations for rehabilitation, if any, should flow logically from the interpretation of neuropsychological data and diagnosis. We strongly encourage neuropsychologists working with children and adolescents to always consider the impact neuropsychological data may have on the child's learning and academic/vocational performance. Recommendations for school programming (if made) should be clear and follow state and federal guidelines. Diagnosis of a learning disorder or developmental disorder should be clearly specified, and follow the Diagnostic and Statistical Manual for Mental Disorders, 4th Edition, text revision (DSM-IV-TR; American Psychiatric Association, 2000) guidelines and/or those of the currently accepted language for state and federal programs. If patients – children and adolescents in particular – meet criteria for accommodations at work or school, we recommend the clinical neuropsychologist specify which program(s) or accommodation(s) the patient is likely to benefit from. At present, the current national standards in the U.S. include the Americans with Disabilities Act (1990) and the Individual with Disabilities Education Act. Indeed, such specific recommendations can be crucial for a patient to obtain access to services.

The ADA is a civil rights law forbidding discrimination against persons with disabilities, including learning disabilities. It provides these persons have access and reasonable accommodations in (but not limited to) areas of employment, education, transportation, as well as access to state and local government activities and communication. The IDEA is a federal law specifying how public agencies (federal, state, and local agencies) provide early intervention and special education services to children with identified disabilities. Thus, the IDEA provides rules for addressing the educational needs of children from birth to age 21. The IDEA requires that public schools create an Individual Education Program (IEP) for each student who is found to be eligible under this law, with the specified goal of children being prepared for employment and independent living. In addition, accommodations for older students pursuing college should be requested through the office of student services or the equivalent office.

Rule of thumb: Conclusions and recommendations

- Conclusions and recommendations should be clearly specified in the body of the report.
- Conclusions section should clearly specify if the study is normal, equivocal, or abnormal.
  - Neuropsychological deficits are often associated with functional neuroanatomical correlates.
- Conclusions section general should include diagnosis(es)
- Recommendations, if applicable, should always answer referral question and be concise and clearly state need.

Providing Results to the Patient and Other Users of the Data

In most situations, the patient is the focus of the evaluation, and neuropsychological services are provided to improve the health of the patient. The conclusions (interpretation of the data) of the neuropsychological evaluation should be communicated to the patient's referring provider/entity and to the patient. Without violating HIPAA privacy rules, it is desirable for the neuropsychologist to provide necessary information gained from the neuropsychological evaluation to all those who will be making treatment decisions about the patient. This commonly includes communicating results to the patient's treating physicians and/or other treatment team members. In the case of children (those under the legal age of majority within the neuropsychologist's licensing board or region), results should be communicated to the patient's parents or legal guardian. It is often the case that discussion with the parents about the results will provide a framework in which to provide feedback when the patient is a minor.

When providing results for children to parents (legal guardian), we recommend information be provided that includes:

1. Child's cognitive strengths and weaknesses.
2. Diagnosis(es).
3. Treatment recommendations/treatment plan (if relevant).
4. If other consultation service experts will be recommended to provide additional information and/or clinical correlation to neuropsychological findings.
5. Provide information to parents about short- and long-term potential prognosis.
6. Educate parents about potential local, regional, and/or national resources available to their child.
7. Implications of the findings to the child's academic functioning and any recommendations for school programming. These may then be, if desired by the patient's legal guardian, disclosed to the patient's school/teachers. While the neuropsychologist should clearly identify the child's weaknesses/deficits, emphasis on strengths should be made. If the child meets criteria for learning disorder or qualifies for services through Americans with Disabilities Act or other state or federal rule, this should also be specified.
8. Recommended limitations, if any, for the child. This should include potential risks or impact of comorbid conditions on the child's functioning.

Rule of thumb: Providing recommendations

- In most cases, we advocate the report include a summary of the scores that were used to derive the conclusions and recommendations for care.
  - The inclusion of standardized scores and/or percentile scores can be helpful, while providing raw scores are likely less helpful, except in some cases.
- Evaluations completed as part of independent medical evaluation (IME) and/or court ordered evaluation often may not be released directly to the claimant, but must come from the insurance company or legal entity that requested and paid for the evaluation.
- In medico-legal contexts, the claimant should be fully informed regarding the confidentiality of information that is provided by him/her, and the restrictions on release of the information, including those parties who will have access to the report. Claimant should also be informed that the usual doctor–patient relationship is not established during the course of an IME.
- The claimant should also be informed regarding procedures for requesting a copy of the results.

Releasing the Report/Data

A copy of the report should be included in the patient's chart, and a copy sent to the referring provider/entity. A copy of the report may (and often is) provided to the patient (and in almost all cases, must be if a patient requests it). As part of routine practice, we ask if the patient would like a copy of the report. Under federal and most state laws, the patient (or the patient's lawful health decision maker, if the patient is under the age of majority or found to be unable to make medical decisions) has access to the neuropsychological report, and in most cases, the test scores. While debate continues with respect to what counts as "raw data," it is generally agreed the patient (and/or health decision maker) have access to the test scores. With appropriate release authorization, the patient's report and his/her scores may be released to the patient and/or someone the patient designates.

In medico-legal contexts, and in cases of independent medical evaluations (IMEs), the individual having the neuropsychological evaluation may *not* be the owner of the data. In these instances, the technical owner of the report is the referring agent, be they an attorney, judge, or other agency, and the claimant should be informed before the evaluation that they will not receive a copy of the report from you (assuming no superseding state or federal laws), but rather must solicit a copy from the referring entity/individual. In these cases, a doctor–patient relationship has not been established, and the individual may be denied a copy of the report by the neuropsychologist. Often, the claimant should be directed to the requesting party (e.g., IME business or attorney) to obtain a copy of the report.

Medico-Legal Considerations in Neuropsychological Reports

Neuropsychological evaluations are increasingly requested in legal contexts both criminal and civil. Neuropsychological reports may be requested for the purpose of supporting litigation from the litigant, defense or the court. In these contexts, it is important to remember the goal of evaluation is often greater than providing input into patient care and management, and is used for assignment of damages or attributions of cause of injury or responsibility for criminal behavior. We suggest adopting an approach that considers any neuropsychological evaluation report or consultation possibly becoming an integral part of a legal proceeding, even if it was not expressly so from the initiation of the evaluation. For this reason, we recommend that evaluations address anticipated legal issues in a straightforward and direct manner. We advise asking directly if there are any legal issues pending or anticipated in most cases and, if so, what those issues might be. We caution against going beyond the existing data and/or research literature in making statements regarding the patient's current or expected functioning. The neuropsychologist should be careful to avoid the impression of over reliance on a single piece of data and be considerate of all the data at their disposal when making summary statements and providing recommendations. Issues that may have legal ramifications are considered below.

Rule of thumb: Medico-legal issues in neuropsychology

- The claimant should be informed that the usual treating/evaluate doctor-patient relationship is not established during the course of an Independent Medical Evaluation (IME) and most other forensic settings.
- In medico-legal contexts, the claimant should be fully informed regarding the limits of confidentiality of information that is provided by him/her, and the restrictions on release of the information, including those parties who will have access to the report.
- The claimant should be advised that evaluations completed as part of an IME and/or court ordered evaluation often may not be released directly to the claimant, and release of results/conclusions and/or test data must come from the insurance company or legal entity that requested and paid for the evaluation.
  - In general, we recommend the claimant be informed regarding procedures for requesting a copy of the results.

Issues of Decision-Making Capacity and Competence

Neuropsychological assessment is frequently used to determine decision-making capacity in several areas of functioning. Unlike in legal proceedings in which competence is an absolute issue (and decided by a judge or jury), in neuropsychological assessment, the clinician can often provide opinions about decision-making capacity, which varies by degree and often by function. While a neuropsychologist can assess overall decision-making capacity, and assist the court in making a determination of competence, the issue for the neuropsychologist is rarely absolute. Neuropsychological assessment can often determine decision-making capacity to manage one's own affairs in a legal, medical or financial context and take into consideration the impact of cognitive, behavioral and emotional factors assessed in the neuropsychological evaluation in determining the ability for decision making. It is often the case that while patients retain the basic understanding necessary to participate in decisions within these realms, their cognitive compromises impair their insight into their deficits, which in turn, affects their decision-making capacity. Thus, the presence of neuropsychological deficits adversely affect a patient's ability to appreciate the extent of their neuropsychological deficits, and this anosognosia limits their insight and judgment. For example, a patient with no, or relatively minor, reasoning difficulties but severe memory problems may not be able to enter into legal agreements or make medical decisions without the assistance of others, but is able to fully understand the ramifications of such decisions at the time the decision(s) is/are made.

Issues of Functional Capacities

Neuropsychological evaluations are also crucial in determining multiple functional capacities including driving, working, living independently and management of activities of daily living (dressing, meal preparation, hygiene, medication management, etc.) and instrumental activities of daily living (transportation, financial management, budgeting/shopping, scheduling, etc.). These functional capacities are often the predominant reason for evaluation, and can have significant impact on the patient and their family and support network. The functional capacities in any of these realms can be negatively impacted by cognitive, behavioral or emotional factors assessed in the neuropsychological evaluation and these issues should be addressed directly. The overriding concern in this regard is balancing patient safety, public safety and the rights of the patient to have the least restrictive environment that provides for their needs. The functional capacities of the patient should be evaluated in the context of their available resources and support network. For example, a patient with good insight into their deficits and a compliant history may be able to continue to live independently with only daily supervision and restrictions on travel, cooking and oversight of finances. Similarly, a patient with limited insight and a recent history of poor judgment may need to live in a 24-hours supervised environment with suspension of driving/transportation, provision of meals and assistance with medication compliance and finances. These capacities should be addressed directly and explicitly in the context of the summary and recommendations section of an evaluation. It is often helpful to address these issues categorically as legal, medical, financial, independent living, medication management and driving capacities.

Rule of thumb: Medico-legal evaluations

- Write reports like you mean it.
- Do NOT offer conclusions (interpretation) and/or recommendations that extend beyond the data
  - Provide conclusions, diagnosis, and recommendations which are supported by the obtained data
- Neuropsychological assessment is increasingly important in medico-legal proceedings and many evaluations that are conducted for clinical purposes eventually become evidence in legal proceedings. It is best to write reports assuming they may eventually become part of a legal proceeding.
- Questions about decision making capacity and functional ability are common.
  - Decision making capacity domains often include the ability to independently make: (1) medical, (2) financial, and legal decisions
- Functional capacity often includes questions about living independently, managing medications, and driving.
  - Driving is not well correlated with individual neuropsychological measures
    - Aspects of driving ability are associated with overall cognitive functioning, attentional/executive functions, processing speed (reaction time), visuoperceptual, and motor skill and neuropsychological assessment is helpful in assessing these domains.

Part II: Perspectives for Physicians, Medical Students/Residents/Fellows: The Neuropsychology Referral

This section is designed to help referring physicians in general, and medical students, residents, and fellows in particular, understand the types of information a clinical neuropsychological evaluation provides, optimize how one may request the specialized skills and knowledge set of clinical neuropsychologists, and aid in the provision of feedback to patients from results obtained from the neuropsychological consult report.

A prerequisite to understand the scope and power of a neuropsychological evaluation is to present a brief overview of key concepts in neuropsychology (see also Chap. 31 and 32 for additional details). Readers of the chapter will appreciate two things about clinical neuropsychology; (1) neuropsychology is a science and a discipline, and (2) the determination of neuropsychological abnormality is based upon deficit measurement. As a science, neuropsychology is studied by many disciplines of the neurosciences. Aspects of neuropsychological assessment are usually included into a typical patient encounter. For example, when one assesses the orientation and basic mental functions of a patient, this process involves some assessment of neuropsychological functions (e.g., assessing basic receptive and expressive speech functions). However, as a subspecialty, the clinical neuropsychologist assesses neuropsychological function in more detail, often using psychometric-based tests that allow for the quantification of specific neuropsychological deficits. As a discipline, the clinical neuropsychologist is a subspecialist with a doctorate degree in psychology who has specialized training in the science of brain–behavior relationships. The discipline is based on the science of measuring brain–behavior relationships, and incorporates knowledge of neuroanatomy, neuropathology, behavioral neurology, psychometrics/statistics, psychiatry, and psychology (e.g., Hannay et al. 1998). Second, neuropsychological evaluation requires establishment of a comparative standard to allow for *deficit measurement*.

Neuropsychology is the science of brain–behavior relationships, and is not limited to the clinical neuropsychologist. Indeed, many health professionals measure neuropsychological function by various means as part of routine patient care. Completing a neurological exam and mental status exam incorporate a screening of basic Neuropsychological functions (e.g., attention/executive, language, visuoperceptual functions and remote and recent memory). However, a clinical neuropsychological evaluation is distinguished from these more cursory reviews of neuropsychological function by the inclusion of a detailed, systematic assessment using psychometric tests with known standardized assessment procedures and normative performance data. Thus, the neuropsychological evaluation can provide a detailed description of a patient's cognitive functioning that is referenced to a comparison standard (see below for details). When integrated with specialized training, the clinical neuropsychologist can provide a unique contribution to the evaluation and management of patients with known or suspected central nervous system dysfunction (see Heilman and Valenstein 2003; Lezak et al. 2004, for reviews).

The concept of *deficit measurement* is an essential principle in neuropsychology. The basic premise in deficit measurement dictates that an observation of a patient's function must be compared against some standard, termed a *comparison standard*, to identify if a change in neuropsychological function has, in fact, occurred. Thus, the comparison standard serves as a benchmark against which current performance is compared against to evaluate if a decline or increase (i.e., deficit or improvement) in neuropsychological functioning has occurred. This same principle also applies in medicine, but the emphasis of the comparison standard is often different. Two general comparison standards are: (1) normative comparison standards, and (2) individual comparison standard.

Normative comparisons include species-specific and population average comparison standards. Species-specific comparison standards reflect species-wide capacities. As an example, in deciding if a deep tendon reflex is abnormal, the comparison standard is a species-based comparison standard. That is, it is known what the normal reflex is for an intact adult human nervous system, and differences from this norm reflect "abnormality." Population averages reflect the average performance of a large sample of individuals on a particular cognitive (or behavioral) test. When using population normative-based information, a patient's performance is compared to standardization data from a known (often healthy) population whose distribution of scores is assumed to approximate a normal curve, but is sometimes negatively skewed (that is, most individuals' performance on a neuropsychological test is close to the highest score possible, with few individuals performing below this level). Using the central limit theorem, we can statistically calculate the position on the normal curve where a patient falls. As a standardized score, the neuropsychologist can provide a percentile score(s) identifying how the particular patient's performance compared against a normative population.

The central limit theorem states many human characteristics in a population are distributed in a manner such that plotting them would represent a normal or bell-shaped curve. This curve would have many people in the average range and fewer and fewer people as we progress farther (higher or lower) from the average (mean). This comparison allows us to more definitively make decisions about the presence of brain dysfunction, the location of brain dysfunction, and gauge the severity of brain dysfunction more precisely. As an example, suppose we measured a male's height as 6′3″ and we want to know how his height compares to the general male population in the U.S. If we know the average male height in the USA is 5′9″ and that the standard deviation for height in males is 3″, then we would know that our 6′3″ person is two standard deviations above average in height, which falls at the 98th percentile (97.72 to be exact) on the normal curve. An example in neuropsychology is an IQ score. This method utilizes statistical properties of the normal population for comparison, while also taking into consideration research findings from patients with specific anatomical lesions and their associated functional deficits. A similar use of population normative comparison standards are used for many laboratory tests in medicine. The laboratory values for identifying abnormal levels are frequently set by a specific laboratory based on reference values obtained within a particular healthy reference population. Therefore, one must either know the laboratory and equipment value or have the laboratory provide the range of normal values and flag an abnormal value within the report. Applying this approach to neuropsychological deficit measurement, if we observe a patient scored two standard deviations below the normal population on a test of verbal memory (2nd percentile), this score would be considered very unusual. If verbal memory was the patient's only low score(s), and the testing was valid, the pattern might be interpreted as a deficit that reflects brain dysfunction. However, it is important to rule out other explanations for an observed significant weakness in verbal memory for a particular patient.

A population normative comparison does *not* provide information sufficient to identify a specific deficit *within an individual*. To highlight the limitation of population-based normative comparison standards, let us say a neuropsychologist finds that a patient scored at the 25th percentile compared to other healthy adults on a measure of memory. Is this score normal or abnormal? The answer is, such a score may be an abnormal or normal performance, depending upon the patient's original (premorbid) level of function. Thus, the individual comparison standard allows the determination that a particular patient's obtained score represents a deficit (decline from previous ability) or is normal (no decline from previous ability). Developing an individual comparison standard requires one to estimate an individual's premorbid level of ability.

Rule of thumb: Perspective from referring providers

- Neuropsychological evaluations provide unique information regarding an individual's cognitive, emotional, and behavioral functioning
- Neuropsychological evaluation can be crucial for diagnosis, predicting outcome, and patient management for individuals with diseases that affect the central nervous system (e.g., brain tumors, epilepsy, dementias, Hepatitis C, etc.)
- Neuropsychological evaluation is often helpful to hospital staff and families in patient management such as level of supervision needed and planning for future care
- Repeated evaluations over time can document improvement or decline in function, assist in evaluating treatment effectiveness, and/or monitor for what type and/or power/intensity of an intervention (e.g., educational programming, assisted living, etc.) might be needed.

Establishing Premorbid Cognitive Ability: The Comparison Standard

Individual comparison standards require the person's level of ability before the onset of known or suspected disease (premorbid functioning) be determined, and compared against current performances. The individual comparison standard may be developed from estimates (often derived from various psychometric methods) or obtained from historical records (e.g., previous cognitive testing, academic records, or vocational indices) and/or behavioral observations (see Lezak et al. 2004; Strauss et al. 2006, for reviews). While establishing a comparison standard using historical records (e.g., prior cognitive test scores) reduces the chance for error in determining change, such historical information is rarely available in the time frames necessary for most clinical neuropsychology services. Thus, clinical neuropsychologists often estimate premorbid ability using a variety of methods, often based on demographic variables (age, education level, occupational history) as well as performance at the time of the evaluation (current performance) on various neuropsychological functions thought to be relatively resistant to effects of brain dysfunction and/or aging (e.g., word recognition, vocabulary knowledge, etc.) (see Lezak et al. 2004, for review). Other techniques have endeavored to decrease errors in estimating premorbid cognitive function by combining demographic-based approaches with current performance on cognitive tests (e.g., reading words or evaluation of known vocabulary). A detailed review of methods to predict premorbid functioning is beyond the scope of this book. However, the reader of the neuropsychological report will often identify the level of functioning the neuropsychologist has established for the patient within the body of the report, often labeled as "estimated premorbid functioning" or something similar. By developing an individual comparison standard, the presence of cognitive or behavioral deficits can be appreciated at the individual level [rather than the nomethetic (i.e., group) level]. If for example, our hypothetical person who scores at the 25th percentile had a 10th grade education and was estimated to be functioning in the normal range, no negative change would be inferred; however, if the person's ability was estimated to be at the 99th percentile of ability, a decline in function is inferred. With an understanding of some basic caveats in neuropsychological evaluations, we turn to the features of the neuropsychological referral.

Rule of thumb: Deficit measurement and comparison standard

- Neuropsychological evaluation is based on deficit measurement using an established comparison standard
- Comparison standard may be established by normative comparisons or individual comparisons
  - Normative comparison standard based on species-wide performance (e.g., development of language, bipedal gait) or population averages (i.e., cognitive and behavioral functions that develop through childhood such as attentional capacity or memory)
    - A patient's performances (test scores) would be compared to species-wide behavior/skill or average of population.
  - Individual comparison standard based on individual history, characteristics, or other data (e.g., educational/occupational history, school records, previous cognitive test scores, etc.). For efficiency, premorbid level sometimes estimated by a variety of demographic variables and/or functional abilities thought to be resistant to effects of aging and brain disease (e.g., word reading ability)
    - A patient's performance (test scores) would be compared to a premorbid estimate of that particular individual's level of cognitive functioning thought to be present before onset of known or suspected neurological dysfunction

What Can You Ask a Neuropsychologist About a Patient?

The neuropsychological referral can provide crucial information to assist in the health care of individuals as reviewed at the beginning of this chapter. As some practical examples, common referral questions might involve the following: (1) identifying the existence of brain dysfunction (e.g., differentiating brain dysfunction from psychiatric diagnosis), (2) describing cognitive and behavioral status for treatment planning or resource utilization decisions; (3) predicting outcome from medical or surgical treatments; (4) identifying change in cognitive function over time (often to monitor status of known or suspected disease or syndrome or to monitor the effect of treatment on a disease or syndrome); (5) evaluating cognitive capacity to make medical, financial, or legal decisions; and/or (6) assist the trier of fact (e.g., a judge or, more often, a jury) in legal proceedings in which the existence, proximate cause, decision-making capacity, and/or likely functional outcome from a known or suspected brain injury is being evaluated. The more detailed referral question(s) you ask, the more likely you will be provided with direct and useful answers from the clinical neuropsychologist.

Neuropsychological data can be crucial to diagnose cognitive disorders (e.g., Mild Cognitive Impairment, HIV-associated cognitive impairment), identify presence of cognitive dysfunction in diseases (e.g., systemic lupus erythematosus, movement disorders, etc.), plan and evaluate treatments (medical, behavioral, surgical, etc.), and to predict recovery patterns. An unfortunately vague referral question that is to "evaluate for 'organicity.'" occurs all too often. By reading chapters such as this one that outline the structure, function and basis of neuropsychological evaluation, it is our hope that our referral sources can become better consumers of neuropsychological evaluations and gain clinically valuable information. The importance of specificity in referral questions cannot be understated (see common referral domains earlier in this chapter). Review of this chapter establishes how neuropsychological evaluations can provide important diagnostic and treatment information. Perhaps more importantly, however, regardless of the sophistication of future neuroimaging technologies, the neuropsychological evaluation is uniquely able to provide the health provider(s) with information about *how* a particular disease, lesion, or treatment is affecting the cognitive and behavioral functions of the individual. The determination of cognitive or behavioral effects of diseases, lesions, or treatments has been shown to be related to quality of life, and can be helpful in understanding how the patient is likely to perform activities of daily living. Dr. Mortimer Mishkin famously said "[neuro]imaging is not enough." To wit, it is well recognized that patients with very similar imaging findings (e.g., left hemisphere stroke or diffuse white matter changes) can present with strikingly different cognitive and behavioral symptoms of varying severity and display marked dissimilarities in their patterns of recovery (e.g., Heilman and Valenstein 2003; Lezak et al. 2004, for reviews).

Overview and Description of Neuropsychological Evaluation Procedures

The neuropsychological evaluation will typically evaluate the following functional domains: (1) Attention/Executive, (2) Learning/Memory, (3) Language/Speech,

(4) Visuoperceptual/visuoconstructional, and (5) Emotion/mood/personality. Additionally, evaluation of general cognitive ability (IQ), academic skills (reading, spelling, writing, arithmetic), and/or quality of life as well as sensory and motor function can be included in the neuropsychological evaluation. Depending upon the referral question, the five areas above may be more thoroughly assessed or, in other cases, given a very limited assessment or, in some cases (e.g., research-based neuropsychological assessment protocols, acute or post-acute assessments) not assessed at all.

From the patient's perspective, the neuropsychological evaluation will typically involve meeting with the licensed neuropsychologist for some period of time to discuss problems/symptoms and provide history. In some cases, a spouse, family member, or close friend may also be requested to interview with the neuropsychologist to provide collateral information. The patient will then complete neuropsychological testing. The patient may be tested by the clinical neuropsychologist and/or a psychometrician. The psychometrician is a technician having training in how to administer and score tests under the supervision of the neuropsychologist. Neuropsychological tests include administration of paper-and-pencil tests, answering questions presented orally, and/or responding using a computer interface.

The time duration of a neuropsychological evaluation can vary substantially based on the referral question(s), the patient's presenting symptoms, and the neuropsychologists' training. In our experience, patients will generally spend 3–8 hours at the clinic to complete a typical outpatient neuropsychological evaluation. Increasingly, shorter evaluations are being completed, and evaluations of 4 hours or less are increasingly popular. This includes time registering in the clinic, interviewing with the neuropsychologist as well as time actually taking the neuropsychological tests. Shorter evaluations lasting less than an hour (some taking less than 30 min) and longer evaluations that may require 2 days of testing may be conducted. The duration of the evaluation is determined by the referral question(s)/needs [i.e. immediate patient management, pre-surgical planning, differential diagnosis (MCI vs Dementia), competency determination, etc.] and patient variables (i.e. age, fatigue, comorbid medical conditions, acuity of injury, questions patient may have regarding their health). There is a trade-off in terms of the depth and breadth of an evaluation and the time it takes to administer, score and analyze data. Longer evaluations allow for more in-depth study of neuropsychological functions, while shorter evaluations limit the detail in which some neuropsychological functions can be assessed. The neuropsychological evaluation is often completed in one day, but in some cases, may be completed over two or more days. Breaks are usually anticipated during longer neuropsychological assessment batteries. Depending upon referral question(s), practice patterns of the referring provider, neuropsychologist's practice pattern, institutional practices, and state licensing laws; the neuropsychologist may provide initial results to the patient on the same day of the evaluation. Alternatively, results may be conveyed to the patient after the evaluation report is completed, which, in our experience, is usually in 3–10 working days. The feedback may include discussion of strengths and weaknesses of cognitive/neuropsychological functions, mood, diagnosis, and opinions to answer the referral question(s) and provide recommendations for the patient's care. In most cases, the neuropsychological evaluation is a procedure that is covered (paid for) by insurance companies. Some exceptions do, however, occur; and some evaluations must be self-paid. This is more common for educational/learning disability evaluations. Pre-authorization for the neuropsychological evaluation from the patient's insurance company (if available) is often obtained by the neuropsychologist's office. Some examples of commonly used neuropsychological tests for each domain are provided in Table 1.1 (see also Chaps. 14–32, this volume for other examples).

Table 1.1 Examples of neuropsychological tests used to assess selected neuropsychological domains

Neuropsychological domain	Examples of neuropsychological tests
General cognitive (IQ), academic achievement	Differential ability scales (children/adolescents)
	Kaufman-ABC
	Neuropsychological assessment battery
	Peabody individual achievement tests
	Reynolds intellectual assessment scales
	Reynolds intellectual screening test
	Wechsler individual achievement test
	Wechsler intelligence tests (adult, child, abbreviated versions)
	Wide range achievement tests
	Woodcock-Johnson – 3rd Ed. NU (tests of cognitive abilities and tests of achievement)
Attention	Brief test of attention
	Color trail making test
	Conners' continuous performance test
	Symbol digit modalities test
	Trail making test, Parts A & B
	Wechsler intelligence tests index scores (working memory index, processing speed index, etc.) and selected subtests (i.e., digit span, letter-number sequencing, coding, digit symbol, symbol search, arithmetic, etc.)
Executive Functions	Booklet category test
	Delis-Kaplan executive function system
	Frontal systems behavior scale
	Ruff figural fluency test
	Stroop color-word test
	Verbal fluency tests
	Wechsler intelligence test subtests (matrix reasoning, similarities, visual puzzles, comprehension, etc.)
	Wisconsin card sorting test
Language tests	Boston diagnostic aphasia exam (BDAE)
	Columbia auditory naming test
	Gray oral reading test – 4th Ed. (GORT-4)
	Multilingual aphasia exam (MAE)
	– Controlled Oral Word Association Test (COWAT)

(continued)

Table 1.1 (continued)

Neuropsychological domain	Examples of neuropsychological tests
	Neuropsychological assessment battery (NAB)
	Peabody individual achievement test – revised (PIAT-R)
	Peabody picture vocabulary test – 4th Ed. (PPVT-4)
	Semantic verbal fluency test (e.g., Animals)
	Woodcock-Johnson psychoeducational battery – 3rd Ed. (WJ-III)
	Western aphasia battery (WAB)
	Wide range achievement test – 4th Ed.
Visuoperceptual/ visuoconstructional	Benton line orientation test
	Beery-Buktenica developmental test of visual-motor integration – 5th Edition
	Benton line orientation test
	Line bisection test
	Hooper visual organization test
	Neuropsychological assessment battery
	Rey-Osterreith complex figure test
	Taylor complex figure test
	Wechsler intelligence tests indexes (perceptual reasoning index) and subtests (e.g., block design, matrix reasoning, picture completion, etc.)
	Wide range assessment of visual motor abilities
Mood/Emotion/ Personality	Beck anxiety inventory
	Beck depression inventory
	Beck youth inventory
	Center for epidemiologic studies depression scale
	Child behavior checklist (CBCL)
	Geriatric depression scale
	Hamilton anxiety rating scale
	Hamilton depression rating scale
	Millon adolescent clinical inventory
	Millon clinical multiaxial inventory – 3rd Ed. (MCMI-III)
	Minnesota multiphasic personality inventory – 2nd Edition (MMPI-2)
	Personality assessment inventory
	Yale-Brown obsessive compulsive scale
	Zung self-rating depression scale

Making the Referral for a Neuropsychological Evaluation

The manner in which the physician (or other health care provider) makes a referral for neuropsychological evaluation can have important implications. There are three issues: (1) specify the referral question(s) you would like answered (see above); (2) providing any previous medical records of the patient documenting or summarizing other evaluation(s) to diagnose and treat the patient's symptoms; and (3) establishing expectations for the patient regarding the neuropsychological evaluation. As detailed above, clarifying the referral question(s) is (are) essential. Like any other specialist in medicine, the neuropsychologist will benefit from the referral accompanied by previous medical records of any other studies completed to evaluate the patient's symptoms (e.g., neuroimaging results, laboratory studies, results of electroneurophysiology studies). The third aspect of the referral can be crucial. A sound referral is one wherein the *referring* clinician provides the patient with a brief explanation of the purpose of the evaluation, what to expect as part of a neuropsychological evaluation, how the information will be used for the patient's care, and the potential risks and benefits of the evaluation. For the clinical neuropsychologist, the referral will be received, and the patient you referred may receive an informational letter, history form, or other information as provided by any other specialty physician. Once you make a referral, you will receive a neuropsychological evaluation report, to which we now turn.

Rule of thumb: Making a referral for neuropsychological evaluation

- Specify, as detailed as possible, questions desired to be answered by neuropsychological evaluation
- Provide previous medical and psychiatric history and/or laboratory study results when available
- Review purpose of neuropsychological referral to patient, and importance of the study in assisting in managing the health care of the patient

---

Understanding the Neuropsychological Report

The neuropsychological report can be somewhat confusing to physicians not accustomed to clinical neuropsychology consult services. While there is considerable variability, the neuropsychological report will often include the typical information of most consultations (e.g., referral question, patient complaints, relevant history, list of medications, mental status exam, and conclusions and recommendations). The more unique aspect of the neuropsychological evaluation is typically the inclusion of a list of either scores (may be standard or percentiles, sometimes raw scores) or description of neuropsychological test scores. Test scores are based on a normative comparison standard, with the 50th percentile being the population average. Multiple different normative groups have been developed, such that normative comparisons are often provided for individuals of similar age, level of education, and in some cases, gender and ethnicity. Then these are adjusted for individual level comparisons, and evaluation of performances are provided in terms of descriptors (low average, average, high average, etc.) and/or percentiles or, in some cases, standardized scores. A listing of qualitative descriptors and approximate corresponding percentiles is provided in Chap. 31. A brief summary is provided below for convenience in Table 1.2.

The clinical neuropsychologist will summarize the cognitive and behavioral data, answer the referral question(s), and, if indicated, provide recommendations for the patient's care. The clinical neuropsychological consult report is often similar to reports provided by other medicine subspecialists who provide a clinical encounter report rather than a technical consult/procedure report (e.g., MRI study report of a radiologist). While the neuropsychological report will typically follow

Table 1.2 Typical descriptors and percentiles in neuropsychological reports

Descriptor	Typical referent percentile range
"Above average"	Scores between 68th to 82nd percentiles
	May also describe obtained scores above the average score of the normative group (i.e., scores 51st percentile or greater)
"Average"	Scores between 25th to 74th percentiles
	May also describe scores 30th to 66th percentiles
"Below average"	Term describing scores 16th to 27th percentiles.
	May also be used to describe scores below the average of the normative group (i.e., scores 49th percentile or less)
"Borderline"	Typically scores between 6th to 15th percentiles
"Borderline low average"	Not common term, typically describing scores 6th to 15th percentiles
"Extremely low"	Scores less than or equal to 2nd percentile
"High average"	Scores between 75th to 90th percentiles
"Impaired"	Typically, scores less than 16th percentile
	May also apply to scores less than or equal to 9th percentile
"Low average or Low normal"	Typically, scores between 16th to 24th percentiles
"Mildly impaired"	Typically, scores between 6th to 15th percentile
	May also refer to scores between 6th and 9th percentiles
"Mildly-to-moderately impaired"	Scores between 2nd and 5th percentiles
"Moderately impaired"	Typically, scores between 1st and 5th percentiles. More recently, scores between 0.6th to 1.9th percentiles.
	Can be subdivided into "mild-to-moderately impaired" and "moderate-to-severely impaired"
"Moderately-to-severely impaired"	Scores between 0.13 to 0.59 percentiles
"Severely impaired"	Typically, scores less than 1st percentile
	More recently, defined as at or below 0.12 percentile.
	However, has been used for scores equal to, or less than, 1st percentile
"Superior"	Scores between "91st to 97th percentiles
"Unusually low"	Scores between 3rd to 9th percentiles
"Very superior"	Scores equal to or above 98th percentile
"WNL or Within normal limits"	Typically scores falling within expectations for the individual or equal to or above the 16th percentile (e.g., 16th percentile or greater)

a typical outline as other clinical encounter reports (history, meds, mental status, procedures, exam/findings/results, conclusions/diagnosis, plan/recommendations), the determination of whether the study is abnormal or normal may be presented in terms of the patient's neuropsychological strengths and weakness or presence (or absence) of neuropsychological deficits (see Reading Between the Lines section below). In general, the report will typically make recommendations for the patient's neuropsychological health. Recommendations may include initiating pharmacological treatment (if otherwise medically indicated), obtaining further clinical correlation for identified neuropsychological deficits, along with other important components of treatment planning (i.e., psychological treatment, rehabilitation, surgical candidacy, educational programming, driving cessation, etc.). Currently, clinical neuropsychologists have prescription authority in two states (New Mexico and Louisiana). In these cases, a clinical neuropsychologist with prescription authority will also communicate if any medications were prescribed. Examples of neuropsychological evaluation reports are provided in the Appendices below. If you are unable to find desired information quickly in the neuropsychological consult report, we encourage you to call or email the consulting clinical neuropsychologist for clarification.

Reading Between the Lines: Appreciating Subtlety in Neuropsychological Consult Reports

We provide this section to inform our referring physicians, and as a notice to our colleagues to assure the neuropsychological evaluation clearly answers the referral question(s). Neuropsychologists are trained from a philosophy of science background, and this training background often imbues the neuropsychological report. Within this tradition, scores or data obtained from a person cannot "prove" the existence of dysfunction, but rather allows the clinician to reject a null hypothesis (rule out a potential cause for the observation). Within the neuropsychological evaluation, the null hypothesis is that the patient's cognitive function is normal. Clinical neuropsychologists often provide extensive data (scores or behavioral observations) in support of an opinion regarding the patient's functioning status. The opinion itself is often expressed in language such as "The neuropsychological study found deficits in _____" or "Neuropsychological data are most consistent with _____." It may be frustrating to read a detailed analysis of an individual's function and not have a definitive conclusion clearly specified as may be the norm in some other consult specialties (such as "The neuropsychological study was abnormal likely due to Alzheimer's disease."). Yet neuropsychological evaluations directly answer the referral question, based on language supporting one hypothesis over another; but it is sometimes a matter of reading between the lines. Table 1.3 provide some common terminology used in neuropsychological reports and research, and a practical description of these terms.

Table 1.3 Common neuropsychological terminology in neuropsychological evaluations

Phrase or term in neuropsychological report:	Neuropsychological term/phrase means:
Attention/executive dysfunction	Impairment in attention/concentration as well as problem solving, sequencing, planning, reasoning, insight, judgment, and inhibition. Localization frequently refers to frontal lobe function and/or fronto-striatal impairment
Below expectations	Test performance is impaired based on determination of patient's likely premorbid level of ability
Data *not* consistent with neurological dysfunction	Study is normal. Often followed by explanation the study quality was either poor due to lack of adequate patient effort and/or psychiatric overlay
Data consistent with [focal, diffuse, or lateralized] brain dysfunction	Phrase to describe where dysfunction occurs. Frequently followed by opinion as to where neurological dysfunction is present and/or etiology
Phrase describing the domains of neuropsychological function that were impaired. Can be followed by determination of localization or lateralization of brain dysfunction	
Neuropsychological impairments were found in [attention, memory, language, visuoperceptual/visuoconstructional, and/or executive functions]	
Data consistent with expectations	Study is normal
Data [most] consistent with brain dysfunction	Study is abnormal. Complaints not due to psychiatric function
Insufficient [effort, task engagement, attention to testing, etc.]	Insufficient patient effort on testing procedures. Quality of study is poor. Question (or diagnosis) of malingering, dissimulation, or somatoform disorder frequently raised/made
Language	Refers to expressive and receptive language skills, inclusive of repetition, writing, reading, and prosody. Not limited to "speech" per se, which is a term to describe the quality of a patient's ability to speak
Memory (and/or learning)	Most commonly refers to declarative memory systems
Neuropsychological deficits present. Etiology unknown, but most likely are/is [presented in order]	Abnormal study. Likely disease or condition is specified. Other possibilities are often provided
No clear deficits	Study is normal. Complaints due to psychiatric variables and/or lack of adequate patient effort
No significant neuropsychological impairment	Study is normal
Overlay of [depression, anxiety, mood, worry, psychiatric disease, etc.]	Study is normal. Complaints due to psychiatric variables
Quality of study is poor [sometimes followed by description of why study quality was poor]	Frequently, this identifies insufficient patient effort on testing procedures. Question (or diagnosis) of malingering, dissimulation, or somatoform disorder frequently raised/made
Task engagement was [poor, inadequate, variable, below criteria, etc.]	Insufficient patient effort on testing procedures. Quality of study is poor. Question (or diagnosis) of malingering, dissimulation, or somatoform disorder frequently raised/made

(continued)

Table 1.3 (continued)

Phrase or term in neuropsychological report:	Neuropsychological term/phrase means:
Validity (or symptom validity) was [descriptor term here] May also be summarized as "The study is valid."	Refers to patients' effort to perform at his/her best ability. Validity may be interpreted to be adequate or good or poor or insufficient. Frequently also incorporates testing environment information and procedures which can adversely affect the validity of the test data, such as insufficient lighting, noise level, participation of third party observers, etc
Visuoperceptual, Visuoconstructional, Visuospatial	Cortical visuoperceptual and visuoconstructional functions such as accurately perceiving objects, visual organization and synthesis of visual material, and being able to accurately draw or reconstruct viewed models (2 or 3 dimensional)

Rule of thumb: Understanding the neuropsychological report

- Neuropsychological reports are often detailed and include a description of how a patient is functioning across many neuropsychological domains (i.e. attention/executive, learning/memory, language, visuoperceptual/visuo-constructional as well as behavior/personality/psychological functions).
- Interpretation is typically given in the summary/conclusions/recommenda-tions section where the test performance results previously described are used to answer the referral question(s) and often providing an opinion regarding diagnosis, neuroanatomic correlates of neuropsychological find-ings, expected disease course, determination of change in function over time (if applicable), and/or answer questions about functional capacity (i.e., driv-ing, living independently, managing medications, and decisional capacity).
- Qualitative description of neuropsychological function follow general guidelines, but variability exists.
- Neuropsychological conclusions are often stated in terms of supporting or refuting a diagnosis/etiology.
  - If conclusions not clear, contact clinical neuropsychologist for clarification

Summary

Neuropsychology is the study of brain–behavior relationships, and the clinical neuropsychologist is a licensed psychologist with specialty training in the clinical neurosciences. Neuropsychological evaluations are a powerful tool to objec-tively assess the cognitive and behavioral functioning of patients. This information cannot be obtained by other means, and empirical evidence continues to demonstrate an evidence base for neuropsychological evaluation in the health care of patients with known or suspected neurological dysfunction. Neuropsychological evaluations can be crucial for the management of a patient, including making diagnoses, evaluate treatment effectiveness, predict outcome from treatment (or disease course), delineate treatment needs and/or develop treatment programming. For the practicing neuropsychologist, the referral is the first and perhaps most important step in providing a neuropsychology service, whether that be a request for an outpatient neuropsychological evaluation, inpatient consult, or providing cognitive rehabilitation. There are several aspects of the referral which are important, both for the neuropsychologist and the referring provider to consider. The referral question(s) should be well delineated, as the question(s) will guide the type and timing of the neuropsychological consult.

References

Achiron, A., Polliack, M., Rao, S. M., Barak, Y., Lavie, M., Appelboim, N., et al. (2005). Cognitive patterns and progression in multiple sclerosis: Construction and validation of percentile curves. *Journal of Neurology, Neurosurgery, and Psychiatry, 76*, 744–749.

American Psychiatric Association (2000). *Diagnostic and statistical manual of mental disorders* (4th ed.). Text Revision (DSM-IV-TR). Washington DC, Author.

Busch, R. M., Frazier, T. W., Haggerty, K. A., & Kubu, C. S. (2005). Utility of the Boston Naming Test in predicting ultimate side of surgery in patients with medically intractable temporal lobe epilepsy. *Epilepsia, 46*, 1773–1779.

Chelune, G. J. (1995). Hippocampal adequacy versus functional reserve: Predicting memory functions following temporal lobectomy. *Archives of Clinical Neuropsychology, 10*, 413–432.

Chelune, G. J. (2010). Evidenced-based research and practice in clinical neuropsychology. *The Clinical Neuropsychologist, 24*, 454–467.

Chelune, G. J., & Najm, I. (2001). Risk factors associated with postsurgical decrements in memory. In H. O. Luders & Y. Comair (Eds.), *Epilepsy surgery* (2nd ed., pp. 497–504). New York: Lippincott Williams & Wilkins.

Chelune, G. J., & Stone, L. (2005). Risk of processing speed deficits among patients with relapsing and remitting and secondary progressive multiple sclerosis. *Journal of Clinical and Experimental Neuropsychology, 11*, 52.

Drane, D. L., Lee, G. P., Cech, H., Huthwaite, J. S., Ojemann, G. A., Ojemann, J. G., et al. (2006). Structured cueing on a semantic fluency task differentiates patients with temporal versus frontal lobe seizure onset. *Epilepsy and Behavior, 9*, 339–344.

Dujardin, K., Defbvre, L., Duhamel, A., Lecouffe, P., Rogelet, P., Steinling, M., et al. (2004). Cognitive and SPECT characteristics predict progression of parkinson's disease in newly diagnosed patients. *Journal of Neurology, 251*, 1432–1459.

Fleisher, A. S., Sun, S., Taylor, C., Ward, C. P., Gamst, A. C., Petersen, R. C., et al. (2008). Volumetric MRI vs clinical predictors of Alzheimer disease in mild cognitive impairment. *Neurology, 70*, 191–199.

Heilman, K. M., & Valenstein, E. (2003). *Clinical Neuropsychology*(4th ed.). New York: Oxford University Press.

Hermann, B., Davies, K., Foley, K., & Bell, B. (1999). Visual confrontation naming outcome after standard left anterior temporal lobectomy with sparing versus resection of the superior temporal gyrus: A randomized prospective clinical trial. *Epilepsia, 40*(8), 1070–1076.

Individuals with Disabilities Act (IDEA) (1990). Pub. L. No 101–336, S2, 104 Stat. 328.

Individuals with Disabilities Act (IDEA) (2004). Pub. L. No 108–446, S2, 647 Stat. 118.

Lezak, M. D., Howieson, D. B., & Loring, D. W. (2004). *Neuropsychological assessment* (4th ed.). New York: Oxford University Press.

Lineweaver, T. T., Morris, H. H., Naugle, R. I., Najm, I. M., Diehl, B., & Bingaman, W. (2006). Evaluating the contributions of state-of-the-art assessment techniques to predicting memory outcome after unilateral anterior temporal lobectomy. *Epilepsia, 47*(11), 1895–1903.

Mesulam, M. (2000). *Principals of behavioral and cognitive neurology* (2nd ed.). New York: Oxford University Press.

Ponsford, J., Draper, K., & Schonberger, M. (2008). Functional outcome 10 years after traumatic brain injury: Its relationship with demographic, injury severity, and cognitive and emotional status. *Journal of the International Neuropsychological Society, 14*, 233–242.

Ropper, A., & Samuels, M. (2009). *Adams and victor's principles of neurology* (9th ed.). NY: McGraw Hill.

Sawrie, S. M., Martin, R. C., Gilliam, F. G., Roth, D. L., Faught, E., & Kuzniecyk, R. (1999). Contribution of neuropsychological data to the prediction of temporal lobe epilepsy surgery outcome. *Epilepsia, 39*, 319–325.

Seidenberg, M., Pulsipher, D. T., & Hermann, B. (2007). Cognitive progression in epilepsy. *Neuropsychology Review, 17*(4), 445–454.

Sherer, M., Novack, T. A., Sander, A. M., Struchen, M. A., Alderson, A., & Thompson, R. N. (2002). Neuropsychological assessment and employment outcome after traumatic brain injury: A review. *The Clinical Neuropsychologist, 16*, 157–178.

Stroup, E., Langfitt, J., Berg, M., et al. (2003). Predicting verbal memory decline following anterior temporal lobectomy (ATL). *Neurology, 60*, 1266–1273.

Whyte, J., Cifu, D., Dikmen, S., & Temkin, N. (2001). Prediction of functional outcomes after traumatic brain injury: A comparison of 2 measures of duration of unconsciousness. *Archives of Physical Medicine and Rehabilitation, 82*, 1355–1359.

Appendix 1

Example of Inpatient/Screening Neuropsychological Consult Report

NEUROPSYCHOLOGY SERVICE
Neuropsychological Consultation

NAME:	XXX, XXXX	**PATIENT #:**	
BIRTH DATE:		**EDUCATION:**	X years

EXAM DATE: [Must document date and time of evaluation and time spent with patient]

REFERAL SOURCE:

REFERRAL INFORMATION AND RELEVANT HISTORY:

[Brief summary of presenting history and reason for referral. Should include symptoms/diagnosis warranting neuropsychological consult]

[Brief summary of presenting patient complaints, if any. The history of complaints, when the symptoms started, severity, and course should be specified].

Example might be: "Patient is a 30-year-old right handed Caucasian male status-post left middle cerebral artery ischemic stroke (date) with mild right hemiparesis and language problems referred to assist with diagnosis and treatment planning. The patient may be a candidate for a community re-integration program. Patient complained of memory and language problems and symptoms of depression."

MENTAL STATUS AND [BEHAVIORAL OBSERVATIONS OR GENERAL CONSTITUTION]

[Detail the patient's mental status. At a minimum, the patient's level of arousal and orientation should be noted along with behavioral observations (gait, tremor, etc.). Quality of speech should be reviewed along with mood and affect. Presence/absence of suicidal and/or homicidal ideation, intent or plan along with hallucinations or delusions should be specified. The patient's cooperation with the evaluation should be noted. Example provided below.]

"Patient was AAOx3 and appropriately groomed. Made good eye contact. Speech articulation, rate, rhythm, and prosody was WNL. Speech content was appropriate. Speech process was linear. Mood was euthymic and effect was full. No suicidal/homicidal ideation, plan or intent (no SI/HI, plan, or intent). No delusions or hallucinations. Insight and judgment WNL. Study is valid."

ASSESSMENT PROCEDURES

[Specified the assessment procedures including what tests were administered. We advise the clinician to specify inclusion of symptom validity measures as such, and not identify specific test names in keeping with recent recommendations.]

NEUROPSYCHOLOGICAL FINDINGS

[Provide results of test scores here. May be separated into major domains or a brief summary. See examples below. We recommend results provided as advised in Chelune (2010).

Examples
Paragraph Format

The patient exhibited deficits in areas of attention/executive functions, verbal memory, and language functions. Specifically, the patient exhibited mild to moderate deficits in complex focused and divided attention tasks. Verbal immediate and delayed memory scores were mildly impaired. Language screening was functional, but there were deficits in confrontation naming and verbal fluency. Strengths were basic span of attention, gross receptive and expressive language functions, and visuo-perceptual skills. Discrepancy among scores were rare in a normal population.

Bulleted Format

Attention: Intact for basic functions. Impaired for complex attention
Memory: Impaired verbal memory. Intact visual memory.
Language: Impaired confrontation naming and verbal fluency. Unable to follow 3-step instructions. Otherwise receptive and expressive speech grossly intact. Repetition intact. No alexia or agraphia.
Visuoperceptual/visuoconstructional: Grossly intact. No constructional apraxia
Executive functions (insight, judgment, reasoning): Insight and judgment [intact, poor, etc.]. Sequencing, set-shifting, problem solving scores were normal.
Personality/psychological/emotional functioning: [brief summary of results of any personality/psychological functioning. May also include quality of life variables, as well as any behavioral apathy and other neurovegetative symptoms.

CONCLUSIONS AND RECOMMENDATIONS

[Interpretation of neuropsychological results. Statement(s) to answer the referral question(s) should be clearly specified. Diagnoses should be listed. If combined with recommendations, recommendations should flow from interpretation.] See example below, and Chelune (2010).

Neuropsychological study was [abnormal, equivocal, normal].

[If relation to neuroanatomical function is needed, specify here. For example: Data suggest left frontotemporal dysfunction, and consistent with reported left MCA stroke.]

[If surgical candidacy is a referral question. For example: *Surgical candidacy*: From a neuropsychological standpoint, the patient is a (poor, fair, good, excellent) candidate for (left, right, extratemporal, multilobar, corpus callosotomy, DBS, VNS, CABG, renal/hepatic transplantation, spinal fusion, morphine pump, etc.…). The patient is at (low, medium, high) risk for post-surgical (language, memory, attention/executive, psychiatric, etc.) problems.

[If feedback notation is included in same report. For example: Initial results of the neuropsychological evaluation were reviewed with _____ [as much detail as is necessary].

Diagnostic impressions: [List diagnostic conditions here. Should follow ICD-9 or DSM-IV diagnostic codes].

Recommendations

[List recommendations here].

We recommend including time spent with patient completing neuropsychological evaluation. Example may be "A total of __ hours of neuropsychological services (including interviewing, administering, scoring, interpretation, and report writing) completed by Dr. ____.

Appendix 2

Example of Outpatient Comprehensive Evaluation Report

NEUROPSYCHOLOGY SERVICE
Neuropsychological Evaluation

NAME: XXX, XXXX   PATIENT #:
BIRTH DATE: ETHNICITY:
EXAM DATE: EDUCATION: X years
REPORT DATE: OCCUPATION:
REFERAL SOURCE:

REFERRAL INFORMATION

[One or two sentences describing reason for referral. Should include symptoms/diagnosis warranting neuropsychological consult]

[OPTIONAL SECTION – RESULTS SUMMARY: [one or two sentences summarizing findings of neuropsychological evaluation. For example: Neuropsychological evaluation was abnormal with deficits in memory and language. (if surgical patient: Patient is a (fill in appropriate descriptor – poor/fair/good surgical candidate) (if dementia patient: Data consistent with (fill in likely etiology)]

CURRENT COMPLAINTS AND HISTORY

[Specify where data was obtained, e.g., patient and spouse]

[Brief summary of presenting complaints, if any. The history of complaints, when the symptoms started, severity, and course should be specified].

Example – bullet format:

1. Seizures/Epilepsy. Patient has a history of seizures since childhood. Seizures medication refractory. Seizures occur 2/month on average. Last known seizure was _____.
2. Attention, memory, and language problems past 2 years. Increasing problems concentrating the past 2 years. Forgets details of recent events, appointments, and repeats self. Increasing dysnomia the past 2 years. Speech problems past ____.
3. Depression for past year. Symptoms of depression more often than not the past year. Denied anxiety symptoms. Sleep and appetite were _____. Difficulty falling asleep and his/her appetite has decreased with loss of 15 pounals past 6 months without dealing. Energy level was _____.

MEDICAL AND PSYCHIATRIC HISTORY: [Relevant medical and psychiatric history specified. This may only be noted as "unremarkable" or "noncontributory" but may also include information about neurological exam, laboratory studies, EEG, MRI, CT, surgical/operative notes, consulting notes of other health care providers, previous diagnosis(es) and treatments (successful or unsuccessful). Allergies may also be stated.).

[Review of developmental, social, educational, occupational history provided. One may also make a statement about patient's ability to complete activities of daily living (ADLs). Can be brief, for example "Patients medical and psychiatric history was reviewed and detailed in chart. Otherwise unremarkable. Developmental history unremarkable. Patient worked as an engineer and retired in 2003. Patient is independent in ADLs and is driving.]

CURRENT MEDICATIONS: [list medications and dosages]

MENTAL STATUS AND GENERAL CONSTITUTION

[Detail the patient's mental status. At a minimum, the patient's level of arousal and orientation should be noted along with observations about gait and station, stature, and hygiene. Quality of speech should be reviewed along with mood and affect. Presence/absence of suicidal and/or homicidal ideation, intent or plan along with hallucinations or delusions should be specified. The patient's cooperation with the evaluation should be noted.]

[A comment about task engagement or validity of the study may be made here or in the neuropsychological results section. An example is given below.]

Appearance: well groomed. Appeared stated age. Of normal height and build.
Gait/station: normal.
Tremor: No obvious tremor observed.
AAOx4: Yes
Speech: articulation and rate, rhythm, intonation, and prosody WNL.
Speech Content: generally appropriate to context.
Speech Process: organized and goal-directed.
Mood: euthymic
Affect: consistent with mood
Suicidal/Homicidal Ideation Plan or Intent: denied
Hallucinations/Delusions: None
Judgment: within normal limits
Insight: within normal limits
Test Taking Behavior: Cooperative and appeared to give adequate effort. *Study is valid.*

ASSESSMENT PROCEDURES

[Specified the assessment procedures including what tests were administered. We advise the clinician to specify inclusion of symptom validity measures as such, and not identify specific test names.]

SENSORY/MOTOR AND PERCEPTUAL FUNCTIONING

[Results from sensorimotor and perceptual testing, if completed, specified here. This may also include results from neurological exam, if completed. Presence of finger agnosia, visual field defects, etc. and motor exam (motor speed, dexterity, and/or grip strength.] Example is below.
Sense of smell: intact to several common scents.
EOM: appeared grossly intact.
Visual fields: grossly full to confrontation.

Light touch: Sensation intact in face and hands, and no extinction with bilateral simultaneous stimulation.

Auditory: intact, bilaterally

Ideomotor apraxia: None (or Yes, present)

Agraphasthesia: None (or Yes, present)

Finger agnosia: None (or Yes, present)

R/L orientation: Intact (or Impaired)

Grip strength: [description of performance. Example "Average, bilaterally."]

Finger tapping speed: [description of performance]

Manual dexterity: [description of performance]

NEUROPSYCHOLOGICAL FUNCTIONING [OR RESULTS]

[Provide results of test scores here. May be separated into major domains or a summary of performances provided]. See examples below. We recommend the inclusion of a summary table of neuropsychological scores (including standardized scores) be included in most neuropsychological reports either imbedded or as an appendix. Base rate information regarding the frequency in which score differences are observed in healthy samples and/or if results exceed reliable change scores (if known) may be included. No references needed. [Note: the reporting base rate and/ or discrepancy information provided following recommendations for evidenced-based neuropsychology practice (Chelune 2010)].

Paragraph format

Premorbid functioning estimated to be high average to superior. General cognitive functioning was average. The patient exhibited deficits in areas of attention/executive functions, verbal memory, and language functions. Specifically, the patient exhibited mild to moderate deficits in complex focused and divided attention tasks. Verbal immediate and delayed memory scores were mildly impaired. Language screening was grossly functional, but there were deficits in confrontation naming and verbal fluency. Strengths were basic span of attention, receptive and expressive language functions, and visuoperceptual skills.

Bulleted format

Premorbid functioning: Estimated to be high average to superior in general cognitive ability.

General Cognitive: High average compared to age-matched peers. Indices of verbal and nonverbal abilities were high average and average, respectively (Verbal Comp.= 115, 84th %; Perceptual Reasoning=100, 50th %).

Processing Speed: WNL.

Attention: Intact for basic functions. Impaired for complex attention

Memory: Impaired verbal memory. Intact visual memory. Differences in scores infrequent in healthy sample.

Language: Impaired confrontation naming and verbal fluency. Unable to follow 3-step instructions. Otherwise receptive and expressive speech grossly intact. Repetition intact. No alexia or agraphia.

Visuoperceptual/visuoconstructional: Grossly intact. No constructional apraxia
Executive functions (insight, judgment, reasoning): impaired. Insight and judgment
[intact, impaired, etc.]

Brief Results Section Example
The patient exhibited deficits in areas of attention/executive functions, verbal memory,
and language functions. Specifically, the patient exhibited mild to moderate deficits
in complex focused and divided attention tasks. Verbal immediate and delayed
memory scores were borderline to impaired compared to age-matched peers.
Language screening was functional, but the patient exhibited deficits in confrontation
naming (BNT = 38/60) and phonemic and semantic verbal fluency scores.

Strengths were in basic attention functions, general cognitive (intellectual) functioning was average, and visuoperceptual and visuoconstructional skills were
entirely intact.

PSYCHOLOGICAL AND PERSONALITY FUNCTIONING

[Provide results of any psychological or personality testing done. See example below]
The patient completed the BDI-2 and STAI. He reported mild to moderate symptoms of depression and anxiety. The patient denied rumination and appeared well
adjusted.

CONCLUSIONS AND DIAGNOSTIC IMPRESSIONS

[Interpretation of neuropsychological results. Statement(s) to answer the referral
question(s) should be clearly specified. Diagnoses should be listed. If combined
with recommendations, recommendations should flow from interpretation.] See
example below.

Neuropsychological study was [abnormal, equivocal, normal]. [If abnormal,
describe what was abnormal].

For example: The study was abnormal due to deficits in attention/executive
functions, verbal memory, and language functions. There were mild to moderate
symptoms of depression. Strengths included the patient's basic span of attention,
nonverbal "visual" memory, visuoperceptual and visuoconstructional skills.

[If relation to neuroanatomical function is needed, specify here. For example:
Assuming normal neuroanatomical functional organization, data suggest left frontotemporal dysfunction, and consistent with history of left temporal mesial temporal
sclerosis.] [In dementia example. Neuropsychological data are generally consistent
with a dementia of the Alzheimer's type. A less likely possibility is a frontotemporal
dementia (FTD) process. History of symptoms argues against FTD].

[If surgical candidacy is a referral question, clearly specify neuropsychological
opinion. For example: *Surgical candidacy*: From a neuropsychological standpoint, the
patient is a (poor, fair, good, excellent) candidate for (left, right, extratemporal,
multilobar, corpus callosotomy, DBS, VNS, CABG, renal/hepatic transplantation,
spinal fusion, morphine pump, etc.]. The patient is at (low, medium, high) risk for
post-surgical (language, memory, attention/executive, psychiatric, etc.) problems.

The patient is likely a good candidate for [additional diagnostic/laboratory procedures to further evaluate for potential risks to the patient.].

[If feedback notation is included in same report. For example: Initial results of the neuropsychological evaluation were reviewed with the patient, and all questions were answered to his/her/their satisfaction. As much detail as is necessary is appropriate here.].

Diagnostic Impressions: [List diagnostic conditions here. Should follow ICD-9 or DSM-IV diagnostic codes].

RECOMMENDATIONS

[List recommendations for the patient's care here.] These will vary widely depending upon the individual patient. However, some common domains for recommendations are provided below:

1. Referral for further work-up of condition.
2. Recommend consultation by another specialist/subspecialist
3. Initiate treatment for psychiatric/psychological symptoms
4. Initiate treatment/rehabilitation for cognitive deficits
5. Cognitive ability to make medical, legal, and/or financial decisions (capacity is a legal term and decided by a court – not a neuropsychologist).
6. Cognitive and/or behavioral prognosis based on available data
7. Rehabilitation/treatment recommendations

   - Summary of deficits with prognosis for recovery
   - Participate in medical treatment
   - Behavioral management
   - 1:1 Supervision/therapies
   - Suicide precautions
   - Escort to and from all activities
   - Relaxation
   - Minimal stimulation
   - Shortened therapy sessions
   - Cognitive rehab.
   - Neglect training
   - Attentional training
   - Orientation group/training
   - Memory notebook training
   - Problem solving training

8. Occupational recommendations/driving restrictions

   - Capacity to return to work (school if child)
   - Schedule to return if unable to return to full time work
   - Accommodations necessary for successful re-integration

9. Reference of local, state, regional, national, or international support and advocacy groups of any known disorders/conditions.

10. Specify diagnosis for Americans with Disabilities Act (ADA) and/or Individuals with Disabilities Education Act (IDEA 2004).

    - Specify need for IEP (based on diagnosis/diagnoses)
    - Specify what accommodations and/or adaptations may be helpful to the patient academically, socially, emotionally, and/or vocationally.

11. [If appropriate, make statement(s) about return to work/school. If not return to work/school now, when, and if accommodations (as above) are likely to be needed.].

12. [Specify if follow-up is needed].

[Closure of report and include information, if appropriate, for further contact and information if desired. Include information about services provided [Services included: Neuropsychological evaluation (_____ hours including administering, scoring, interpretation and report writing). Psychometrician-based neuropsychological assessment (_____ hours).]

Chapter 2
Deconstructing the Medical Chart

Alan J. Lerner and Mike R. Schoenberg

Abstract This chapter provides an overview of the medical chart, and its sections. The neuropsychologist will be provided with detailed information about how to decipher some of the many abbreviations, and we also provide the neuropsychologist, who may not be familiar with common lab values with descriptions of the neurologic examination common grading systems such as motor and sensory functions. In addition, this chapter provides a brief overview of neurologic terms commonly encountered in general medical and more detailed neurological examinations along with figures and illustrations of some of these terms.

Key Points and Chapter Summary

- The medical chart has several components and familiarity with the basic structure of each section is important to both effective patient management and quality care
- The History and Physical (H&P) is the initial evaluation of a patient upon admission to a hospital, service, or transfer, and is often the most comprehensive source of current patient information
- While the basic structure of a H&P is similar across medical disciplines/specialties, elaboration within different sections is often discipline/specialty-specific

---

The Medical Chart

The quality of care rendered by medical personnel is proportional to the quality of the assessment, diagnosis and management of the patient. While the point of medical training is to ensure consistent high quality patient care, certain variables such as

A.J. Lerner (✉)
Memory and Cognition Center, University Hospitals Case Medical Center and Case Western Reserve University School of Medicine, Cleveland, OH, USA
e-mail: Alan.Lerner@UHhospitals.org

M.R. Schoenberg and J.G. Scott (eds.), *The Little Black Book of Neuropsychology:*
A Syndrome-Based Approach, DOI 10.1007/978-0-387-76978-3_2,
© Springer Science+Business Media, LLC 2011

the information available to assist in this process often remain beyond our control. Good assessment and consultation often start with a review of the existing medical chart and records. In this chapter, a practical method for extracting information from often complex, chaotic medical records is reviewed with particular emphasis on information relevant for neuropsychological evaluation (see also Lezak et al. 2004; Victor and Ropper 2001; Zaidat and Lerner 2008, for review).

Inpatient Chart

Various state and federal guidelines mandate the prompt evaluation of an individual admitted to a hospital or longer-term health care facility. The admission note is often the most detailed source of information available in an entire chart, and therefore bears special scrutiny in helping with neuropsychological assessment. The basic form of the admission History and Physical includes the following sub-sections

Chief complaint. This is usually in the form of a succinct sentence often or ideally in the patient's own words such as "shortness of breath" or "change in mental status" or "admitted for elective cardiac surgery." The chief complaint encapsulates the reason for admission, at least on the initial basis.

1. *History of present illness.* This forms the main narrative of the admission history and physical and often starts with a brief review of past medical history. An example of this might be a "Chief complaint of left-sided weakness" followed by "The patient is a 68-year-old right-handed man with a history of hypertension, diabetes, coronary artery disease admitted for left-sided weakness of 1 day's duration."

   The History of Present Illness often contains additional important information such as who provided the history; whether it was the patient or family or other medical personnel. It may also contain cross-references to other portions of the medical chart such as records obtained from the Emergency Medical Services. More importantly, one needs to scrutinize the History of Present Illness section for what it does *not* contain, such as important demographic information or vague statements that need to be considered in making one's own evaluation at a later date.

2. *Past medical history.* Typically, this is a listing of medical conditions, frequently abbreviated. Regulatory agencies such as JCAHO have rightly criticized the practice of abbreviations in medical charts as they can be confusing or ambiguous, and this may impact patient quality of care. Caution should be given in considering the source of medical history and confirming the list of critical past illnesses, as these can be in error and, if so, may lead to erroneous conclusions about contributing factors in the patient's current condition. For example, a patient with an erroneously reported history of Diabetes, Hypertension, or Coronary Artery Disease may be evaluated differently when presenting with stroke symptoms only to find out they have blood clots (phlebitis) after a long journey in a sedentary position.

Table 2.1 Abbreviations for common medical diseases, conditions, and terms

Abbreviation/Acronym	Medical Term, Condition, Disease
AD	Alzheimer's disease OR Attachment disorder
ADD(-R)	Attention deficit disorder(-resistant)
ADEM	Acute disseminated encephalopathy
ADHD	Attention deficit hyperactivity disorder
AF	Atrial fibrillation
AIDS	Acquired immune deficiency syndrome
ALS	Amyotrophic lateral sclerosis (Lou-Gehrig's disease)
APS	Antiphospholipid syndrome
ARDS	Acute respiratory distress syndrome
ASD	Autism spectrum disorders (see also PDD)
AVM/ AVMs	Arteriovenous malformations
BEB	Benign essential bepharospasm
BPH	Benign prostatic hyperplasia
BSE	Bovine spongiform encephalopathy
CAD	Coronary artery disease
CADASIL	Cerebral autosomal dominant arteriopathy with sub-cortical infarcts and leukoencephalopathy
CAT	Computerized axial tomography study
CCU	Critical care unit OR Coronary care unit
CF	Cystic fibrosis
CFS	Chronic fatigue syndrome
CH	Cluster headache
CHD	Congenital heart disease OR Coronary heart disease OR Congenital hip dysplasia
CHF	Congestive heart failure
CICU	Cardiac intensive care unit
CIPD	Chronic inflammatory demyelinating polyneuropathy
CJD	Creutzfeldt-Jakob disease (see also SSE)
COPD	Chronic obstructive pulmonary disease
CRF	Chronic renal failure
CSA	Central sleep apnea
CSF	Cerebrospinal fluid
CT	Computerized tomography study
CVD	Cardiovascular disease
DM (I or II)	Diabetes mellitus, [Type I (juvenile); Type 2 (acquired)
DLB	Dementia with Lewy bodies (also DLBD)
DTs	Delirium tremens
ED	Emergency department OR emotionally disturbed
EDS	Ehlers-danlos syndrome OR excessive daytime sleepiness
EMR	Electronic medical record
EPS	Extrapyramidal symptoms
ESRD	End state renal disease
FAE	Fetal alcohol effects
FAS (FASDs)	Fetal alcohol syndrome (Disorders)
FMA	Focal muscular atrophies
FMLA	Family medical leave act
FXS	Fragile X syndrome

(continued)

Table 2.1 (continued)

Abbreviation/Acronym	Medical Term, Condition, Disease
GAD	Generalized anxiety disorder
GAS (disease)	Group A streptococcal disease
GBS (disease)	Guillain-barre syndrome OR Group B streptococcal (disease)
GD	Gestational diabetes
GERD	Gastroesophageal reflux disease
HA (H/A)	Headaches
HD	Huntington's disease
HTN	Hypertension
HPV Infection	Human papillomavirus infection
HSV (infection)	Herpes Simplex Virus
IBD	Inflammatory bowel disease OR Ichthyosis bullosa of siemens
IS	Infantile spasm
JRA	Juvenile rheumatoid arthritis
LD	Learning disability OR Legionnaires' disease
LKS	Landau-Kleffner syndrome
LP	Lipoid proteinosis OR Little Person
MD	Muscular dystrophy
MMR(V)	Measles, mumps, rubella (varicella)
MND	Motor neuron disease
MPS (I to VII)	Mucopolysaccharoidosis (Type _)
MR(/DD) (MRDD)	Mentally retarded/Developmentally disabled
MRI	Magnetic resonance imaging
MS	Multiple sclerosis
NCL	Neuronal ceroid lipofuscinosis
NF (1 or 2)	Neurofibromatosis (type __)
NICU	Neonatal intensive care unit
NLD (NVLD)	Nonverbal learning disorder
NP (NPC1)	Niemann-pick disease (type C1)
NPH	Normal pressure hydrocephalus
NSU	Neurosciences (Neurological) intensive care unit
OCD	Obsessive-compulsive disorder
ODD	Oppositional defiant disorder
OPCA	Olivopontocerebellar atrophy
OSA	Obstructive sleep apnea
PACU	Post anesthesia care unit
PCP	Primary care physician
PD	Parkinson's disease
PICU	Pediatric intensive care unit
PDD (NOS)	Pervasive developmental disorder (Not Otherwise Specified)
PML	Progressive multifocal leukoencephalopathy
PMS	Premenstrual syndrome
POTS	Postural orthostatic tachycardia syndrome
PSP	Progressive supranuclear palsy
PVL	Periventricular leukomalacia
RA	Rheumatoid arthritis
RIND	Reversible ischemic neurologic deficit

(continued)

Table 2.1 (continued)

Abbreviation/Acronym	Medical Term, Condition, Disease
RLS	Restless legs syndrome
ROP	Retinopathy of prematurity
RSD	Reflex sympathetic dystrophy
RTI	Respiratory tract infection
SARS	Severe acute respiratory syndrome
SB	Spina bifida
SBS (SIS)	Shaken baby syndrome (Shaken infant syndrome)
SIDS	Sudden infant death syndrome
SLE	Systemic lupus erythematosus
SMA	Spinal muscular atrophy
SPS	Stiff person syndrome
SSE	Subacute spongiform encephalitis
SSPE	Subacute sclerosing panencephalitis
STD	Sexually transmitted disease
SWS	Sturge-weber syndrome
TB	Tuberculosis
TBI	Traumatic brain injury
TCS	Tethered cord syndrome
TIA	Transient ischemic attack
TMJ (TMD)	Temporomandibular joint disorder
TS	Tourette syndrome OR Tuberous sclerosis
TSC	Tuberous sclerosis
TSE	Transmissible spongiform encephalopathies
UTI	Urinary tract infection
VD	Venereal disease
VHF	Viral hemorrhagic fever
VSD	Ventricular septal defect
WD	Wilson's disease

3. *Family and social history.* Although this is usually a very truncated section of the history and physical, it is of importance in interpretation of any neuropsychological testing. This is one of the few sections that actually gives a sense of the person as living on a day-to-day basis. It will frequently contain information such as marital status or gender, tobacco, alcohol, and drug abuse. It may also contain information about the number of children, although in an inpatient setting this is often not specified. Of special importance is the patient's educational history and primary language (if specified), as many neuropsychological skills and test performances vary considerably with education, and consideration should be given to evaluate a patient in his/her primary language. For example, the same memory capacity would not be expected of someone with 4 years of education compared to someone with a graduate degree. If not a Fluent English speaker, performances and expectations should be altered. For practitioners who do not speak the language of the patient, options may include identifying another practitioner who does speak the language or finding an interpreter (caution should be taken if a family member or friend of the patient is used as this may

introduce bias). If unavailable basic cognitive testing using nonverbal tasks/tests may provide some useful information, but interpretation and conclusions should be viewed with caution.

4. *Review of systems.* The review of systems should ideally complement previous medical history. A complete review of systems encompasses constitutional symptoms as well as up to about 15 bodily systems. Frequently, this may be just marked as NC for noncontributory.

5. *Vital signs.* Typically, this would include Temperature (recorded either in Centigrade or Fahrenheit), Pulse (per minute), Respirations (per minute) and Blood Pressure with systolic recorded over diastolic. In charting, these are often abbreviated as T, P, R, B/P, and often noted as numbers in that order. Caution is again warranted as the information provided here may have been copied from earlier in the chart (or another chart), such as the evaluation in the emergency room, and may not reflect information at the time of the writing of the admission History and Physical. It is also not uncommon in a busy inpatient hospital setting for the actual writing of the admission History and Physical to be delayed for several hours following the actual examination.

Rule of thumb: Outline of the H&P

- Chief Complaint
- History of Present Illness
  - Current medications
- Past History
  - Medical history (including Psychiatric)
  - Family and Social history
- Review of Systems
  - Head, Eyes, Ears, Nose and Throat (HEENT)
  - Neck
  - Lungs
  - Cardiovascular
  - Abdominal
  - Extremities
  - Back
  - Genito-urinary
  - Neurologic
    - Cranial Nerves
    - Mental Status
    - Motor
    - Sensory
    - Gait/Station
- Laboratory

The following subsections of the Review of Systems are often found:

HEENT. This stands for Head, Eyes, Ears, Nose, and Throat. A frequent abbreviation is NC/AT which stands for Normocephalic, Atraumatic. Ideally, this section will identify any observed defects and state of the skin, oral mucosa, dentition, use of hearing aides, or glasses. However, this information is often omitted. Again, cross-reference with the history as described above is often useful. Gross vision problems may be noted here (or in CN exam section), including strabismus, exotropia, esotropia, or ambylopia. Strabismus is the lack of muscle co-ordination between the eyes. Exotropia refers to an eye being deviated away from midline (deviated outward), and is a form of strabismus. Esotropia refers to an eye being deviated towards the midline (deviated inward), and is a form of strabismus. Amblyopia refers to when the brain does not process visual signals of a misaligned eye (the eye that is exotropic or esotropic), resulting in vision being based on one eye and a patient losing depth perception. Strabismus refers to the condition of misaligned eyes when looking ahead.

Neck. This is often described as supple, a rigid neck being a concerning finding regarding the possibility of meningitis in a patient particularly who is febrile. There may be referral to nuchal (neck) rigidity which may be accompanied by a Brudzinski's sign (raising of the legs towards the chest when the head is bent forward at the neck) often associated with meningeal irritation or inflammation. Other abbreviations seen here would be JVD, standing for jugular venous distention, which may be increased with right heart failure as with pulmonary hypertension, for example. There may also be references to the size of the thyroid as well as the presence or absence of carotid bruits (an abnormal sound made by blood in the carotid arteries when it swirls past a stenotic or ulcerative plaque).

Lungs or chest. This may or may not include a breast examination. A variety of maneuvers are taught to medical students to describe chest findings. The most common abbreviation here is CTA (Clear To Auscultation) meaning the quadrants of the chest do not demonstrate any abnormal (i.e. different or atypical) sound when thumped or listened to (ausculated). It is less likely, particularly with more senior clinicians, to have a detailed chest examination unless they are performed by a pulmonologist or a cardiologist. Other findings of note may include findings suspicious for a pleural effusion such as dullness at the base or evidence for pneumonia such as crackles or decreased breath sounds. The presence of wheezes suggestive of obstructive airway disease is sometimes noted as well. These comparisons are often reported by chest or lung quadrant indicating a more precise area of abnormal findings.

Cardiovascular. This refers primarily to the heart sounds on auscultation, but may also contain information regarding peripheral arterial disease. Most commonly, it may say normal $S_1 S_2$ (S refers to sound and S_{1-4} refers to the 1st through 4th heart sounds in a normal heart beat) referring to the normal opening heart sounds. The presence of additional heart sounds which are nonspecific findings include the possibility of an abnormal S_3 or S_4. The presence of murmurs is often noted, and this may be abbreviated as an M. Pulses may also be included under cardiovascular. The dorsalis pedis pulse (or pedal pulse) is abbreviated as DP and often will be marked as +/+; the initial + referring to their right side and the second + to the left side.

Abdomen. Frequently abbreviated as ABD. The most common abbreviations here are BS for bowel sounds and NT for non-tender. Also noted is focal tenderness or masses, and sometimes the presence of an aortic or femoral bruit may be located here rather than under the cardiovascular examination.

Extremities. Frequently abbreviated as EXT. The most common abbreviation is C/C/E standing for cyanosis, clubbing, or edema. The presence of osteoarthritic changes may be noted here, as may be congenital or acquired deformities such as an amputation. This is sometimes accompanied by a drawing of an affected or infected extremity. Frequently, the pulse is recorded and relevant here, and may be obtained from two extremities (e.g., the dorsalis pedis pulses may be recorded here rather than under the cardiovascular examination). Evaluation is based not only on recording abnormalities but also symmetry. Differences in symmetry in either palor, size or functionality may be noted here. Limitations in movement, such as inability to abduct or adduct a limb may be noted here. Abduct(ion) is action that moves a body part away from the midline or center axis along an horizontal plane. Adduct(ion) is action moving a body part toward the midline or center axis.

Back. This may or may not be present. A common abbreviation is CVA or costovertebral angle (this refers to the angle of the spine and ribs) or CVAT for costovertebral angle tenderness which may or may not be present. The presence of scoliosis or kyphosis may also be noted here. Also noted here may be any complaints of pain and the distribution of the region of the pain, which may be helpful in differentiating central and peripheral from referred pain that may be associated with organ dysfunction.

Rectal. This may be included under the abdominal examination or it may be deferred. Often times, abbreviations here refer to the presence or absence of occult blood such as determined with the guaiac screening card or the presence of normal rectal reflexes indicative of normal sacral spinal cord function.

Genitourinary. Abbreviated as GU. This would include vaginal or external male genitalia examination including the penis, scrotum, and testes. This examination may also be deferred in inpatient evaluations.

Neurological. The neurologic examination is frequently replete with abbreviations. The importance of the neurologic examination to neuropsychological evaluation cannot be overstated. The most important piece of information available to the consulting neurologist or neuropsychologist is a prior neurological examination noted in sufficient depth to reassure the examiner that it was performed with more than cursory inspection. The components of the Neurologic examination are elaborated below.

Mental status. This is frequently abbreviated as AO × 3 standing for alert, oriented to person, place, and time. Occasionally one may see orientation described as AO × 4 with the "4" referring to situation or circumstances. Just as commonly, one will see AAO × 3 (or AAO × 4) which stands for *Awake*, Alert and Oriented to person, place, and time (and circumstances/ situation). A more detailed listing of specific findings such as a score obtained for the Mini-Mental State Exam (MMSE; Folstein et al. 1975) may be found (e.g., 30/30), as well as descriptions of which items the patient failed. This section should include observations regarding attention, language, memory and insight/awareness of any current problems. Notation of defects in orientation, language problems (dysarthria, expressive/receptive aphasia, paraphasias) may be reported here. This section may also report about the patient's mood and affect along with presence of hallucinations or delusions and risk of harm to self or others. The presence of more specific observations indicates the person was examined in depth, since the designation of "AO × 3 or AAO × 3" does not indicate a full or detailed exam was performed.

Cranial nerves. These are often summarized as "CN II-XII intact." Cranial nerve I (olfactory nerve) is generally not tested. As with mental status, it is not always clear when this is a cursory evaluation versus a summation of a detailed examination. See Chap. 3 for review of anatomy of Cranial Nerves, and Chap. 4 for list of the Cranial Nerves and methods for assessment. Neurologists will often group cranial nerves into functional clusters including smell, taste, vision and eye movement, hearing, swallowing, and facial and neck strength and sensation. Sometimes, one will see "CN I–XII were intact (or WNL)," indicating sense of smell was evaluated. However, a more detailed exam will provide clear indication how the CN's were tested (e.g., "each nostril tested separately, and pt. able to identify several common scents.").

Motor examination. This includes muscle tone (resistance to passive movement), bulk, strength, often expressed according to the 0–5 Medical Research Council (MRC) grading scale (Table 2.2). Deep tendon reflexes (DTRs) should be noted here. Frequently, these are provided along with a stick drawing of a person with reflexes noted (see Fig. 2.1 and Table 2.3). Plantar responses may also be provided here, and may be noted along with DTRs (see Fig. 2.1). Figure 2.2 illustrates how the plantar response can be elicited.

The presence of a abnormal movements/movement disorder (e.g., tremor, jerks, incoordination), apraxia, ataxia, hypertonicity (rigidity), hypotonicity (flaccidity) or other abnormalities of gait and station are also often noted here. Tremor

Table 2.2 Grading of muscle strength (MRC scale)

Grading of muscle strength	Qualitative descriptor of muscle grading
0	No palpable muscle contraction
1	A flicker or trace of contraction
2	Active movement with gravity eliminated
3	Movement against gravity but not resistance
4–	Active movement against gravity and slight resistance
4	Active movement against gravity and resistance
4+	Active movement against gravity and strong resistance
5	Full active range of motion and normal muscle resistance

A muscle grading of 0 is verbally discussed as "muscle strength is/was zero or zero out of five".

Fig. 2.1 Common notation used to record reflexes as part of a neurological exam

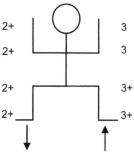

Note: Illustration for left sided increased deep tendon reflexes (i.e. left hyperreflexia). Note also the Plantar flexor noted for abnormality.

Table 2.3 Grading of deep tendon reflexes (DTRs)

Grading of DTRs	Qualitative descriptor of reflex grading
0	Not present, even with facilitory procedure
1	Present but reduced or weak
2	Normal
2+	Normal, but somewhat brisk (high normal)
3	Brisk
3+4 (or 3+)	Very brisk, but no clonus
4	Pathologically brisk with clonus

Reflex grading of 2+ throughout, is discussed as "reflexes were 2+ throughout".

Fig. 2.2 Illustration of the Plantar (Babinski) reflex

Babinski's Response

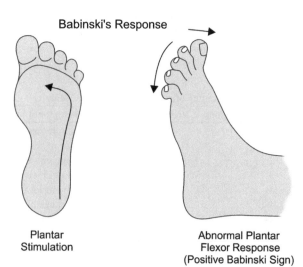

Plantar
Stimulation

Abnormal Plantar
Flexor Response
(Positive Babinski Sign)

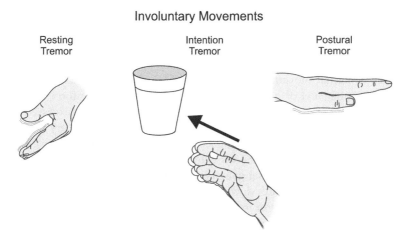

Fig. 2.3 Illustration and descriptions for common types of tremors

description should indicate where the tremor is present (e.g., upper extremity, lower extremity, head), when it is present (i.e., continuous, under stress, only at rest), and the severity of the tremor (see Fig. 2.3 for illustration of tremors). A variety of terms may be used to describe when it is present, but the most common will be *action tremor* (including postural, kinetic, physiological, and intention tremors) or *resting tremor* (classically, Parkinsonian tremor). Among action tremors, the most common clinically diagnosed type is *essential tremor* (ET), which is a tremor of 4–8 Hz most predominant when a static limb posture is maintained, but may also be evident when moving (intention tremor). Classically, it affects the upper limbs bilaterally, but may present worse in one limb (typically dominant hand). It may also involve the head, termed titubation, with a nodding type of movement. Involvement can include jaw, lips, and larynx, such that the patient's voice has a quavering quality. It is uncommon for lower extremities to be markedly affected by ET. It can progress to be disabling, making writing illegible and preventing a patient from holding a cup of water to drink (see also Chap. 19, this volume, for further review of ET and other movement disorders). Physiological tremor is present in all normal individuals, and is of high frequency (8–13 Hz) and low amplitude such that it is not seen by the naked eye nor appreciated by most people. When exaggerated, termed Enhanced Physiological tremor, by fright, anxiety, extreme exertion, withdraw from alcohol, toxic effects from some chemicals (caffeine, lithium, etc.) or metabolic dysfunction (e.g., hyperthyroidism or hypoglycemia), the physiological tremor increases to be seen and to disrupt routine activities. Enhanced physiological tremor can appear like ET, and is most easily appreciated when holding arms out with fingers outstretched. Intention tremor refers to a tremor distinguished from other action or postural tremor by its form and associated features. Intention tremor is absent at rest and the initial start of a movement. However, as increasingly fine movement is needed for an act (i.e., picking up a full cup of water), the tremor becomes present with a sideways oscillation at about 2–4 Hz of increasingly large amplitude that often continues after the target is reached. Intention tremor is always associated with cerebellar ataxia.

Other abnormal movements, such as chorea, athetosis, dystonias, ballismus (often hemiballismus) or akinesia, are often noted here. Choreiform movements may involve the proximal or distal muscles and are involuntary, excessive, jerky, irregularly timed, and randomly distributed. These movements can vary from subtle (appearing as "restlessness" to unstable dance-like gait while walking), to more severe (disabling flow of continuous extreme and violent movements). They are frequently associated with basal ganglia diseases. Athetosis describes slow writhing-like movements that are slower than choreiform movements, but may be described as "slow choreiform movements." Choreoathetosis is an "intermediate" form of choreiform movements. Ballismus describes an extreme of choreiform movement in which motor movements are rapid and include violent flinging movements. It typically involves an involuntary, continuous, uncoordinated movement involving proximal and distal muscle groups resulting in a limb being "flung out." It typically involves one side of the body, termed hemiballismus, but bilateral paraballismus has been reported. Ballismus is considered an extreme choreiform motor movement. Akinesia is lack of movement.

Motor abnormalities of hypertonicity/rigidity [e.g., spasticity, cogwheel rigidity, lead pipe rigidity, paratonia (gegenhalten), etc.] or hypotonicity are also frequently noted here. Hypertonicity refers to excess motor tension, presence of spasticity, lead pipe rigidity (rigidity of a limb maintained during and after passive movement of muscle), cogwheel rigidity (passive movement results in a cogwheel or ratchet like catching and quickly releasing as limb moves), and paratonia (involuntary variable resistance to efforts at passive movement of a muscle, like a limb) (see Chaps. 10 and 19, this volume, for more details).

The presence of apraxia, ataxia and/or disorders associated with cerebellar function, such as dysmetria or dysdiadochokinesia, may be identified here or in the Gait and Balance section below. Apraxia refers to the loss of ability to complete previously learned purposeful motor movements, not due to motor weakness (see Chap. 9 for additional review). Examples include ideomotor and ideational apraxia. Ataxia refers to inability to coordinate muscle movements that is not due to motor weakness. Muscle movements will appear clumsy or "jerky." Ataxia is typically associated with lesions to the cerebellum leading to gait abnormalities (see below), but may also occur due to sensory ataxia from damage to proprioception sensory pathways. Optic ataxia is the inability to coordinate eye–hand motor movements and is observed with Balint's syndrome (see Chap. 9, this volume). Ataxic respiration is the poor coordination of muscles in chest and diagram, related to damage of the respiratory centers in the medulla oblongata or associated pathways.

Gait and balance. Sometimes included under the motor system, this includes rapid alternating movements (RAM), finger to nose testing (FTN), Romberg testing, and other gait and balance descriptions. Observations of ataxia (e.g., dysmetria, dysdiadochokinesia) may be noted here. Dysmetria is abnormal movements associated with cerebellar damage, and involves dysfunction in the ability to accurately control the range of movement needed for a muscular action. Dysmetria is commonly tested with finger-to-nose testing. The individual with dysmetria will be unable to guide his/her finger to the examiners finger or nose, in which the target is under- or overshot, with attempts at corrections which have a 'jerky' quality and overcorrection is often present. Dysdiadochokinesia is the inability to complete rapid alternating movements associated with cerebellar ataxia, and is often tested by having a patient rapidly alternate slapping the palm of each hand and back of the hand on a stable surface (i.e., pronation/supination test). Gait may be described with various terms, but some of the more common include: normal, spastic, apraxic (wide-based), ataxic (also wide-based), parkinsonian, steppage, or scissored gait (see Fig. 2.4 for illustration and summary description of common gait abnormalities).

Sensory. Basic sensory modalities include light touch, pain sensation, vibratory sensation and joint position testing. "Higher order" sensory testing such as two point discrimination, sensory extinction, and/or graphesthesia may be included here. Figure 2.5 illustrates a bedside neurological examination to assess for graphesthesia. While this illustrates using the patient's palm, it may also be tested on the patient's finger tips. Presence of agraphasthesia is associated with contralateral parietal lobe damage.

Laboratory evaluations. Frequently listed after the physical examination in both the admission note and daily progress notes, laboratory evaluations include many abbreviations and common ways of recording the results. Tables 2.4–2.6 provide the abbreviations, descriptors, and purpose or function of common laboratory tests. Figures 2.6 and 2.7 illustrate how common laboratory values are diagramed in a chart.

Outpatient Medical Chart

The outpatient medical chart is often very similar to the inpatient chart, although follow-up visit notes may note less detail than above for some medical subspecialties. However, like the inpatient medical chart, the beginning consultation (office visit) report generally will include a detailed written report of the patients presenting history and medical evaluation similar in format (often identical to) that reviewed above for the inpatient medical record. However, return office visits may not re-review all the patient's history again and note changes in the patient's history as necessary for the patient's ongoing care with the treatment provider. Thus, we will not re-review the sections noted above.

Abnormalities of Gait and Posture

Spastic Hemiparesis

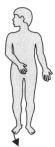

Gait resulting from upper motor neuron disease. Arm of affected side is held immobile and close to the body. Elbow, wrist, and finger joints often flexed. Leg is 'stiff' and extended. The foot is also often flexed out (plantor flexion). When walking, the affected leg is often circumducted (swung in a side ways arc motion). The toe may drag along the ground during this movement.

Scissors Gait

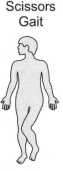

Gait resulting from spastic paresis of both legs (bilateral upper motor neuron dysfunction affecting legs). Gait appears stiff and with each advancing step, the thigh will cross over in front of the other thigh. Steps are short. One may hear the thighs rubbing together. May appear as if person is walking through deep water.

Abnormalities of Gait and Posture

Sensory Ataxia

Closed Eyes

Open Eyes Watching the Ground While Walking

Wide Stance

1. Heel Hit Ground

2. Toes Hit the Ground

Gait resulting from deficient sensory input due to polyneuropathy or damage to dorsal column (medial leminiscus tract). Gait is unsteady and wide based. Feet appear 'thrown forward' and then down to the ground, heals first. Patients watch the floor for visual guidance. When eyes are closed, gait worsens with more exagerated stagering and the patient may fall. Patients are also unable to stand with feet together and eyes closed (positive Romberg sign).

Fig. 2.4 Illustration and description of common gait abnormalities

Abnormalities of Gait and Posture

Steppage Gait

Parkinsonian Gait

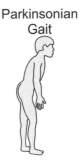

Gait resulting from when a foot (or both feet) are weak, resulting in so-called "foot drop." Classically, the patient will lift up leg(s) high (as if climbing up stairs). When the patient puts a foot down, the foot 'slaps' the ground, which can often be heard. Patients unable to walk on heels.

Gait is characteristically slow and shuffling with short steps (festinating gait), and the person is often stooped over. Arm swing is diminished and may be absent. Patient can have difficulty taking a step (start hesitation or freezing), and sometimes a verbal cue ("ready, go!") or placing an object in front of the patient to step over can start (resume) walking. Turns are made "en bloc," in which turns are made with a number of small steps.

Abnormalities of Gait and Posture

Cerebellar Ataxia

Open Eyes or Closed

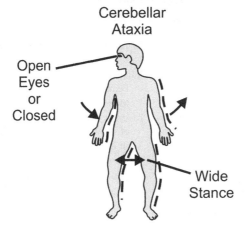

Wide Stance

Gait resulting from damage to cerebellum or associated motor tracts. Gait is unsteady and wide based. Turning is completed with difficulty. Gait does not worsen when eyes are closed. A positive Romberg sign is present, eyes open or closed.

Fig. 2.4 (continued)

Fig. 2.5 Bedside procedure
to assess graphesthesia

Graphesthesia

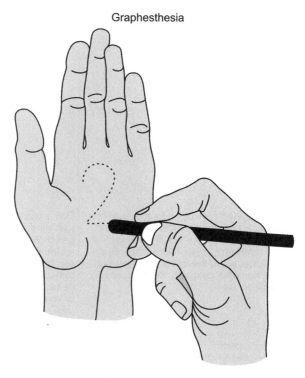

Table 2.4 Blood count and coagulation descriptors and abbreviations

Laboratory abbreviation	Laboratory term	Purpose of function of test (what abnormal value may mean)
Complete blood count		
Hb	Hemoglobin	To assess for anemia. Transports O_2 to cells and CO_2 away Adult Reference Ranges: – Females = 12–16 g/dL – Males = 13–18 g/dL
Hct	Hematocrit	To assess for anemia; Hematocrit is the percentage of blood volume occupied by cells Adult Reference Ranges: – Females = 35–48% – Males = 39–54%
Plt	Platelet count (in thousands)	Primary hemostasis. Initial blood clotting ability
RBC	Red blood cells	Density of Red Blood cells. Scales with Hb and Hct Adult Normal Range: Males = 4.2–5.4 × $10^6/\mu L$ Females = 3.6–5.0 × $10^6/\mu L$
WBC	White blood cell count	Assessment for infection; > 11,000/μL very elevated, can reflect infection, bone marrow disease (leukemia), trauma, etc.; <4,300/μL very low, can reflect bone marrow disease (leukemia), infection, chemotherapy, etc.

(continued)

Table 2.4 (continued)

Laboratory abbreviation	Laboratory term	Purpose of function of test (what abnormal value may mean)
Coagulation/sedimentation		
INR	International normalized ratio	Measure of anticoagulation (normal = 1.0) based on PT
PT	Prothrombin time	Measures function of vitamin K dependent clotting factors
PTT	Partial thromboplastin time	Measure of clotting function; measured with PT Adult reference range: 25–41 s
ESR	Erythrocyte sedimentation rate	Measure of rate RBC's settle out of whole blood in 1 h Adult reference ranges: – Females = 1–20 mm/h – Males = 1–13 mm/h

Table 2.5 Chemistry (routine) laboratory descriptors and abbreviations

Laboratory abbreviation	Laboratory term	Purpose or function of test
Alb	Albumin	Major protein found in blood. Diminished with severe illness, kidney or liver dysfunction. Often measured with TP and Glob Adult reference range: 3.5–5.0 gm/dL
ALK or ALK Phos	Alkaline Phosphatase	Liver function. Elevated in conditions with increased bilirubin and in some bone diseases (e.g., Paget's disease)
ALT	Alanine Aminotransferase	Liver function. Also found in cardiac and skeletal muscle. Elevated with liver damage Adult reference range: 1–21 units/L
AST	Aspartate Aminotransferase	Same purpose as ALT Adult reference range: 7–27 units/L
Bili	Bilirubin (total, direct, or indirect may be specified)	Bilirubin forms bile and is increased with cholestasis (blockage of bile excretion) Adult reference range: Total: 0.3–1.0 mg/dL
BUN	Blood urea nitrogen	Measures kidney function. Increased with kidney failure. Associated with Cr Reference ranges: – Adults = 6–20 mg/dL – Higher in elderly (i.e., 8–23), lower in kids (5–18)

(continued)

Table 2.5 (continued)

Laboratory abbreviation	Laboratory term	Purpose or function of test
Ca (Ca^{+2})	Calcium	Involved in neural transmission and muscle function
		Adult reference range:
		8.5–10.5 mg/mL
Cl (or Cl$^-$)	Chloride	Major anion in body fluids. Often abnormal when sodium or potassium abnormal
		Adult reference range:
		98–106 mEq/L
Cr	Creatinine	Measure of renal (kidney) excretion. Produced as part of energy metabolism in muscle
		Adult reference ranges:
		0.6–1.2 mg/dL
GGT	Gamma Glutamyl transpeptidase	Abnormal with cholestasis; elevated in alcoholism
Glob	Globulins	Measure of antibodies. Associated with TP and Alb
		Adult reference range:
		2.3–3.5 gm/dL
HCO3 (or HCO$_3$)	Bicarbonate	Measure of acid – base balance
		Adult reference range:
		18–23 mEq/L (CO$_2$ content)
K (or K$^+$)	Potassium	Involved in muscle contraction and function. Extreme low or high levels may be life threatening
		Adult reference range:
		3.5–5.0 mEq/L
Na (Na$^+$)	Sodium	Involved in muscle and nerve function. Low levels may be associated with seizures
PO$_4$ or Phos	Phosphorus	Associated with bone metabolism and excreted renally. Related to calcium levels
		Adult reference range:
		3.0–4.5 mg/dL (inorganic)
T4	Thyroxine	Thyroid hormone level.
		Adult reference range:
		4.6–12.0 μg/dL
TP	Total protein	Sum of albumin and globulin concentration.
		Adult reference range:
		6.0–8.4 gm/dL
TSH	Thyroid stimulating hormone	Pituitary hormone whose levels are inversely related to thyroid function.
		Adult reference range:
		0.5–5.0 microlU/mL

Table 2.6 Cerebral spinal fluid and other body fluid laboratory descriptors and abbreviations

Laboratory abbreviation	Laboratory term	Purpose or function of test
Cell ct	Cell count	Increased in meningitis or cerebral hemorrhage
Diff	Differential	Assesses for type of white blood cells found in body fluid (blood, CSF, etc.)
Prot	Protein	In CSF, elevations are nonspecific; elevated with neuropathy, stroke, MS and other conditions
Glu	Glucose	Low levels seen with bacterial meningitis. Usually 60% of serum value
		Adult Reference Range:
		70–110 mg/dL (fasting)
U/A	Urinanalysis	Screen for urinary tract infection, and measure of kidney function
C + S	Culture and sensitivity	Identification of pathogens (usually bacterial)
Cx	Culture	As above
14-3-3 protein		used for evaluating for prion disorders
Oligoclonal bands	Antibodies that appear as discrete "bands" on staining	Evaluates for inflammatory conditions (such as Multiple Sclerosis, but are *non-specific*)

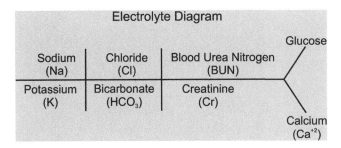

Fig. 2.6 Basic chemistry notation diagram(The serum glucose is often appended at the right hand side of this figure as illustrated)

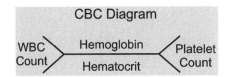

Fig. 2.7 Basic Blood Chemistry diagram

References

Folstein, M. F., Folstein, S. E., & McHugh, P. R. (1975). "Mini-mental state". A practical method for grading the cognitive state of patients for the clinician. *Journal of Psychiatric Research, 12*, 189–98.

Lezak, M. D., Howieson, D. B., & Loring, D. W. (2004). *Neuropsychological assessment* (4th ed.). New York: Oxford.

Victor, M., & Ropper, A. H. (2001). *Adams and Victor's principals of neurology* (7th ed.). New York: McGraw-Hill.

Zaidat, O. O., & Lerner, A. J. (2008). *The little black book of neurology* (5th ed.). Philadelphia: Elsevier Health Sciences.

Chapter 3
Neuroanatomy Primer: Structure and Function of the Human Nervous System

Mike R. Schoenberg, Patrick J. Marsh, and Alan J. Lerner

Abstract This chapter is provided as a general primer for the neuropsychologist and others interested in functional neuroanatomy. This chapter is not meant as a detailed examination of the nervous system, and readers are encouraged to review comprehensive texts in the area for further detail (e.g., Blumenfeld H, Neuroanatomy through clinical cases, 2nd edn. Sinauer Associates Inc., Sunderland, 2010; Fix JD, Neuroanatomy, 4th edn. Lippincott, Williams, & Wilkins, Philadelphia, 2008; Heilman KM, Valenstein E, Clinical neuropsychology, 4th edn. Oxford University Press, New York, 2007; Kolb B, Whishaw I, Fundamentals of human neuropsychology, 6th edn. W.H. Freeman, New York, 2009; Lezak MD, Howieson DB, Loring DW, Neuropsychological assessment, 4th edn. Oxford University Press, New York, 2004; Mesulam MM, Principles of behavioral and cognitive neurology, 2nd edn. New York: Oxford University Press, 2000; Victor M, Ropper AH, Adams and Victor's principals of neurology, 7th edn. McGraw-Hill, New York, 2001).

The primer is organized into two sections. "Introduction to the Human Nervous System" provides an overview of the anatomical structure of the human nervous system. "Functional neuroanatomy: Structural and Functional Networks" provides a primer on functional neuroanatomy. While neuropsychologists are generally well versed in aspects and organization of the central nervous system, particularly the cerebral cortex, less attention is given to the spinal cord, brain stem, diencephalon, and peripheral nervous system. This chapter will also provide a brief overview of gross pathology of the skull, meninges, cerebral spinal fluid, and important afferent and efferent pathways of the human nervous system. We begin with a review of some important terms and definitions.

M.R. Schoenberg (✉)
University of South Florida College of Medicine,Tampa, FL, USA
e-mail: mschoenb@health.usf.edu

M.R. Schoenberg and J.G. Scott (eds.), *The Little Black Book of Neuropsychology:*
A Syndrome-Based Approach, DOI 10.1007/978-0-387-76978-3_3,
© Springer Science+Business Media, LLC 2011

Key Points and Chapter Summary

- Central nervous system includes the brain and spinal cord.
- Neurons process information by electrochemical process in which "communication" between neurons (and some glial cells) occurs with release of neurotransmitters.
- Neurotransmitters are small molecules (ex. Glutamate, GABA) that are released pre-synaptically and facilitate action potentials that excite or inhibit synapsing neurons
- Peripheral nervous system includes cranial nerves, spinal nerves (motor and sensory), and autonomic nervous system
- Autonomic nervous system includes the parasympathetic and sympathetic divisions. The parasympathetic nervous system maintains consistent homeostasis while the sympathetic nervous system involves the changes necessary to respond to threats.
- Major afferent (sensory) system is dorsal (posterior) column-medial lemnniscus (vibration, two-point discrimination, proprioception) and spinothalamic (pain, temperature, and deep/crude touch).
- Major efferent (motor) system is corticospinal (corticobulbospinal) pathway
- Cerebrovascular supply is from paired internal carotid arteries for anterior supply and paired vertebral arteries for posterior supply
- Major regions of the brain include Medulla, Pons, Cerebellum, Midbrain, Thalamus, Basal ganglia, and cerebral cortex
- Medulla and Pons are associated with basic life functions
- Cerebellum is associated with balance, posture, motor coordination, implicit learning
- Cerebral hemispheres are divided into Frontal, Parietal, Temporal, Occipital lobes and insular cortex (lobe).
- Frontal lobes are associated with motor functions, expressive language, "executive" functions (e.g., behavioral planning, monitoring/regulation, inhibition, motivation, judgment), and mood/affect (emotional regulation). Also includes olfactory cortex.
- Parietal lobe function is associated with somatosensory functions, spatial awareness/attention and complex visuoperceptual processing (reading and shape orientation/direction)
- Temporal lobe associated with receptive language, primary auditory cortex, declarative memory, visuoperceptual processing (form/shape integration), mood/affect, and olfactory cortex.
- Occipital lobe associated with primary and secondary visual processing.
- Neuropsychological functions involve distributed networks of cortex involved in processing one stimuli along with cortex involved in integrating functions.

Definitions and important terms

Action potential	A transient voltage change that occurs when excitatory synaptic inputs combine with endogenous transmembrane currents to sufficiently excite a neuron. Lasts about 1 ms and can travel rapidly throughout the length of a neuron at rates up to around 60 m/s. Classically, they travel from the dendritic end of a neuron along its axon to reach presynaptic terminals, and are often coupled to neurotransmitter release from the presynaptic terminal.
Afferent (see also efferent)	Pathway carrying signals *to* a Central Nervous System (CNS) structure. For example sensory pathways are afferent, sending sensory information to the brain. Often termed as afferents or afferent (fibers, pathways, or tracts).
Basal ganglia	Term used to describe a cluster of nuclei lying in the deep white matter under the cerebral cortex. It includes the caudate nucleus putamen, and globus palidus.
Cingulum (cingulate gyrus)	Means "girdle" or "belt," and is a medial cortical gyri which is immediately superior to the corpus callosum. Part of the limbic system.
Commissure	White matter pathway connecting analogous structures between the right and left hemispheres of the brain. There are the anterior commissure and posterior commissure.
Corpus callosum	Main bridge/pathway between the two cerebral hemispheres. The corpus callosum is divided into four sections: *rostrum*, *genu*, *body*, and *splenium*.
Cuneus ("wedge")	Portion above the calcarine fissure in the visual cortex.
Decussate/decussation	Term used to describe the "crossing" of a fiber tract. Most of the motor tracts and some of the sensory pathways decussate in the pyramids of the brain stem and gives the CNS its "crossed" (right brain–left body: left brain–right body) characteristic.

Efferent (see also afferent)

Pathway carrying signals *away* from a CNS structure. Classically motor pathways are frequently thought of as taking motor signals from the brain to muscles, and are termed efferents or efferent (fibers, pathways, or tracts).

Fascicle/fasciculus (see also fiber)

White matter tract connecting areas within a hemisphere. May connect neighboring gyri (arcuate or U-fibers) or more distal areas (e.g., Arcuate fasciculus connects expressive and receptive language areas in the left hemisphere and is considered part of the superior longitudinal fasciculus, which runs from the frontal to occipital lobes).

Fiber (also termed bundle fascicle, lemniscus, or tract)

Names for white matter pathways. Fibers have been classified as association, commissural, or projection. Association fibers connect cortical areas in each hemisphere. Commissural fibers connect homogulus areas between hemispheres. Projection fibers connect cortical areas with deep brain nuclei.

Ganglia

A cluster of neuronal cell bodies often applied to "basal ganglia" (see above).

Gyri

Bumps or ridges between sulci giving the cortex its characteristic wrinkled appearance. The folding of tissue allows for more surface area.

Gyrus rectus

("Straight gyrus")

Insular cortex

Cortical structure located between the temporal and frontal lobe deep within the lateral fissure.

Lemniscus (see also tract fascicle, fiber, and bundle)

Names for white matter pathways.

Lingula ("little tongue")

Portion of the medial occipital lobe below the calcarine fissure.

Longitudinal fissure (or interhemispheric fissure)

Midline fissure separating the two hemispheres.

Myelin sheath

Insulating lipid layer of an axon formed by specialized glial cells speeds the rate of action potential conduction.

Nodes of Ranvier	Short exposed segments of axon where voltage-gated ion channels are concentrated conduction from node to node occurs rapidly by a process called *salutatory conduction.*
Nuclei	Large cluster of neurons within the CNS.
Oligodendrocytes	Myelin-forming glial cells in the CNS. In the PNS myelin is formed by Schwann cells.
Operculum	"Lip", the folds from the frontal, parietal, and temporal lobes of the cerebrum overlying the insular cortex.
Schwann cells	A specialized cells in the PNS, which support the neurons. Schwann cells wrap around the axons of neurons to form the myelin sheath for nerves which increases speed of neuronal transmission via salutatory conduction.
Somatotopic	Related to point-to-point correspondence between a body part (e.g., finger, hand, arm, etc.) and its representation in the brain. The primary motor and sensory cortices of the brain are arranged somatotopically.
Sulci	Crevices/infolds of brain. Sulci that are deep valley's between the folds, and are termed *fissures.*
Synapse	Gap or space between two neuron structures in which neurotransmitter substances are transferred and cellular communication occurs.
Tract (see also fascicle fiber, lemniscus, and bundle)	Names for white matter pathways.

Introduction to the Human Nervous System

The human nervous system is grossly organized into the central and peripheral nervous systems (see Fig. 3.1). The central nervous system (CNS) is defined as the brain and the spinal cord. The brain is a three-pound organ encased in the skull while the spinal cord is located in the spinal canal within the vertebrae. The peripheral nervous system (PNS) includes the nerves of the body that are not the brain or spinal cord. Said another way, the PNS is the nerves outside of the dura matter. The PNS has three main components: (1) somatosensory (afferent)

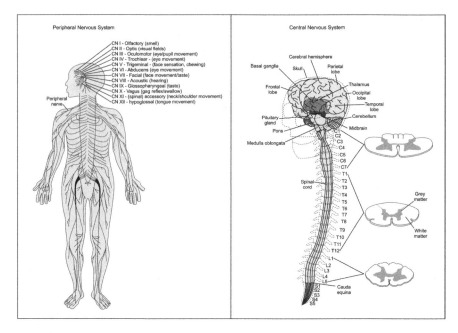

Fig. 3.1 Overview of human central nervous system and peripheral nervous system

---

Rule of thumb: Human nervous system

- Central Nervous System
  - Brain
  - Spinal cord (cervical, thoracic, lumbar, sacral, and coccyx)

- Peripherial Nervous System
  - 12 paired cranial nerves
  - Spinal nerves (sensory and motor)
  - Autonomic nervous system

    □ Parasympathetic – "rest and digest"
    □ Sympathetic – "fight or flight"
    □ Enteric – controls peristalsis and gastrointestinal secretion

---

nerves, (2) motor (efferent) nerves, and (3) autonomic nervous system. The autonomic nervous system is composed of three systems: (a) the sympathetic nervous system, (b) the parasympathetic nervous system, and (c) enteric nervous system (see PNS description below for more details). The PNS includes the paired 12 cranial nerves. The cranial nerves include somatosensory and motor functions, and a description of the function and assessment of each cranial nerve is provided in Chap. 4.

The Central Nervous System

The brain is encased in the skull, which consists of 22 individual bones. Fourteen of the bones make up the facial structures of the skull and 8 cranial bones house the brain. The cranial bones include: Parietal, Temporal, Occipital, Frontal and right and left Ethmoid and Sphenoid bones (see also Fig. 3.9). Figure 3.2 illustrates a cut-away view of the anatomy from the scalp to the brain, inclusive of the skin layers, skull, layers of meninges, and brain surface. The meninges surround the entire brain and spinal cord, and are composed of three different membranes: Dura mater, Arachnoid mater, and Pia mater. Adherent to the inside of the cranial bones and surrounding the entire brain is the Dura mater. The dura is a somewhat shiny, inelastic membrane. In addition to surrounding the brain, the dura folds to divide the cranium into separate compartments and create the venus sinuses which drain blood from the brain. The dura creates three named falx. The falx cerebri divides the cranium vertically into right and left compartments housing the right and left hemispheres of the brain. The tentorium cerebelli supports the occipital lobes horizontally and separates them from the cerebellum. The falx cerebelli is analogous to the falx cerebri and separates the left and right hemispheres of the cerebellum. The next layer is the arachnoid, which is an elastic and fibrous two-layered membrane lining the inner surface of the Dura mater. Between the dura and the arachnoid mater is a non-communicating space called the subdural space. Subdural veins with very little mechanical support traverse the subdural space and are susceptible to mechanical injury (subdural hemorrhage). Because the subdural space is non-communicating (closed space), bleeding from a subdural vein accumulates to create a subdural hematoma. Subdural hematomas can become large and exert pressure on brain structures necessitating external drainage through the skull (see Chap. 21 for more details of traumatic hemorrhages). Inferior to the arachnoid mater is a fine membrane rich in blood supply called the pia mater. The pia mater is intimately associated with the brain surface, following all the sulci, gyri and conformations of

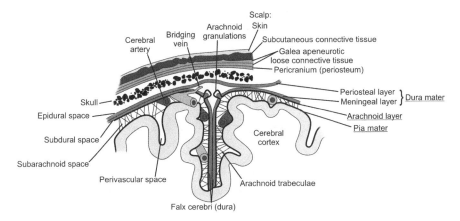

Fig. 3.2 Illustration of components of dura matter and falx cerebri

> **Rule of thumb: Layers of meninges**
>
> - Dura mater
> - Subdural space
> - Arachnoid matter
> - Subarachnoid space
> - Pia mater

the brain surface. Between the arachnoid mater and the pia mater is the subarachnoid space. The subarachnoid space is a spongy area containing cerebrospinal fluid. Damage to blood vessels here results in subarachnoid hemorrhages, which may result in blood products entering the spaces of the cerebrospinal fluid.

Brain Anatomy Overview

The brain is divided into Hindbrain (Rhombencephalon), Midbrain (Mesencephalon) and Forebrain (Prosencephalon) based on anatomic location and embryologic origin of the tissues which make up each division (see Fig. 3.3). The hindbrain and midbrain contain nuclei essential for sustaining life and homeostasis. The forebrain includes the basal ganglia, white matter, and neocortex traditionally associated with complex behaviors and cognition. The neocortex is divided into four "lobes" or areas: frontal, parietal, temporal, and occipital (some argue the insula is the 5th lobe).

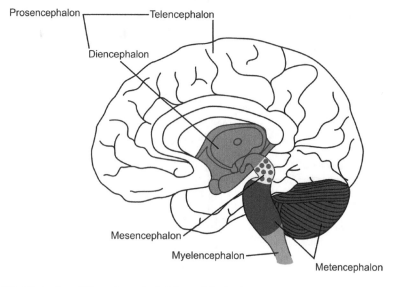

Fig. 3.3 Illustration of the embryonic divisions of the brain

We now turn to reviewing the anatomy of functions of the major components of the central nervous system.

The *Hindbrain (Rhombencephalon)* is composed of the Medulla, Oblongata, Pons and Cerebellum. The *medulla oblongata* (or medulla) is the most rostral portion of the brain and continues to form the spinal cord as it exits the skull. It mainly is a functional center for the crossing (i.e. decussation) of the afferent and efferent pathways leaving or entering the brain. The medulla also contains the nuclei of the cranial nerves IX–XII, Glossopharnygeal, Vagus, Acressory, and Hypoglossal (see Fig. 3.1 and Chap. 4 for review of function and bedside assessment). Centers for respiration, vasomotor and cardiac control, as well as many mechanisms for controlling reflex activities such as coughing, gagging, swallowing and vomiting, are located in the medulla.

The *pons* is a bridge-like structure which links the medulla and midbrain. The large body of the pons is made up of axons entering the cerebellum. These axons or fiber tracts are referred to as the cerebellar peduncles. The pons contains nuclei for cranial nerves V–VIII (trigeminal, abducens, facial and vestibulochochlear nuclei, respectively). A group of neurons referred to as the pontine respiratory group, which influences the rate of breathing, is located in the upper pons. In addition to respiration, the pons is associated with sensory (crossed afferent pathways) and motor functions (crossed efferent pathways) and arousal and attention due to function of locus cerelus and general projection of norepinephrine throughout brain (see below).

The *cerebellum* is a structure attached to the brain stem via the cerebellar peduncles that appears like a second smaller brain. It is divided into right and left hemispheres with a midline structure referred to as the vermis. The cerebellum ("little brain") has convolutions similar to those of the cerebral cortex, called folia. The folds of the cerebellum are much smaller. Like the cerebrum, the cerebellum has an outer cortex, an inner white matter, and deep nuclei below the white matter. The traditional function of the cerebellum has been considered coordination of voluntary motor movement, balance and equilibrium, and muscle tone. However, more recently, the cerebellum has been shown to be involved in some types of learning (nondeclarative or implicit learning). The cerebellum receives indirect input from the cerebral cortex, including information from: (1) sensory areas of the cerebral cortex, (2) motor areas, (3) cognitive/language/emotional areas of the cortex and thalamic nuclei.

Rule of thumb: Hindbrain (Rhombencephalon)

- Medulla (oblongata) – life-support functions (heart rate, blood pressure, gag reflex, etc.) and area where afferent (sensory) and efferent (motor) pathways decussate
- Pons – life-support (sleep, heart rate, breathing), arousal (reticular activating system), and crossed afferent (sensory) and efferent (motor) pathways.
- Cerebellum – motor control and coordination, balance, posture/equilibrium as well as implicit learning and memory (motor actions)

The *Midbrain* (*Mesencephalon*) is composed of the Tectum, Cerebral peduncles, Tegmentum, Pretectum, and Mesencephalic duct (aka aqueduct of Sylvias) (see Figs. 3.1 and 3.3).

The dorsal surface of the midbrain forms the *tectum,* meaning "roof." It consists of the superior colliculi and inferior colliculi. The superior colliculus is involved in preliminary visual processing and control of eye movements (automatic/unconscious visual orientation). The inferior colliculus is involved in automatic (e.g., unconscious) orientation to auditory stimuli, and receives auditory input from various brain stem nuclei. Afferent fibers than project to the thalamus to relay auditory information to the primary auditory cortex.

Rule of thumb: Mnemonic for superior coliculus

- Superior coliculus is for See (automatic visual orientation)

The term *cerebral peduncle* denotes the white matter tracts, which contain the efferent axons of the cerebral cortex that project to the brainstem and spinal cord. The cerebral peduncles are the part of the midbrain that links the remainder of the brainstem to the thalami. They form the walls of the fourth ventricle.

The midbrain *tegmentum* is the part of the midbrain extending from the substantia nigra to the cerebral aqueduct in a horizontal section of the midbrain, and forms the floor of the midbrain which surrounds the cerebral aqueduct. The midbrain tegementum contains cranial nerve nuclei III, IV, and two important nuclei complexes of the motor system, the red nucleus and the substantia nigra. Running through the midbrain tegmentum is the reticular formation, which is integrally involved in maintenance of arousal and the conscious state. The ventral tegmental area has a concentration of dopaminergic neurons which project to the nucleus accumbens, limbic structures, and frontal lobes. This structure and dopaminergic pathway is associated with feelings of pleasure, and is a so-called "pleasure center" of the brain along with the nucleus accumbens and other limbic structures.

Rule of thumb: Midbrain

Associated with afferent (sensory) and efferent (motor) pathways, motor control (part of basal ganglia and substantia nigra), eye movements, auditory relay area, arousal/attention (superior part of Reticular Activating System) and "pleasure center" of brain (ventral tegmental area)

- Inferior colliculus – auditory attention
- Superior colliculus – visual attention/reflexes
- Cerebral peduncles/red nucleus – projections to and from cerebrum to cerebellum
- Tegmentum – arousal and ventral tegmentum area part of "pleasure center" of brain

---

The midbrain *Pretectum* is a group of neurons found at the border of the midbrain and the thalamus. The pretectum receives input from retinal cells, and is responsible for the pupillary light reflex. The *Mesencephalic Duct (aqueduct of Sylvius)*, connects the third and fourth ventricles.

Forebrain (Procencephalon). Embryonic term referring to the Diencephalon and Telencephalon.

Diencephalon. Term to describe a part of the brain that includes the Epithalamus, Thalamus, Hypothalamus, Subthalamus, Pituitary gland, Pineal gland, and the Third ventricle (see Figs. 3.1, 3.4, 3.5, and 3.8).

Thalamus. The thalamus is a roughly football-shaped pair of structures at the top of the midbrain. All afferent somatosensory neurons, except olfaction (smell), synapse at thalamic nuclei prior to reaching the cerebral cortex. Efferent motor commands are processed by thalamic nuclei as well, prior to being acted on.

The thalamus serves as a major "relay" station for sensory input into the brain (see Fig. 3.4). In addition to senses, the thalamus receives input from the cerebral cortex, basal ganglia as well as brain stem/cerebellum nuclei (see Fig. 3.4) and is involved in motor behaviors as well as cognition/emotional processes. The thalamus has been divided into five nuclear groups, based partly on a "Y"-shaped white matter tract through the thalamus called the internal medullary lamina. The "Y"-shaped white matter tract divides the thalamus into three broad areas, anterior, lateral, and medial. The fourth nuclear group is a series of nuclei that lie within the internal medullary lamina termed the intralaminar nuclei. The fifth thalamic nuclear group, a thin wall of neurons covering the lateral aspect of the thalamus, is termed the reticular nucleus.

The nuclei of the thalamus are of three types: Relay, Association, and Nonspecific nuclei. Relay nuclei have well-defined afferent projections and relay this to functionally distinct cerebral cortex areas (see Table 3.1). The Relay nuclei include the primary sensory nuclei (VPL, VPM, LGN, MGN) and motor functions (VL and VA). These nuclei maintain a somatotropic organization from afferent to efferent projections. The LGN is a major pathway for vision (to remember LGN is for vision, remember *L* in *LGN = Look*), while the MGN is for auditory inputs from the inferior colliculus, and these nuclei are thought to be involved in orienting behaviors to these sensory stimuli that are out of conscious control (e.g., reflexive movements). Association nuclei receive afferents (input projections) from the cerebral cortex and project back to association cortex [e.g., Pulvinar, Lateral posterior (LP), Medial Dorsal (MD), Lateral Dorsal (LD)]. The nonspecific nuclei receive diffuse inputs from the ascending reticular activating system/reticular activating system (ARAS), cerebral cortex and other thalamic nuclei, and have diffuse projections throughout the cortex (intralaminar and reticular nuclei). Figure 3.4 highlights the afferent/input (gray arrows) and efferent/outputs (black arrows) for the major thalamic nuclei. All thalamic nuclei have reciprocal projections to and from the reticular nuclei of the thalamus and associated cortical regions. Table 3.1 provides a list of the presumed behavioral function of the major thalamic nuclei.

Clinically, lesions to the thalamus are typically associated with marked neurologic impairment (e.g., hemi-sensory loss, hemi-neglect), but can also result in marked neuropsychological deficits (amnestic syndrome). Symptoms can include hemi-neglect (sensory and/or motor), hemi-anesthesia, apraxis, amnesia, and aphasias.

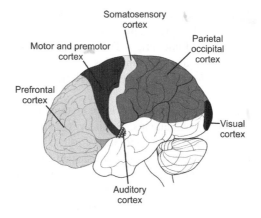

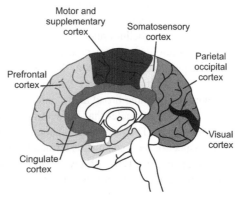

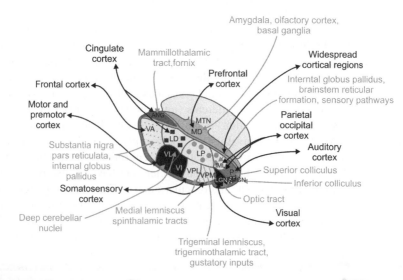

Fig. 3.4 Major thalamic nuclei with afferent and efferent pathways identified with associated cerebral cortex projection areas

Table 3.1 Thalamic nuclei, afferents, efferents, and function

Nuclei	Afferent (input)	Efferent (output)	Function
Anterior nuclei group			
Anterior nucleus	Hippocampus/fornix, mammilary bodies	Cingulate gyrus	Explicit memory
Intralaminar nuclei			
Centromedian	Globus palidus, ARAS, sensory pathways	Striatum, cerebral cortex	Motor function. Relay for basal gangalia to cerebral
Lateral nuclei group			
Lateral geniculate nucleus (LGN)	Retina	Primary visual cortex	Visual input to primary visual cortex
Medial geniculate nucleus (MGN)	Inferior colliculus	Primary auditory cortex	Auditory inputs to primary auditory cortex
Pulvinar	Tectum (extra lateral geniculate visual pathway)	Parietal, occipital, temporal heteromodal association cortex	Behavioral orientation to visual (and other sensory) stimuli
Ventral anterior nucleus (VA)	Substantia nigra pars reticulata, globus palidus interna, cerebellar nuclei	Frontal cortex, particularly pre-motor/ supplementary motor and prefrontal regions	Relay loop of basal ganglia and cerebellar inputs to cortex. Awareness and control of body movements/ coordination
Ventral lateral nucleus (VL)	Globus palidus interna, substantia nigra pars compacta, cerebellar nuclei	Motor, premotor, and supplementary motor cortex	Relay loop for basal ganglia and cerebellum to cortex
Ventral posterior lateral nucleus (VPL)	Medial lemniscus/ dorsal columns, spinothalamic tract	Parietal somatosensory cortex	Somatosensory inputs to cortex
Ventral posteromedial nucleus (VPM)	Trigeminal lemniscus, trigeminothalamic tract, gustatory inputs	Parietal somatosensory cortex	Somatosensory cranial nerve inputs (including taste) to cortex
Lateral dorsal nucleus (LD)	Substantia nigra pars reticulata, globus palidus interna, cerebellar nuclei	Frontal cortex, particularly pre-motor/ supplementary motor and prefrontal regions	Relay loop of basal ganglia and cerebellar inputs to cortex. Awareness and control of body movements/ coordination
Lateral posterior nucleus (LP)	Tectum (extra lateral geniculate visual pathway)	Parietal, occipital, temporal heteromodal association cortex	Behavioral orientation to visual (and other sensory) stimuli
Ventral medial nucleus (VM)	Reticular formation (midbrain)	Diffuse afferents to cortex	Likely involved in maintaining awake conscious state

(continued)

Table 3.1 (continued)

Nuclei	Afferent (input)	Efferent (output)	Function
Medial nuclear group			
Mediodorsal (MD)	Amygdala, limbic basal ganglia, olfactory cortex	Frontal cortex	Cognition (attention/ memory), emotional functions. Major limbic/frontal relay pathway
Midline nuclei			
Internateromedial, intermediodorsal, paraventricular, parataenial, etc.	Amygdala, basal forebrain, hippocampus, hypothalamus	Amygdala, hippocampus, limbic cortex	Limbic pathways
Reticular nucleus			
Reticular nucleus	Cerebral cortex, thalamic, all other thalamic nuclei, ARAS	All thalamic nuclei	Appears to regulate other thalamic nuclei

ARAS = ascending reticular activating system.

Rule of thumb: Thalamic nuclei

- Anterior nuclei group
  - Anterior nucleus – memory input from hippocampus/mamilary body to cingulate gyrus
- Lateral nuclei group
  - LGN – visual input from retina to primary visual cortex
  - MGN – auditory input from inferior colliculus to auditory cortex
  - Pulvinar – visual input from tectum to diffuse association cortex.
  - VPL – sensory from dorsal (posterior) column-medial lemniscus to primary sensory cortex
  - VPM – sensory from trigeminal lemniscus/taste to primary sensory cortex
  - VL – motor from basal ganglia and cerebellum to motor cortex
  - VA – motor from basal ganglia and cerebellum to diffuse frontal cortex
- Medial nuclei group
  - Affective/mood and cognition input from amygdale, olfactory (piriform) cortex, nucleus basalis of meynert to frontal cortex.
- Intralaminar nuclei group
  - Centromedian nucleus – motor, arousal, sensory input to basal ganglia and cortex
- Reticular nuclei
  - From diffuse thalamic relay to cortex

Lesions to the language dominant thalamus can result in transient aphasia syndromes, most commonly presenting as a mixed transcortical aphasia (see Chap. 7), but also stuttering as well as hypophonia and dysarthria. The aphasic symptoms tend to resolve after a few weeks, with poor expressive speech, reduced auditory comprehension (although reading is often preserved), intact repetition (and writing to dictation, but poor spontaneous writing), and anomia. Memory deficits limited to impaired verbal memory (see Chap. 8) has been reported with unilateral language dominant (left) thalamic lesions involving the anterior (and also often including the medial nuclei). Left thalamic lesions to the lateral nuclei often result in sensory loss without gross cognitive impairment (so-called "pure sensory stroke," see Chap. 13).

Nondominant (right) thalamic lesions typically result in pronounced hemineglect to sensory but also motor functions and a constructional apraxia (see Chap. 9). The right thalamic lesion can also exhibit anosognosia and asomatognosia (lack of awareness of a part or whole body). Visual (spatial) memory impairments have been reported with unilateral nondominant thalamic infarcts. The clinically most relevant thalamic nuclei to the neuropsychologist are major sensory relay nuclei (VPL, VPM) as well as the anterior nucleus and mediodorsal (MD) nucleus. Lesions of the sensory relay nuclei are associated with loss of sensory function (and sometimes thalamic pain syndrome with lesions to the VPL). As noted above, damage to the anterior nucleus results in a dense amnestic syndrome, in which episodic memory is lost (anterograde amnesia), but semantic knowledge and implicit memory remains intact. Damage limited to the MD nucleus results in a clinical presentation of severe inattentiveness, confusion (disorientation to time and place), and lethargy. Memory loss can also be present, and may or may not improve, depending upon the extent of the lesion. Damage to the MD nucleus results in EEG changes similar to that seen in Wernicke's encephalopathy (inability to generate EEG sleep patterns). In addition, damage to the intralaminar and/or reticular thalamic nuclei result in lethargy and coma, thought to reflect the diffuse reciprocal projections from the ascending reticular activating system (ARAS) and the cortex.

Hypothalamus. The hypothalamus is located at the most inferior portion of the thalamus. The hypothalamus, together with the pituitary and adrenal glands, play a major role in whole-body homeostasis and control and regulation of the autonomic nervous system. The hypothalamus is involved in the regulation of appetite and thirst as well as the body's efforts to regulate temperature. The hypothalamus is also involved in regulating sexual arousal as well as behaviors associated with fear and rage reactions. Together, the hypothalamus–pituitary–adrenal (HPA) axis (described in detail below) has also been implicated in the development and maintenance of mood disorders. Secretions from hypothalamic neurons regulate a number of physiological functions (see Table 3.2). The hormones involved in the HPA are detailed in Table 3.3.

Pituitary gland. The pituitary gland is about the size of a pea and located inferior (underneath) of the hypothalamus. A small funnel-shaped fiber tract called the infundibulum or infundibular stalk connects the pituitary gland to the base of the hypothalamus. The pituitary gland is referred to as "the master gland," because of its control of other endocrine organs. Hormones released from the pituitary gland regulate endocrine organs and processes throughout the body. See Table 3.3 for a summary of the hormones and function excreted by the pituitary gland.

Table 3.2 Major hypothalamic nuclei and associated hormone

Hypothalamic nucleus	Releasing hormone
Supraoptic	Oxytocin, vasopressin/ADH
Paraventricular	Oxytocin, vasopressin/ADH
Preoptic, Septal	GnRH
Arcuate	GnRH, GHRH, PIH
Periventricular	TRH, GHIH

Table 3.3 Hormone and related function of the pituitary gland

Hormone	Function
ACTH (adrenocorticotropic hormone)	Adrenal glands – released during arousal or stress. Causes production/release of adrenalin to increase metabolic availability
CRH (corticotropin releasing hormone)	Stimulates adrenocorticotropic (ACTH) and sex hormone production, can act as a neurotransmitter, regulates neuroendocrine stress response
FSH (follicle-stimulating hormone)	Ovaries and testes – regulates hair growth
GHIH (growth hormone inhibitory hormone or somatostatin)	Reduces growth at epiphyseal centers of cartilage
GnRH (gonadotropin releasing hormone)	Controls the development and maintenance of reproductive maturation/function
Growth hormone	Stimulates cell production and growth
LH (luteinizing hormone)	Ovaries and testes
Melanocyte-stimulating hormone	Control skin pigmentation
Oxytocin	Contract the uterus during childbirth and stimulate milk production
PIH (prolactin inhibitory hormone, dopamine)	Inhibits lactogenesis
PRH (prolactin-releasing hormone)	Stimulates lactogenesis
Prolactin	Stimulates milk production after giving birth
Vasopressin = ADH (antidiuretic hormone)	Increase absorption of water into the blood by the kidneys
TSH (thyroid-stimulating hormone)	Thyroid gland – causes release of thyroid hormone and affects metabolism rate

Stress and the Hypothalamus–Pituitary–Adrenal Axis

The hypothalamus–pituitary–adrenal (HPA) axis is a neuroendocrine control system for initiating, regulating and terminating the secretion of glucocorticoids in response to physical and psychological stressors. Glucocorticoids are cholesterol-derived hormones which travel through the blood stream and interact with glucocorticoid receptors to influence metabolic and inflammatory processes. Figure 3.5 summarizes the major afferent and efferent pathways of the HPA axis. The paraventricular nucleus (PVN) of the hypothalamus receives input from ascending brain systems in response to stress. Input to the PVN comes from brain stem aminergic and petidergic systems in the nucleus of the solitary tract and the ventrolateral medulla and limbic system

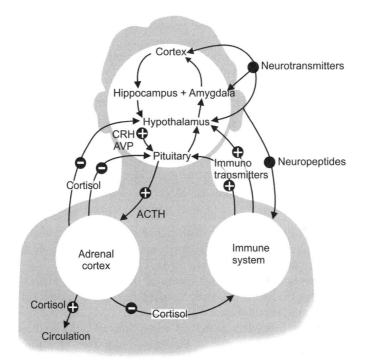

Fig. 3.5 Illustration of the hypothalamus–pituitary–adrenal axis function. *Note*: ACTH = adreno-corticotropic hormone; AVP = vasopressin; CRH = corticotropin releasing hormone

associated regions including the pre-frontal cortex, the hippocampus and the amygdala. The hippocampus projections to the PVN are inhibitory while projections from the amygdala are excitatory. In addition, local hypothalamic interactions influence hormone release (see Table 3.2). These inputs trigger the release of corticotrophin-releasing hormone (CRH) and vasopressin. These hormones act on the pituitary gland causing the release of adrenal corticotropic hormone (ACTH) which, in turn, travels through the blood and acts on the adrenal cortex causing the rapid release of corticosteroids (glucocorticoids) such as cortisol into the bloodstream. Cortisol affects various organ systems to promote homeostasis but also provides negative feedback to the hypothalamus and the pituitary gland. The net effect of the cortisol inhibitory effect on the hypothalamus and pituitary gland is a reduction in the production of CRH, vasopressin (AVP) and ACTH. Chronic stress has been shown in animals and some human experiments to result in chronically elevated cortisol levels. Chronic stimulation of the HPA axis in response to stress has been argued to adversely affect the function of the HPA axis as well as associated interconnected brain areas (neocortex, hippocampus, and amygdala). This dysfunction is thought to play a role in the development of symptoms in depressive and anxiety disorders (Tsigos and Chrousos 2002).

Epithalamus. The epithalamus includes the *Pineal Gland* and the habenular nuclei. The function of the pineal gland in humans is not entirely clear, but is thought to be associated with the regulation of the circadian rhythm.

Third ventricle. Ventricle located between the lobes of the thalamus (see Fig. 3.8). It is connected to the lateral ventricles via the foramin of Monroe (Interventricular Foramin) and with the fourth ventricle via the aquaduct of Sylvius (cerebral aqueduct).

Rule of thumb: Hypothalamus, pituitary, and HPA axis

- Hypothalamus – regulation of thirst, appetite, temperature sexual arousal, and fear/rage behaviors as well as affect activity of pituitary gland
- Pituitary gland – regulation of endocrine functions

Telencephalon. Embryonic term that includes the following structures of the brain: Rhinencephalon, Amygdala, Hippocampus, Basal ganglia, Neocortex, and the Lateral ventricles (see Figs. 3.3 and 3.8).

The *Rhinencephalon* (also called piriform, pyriform, or olfactory cortex) in humans is responsible for olfaction and includes the olfactory nerve, bulb, stria and tract and a portion of the amygdala.

Amygdala. Almond-shaped groups of nuclei located deep within the medial temporal lobes and just anterior to the hippocampi (see also Fig. 3.3). The Amygdala receives input from somatosensory areas as well as limbic structures, and is thought to be primarily involved in processing emotional states and associates memory with emotional functioning (i.e., involved in state-dependent learning; see Kendel et al. (2000), for review).

Hippocampus. The hippocampi structures make up part of the mesial temporal lobes, and are located beneath the cortical surface of the parahippocampal gyrus and just posterior to the amygdala. The hippocampus takes the form of an elongated tube thicker at its anterior end and becoming thin at its posterior (tail) end (see Fig. 3.3). The hippocampus plays a significant role in long-term memory formation and spatial navigation (see Sect. II below, and Chap. 8 for more details).

Basal Ganglia. Term to describe a group of nuclei beneath the cortex white matter, and including: caudate nucleus, putamen, globus pallidus external and internal (GPe and GPi), substantia nigra pars reticulata and pars compacta (SNr and SNc) and subthalamic nucleus (STN). The nucleus accumbens is also generally included in the basal ganglia (see Chap. 19 for detailed review of the structure and function of the basal ganglia). In general, the basal ganglia reflects a system of control and mediation of motor function between the cortex, thalamus and cerebellum. The major input to the basal ganglia is the striatum (caudate nucleus, putamen, and nucleus accumbens). The SNr and GPi are the major output nuclei. Traditionally, the basal ganglia functional processes is presented as consisting of two pathways, a "direct" and "indirect" pathway. While overly simplistic, the traditional perspective is provided here as a foundation (see Chap. 19). The "direct" pathway serves to increase (excite) the activity of the thalamus, thereby increasing cortical motor activity. Alternatively, the "indirect" pathway, which serves to decrease activity of the thalamus, inhibits cortex activity (indirect inhibits).

Once considered limited to purely motor control, the basal ganglia is recognized as having at least five major channels that run parallel using related but separate nuclei and fibers, but also have areas where these pathways intermingle: (1) motor, (2) ocular motor, (3) dorsolateral, (4) orbitofrontal, and (5) anterior cingulated/limbic/affective. Each component or channel maintains a somatotropic organization through the basal ganglia along with input and output cortices. The motor channel is the traditionally recognized function of the basal ganglia, and receives inputs from somatosensory and motor cortex to the putamen, which projects to the GPi/SNr (direct pathway) or projects to the GPe, then to the STN and then to the GPi/SNr (indirect pathway). Projections of the GPi/SNr go to the VL/VA of the thalamus and then to the motor cortex (primary, pre-, and supplementary). The ocular motor channel receives input from frontal and parietal cortex to the caudate nucleus (body), which then project to the direct and indirect pathways and the GPi/SNr flow to the MD and VA thalamic nuclei than to the frontal eye fields. The dorsolateral prefrontal channel receives inputs from dorsolateral prefrontal as well as some motor and parietal cortex and project to the caudate nucleus (head) with the primary outputs (GPi/SNr) coursing to the MD and VA thalamic nuclei which then projects to the dorsolateral prefrontal cortex. The orbitofrontal component is similar to the dorsolateral, except the input fibers are mostly from the lateral orbitofrontal region as well as some from the anterior temporal lobes. These cortical areas project to the caudate nucleus (head) and project to MD and VA thalamic nuclei, which then courses back to the orbitofrontal regions. The anterior cingulate/limbic channel receives inputs from the anterior cingulate and temporal cortices (amygdala and hippocampus), sending fibers to the nucleus accumbens and ventral caudate nucleus. Output from the basal ganglia is via the ventral pallidum that project to the MD thalamic nuclei. This information is then projected to the anterior cingulate and orbital frontal cortex.

Rule of thumb: Basal ganglia

- Basal ganglia include the major input nuclei of the striatum (caudate nucleus, putamen, and nucleus accumbens), the globus palidus externa and substantia nigra pars compacta, and major output nuclei (globus palidus interna and substantia nigra pars compacta)
- Two major pathways: direct and indirect
    - Direct: "excites", and main effect is to excite activity of cortex
    - Indirect: "inhibits" and main effect is to inhibit activity of cortex
- Major channels of basal ganglia
    - Motor
    - Occular-motor
    - Dorsolateral prefrontal
    - Lateral orbitofrontal
    - Anterior cingulate/limbic/affective

Neocortex. Term defining the outermost layers (6, see below) of neurons and underlying white matter. The neocortex is the newest part of the nervous system to develop, and serves as the center of all higher mental functions such as speech and language, declarative memory (see Chap. 8), visuoperceptual/visuospatial skills and conscious thought. The neocortex is divided into right and left cerebral hemispheres by the longitudinal cerebral fissure. Information is passed directly between the two hemispheres via a massive collection of axons called the corpus callosum. The embryologic development of the cerebral hemispheres results in a wrinkled or folded appearance. The convex portions of the cerebral cortex are referred to as gyri, and the concave portions are referred to as sulci. While there are no two brains that have the exact same pattern of gyri and sulci, there are some gyri and sulci that are consistently maintained (central sulcus, Sylvian fissure), and form the basis for named landmarks that are used to divide the cerebral cortex into the frontal, parietal, temporal, and occipital lobes. The region between the frontal and temporal operculum (a series of gyri and sulci lying underneath the frontal and temporal lobes) is identified as the insular cortex or lobe (see Figs. 3.1, 3.3, 3.6, and 3.7).

Each hemisphere of the neocortex is divided into four traditional "lobes": Frontal, parietal, temporal, and occipital. The insular region (or cortex) is cerebral cortex underlying the frontal and temporal operculum (making the "floor" of the sylvian fissure), and is sometimes referred to as a "fifth" lobe of the human brain (see below). The frontal cortex is divided from the parietal by the central sulcus. The frontal lobe is separated from the temporal lobe by the Sylvian fissure. The parietal and occipital lobe are separated by the parieto-occipital sulcus. The inferior portion of the parietal cortex is divided from the temporal cortex by the posterior portion of the sylvian fissure (see Fig. 3.6).

Cerebro-Spinal Fluid

The entire central nervous system is bathed and suspended in a clear colorless fluid called Cerebrospinal Fluid (CSF). The CSF occupies the space between the arachnoid matter and pia matter surrounding the brain, and also fills the spaces within the brain formed by the ventricles, cisterns, sulci, and the central canal of the spinal cord (see Fig. 3.8). The total volume of CSF in an adult human is about 125–150 mL. While the weight of the brain is anywhere from 1,100–1,400 g, the effective weight of the brain while suspended in CSF encased in the skull is decreased to about 50 g. CSF is produced by the choroid plexus in the lateral, third, and fourth ventricles at a rate of about 400–700 mL/day (average is 500 mL/day) or about 20–22 mL/h, allowing for the "turn over" of all CSF fluid 4–5 times per day. Figure 3.8 illustrates the circulation of CSF beginning in the lateral ventricles, through the Foramen of Monro to the 3rd ventricle then through the aqueduct of sylvius to the 4th ventricle and the foramina of Magendie (medial) or Luschka (lateral) to the subarachnoid space, where it flows around the brain stem and spinal cord and is reabsorbed by

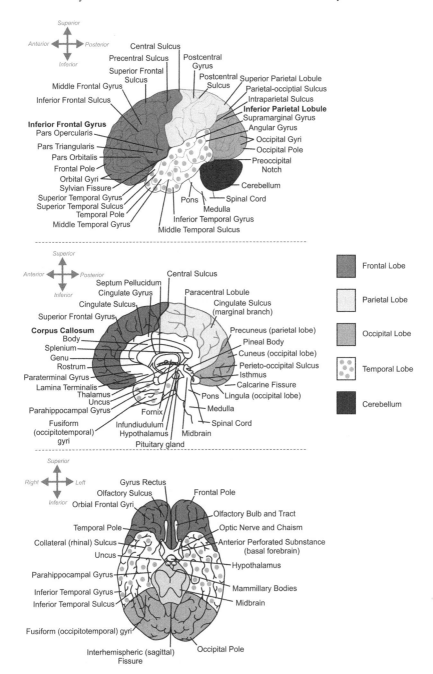

Fig. 3.6   Surface anatomy of the lateral, midsagital, and inferior views of the brain

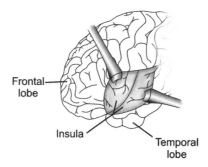

Fig. 3.7 Frontal and temporal operculum pulled back to show the underlying insular cortex (lobe)

the arachnoid granulations that contain the arachnoid villus. Because the brain and spinal cord are encased in the skull and the spinal canal is surrounded by the meninges; changes in the volume of the brain, blood, or cerebrospinal fluid will result in increased intracranial pressure (ICP). In adults, normal CSF pressure is 150–180 mm H_2O (or 8–14 mmHg), and is lower in children (30–60 mm H_2O).

There are a several common mechanisms of increased intracranial pressure, including (1) space occupying lesion, (2) generalized brain swelling, (3) increased venous pressure (e.g., cerebral venous thrombosis or obstruction of jagular vein), (4) obstruction of the flow or absorption of CSF, or (5) process increasing CSF volume (e.g., tumor increasing CSF production). The aspects of increased intracranial pressure due to the first three are reviewed in Chaps. 13 and 21. Interruptions in the flow or re-absorption of CSF can result in increased CSF pressure termed hydrocephalus. There are two general types of hydrocephalus, (1) communicating and (2) noncommunicating (obstructive) hydrocephalus. Communicating hydrocephalus is a term used to describe hydrocephalus not due to blockage of the CSF flow through the brain, but rather due to disrupted re-absorption of CSF. Noncommunicating (obstructive) hydrocephalus is a term used to describe increased CSF pressure when the flow of CSF fluid is obstructed. Common areas for obstructed flow is the foramen of Monro (between lateral and 3rd ventricle), the aqueduct of Sylvias (between 3rd and 4th ventricles) or the result of fibrosing meningitis due to infection or subarachnoid hemorrhage (see also Chap. 14).

Rule of thumb: Cerebrospinal fluid (CSF)

- Produced by choroid plexus in lateral, third, and fourth ventricles
- CSF produced 20–22 mL (20–22 cm³) per hour
- Total CSF volume is 125–150 mL (125–150 cm³)
- Provides buoyancy to brain

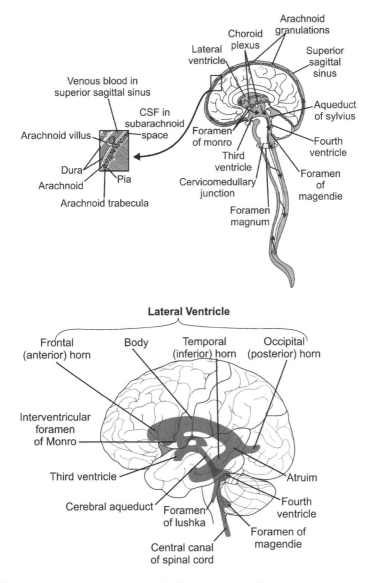

Fig. 3.8 Cerebral ventricles, cerebrospinal fluid production and flow

Spinal Cord

The bony skull attaches to the spinal column at the base of the skull by means of a series of dense fibrous ligamentous attachments. There are 33 vertebrae which make up the spinal column, and are divided into 7 cervical, 12 thoracic, 5 lumbar, 5 fused sacral and 4 fused coccygeal vertebrae (see Figs. 3.1 and 3.10). The bony

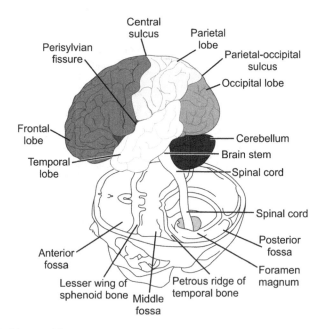

Fig. 3.9 Skull base and foramen magnum

spinal column houses the spinal cord. The spinal cord begins at the base of the skull where it is the continuation of the medulla oblongata. The spinal cord exits the skull through the foramen magnum (Fig. 3.9), and 31 pairs of spinal nerve roots exit the spine at each vertebral level between vertebral processes. The nerve roots derived from the dorsal aspect of the spinal cord make up the spinal *sensory nerve roots*. The nerve roots derived from the ventral aspect of the spinal cord make up the spinal *motor nerve roots*. The body of the spinal cord terminates at lower border of the first lumbar vertebrae, L1, into the conus medularis. The conus medularis terminates as the cauda equina, a filamentous structure which gives rise to the lumbar, sacral and cocygeal spinal nerve roots. The spinal cord itself generally ends around the L1 vertebral body, so one needs to distinguish between spinal cord level (such as neurons affecting L3 nerve root, and the vertebral level, as this dissociation occurs with development with elongation of the spine relative to the spinal cord.

Figure 3.10 provides an overview for the organization of the spinal cord. Unlike the brain with gray matter (neurons) on the exterior and white matter on the interior, the organization of the spinal cord has gray matter (neurons) on the interior and white matter (axons) on the periphery. The major afferent (sensory) and efferent (motor) pathways are discussed in detail below. For now, we direct the reader to appreciate that the sensory pathways are generally in the dorsal (posterior) aspect of the spinal cord while the motor afferents are generally in the ventral (anterior) area of the spinal cord.

Rule of thumb: Spinal cord

- Dorsal (towards back) root is sensory
- Ventral (towards stomach) root is motor
- Clinically important reflex levels
  - C5/6 – Biceps and Brachioradialis
  - C7 – Triceps
  - C8 – Finger flexors
  - L3 – Knee
  - S1 – Ankle
- Clinically important dermatomes
  - C2/3 – Posterior head and neck
  - C5 – Anterior shoulder
  - C6 – Thumb
  - C7 – Index and middle fingers
  - C7/8 – Ring finger
  - C8 – Pinky (little finger)
  - T1 – Inner forearm
  - T2 – Upper inner arm
  - T4/5 – Nipple
  - T10 – Umbilicus
  - L2 – Anterior upper thigh
  - L3 – Knee
  - S1 – Toes, 4th and 5th toes

Peripheral Nervous System (PNS)

The peripheral nervous system innervates the organs and muscles of the body and is classically divided into the motor and sensory components, which applies both to segmental nerve roots from the spinal cord as well as the cranial nerves (see Fig. 3.11). The sensory and motor components incorporate what is termed the autonomic nervous system.

Components of the Peripheral Nervous System

Cranial Nerves are part of the PNS. There are 12 paired cranial nerves. These are illustrated in Fig. 3.1 with respect to the overall organization of the PNS. The function and assessment of the 12 cranial nerves are reviewed in Chap. 4.

Dorsal nerve roots carry afferent sensory information from the peripheral nervous system to the sensory neurons of the spinal cord (CNS). The neurons that make up the dorsal root ganglia, the primary sensory neurons, are outside the CNS,

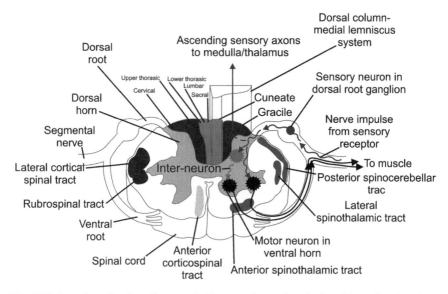

Fig. 3.10 Location of major afferent and efferent pathways in spinal cord including dorsal and ventral roots

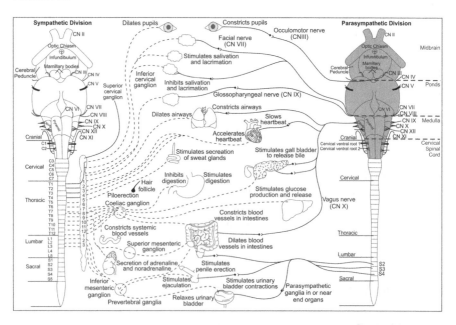

Fig. 3.11 Sympathetic and parasympathetic divisions of the peripheral nervous system *Note:* The sympathetic nervous system is mostly associated with "flight or fight" responses, while the parasympathetic nervous system is involved in "rest and digest" functions

but have axon processes that enter and ascend in the spinal cord to synapse with secondary sensory neurons (see Fig. 3.26).

Ventral nerve roots carry efferent motor information from the upper motor neurons (e.g., corticospinal tract) to the endings in skeletal muscle.

Plexus is a term that refers to an elaborate meshwork of peripheral nerves [e.g., brachial plexus (arm) or lubmosacral plexus (leg)] where axons from several adjacent nerve roots (e.g., c5 to T1 in the brachial plexus) are recombined into named peripheral nerves, such as the median nerve which contains motor axons from several nerve roots.

Autonomic Nervous System

The autonomic nervous system is divided into the *sympathetic* and *parasympathetic* nervous system. The sympathetic nervous system arises from thoracic and lumbar spinal levels and releases *norepinephrine* onto end organs. The sympathetic nervous system is involved in "fight or flight" functions. The parasympathetic nervous system is the "counterpart" to the sympathetic nervous system. The parasympathetic nervous system is associated with "rest and digest" functions, such as increasing gastric secretions and peristalsis, slowing heart rate, and decreasing pupil size. The parasympathetic nervous system arises from the cranial nerves and from the sacral spinal levels (S2–S4) and primarily utilizes the neurotransmitter *acetylcholine* for its actions on the end organs. While a comprehensive description of the actions of the parasympathetic and sympathetic nervous system is beyond the scope of this chapter, Fig. 3.11 provides a detailed illustration of the actions of the parasympathetic and sympathetic systems on organs and tissues.

Rule of thumb: Peripherial nervous system

- Cranial nerves
  - 12 pairs (eyes, vision, face, hearing, tongue, larynx, pharynx, heart)
- Spinal cord
  - Sensory (dorsal) component
  - Motor (ventral) component
- Autonomic nervous system (ANS)
  - Parasympathetic nervous system
    - □ "Rest and digest" functions
    - □ Arises from cranial nerves and sacral (S2–S4) spinal levels
    - □ Acetylcholine neurotransmitter on end organs.
  - Sympathetic nervous system
    - □ "Flight or fight" functions
    - □ Arises from thoracic and upper lumbar (T1 to L2) spinal levels
    - □ Norepinephrine neurotransmitter on end organs
  - Enteric nervous system
    - □ Inervates walls of digestive tract
    - □ Controls peristalsis and gastrointestinal secretion with other ANS

Cerebrovascular System Overview

The blood supply to the brain is provided by two paired sets of arteries, forming an anterior and posterior circulatory system to the brain (see Fig. 3.12) (see also Chap. 13 for further details). The paired internal carotid arteries (ICA) arise from the common carotid artery on each side. The ICA enters the skull through the carotid canal and supplies blood to the anterior portion of the brain and intracranial structures. The major arteries providing vascular supply to the brain derived from the ICA include the anterior cerebral artery, middle cerebral artery and the posterior communicating artery (see Chap. 13 for further details). The MCA provides blood to most of the basal ganglia through a variety of small penetrating arteries termed lenticulostriate arteries (see Fig. 3.13). The ophthalmic artery and the anterior choriodal also originate from the ICA.

Rule of thumb: Mnemonic for arteries that originate from the internal carotid artery (proximal to distal): OPAAM

- *O*phthalmic artery
- *P*osterior communicating artery (PCoA)
- *A*nterior choroidal artery
- *A*nterior cerebral artery (ACA)
- *M*iddle cerebral artery (MCA)

The *vertebral artery* supplies the posterior portion of the brain (see Fig. 3.14). The vertebral artery is a branch of the subclavian artery which ascends through the foramina of the transverse processes of the upper six cervical vertebrae, winds behind the articular process of C1 and enters the skull through the foramen magnum. The paired vertebral arteries traverse across the anterior surface of the medulla oblongata and join at the pontomedullary junction (base of the pons) to form the single basilar artery. Along the course the vertebral arteries give off three primary branches which provide blood supply to the brain stem and cerebellum: (1) posterior spinal artery, (2) anterior spinal artery, and (3) posterior inferior cerebellar argery (PICA). The posterior spinal arteries (not shown) provides blood supply to the posterior 1/3 of the spinal cord (one side of the cord for each posterior spinal artery). The anterior spinal artery runs along the ventral midline of the spinal cord and supplies the anterior 2/3 of the spinal cord. The PICA provides blood to the lateral medulla and inferior surface of the cerebellum. The basilar artery gives rise to short paramedian arteries as well as the Anterior Inferior Cerebellar artery (AICA) and the Superior Cerebellar artery (SCA) before bifurcating to form the two Posterior Cerebral arteries (PCA). The two AICAs supply the anterior portions of the ventral surface of the cerebellum (e.g., flocculus) and the caudal pons. The SCAs perfuse the remaining superior surface of the cerebellum, rostral pons, and caudal midbrain. The PCAs perfuse primarily the mesial temporal lobes and

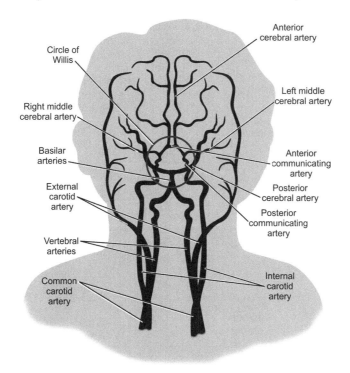

Fig. 3.12 Blood supply to the brain

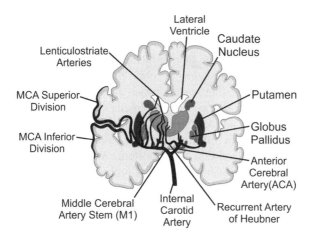

Fig. 3.13 Coronal view of MCA Inferior and superior divisions and lenticolostriate arteries

occipital (mesial and lateral) lobes. The PCAs can also provide blood flow to the occipitotemporal and occipitalparietal cortices. Branches of the PCA perfuse the subthalamic nucleus, posterior thalamus, hypothalamus, and splenium of the corpus collosum (see Fig. 3.12 and Chap. 13).

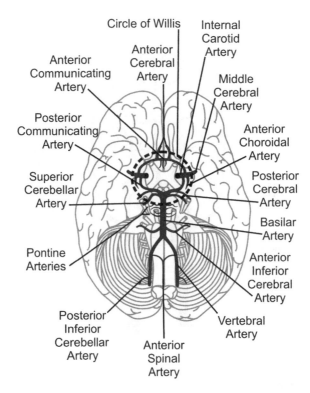

Fig. 3.14 Cerebral vasculature and the circle of Willis

The major branches of the internal carotid artery and the basilar artery combine to form a structure referred to as the *Circle of Willis* (see Fig. 3.14). The Circle of Willis is a ring of blood vessels surrounding the optic chiasm and pituitary stalk. It consists of the posterior communicating arteries which arise from the ICA and connect the posterior cerebral arteries to the anterior circulation. The anterior communicating artery connects the right and left anterior cerebral arteries. The posterior cerebral arteries are connected at the bifurcation of the basilar artery. A complete circle of Willis allows collateral blood flow to the posterior and anterior cerebrovascular systems. However, there is substantial variability to the circle of Willis, and a hemodynamically complete circle of Willis is found in 21–52% of healthy subjects.

Venus System of the Brain

The veins of the brain carry away deoxygenated blood, and flow into a series of sinuses formed by spaces left between the meninges (dura). Cortical veins drain tverse sinuses are at the junction of the tentorium cerebelli and the dura. The transverse sinuses flow along the occipital bone to the petrous bone. At the petrus bone, the two transverse sinuses form the sigmoid sinus which makes an "S" shape

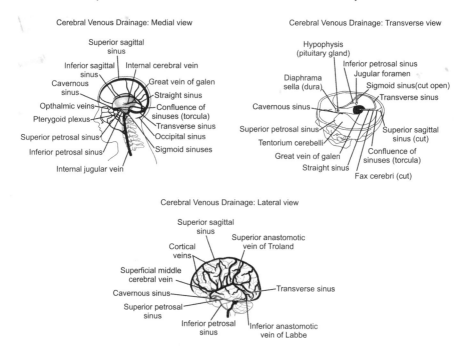

Fig. 3.15 Venus system of brain including sinuses

through the skull to form the internal jugular vein (see Fig. 3.15). The inferior sagital sinus lies at the inferior edge of the falx cerebri, and drains the mesial brain structures. The flow of the inferior sagital sinus is anterior (rostral) to posterior (caudal) and then forms the straight sinus which runs directly posterior and connects with the superior sagital sinus and the two transverse sinuses at the sinus confluence (Torcula). The superior sagital sinus lies in the interhemispheric fissure and flows posteriorily to the sinus confluence. The straight sinus also receives blood from the great vein of Galen, which drains blood from the basal ganglia and thalamus. The cavernous sinus is at the base of the brain (anterior portion) and lies in the sella turcica. The cavernous sinus drains blood posterior to the superior and inferior petrosal sinuses which then drain into the transverse sinus.

Rule of thumb: Venous system of brain

- Reflects the network of veins and sinuses to carry venus blood to heart
- Sinuses formed by spaces in dura.
- Sinuses drain both midsagitally (superior sagital sinus) and laterally (transverse sinuses)
- Transverse sinuses form sigmoid sinus which forms the Jugular vein

It has been estimated the human brain consists of about 100 billion neurons, which have unique characteristics allowing the cells to alter their function and activity in response to stimuli from other neurons and supporting cells called glial cells. A neuron consists of (1) cell body (soma), (2) dendrites, and (3) an axon (see Figs. 3.16 and 3.17). The *soma* contains the nucleus of the cell, which contains the genes and chromosomes of the cell. The soma also includes the *endoplasmic reticulum* where proteins are synthesized, and the *Golgi bodies* that package proteins for

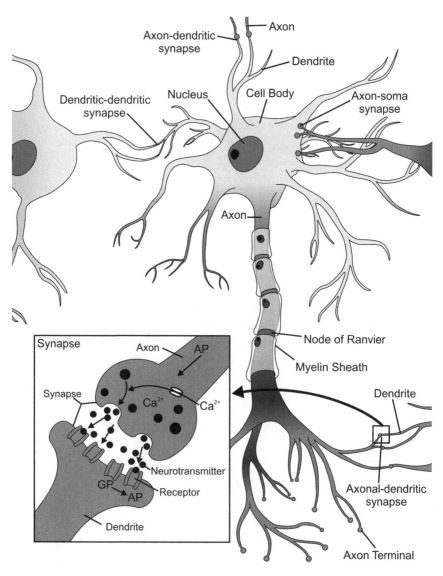

Fig. 3.16 Components of neuron and common types of synapses

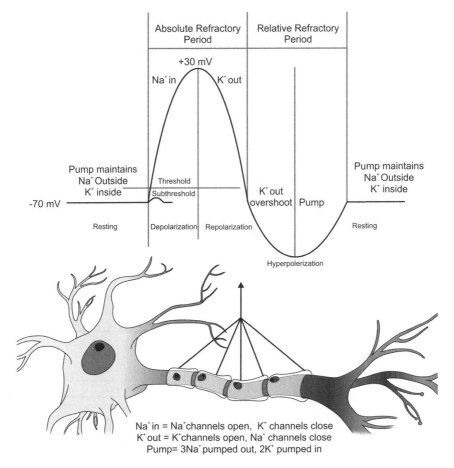

Fig. 3.17 Resting potential and initiation of action potential in a neuron

transportation via *microfilaments* (tiny microtubules making up a "transportation" network) to all areas of the cell. The powerhouse of neurons, like all cells, are the *mitochondria*. *Dendrites* are branchlike processes of the neuron that receive most electrochemical inputs into a neuron. Dendrites have tiny protrusions along the surface called *dendritic spines*, which increase the surface area of the dendrites. The *axon* is a process beginning as a slight swell in the neuron called *axon hillock*, which provides most electrochemical output of the neuron. Most axons branch extensively, which are termed *axon collaterals*. Toward the end of the axon, smaller branches may occur, called *teleodendria*. At the end of the axon (teleodendria) are the axon terminals (or *terminal buttons*) (see Fig. 3.16). Neurons may be multipolar, bipolar, or, rarely in vertebrates, unipolar. Multipolar neurons are the most common in humans, and have one axon hillock, but have multiple dendrites originating from the cell body. A bipolar neuron has one axon and only one primary dendrite, and are typically found in sensory processes (e.g., vision, olfaction, hearing). Unipolar are mostly in invertebrates and have only one extension from the cell body (soma) which is a dendrite and axon.Glial cells provide structure and serve important functions in the nervous system, and include macro- and microglial cells (see Table 3.4). Macroglial cells have been classically described as providing structure and nutrients for neurons and form myelin in the nervous system, it is now clear macroglial cells are involved in homeostasis and neuronal processing activities of the nervous system. As an example, macroglial cells have receptors for various chemicals that affect the function of neurons and/or neurotransmitters (such as ATP) and release neurotransmitters themselves. Macroglial cells are involved in aspects of the neuroregulation of neuronal systems and in the nervous systems response to stress and/or damage.

Rule of thumb: Neurons

- ~100 billion neurons in brain
- ~300 billion glial cells
- Neuron cells made of soma, axon, and dendrites

Table 3.4 Types of glial cells

Location	Cell type	Cell name	Cell description
CNS	Macroglial	Astrocytes	Most numerous macroglial cell, forming the "building block" of the nervous system. Provides support and immediate extracellular environment of neurons.
CNS	Macroglial	Oligodendrocytes	Provide a specialized cell membrane to axons and dendrites of neurons called myelin, which form the myelin sheath. Myelin is a lipid layer surrounding an axon which increases the speed an action potential progresses based on the principal of salutatory conduction.
CNS	Macroglial	Ependymocytes	Produce Cerebral Spinal Fluid (CSF) and are found in the lateral and 3rd ventricle. These cells form the choroids plexus and move long cilia to help move the CSF throughout the CSF space.

(continued)

Table 3.4 (continued)

Location	Cell type	Cell name	Cell description
CNS	Macroglial	Radial cells	In mature brains, only found in cerebellum (Bergmann glia) and retina (Muller glia). In developing nervous system (e.g., before birth), found throughout nervous system and provide for neurogenesis.
CNS	Microglia	Ameboid	Present during perinatal period in the white matter of the corpus callosum.
CNS and PNS	Microglia	Quiescent cells	A "resting" microglial cell not currently engaged in clearing cellular material from nervous system.
CNS and PNS	Microglia	Activated non-phagocytic	Part of the microglial cell response to damage. These cells cannot phagocytose cellular debris or foreign bodies, but do express immunomolecules and secrete pro-inflammatory and pro-cytotoxic factors.
CNS and PNS	Microglia	Activated phagocytic cells	Most immune responsive microglia cell. Have qualities of Activated Non-Phabocytic cells and also actively phagocytose cellular debris and foreign bodies.
CNS and PNS	Microglia	Gitter cells	Resulting cell after microglial cell can no longer phagocytose any more cellular/foreign material. Also called granular corpuscle.
CNS and PNS	Microglia	Perivascular cells	Microglial cells found in the walls of blood vessels. Essential in the repair and/or formation of new vessel walls.
CNS and PNS	Microglia	Juxtavascular cells	Microglial cells found making direct contact with the walls of blood vessels (but not inside the walls like perivascular cells).
PNS	Macroglial	Satellite cells	Cover the exterior of PNS axons and regulate the PNS extracellular environment.
PNS	Macroglial	Schwann cells	The oligodendrocytes of the PNS, Schwann cells form the myelin sheath for axonal and dendritic pathways (fibers). Schwann cells also remove cellular debris.

CNS central nervous system, *PNS* peripheral nervous system

Microglia incorporate about 20% of all glia and provide an important component of the immune response in the CNS. The cells subserving myelination in the CNS are oligodendrocytes (see Fig. 3.16) and Schwann cells in the PNS. The spaces between oligodendrocytes (and Schwann cells) are called nodes of Ranvier and are important in saltatory conduction (see Fig. 3.17).

Neurophysiology and Neurochemical Activity of the Nervous System

The inside of a neuron has a weak negative electric charge at rest (−70 millivolts, mV) compared to the outside of the cell (extracellular space). This resting negative state, termed resting potential, is maintained and regulated by a combination of the cellular membrane (ion channels), Na^+ gates, and the $Na^+ \mid K^+$ pump (see Fig. 3.16). There is a larger concentration of Na^+, Cl^- and Ca^{2+} ions extracellularly, while there is a greater concentration of K^+ intracellularly.

Neurotransmitters are a group of endogenous chemicals responsible for signaling between neurons and other cells (there is very little direct "electrical" connection between neurons). Thus, signaling of the nervous system is a bioelectrochemical process affected by neurotransmitters. Neurotransmitters act on proteins called neurotransmitter receptors, which are found on cell membranes in synapses. Synapses are very narrow gaps (20–50 nm) between neurons allowing for chemical transmission via neurotransmitters. The binding of neurotransmitters to pre- and post-synaptic receptors results in changes in the polarization of the cell. Neurotransmitter actions that increase the likelihood of initiating an action potential are called excitatory postsynaptic potentials (EPSPs) while those that reduce the likelihood of an action potential are termed inhibitory postsynaptic potentials (IPSPs). Neurotransmitter receptors may be located before the synapse (termed pre-synaptic) or after the synapse (termed post-synaptic) (and also identified on some glial cells). Synapses may occur between an axon (terminal button) and a dendrite (axon-dendritic), axon and an axon (axon-axonal), axon and a cell body/soma (axon-somatic), or dendrite to a dendrite (dendo-dendritic) (see Fig. 3.16). Receptor binding results in many of these IPSPs and EPSPs occurring every second, and the acute action of these lead to fluctuations in the intracellular resting potential. If enough EPSPs occur to raise the resting potential to around −50 mV, termed the threshold potential, an action potential will occur (see Fig. 3.17). This action potential is a positive charge of about +30 mV that runs the length of the axon at speeds ranging from 1 to 110 m/s (see Table 3.5 for description of the major motor and sensory fibers). Action potentials are faster for axons that are myelinated due to saltatory conduction. Saltatory conduction allows for an increase in action potential, as the action potential occurs at each node of Ranvier, "skipping" along the axon as opposed to a steady wave in nonmyelinated axons. During an action potential, a neuron is unable to produce another action potential, and this time is termed the absolute refractory period. The relative refractory period refers to the time the neuron is hyperpolarized, when only a very large stimulus will result in an action potential. During the refractory period, the $Na^+–K^+$ pump works to reinstate the resting potential.

Table 3.5 Types of motor and sensory fibers

Type	Diameter (μm)	Velocity (m/s)	Myelinated
Motor			
Alpha motor neuron	13–20	80–120	Yes
Gamma motorneuron	5–8	4–24	Yes
Sensory			
1a	13–20	80–120	Yes
1b	13–20	80–120	Yes
II	6–12	33–75	Yes
A delta	1–5	3–30	Yes, thin
C	0.2–1.5	0.5–2.0	No
Autonomic			
Preganglionic	1–5	3–15	Yes
Postganglionic	0.2–1.5	0.5–2.0	No

Rule of thumb: Neuronal neurophysiology and Saltatory conduction

- Resting potential of neurons is −70 mV
- At rest, neurons have greater concentration of Na^+, Cl^- and Ca^{2+} outside cell, and K^+ inside cell.
- Action potentials start at axon hillock and able to "skip" or "jump" from one node of Ranvier to the next on myelinated axons.

Major Neurotransmitter Systems of the CNS

Hundreds of chemicals have been identified that satisfy the definition of a neurotransmitter; however, some are much more abundant and have had more research as playing a significant role in cognitive and mood/behavioral functions. Common neurotransmitters can be classified into those of small molecules [acetylcholine, Gama Amino Butyric Acid (GABA), Glutamate, and Glycine], catecholamines, (e.g., dopamine, epinephrine, histamine, norepinephrine, and serotonin), and neuropeptides [e.g., calcitonin gene-related peptide (CGRP), endorphins, enkephalins, and substance P]. Currently, the neurotransmitters with the most research include: acetylcholine, dopamine, norepinephrine, serotonin, GABA and glutamate. Small molecule neurotransmitters are the most plentiful in the nervous system, and are primarily excitatory (glutamate) or inhibitory (GABA and glycine). Acetylcholine (Ach) appears to have both excitatory and inhibitory effects. It is excitatory in the CNS and neuromusculature junction and inhibitory on smooth muscle. Catacholamines are involved in mood modulation and stabilization, and have both excitatory and inhibitory processes. Neuropeptides form a large class of neurotransmitter substances (over 100), but their effects appear to be through second messenger systems. Neurotransmitters are typically produced in the soma (or at the terminals), and are released at synapses to exert their influence.

Rule of thumb: Neurotransmitter actions

- Neurotransmitters "communicate" between neurons by binding to receptors
- Receptors are located in chemical synapses
- Chemical synapses are where many clinical disorders are expressed either in abnormalities in the receptor binding or the production or release of neurotransmitters
- Chemical synapses are the site of action for the behavioral effects of drugs
- Receptors may have multiple binding sites for multiple neurotransmitters
- Neurotransmitter actions are either "fast acting" or neuromodulatory
    - Fast acting is binding that generally results in EPSP or IPSP within milliseconds via ligand-gated ion channels
    - Neuromodulatory effects occur within seconds to minutes of binding, and can alter the structure, function, and expression of the neuron, often via G-protein-coupled receptors and activation of 2nd messenger systems

Small Molecule Neurotransmitters

Acetylcholine acts as a neuromodulator in the CNS, generally having an inhibitory influence. Acetylcholine is also thought to play a major role in memory functioning, with reduced concentration of aceylcholine thought to account for some of the cognitive loss associated with Alzheimer's disease. Furthermore, medications with an anticholineragic effect (e.g., tricyclic medications) are known to adversely affect learning and memory, particularly among older adults. The Nucleus Basalis of Meynert is a major source of acetylcholine producing neuronal projections to the neocortex. It is a collection of neuronal cell bodies located within the substantial inomminata (see Fig. 3.18).

GABA is the primary inhibitory neurotransmitter in the human CNS, and is found in all brain regions (see Fig. 3.19). GABA action tends to be "fast" inhibition, most commonly through the $GABA_A$ receptors but also through $GABA_B$ receptors. Activation of the GABA receptor lead to an influx of Cl^- and other anions which hyperpolarize the neuron (reduce the negative charge) such that action potential generation is unlikely (IPSP). The action of GABA can be thought of as counteracting the principal excitatory neurotransmitter *glutamate* (see below). There are 20 subtypes of $GABA_A$ receptors identified, and can be found in the synapse and post-synaptic membranes on dendrites.

Glutamate is always excitatory in the human nervous system, and plays a central role in long-term potentiation in the hippocampus and neocortex. Glutamate binds to at least four different receptors. Three are traditionally described as shorter acting receptors, while a fourth, NMDA, initiates a second messenger system termed long-term potentiation, which is a cellular process thought to account for the cognitive functions of learning and memory. Glutamate is also a neurotoxin when in excess, believed to be due to a cascade which leads to excess Ca^{2+} ions and lead to neuronal death. Glutamate is synthesized throughout the CNS (see Fig. 3.20).

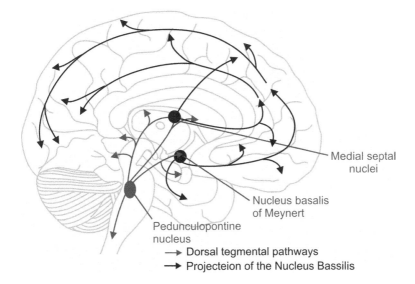

Fig. 3.18 Acetylcholine system

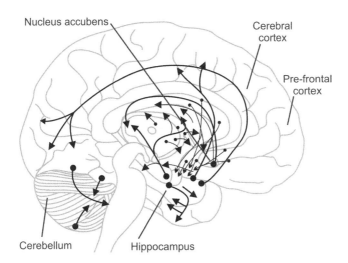

Fig. 3.19 GABA system

Catecholamine Neurotransmitters

Dopaminergic neurons originate in substantia nigra pars compacta, ventral tegmental area (VTA), and hypothalamus. Dopaminergic neurons project throughout the CNS through four major pathways: the mesocortical and mesolimbic pathways, the nigrostriatal pathway and the tuberoinfundibular pathway (see Fig. 3.21). Mesocortical dopamine neurons project from the ventral tegmental area to the pre-frontal cortex. Mesolimbic dopamine neurons project from the ventral tegmental

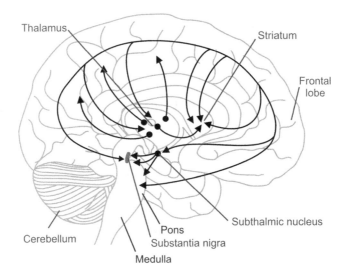

Fig. 3.20 Glutamate system

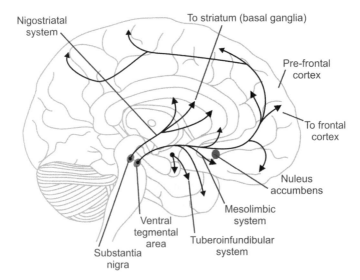

Fig. 3.21 Dopamine system

area to the nucleus accumbens via the hippocampus and amygdala. The nigrostriatal pathway is neurons in the substantia nigra that project to the caudate and putamen. The tuberoinfundibular dopamine neurons project from the hypothalamus to the pituitary gland.

Norepinephrine (noradrenergic) neurons originate both in the locus coeruleus and the lateral tegmental area (see Fig. 3.22). The noradrenergic neurons in the locus coeruleus project to many areas of the brain. The lateral tegmental noradrenergic

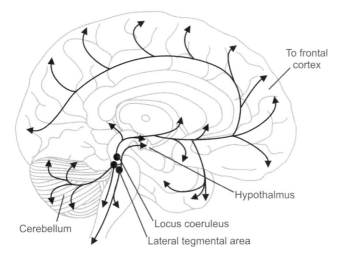

To frontal
cortex

Hypothalmus

Locus coeruleus

Lateral tegmental area

Cerebellum

Fig. 3.22 Norepinephrine system

neurons mainly project to the hypothalamus. The noradrenergic system in the brain affects alertness and arousal, and influences the reward system.

Serotonin (also known as 5HT for 5-hydroxytryptamine) is a monomine synthesized from tryptophan. A major source of 5HT is from the neurons of the raphe nuclei. The raphe nuclei are centered around the reticular formation, grouped and distributed along the entire length of the brainstem. Axons from these neurons reaching almost every part of the central nervous system. Neuron projections in the lower raphe nuclei terminate in the cerebellum and spinal cord while the projections of the higher nuclei spread throughout the entire brain (see Fig. 3.23). Serotonin has a poorly understood neuromodulation effect on the CNS, which appears to be related to affects of 5HT binding to 15 serotonin-activated G-Protein-Coupled Receptors (GPCRs). Activation of 5HT GPCRs can inhibit and/or excite the release of neurotransmitters, lead to general hyperpolarization or depolarization of associated neurons, and can alter intracellular enzymes and gene expression.

Rule of thumb: Neurotransmitters

- Acetylcholine – diffuse. Major projection area is nucleus basalis of Meynert
- Glutamate – excitatory. Diffuse through nervous system
- GABA – inhibitory. Diffuse through nervous system
- Dopamine – neuromodulatory. Major projection areas are SNc, ventral tegmental area, hypothalums
- Norepinephrine – neuromodulatory. Major projection areas are locus coeruleus and lateral tegmental area
- Serotonin – neuromodulatory. Major projection area is raphae nuclei.

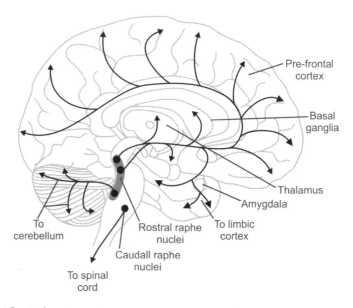

Fig. 3.23 Serotonin system

Cellular Organization of the Cortex

The outer layer of the cerebral cortex is composed of six quite distinct layers identified by the different density and type of neurons that make up each cell layer (see Fig. 3.24). The principal neuronal cell type found in the gray matter is the pyramidal cell. Pyramidal cells extend axons out of the grey matter to remote portions of the nervous system forming the white matter projection fibers making up the subcortical white matter. The neurocortical cell layers are labeled from the surface of the brain inward, and are as follows:

- Layer I (molecular layer) dendrites and axons from other layers
- Layer II (small pyramidal layer) cortical–cortical connections
- Layer III (medium pyramidal layer) cortical–cortical connections
- Layer IV (granular layer) receives inputs from thalamus
- Layer V (large pyramidal layer) sends outputs to subcortical structures (other than thalamus)
- Layer VI (polymorphic layer) sends outputs to the thalamus.
- The thickness of the cell layers varies according to the function of that area of the cortex. Primary motor cortex has a thicker layer V, because there are many more cell bodies than, say, layer IV. However, layer IV is thicker in a sensory area, such as primary visual cortex.

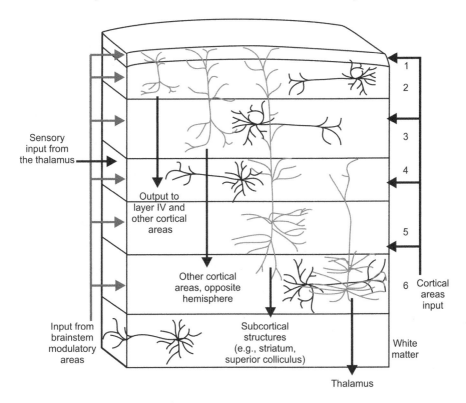

Fig. 3.24 Cellular organization of neocortex

Structural Classification of the Neocortex: Cytoarchitecture

The regions of the cerebral cortex were divided into discrete regions by Korbinian *Brodmann* in 1909 based on *cytoarchitectonic areas* (areas based on the microscopic appearance (cellular layer distribution) of different regions of the cerebral cortex) reviewed above. Often referred to as "Brodmann's Areas" (BA), the areas identified by Brodmann are sometimes used to describe specific functional regions of the brain (e.g., Brodmann's area 44 is often used to identify Broca's area, although Broca's area also includes BA 45). While potentially useful, the structural designation of areas is problematic in variation from individual to individual. Figure 3.25 provides a lateral and midsagital view of the brain that identifies the location of each of Broadmann's areas as well as a general description of its function (e.g., motor, sensory, cognition, emotion, etc.). A more detailed description of each of Brodmann's areas is provided in Table 3.6.

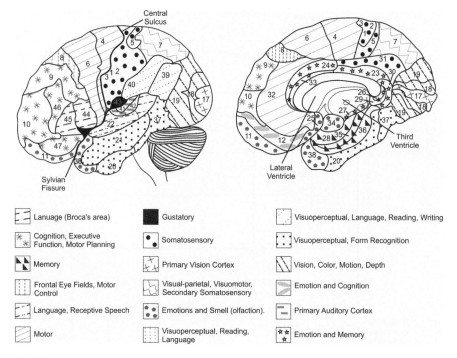

 (figure legend contained within)

Central Sulcus

Sylvian Fissure

Lateral Ventricle

Third Ventricle

Lanuage (Broca's area)	Gustatory
Cognition, Executive Function, Motor Planning	Somatosensory
Memory	Primary Vision Cortex
Frontal Eye Fields, Motor Control	Visual-parietal, Visuomotor, Secondary Somatosensory
Language, Receptive Speech	Emotions and Smell (olfaction).
Motor	Visuoperceptual, Reading, Language

Visuoperceptual, Language, Reading, Writing

Visuoperceptual, Form Recognition

Vision, Color, Motion, Depth

Emotion and Cognition

Primary Auditory Cortex

Emotion and Memory

Fig. 3.25 Brodmann's areas and associated function

Rule of thumb: Broadmann's areas important in neuropsychological evaluations

- 1–3 (primary somatosensory cortex of postcentral gyrus)
- 4, 6 (primary motor and supplemental motor)
- 5 (tertiary somatosensory area)
- 7 (heteromodal visuomotor, visuoperceptual function)
- 8 (frontal eye fields)
- 9–12 (prefrontal association areas)
- 17–19 (primary and secondary visual cortex)
- 20–21 (visual inferiorotemporal area for recognition of visual forms)
- 22 (Wernicke's area/higher order auditory cortex)
- 23–27 (limbic/emotional functions)
- 39 (parietal-temporal-occipital heteromodal association cortex for higher order vision/reading/speech)
- 41 (Primary auditory cortex/Heschl's gyrus)
- 44 (Broca's area/motor speech area)
- 45–47 (prefrontal heteromodal association cortex for behavioral planning, reasoning, etc.)

Table 3.6 Brodmann's area, presumed function, and functional area

Brodmann's area	Function	Functional area	Location
1, 2, 3	Two-point discrimination, vibration sense/light touch	Primary somatosensory area	Postcentral gyrus
4	Voluntary motor movement	Primary motor cortex	Precentral gyrus
5	Stereognosis, tactile agnosia, apraxia	Secondary somatosensory cortex (posterior parietal association area). Part of visual dorsal stream.	Superior parietal lobule
6	Motor planning and movement (limb and eyes)	Supplementary motor cortex, premotor cortex, frontal eye fields	Precentral gyrus and rostral cortices.
7	Visuomotor function, and visuoperceptual skills	Posterior parietal association area. Part of visual dorsal stream.	Superior parietal lobule
8	Eye movements (saccades)	Frontal eye fields	Superior frontal (middle) gyrus (medial frontal lobe)
9, 10, 11, 12	Planned movement, problem solving, organization	Prefrontal association cortex	Superior and middle frontal lobe (rostral to frontal eye fields)
13, 14, 15, 16	Psychic awareness of viscero-sensory feelings, stomach/gastric sensations, emotional aspect to sensory feelings, heart rate/blood pressure perception, psychic evaluation of temperature and body states	Limbic cortex, heteromodal association cortex	Insular cortex
17	Visual perception	Primary visual cortex (V1)	Calcarine fissure
18	Depth perception, vision	Secondary visual cortex (V2)	Medial and lateral occipital gyri
19	Color, depth perception, motion	Associative visual cortex (V3)	Medial and lateral
20, 21	Visual naming, auditory naming, visual perception of form	Inferotemporal cortex	Inferior and middle temporal gyrus
22	Auditory perception/speech sounds	Auditory association cortex (Wernicke's area)	Superior temporal gyrus

(continued)

Table 3.6 (continued)

Brodmann's area	Function	Functional area	Location
23–27	Emotional regulation/perception, memory	Limbic association cortex, subgenual cingulate, part of hippocampal formation	Cingulate gyrus, BA 25 in caudal orbitofrontal area, Rostral parahippocampal gyrus (presubiculum)
28	Memory, emotional experience, smell	Limbic cortex, olfactory cortex	Parahippocampal gyrus (entorhinal cortex)
29–33	Emotional experience, memory	Limbic association cortex	Cingulate gyrus retrosplenial area,
34–36	Memory, emotions, olfactory (smell)	Limbic cortex, olfactory cortex	Parahippocampal gyrus
37	Reading, speech, vision	Parietal–temporal–occipital association cortex	Middle and inferior temporal gyri at temporo-occipital junction
38	Smell, emotions, speech/naming	Primary olfactory cortex, limbic association cortex	Anterior temporal pole
39	Reading, speech, vision, dysgraphia, dyscalculia, visual working memory	Parietal–temporal–occipital heteromodal association cortex	Inferior parietal lobule (angular gyrus)
40	Reading, speech, vision, dysgraphia, dyscalculia, visual working memory	Parietal–temporal–occipital heteromodal association cortex	Inferior parietal lobule (supramarginal gyrus)
41	Perception of sound	Primary auditory cortex	Heschl's gyrus and superior temporal gyrus
42	Hearing of speech sounds	Secondary auditory cortex	Medial Heschl's gyrus and superior temporal gyrus
43	Taste	Gustatory association cortex	Insular cortex, frontoparietal operculum
44	Expressive speech	Broca's area, lateral premotor cortex	Inferior frontal gyrus (frontal operculum)
45	Expressive speech, planning, reasoning	prefrontal association cortex	Inferior frontal gyrus (frontal operculum)
46	Planning, reasoning, sequencing, abstraction	frontal heteromodal association cortex	(Middle frontal gyrus) Dorsolateral prefrontal cortex
47	Judgment, insight, reasoning, altering behavior with feedback	Ventrolateral prefrontal cortex	Inferior frontal gyrus (frontal operculum)
48	Likely multimodal	Association cortex	Medial surface of temporal lobe
52	Likely multimodal	Association cortex	Parainsular area between temporal lobe and insula

Functional Classification of the Neocortex

The areas of the cerebral cortex can also be divided in terms of functional subtype areas. While several different terms have been used, these generally reflect efforts to describe regions of the brain in terms of the behaviors or level of processing that may occur within the region. Five main functional subtypes have been identified: Limbic, Paralimbic, primary sensory-motor, primary association, and heteromodal (multimodal) association cortex.

Limbic cortex includes cortical zones termed "corticoid" and allocortex. The limbic cortex zone includes portions of the basal forebrain and amygdala, piriform (or pyriform) cortex (also identified as olfactory cortex). The basal forebrain structures (septal region, substantia innominata) and amygdala, and part of the olfactory cortex are designated corticoid since the organization of neurons is not well differentiated, and no clear layers can be identified. The hippocampus and piriform/pyriform cortex (also known as paleocortex) are the two areas of the cortex having two bands of neurons and has been termed allocortex. The piriform/pyriform cortex is localized to the most rostral part of the parahippocampal gyrus and the dorsal part of the uncus. The hippocampus complex is posterior (caudal) to the piriform cortex in the parahippocampal gyrus. The limbic zone is associated with function of the hypothalamus, and is associated with regulation of autonomic functions, emotions, hormonal balance, memory, and motivation.

Paralimbic cortex (also known as mesocortex) has an increased structural complexity over the limbic cortex, but does not have the six-layer cortical organization of the neocortex. The paralimbic cortex reflects a "transition area" of cortex between limibic and associative cortex and involves five regions: (1) orbitofrontal cortex, (2) insula cortex, (3) temporal pole, (4) parts of the parahippocampal gyrus (e.g., entorhinal area), and (5) the cingulate gyrus. The functional aspects of the paralimbic cortex are associated with primary limbic functions, including autonomic function perception, emotions, hormonal functions, memory, and motivation.

Primary sensory-motor cortex refers to the cortex where primary auditory, motor, and somatosensory functions occur. Primary auditory cortex refers to Heschl's gyrus in the Sylvian fissure. Primary motor refers to cortex of the precentral gyrus. Primary somatosensory cortex is cortex of the postcentral gyrus. Primary visual cortex (striate or calcarine cortex) refers to the cortex on the sides of the calcarine fissure in the occipital lobe. These primary sensory-motor cortex areas project to unimodal and heteromodal (multimodal) cortex areas.

Unimodal cortex is composed of six-layered cortex that is modality specific. This area of the cortex have neurons that respond to stimulation of a single sensory modality, and afferents to this cortex only come from primary sensory (or motor) cortex and/or other unimodal cortex.

Heteromodal cortex refers to cortex that receives afferent (input) from multiple sensory (or motor) unimodal (or other heteromodal) cortex. Neurons in heteromodal cortex respond to multiple sensory (and/or motor) stimuli. Damage to heteromodal cortex results in disruptions of functions not confined to one sensory (or motor) modality (e.g., not just deafness or blindness).

Functional Neuroanatomy: Structural and Functional Networks

Below, we provide a brief overview of the functional neuroanatomy of the central nervous system. We first review the major afferent (sensory) and efferent (motor) systems. We then review the major divisions of the neocortex (frontal, occipital, parietal, and temporal lobes). The reader is also directed to review chapters that identify neuropsychological functions for more detailed description of the functional neuroanatomy.

Major Afferent (Sensory) and Efferent (Motor) Pathways. The spinal cord has afferent (sensory) and efferent (motor) pathways. In general, motor pathways are anterior or lateral. Sensory pathways are lateral and ventral (see Fig. 3.9). Below, we summarize the major efferent (sensory) pathways, followed by afferent (motor) pathways through the central nervous system.

Major Sensory (Afferent) Pathways

There are two principal somatosensory pathways. The rapidly conducting and highly localized dorsal column–medial lemniscus system and the slowly conducting and diffuse, anterolateral system. Both convey information from a peripheral receptor to the cortex via three neurons. The primary afferent has a specialized peripheral termination which is the sensor. The soma of the primary afferent is located in the dorsal root ganglion and makes a synaptic connection with a secondary neuron in the ipsilateral spinal cord. The secondary neuron axon crosses the midline and terminates in the thalamus. The tertiary neuron makes synaptic connection with the secondary neuron in the thalamus and projects to layer IV of the cortex.

Dorsal column-medial lemniscus. The dorsal column is the rapidly conducting system which carries fine tactile sensation (e.g., two-point discrimination), vibration, and proprioception (see Fig. 3.26). The dorsal columns can be divided into the cuneate and gracile pathways. The gracile pathway carries information from the legs and trunk, while the cuneate tracts carry signals from the upper extremities (see Fig. 3.10). The primary afferent neurons form synaptic connections with the second order neuron in the gracile and cuneate nuclei in the dorsal medulla. The second order neurons then cross the midline as the internal arcuate fibers and become the medial lemniscus. The medial lemniscus continues anteriorly towards the ventral posterior lateral (VPL) nucleus of the thalamus. Fibers of facial sensation from the trigeminal nerve join the medial lemniscus and project to the thalamic ventral posterior medial (VPM) nucleus. From the thalamus, sensory information is projected to somatosensory cortex (Brodmann's areas 3, 1, and 2, where area 3 gets most of the projections). Projects to cerebral cortex are primarily to level IV (granular layer).

Anterolateral system. The sensory neurons in the joints, muscles, organs, and skin project to the lateral and anterior tracts (spinothalamic tract, spinomesenthalamic, spinoreticular tract) in the spinal cord, carrying information about *pain, temperature,*

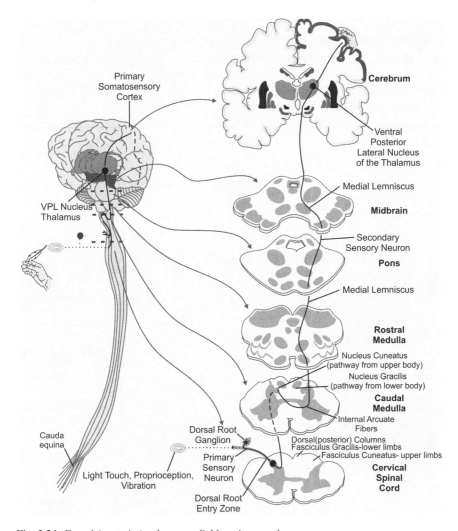

Fig. 3.26 Dorsal (posterior) column-medial lemniscus pathway

and "*crude*" *touch*. These pathways project primarily to ventral posterior lateral (VPL) nuclei of the thalamus, but also to intralaminar thalamic nuclei, and the reticular formation (see Fig. 3.27). While many of the anterolateral sensory fibers do *not* project to the parietal cortex, terminating in the basal ganglia, midbrain, and/or thalamus, some thalamic fibers do project via the posterior limb of the internal capsule to the somatosensory area of the parietal cortex. Fibers of the anterolateral system are small and have slower conduction rates than the large fibers making up the medial lemniscus (see Table 3.5 for review). Analogous fibers subserving pain and temperature from the face enter the CNS through the trigeminal nerve, then descend in the spinal trigeminal tract. These fibers project to the VPM thalamic nucleus, with projections to primary somatosensory cortex for the third order neurons.

Rule of thumb: Major afferent (sensory) pathways

- Dorsal (Posterior) Column/Medial Lemniscus – decussates at medulla. Conveys vibration sense, proprioception, and light touch
- Anterolateral – decussates close to level of entry in spinal cord. Conveys pain, temperature, and "crude" touch

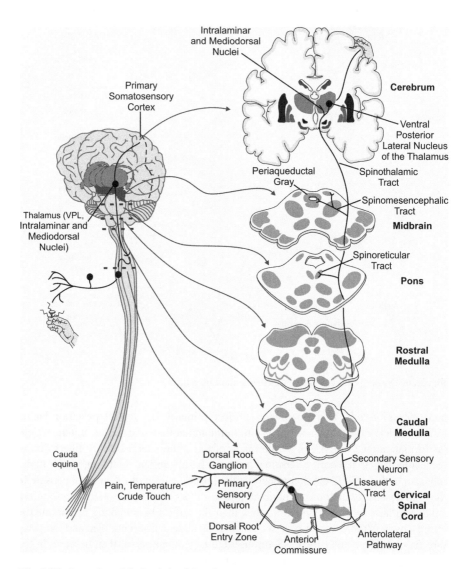

Fig. 3.27 Anterolateral (spinothalamic) pathway

Motor (Efferent) Descending System Pathways

The descending motor pathways are organized into four sets of tracts based on the origin of cell bodies. The four tracts are; the corticospinal (also called corticobulbospinal), the rubrospinal, the reticulospinal and the vestibulospinal (see Figs. 3.28 and 3.29).

Corticobulbospinal tract. The corticobulbospinal (corticospinal) tract originates from neurons in the primary motor cortex as well as from some neurons in the supplementary motor and the posterior parietal cortex. Axons from these neurons

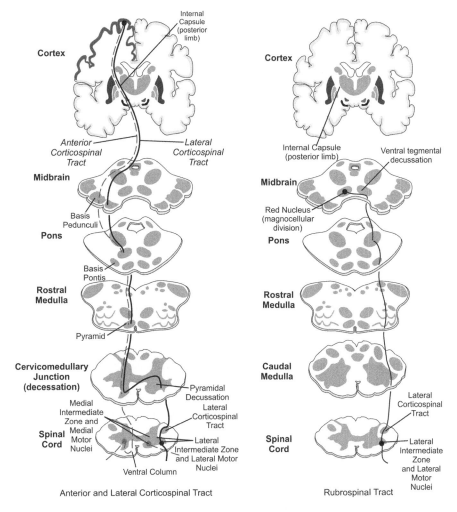

Fig. 3.28 The lateral corticospinal (corticobulbospinal) and rubrospinal pathways. *Note*: The lateral corticospinal illustration incorporates the anterior corticospinal tract as a subsystem of the lateral corticospinal tract that does not decussate

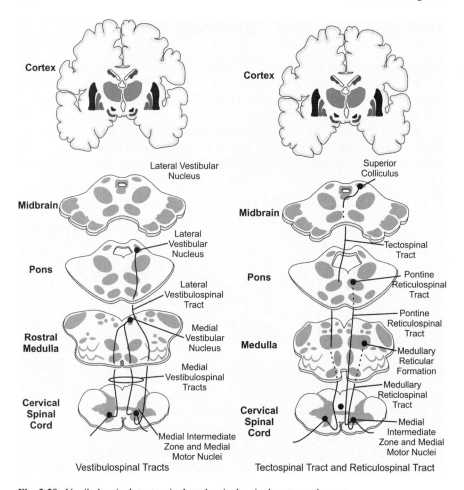

Fig. 3.29 Vestibulospinal, tectospinal, and reticulospinal motor pathways

project to the brain stem and spinal cord (see Fig. 3.28). This tract comprises the entire voluntary cortical drive to brain stem and spinal motor systems. The system is traditionally divided into a corticospinal (limbs) and corticobulbar (head) tract. Axons collect together forming the corona radiata and then become increasingly closely bundled forming part of the posterior limb of the internal capsule. Axons of the corticobulbar division synapse in the red nucleus and the various motor nuclei of the cranial nerves. The majority of the axons of the corticospinal division cross at the pyramidal decussation, becoming the *lateral corticospinal tract*. About 10% of the corticospinal neurons continue uncrossed as the *anterior corticospinal* tract but cross the midline at the level of their termination. Corticospinal neurons terminate primarily on interneurons of the spinal cord.

Rubrospinal tract. Beginning with axons in the red nucleus, axons cross the midline immediately after leaving the red nucleus and descend through the brain stem and form a pathway just ventral to the corticospinal tract (see Fig. 3.28). The rubrospinal tract mediates mainly voluntary control of large muscles in the upper extremities.

Reticulospinal tract. The reticulospinal tract has two subdivisions: the pontine and medullary reticulospinal tracts (see Fig. 3.29). The pontine division descends in the medial cord to facilitate extensor motor neurons and inhibit flexor motor neurons of the limbs. The medullary division descends in the anterolateral column of the spinal cord. It functions to inhibit extensor and facilitate flexor motor neurons.

Vestibulospinal tracts. Four tracts originating from the superior, lateral, medial and

---

Rule of thumb: Major efferent (motor) pathways

- Cortico(bulbo)spinal – motor output to limb muscles
- Rubrospinal – motor output to upper extremities
- Reticulospinal – motor output for extensor and flexor muscles
- Vestibulospinal – divided into four subdivisions for vestibular function for maintaining balance and posture and a stable platform for vision when running, etc.

---

inferior vestibular nuclei, all of which receive afferent connections from the vestibular nerve. The lateral and medial vestibulospinal tracts are descending motor tracts (Fig. 3.29). The medial vestibulospinal tract descends only to cervical and high thoracic levels and synapses on neurons innervating the muscles of the head and neck. The principal function is to provide a stable platform for the eyes. The lateral vestibulospinal tract descends to all levels of the spine in the ipsilateral ventral medial funiculus. The lateral vestibulospinal tract primarily regulates posture and balance.

Injuries to the spinal cord result in readily identifiable spinal cord syndromes (see Fig. 3.30). While these spinal cord syndromes do not adversely affect neuropsychological function, they are summarized briefly below to highlight the consistent organization of the sensory and motor pathways in the spinal cord.

Complete transaction of the cord. Somatosensory and motor function below the neurologic level of the injury is lost. Injury to the cord at or above C3 also typically results in loss of diaphragm function and necessitates the use of mechanical ventilation for breathing.

Central cord syndrome. Hyperextension injuries to the spinal cord can result in hemorrhage, edema or ischemia to the central portion of the spinal cord. The result is greater loss of upper limb function compared to lower limb because of the anatomical arrangement of the corticospinal tract with the arm fibers medially and the leg fibers laterally.

Brown-Sequard syndrome. Unilateral hemisection of the spinal cord will disrupt fine tactile, proprioception and vibratory fibers on the same side of the body as the injury as well as pain and temperature sensing fibers on the contralateral side. Descending motor tracts on the same side as the injury will also be disrupted. This results in weakness and loss of proprioception on the ipsilateral side and loss of pain and temperature sensation on the contralateral side.

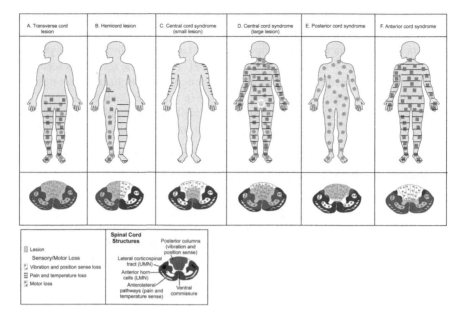

Fig. 3.30 Spinal cord syndromes

Anterior cord syndrome. Lesion to the anterior aspect of the cord interrupts the descending motor fibers as well as the fibers carrying pain and temperature sensation below the site of injury. The posterior fibers which carry fine touch and proprioceptive sense are intact. Clinically, the presentation is weakness and loss of pain and temperature sensation below the injury site, while proprioceptive sense is maintained.

Tabes Dorsalis. Clinical syndrome due to degeneration of the posterior column of the spinal cord, classically from tertiary syphilis. Clinically, sense of touch and proprioceptive sensation is lost below the site of lesion on both sides of the body (assuming bilateral dorsal column injury). If only one side is injured, loss of proprioception, vibration, and two-point discrimination occurs ipsilaterally to the spinal cord injury. Similar findings can occur with other causes of dorsal column-medial lemniscus pathway injury, such as Multiple Sclerosis.

Cortical Functional Neuroanatomy

Frontal lobe. The functional neuroanatomy of the frontal lobe is detailed in Chap. 10, and is briefly reviewed here for convenience. The neuroanatomical organization of the frontal lobe includes all the brain tissue anterior (rostral) to the central sulcus, which makes up about 40% of the cerebral cortex. The functional aspects of the frontal lobe can be divided into three broad areas/functional systems: (1) Motor, (2) Premotor, and (3) Prefrontal. The prefrontal region has been divided into several distinction regions, and we believe the division of the prefrontal into the (a) dorsolateral (BA 9 and 46), (b) orbitofrontal (also called the inferior ventral frontal) (BA 11, 12, 13, and 14), and (c) medial frontal/cingulate gyrus (BA 25 and 32) has utility (although see also Mesulam 2000).

Motor cortex. The motor cortex is principally the precentral gyrus (BA 4). The motor cortex is primary motor cortex and neurons composing this area of the cortex forms the neurons of the corticobulbospinal tract for the control of motor movement. Projections from BA 4 neurons also extend to basal ganglia and from there extend to thalamic and sucortical nuclei (e.g., red nucleus) for fine motor coordination, correction, and planning as well as vestibular and balance functions.

Premotor cortex. The premotor cortex includes the regions anterior (rostral) to the precentral gyrus, and includes BA 6 and 8. The areas of BA 6 and 8 have been further subdivided into the premotor and supplementary motor cortices. Lateral BA 6 is premotor cortex while medial BA 6 is supplementary motor cortex. BA 8 is the frontal eye fields while the more lateral aspects are supplementary eye fields. The premotor areas are heteromodal cortex, receiving inputs from parietal association cortex (BA 5 and 7), and projecting axons to the primary motor cortex as well as directly to the corticobulbospinal (corticospinal) pathways. The premotor and supplementary motor cortices are involved in motor planning.

Prefrontal cortex. In general, the prefrontal cortex is involved in planning, organizing, executing, initiation, inhibiting, and/or selecting behaviors. In addition, areas of the frontal lobe are also associated with processes of speech production, maintaining vigilance and working memory, as well as learning and memory. Each of the three prefrontal regions have classic characteristics that are summarized below.

Dorsolateral Prefrontal (dysexecutive syndrome). The dorsolateral prefrontal area is involved in reasoning, problem solving, sequencing, and maintenance of behaviors (persistence). Problem solving and reasoning is concrete with patients having more difficulty with divergent reasoning tasks (requiring many solutions to a problem) than convergent reasoning tasks (drawing similarities or solutions from two or more things). Furthermore, insight and judgment is often poor. Patients may exhibit environmental dependency and memory problems. Learning rate is often slow, and memory may be disrupted due to reduced working memory/attention as well as problems with efficient retrieval. Additionally, deficits in remembering the temporal sequence of when events occurred (as opposed to forgetting altogether that something occurred) may be present. Finally, disruption in emotional functioning can also occur, in which the effect is generally blunted/apathetic, but intermixed with episodes of anger outbursts when emotionally aroused. Expressive aphasia occurs with involvement of BA 44/45, but spontaneous speech can be generally reduced.

Orbitofrontal or inferior ventral frontal (pseudopsychopathy or pseudodepressed syndrome): The obitofrontal (inferior ventral) part of the prefrontal cortex is involved in behavioral inhibition and emotional regulation as well as olfaction. In general, patients with orbitofrontal lesions often appear disorganized, behaviorally disinhibited, impulsive and emotionally dysregulated. Anosmia is not uncommon. Behavior inhibition is reduced, so individuals will behave hedonistically, often appearing to have no concern for the feelings or rights of other people.

The orbitofrontal region is associated with conscious control of behavior through the evaluation of punishment (lateral orbitofrontal) and reward value of reinforcing (desirable) stimuli (medial orbitofrontal). Memory is *only* disrupted *if* the basal forebrain/septal area is damaged, which results in a dense antegrade amnesia (poor declarative memory) and a temporally graded retrograde amnesia. *Witzelsucht,* a term to describe "hollow" or inappropriate jocularity (laughing at a funeral), may be present.

Mesial Frontal/Anterior Cingulate (*akinetic syndrome*). The medial frontal/ anterior cingulate cortex is associated with attention, behavioral inhibition, initiation and motivation, motor function (lower extremities), social cognition, including Theory of Mind, memory, mood, and autonomic (visceral) systems. Damage to the orbitofrontal/anterior cingulate can result in akinesia, lethargy, lack of self initiation of behavior, and a dense antegrade amnesia (impaired explicit memory). Bilateral lesions can result in an akinetic and mute state. Unilateral lesions are less devastating, and the patient may engage in some self-initiated behaviors. Lesions affecting the language dominant hemisphere can result in a transcortical motor aphasia. Emotional functioning is generally blunted, with little insight or judgment. Damage to the medial motor cortex results in a contralateral hemiparesis of the lower extremity (extremities if bilateral lesions).

Insular Cortex (*lobe*). The insular cortex is a small area of cortex underlying the frontal and temporal operculum and lies deep within the Sylvian (lateral) fissure (see Fig. 3.7). Some believe the area should be labeled as a distinct lobe in the brain. The insular cortex is divided into two regions, a larger anterior region and a smaller posterior region. Less is known about the functional neuroanatomy of the insular cortex, but structurally, the insular cortex (lobe) has an extensive network of pathways with connections to auditory cortex (primary and secondary), amygdala, entorhinal cortex, hippocampus, motor cortex, prefrontal cortex (anterior cingulate gyrus, dorsolateral and orbitofrontal), frontal operculum, olfactory cortex/bulb, parietal operculum, the temporal pole and superior temporal gyrus, and somatosensory association cortices (primary and secondary).

While details remain to be delineated, the insular cortex appears to be involved in: motor control, homeostasis, interceptive awareness and association with somatosensory experiences, cognitive functions including self-awareness and social emotional processing, as well as complex somatosensory association experiences. Motor control function includes association for the coordinated movement of hand and eyes, swallowing, speech articulation, and motor activities of the gastrointestinal (GI) tract. Homeostatsis functions include the control and monitoring of the autonomic nervous system. Interceptive awareness refers to being aware of internal body states, and the insular cortex (lobe) appears to be a center for the conscious appreciation of cardiovascular function (heart beat and blood pressure), pain, temperature, and GI sensations. Indeed, the insular cortex has a "command center" for increasing heart rate and blood pressure with exercise. Right (nondominant) insular cortex has been associated with conscious perception of heart rate. The judgment as to the degree or severity of pain as well as the subjective grading of nonpainful coldness or warmth involves the insula. Conscious perception of visceral organs (distension of stomach or bladder) is also associated with the insular cortex. Relatedly, the insular cortex is associated with the limbic system, and involved in the integration of sensory inputs with limbic and body visceral states in higher cognitive order processing and perception. This process is thought to unite limbic and sensory processes to memories and associate these with interpersonal relationships and events (e.g., stomach in knots when thinking about a particular person or event). The insular cortex appears to have an important role as an area for integrating multiple sensory (auditory, gustatory, olfactory, tactile, vestibular, and visual) information. Recently, it was found that synaesthesia (perception of one sensory modality as another, for example hearing colors or seeing music) is associated with disruptions of the insular cortex. Food and drug craving has been associated with the insular cortex. Emotionally, the insular cortex is involved in processes for anger, fear, disgust, happiness, and sadness. The insular cortex is involved in the association of disgust to both olfactory inputs and/or visual images of mutilation and contamination or putrification. Imagination of these inputs is sufficient for similar brain activation and insular cortex activity. Finally, emotional salience, that is, attending to and making decisions about, the subjective importance of stimuli, is associated with the insular cortex (along with the cingulate gyrus and connected orbitofrontal cortex).

Occipital lobe. The occipital cortex is traditionally identified as integral for visual processing. Visual processing is a distributed hierarchical organized process. Primary visual processing begins in the calcarine sulcus (striate cortex or BA 17 or V1), and more complex visual processing occurs in associated anterior (rostral) areas (e.g., BA 18 and 19 or V2). The lateral geniculate nucleus (of the thalamus) projects to V1. Neurons of V1 project to other visual unimodal and heteromodal cortex (V2, V3, etc.). Neurons in V2 also project to other visual unimodal and hetermodal cortex. Beginning after V2, there are three distinct visual processing systems: (1) dorsal stream, (2) ventral stream, and (3) a superior temporal sulcus (STS) stream. The dorsal stream and the ventral stream have been well described while the third stream, the STS stream, is less well described (see Fig. 9.4).

The region of V4 is specialized to appreciate color, although cells here also respond to color/form combinations. Lesions to V4 result in inability to see color and are unable to "think" in color. This reflects loss not of color perception but of color knowledge. The area described as area V3 appears to be sensitive to processing the object of shapes in motion (Kolb and Whishaw 2009). Area V5 is also concerned with the perception of objects in motion. Lesions to area V5 can result in the inability to see objects when they are moved, while still retaining the ability to see the objects when they are stationary.

The dorsal pathway is primarily involved in identifying where objects are in space and the relative distances from one another and the person as well as guiding body movements by vision, which runs from the occipital cortex to the parietal cortex. The ventral pathway processes the object forms and the associated semantic network for recognizing objects in space. This system runs from the occipital cortex to the temporal cortex (see Chap. 9, this volume, for more details). The STS pathway appears to be specialized for the categorization of stimuli as well as the detection of motion of body parts (e.g., hands) thought to be involved in the perception of social nonverbal communication cues.

Parietal lobe. The parietal cortex is demarcated by the cortex posterior to the central sulcus and anterior to the parietoccipital sulcus and ventral (superior) of the sylvian (lateral) fissure. It also includes the cortex and underlying white matter from the interhemispheric fissure to the cingulate gyrus. The parietal lobe includes BA 1, 2, and 3 (postcentral gyrus), BA 5 and 7 (superior parietal lobule), BA 39 (angular gyurs), BA 40 (supramarginal gyrus), and BA 43 (parietal operculum).

Functionally, the parietal cortex may be divided into two broad functions: somatosensory processing and sensory integration for motor control. The anterior parietal areas (BA 1, 2, 3, and 43) is primarily involved in somatosensory processing, and includes primary sensory and unimodal association cortex in the postcentral gyrus. The posterior parietal cortex includes BA 5, 7, 39, and 40 which are involved in the dorsal pathway of visual processing (see Occipital lobe above).

The anterior parietal area reflects primary and unimodal somatosensory cortex, and processes information about tactile, muscle, joint, vibration, vestibular, and two-point discrimination information. The primary and unimodal association cortex project to posterior parietal regions in BA 5 and 7 as well as supplementary and premotor areas, which are unimodal and heteromodal cortex. Projections of BA 5 go to the posterior parietal regions (BA 7) as well as supplementary and premotor areas. Additionally, BA 7 receives input from primary somatosensory cortex, motor and premotor cortex and some inputs from visual occipitoparietal regions. There are reciprocal connections between areas of BA 7 and the dorsolateral prefrontal cortex (BA 8 and 46). The posterior parietal cortex is involved in the integration of sensory inputs (somatosensory, visual, auditory, etc.) for the control of movement and processing of visual word information (reading). As discussed in the occipital lobe functional neuroanatomy, the visual pathways of where objects are in space (dorsal pathway) are processed in the hetromodal cortex of the superior parietal lobe (BA 5 and 7), making a part of the *dorsal visual stream* (see Chap. 9, this volume). Together, BA 5 and 7 are involved in guiding movement and some processing of spatial working memory. BA 39 and 40 are involved in high level integration of visual stimuli and language functions in association with reading. In addition, arithmetic functions, particularly those involved in more complex arithmetic requiring "borrowing" or other mathematical operations requiring a spatial aspect, have been associated with posterior parietal regions, particularly the inferior parietal lobule.

Lesions of the postcentral gyrus that disrupt the connections between primary and unimodal association cortex areas result in *astereognosia* (inability to recognize objects by feel/palpitating them but not seeing them). Damage also frequently results in *agraphesthesia*, which is the inability to identify letters or numbers written on the palm of the hand or finger tips. Other associated agnosias include *atopognosia* (inability to localize touch) and *abarognosia* (the inability to discriminate weights). Lesions to the medial parietal area [medial parietal region (MPR)] and posterior cingulate gyrus results in poor spatial navigation. Spatial rotation appears to include the interparietal sulcus.

Temporal lobes. The temporal lobe is most commonly associated with receptive language functions (BA 41, 42, and 22) and probably memory (parahippocampal gyrus, BA 28, 35, and 36). However, the temporal lobe is also involved in considerable visual processing, and makes up the ventral visual pathway (BA 20, 21, 37, and 38), which allows for the processing of "what" visual percepts are and associating these with a semantic memory network that is thought to include portions of the temporal lobe, including the anterior tip. In fact, the temporal lobe has (at least) five distinct neuroanatomic pathways: (1) sensory pathways of auditory and visual information; (2) auditory dorsal pathway; (3) polymodal/heteromodal processing/STS visual processing pathway; (4) memory/mesial temporal pathway; and (5) affective/emotional processes and movement control/frontal lobe pathway. We briefly summarize the functional anatomy of each below.

Sensory pathways of auditory and visual information. The temporal lobe includes primary sensory and association cortex for auditory stimuli as well as association cortex for visual information. These are discussed separately below.

Auditory processing. The dorsal (superior) aspect of the temporal lobe includes Heschel's gyrus (BA 41 and 42), which lies in the Sylvian fissure and is primary auditory cortex. Cells in the left (language-dominant) hemisphere within Heschel's gyrus are disproportionately sensitive to sound frequencies associated with human speech, while cells in the right (nonlanguage-dominant) hemisphere are sensitive to the pitch, timbre and melodies of music. The primary auditory sensory cortex projects to hierarchical auditory association cortex (Wernicke's area, BA 22) classically associated with verbal comprehension (or spoken and written language) in the language-dominant hemisphere. Projections from BA 22 radiate anteriorly along the superior aspect of the temporal lobe towards the temporal pole. There is also a dorsal projection of BA 22 posteriorly to the angular gyrus in the temporoparietal region (described below).

Visual processing. The temporal lobe includes the visual association cortex receiving projections from the primary visual cortex (BA 17, 18, 19) involved in the ventral visual processing pathway for object recognition. In addition, the temporal lobe includes (at least) two special visual perception regions, the fusiform face area (FFA) and the parahippocampal place area (PPA). The FFA is differentially active while viewing faces, and reflects a unique processing area and pathway for the perception of faces. The activation of this region is specific to faces, and is active despite variability in the presentation of faces (having glasses, a beard, a hat, etc.). The FFA is active regardless if the face is directly "facing" the viewer or is it some other angle (e.g., from the side). However, the FFA is *not* active if a face is viewed "upside down". The right hemisphere is more sensitive to facial perception than the left hemisphere. Additionally, the unique pathway for processing of human faces also includes input from the STS pathway, which provides input as to facial movements important for conveying nonverbal communication cues as to mood/affect and social-emotional functioning. The PPA is preferentially active when the visual stimuli is a geographic scene (e.g., picture of your town or Central Park in New York, NY).

The neurons making up the cortex of the inferior temporal lobe activate to complex visual features, and cells having similar but not identical selectivity for activation to particular complex visual stimuli are organized together in columns. The columnar organization of neurons responding to similar, but not identical, complex visual features allows these areas to activate despite slight variations in the visual properties of the stimuli. In so doing, this organization allows for learning visual categorization based on similarity of a complex series of features.

Auditory dorsal pathway. A processing pathway projecting posterior and dorsally to the parietal cortices thought to be involved in semantic knowledge of words and word reading, and related to aspects of directing movements that are related to auditory sensory information. Since BA 39 is involved in reading, some aspects of discerning the visual aspects of language, or perhaps semantic knowledge of words (e.g., word identification and meaning) have been associated with processing of the superior temporal lobe and angular gyrus.

Polymodal/heteromodal processing/STS visual processing pathway. Described above briefly as part of the occipital lobe, the STS visual processing pathway includes a series of parallel projections from visual and auditory association cortices converging largely in the superior temporal sulcus and running posteriorly towards the temporal pole. It is complex heteromodal/multimodal association cortex and has a role in associating visual and auditory information for categorization (associating sounds with certain objects). This region is also involved in the perception of different facial features and body movements with nonverbal communication cues and social behaviors (e.g., recognizing a smirk while telling a joke).

Memory/mesial temporal pathway. The projections of the auditory, visual and other somatosensory information is projected towards the parahippocampal gyrus where information is "funneled" to the perirhinal cortex and then entorhinal cortex along to the hippocampal formation and/or amygdala. Efferent projections from the hippocampus form the perforant pathway which form part of the Papez circuit involving the limbic cortex. The mesial temporal lobe structures (perirhinal and entorhinal cortices and hippocampus) are involved in declarative memory, particularly episodic (time and person specific) memory (see Chap. 8 for details) for objects, spatial information, and verbal/auditory information.

Affective/emotional aspects to memory and movement control/frontal lobe pathway. The temporal lobe has projections to the frontal lobe, both the dorsolateral and the orbitofrontal lobe based on fibers from the inferior longitudinal fasciculus and the uncinate fasciculus that is primarily involved in affective/emotional processing, short-term memory, and aspects of movement control. The emotional processing is associated with connections of the amygdala and orbitofrontal connections, inclusive of olfactory processing and affective/emotional processing. One function of the amygdala is to "tag" affective/emotional features to visual and/or auditory information, which increases the encoding (learning) of material and provides a neuroanatomic pathway for state dependent learning. An example of state dependent learning is that being in a similar affective state can enhance retrieval (memory). The associative information for categorizing information, including the body movements that have implications for emotional/social communication is processed in the STS pathway and also areas of the dorsolateral and orbitofrontal lobes. The recognition of body movements as having emotional/social communication implications has been associated with the "theory of mind", and is thought to be involved in the "theory of mind" (see Chap. 10). Briefly, theory of mind refers to the ability of a person to theorize about other individuals' feelings, thoughts, and the intentions of their behaviors.

After summarizing the five different neuroanatomic projection pathways in the temporal lobe, there are nine neuropsychological symptoms frequently associated with temporal lobe lesions, which include impaired:

1. Auditory sensation or perception (cortical deafness to receptive aphasia)
2. Perception of visual features (visual object agnosias, prosapagnosia, alexia, and appreciation of social facial/body part cues). Alexia has been associated with lesions to BA 39 (angular gyrus) as well as a region on the inferior occipitotemporal gyurs. Patients with right temporal resections fail to exhibit the left visual field bias in viewing faces that is normal.
3. Perception of music (amusica)
4. Auditory and/or visual selective attention
5. Categorization of visual or auditory stimuli (poor semantic organization)
6. Use of contextual information
7. Declarative (particularly episodic) memory
8. (Altered) personality and/or affective behavior. Patients may exhibit an increased focus on minutiae, particularly details of personal problems, have religious preoccupation, paranoia, and increased aggressiveness associated with the so-called temporal lobe or Geshwind personality. However, these features are rarely all present, and there are no consistent data supporting the temporal lobe personality. Nonetheless, personality change has been associated with temporal lobe damage, more often with right temporal lobe injury.
9. (Altered) sexual behavior (associated with Kluver-Bucy syndrome)

Distributed and Parallel Processing Networks: Structural and Functional Components

In the discussion above, we provided an overview of functions traditionally associated with a region of the cerebral cortex (e.g., frontal lobe); however, the discussion of cytoarchitecture and functional divisions of the cortex highlights the function of the nervous system (and production of behaviors) is based on complex systems of distributed and parallel processing networks that can be demonstrated both in terms of structural neuroanatomy as well as functionally in terms of neurophysiological mechanisms and effectors acting on associated brain areas (e.g., neurotransmitter actions). The neuroanatomic organization of the brain into networks can be appreciated at a cellular level, discussed above in terms of the extensive connections of each neuron with other neurons (one neuron may synapse to 1,000 or more other neurons via axons and dendrites) as well as the hierarchical and integrative networks displayed by the cytoarchitecture or the functional cortical areas organized hierarchically to process single sensorimotor stimuli projecting to more complex heteromodal/multimodal association cortex. At a larger neuroanatomical level, the complex processing networks of the brain can be readily appreciated by the intricate network of white matter tracts (bundles, fibers, and fasciculi) projecting throughout the cortex and to other regions of the CNS. Fibers (bundles of axons) may project from one closely associated region to another (neighboring gyri) with arcuate fibers (also called U-fibers) or to regions quite distant from each other via fasciculi. Figure 3.31 illustrate some of the major fasciculi of the neorcortex. Table 3.7 identifies the major fasciculi and the association areas connected.

The multiple processing networks involved in many behaviors/cognitions are illustrated by two examples. Figure 3.32 illustrate a complex widely diffuse distributed network thought to account for semantic memory (conceptual knowledge). Recall that semantic memory (conceptual knowledge) refers to one's memory for facts and knowledge and is not specific to time or place (autobiographical), and is cultural in nature (e.g., knowing the capital cities of the 50 states in the USA) (see also Chap. 8). The two theories accounting for semantic memory reflect a distributed network model and a distributed network-plus-hub model. The later model includes a distributed network of modality specific cortex processing areas (e.g., visual form, movement, language, tactile features, etc.) as in the distributed network model, but also includes a nondomain-specific processing center (or perhaps more correctly a multimodal processing center) which processes the many different domain-specific information by a common set of neurons. The distributed network-plus-hub model is garnering increasing support, but there remains debate as to the location and importance of these nondomain-specific hub area(s). While the debate continues, neuropsychological processes clearly involve a distributed network of areas, many with "hub" areas which are highly efficient at integrating stimuli for the neuropsychological functions reviewed in this book.

The second example is the complex parallel distributed network needed for speech, which is presented in detail in Chap. 7 (see Fig. 3.1). The distributed network includes hubs for expressive (BA 44/45) and receptive language (BA 22, 41/42), which network with other regions of the frontal (e.g., BA 6), temporal (BA 38, 20, 21, and 37), parietal (BA 39 and 40), and occipital (BA 17, 18, 19) cortices to allow for effortless language functions. Note the production of speech requires activation of brain regions outside the traditional language areas (BA 44/45; Broca's area), such as the facial area of the premotor cortex (BA 6, inferior portion). Similarly, reading involves primary and associative visual cortex (BA 17/V1, BA18/V2, BA19/V3) in processing letters/words. The semantic association of words (i.e., mental representation of a "canary," which is a unit of the semantic class of birds) involves areas of the occipital, occipito-temporal and inferior parieto-temporal cortices (BA 19, 21, 37, and 39) and left frontal regions (note these areas are part of the semantic memory network reviewed above). In addition, motor and premotor areas are involved in reading and writing, respectively, along with the corticobulbar tracts and cranial nerves. Chapter 7 reviews the analogous areas in the nondominant hemisphere involved in language prosody functions. Clearly, there is

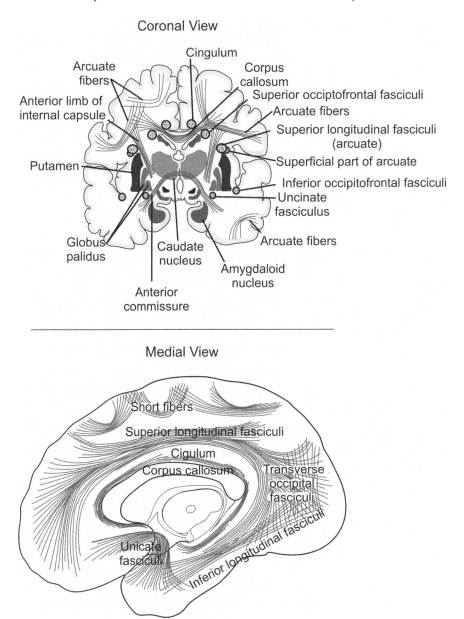

Fig. 3.31 Fasciculi and fibers of cerebral cortex

a distributed network to read, understand, or produce speech. Similarly, there are distributed and parallel networks involved in the neuropsychological functions reviewed in this book, including alertness/arousal (Chap. 5), attention/concentration (Chap. 6), visuoperceptual/visuoconstructional skills (see above and Chap. 9),

Table 3.7 Major fasciculi of the brain with associated connected areas

Fasciculus name	Areas connected	Function
Arcuate fasciculus (now considered part of superior longitudinal fasciculus)	Temporal and frontal lobes	Language functions associating receptive and expressive areas
Inferior longitudinal (occipitotemperal)	Occipital and temporal lobes	Semantic language, memory, visual processing
Superior longitudinal	Occipital, parietal, temporal, and frontal lobes	Regulate motor movement, spatial orientation, spatial perception, working memory, language
Inferior occipitofrontal	Occipital, temporal and frontal lobes	Visual processing, semantic memory?, language processes?.
Superior occipitofrontal	Occipital, parietal, temporal and frontal lobes. Fibers project to thalamus	Visual processing, motor control, language functions, semantic memory?
Uncinate	Orbitofrontal regions to anterior temporal	Affective (emotion), memory, cognition?
Anterior commissure	Left and right anterior temporal/olfactory bulb/ basal frontal areas.	Olfactory functions?, affective/emotional processing?
Cingulum (bundle)	Cingulate gyrus to frontal lobe, amygdala, nucleus accumbens, and thalamus	Cognition (including alertness/attention) and affective/emotional processes
Corpus colossum	Left and right hemispheres	Broad connections for motor, sensory and cognitive processes
Posterior commissure	Left and right pretectal nuclei	Pupil light reflex

memory (see Chaps. 8 and 10), motor control (above and Chaps. 10 and 19), executive (Chap. 10) and affective/emotional functions (Chaps. 10 and 11). The distributed networks include cortical areas involved in more integrative functions and interconnected with cortical areas that are highly specialized and efficient at processing specific types of information. We know turn to further evaluating the cerebral and cortical specializations in behavior.

Cerebral Asymmetry

While the brain has two hemispheres that, on gross examination, appear very similar, decades of research have documented asymmetry in the structure and function of the human brain. Below, we summarize some anatomic and functional differences.

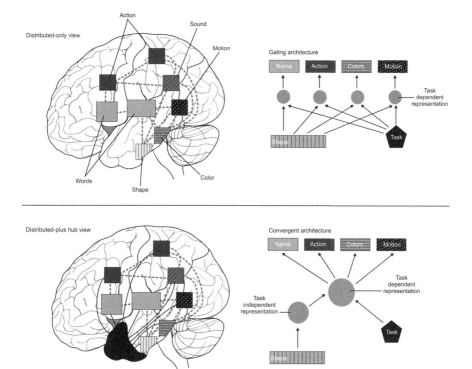

Fig. 3.32 Models of distributed network and distributed network-plus-hub for semantic memory

Anatomic cerebral asymmetry. As early as the 1860s, the asymmetry of the cerebral cortex has been appreciated (Kolb and Whishaw 2009, for review). Some common anatomical asymmetries of the cerebral hemispheres are summarized below:

Asymmetry Favoring the Dominant (Left) Hemisphere

- Left hemisphere is denser and has more gray matter relative to amount of white matter
- Frontal operculum total area larger due to more surface area in sulcus.
- Inferior parietal lobule larger
- Insula is larger
- Medial temporal lobe larger
- Neocortex is thicker
- Occipital lobe wider
- Occipital horn of lateral ventricle longer
- Planum temporale (Wernicke's area/BA 22) larger
- Sylvian fissure is longer
- Temporoparietal cortex larger in some areas

Table 3.8 Functional asymmetries of the human brain

Function	Left dominant	Right dominant
Attention	Speech sounds (see below)	Left hemispace for visual, auditory, somatosensory stimuli
Auditory system	Language/speech related sounds	Music Nonlanguage sounds
Language/speech	Expressive and receptive speech: • Verbal comprehension • Spontaneous speech • Repetition • Reading • Writing	Prosody of speech • Comprehension of prosody • Expressive prosody • Repetition of prosody
Memory	Verbal memory • Word lists • Stories • Word-pairs	Spatial/"visual" memory[a] • Faces • Spatial locations
Motor/movement	Right side of body Mouth movements	Left side of body
Visual/spatial processing	Printed letters/words	Faces Geometric patterns Geometry Mental rotation of shapes Spatial orientation

[a]Determination of right hemisphere material specific memory dominance for "spatial/visual memory" has not been consistent

Table 3.9 Visual processing regions of the posterior neocortex (Adapted from Kolb and Whishaw 2009)

Pathway	Function	Cerebral localization
Dorsal (where)	Eye movements (voluntary)	Lateral intraparietal sulcus
	Visual motor guidance and grasping	Ventral and anterior intraparietal sulcus
	Visually guided reach	Parietal reach region
Ventral (what)	Body analysis	Extrastriate and fusiform body areas
	Face analysis	Fusiform face area
	Landmark analysis	Parahippocampal place area
	Object analysis	Lateral occipital
STS (specialized where/what)	Analysis of body movements for nonverbal communication	Superior temporal sulcus
	Analysis of moving body	Superior temporal sulcus

Asymmetry Favoring the Nondominant (Right) Hemisphere

– Right hemisphere is larger and slightly heavier
• Heschle's gyri is larger

- Convexity of frontal operculum (due to larger gyrus) larger
- Frontal lobe wider
- Medial geniculate nucleus larger (auditory)

Functional cerebral asymmetry. Study of the asymmetry of the brain has a long history, predominately with patients whom suffered lateralized lesions (Kolb and Whishaw 2009; Lezak et al. 2004). Some functional asymmetries of the cerebral hemispheres are provided in Tables 3.7, 3.8, and 3.9.

Summary

The nervous system is composed of the central nervous system (brain and spinal cord) and the peripheral nervous system (motor and sensory nerves outside the CNS, including the cranial nerves). There are about 100 billion neurons and about 300 billion supporting glial cells, allowing for 60–240 trillion synapses in the adult human brain. The trillions of synapses form complex distributed, parallel and hierarchical networks to process sensory stimuli in order to affect behavior. The complex neurochemical process involving neurotransmitters provides the neuro-physiological basis in the function of the nervous system. The major afferent (sensory) and efferent (motor) pathways maintain a somotropic organization in which sensory functions tend to be caudal/dorsal/posterior (towards the back) while motor functions tend to be rostral/ventral/anterior (towards the nose). Lesions produce well-defined clinical syndromes. The thalamus is a major relay station for sensorimotor- and cognitive-based pathways, and is interconnected with the basal ganglia to have extensive interconnections with both afferent (sensory) and efferent (motor) functions of the brain and spinal cord. While the review

---

Rule of thumb: Cortical functional neuroanatomy

- Frontal Lobe – "executive functions" planning, organizing, monitoring, inhibiting behavior, motor function, motor speech area, orbital and mesial frontal areas involved in affect and personality
- Temporal lobe – memory, affect/mood, olfactory and gustatory process
- Parietal – somatosensory perception, spatial awareness/attention, and complex visuoperceptual processing (letter/word identification and shape orientation/direction)
- Occipital lobe – primary and secondary visual processing
- Insular cortex (lobe) – emotions and association with sensory information, homeostasis, motor control, self-awareness, cognitive function and social-emotional experiences

of functional neuroanatomy has suggested some localized areas important in sensory or motor functions, the complex organization of the brain cannot be overstated. These networks should be appreciated when evaluating each patient's neuropsychological functioning, and the determination of neuropsychological (brain) dysfunction is best made when the identified patterns of neuropsychological deficits can be appreciated in the context of functional neuroanatomy and known neuropathology. That is, recognition of the patterns of neuropsychological deficits that can be expected to present together versus a distribution of poor neuropsychological test scores that cannot be reasonably associated with known functional neuroanatomy. Other chapters in this book provide more detailed functional neuroanatomical reviews when appropriate.

References and Suggested Readings

Blumenfeld, H. (2010). *Neuroanatomy through clinical cases* (2nd ed.). Sunderland: Sinauer Associates Inc.

Fix, J. D. (2008). *Neuroanatomy* (4th ed.). Philadelphia: Lippincott, Williams, and Wilkins.

Heilman, K. M., & Valenstein, E. (2007). *Clinical neuropsychology* (4th ed.). New York: Oxford University Press.

Kendel, E. R., Schwartz, J. H., & Jessell, T. M. (2000). *Principals of neural science* (4th ed.). New York: McGraw-Hill companies.

Kolb, B., & Whishaw, I. (2009). *Fundamentals of human neuropsychology* (6th ed.). New York: W.H. Freeman press.

Lezak, M. D., Howieson, D. B., & Loring, D. W. (2004). *Neuropsychological assessment* (4th ed.). New York: Oxford University Press.

Mesulam, M. M. (2000). *Principles of behavioral and cognitive neurology* (2nd ed.). New York: Oxford University Press.

Tsigos, C., & Chrousos, G. P. (2002). Hypothalamic-pituitary-adrenal axis, neuroendocrine factors and stress. *Journal of Psychosomatic Research, 53*, 865–871.

Victor, M., & Ropper, A. H. (2001). *Adams and Victor's principals of neurology* (7th ed.). New York: McGraw-Hill.

Chapter 4
Components of the Neuropsychological Evaluation

James G. Scott

Abstract Neuropsychological evaluation examines brain–behavior relationships as they pertain to cognitive, emotional and behavioral manifestations of central nervous system trauma, disease or dysfunction. Neuropsychological evaluation includes examination of sensory, motor and perceptual functioning as prerequisite for evaluation of increasingly complex cognitive, emotional and behavioral functions. Evaluation is typically on an ordinal scale (i.e., impaired/non-impaired) for sensory and perceptual skills and progresses to an integral scale for more complex functions (i.e., percentile relative to normative group). Rapid bedside or interview assessment of functions such as attention, language and memory can be done; however, it is important to note a brief evaluation will yield less precise information than formal testing. Brief evaluation has several advantages. These evaluations are quick to perform and can be repeated as necessary to mark progress or suspected deterioration. Information from such evaluations are typically used to assist in patient management, set immediate goals and assist in treatment planning. In later chapters, we discuss brief assessment methods in each domain of cognition.

Further details regarding the interpretive process, prerequisite knowledge base for adequate neuropsychological evaluations, psychometric principles guiding interpretation of neuropsychological psychometrically-derived data, and common errors in interpretation can be found throughout this book, but particularly Chapters. 1, 2, and 29–31). Sample neuropsychological reports are provided in Chapter. 1, Appendix A.

J.G. Scott (✉)

Department of Psychiatry and Behavioral Sciences, University of Oklahoma Health Sciences Center, Oklahoma City, OK, USA

e-mail: jim-scott@ouhsc.edu

M.R. Schoenberg and J.G. Scott (eds.), *The Little Black Book of Neuropsychology: A Syndrome-Based Approach*, DOI 10.1007/978-0-387-76978-3_4, © Springer Science+Business Media, LLC 2011

Key Points and Chapter Summary

- Neuropsychological evaluation uses a biopsychosocial model in assessing Brain–Behavior Relationships
- Assessment progresses from simple sensory and motor functions to complex integrative cognition and/or behaviors (including affective/mood) such as language, memory, visuoperceptual/visuoconstructional, executive (reasoning, problem solving, insight, judgment, etc.), and mood/personality functioning
- The foundations of Neuropsychological Assessment include a knowledge of neuropsychology, psychology, functional neuroanatomy, neuropathology, and psychometric principles of tests and measurements
- Neuropsychological assessment of cognitive skills can range from rapid bedside qualitative assessment in consultation to lengthy formal psychometric evaluation
- The decision regarding the assessment method, whether brief qualitative evaluation or detailed psychometric assessment is determined by the neuropsychologist by a combination of factors including: (1) the purpose and nature of the referral, (2) the hypothesized etiology of the known or suspected neuropsychological dysfunction, and (3) the time and course of symptoms

Basics of the Neuropsychology Evaluation

The clinical neuropsychologist will integrate the patient's current complaints and history (medical, psychiatric, educational, etc.), with available imaging, laboratory data, knowledge of brain–behavior relationships, functional neuroanatomy, neuropathology, cognitive psychology, psychometrics and test theory, psychopathology, and neurodevelopment. The assessment data obtained are compared against a comparison standard to identify relative neuropsychological deficits. The pattern of deficits manifested by patients are associated with brain function, which guides the answers to the referral questions. This information is integrated into a consultation or more lengthy formal report. This information is helpful to assess acutely the functioning of the patient and assist in guiding nursing staff and hospital staff (i.e., Physical therapist, Occupational therapist, Speech pathologist, etc.) in their expectations and care of the patient. This detailed consultation or formal assessment can also help family in recognizing deficits, adjusting to change in the patient, and in beginning to set expectations for the future functioning and accommodations which may be necessary. Below, we review critical patient history and medical information to be obtained followed by a sequential process of skills and behaviors of increasing complexity, which are essential in evaluating brain function. This sequential process is necessary because each previous process or skill is an essential prerequisite to successful and accurate evaluation of subsequent skills of a higher, more complex level. It does us no good to evaluate memory functioning when arousal is impaired or, taken to its absurd, everyone in a coma is aphasic.

Rule of thumb: Neuropsychological assessment

- Assessment must be sequential and assure integrity of prerequisite skills
- Assessment must take a biopsychosocial perspective including all available information (i.e., etiology, course, medical history, social history, psychiatric history) in the analysis and interpretation of assessment results
- Assessment should be tailored to meet the specific purpose and goals for the assessment and may range from brief consultative assessment to lengthy psychometrically-based evaluation

---

Factors Affecting Neuropsychological Functioning

The clinical neuropsychologist will conduct a review of the patient's records, including medical, psychiatric, and personal history. In addition, basic demographic information is important to obtain to assist in interpretation of any subsequently obtained neuropsychological data. Important demographic information is reviewed first, followed by medical and psychiatric history.

Several patient-specific demographic factors are critical for accurate interpretation of assessment results and must be considered prior to the evaluation. These demographic factors include age, education, gender, socioeconomic status, employment history, and social history such as alcohol use/abuse and other substance use/abuse. In addition, English language proficiency must be considered in persons fluent in another language or who have acquired English as a second language. This is true whether assessment is conducted briefly or with more formal psychometric test instruments.

A thorough understanding of the medical history is also essential. A review of the medical history should be obtained via the patient, collateral informant, and, if at all possible, medical records (as medical records can differ from the patient's report). These issues should cover medical history, family medical (and psychiatric) history, social history, and developmental history as well as factors such as lateral dominance (i.e., handedness, ocular dominance, pedal dominance). Psychiatric history is important to consider, as chronic and acute psychiatric symptoms can influence test or assessment results and have important implications for any interventions or treatments being considered.

A thorough history of the present illness is also critical and will guide evaluation regarding the diagnostic possibilities, cause and expected outcome. This examination should also include current medical factors which may contribute to the present illness such as medication change, toxic exposure, electrolyte imbalances, hormonal deficiencies, previous major surgeries, and other medical factors which may be risk factors for the current illness (e.g., diabetes, hyperlipidemia, hypertension, cardiac arrhythmia, sleep apnea, genetic abnormality, etc.)

Time: An Important Variable in the Neuropsychological Evaluation

The duration of symptoms is an important factor the neuropsychologist should consider when designing the assessment (or treatment program). Time refers not only to the elapsed time since the onset of the symptom but also to the course of the injury and any complications that have arisen. Acute onset or chronic course may result in a neuropsychological evaluation. This should be considered when deciding the type of evaluation to conduct. The neuropsychologist should consider the likely source of the onset of problems and design an evaluation appropriately. For example, a patient sustaining a moderate to severe TBI may be assessed acutely and/or repeatedly with a brief bedside screen to evaluate the severity of their current deficits and gauge recovery. This same patient may need a more formal and thorough evaluation to measure more precisely their functioning when they have stabilized in their recovery, and allow for precise assessment of long-term deficits and functional capacities. In the case of ischemic or hemorrhagic stroke, acute neuropsychological assessment may be used to gauge recovery, but changes in neuropsychological functioning over weeks, days, and even hours may occur. When the presentation is progressive or of insidious a more comprehensive neuropsychological evaluations may be conducted to precisely evaluate current functioning. Duration of complaints, knowledge of the recovery process, and the timing of the assessment thus have a profound impact on the selection of neuropsychological procedures and interpretation of neuropsychological data obtained. We now turn to outlining the hierarchical components of a neuropsychological evaluation.

Assessment of Basic Nervous System Functions (Cranial Nerves, Sensory and Motor Functions)

Pre–requisite Function

Examination of cranial nerve function is important for establishing prerequisite functioning for the remainder of the evaluation. This is especially true in acute hospital settings. The cranial nerves, associated functions, and methods to assess cranial nerve function are provided in Table 4.1.

Table 4.1 Cranial nerve

	Cranial nerve	Function	Abnormality	Assessment
I.	Olfactory	Smell	Anosmia	Test each nostril independently for smell (i.e., coffee) (*Note*: Smell is the only uncrossed sense)
II.	Optic	Vision	Prechiasmic: monocular blindness Postchiasmic: hemi-visual field loss	Test visual fields in each eye and for both eyes simultaneously
III.	Oculomotor	Eyelid retraction Pupilary constriction Medial eye movement	Drooping eyelid Enlarged pupil Deviation of affected eye laterally (outward)	Note ptosis, check pupilary asymmetry and reaction to light and accommodation. Note downward and lateral eye deviation upon fixed forward gaze
IV.	Trochlear	Rotation of eye with head tilt	Compensatory head tilt to reduce diplopia	Note diplopia produced with head tilt. Note which eye does not demonstrate appropriate rotation upon head tilt (*Note*: Often difficult to test without specialized equipment)
V.	Trigeminal	Mastication muscles Facial sensations	Weakness in bite Loss of sensation	Note asymmetry in mastication musculature or facial sensation threshold
VI.	Abducens	Lateral eye movement	Deviation of eye medially (inward)	Note inward deviation of affected eye upon fixed forward gaze
VII.	Facial	Musculature of facial expression Anterior tongue taste	Weakness of facial muscles Loss of taste on anterior tongue (Ageusia)	Note weakness of facial muscles or asymmetry in facial expression. Inquire about loss of sense of taste, particularly sweet sensitivity
VIII.	Acoustic	Hearing	Decreased auditory sensation	Assess symmetry of auditory threshold
IX.	Glossopharyngeal	Taste on posterior tongue Gag reflex	Ageusia Poor gag reflex	Inquire about loss of sense of taste, particularly sour/bitter. Assess gag reflex
X.	Vagus	Motor movement of soft palate Vocal cord innervation	Decreased palate movement Hoarse voice	Assess elevation symmetry of soft palate. Inquire about change in vocal quality
XI.	Spinal accessory	Neck muscles	Weakness of trapezia	Assess symmetry of strength in shoulder shrug
XII.	Hypoglossal	Muscle of the tongue	Weakness or deviation upon tongue protrusion	Assess tongue weakness via sustained tongue thrust and note deviation.

Cranial nerves consist of 12 pairs of nerves that emanate from the brain stem (Medulla, Pons, and Midbrain) and basal forebrain. Cranial nerves project ipsilaterally and produce deficits on the same side as the injury. Anatomically, Cranial Nerves (CN) I–IV originate from the basal forebrain and midbrain, CN V–VIII originate from the pons and CN IX–XII originate from the medulla. Both the laterality and anatomical origination of cranial nerves are important for differentiation of cortical and subcortical injuries and localization of injury. Examination of CN function is a critical part of the neurologic evaluation and establishes the integrity of functions that are prerequisite for any accurate evaluation of subsequent cortical functioning.

Cranial nerve function can be grouped into sensory associations such that smell is attributable to the Olfactory nerve (CN I) and vision is associated with the Optic nerve (CN II). Eye movement is associated with the Occulomotor (CN III), Trochelear (CN IV) and Abducens (CN VI). Similarly, taste is associated with the Facial nerve (CN VII) and Glossopharyngeal (CN IX). Specifically, the facial nerve innervates the tip of the tongue and the perception of predominately sweet taste while the Glossopharyngeal nerve innervates the posterior aspect of the tongue and perception of sour tastes. (Now you know the secret to sweet and sour sauce!) Auditory function is associated with the Acoustic nerve (CN VIII).

It should be noted CN functions are considered part of the peripheral nervous system and that similar deficits can be obtained from cortical or other central nervous system lesions. Lesions produced centrally (cortically) are distinguished by the contralateral nature of the deficit they produce (with the exception of olfaction). For example, deficits to primary auditory cortex on the right will produce primarily auditory deficits in the left ear, while a lesion to the left acoustic nerve (CN VIII) would produce a primary auditory deficit in the left ear.

Sensory Functioning

Sensory testing involves establishing thresholds for vibratory, tactile, and position sensations. Sensation is evaluated for each level of the spinal cord, as well as sensation requiring cortical processing (i.e., graphasthesia, asteroagnosia, and bilateral simultaneous stimulation).

Primary sensory testing involves touch and vibratory sensation thresholds, established for each level of the body from feet to neck (recall sensation above the neck is governed by CN function). Sensation from the cervical spinal region (C2–C8) is in the upper chest and arms. The thoracic region (T1–T12) innervates from the chest to just below the umbilicus, whereas the lumbar spine (L1–L5) innervates the genitalia and legs with the exception of the dorso-lateral aspect and sole of the foot, which is innervated by the sacral region (S1–S2) of the spinal cord.

Secondary sensation involves examination of sensory functions requiring cortical processing beyond basic perception. Such functions involve bilateral simultaneous processing of stimuli, which may indicate a subtle lesion in the sensory cortex of the hemisphere contralateral to the body side on which the sensation was suppressed. In addition, tactile identification of objects (steroagnosis) or the inability to identify tactile information (numbers or letters) written on the palms (graphasthesia) may be impaired, and typically represents right hemisphere parietal lobe lesions. In addition, examination of position sense and joint pressure can be evaluated by manipulation of joint position (toe up or down) and by asking the patient to judge weights held in the hands.

Motor Testing

"Motor Testing" may refer to two different types of assessing the function of a patient's motor system: (1) a neurological-based approach utilizing species-wide normative reference information for motor strength, tone, and deep tendon reflexes, and (2) a clinical neuropsychological-based approach using population normative information to assess motor speed, dexterity and strength.

Neurological-Based Assessment

This assessment approach is not routinely administered by clinical neuropsychologists, but if available, the clinician can (and should) incorporate this information into the more quantitative motor assessment often completed as part of a neuropsychological evaluation. As part of the neurological evaluation, motor function is graded in terms of motor strength, tone, and deep tendon reflexes. In addition, cerebellar functioning and praxis are often evaluated. Motor strength is graded on a 1–5 scale where 1 is paralysis and 5 is full strength. Scores of 2–4 represent graded degrees of paresis (weakness) (see Chapt. 2, Table 2.1 for description of anchor points). Motor strength is evaluated both in lateral plane (right–left) and in terms of proximal–distal (moving away from the center of the body). While the lateral plane is indicative of the side of the lesion (contralateral), the proximal–distal and extensor–flexors are often related to the degree of recovery. Specifically, motor recovery after an injury often progresses from proximal to distal with large muscle groups such as shoulders and hips regaining function before hands and feet. Motor function also typically recovers in a pattern of flexor muscles returning before extensor muscles. This is important for ambulation in that the ability of patients to raise the foot (dorsiflexion) and for manual functioning in the extension of the hand, are often the last motor functions to return following cerebral damage.

Motor tone is graded on a continuum of flaccid to spastic, with muscle wasting and post acute flaccidity being associated with peripheral (lower motor neuron) injury and spasticity being associated with central nervous system (upper motor neuron) injury. While initial response to both peripheral and central nervous system injury results in flaccidity, as time progresses, flaccidity remains in peripheral injury and is replaced by hyper-tonicity in central nervous system injury.

Tone is graded on a scale of 1–4, determined subjectively by muscle stretch reflexes (see Chapter. 2, Table 2.2). Hyper-tonicity (i.e., spastic muscle tone) is associated with central nervous system damage whereas hypo-tonicity (decreased muscle stretch reflex) is associated with peripheral nerve injury. Reflex rating of 2 is normal, with ratings of 3 indicating hyper-reflexia and ratings of 4 indicating hyper-reflexia with clonus (repeated elicitation of stretch receptor reflex after single stimulation). These ratings are sometimes denoted with a plus sign (i.e., 2^+ or 3^+) if they are considered to be in the high end of normal (2^+) or the high end of abnormal but do not elicit clonus (3^+) (see Chapter. 2, Table 2.1).

Neuropsychological-Based Assessment

Evaluation of motor function is often completed as part of the neuropsychological examination. Clinical neuropsychologists will frequently assess motor function using a hand dynamometer, rate of finger oscillations within a specified time, and/or performance completing a timed task of fine motor dexterity [e.g., Grooved Pegboard Test (Klove 1963) or Purdue Pegboard Test (Purdue Research Foundation 1948)]. Unlike neurological examination of motor strength, the comparison standard for these tests are population based, such that age-, education- and gender-demographic-based norms are available. The normative-based motor function assessment, often completed as part of a neuropsychological evaluation, should be incorporated with global ratings of motor function and muscle tone. Patients with clear hemiparesis (e.g., flaccid hemiplegia) often will not require further neuropsychological-based assessment of motor function. Alternatively, patients completing rehabilitation, and having good recovery of motor function to a cursory neurological examination, will often continue to exhibit clear deficits on more detailed neuropsychological-based assessment of motor function, providing helpful information for diagnosis and treatment planning (see Lezak et al. 2004 for review).

Cerebellar and Praxis Examination

Examination of cerebellar functions involves performing tasks of smooth motor pursuit and balance. This is most typically evaluated by having the person perform such tasks as finger to nose in which they alternately touch the examiner's finger and their nose rapidly in succession. Heel-to-toe walking, walking on a straight line, and raising the heel along the shinbone while seated are other common methods of assessing cerebellar function. Each activity is evaluated subjectively on a pass/fail basis.

Praxis evaluation involves performing complex, sequenced motor movements both to command and imitation (see also Chap. 9, this volume, for more details). Cortical damage to the left parietal association area often disrupts such overlearned complex motor tasks and may affect such tasks as grooming, dressing, or feeding behaviors. Damage to the right parietal lobe often is associated with constructional praxis. Praxis is typically evaluated by asking patients to simulate blowing out a match, unlocking a door, using a hammer, or sucking a straw. Patients who are unable to easily simulate these acts spontaneously are then asked to mimic the examiner performing these acts. Individuals suspected of constructional praxis are typically asked to draw a simple object (i.e., house, face, tree) and, if they are unable to draw spontaneously, they are given a design to copy. Failure to spontaneously perform commands or draw is indicative of deficits and should prompt further, more detailed assessment.

"Higher Order" Neuropsychological Function Examination

We now turn our attention to higher level cognitive processing. These skills involve arousal, processing speed, attention and concentration, language, memory, visuospatial/visuoperceptual, executive skills (i.e., reasoning, sequencing, problem solving, judgment, and insight), and mood/affect. In addition, a thorough neuropsychological evaluation will evaluate a patient's effort or motivation to perform to his/her best ability, using a variety of methods that can include stand-alone measures of task engagement (e.g., symptom validity testing), as well as various algorithms and comparisons within and across neuropsychological measures, to assess for consistency and adherence to known neuropathological patterns of performance (see Chapter. 20, this volume, for details). Evaluation of mood is typically completed using a variety of psychological measures, which may be based on the patient's report, the report of collateral informants (i.e., family members, teachers, and perhaps friends or coworkers), and/or ratings by a clinician. In general, we recommend an assessment for symptoms of anxiety and depression at the minimum. More detailed psychological assessment may be needed depending upon the nature of the referral, patient variables, and clinician variables. The potential for suicide/homicide should be included in clinical neuropsychological evaluations (but may not be needed in research settings). Finally, the neuropsychological evaluation will establish a premorbid level of cognitive functioning as a comparison standard.

The neuropsychological functions assessed as part of a comprehensive evaluation are discussed throughout the rest of this book. However, as a process of neuropsychological evaluation, they are mentioned here to highlight the sequential nature of each as an integral part of the assessment of increasingly complex functions. As measurements of cognitive functions get increasingly complex, the lateralizing and localizing nature of them become less certain. For example, the areas that can result in an expressive aphasia are well established, but damage almost anywhere in the brain can produce attentional and information processing deficits. As a process, however, accurate neuropsychological evaluation is dependent on the adequacy of a hierarchical series of prerequisite skills. These skills are presented graphically in a Neuropsychological Evaluation Process Pyramid, with prerequisite skills at the bottom and subsequently more complex skills at the top (Fig. 4.1).

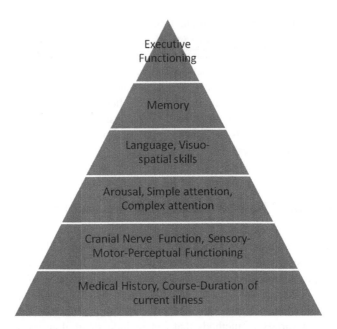

Fig. 4.1 Pyramid perspective for interpretation of neuropsychological evaluation

Assessment of these functions may be brief or extensive. In brief examinations, these areas of more complex and integrative cognitive functioning are assessed at basic levels. Individuals who have acquired these skills are expected to demonstrate very good function on these brief and often simple assessment tasks. In younger patients or those with developmental delays or mental retardation, expectations must be adjusted accordingly. These brief evaluations are limited in that they yield results that allow only ordinal data such as impaired versus normal or mild–moderate–severe impairment continuum. While brief evaluation has the benefit of repeatability, rapid assessment and targeting specific deficits. It also has the draw-backs of being less thorough in the assessment of any given higher cognitive function as well as, not provide a psychometrically-based measurement of the higher cognitive function or integrative skill.

More formal neuropsychological assessment involves measurement of these "Higher Cognitive" functions and comparisons to both known population standards, that are matched as closely as possible to the patient in age, education, gender, and other demographic factors which might have an influence on the function being measured. The patient's performance is also typically evaluated in the light of an individual level comparison standard that is derived from estimates of the individual's premorbid level of cognitive function. Further details of psychometrics and interpretation are covered in Chapter. 1 and Chapters. 29–31 in this volume (see also Lezak et al., 2004 for detailed discussion of interpretation in neuropsychology).

Rule of thumb: Deficit Measurement

- Assessment of change requires a comparison standards be established
- Comparison standards include normative comparison standards or individual comparison standards
    - Normative comparison standard may be species-wide behaviors/skills or population-based normative information on cognitive skills and behaviors
    - Individual comparison standards can include historical information (previous test scores before onset of known or suspected brain dysfunction) or, most commonly, estimated premorbid ability level(s)
- Comparison standard establishes benchmark against which patient's performances are compared to determine if change (deficit or improvement) in neuropsychological function has occurred
- Patterns of neuropsychological deficits are associated with functional neuroanatomy and neuropathology to associate behavior deficits to brain dysfunction

References and Suggested Further Readings

Bonner, J. S., & Bonner, J. J. (1991). *The little black book of neurology* (2nd ed.). Baltimore: Mosby.

Lezak, M. D., Howieson, D. B., & Loring, D. W. (2004). *Neuropsychological assessment* (4th ed.). New York: Oxford University Press.

Chapter 5
Arousal: The Disoriented, Stuporous, Agitated or Somnolent Patient

James G. Scott

Abstract Arousal refers to the maintenance of an appropriate level of cerebral activity to successfully complete the task in which one is engaged. Arousal occurs on a continuum from hypoarousal to hyperarousal and may fluctuate quickly. Appropriate arousal is a necessary prerequisite for consciousness. Arousal is anatomically mediated through the ascending reticular activating system (RAS), which has projections arising from the medulla and pons, projecting to the midbrain, thalamus and hypothalamus (see Chap. 3 for more details). Stimulation of the RAS is essential for maintaining consciousness at a basic neurophysiologic level. Hyperarousal produces states of agitation. States of arousal vary from coma to normal and are typically classified or categorized clinically as below. Table 5.1 presents categorical classification of arousal, response to attempts to influence arousal and course of arousal with varying stimulation.

Key Points and Chapter Summary

- Maintenance of appropriate arousal is a critical prerequisite for assessment of cognition in patients
- Arousal level should be assessed at several points in time as it may fluctuate considerably over time
- Delirium is common in many hospitalized groups and should be monitored frequently
- Delirium in outpatient populations should be an initial focus if acute cognitive and behavioral changes or fluctuations are noted

---

J.G. Scott (✉)
Department of Psychiatry and Behavioral Sciences, University of Oklahoma Health
Sciences Center, Oklahoma City, OK, USA
e-mail: jim-scott@ouhsc.edu

M.R. Schoenberg and J.G. Scott (eds.), *The Little Black Book of Neuropsychology:*
A Syndrome-Based Approach, DOI 10.1007/978-0-387-76978-3_5,
© Springer Science+Business Media, LLC 2011

Arousal Problems: A Behavioral Guide

A symptomatic guide for how problems in arousal typically present is provided below. This is then followed by a list of possible diagnostic or syndromic explanations for the observed problems in arousal (see also Chap. 15, this volume). In general, alterations in a patient's arousal should be considered a serious concern to the clinical neuropsychologist. It often reflects a serious medical condition (Table 5.1).

Table 5.1 Categorization of arousal states

Arousal state	Arousal response	Course
Coma	No response to stimuli	No change
Stupor	Sleepy – awakens to arousal but unable to maintain without stimulation	Fluctuations build or fall as stimulation varies with return to sleep with decreased stimulation
Delirium	Awake with fluctuations in arousal, vacillations from hypo- to hyper-arousal	Fluctuations based on environmental factors and medical factors. Fluctuations may be rapid or prolonged.
Normal	Awakens to stimulation, maintains arousal	Normal sleep–wake cycle established

There are three general patterns of disrupted arousal:

1. Hypoarousal–hypoactive problems

   The patient appears stuporous, sleepy, "hypoalert" or somnolent. The patient may react to auditory or other somatic stimuli (touch, mild pain) by appearing to wake up, may look around the environment, and then fall back asleep. If not "sleeping," the patient will appear "sleepy," often will complain of being tired, may yawn frequently, appear confused, and is easily irritated. Speech may be slurred and/or is often of short phrase length (often one or two word answers to questions). If phrase length is longer, speech content may not be consistent with the situation, with the patient being tangential or incomprehensible. Patients with hypoarousal generally do not exhibit spontaneous speech. The patient may only eat with encouragement and the patient's sleep–wake cycle is likely disrupted. Management of other basic activities of daily living, toileting, bathing, etc. are also likely to be disrupted. Arousal in these patients may be solicited with constant stimulation (i.e., interacting or physical movement), but they quickly revert to hypo-aroused when external stimulation is reduced or withdrawn.

   The patient is likely to have difficulty with attention, and assessing higher cortical functions at this point is not advised. Unlike a patient with problems in attention, but not in arousal (see Ch. 6, this volume), patients with poor arousal have difficulty appearing awake long enough to complete any evaluation. More subtle disruptions in arousal can appear as a problem with attention, but close observation will demonstrate fluctuations in arousal rather than deficits in efforts to sustain or focus attention.

2. Hypearousal–hyperactive problems

   The patient will appear "hyperactive," and may present with delusions, hallucinations, and extreme irritability and agitation. The patient's high energy level is unable to be effectively directed to any task or focused activity. The patient is likely to be agitated and anger outbursts or episodes of aggression may occur. Other affective lability is also possible, with patients crying or laughing easily. While the patient may appear aroused enough to complete testing of higher order cognitive functions, frequently the impairment in arousal will manifest as extreme disruption of attention.

3. Mixed arousal problems

The patient will appear to present with alternating periods of hypoarousal-hypoactivity and hyperarousal-hyperactivity. The fluctuating course can occur over periods of minutes to hours and may be the most frequently seen pattern of arousal deficit seen in acute hospitalization.

Below, diagnostic considerations for altered arousal are provided. In general, there are four broad categories resulting in disrupted arousal: intracranial disease, systemic disease affecting CNS, toxins/metabolic, drug withdraw.

1. Primary intracranial disease (stroke, seizure, intracranial mass). Primary intracranial disease affects the RAS by compression on the brain stem. Frequent causes are uncal herniation or central (foramen magnum) herniation, diffuse increased intracranial pressure, or bilateral diffuse frontal lobe damage.
2. Systemic disease affecting the CNS. Some of the more common are urinary tract infections, sepsis, hepatic failure, and cardiopulmonary diseases. Included in this category are medical procedures which place the patient at high risk such as those resulting in high volume blood loss (i.e., orthopedic surgery) or those requiring extensive time on cardio-pulmonary support (i.e., Cardiac Artery Bypass Grafting, CABG). In addition, those procedures that require extended periods of general anesthesia also place patients at risk for subsequent deficits in arousal.
3. Toxins/metabolic conditions. Exposure to exogenous toxins and drugs (e.g., ETOH) as well as metabolic dysfunction (e.g., hypoglycemia, hyponatremia, etc.).
4. Drug withdraw. Drug exposure and/or withdraw can induce alterations in arousal, and a delirium (e.g., narcotics, sedatives, muscle relaxers, etc.).

Rule of thumb: Assessment of arousal

- Arousal deficits and delirium are a significant risk factor for mortality and should not be dismissed as a normal course of recovery
- Arousal may fluctuate rapidly and necessitates serial assessment
- Causes of arousal deficits and delirium are numerous and complex and require a thorough medical workup to identify contributing factors

Stuporous Conditions Mimicking Coma

Several conditions may present as coma-like with restricted responses to environmental stimuli or attempted arousal. These conditions include akinetic mutism and decorticate state or persistent vegetative state (see also locked-in syndrome below).

A triad of symptoms distinguish the first two from stuporous conditions, including akinesia, mutism, and decreased consciousness. Akinetic mutism and persistent vegetative state result from incomplete disturbance of the reticular activity system and produce varying states of disturbances of arousal. There is controversy regarding these states and whether it is better to categorize them as a continuum of coma states or separate entities. The distinction lies in the presence of visual alertness with spontaneous eye opening and sporatic tracking of auditory, tactile and visual stimulation in the environment. Akinetic mutism results from damage to the sub-thalamic region and septal nucleus, or from bilateral extensive frontal lobe lesions. While some response to arousal occurs, this arousal is not maintained and a return to an akinetic-mute state quickly results. When akinetic mutism is due to bilateral frontal lobe damage, the patient presents as severely abulic with extreme amotiva-tion. Unlike patients with damage to areas around the 3rd ventricle, patients with bilateral frontal lobe lesions are aware of surroundings and can encode new infor-mation. In persistent vegetative states, following a period of coma, diurnal rhythms often re-establish and the individual exhibits spontaneous eye opening and sporadic eye tracking of visual, auditory, or tactile stimulation of their environment. Individuals with diffuse cortical lesions often exhibit eye opening to stimulation with frequently intact brain stem reflexes. These states often are the result of acute diffuse causes such as anoxia/hypoxia, toxic/metabolic, or drug-induced states.

Locked-In Syndrome

In locked-in syndrome, a lesion in the pontine level (tegmental area) effectively blocks descending pathways (complete transaction of the corticospinal and corticobulbar path-ways) while the ascending pathways remain intact. These lesions are often the result of a circumscribed hemorrhagic or occlusive lesion and spare the cortex and cranial nerves I–III, sparing smell, sight and some aspects of eye movement. Thus, a patient with locked-in syndrome may appear in a coma, but these patients' mental status is generally entirely preserved. Locked-in syndrome can be distinguished from stuporous condition or coma in careful examination utilizing eye movements to demonstrate responses to stimuli. These patients are able to communicate only with eye movements, but remain very much conscious, perceive stimulation throughout their bodies, and are aware, despite their inability to speak or produce voluntary movement.

Delirium

Delirium refers to an acutely developing and fluctuating deficit in arousal (see also Chap. 15 for a discussion of confusional states generally, including encephalopathy and delirium). Delirium is common in acute medical settings with estimates of prevalence raging from 10% to 15% of hospital admissions. Increasing risks for delirium are closely associated with the reason for hospitalization and associated

Table 5.2 *Diagnostic and Statistical Manual*, 4th edition: criteria for delirium

Criteria A:	Disturbance of consciousness with reduced ability to focus, sustain or shift attention
Criteria B:	Change in cognition (memory, orientation, language) or development of perceptual disturbance that is not better accounted for by pre-existing dementia
Criteria C:	Development of disturbances over a short period of time (hours to days) and fluctuation during course of a day or over time
Criteria D:	Evidence by history that these changes are associated with the patient's general medical condition

demographic factors. Specifically, individuals undergoing cardiac or orthopedic procedures are especially vulnerable, as are the chronically ill, aged or demented. In addition, these procedures are often associated with high blood volume losses, high use of pain medication and potential hypoxia associated with length of time on heart/lung bypass equipment. Table 5.2 lists the DSM-IV diagnostic criteria for delirium. Table 5.3 lists some of the common medical and demographic risk factors in delirium. The diagnosis of acute delirium is critical as mortality rises dramatically as delirium is prolonged. A useful mnemonic of I WATCH DEATH is presented in Yudofsky and Hales (1992) and adapted below.

Rule of thumb: Mnemonic for medical conditions associated with delirium

Category	Medical factors
*I*nfection	Encephalitis, meningitis, Sepsis
*W*ithdrawal	Alcohol, sedatives, analgesics
*A*cute metabolic	Electrolyte, renal-hepatic failure, acidosis, alkalosis
*T*rauma	Post-surgical, hypo- or hyperthermia
*C*NS pathology	Hemorrhage, hydrocephalus, seizure, tumor, vasculitis
*H*ypoxia	Carbon monoxide poisoning, hypotension, cardiac arrest
*D*eficiencies	B12, thiamin, severe nutritional deficiency
*E*ndocrinopathies	Hyper- or hypoadrenocorticism, hyper- or hypoglycemia
*A*cute vascular	Hypertension, occlusive stroke
*T*oxins or drugs	Medication reaction/change/overdose, toxic exposure
*H*eavy metals	Manganese, mercury

Adapted from Wise and Brandt in Yudofsky and Hale (p. 368)

Table 5.3 Demographic and medical risk factors associated with increased delirium

- Increased age
- Previous cognitive compromise (stroke, dementia, trauma)
- Chronic medical condition (diabetes, hypertension, cardio-pulmonary deficit)
- Prolonged hospitalization
- Sensory deprivation, sleep–wake disturbance
- Medical procedures with high blood volume loss/exchange (transplant, etc.)
- Cardiac procedures with necessary prolonged cardio-pulmonary bypass
- Occupational exposure to toxins
- Use of, or change in, dose of sedative, analgesic medications or reaction to new medication

Assessment of Arousal

Several aspects of arousal can be evaluated in the initial assessment in inpatient and outpatient settings (Table 5.4). Minimal assessment of arousal should include qualitative observation of arousal over time and fluctuations in arousal level across time through serial assessment. Several instruments have been designed to assess arousal and have applications for serial assessment in acute settings such as the Galveston Orientation and Amnesia Test (GOAT; Levin et al. 1979), the Glasgow Coma Scale (GCS; Teasdale and Jennett 1974) and Confusion Assessment Method (CAM; Inouye et al. 1990). The GOAT, GCS, and CAM are presented in Tables 5.5, 5.6, and 5.7. In addition, arousal can be assessed by evaluating the patient periodically throughout the day by observation and rating aspects of arousal (see Table 5.4). Finally, the clinical neuropsychologist observing a patient with disrupted arousal should also observe for cranial nerve abnormalities, hemiparesis, tremor, or signs of decorticate or decerebrate posturing. If not already under a physician's care, we strongly recommend the neuropsychologist immediately refer the patient with suspected altered arousal to a physician or hospital Emergency Department for further evaluation.

Table 5.4 Observational Assessment of Arousal

Feature	Assessment	Grading[a]			
Adaptation to environmental change	Response to new person, verbal or visual stimulation	0	1		
Activity level	Maintenance of appropriate response, avoidance of fluctuations	0	1	2	3
Response latency	Similar reaction time, response latency across tasks and time	0	1	2	3
Task persistence	Persistence on task through completion, minimal redirection needed	0	1	2	3

[a]0, No response/severely impaired; 1, Hypo arousal, minimal impairment; 2, Fluctuations hypo-hyperarousal, normal/impaired; 3, Normal performance

Table 5.5 The Galveston Orientation and Amnesia Test (GOAT)

	Error	Points
Name: _____ Date of test: ____/____/____		
Gender:_____ Time: _____		
Day of the week: _____ Date of injury: ____/____/____		
Date of birth: ____/____/____		
Diagnosis: _____		
1. What is your name? (2)_____	_____	_____
When were you born? (4)_____	_____	_____
Where do you live? (4)_____	_____	_____
2. Where are you now? (5) city_____	_____	_____
(5) Hospital_____	_____	_____
(Unnecessary to state name of hospital)		
3. On what date were you admitted to this hospital? (5) _____	_____	_____
4. What is the first event you can remember after the injury? (5)	_____	_____
_____		
Can you describe in detail (e.g., date, time, and companions) the first event you can recall after the injury? (5)	_____	_____
_____		
5. Can you describe the last event you recall before the accident? (5)	_____	_____
_____		
Can you describe in detail (e.g., date, time, and companions) the first event you can recall before the injury? (5)	_____	_____
_____		
6. What time is it now?_____	_____	_____
(−1 for each ½ hour removed from correct time to maximum of −5)		
7.What day of the week is it now?_____	_____	_____
(−1 for each day removed from the correct day to a maximum of −5)		
8. What day of the month is it now?_____	_____	_____
(−1 for each day removed from correct date to maximum of −5)		
9. What is the month?_____	_____	_____
(−5 for each month removed from correct one to maximum of −15)		
10. What is the year?_____	_____	_____
(−10 for each year removed from correct one to maximum of −30)		
Total error points:	_____	_____
Total GOAT score (100 points minus total error points)		

Table 5.6 Glasgow Coma Scale (GCS) 1974

Eye opening	
1. None	Not attributable to ocular swelling
2. To pain	Pain stimulus is applied
3. To speech	Nonspecific eye opening to speech; does not imply the patient obeys commands
4. Spontaneous	Eyes are open, but this does not imply intact awareness
Motor response	
1. No response	Flaccid
2. Extension	"Decerebrate"; extended arms, internal rotation of shoulder, and pronation of the forearm
3. Abnormal flexion	"Decorticate"; contracted arms, abnormal flexion of wrists and hands
4. Withdrawal	Normal flexor response; generalized withdrawal (non-specific) to pain
5. Localizes pain	Localized withdrawal to painful stimuli, attempts to remove pain source
6. Obeys commands	Follows simple commands
Verbal response	
1. No response	(Self-explanatory)
2. Incomprehensible	Moaning and groaning, but no recognizable words
3. Inappropriate	Intelligible speech (e.g., shouting or swearing), but no sustained or coherent conversation
4. Confused	Responds to questions, but the responses indicate varying disorientation and confusion
5. Oriented	Normal orientation to time, place, and person

Table 5.7 The Confusion Assessment Method (CAM) Diagnostic Algorithm

Feature 1.	Acute onset and fluctuating course
	This feature is usually obtained from a family member or nurse and is shown by positive responses to the following questions: Is there evidence of an acute change in mental status from the patient's baseline? Did the (abnormal) behavior fluctuate during the day, that is, tend to come and go, or increase and decrease in severity?
Feature 2.	Inattention
	This feature is shown by a positive response to the following question: Did the patient have difficulty focusing attention, for example, being easily distractible, or having difficulty keeping track of what was being said?
Feature 3.	Disorganized thinking
	This feature is shown by a positive response to the following question: Was the patient's thinking disorganized or incoherent, such as rambling or irrelevant conversation, unclear or illogical flow of ideas, or unpredictable switching from subject to subject?
Feature 4.	Altered level of consciousness
	This feature is shown by any answer other than "alert" to the following question: Overall, how would you rate this patient's level of consciousness? (alert [normal], vigilant [hyper alert], lethargic [drowsy, easily aroused], stupor [difficult to arouse], or coma [unarousable])

The diagnosis of delirium by CAM requires the presence of features 1 and 2 and either 3 or 4

References and Suggested Further Reading

Inouye, S. K., Van Dyke, C. H., & Alessi, C. (1990). Clarifying confusion: The confusion assessment method (CAM). *Annuals of Internal Medicine, 113*, 941–948.

Levin, H. S., O'Donnell, V. M., & Grossman, R. G. (1979). The Galveston Orientation and Amnesia Test (GOAT): A practical scale to assess cognition after head injury. *Journal of Nervous and Mental Disease, 167*, 675–684.

Lipowski, Z. J. (1990). *Delirium: Acute confusional states*. New York: Oxford University Press.

Teasdale, G. M., & Jennett, B. (1974). Assessment of coma and impaired consciousness. *Lancet, 2*, 81–84.

Yudofsky, S. C., & Hales, R. E. (1992). *Textbook of neuropsychiatry* (2nd ed.). Washington: American Psychiatric Press.

Chapter 6
Attention/Concentration: The Distractible Patient

James G. Scott

Abstract Attention and concentration are simple concepts on the surface but become complex when asked to assess or differentiate among capacities. While, at its most basic, attention refers to an organisms ability to recognize and respond to changes in its environment. The concept of attention when applied in neuropsychology represents a range of behavior which is dependent on functional integrity of many anatomical regions. The range of behavior includes everything from autonomic and reflexive auditory and visual orientation to sound and movement, to the ability to process several stimuli simultaneously or alternate back and forth from competing stimuli (see Kolb B, Whishaw, 2009 for review). While a universally accepted definition of attention and concentration would be broad and potentially unusable, the models of attention typically have common features including orienting, selecting stimuli and maintenance for a necessary time or successful completion of a task. These factors are represented in Fig. 6.1. Attention is typically viewed as a sequence of processes that occur in several different regions of the brain, which are involved with the acquisition and sustaining of attention. Attention is organized hierarchically, usually modality-specific at its origin and then multi-modality or multi-cortically mediated as in rapid alternation or switching of attention or maintenance of concentration.

In addition to attention, concentration refers to two elements: the capacity to sustain attention on relevant stimuli and the capacity to ignore irrelevant competing stimuli. Again, while simple, the concept of concentration is objectively difficult to differentiate in an orthogonal manner, several models of attention and concentration have been proposed and the interested reader is referred to Posner (1990) for elaboration.

J.G. Scott (✉)
Department of Psychiatry and Behavioral Sciences, University of Oklahoma Health
Sciences Center, Oklahoma City, OK, USA
e-mail: jim-scott@ouhsc.edu

M.R. Schoenberg and J.G. Scott (eds.), *The Little Black Book of Neuropsychology*:
A Syndrome-Based Approach, DOI 10.1007/978-0-387-76978-3_6,
© Springer Science+Business Media, LLC 2011

Key Points and Chapter Summary

- Attentional capacity is a prerequisite skill for accurate assessment of more complex neuropsychological functions
- Damage to the frontal lobes is most detrimental to attentional skills, but damage in any part of the brain can compromise attention
- Attention should be assessed at many levels including:
  - Voluntary attention
  - Focused attention
  - Divided attention
  - Sustained attention (concentration)
  - Alternating attention

Initial Attention		Selective Attention		Concentration
Automatic or voluntary orientation to sensory stimuli	→→→	Selection of stimuli from array of competing sensory stimuli	→→→	Maintenance of focus on stimuli to complete task

Fig. 6.1 Common elements in cognitive models of attention and concentration

Anatomy of Attention/Concentration

Attention and concentration is multiply determined from an anatomical perspective and involves many regions of the brain. Broadly speaking, attention and concentration deficits can arise from compromise in virtually any region of the brain; however, certain regions contribute different aspects to the attentional process. Table 6.1 outlines anatomical areas involved in different aspects of attention. For additional review of neuroanatomic correlates of attention, see Chap. 3, this volume (see also Kolb and Whishaw 2009; Lezak et al. 2004 for a thorough review of functional neuroanatomy for attention and concentration).

Table 6.1 Localization and lateralization of attentional deficits

Area	Attentional function
Superior colliculus	Regulates automatic orientation to visual stimuli
Inferior colliculus	Regulates automatic orientation to auditory stimuli
Ascending reticular activating system	Provides activating stimulation to cortex to initiate and maintain arousal necessary for initial and sustained attention
Thalamus	Lesions can produce contralateral inattention, or interfere with transmission of sensory input necessary for sustained or alternated attention
Limbic system (amygadala, cingulate gyrus and hippocampus)	Determines saliency of increasing stimuli, provides emotional tone thus facilitating attention and memory, involved with stimuli detection and appropriate alternation of attentional focus
Parietal lobes	Cross-modality hemispatial attention, with right parietal dominance for hemispace attention
Pre-frontal cortex	Responsible for voluntary initiation and sustaining attention, rapid alternation of attentional focus and shifting of attention
Dorsolateral frontal cortex	Initiation of attentional focus
Orbital frontal cortex	Sustaining of attentional focus

Attention Problems: A Behavioral Guide

Below, we provide a behavioral description of some common types of attention problems followed by a possible diagnostic or syndromic explanation for the observed attention deficits. It is important to note that attention problems may not be apparent in one-on-one situations and/or in highly structured settings where distracting stimuli are minimized and the environment and task are novel. Common symptoms of attention deficits and hyperactivity and impulsivity as listed by the DSM-IV are summarized in Table 6.2.

Table 6.2 Common symptoms of attention deficits, hyperactivity and impulsivity as listed by the DSM-IV

Neuropsychological deficit	Clinical presentation/symptoms
Attention	For DSM-IV diagnostic criteria, must have six (6) or more of the symptoms below for six (6) months in duration of severity that is maladaptive and inconsistent with the patient's developmental level
	• Avoids engaging in tasks that require sustained mental effort
	• Does not listen when spoken to directly
	• Does not follow through on instructions
	• Has difficulty sustaining attention in activities
	• Fails to give close attention to details
	• Has difficulty organizing tasks
	• Loses things necessary for activities
	• Is easily distracted by extraneous stimuli
	• Is forgetful in daily activities

(continued)

Table 6.2 (continued)

Neuropsychological deficit	Clinical presentation/symptoms
Hyperactivity and impulsivity	For DSM-IV diagnosis of hyperactivity/impulsivity type (or combined type) ADHD, patient must have six (6) or more of the following symptoms persisting for at least six (6) months in duration of severity that is maladaptive and inconsistent with the patient's developmental level.
	Hyperactivity
	• Acts as if "driven by a motor."
	• Has difficulty playing quietly
	• Is fidgety
	• Leaves seat when expected to remain seated
	• Runs about in situations in which it is inappropriate
	• Talks excessively
	Impulsivity
	• Blurts out answers before questions have been completed
	• Has difficulty taking turns
	• Interrupts or intrudes on others

A. Problems in attention without hyperactivity

Patients often present as being easily distractible and may have difficulty with compliance to complete some testing due to attention problems. Patients may be distracted by efforts to examine visual fields with confrontation, and will have difficulty maintaining a task if the examiner is making noise or moving around. While common in the general population, these patients frequently report difficulty completing projects they start and start another project before finishing the current project. Patients may also complain of memory problems such as, forgetting to do school or work projects. However, the forgetfulness often reflects a secondary effect of varying attention on consolidation of memory rather than a direct memory failure. These individuals often appear disorganized and inefficient or scattered due to the effect of their attentional difficulties in gathering the necessary prerequisite materials or completing tasks. While overt hyperactivity and impulsivity may not be present, these patients often appear fidgety, restless, or anxious.

B. Problems primarily with impulsivity and/or hyperactivity

Patients often present with a history of rash decisions and impulsive behaviors, that can often threaten their safety. These patients are clearly overactive relative to their peers and are often perceived as disruptive, non-compliant and unruly. They are also often perceived by peers as intrusive or annoying. Patients may complain of difficulty maintaining vigilance (focus) on tasks across environments (home, school, and/or work). Patients often have difficulty keeping still, and will fidget in their chairs or when trying to stand still. Younger patients may exhibit symptoms of conduct disorder and/or mood symptoms of anxiety or depressive symptoms. These patients may describe themselves as "class clowns" and may over-use alcohol and/or drugs. They are often avoidant of situations that require restricted movement or sustained attention (i.e., long travel, classrooms/lectures/meetings).

C. Problems in attention with impulsivity/hyperactive

Patients present with a combination of inattentiveness and impulsivity and hyperactivity. Patients present with being easily distracted, and go from one project to another without finishing the first. Patients also exhibit high energy levels and make rash and impulsive decisions. They often have difficulty learning from past mistakes and appear to impulsively make the same judgment errors repeatedly, despite good ability to verbalize alternative or correct responses and often display true remorse subsequent to their repeated mistakes. Like patients with primarily hyperactive-based attention problems, patients with both attention and hyperactivity/impulsivity may describe themselves as "class clowns" and may over-use alcohol and/or drugs as coping strategies.

D. Problems in maintaining vigilance

Patients having trouble maintaining vigilance may readily engage in a task and indicate an interest in completing the task. Span of attention (e.g., digit span) can be entirely intact, potentially even above average. However, for tasks taking longer times to complete, these patients lose interest in the task and become distracted. Patients typically begin to fidget and can daydream. Other novel stimuli present in the area will frequently distract a patient to move or stop engaging in the task. Patients with deficits in vigilance often avoid and/or complain about engaging in repetitive tasks.

Patients with deficits in vigilance often develop compensatory behaviors and fidget by playing with writing instruments, doodling, shifting position frequently (sitting or standing), and may "tap" their foot or fingers.

While appearing to be entirely inattentive, often when these patients are asked about recent events or details, they can usually respond correctly. Child patients with problems in vigilance deficits are often able to respond correctly to questions posed to them about what had recently transpired in the class-room, despite seemingly attending to doodling, talking to neighbors, and/or fidgeting in their desks.

E. Adult presenting with primary attention problems

The adult patient presenting to the neuropsychology clinic for predominate attention problems poses a significant challenge to the diagnosis and treatment of attention deficits. The diagnosis of Attention Deficit Disorder and Attention Deficit with Hyperactivity Disorder (ADD/ADHD) retrospectively requires a careful and detailed analysis of when symptoms of attention and/or impulsivity/hyperactivity problems began. DSM-IV criteria require onset of attention problems before the age of 7 years old. Onset of attention problems and/or hyperactivity/impulsivity in adulthood (after age 18) generally precludes a diagnosis of ADHD. While changes in attentional capacity are both common in the general population and expected with age, they may be a secondary symptom of developing neurologic or psychiatric disease. Attentional difficulties are a very common symptom across multiple neurologic and psychiatric disorders and thus it is critical that an acute cause be ruled out. In adult patients complaining of attention and/or hyperactivity/impulsivity symptoms, the diagnosis is neurological disease or psychiatric mood disorder until proven otherwise.

Assessment of Attention

The clinical assessment of attention ranges from tasks requiring simple attentional capacities to complex attentional functions involving selection, sustaining and alternating attention as well as inhibiting distraction or avoiding unwanted attentional switching to automatic or overlearned processes (i.e., reading or semantic processing rather than color naming or stating the case a word is printed in). Assessment of attention typically involves assessment of attentional capacity including, *focused attention, sustained attention, divided attention and rapid alternating attention.* In addition, assessment of attention frequently includes an evaluation of ability to inhibit automatic or overlearned responses. Assessment proceeds from the simplest tasks of attentional capacity to more complex tasks of focused, sustained, divided, and rapid attentional alternation. A brief summary is provided below, and bedside assessment examples are discussed in more detail below.

- Simple attentional capacity is a prerequisite skill which must be considered both in the assessment of more complex attentional factors in addition to other higher order cognitive skills (memory, language, visual-spatial reasoning, abstraction, etc.) that are assessed later in the neuropsychological evaluation. Digit span forward is an example of this ability in which patients are asked to repeat a series or random numbers.
- Focused attention (selective attention) refers to the ability to "tune out" or attend to chosen (consciously targeted information) stimuli while simultaneously ignoring other stimuli that are judged less important (i.e., not becoming distracted by competing stimuli). Examples of this are the Wechsler Intelligence tests digit symbol/coding and symbol search tasks and cancelation tasks. Among researchers, there is debate as to whether there is a difference between focused and sustained attention.
- Sustained attention (or vigilance) is the ability to maintain attention to stimuli over an extended period of time, even when stimuli may not be constant. Some would consider sustained attention as *concentration.* Examples include the various continuous performance tests in which attention must be sustained on a computer screen looking for a specified target over an extended time.
- Divided attention (some consider this to reflect working memory) refers to the ability to process more than one (multiple) stimuli (information) at the same time or maintain involvement in more than one task at a time (keeping information from multiple stimuli or tasks "on line" and respond appropriately to several operations of a task simultaneously). An example of this is mental arithmetic and letter–number sequencing tasks.
- Rapid alternating attention refers to the ability to rapidly shift attentional ability between stimuli or tasks. This type of attention is more difficult to evaluate without psychometric instruments. Examples include the Wechsler Intelligence tests digit symbol/coding subtest and symbol search subtest. These tests require rapid alternation of attentional focus, usually for short periods of time (ex. 90 seconds).

Table 6.3 Factors which can negatively effect assessment of attention

Factor	Assessment
Establish sensory thresholds	Assure adequate auditory, visual and tactile sensory thresholds, provide compensation if necessary (i.e., amplifier, large print, etc.)
Medication	Rule out sedative, hypnotic, analgesic, anxiolytic or other medication that affects attention (i.e., antihistamines).
	Examine dose schedules to minimize negative post dose effect.
	Examine medication and dose changes that may indicate magnified effect due to ineffectual habituation.
Fatigue	Examine the individual's activity level on the day of assessment; ask about changes in sleep/wake cycle and quality of rest on previous evening.
	Note the age and general health condition of the individual; examine individual level of fatigue as testing progresses, and note time of day the assessment of attention is occurring.
Environmental factors	Note auditory and visual distractions.
	Note presence of others or any change in environmental stimuli and the individual's response to these changes.

Before discussing the assessment of attention, several factors should be considered which could produce detrimental effects on immediate attention and distort the assessment of attention. These factors include the general medical condition of the patient, with acute patients and those immediately post-procedure likely to display attentional deficits that are varying and transient. Medication can also have a detrimental effect, and it is critical to be aware of the medication the patient is taking, the dosing schedule of medication that potentially affects attention and any recent change in medication, dose or dosing schedule. It is also important to assess the patient's level of fatigue, the extent of previous activity on the day of assessment and to account for the potentially fatigue-inducing effect of your current assessment. In noting fatigue, it is important to consider the time of day in which the assessment occurs, as in many individuals (especially the young and elderly) fatigue effects occur rapidly as the day progresses. An assessment of the environment is also necessary to rule out any extraneous distractions prior to assessing attention. Table 6.3 provides a checklist of pre-testing factors that can affect measured attentional skills.

Methods to Assess Attention and Concentration

As previously discussed, attention varies in complexity from simple to complex attentional abilities. Simple components of attention can be assessed in the interview both informally and formally. Attention should be assessed through observation by noting such behaviors as reciprocal conversation skill, time on task, response time and susceptibility to distraction or environmental change. Assuming that these behaviors are noted to be within normal limits, assessment of attention should progress from simple attention to auditory and visual tasks to more demanding tasks requiring sustained attention, rapid shifting of attention and dual processing of information. Many of these tasks can be administered at the bedside for patient screening or brief assessment while other components of attention are better evaluated in a controlled testing environment. This chapter will focus on brief/bedside evaluation of attention and concentration, but for more structured and elaborate attentional assessment the interested reader is referred to Lezak et al. (2004).

Brief/Bedside Assessment of Attention

Auditory Attention Span. Forward digit span involves the presentation of random single-digit numbers (0–9) to the patient at one per second (e.g., $6 - 4 - 9 - 7 - 2$). The numbers are repeated by the patient and assessed for accuracy. While education does have an impact on performance, age appears to have a minimal effect on digit-span forward (Lezak et al. 2004). The range of repetition of digits forward is traditionally considered to be 7 with an approximate standard deviation of 2 (e.g., correctly repeating 5–9 digits forward is considered normal). Test presentation data and descriptions of performance are presented in Table 6.4. For those patients older than 65, a reduction of 1 digit is appropriate (e.g., 4–8 digits forward). Individuals who have speech production problems can be presented with a page with numbers arranged from 0 to 9 and test stimuli either presented aurally or by pointing to numbers. Similar performance levels should be expected as with aural presentation and verbal response.

Reverse digit span is a slightly more difficulty task requiring patients to listen to digits presented at a rate of one per second (or view as in the case of visually presented stimuli) and then report the sequence of numbers in reverse order. This task is more demanding in that it not only requires short-term attention, but the storage and manipulation of this information prior to repetition of the digits. This task has been

Table 6.4 Digit span forward and reverse[a]

Digits	Forward	Reverse
$2 - 6$	Severely impaired	Moderately impaired
$9 - 3 - 1$	Moderately impaired	Mildly impaired
$5 - 7 - 4 - 8$	Mildly impaired	Borderline
$3 - 9 - 6 - 2 - 5$	Borderline	Low normal
$8 - 3 - 1 - 2 - 9 - 4$	Low normal	Normal
$7 - 6 - 4 - 1 - 3 - 5 - 2$	Normal	High normal
$3 - 9 - 4 - 6 - 8 - 2 - 5 - 1$	High normal	High performance
$5 - 6 - 9 - 2 - 8 - 3 - 5 - 1 - 7$	High performance	Superior

[a]For patients age 65 or older, add one digit to obtained performance to derive normative descriptor

---

Rule of thumb: Bedside Assessment of Attention

- Adequate and sustained arousal is a prerequisite for assessment of attention
- Attentional deficits produce a pattern of variable performance across neuropsychological assessment
- Attention Assessment should include:
  - Sustained attention/Vigilance
  - Attention under distraction
  - Divided attention
  - Rapid alternation of attention focus

---

shown to be much more revealing as to the effects of acute and chronic cortical compromise. In a normal population, the average person should perform one digit less in digits backward than forward (i.e., 6 ± 2). Test data are presented in Table 6.4.

Many other attention span tasks are available that include assessing forward and reverse span including letter span and visual span, and the interested reader is referred to Lezak et al. (2004) for a description of these tests.

Assessment of Vigilance

Vigilance, or the ability to sustain attention voluntarily, is also critical for successful performance on neuropsychological tests and a prerequisite skill in making meaningful interpretation of subsequent neuropsychological test data. It is especially important to assess vigilance periodically in patients who are acutely injured or otherwise believed to experience fluctuations in attentional capacity.

The most direct way to assess vigilance is to ask the patient to perform a task that requires sustaining attention. Vigilance should be sustainable for at least 60–90 seconds without interruption. In the interview, a patient can be asked to point to a series of objects in the room either by mimicking the examiner or by following verbal commands. Such commands can be repeated to ensure that vigilance can be sustained for 60–90 seconds. Such commands or mimicking can include pointing to ceiling, floor, walls, windows, furniture or personal objects in the room. The individual could also be asked to count to 100 or recite the alphabet or read aloud for 60 seconds. The critical element is that the task involves over learned stimuli which require minimal cognitive processing.

More formal bedside assessment of vigilance can be conducted using a letter or digit vigilance task (see Table 6.5 for example). Such tasks require the patient to listen to a series of numbers or letters and respond only to a target letter or number by raising a finger or tapping a table. In such tasks, each number or letter is read at a rate of one per second and performance is evaluated based on omissions errors

Table 6.5 Letter and number vigilance assessment tasks[a]

Digits	Letters
5 3 9 1 5 5 6 7 4 1 8 2 5 6 5	A C R P A A M D Q S D T A B A
5 5 8 3 1 6 4 4 2 7 1 9 4 5 1	A A Z P T M N N E F G B S A L
5 8 6 3 9 5 5 5 2 7 6 1 5 4 2	A S P L R A A A G M C D A D B
2 7 6 5 4 9 3 8 6 4 8 2 5 1 4	B G F A D S T P Z R F T A C F

[a]Digits and letters should be read at one per second. Errors should be noted as commission (c) omission (o) or perseveration (p). Total errors exceeding three indicate impairment. After a patient understands directions, no further assistance is provided during testing

(failing to detect a target), commission errors (falsely reporting a target as presented) and perseverations of response. These tests typically have a one-to-four response items-to-distracter ratio, and minimal total errors are expected in normally functioning patients aged 6 years old and older. Patients with greater than three total errors should be considered to be impaired. Test stimuli are presented in Table 6.5 for both letter and digit vigilance tasks (Target letter A and number 5 in this example). While the assessment of attention should be conducted at the bedside or during interview, assessment of more complex attention and a quantitative assessment of attentional capacities is best done in a formal assessment setting which can control environmental factors and make comparisons to standardized data. The interested reader is referred to Lezak et al. (2004) for a thorough review of attention assessment measures. Common measures to assess for vigilance include continuous performance tests, which require the patient to respond to various stimuli on the screen while not responding to others.

References and Suggested Further Reading

Kolb, B., & Whishaw, I. Q. (2009). *Fundamentals of human neuropsychology* (6th ed.). New York: Worth Publishers.

Lezak, M. D., Howieson, D. B., & Loring, D. W. (2004). *Neuropsychological assessment* (4th ed.). New York: Oxford University Press.

Posner, M. I. (1990). Hierarchical distributed networks in the neuropsychology of selective attention. In A. Caramazzo (Ed.), *Cognitive neuropsychology and neurolinguistics: Advances in models of cognitive function and impairment*. Hillsdale, NJ: Erlbaum.

Strub, R. L., & Black, R. W. (1993). *The mental status examination in neurology* (3rd Ed.). Philidelphia, PA: F.A. Davis.

Chapter 7
Language Problems and Assessment: The Aphasic Patient

James G. Scott and Mike R. Schoenberg

Abstract The singularly most uniquely human attribute is language. Such a bold statement is difficult to make, but profoundly true. Many species possess communication skill and communication among some species is elaborate and facilitates complex social relationships and interactions; however, the extent and sophistication of human use of representational language is truly unique. Language is so intertwined into what it is to be human that its complexity is often overlooked as a prerequisite skill in neuropsychological assessment.

At its simplest, language can be conceptualized as expressive and receptive language functions. While typically residing in the left hemisphere (referred to as the dominant hemisphere because of the propensity of language to develop even if damage occurs to normal language centers), bilateral representation and right hemisphere representation of language occurs both naturally and secondarily in response to early cerebral injury that affects the typically dominant left hemisphere (see (Table 7.1) for relative frequencies of hemispheric language dominance). See also Chaps. 3 and 12.

Table 7.1 Percent of individuals with hemispheric language dominance by handedness

Handedness	Hemispheric language dominance		
	Left	Right	Bilateral
Left	70	15	15
Right	96	4	0

Note: Numbers are percentages

J.G. Scott (✉)
Department of Psychiatry and Behavioral Sciences, University of Oklahoma
Health Sciences Center, Oklahoma City, OK, USA
e-mail: jim-scott@ouhsc.edu

M.R. Schoenberg and J.G. Scott (eds.), *The Little Black Book of Neuropsychology: A Syndrome-Based Approach*, DOI 10.1007/978-0-387-76978-3_7,
© Springer Science+Business Media, LLC 2011

The evaluation of the patient with language deficits first requires a review of the assessment of language and the definition of some terms. We will first review the basic aspects to evaluate speech and define terms describing different types of speech problems. We will then return to evaluating various speech problems commonly encountered in the clinic.

Key Points and Chapter Summary

- The hemisphere that controls language is referred to as the Dominant hemisphere
  - The left hemisphere controls language in the vast majority of people (but not all)
  - Anterior dominant cortex controls expressive language (including writing)
  - Posterior dominant cortex controls receptive language (including reading)
- The right hemisphere plays a significant role in prosodic aspects of language
  - Expressive prosody is controlled by the nondominant anterior cortex
  - Receptive Prosody is controlled by the nondominant posterior cortex
- Language deficits are most commonly produced by focal lesions, but more diffuse lesions can product subtle language deficits in high level language skills such as organization and discourse

---

Overview of Language

Assessment of language can be complex and detailed with many aspects of language being parceled out, but most clinical assessment of language includes basic aspects of expressive language (including writing), receptive language (including reading), repetition, naming and verbal fluency. The acquired inability to read is termed alexia and the acquired inability to write is called agraphia. Developmental deficits in reading (that is, difficulty learning to read, when reading had not been acquired, is termed dyslexia). Another domain frequently assessed is termed language prosody. Prosody refers to the ability to express and interpret vocal tone, inflection and other nonlanguage auditory cues and extract meaning that facilitates communication. The quality of an increased tone at the end of the sentence, "Here he comes," distinguishes that it was a question rather than an affirmative statement. Similar auditory cues are used in detecting sarcasm, irony, innuendo, and many other aspects of communication.

Assessment of language functions should differentiate deficits in the language process from articulation and other oral motor deficits that may significantly impact speech production. For example, patients can develop oral apraxias, which reflect inability to appropriately move the musculature of the mouth, tongue and larynx. The motor apraxias can be distinguished from aphasias by the fact that difficulty in moving the musculature of the mouth, tongue and larynx will also be present with tasks other than talking, such as swallowing, using a straw, trying to whistle, or chewing. Patients with oral apraxias may also have difficulty smiling appropriately to conscious effort (a good joke, however, will allow the patient to smile spontaneously). Note, however, there may be motor weakness (e.g., hemiparesis) associated with a contralateral cortical lesion or ipsilateral lesion of the cranial nerves innervating the face, lips, and tongue. Likewise, evaluation of basic hearing and vision functions should precede any evaluation to assess for language comprehension.

Anatomical Correlates

We briefly review anatomic correlates for language below for convenience. Readers are also directed to Chaps. 3 and 12 for additional review.

Language function is traditionally described as inclusive of the perisylvian area (cortex around the sylvian fissure or lateral fissure) of the dominant (left) hemisphere. Analogous representation of prosodic language function has been proposed for the nondominant hemisphere (e.g., Ross 1997). Language function can be divided into two broad neuroanatomical zone, an anterior expressive language zone and posterior receptive language zone. Expressive language is strongly associated with function of the left posterior frontal cortex, typically referred to as Broca's area, and corresponds to Brodmann's area (BA) 44 (along with BA 45) (see Fig. 7.1). Receptive language (comprehension) is associated with the left posterior temporal–parietal area, in which Wernicke's area (BA 22) is classically identified as the neuroanatomic localization for receptive language (see Chap. 3, Fig. 3.25 for detailed cortical map of Brodmann's areas).

Figure 7.1 highlights the cortical regions involved in expressive (spoken and writing) and receptive (aural and reading) language functions. The numbers correspond to Brodmann's areas involved in the left hemisphere. The illustration includes areas of the cortex not traditionally considered to be involved in language (e.g., visual cortex of BA 17, 18, and 19), but are included here to provide the reader with a better appreciation for the complex distributed network involved in language processes (see also Chap. 3). Broca's area is the expressive language hub, and integrally involved in expressive language (speech and writing). In addition, BA 6 (premotor area) is also involved in expressive language, including motor planning in speech articulation of the face, tongue, lips, pharynx/lanrynx, etc. The production of speech includes the corticobulbar tracts and cranial nerves involving the motor/sensory function of the mouth, tongue, and larynx as well as control of the diaphragm in order to produce speech. Receptive language

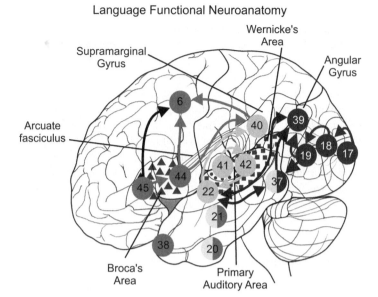

Fig. 7.1 Neuroanatomy of language

(comprehension and reading) is strongly associated with BA 22 (Wernicke's area), BA 41 and 42 (primary auditory sensory cortex), and BA 39 (angular gyrus). Primary auditory cortex anatomically corresponds to Heschl's gyrus, which is a part of the temporal lobe located in the Sylvian fissure. The projections from BA 41 and 42 to BA 22 (Wernicke's area) are integral in the perception of auditory sensory stimuli. Wernicke's area (BA 22) is identified as the central receptive language area, which is involved in comprehension of oral and written language. Brodmann's area 39 (angular gyrus) is a central area in the processing of written language. Semantic association of words (i.e., mental representation: canary is a bird) involves the occipitotemporal cortex (BA 21 and 37). Note that reading involves visual stimuli projected first to primary and associative visual cortex (BA 17/V1, BA18/V2, BA19/V3), which is then projected to language areas (BA 37, 22, and 39). In addition, the frontal eye fields (BA 8) are also involved (not shown). Receptive and expressive speech also activate BA 21. The arcuate fasciculus (part of the superior longitudinal fasciculus) underlying BA 39 and 40 and projecting to BA 44/45 is necessary for intact language, traditionally associated with the ability to repeat what is heard. Naming functions have been associated with the anterior superior and middle temporal gyri (BA 38, 21, and 22) as well as the left anterior cingulate, left ventral frontal lobe, and left medial occipital regions (not shown). Naming persons is associated with BA 38. Areas BA 20 and 37 have been implicated in naming animals (also left medial occipital lobe) and tools (also left premotor frontal lobe), respectively. Auditory naming (i.e., tell me the name for a doctor that takes care of children) tends to involve the anterior temporal regions (BA 38 and anterior BA 22, 21, and 20), while visual naming tends to involve the middle and posterior temporal areas (posterior BA 22, 21, 20, and 37). Disruption in receptive naming (being unable to name auditory descriptions) has been localized to the superior temporal gyrus (BA 22) while expressive auditory naming is associated with posterior middle temporal gyrus (BA 21) and temporo-parietal areas (BA 37 and 39). Finally, writing also involves motor and premotor cortex of the arm/hand (BA 4 and 6), basal ganglia and cerebellum (not shown).

Large lesions in the left hemisphere frequently produce both verbal expressive and auditory receptive language deficits such that reading and writing are also impaired (see Fig. 7.2). Focal damage to BA 44/45 produces a gross decrease in expressive language. However, lesions to BA 6 also result in impaired speech production beyond motor paresis, and BA 6 is involved in expressive speech (see Chap. 12). Lesions affecting primary auditory cortex (BA 41 and 42) result in deficits in auditory sensory perception (e.g., cortical deafness, auditory verbal agnosia, etc.; see Chap. 12). Injury to BA 22 results in deficits of language comprehension, including reading. The basic aphasias are presented in Table 7.2 along with their typical lesion location. See Chap. 12 for detailed review of aphasic syndromes.

Prosodic functions are similarly represented as Expressive and Receptive language functions in the left hemisphere, with expressive prosody functions being associated with right anterior (frontal) areas and receptive prosody being associated with right posterior (temporoparietal) regions. The effect of prosody deficits in communication can be profound, leading to literal, inefficient communication, which has a significant impact on communication of emotional information. Individuals with expressive aprosody are often viewed by others as dull, emotionless, and lacking compassion and empathy. Their verbal output is

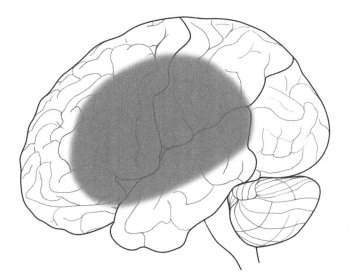

Fig. 7.2 Large left hemisphere damage resulting in global aphasia

Table 7.2 Types of aphasias and associated deficits

	Anatomical association	Speech	Comprehension	Reading	Writing	Repetition
Expressive (Broca's) aphasia	Left posterior frontal (Broca's area)	Impaired	Grossly intact	Grossly intact	Impaired	Impaired
Receptive (Wernicke's) aphasia	Left posterior temporal/parietal (Wernicke's area)	Fluent, but non-sensical	Impaired	Impaired	Grossly intact	Mildly impaired, paraphasic
Global aphasia	Left anterior and posterior	Impaired	Impaired	Impaired	Impaired	Impaired
Mixed transcortical aphasia	Left anterior and posterior sparing Broca's and Wernicke's areas	Impaired	Impaired	Impaired	Impaired	Intact
Transcortical motor aphasia	Left anterior frontal with relative sparring of Broca's area	Impaired	Typically intact	Typically intact	Impaired	Typically intact
Transcortical sensory aphasia	Posterior parietal/temporal cortical lesion with sparring of Wernicke's area	Impaired	Impaired	Impaired	Typically intact	Typically intact
Conduction aphasia	Lesion of the arcuate fasiculus which connects Broca's and Wernicke's areas	Mildly impaired – frequent paraphasias	Intact	Intact – for comprehension. Oral reading poor due to paraphasias	Typically impaired. Poor spelling/paraphasias	Impaired, even for single words

frequently monotone, flat, and lacking the tone and inflection that communicates the appropriate emotional state. When asked directly, they are often able to verbalize the presence of emotional states that they are not able to display adequately in their verbal tone and inflection. Similarly, individuals with receptive aprosodies are often viewed as emotionally unavailable, lacking insight into others' emotional states or uncaring. They often miss verbal cues that would communicate the emotional states of others. This in turn leads to a decrease in appropriate emotional responsiveness and a generally literal interpretation of what is verbally said with little appreciation for the way it was verbalized or the context in which it occurred. Table 7.3 lists the major Aprosodies and their anatomical correlates. See Chap. 12 for a detailed review of common aphasia and aprosody syndromes.

Rule of thumb: Language anatomical correlates:

- Broca (Brodmann area 44) is twice Wernicke's (Brodmann area 22)
- Language arc: in to Wernicke's area project via Arcuate fasciculus to Broca's area
- Written language needs Brodmann area 39 (angular gyrus)

Receptive Language and Receptive Aprosodies

Examination of receptive language includes aural and written receptive communication as well as examination of receptive prosody. These basic functions are prerequisite skills to the assessment of both higher and more difficulty aspects of language (phonemic or semantic fluency) and verbal reasoning. The appendix demonstrates items which assess a progression of receptive language skills from simple to complex. Each item should be passed easily by intact individuals, but additional items of similar complexity can be administered to assess degree and consistency of deficit in the assessed area of functioning.

Expressive Language and Expressive Aprosodies

Expressive language should be assessed both verbally and in writing. Similarly, expressive language should be assessed in both simple and gradually more complex functions. Appendix A includes a section for assessing expressive language functions. Assessment should include both responses to simple questions and responses to more unstructured, open-ended questions. Again, emphasis should be taken to note any paraphasic errors of either phonemic or semantic type as well as any articulation or oral motor deficits.

Table 7.3 Types of aprosodies and associated deficits

	Anatomical location	Verbal (expressive) prosody	Aural (receptive) prosody	Gestural receptive prosody	Gestural expressive prosody
Expressive aprosody	Right lateral frontal lobe, superior anterior temporal lobe	Severely impaired	Grossly intact	Grossly intact	Moderately impaired
Receptive aprosody	Right posterior temporal lobe, inferior parietal/temporal lobe juncture	Grossly intact	Severely impaired	Moderately impaired	Grossly intact
Global aprosody	Right anterior and posterior lesion	Severely impaired	Severely impaired	Moderately impaired	Moderately impaired

Recovery of Language Function

It is important to note that lesions that result in language deficits acutely may resolve substantially over the course of the first few weeks to months post-injury. In most cases, the most recovery occurs in the first 3 months after insult. Thus, assessment must consider the time since injury carefully as a critical factor in expected future functional language deficits and treatment programming (see also Chap. 1 for related issues in referral timing). Often, individuals having acquired broad language deficits (receptive and expressive speech is impaired) will exhibit recovery, but less recovery of language function than individuals with less disrupted language functions. As an example, individuals with language deficits in which receptive speech remains intact while expressive speech and repetition are impaired (Broca's aphasia) will often have recovery of language function such that repetition improves, and expressive language improves to include consistent simple one or two word utterances that enhance functional communication. A patient with pronounced acute expressive deficits may present in the neuropsychology clinic months later with subtle deficits of reduced phrase length, dysnomia, and dysgraphia. Conversely, patients with moderate to severe receptive language deficits may recover concrete receptive language skills, with only subtle residual deficits. Global aphasias recovery is generally to a Broca's (expressive) aphasia while Wernicke's (receptive) aphasias will recover to a conduction or anomic aphasia. Recovery may be so complete that deficits remain only in complex receptive language and are only detectible with detailed, in-depth testing of language skills. Unfortunately, patients with global deficits acutely often do not have good functional language outcomes and remain profoundly impaired.

We turn now to descriptions of various language problems one might encounter in the clinic setting. For the sake of description, subtle impairments which may be present are not reviewed, and the following is limited to description of language problems that may be readily identified by a detailed bedside evaluation of language functions.

Rule of thumb: Recovery of language

- Lesions in the dominant hemisphere are much more likely to produce permanent language deficits
- The size of the lesion is significantly related to the extent and persistence of the language deficit
- Most language recovery occurs rapidly in the first 1–3 months following an injury
- Expressive, receptive and repetition language deficits are anatomically separate
- Expressive deficits generally include written and spoken modalities equally
- Receptive deficits generally include auditory and reading modalities equally

Language Problems: A Behavioral Guide

Below, we provide a symptomatic description of various common language problems followed by a possible diagnostic or syndromic explanation for the observed language deficits. Further details of the identified aphasia syndrome and associated neurological and neuropsychological deficits can be found in Chap. 12.

Nonfluent Speech Problems: Speech Is Generally Nonfluent

The patient is unable to speak or speech is halting or limited to a few words and/or may be of shorter phrase length in less severe cases.

1. The patient is unable to speak, repeat what he/she hears or comprehend speech. The patient is unable read or write. The patient is observed to be able to swallow and eat without choking. Naming is impaired. The tongue is not significantly weak, although some weakness of the lower face and limbs is to be expected.
   - Suggests a *global aphasia*. Commonly associated with large left hemisphere lesions affecting left frontal, parietal, and temporal lobes (MCA stem infarct). A lesion affecting the left frontal lobe that extends mesially to insular region and basal ganglia can result in global aphasia, which may improve to a Broca's aphasia.
2. The patient is unable to speak, repeat, or comprehend speech. The patient is able to write. The patient is able to read. Weakness may or may not be present.
   - This pattern is not associated with known neurological etiology and reflects a psychiatric syndrome.
3. The patient is unable to speak, or speech is labored with a few words (telegraphic) that are typically nouns. Prosody and intonation impaired (dysprosody). Repetition is disrupted. Comprehension is grossly intact. The patient is able to follow basic commands and understand simple sentences, but some difficulty with grammatically complex sentences. Writing impaired with poorly formed letters and few if any words. Frequently has right hand hemiparesis, forcing patient to hold pen with nondominant (left) hand. The patient can comprehend simple words as indicated by motor or gestural responses and reading comprehension is often intact for simple commands. There are paraphasias. While nearly mute, patients may be able to blurt out words of profanity when upset or irritated. Patients may also be able to sing well-known songs. Naming generally impaired. Improved with phonemic cues.
   - Suggests a *Broca's aphasia*. Commonly associated with left inferior frontal lobe lesions. More extensive lesions affecting the left inferior gyrus and extending beyond central sulcus along the Rolandic fissure in which underlying white matter is affected results in more extensive and long-lasting Broca's aphasia features. Smaller lesions, affecting only left inferior frontal gyrus area (Broca's area), results in temporary mutism followed by mild transcortical motor aphasia (see below). Lesions limited to precentral gyrus result in aphemia.

4. The patient is unable to speak, or speech is labored and effortful with few words and/or paraphasias. Echolalia can be present. Less telegraphic speech (speech grammar is better than in Broca's aphasia). Speech prosody is poor (dysprosody). Repetition is grossly intact, and patient able to repeat single words and short sentences. Comprehension is intact. Writing is impaired with poorly formed letters. Reading comprehension is intact. Reading out loud is disrupted, effortful, and paraphasias and echolalia may be present. Naming is variable, but may be intact.
   - Suggests a *transcortical motor aphasia.* Commonly associated with left frontal lesions anterior and superior to Broca's area, which is spared. Generally, involves anterior dorsolateral cortex, but may also occur with mesial frontal lesions affecting anterior cingulate and supplementary motor area fibers. Lesions affecting basal ganglia of the left (dominant) hemisphere also associated with this aphasia syndrome. The patient is likely able to blurt out words of profanity when upset or irritated. Patients may also be able to sing over-learned songs (e.g., "Happy Birthday").
5. The patient's speech is mildly disrupted with short phrase length (commonly less than 6–7 words per sentence). Phonemic paraphasias often present. Repetition is grossly intact. The patient is able to repeat short phrases. Comprehension is intact. The patient can follow basic commands. Reading may be intact for simple words. Writing may be mildly disrupted, with misspelling and frequently short sentences. Naming grossly intact.
   - Suggests a resolving *transcortical motor aphasia.*
6. The patient is unable to speak, or speech is labored and effortful with few words and/or paraphasias. Repetition is intact. The patient may be able to repeat surprisingly long sentences accurately. Comprehension is impaired, and frequently unable to follow basic commands. Writing is impaired. Reading comprehension is impaired. Reading aloud is impaired. Naming is impaired.
   - Suggests a *mixed transcortical aphasia.* Commonly associated with diffuse left hemisphere lesions that spare the perisylvian fissure with lesions affecting both anterior and posterior regions. Most often caused by watershed infarcts of the ACA–MCA and MCA–PCA territories.

Rule of thumb: Nonfluent speech problems

Nonfluent speech is generally effortful and labored, and can consistent of no spoken or written words. Words of profanity may be elicited when upset. May be able to sing.
- *Global aphasia*: Often mute (but may have few words and is effortful). Repetition impaired. Comprehension impaired. Reading impaired. Writing impaired.
- *Broca's aphasia*: May be mute or speech is limited with few words and effortful. Repetition impaired. Comprehension intact. Reading comprehension intact. Writing impaired.

(continued)

> **Rule of thumb: Nonfluent speech problems** (continued)
> - *Transcortical motor aphasia*: Speech is limited with few words and effortful. Repetition grossly intact. Comprehension intact. Reading comprehension intact. Writing impaired.
> - *Mixed transcortical aphasia*: Speech is limited with few words and effortful. Repetition intact for even complex sentences. Comprehension impaired. Reading impaired. Writing impaired (can copy written sentence).

Fluent Speech Problems: Speech Is Fluent, but Is Unintelligible

The extent of unintelligibility will vary from extensive to mild. At the extreme, the patient may emit sounds fluently, but speech sounds do not correspond to recognized words. Mild cases will reflect fluent speech in which paraphasias and/or neologisms are present and/or speech (writing) grammar and syntax structure is poor.

1. The patient's speech is fluent but unintelligible. Words are paraphasias or neologisms (e.g., "whifel da pora at da sefa be fod the no…"). Prosody and intonation intact. Repetition is impaired. Comprehension is impaired. Patient is unable to follow basic commands. Reading is impaired. Writing is impaired, consisting of well-formed letter(s) and paraphasias and/or neologisms that does not make sense. Few if any real words. Naming is impaired.
   - Suggests a *Wernicke's aphasia*. Commonly associated with left posterior lesions affecting Wernicke's area and superior temporal lobe (e.g., superior temporal gyrus) and, often, extending to left parietal supramarginal and/or angular gyrus while anterior persylvian fissure remains intact. Underlying white matter damage result in more classic Wernicke's aphasia symptoms and more persistent aphasia.
2. The patient's speech is fluent, but generally unintelligible. Some distinct words may be appreciated, but most words are paraphasias and/or neologisms (e.g., "why da pora at be thing over the tretka…"). Words of profanity can be blurted out when upset or irritated. Prosody and intonation intact. Repetition may be surprisingly intact, even for long and complex sentences. Comprehension is impaired, but patient may be able to respond correctly to simple yes/no questions and/or follow simple one-step commands ("close your eyes"). Reading is impaired. Writing is nonsensical, and composed of well-formed letters and frequent paraphasias and neologisms. Some real words may be present. Naming is impaired.
   - Suggests a *transcortical sensory aphasia*. Commonly associated with left posterior hemisphere lesions typically including left temporo-occipital or left temporo-parietal. Brain structures of Wernicke's area and forward are persevered.
3. The patient's speech is generally fluent and grossly intelligible, although frequent phonemic paraphasias are usually present, which does decrease ability to understand the patient. Some pauses for naming (dysnomia) may also be present. Repetition is markedly impaired, and the patient may have difficulty repeating

even single words. Comprehension is intact. Reading comprehension is generally intact, but reading aloud is somewhat impaired, with frequent phonemic paraphasias. Writing is generally impaired with frequent phonemic paraphasias (poor spelling) and confused word order. Naming is mild to moderately impaired.

- Suggests a *conduction aphasia*. Commonly associated with lesion of the left (dominant) temporoparietal area, particularly the supramarginal area and underlying white matter. Arcuate fasciculus is classically involved; however, damage to arculate fasciculus itself need not occur, as conduction aphasia is possible with damage to left insular region and associated white matter. Overlying cortex of arcuate fasciculus damage can also lead to conduction aphasia symptoms.

4. The patient's speech is generally fluent and intelligible. Some paraphasias or pauses in speech is present when the patient appears to be searching for a word. Phonemic cues often help the patient retrieve the word during a pause in speech. Repetition is intact, even for long phrases. The patient's comprehension is intact. Able to follow three-step commands without difficulty. Reading is intact. Writing is intact. Naming is impaired.

- Suggests an *anomic aphasia*. Can be associated with residual deficit from a previous left hemisphere stroke that had resulted in more extensive aphasia syndrome. Acute anomia associated with small inferior temporal or angular gyrus dysfunction of dominant (left) hemisphere. However, is also frequently found among patients with neurodegenerative disorders with more diffuse brain dysfunction, such as Alzheimer's disease, fronto-temporal dementia, and Parkinson's disease dementia. Damasio et al. (1996) found anterior temporal tip most associated in naming famous faces/people. The inferior temporal lobe was most strongly associated with inferior temporal lobe, while tool naming was associated with left posterior lateral temporal lobe.

Rule of thumb: Fluent speech problems

Speech is rapid and effortless, but speech will not make sense with paraphasias and neologisms.

- Wernicke's aphasia: fluent speech that does not make sense. Repetition impaired. Comprehension impaired. Reading impaired. Writing impaired.
- Transcortical sensory aphasia: fluent speech that does not make sense. Comprehension impaired. Repetition intact. Reading is impaired. Writing somewhat impaired.
- Conduction aphasia: fluent speech that makes some sense, but frequent phonemic paraphasias and some neologisms decrease intelligibility. Repetition impaired. Comprehension intact. Reading comprehension intact. Writing impaired.
- Anomic aphasia: Speech effortful with pauses and some paraphasias. Repetition intact. Comprehension intact. Reading intact. Writing intact.

Other Types of Speech/Language Problems

1. The patient's speech is generally fluent and intelligible. Some paraphasias or pauses in speech is present. Repetition is intact, even for long phrases. Comprehension is intact. Able to follow three-step commands. Reading is markedly impaired (alexia). Writing is impaired (agraphia). Naming is frequently reduced, but no frank impairment.
   - Suggests an *alexia with agraphia.* Commonly associated with discrete lesion of the left (dominant) temporo-parietal angular gyrus or underlying white matter.
2. The patient's speech is generally fluent and intelligible. Some paraphasias or pauses in speech may be present or may not be. Repetition is intact, even for long phrases. Comprehension is intact. Able to follow three-step commands. Reading is markedly impaired (alexia). Writing is intact. Naming is generally intact.
   - Suggests *alexia without agraphia.* Classically associated with discrete lesion of the dominant (left) hemisphere involving the white matter of the posterior corpus collosum which underlies the occipital lobe. Can also be associated with discrete lesion involving the posterior dominant (left) inferior temporal gyrus.
3. The patient is unable to speak or speech is effortful with few words. Speech articulation can be poor or the patient may sound as if he/she is speaking with an unusual accent. Repetition is intact, even for long phrases. Comprehension is intact. Able to follow three-step commands. Reading is intact. Writing is intact. Naming is poor, but patient able to accurately write out objects. This condition may be acquired or it maybe present since early development.
   - Suggests *aphemia* (verbal apraxia in childhood). Commonly associated with discrete lesion of the dominant (left) frontal lobe affecting precentral gyrus involving primary motor and premotor areas.
4. The patient's speech articulation is poor. Speech may sound as if the patient is mumbling, slurring, and/or has "marbles in his/her mouth." Speech rate is often slowed and may have a labored aspect. Paraphasias can be present. Repetition is intact. Comprehension is intact. Able to follow three-step commands. Reading is intact. Writing is intact (however, writing size may be very small in some cases). Naming is reduced secondary to poor articulation or slurring and/or mumbling.
   - Suggests speech *dysarthria.* May be due to Parkinson's disease but also found following lesions to the corticobulbar tracts, including brain stem lesions.
5. The patient's speech is fluent and articulate. Comprehension is impaired for words presented orally (can repeat written words and sentences). Repetition is impaired for materials presented orally (but can repeat written words and sentences). Reading is intact. Writing is intact. Naming is intact. The patient is unable to respond appropriately to other sounds (appears deaf).
   - Suggests *cortical deafness.* Classically associated with bilateral lesions to Heschl's gyrus.

6. The patient's speech is fluent and articulate. Comprehension is impaired for words presented orally (can repeat written words and sentences). Repetition is impaired for materials presented orally (but can repeat written words and sentences). Reading is intact. Writing is intact. Naming is intact. The patient is able to respond appropriately to other sounds (does not appear deaf to other sounds).
   • Suggests *pure word deafness* (also known as *verbal auditory agnosia*). Classically associated with discrete lesion of the dominant (left) temporal lobe Heschl's gyrus that extends to the underlying white matter to prevent input from the contralateral hemisphere primary auditory cortex.

7. The patient's speech is fluent and articulate. Comprehension is intact. Repetition is intact. Reading is intact. Writing is intact. Naming is intact. The patient is unable to respond appropriately to other sounds (appears deaf to sounds, except for spoken words).
   • Suggests *nonverbal auditory agnosia*. Rare, but classically associated with discrete lesion of the nondominant (right) Heschl's gyrus. Recovery is often complete in days to weeks.

Prosodic Speech Problems

In general, the description below describes patients' with intact basic speech. That is, the patient can both follow directions and speech is articulate and reasonably fluent. The deficits in language may only be appreciated with an examiner's appreciation of a speaker's monotone by careful evaluation for prosody, intonation, and inflection. The patient's speech may be monotone voice (almost robotic in quality), and with careful assessment for difficulties in appreciating the nonverbal aspects of speech (prosody, intonation, inflection).

1. The patient is unable to appreciate or express mood in speech. While speech production and comprehension is generally intact, the patient's speech output is monotone. Repetition for prosodic inflection is impaired. Able to follow three-step commands. Reading, writing, and naming are intact.
   • Suggests a *global aprosody*. Commonly associated with large lesion involving the right (nondominant) hemisphere.
2. Receptive prosodic deficits. Inflection and tonal quality of emotions can be expressed. However, the patient is unable to appreciate tonal inflections in speech. Repetition for prosodic inflection may be impaired.
   • Suggests *receptive aprosody*. Classically associated with lesion of the nondominant (right) hemisphere involving the temporoparietal area and/or underlying white matter.
3. Expressive prosodic deficits. Inflection and tonal quality of emotions cannot be expressed. Speech is likely to sound monotone (although rate can vary).

Repetition for prosodic inflection and intonation may be impaired. The patient is able to appreciate prosodic inflection and intonation of other's speech.

a. Suggests an *expressive aprosody*. Commonly associated with lesion of the nondominant frontal region homologous to the left hemisphere Broca's area, including underlying white matter.

Bedside Assessment of Language

For most clinical evaluations, language assessment serves two functions – first as a screening for language impairment and secondly as an assessment of prerequisite skills necessary for language-dependent aspects of the remainder of the neuropsychological examination. Language assessment should be conducted systematically to evaluate for deficits in receptive (comprehension and reading), expressive (speech output and writing), repetition, and naming. In addition, careful observation of word finding deficits, semantic or phonemic paraphasic errors and articulation difficulties should be noted. The quality of language organization and completeness of responses in reciprocal conversation should be evaluated relative to common expectations or in conjunction with collateral confirmation of a change. We have included a bedside-based screening form for the assessment of language in Appendix A.

The brief assessment below begins with receptive language in both auditory and written modalities. Auditory comprehension starts initially with simple yes/no questions and progresses to more complex yes/no questions and multi-step commands in congruent sequence and reversed sequence. Note that comprehension

---

Rule of thumb: Language assessment

Language assessment should include
- – Expressive skills
  - • Fluency
  - • Articulation
  - • Organization
  - • Writing
- – Receptive skills
  - • Naming
  - • Aural comprehension
  - • Reading
- – Repetition
- – Prosody
  - • Expressive prosody
  - • Receptive prosody

need *not* be illustrated by the patient speaking or writing. Indeed, questions should be posed such that responses can be elicited by movement of eyes, eye blink, etc. among patients who have expressive language or motor paresis. Basic comprehension testing may then be followed by increasingly more complex receptive language skills involving both auditory and reading skill. Questions such as "Is my hair on fire?," "Do airplanes eat their young?" and "Does two pounds of sugar weigh more than one pound of sugar?" are sensitive to mild deficits in comprehension. This gives us a brief understanding of comprehension in both auditory and written modalities, which is essential in managing patient care. Additionally, receptive prosody is assessed by making statements emphasizing different emotions which use the exact same words. Patients should be able to identify the emotional tone implied in the way the phrase was spoken with little difficulty as long as they are presented in exaggerated fashion by the examiner. When assessing for prosody, the examiner may wish to have the patient close his/her eyes and/or turn from the patient to prevent the examiner from providing visual cues as to the emotional content of the prosody stimulus if the examiner accidently exhibits a facial expression along with the auditory stimuli.

Expressive language is subsequently assessed by asking the patient to name objects of increasing detail from general objects such as a shirt to parts like sleeve, cuff or collar. While patients are often able to name whole objects (pen), requesting them to name parts of objects (clip) often elicits naming deficits which might otherwise go undetected. Additionally, patients are asked to repeat words and phrases of increasing complexity to assess repetition which may be impaired independently from both receptive and expressive language functions. Expressive prosody is assessed by asking patients to make statements as if they were mad, happy or sad.

Lastly, language should be assessed for organizational quality and discourse. Any suspected tangentiality, circumloquaciousness, or halting or incomplete expression patterns should be noted. This is typically done by providing stimuli such as a picture or scenario and asking an open ended question requiring the patient to organize and structure a response that is reasonably complete. Note should be taken to describe the quality of organization, completeness of the response and the patient's ability to both expect and respect reciprocal conventions in communication such that a conversation occurs naturally and speech is not pressured in a way that might belie great effort in getting words out before they are lost.

Psychometric Based Assessment of Language

Many excellent comprehensive batteries are available for the assessment of language such as the Boston Diagnostic Aphasia Examination – 3 (Goodglass et al., 2000), Neurosensory Center Comprehensive Examination for Aphasia (Spreen and Strauss, 1991), Multilingual Aphasia Examination (Benton and Hamsher, 1989), and the Western Aphasia Battery (Kertesz, 1982) (see Strauss et al., 2006 or Lezak et al.,

2004, for detailed review and description of these and other language tests.) These batteries examine aspects of language in greater depth than conventional bedside clinical evaluations, and offer a more comprehensive quantification and description of language deficits.

In general, the advantage of detailed neuropsychological assessment of language functions allows for quantification of language function in terms of performance compared to population normative data, which may be expressed in terms of percentiles. Such a detailed assessment allows for the identification of subtle expressive and/or receptive language deficits that may not be appreciated in a bedside assessment. We recommend an outpatient neuropsychological evaluation to assess expressive and receptive speech along with repetition and naming. Common measures of expressive speech include carefully listening to the patient describe his/her problems or history, and various oral or written verbal fluency tests. Typical measures include phonemic verbal fluency and semantic verbal fluency tests. Naming is commonly assessed with visual or auditory confrontation naming tests. Comprehension can be assessed with measures assessing increasing complex directions. See Chap. 12 this volume and Heilman and Valenstein, 2003; Lezak et al., 2004; Mesulam, 2000; and/or Strauss et al. 2006 for detailed reviews.

References

Benton, A. L., & Hamsher, K. (1989). *Multilingual aphasia examination*. Iowa City: AJA Associates.

Cermack, L. (2000). *Language and the brain: Representation and processing*. New York: Academic.

Damasio, H., Grabowski, T. J., Tranel, D., Hichwa, R. D., & Damasio, A. R. (1996). A neural basis for lexical retrieval. *Nature, 380*, 499–505.

Goodglass, H., Kaplan, E., & Barresi, B. (2000). *The Boston diagnostic aphasia examination (BDAE-3)* (3rd ed.). Philadelphia: Lippincott Williams & Wilkins.

Heilman, K. M., & Valenstein, E. (2003). *Clinical neuropsychology* (4th ed.). New York: Oxford University Press.

Kertesz, A. (1982). *Western aphasia battery*. San Antonio: Psychological Corporation.

Kolb, B., & Whishaw, I. (2009). *Fundamentals of human neuropsychology* (6th ed.). New York: W.H. Freeman press.

Lezak, M. D., Howieson, D. B., & Loring, D. W. (2004). *Neuropsychological assessment* (4th ed.). New York: Oxford University Press.

Mesulam, M. M. (2000). *Principles of behavioral and cognitive neurology* (2nd ed.). New York: Oxford University Press.

Ross, E. D. (1997). The aprosodies. In T. E. Feinberg & M. J. Farah (Eds.), *Behavioral neurology and neuropsychology* (pp. 699–717). New York: McGraw-Hill.

Spreen, O., & Straus, E. (1991). *A compendium of neuropsychological tests: Administration, norms, and commentary*. New York: Oxford University Press.

Straus, E., Sherman, E. M. S., & Spreen, O. (2006). *A compendium of neuropsychological tests: Administration, norms, and commentary* (3rd ed.). New York: Oxford University Press.

Appendix A

Acute Assessment of Language and Prosody

Receptive language and prosody	Response	Correct
Simple receptive language		
Simple Yes/No question		
Is it winter?	_____	_____
Are you in a hospital?	_____	_____
Complex Yes/No question		
Are cows carnivorous?	_____	_____
Would a nice person express complements?	_____	_____

Receptive comprehension of commands

Simple
  one Step
  Point to the door _____ _____
  two Step
  Look up and then look down _____ _____

Complex
  Sequenced
  Touch your arm and then touch your ear _____ _____
  Reversed
  Point to the door after you point to the chair _____ _____

Reading (Read and/or comply)

I feel good today	_____	_____
Point to each person in the room	_____	_____

Prosody

Simple Prosody (statement or question)
  I'm going to town! (spoken as a statement) _____ _____
  I'm going to town? (spoken as a question) _____ _____
Emotional Prosody (expressed emotion)
  That is wrong. (Spoken Angrily) _____ _____
  That is wrong. (Spoken sadly) _____ _____
  That is wrong. (Spoken happily) _____ _____

Expressive language and prosody

Naming
    Simple objects
        What is this? (Point to shirt)   _____   _____
        What is this? (Point to pen)   _____   _____
    Complex naming
        What is this? (Point to sleeve or cuff of shirt)   _____   _____
        What is this? (Point to point or tip of pen)   _____   _____

Repetition
    Single word
        Desk, chair, light   _____   _____
    Simple Statement
        I would like some ice cream   _____   _____
    Complex Statement
        No ifs, ands or buts   _____   _____

Writing
    Simple
        Write his/her name   _____   _____
        Write name of watch   _____   _____
        Write a sentence   _____   _____

Verbal Fluency (60 seconds, record number)
        Phonemic fluency (ie. words beginning with the letter r)   _____   _____
        Semantic fluency (ie. Animals)   _____   _____

Expressive Prosody
        Say, "I'm going to work."
        Phrase as if sad   _____   _____
        Phrase as if angry   _____   _____

Discourse/spontaneous expressive speech
Structured
        Show a picture; ask patient to describe what is happening   _____   _____
Unstructured
        Ask patient what he/she did/does
        for work and give the details.   _____   _____

Chapter 8
Memory and Learning: The Forgetful Patient

James G. Scott and Mike R. Schoenberg

Abstract The capacity to encode, retain and retrieve information is essential to the evolution of all living animals. From the ameba to ourselves, learning from interaction with our environment is critical to adaptation to the stimuli that influence our well being. The human brain is masterful at recognizing patterns of recurrence, be they sensory, motor or cognitive. This process of pattern recognition produces engrams which are the building blocks of concepts and organization which facilitate retrieval. Through this chapter, we will discuss models of processing and outline the essential elements for memory. We will discuss the anatomical correlates of memory and discuss how damage to many parts of the brain can have a direct or secondary effect on memory functioning. Several syndromic patterns of memory loss are reviewed below and recommendations given regarding possible etiologies for these observed memory scores. The factors which influence memory including encoding, storage and retrieval will be addressed. Finally, in this chapter we will discuss how to perform an assessment of memory functions which will allow the clinician to determine if problems in memory are present and if more detailed assessment of memory functions is indicated. Additional detailed information regarding the impact that different etiologies can have on memory functioning are discussed throughout this text.

As with many cognitive functions beyond the basic sensory, perceptual and motor systems, memory is dependent on prerequisite skills for accurate assessment and determination of the etiology of a deficit. Accurate assessment of memory hinges on the adequacy of sensory input, perceptual skill, motor output and attentional capacity. Factors which influence these prerequisite skills can produce a profound impact on memory. In addition, some internal cognitive aspects of functioning such as reasoning and organization produce secondary effects on measured memory skills. In addition to these factors, assessment of memory must consider the emotional functioning of the person being assessed. Severe psychopathology such as schizophrenia or bipolar disorder can have an obvious and profound effect on memory; however,

J.G. Scott (✉)
Department of Psychiatry and Behavioral Sciences, University of Oklahoma
Health Sciences Center, Oklahoma City, OK, USA
e-mail: jim-scott@ouhsc.edu

M.R. Schoenberg and J.G. Scott (eds.), *The Little Black Book of Neuropsychology:*
A Syndrome-Based Approach, DOI 10.1007/978-0-387-76978-3_8,
© Springer Science+Business Media, LLC 2011

even mild depression and situational anxiety can produce subtle but predictable effects on memory performance which may be detrimental or enhancing.

Key Points and Chapter Summary

- Memory includes encoding, storage and retrieval and memory deficits can be caused by impairment at any level in the process
- Intact sensory, motor, arousal and attentional skills are prerequisite for memory assessment
- Memory capacities change considerably with ageing and assessment must consider age in evaluating performance to improve accuracy in detecting deficits or change
- There are many individual- (i.e., age, education), anatomical- (i.e., Temporal, Frontal, Somatosensory) and material (i.e., Verbal, Visual)-specific factors that affect memory performance and these vary across individuals and etiology
- Memory assessment should include evaluation of recent memory and remote memory as the pattern of memory impairment is related to the anatomy and etiology of impairment

---

A Model of Memory

The act of turning an experience into a memory appears simple at first glance, but involves a complicated series of processes, which are dependent on the integrity of many brain functions. While there are several models, common themes include three stages involving encoding, storage and retrieval. The process by which information is transferred from encoding to storage depends on the nature of the material which is to be recalled. There are three basic memory stages: sensory storage, short-term memory, and long-term memory. Each has been subdivided into more refined aspects of memory systems, and briefly reviewed below.

Rule of thumb: General memory functioning

- Memory processes can be divided into Encoding, Recall and Recognition Phases
- Recognition should almost always be better than encoding and recall unless motivational factors are responsible
- The number of repetitions in learning trials (overlearning) improves recall for almost all people, but does not facilitate delayed recall in persons with neurologic memory impairment
- Memory impairment typically is either from a discrete injury point forward or a gradual decline from a past point. Even in neurologic conditions, remote memory is almost always better than recent memory.
- Except for the immediate period of trauma or injury, memory impairment rarely if ever is for a discrete point of time.

Sensory Storage (Sensory Registration)

The first stage of memory is typically referred to as the sensory storage or sensory registration stage. It refers to the point of time that auditory, visual, gustatory, tactile or olfactory information is initially registered as a conscious phenomenon. This stage of memory is very short in duration, lasting milliseconds to seconds, and decays rapidly if no further attending to the stimuli is done. The information in sensory storage must be attended to before being transferred to short-term memory.

Short-Term Memory

Short-term memory is frequently referred to as working memory. The average capacity of short-term memory in humans is typically seven items ±2. This capacity can easily be expanded through superimposing organization such as chunking. For example, the letters in the 4×4 array below can be recalled much more easily if organized thus turning 16 individual items into 6 items (Fig. 8.1). The array of letters on the left may appear as 16 individual bits of information and difficult to memorize while the array on the right has been altered to facilitate semantic clustering thus the number of items to be recalled is reduced to 7. Without imposing some process such as organizing or rehearsal, information in short-term memory is quickly forgotten.

Fig. 8.1 Facilitation of memory by chunking

A B C I	A B
A F B I	CIA
N O W S	*FBI*
P C A I	N O W
	SPCA
	I

Long-Term Memory

Long-term memory refers to information which is relatively permanent and can be retrieved volitionally. Several processes facilitate the consolidation of information into long-term memory. The simple act of rehearsal facilitates transfer to long-term memory, but the emotional strength of the material also facilitates consolidation. Material which is associated with emotional experiences (positive or negative) is more easily encoded and facilitates retrieval. The level at which information is processed makes encoding information more efficient. For example, retrieval of words is facilitated when individuals are asked if the words describe themselves compared to being asked if the word was a positive or negative characteristic. Elaborating the material to be learned also associates it with previously acquired information and again facilitates transfer to long-term memory. Yet other processes can affect memory consolidation, including state and environmental learning. State-depending learning reflects improved learning and recall when the emotional and physical state of the individual are congruent. Additionally, the saliency of the material to be recalled influence encoding and retrieval. For example, material which is learned in one physical environment is recalled much better in the same environment or a highly similar environment. This phenomenon is appreciated when examining the discrepancy when recalling high school events while at your old high school (i.e., names, events, faces) compared to recall of the same material while at home. Similarly, the state (i.e., physical state such as inebriation or emotional state such as sadness) facilitates recall of information encoded while in such states.

The graph below demonstrates the stages of memory and processes by which information is transferred from one stage to another and notes some of the factors which impact consolidation of information into long-term memories (Fig. 8.2).

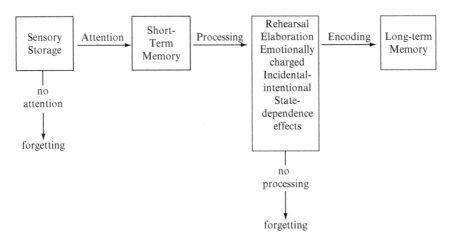

Fig. 8.2 Stages of memory

Types of Memory

Many types of memory have been described (for example, see Kolb and Whishaw 2009; Squire and Zola 1996, for reviews), but heuristically two predominant types of memory, each having unique associated anatomical and phenomenological characteristics, have remained robust. These memory types are referred to as *Declarative* (or *Explicit*) memory and *Non-declarative* (or *Implicit*) memory. While these types of memory have been given various names (see Table 8.1, common terms for Declarative and Nondeclarative memory), the characteristics of each have been well established.

Table 8.1 Common terms for declarative and nondeclarative memory (Adapted from Squire, 1987)

Declarative memory	Nondeclarative memory
Who, What, When, Where Memory	Classical Conditioning
Conscious Memory	How Memory
Visual Memory[a]	Motor Memory
Verbal Memory[a]	Automatic Memory
Explicit Memory	Subconscious Memory
Autobiographical Memory[b]	Perceptual Memory
Episodic Memory[c]	Habit Memory
Semantic Memory[c]	Procedural Memory
Prospective Memory	

[a]Terms describe components of declarative memory often seen in neuropsychological reports
[b]Autobiographical memory is a term to describe components of Episodic memory
[c]Episodic and Semantic memory are two major divisions of Declarative (Explicit) memory

Declarative (Explicit) Memory

Declarative memory refers to those things which we recall including, people, names, faces, events, facts and places, etc. This type of memory is also termed Explicit memory, and the two terms (declarative and explicit are often used interchangeably). Declarative (or explicit) memory is divided into *Episodic memory* and *Semantic memory* (Squire and Zola 1996).

- *Episodic memory* is an autobiographical memory, and recalls the personal events and facts which are bound in time and place. This is the memory for what you did yesterday, where you went on your first date, or your first car.
- *Semantic memory* is composed of facts and knowledge. This type of memory is not time dependent. Semantic memory is knowing which city is the capital of the USA, the multiplication tables, how many dimes make a dollar, or which countries border France.

Episodic memory is the active recall of the learning event, while semantic memory recall is retrieval of a fact, and does not require one to recall the autobiographical event when the material was learned. Semantic memory is unable to determine a particular place and time the information was learned. The unique aspects of this remembered material is the conscious effort involved in the learning and retrieval process. This is the conscious material that can be recalled which is unique to the experiences of the individual. Declarative memory is frequently divided into categories, such as verbal–visual, intentional–incidental, recent–remote, etc. Declarative memory is the type of memory which we most commonly refer to when discussing memory in a clinical setting. And it is episodic memory which is of particular emphasis in neuropsychological assessments. Episodic memory is also frequently disrupted by injury or diseases such as anoxia, traumatic brain injury and Alzheimer's. The anatomical disassociation will be outlined later in this chapter.

Nondeclarative (Implicit) Memory

Nondeclarative memory refers to memory for skills and procedures which are learned and recalled. Evidence for such a memory system is found by the efficiency and skill gains which accumulate for even complex activities. The origins of the learning process are often lost such as learning to speak or riding a bicycle, but the transfer of learning must occur for such behaviors to be demonstrated and recalled. Nondeclarative memory includes a number of acquired motor skills, but also includes a great number of very complex behaviors such as playing a musical instrument or driving a car. The adaptation of humans to perform repetitive skills with precision and very little conscious processing is astounding. This memory system is often preserved in injury and disease states.

    The next section provides an overview of common terms used to describe memory problems followed by a brief review of neuroanatomical correlates of memory.

Terms of Memory Impairment

The loss of memory is called *amnesia*. Classically, amnesia describes the loss of memory while other neuropsychological functions remain intact. The individual exhibits a profound inability to learn new material, in which declarative memory functions are largely lost. Alternatively, non-declarative (implicit) memory is often preserved. Individuals may have anterograde amnesia and/or retrograde amnesia.

Anterograde Amnesia

Anterograde amnesia describes the inability to encode new material since the event onset or injury. With pure anterograde amnesia, the individual is able to recall previous events, up to very close to the time of the event leading to anterograde amnesia (see below for common causes of anterograde amnesia).

Retrograde Amnesia

Retrograde amnesia refers to loss of memory for events that occurred prior to the event leading to an amnesia syndrome. The most common is an inability to recall immediate previous information from before the event. Retrograde amnesia is frequently temporally graded, such that memories immediately before the event leading to amnesia are markedly poor while memories farther removed from the event (moving increasingly early in recent experience) may be better recalled.

Typical Patterns of Memory Loss

A typical pattern for amnesia is for anterograde to predominate while retrograde amnesia is temporally graded by hours, days, weeks, months, or rarely years. The extent of retrograde amnesia is often dependent upon the extent of damage. Anterograde amnesia may be temporally limited, that is recovery of normal memory functions after a period of hours, days, weeks, or rarely months to years. Alternatively, some conditions can result in a permanent amnestic syndrome involving anterograde amnesia and usually some retrograde amnesia. Cases of predominate retrograde amnesia with preserved anterograde amnesia are very rare, but have been reported. However, the loss of memory is typically not relegated to one aspect of one's life (e.g., remembering starting a new job and meeting new friends, but forgetting you got married or had children during this time frame).

Neuropsychological assessment includes assessment of various components of (mostly) declarative memory, but some aspects may also assess nondeclarative memory function. Common terms to describe domains of memory that may be impaired within a neuropsychological evaluation include: recent memory, remote memory, long-term memory, short-term (immediate) memory, working memory, and semantic memory. An overview of what these terms measure is provided below.

Memory Terms: A Brief Review

Delayed recall (recall of a previously exposed material after some period of delay, typically less than 1 hour)
Delayed recognition (refers to recognition of stimuli previously presented).
Learning over trials (*LOT*) describes successive performance of immediate recall of material presented over successive trials.
Recent memory is a term to describe memory for events that occurred within the past few days; however, there is disagreement as to the demarcation of recent and remote memory
Remote memory describes memory for events that occurred before the present. Traditionally, this term may be used to describe the memory of events or experiences of

an individual in the distant past; however, as noted above, the demarcation regarding how far in the past is a matter of debate.

Long-term memory in neuropsychological reports refers to memory scores obtained after a delay of usually 30–40 minutes. Performance after a 30-minute delay is highly correlated with memory function after days to weeks, although some temporal forgetting or decay does occur.

Short-term memory describes memory scores obtained usually after a proceeding recall trial.

Immediate memory refers to recall of material immediately after presentation. Material to be learned must exceed attention span. The material to be learned may be either verbal or visual (nonverbal).

Working memory is a term to describe immediately processed information before it is sent to short term memory.

Encoding refers to the process of learning material.

Consolidation refers to the process of transferring information from immediate (short-term memory) to long-term memory.

Retrieval refers to the process of retrieving information from long-term memory; that is, conscious recollection.

Primacy effect refers to the observation of recalling the first part of to be learned material. May reflect learning the first initial items in word list or the first part of a verbal story or the first series of pictures or presented figures in a series of to be learned material.

Recency effect refers to the enhanced recall of the last part (most recent) of to be learned items. The recency effect is easily observed in learning a list of words or a short story with the recall of the last part of a list of words (the last set of words, commonly the last 3–5 words presented in a list of words) or the last part of a story that was presented.

Verbal Semantic Memory (also termed *Verbal Contextual memory*) describes memory for short stories that are typically auditorily administered (read out loud). There are typically immediate and delayed recall trials.

List Learning refers to immediate and delayed recall for a rote memorization of a word list. The word list may have words that are part of several semantic clusters (e.g., furniture, animals, things you can do at a beach, etc.), or the list may have words unrelated to each other.

Visual Memory (also termed *NonVerbal memory*) describes memory for nonverbal material developed to avoid being easily verbally encoded such as faces, geometric figures, or spatial locations. Visual memory typically includes immediate memory and delayed recall of nonverbal material.

Neuropsychological Assessment of Memory Problems

Evaluation of memory processes must include assessment of (1) learning, (2) immediate memory, (3) delayed memory, and (4) recognition formats. Evaluating the difference between immediate memory trials and delayed memory provides an index of the efficiency of consolidation (or retention). Including recognition format after delayed recall allows for assessment of retrieval deficits accounting for poor memory. Relatively preserved recognition (true hits without false positives) in the presence of deficient spontaneous recall implicates faulty retrieval processes with intact encoding.

Memory Deficits/Complaints: A behavioral Guide

While the performance of individuals suspected of memory loss can reflect numerous patterns of performance, several common patterns of memory deficits are listed below, along with some possible hypotheses that may account for these observations.

1. Very poor encoding, delayed recall and recognition: Patient's learning is deficient with a flat learning curve. No gain in memory with repeated presentation of the to be learned material. Frequent perseverations and/or intrusions. Immediate memory and delayed recall are deficient, and recognition cues do not improve recall (false positive hits and some false negative hits). This is common in diseases which impair encoding and consolidation such as bilateral frontal lobe lesions affecting orbitofrontal and medial frontal structures, medial diencephalic lesions or bilateral mesial temporal damage found in patients with severe traumatic brain injuries or severe Alzheimer's disease.
2. Poor encoding, severe delayed recall impairment and mildly impaired recognition: Patient's immediate learning is deficient, but some learning may be present (learning curve not flat). Immediate memory is mildly impaired. Delayed memory is markedly deficient. Recognition is impaired although better than recall. This pattern is highly suggestive of deficits in consolidation and rapid forgetting and is classically observed in initial stages of dementia of the Alzheimer's type and bilateral mesial temporal dysfunction.
3. Normal encoding, poor recall, and good recognition: Patient's initial learning is normal or nearly normal. Delayed memory is deficient. Recognition is normal. This pattern is highly suggestive of deficits in retrieval and is classically observed in sub-cortical or vascular dementias.
4. Variable encoding, variable recall and good recognition: Patient's learning is variable across trials and may be mildly impaired overall. Immediate memory is variable. Perseverative responses and intrusions may occur. Delayed memory recall is variable and often similar to immediate recall score (no forgetting). Recognition is improved with cues, but patient may exhibit confabulation and/or make high number of false positive errors from any material previously presented to him/her (i.e., interference). Memory of semantically organized information (e.g., stories that make sense) better recalled than word lists of unrelated material. Reflects inefficient encoding with intact consolidation. Common in dementias affecting frontal lobes or etiologies affecting attentions such as traumatic brain injuries.
5. Normal encoding, Normal recall, Impaired Recognition: Patient's learning is normal or nearly normal learning with normal or nearly normal delayed memory

recall, but marked and disproportionately deficient recognition. This pattern is irregular and may reflect inattention and/or variable motivation. Non-neurological memory impairment.

6. Material-specific encoding discrepancy, Material-specific recall discrepancy, and Material-specific recognition discrepancy: Patient exhibits learning that is normal or nearly normal for one type of material but deficient for another type of material (e.g., verbal memory is impaired while recall of visual, "nonverbal" learning is normal or nearly normal). Consolidation and retrieval 'lateralized'. Commonly found in lateralized neurological lesions such as focal epilepsy and/ or focal strokes resulting in unilateral mesial temporal lobe or, less often, thalamic or frontal lobe lesion.

7. Poor initial encoding with appropriate improvement across repeated trials, Variable recall and Normal Recognition: Patient's learning slow and/or variable (patient may recall more and then less material with repeated learning trials). Immediate recall mildly impaired. Patient frequently says "I don't know." Delayed recall is variable or mildly impaired and may not differ substantially from immediate delayed memory. Recognition memory is normal. No false positive errors, but false negative error bias may occur (i.e., "I don't know"). This pattern can be seen among individuals with severe depression or anxiety.

Learning Curve Patterns

Below, we provide a brief review of some common patterns to learning. This is particularly true for tests of verbal memory using a word list that is presented multiple times. Normal recall patterns in a word list learning test include improved recall for both the first words and last words in a list. Recall of words in the first third of the list is called the Primacy Effect while recall of the words in the last third of a list is referred to as the Recency Effect. Normal performance in a list learning test is to recall a greater percentage from the Primacy and Recency regions of a list on initial trials with gradual inclusion or recall of the middle third of the list on subsequent repeated recall trials. While deviations from this pattern can be produced by the patient deciding to apply different strategies, deviation from this pattern can indicate important information regarding memory processes. Retention of only the primacy or recency region with little improvement across repeated trials is typically indicative of a primary amnestic disorder. Inclusion of words from both the primacy and recency regions with additional improvement across trials from words in the middle region is a normal memory pattern. Recall of words randomly from all regions (an absence of Primacy or Recency effects) is typically associated with secondary factors that affect learning efficiency such as frontal lobe deficits or attentional deficits or may indicate poor motivation or effort.

As can be seen above, a systematic evaluation of memory processes can help to reveal the mechanisms responsible for observed deficits in memory complaints and can be crucial in the differential diagnosis of syndromes associated with amnesia.

Anatomy of Memory

Multiple brain regions are involved in the functioning or process of memory. We previously noted the prerequisite skills of arousal, sensory, motor or perceptual integrity, and attentional capacity which are necessary components for efficient encoding of information or transfer of stimuli from one stage of memory to another (for declarative memory functions). Assuming that these prerequisite functions are intact, areas that are involved in memory include the medial temporal lobes, entorhinal cortex, hippocampus and amygdala, cingulate cortex, basal forebrain, and diencephalic structures (see Fig. 8.3 and Chap. 3). Classically, there are two well-described circuits underlying memory functions: Papez circuit and the amygdaloid circuit.

The Papez circuit is involved in forming new autobiographical memories, and in declarative (explicit) memories in general. Figure 8.3 illustrates the basic projection path of the Papez circuit, which makes a functional loop. Input from multimodal association cortex of the brain (frontal, parietal, occipital, and temporal lobes) flows to perirhinal and parahippocampal cortices and is relayed to the entorhinal cortex. The entorhinal cortex is the primary input (and an important output) pathway of the hippocampal formation, with projections to the dentate gyrus and hippocampus. Projections from hippocampus structures from the subiculum form the fornix which projects to the mammilary bodies. Output fibers from the mammilary bodies (the mammillothalamic tract) go to the anterior thalamic nuclei, then project to the cingulate gyrus. The cingulate gyrus projects back to parahippocampal gyrus and entorhinal cortex via the cingulum (or cingulate bundle) completing the loop.

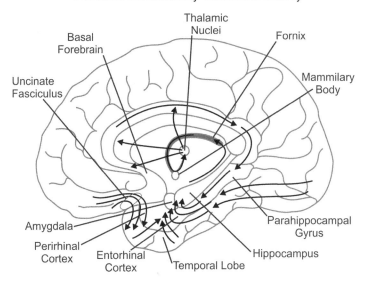

Functional Neuroanatomy- Declarative Memory

Fig. 8.3 Neuroanatomy of memory figure

The amygdaloid circuit includes the amygdala, thalamic nuclei (mediodorsal or pulvinar), orbitofrontal cortex, olfactory piriform cortex, insula (gustatory and somatosensory information), hypothalamus, limbic striatum and nucleus basalis of meynert. Another important output pathway of the hippocampus and dentate gyrus is the projections from the subiculum back to the entorhinal cortex where projections to parahippocampal association cortex and other multimodal association cortex of the frontal, parietal, occipital and temporal areas occur. Figure 8.3 illustrates potential input pathways from frontal (uncinate and anterior cingulate), parietal, occipital, and temporal cortex. The uncinate fasciculus connects the amygdala with the orbital frontal and cingulate cortices.

The diencephalic structures implicated in memory include thalamic nuclei (anterior, dorsomedial, laterodorsal, pulvinar and other intralaminar), fornix, and mammilary bodies (hypothalamus). The cerebellum has also demonstrated roles in memory, particularly for nondeclarative memory functions. These neuroanatomic structures have connections to and from temporal and frontal areas such that damage to diencephalic structures can profoundly affect memory (see Chap. 3).

Temporal Lobe and Memory

While many other brain structures have been implicated in the formation of memories, no other brain structure has demonstrated the importance in memory function compared to the temporal lobes. Specifically, the anterior temporal cortex and underlying structures of the hippocampus, parahippocampal gyrus, and entorhinal cortex are critically involved in the formation of new memories. This relationship has been repeatedly demonstrated using animals and patient populations (i.e., epilepsy, tumor patients and accident victims). Critical cortical areas in the temporal lobe include the entorhinal cortex which resides in the anterior, medial and inferior aspect of the temporal lobe. The temporal lobe has many afferent and efferent projections to somatosensory cortex (i.e., sight, hearing, tactile, etc.). The hippocampus and its subsections (entorhinal cortex) are the primary areas implicated in amnestic disorders such as Alzheimer's disease or anoxia. The amygdala lies in the anterior aspect of the hippocampus. The amygdala plays a significant role in the impact of emotion on memory encoding as well as retrieval.

Diencephalon and Memory

In addition to the prominent role of the temporal lobes and underlying structures in the formation of memories, several diencephalic (medial subcortical) structures play significant roles in memory formation. The predominant structures in the diencephalon are the thalamus and hypothalamus. The supporting evidence for involvement of these structures in memory comes from the study of patients with discrete lesions in these areas which produce profound amnesic conditions. The debate continues as to the extent and permanence of damage necessary in the anterior nucleus of the thalamus, the mediodorsal (MD) nuclei of the thalamus and mammilary bodies to produce such amnestic conditions. Recent research suggest it is the degeneration of the anterior nucleus of the thalamus that is necessary and sufficient for onset of the amnestic syndrome seen in Korsakoff's syndrome.

Frontal Lobes and Basal Forebrain and Memory

The role of the frontal lobes and basal forebrain in the formation of memories is extended from the finding of memory impairment in dementia and stroke patients that involve the frontal lobes and/or parts of the basal forebrain. Frontal lobe areas affecting memory can include the orbitolateral (ventral) frontal lobe, medial frontal, and some memory dysfunction associated with dorsolateral frontal lobe damage (see Chaps. 3 and 13). The basal forebrain describes the septal nuclei, nucleus basalis of Meynert, substantia innominata, and the amygdala. In conditions such as anterior communicating artery aneurysms ruptures or Alzheimer's disease, extensive damage to acetylcholine-producing regions such as nucleus accumbens and septal nucleus that then project to basal forebrain are damaged and can produce profound effects on memory. The issue of whether it is damage specifically to these areas or the secondary loss of acetylcholine production in these areas that is the primary reason for the amnestic effect remains to be settled (see Kandel 2007, for review).

Laterality and Memory

Evidence for the lateralized effect of memory comes primarily from studies of accident victims and neurosurgery patients (most specifically unilateral temporal lobectomy). Evaluation of these individuals' memory functioning indicates a significant, although far from perfect, lateralizing effect where memory for stories, words and numbers is most commonly disrupted by left temporal lobe damage and memory for figures, faces and tunes is more frequently impaired in those with right temporal lobe damage. A note of caution is in order, as the lateralized effect of memory material is not definitively dissociative. The process by which the active learner attempts to organize or encode the stimuli to be learned impacts which side of the brain is involved and thus potentially affects the outcome. There is also an interactive effect of the age at which a lesion is acquired and the length of time since the injury that can produce either a re-organizational effect or a compensatory effect which obscures lateralizing signs in memory.

In addition to material specific memory differences (verbal versus visual or nonverbal memory) between the left and right hemispheres noted above, other hemispheric differences have been identified (see Kandel 2007; Lezak et al. 2004;

Tulving et al. 1994, for reviews). Sometimes termed *Hemispheric Encoding and Retrieval Asymmetry* (HERA; see Tulving et al. 1994), studies suggest the left prefrontal cortex is more involved during encoding of episodic and semantic memory material and less involved during retrieval. The right prefrontal cortex (and insula and parietal cortices) are thought to be more involved in retrieval of episodic memories. Finally, retrieval of semantic memory material appears to preferentially involve the dominant (left) inferolateral prefrontal and temporal lobe, while the right hemisphere may be more involved in episodic (autobiographical) memory retrieval.

Storage and Retrieval in Memory

While the role of the temporal lobe and associated subcortical structures is demonstrated in the formation or encoding of memories, the role of structures in the retrieval process is less clear. While it is likely that cortical areas play a more significant role in recall of declarative memory, these areas are likely to be widely dispersed and interactive. Theories of how memories are stored involve associative networks that are formed between the sensory, emotional, behavioral and cognitive elements that represent those particular declarative stimuli (i.e., word, face, event, etc.). The strength of a memory would be associated with the relative strength of each of these component influences. For example, the recall of a person's name might be facilitated if it were presented in multiple sensory modalities, with emotional content, with behavioral cues and cognitive processing or elaboration. Such a process can be achieved by introducing yourself, asking the patient to repeat your name, notice some distinguishing characteristic, asking about an emotional association, and then asking questions requiring some cognitive association or processing. An example is given in Table 8.2 that might be used in an interview or bedside evaluation of a patient. The cues can be given as necessary to assess the level of cueing needed to retrieve information if the patient does not recall your name spontaneously when asked.

Once memories are encoded, they are typically retained with a decaying degree of accuracy over time. Even highly encoded memories which maximize encoding

Table 8.2 Facilitation of learning in interview or bedside evaluation

	Interviewer behavior	Facilitating process
a.	My name is Dr. Herman Jones.	Auditory presentation
b.	Repeat my name.	Cognitive/Auditory repetition
c.	I'm the only doctor you know with a bald head and pug nose.	Associating visual characteristics
d.	How many other Hermans do you know?	Cognitive elaboration
e.	Am I the most handsome Herman you know?	Cognitive/emotional elaboration
f.	Feel my handsome face.	Behavioral/motor elaboration
g.	Now remember my name.	Intentional encoding

facilitators such as those mentioned above demonstrate decay over time without repeated refreshing of the same or highly similar information. The reconstructive nature of many memories does allow people typically to be more confident in the completeness and accuracy of their perceived recall.

Nondeclarative memory is typically better preserved than declarative memory across both aging and injury. The motor and repetitive nature of nondeclarative memory is a distinct system that is less affected by temporal lobe and medial temporal structures. While the debate regarding the area of short-term storage of nondeclarative memory rages on, the presumed area of storage for long-term declarative memory is likely to reside in the cerebellum, basal ganglia, pre-motor and parietal-temporal-occipital association center of the angular and supramarginal gyri. These areas have been shown to be involved in apraxias such as grooming, dressing or feeding oneself. The dissociation of declarative and nondeclarative memory systems can be seen clearly to go beyond simple or repetitive motor tasks in the performance of severely amnestic patients in playing novel music, playing bridge or other skilled games. While typically preserved long after the impairment of declarative memory, even nondeclarative memory fails in late stages of degenerative disorders or severe brain injuries.

Assessment of Memory

The assessment of memory is necessary in many clinical settings from acute assessment to precise laboratory assessment in stable populations. This need for memory assessment in such varied settings requires flexibility in assessment approach and subsequently involves a trade off between the brevity of assessment and the reliability of the results. Brief assessment in acute populations should be reviewed as a snapshot of a moving target which is likely related to the ultimate outcome, but should be viewed with appropriate reservations. This assessment is the least standardized but may yield important information about current impairment. While the lack of stability across assessment in acute populations may give concern to more psychometrically oriented neuropsychologists, its value should not be ignored. Intermediate memory assessment involves more structured and standardized assessment of memory, but continues to make a compromise on the brevity–precision continuum. Lastly, laboratory or standardized assessment yields the most reliable assessment of memory, but does take considerable time and resources to collect the data necessary for such an assessment.

Assessment of memory across stages of illness or trauma must include both immediate recall and spontaneous delayed recall in addition to assessing recall with cues and recognition. Assessing these aspects of memory yields much information about the memory process across encoding and retrieval and can also produce beneficial patient management and safety information. Assessment across all stages also typically includes the use of verbal and nonverbal information. Verbal information is further subdivided into semantic and word list material.

Brief Bedside (Acute) Assessment of Memory

An initial assessment of memory can be done in an interview format as part of an extended mental status examination. This type of assessment relies on environmental factors and is intended to gather information about current memory functioning. Specific accident and/or illness factors are likely to be large influential considerations and statements about functioning garnered from this type of assessment must include the possibility of rapid change. Such an assessment is easily conducted in a nonthreatening manner and can yield very useful information that assists in establishing a baseline, indicating the need for ongoing or future assessment and providing information about the current level of independence or supervision necessary. Table 8.3 lists methods for acute assessment. These items should be recalled with nearly complete accuracy. This assessment yields information about remote and recent memory as well as memory across visual, semantic and verbal domains. While it is not appropriate to assign quantitative levels of performance to such an examination, useful information is gathered about current functioning which serves a baseline function, indicates the need for future assessment, and is helpful in managing patients or providing the degree of supervision necessary to meet their needs.

Intermediate/Bedside Assessment of Memory

Several methods can be used to briefly assess memory functioning in a systematic and structured manner. These methods focus on list-learning tasks, semantic memory tasks and visual memory tasks. The following three-component memory assessment task is offered for an expedient assessment of memory with guidelines provided for interpretation. Caution should be used when applying such interpretation, as many factors influence memory performance and should be considered. This type of assessment of current memory function is not intended to substitute for a more thorough assessment of memory, but rather is offered to assess memory in acute or medical office settings and determine if referral for further assessment is indicated. The guidelines for levels of impairment are also offered for clinical purposes and recognition that these guidelines for levels of performance are not rigid and are certainly affected by age and educational factors. With these cautions in mind, the following Ten-minute Intermediate Memory Evaluation (TIME) is described in Table 8.4. The word list consists of five unrelated words which are presented three times while patients are told which words they forgot in the immediate recall phase. They are reminded that they will be asked to recall these words later. Their immediate spontaneous recall across the three trials is recorded. A semantic message which contains five elements is then related and immediate recall is requested. The message is repeated twice, and the subject is told that they will be asked to recall the story in verbatim detail later. Subsequently, the subject is shown a drawing with five elements and requested to look at the drawing and

Table 8.3 Acute/interview assessment of memory

	Item	Example	Area assessed	Record response/accuracy
1.	Self-introduction	I'm Dr. Herman Jones	Auditory registration	
	• Ask them to repeat.	My name sounds like _____.	• Repetition	
	• Give multiple cues.	I look like _____.	• Cued recall	
		Touch my pretty face.		
		How many pretty Hermans do you know?		
	• Tell them you will ask them your name later.		• Intentional recall	
2.	Ask why they are here.	What happened?	• Remote memory/Orientation	
		Last memory prior...	• Retrograde amnesia	
		First memory after...	• Anterograde amnesia	
	• Provide info if necessary	You are here because...		
		You have been here...		
3.	Ask about family	Who lives with you?	• Autobiographical information	
		Describe your family.	• Personal facts	
		Who lives in the area, where, when?	• Remote memory	
4.	Contemporary information	How about the Middle East?	• Recent memory	
		What can be done about terrorists, etc.?	• Intentional semantic memory	
	• Tell them you will ask about this topic later.	What issues are politicians focused on?		
5.	Intervening conversation	What is your doctor's name?	• Recent memory	
		Is he/she your regular doctor?		
		What medications do you take?		
		What do you do to stay healthy?		
6.	Close your eyes and tell me		• Incidental visual memory	
	a. Items patient is wearing	• Item, color, description		

(continued)

Table 8.3 (continued)

Item	Example	Area assessed	Record response/accuracy
b. What you (the interviewer) are wearing	• Shirt or other prominent item		
c. Where items are in room	• Furniture, door, window, TV		
7. Show them 3 items and ask patient to remember them. • Tell patient you will ask again later.	• Cup, paper clip, coins, pen	• Immediate intentional visual memory	
8. Ask them to recall your name.	• I'm Dr. _____. • Provide previous cues as necessary.	• Intentional verbal recall • Cued facilitation	
9. Ask patient to recall items previously shown.	• Coins, paper clip, pen • Provide cues if necessary • Office supply • In my pocket	• Intentional visual recall	
10. Ask patient to recall topic previously discussed.	• Babies, politics, terrorism • Recall accident facts	• Intentional verbal semantic recall	

Table 8.4 Ten-minute Intermediate Memory Evaluation (TIME)

Learning Trials

	Trial 1	Trial 2	Trial 3	Recall	Cue	Recognition	
Horse	___	___	___	___	Animal ___	Cow ___	Car ___
Bus	___	___	___	___	Transportation ___	Bug ___	Horse ___
Fly	___	___	___	___	Insect ___	Bus ___	Nurse ___
Nurse	___	___	___	___	Occupation ___	Doctor ___	Stove ___
Phone	___	___	___	___	Appliance ___	Phone ___	Fly ___

Learning Trials

	Trial 1	Trial 2	Recall	Cue	Recognition (read **Pair** and **circle response**)	
Angela	___	___	___	Who called ___	Maria	Angela
called home	___	___	___	Called where ___	Home	Work
tied up	___	___	___	Why ___	Sick	Tied up
at work	___	___	___	Where ___	School	Work
late	___	___	___	When ___	Late	Absent

Angela called home to say she was *tied up at work* and would *be late.*

Items	Recall	Recognition
Circle	___	correct ___
Chimney	___	incorrect ___
Door	___	
Window	___	
Horizontal	___	
dissection line		

Recall Item   Recognition Items

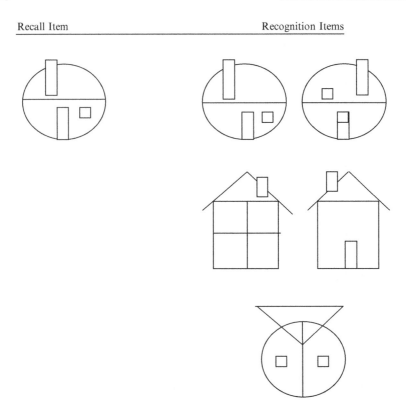

remember the elements as precisely as possible. The drawing is exposed for 10 seconds and then removed from sight. This is succeeded with spontaneous free recall of the five words and a recall of the story. Cued recall and recognition recall of the words and story are attempted following spontaneous recall trials. Then the spontaneous recall of the figure is requested, followed by recognition of the figure from among five designs. Table 8.5 offers qualitative evaluation descriptors of performance on the TIME. Again, caution should be used when interpreting performance and these descriptors are offered as guidelines and should not be considered an adequate replacement for a thorough memory assessment in a stable neurologic population.

Several screening batteries which incorporate a memory component are available and can often be used in both inpatient and outpatient populations. These measures have the added benefit of briefly assessing other areas of functioning in addition to memory such as attention, language and visuospatial skills. These measures usually take 30 min to 1 hour to administer. Examples of such measures incorporating memory assessment that may be used for bedside assessment include *Dementia Rating Scale – 2nd Ed.* (DRS-2, Mattis 2001), Repeatable Battery for the Assessment of Neuropsychological Status (RBANS, Randolph 1998), and Cognistat (Kiernan et al. 1995) among others (see Lezak et al. 2004 for review).

Table 8.5 Qualitative assessment of 10-min intermediate memory evaluation (TIME)

	≤60				>60			
	Normal	Mild	Moderate	Severe	Normal	Mild	Moderate	Severe
List recall								
Total of 3 trials	12–15	6–9	3–5	<3	9–15	6–8	3–5	<3
Delayed recall	4–5	2–3	1	0	3–5	2–3	1	0
Recognition	9–10	8	7–8	5	8–10	7–8	6	5
Message recall								
Total of 2 trials	8–10	7–8	5–6	<5	7–10	6–7	4–5	<4
Delayed recall	4–5	3	2	<2	3–5	2	1	0
Recognition	9–10	8	6–7	5	8–10	7–8	6	5
Figure recall								
Recall	4–5	3	2	1	3–5	2	1	0
Recognition	5	4	3	2	5	4	3	2

Comprehensive/Outpatient Laboratory Assessment of Memory

There are a vast array of neuropsychology memory tests, ranging from stand alone memory tests [e.g., Rey Auditory Verbal Learning Test (AVLT or RAVLT, Rey 1964), *California Verbal Learning Test – 2nd Ed.* (CVLT-2, Delis et al. 2000), and *Hopkins Verbal Learning Test* – Revised (HVLT-R, Benedict et al. 1998) to comprehensive memory batteries (e.g., *Wechsler Memory Scale – 4th Ed.* (WMS-IV, Wechsler 2008); *Children's Memory Scale* (CMS, Cohen 1998), *Wide Range Assessment of Memory and Learning, 2nd Ed.* (WRAML-2, Sheslow and Adams 2004)]. A review of these instruments is beyond the scope of this book. Selection of the appropriate measure(s) of memory will reflect the purpose of the referral, patient variables, and expertise and training of the clinician. As specified above, we strongly advocate assessment of learning over trials, immediate (short-term) memory, delayed memory, and recognition. We also recommend inclusion of a measure allowing for assessment of proactive and retroactive interference effects. Typically, neuropsychological assessment of memory will also include more than one verbal memory test and more than one non-verbal (visual) memory test. Neuropsychological assessment protocols have been established or recommended for several different disease entities [e.g., Consortium to Establish a Registry for Alzheimer's Disease (CERAD, Rosen et al. 1984; Morris et al. 1989) and schizophrenia)], and work is currently underway to identify a series of tests that may be used across a variety of research fields supported by the National Institute of Health. Recommendations are also provided in this volume for various neurological diseases and syndromes.

References and Suggested Further Reading

Benedict, R. H. B., Schretlaen, D., Groninger, L., & Brandt, J. (1998). Hopkins Verbal Learning Test – Revised: Normative data and analysis of inter-form and test-retest reliability. *The Clinical Neuropsychologist, 12*, 43–55.

Cohen, M. (1998). *Children's Memory Scale*. San Antonio, Texas, Psychological Corporation.

Delis, D. C., Kramer, J. H., Kaplan, E., & Ober, B. A. (2000). *California verbal learning test (CVLT-II)* (2nd ed.). San Antonio: Pearson.

Kandel, E. (2007). *In search of memory: The emergence of a new science*. New York: W. W. Horton.

Kiernan, R. J., Mueller, J., & Langston, J. W. (1995). *Cognistat (neurobehavioral cognitive status examination)*. Lutz: Psychological Assessment Resources.

Kolb, B., & Whishaw, I. (2009). *Fundamentals of human neuropsychology* (6th ed.). New York: W. H. Freeman.

Lezak, M. D., Howieson, D. B., & Loring, D. W. (2004). *Neuropsychological assessment* (4th ed.). New York: Oxford University Press.

Mattis, S. (2001). *Dementia rating scale* (2nd ed.). Lutz: Psychological Assessment Resources.

Mesulam, M. (2000). *Principals of behavioral and cognitive neurology* (2nd ed.). New York: Oxford University Press.

Morris, J. C., Heyman, A., Mohs, R. C., et al. (1989). The Consortium to Establish a Registry for Alzheimer's Disease (CERAD). Part 1. Clinical and neuropsychological assessment of Alzheimer's disease. *Neurology, 39*, 1159–1165.

Randolph, C. (1998). *Repeatable battery for the assessment of neuropsychological status*. San Antonio: The Psychological Corporation.

Rey, A. (1964). *L'examen Clinique en psychologie*. Paris: Presses Universitaires de France.

Rosen, W. G., Mohs, R. C., & Davis, K. L. (1984). A new rating scale for Alzhiemer's disease. *The American Journal of Psychiatry, 141*, 1356–64.

Sheslow, D., & Adams, W. (2004). *Wide range assessment of memory and learning (WRAML-2)* (2nd ed.). Cheektowaga: Multi-Health Systems.

Squire, L. R. (1987). *Memory and Brain*. New York, Oxford Press.

Squire, L., & Schacter, D. (2003). *Neuropsychology of memory* (3rd ed.). New York: Guilford.

Squire, L., & Zola, S. M. (1996). Structure and function of declarative and nondeclarative memory systems. *Proceedings of the National Academy of Sciences of the United States of America, 93*, 13515–13522.

Tulving, E., Kapur, S., Craik, F. I., Moscovitch, M., & Houle, S. (1994). Hemispheric encoding/retrieval asymmetry in episodic memory: Positron emission tomography findings. *Proceedings of the National Academy of Sciences of the United States of America, 91*, 2016–2020.

Wechsler, D. (2008). *Wechsler memory scale (WMS-IV)* (4th ed.). San Antonia, TX: Pearson.

Chapter 9
Deficits in Visuospatial/Visuoconstructional Skills and Motor Praxis

James G. Scott and Mike R. Schoenberg

Abstract Visuospatial and visuoperceptual skills play a role in every day functioning; however, they are typically automatic. We process information visually and make identifications and analyze complex visual stimuli and are largely unaware of the visuoperceptual process involved or complexities of the stimuli that were analyzed. As an example, assume that you have purchased a new car and now suddenly that make and model seems to be everywhere. You suddenly notice the different colors in which the car comes, the different trim packages, and optional equipment (i.e., roof racks, spoiler, etc.). Soon you find yourself distinguishing among similar year models based on detail changes such as tail light configuration or color-matching door hardware. You can also identify this car from multiple angles (front, side, rear, corner, etc.) These complex stimuli are typically automatically perceived, poorly verbally labeled, yet precisely and accurately analyzed and identified. The centers in the brain that process such information are ever vigilant to visual and visuospatial stimuli and organized to simultaneously and sequentially take that information and transform it into usable, salient information or associated knowledge. All this occurs in a split second and typically below our level of awareness. While this process can certainly be consciously controlled, typically in novel learning or acquisition stages, our nature is to use repetition, familiarity or repeated recurrence to allow for more automatic processing and save the conscious and effortful processing capacities for the novel or necessary tasks at hand.

If this process is impaired, many types of deficits occur, from failure to process basic elements in the visual stimuli (i.e., color, lines, orientation) to more complex and integrative features such as object identification, faces or familiar scenes. These deficits can include phenomena such as *visual neglect* and *hemi-inattention* or more dramatic *visual agnosias* or *prosopagnosia*. This impairment may include what is referred to as disconnection syndromes in which centers of basic visual sensory

J.G. Scott (✉)
Department of Psychiatry and Behavioral Sciences, University of Oklahoma
Health Sciences Center, Oklahoma City, OK, USA
e-mail: jim-scott@ouhsc.edu

M.R. Schoenberg and J.G. Scott (eds.), *The Little Black Book of Neuropsychology: A Syndrome-Based Approach,* DOI 10.1007/978-0-387-76978-3_9,
© Springer Science+Business Media, LLC 2011

functions are dissociated or disconnected from association cortex areas that allow for synthesis or analysis necessary to recognize the sensory stimuli as a specific object.

Key Points and Chapter Summary

- Visuospatial and visuoconstructional deficits are much more likely with right-sided parietal lobe damage especially to the angular gyrus and supramarginal gyrus
- Much of visuospatial and visuoconstructional processing occurs automatically and may not be evident to the patient or family
- Praxis deficits can occur in many motor functions including feeding, dressing, tool use, drawing, and complex skills such as mechanical skill or musical skill
- Hemi inattention or neglect is
  - Hemi-inattention involves only one modality. Hemi-neglect involves more than one sensory modality.
  - Most frequently associated with right parietal lobe damage but can occur with left parietal lobe damage
  - Is often severe acutely and may involve vision, hearing and tactile sensation.
  - Hemi-neglect or hemi-inattention does demonstrate a tendency decrease over time (usually a few months)
  - In the case of hemi-neglect, resolution usually remits across tactile modalities first, auditory modalities second, and vision last.

Anatomy of Visual and Visuospatial Processing

Visual and visuospatial processing involves many area of the cortex as well as subcortical areas depending on the functional aspect of visual processing that is to occur. The occipital lobe contains the primary visual cortex and performs many basic visual functions. The right hemispace or visual field is generally processed by the left occipital lobe while the left visual field is processed by the right visual cortex. In relation to the calcarine fissure (see Fig. 9.1), the processing of information from the perceivable visual field is most easily understood as upside down and anteriorly to posteriorly backward. Thus, the upper half of the visual field is processed by the gyri below the calcarine fissure while the lower half of the visual field is processed by the gyri superior to the calcarine fissure. Similarly, stimuli in the center of the visual field are processed by the cortex in the posterior visual cortex while stimuli from the periphery of the visual field are processed by cortex of the anterior occipital lobe medially to the calcarine fissure.

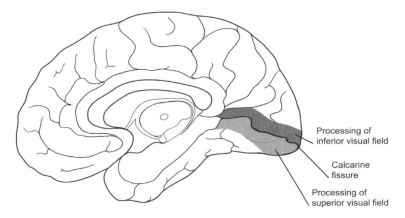

Processing of
inferior visual field

Calcarine
fissure

Processing of
superior visual field

Fig. 9.1   Medial picture of brain illustrating primary visual cortex above/below calcarine fissure

---

Rule of thumb: Organization of retinocortical map for primary visual cortex

- Upside down and backwards
  - Upper halves of visual fields are processed by the gyri below the calcarine fissure
  - Lower halves of the visual fields are processed by the gyri above the calcarine fissure.
  - Visual information from the center is processed by primary visual cortex closest to the occipital pole (posterior visual cortex).
  - Visual information from peripherial vision processed by occipital lobe closest to the calcarine fissure and anterior to the occipital pole

---

In processing visual stimuli, information that provides stimulation to the retinas is transferred via the optic nerve, primarily either to the primary visual cortex or lateral geniculate body. Both these areas have similar topographic organizational representations (i.e., upside down and backward) throughout the visual system. In addition, some visual information is projected to the superior colliculus which is instrumental in visual orientation to movement within the visual field. Figure 9.2 depicts the visual system and process of visual sensation from perception of stimuli to transfer to the visual cortex.

As visual stimuli are processed, their basic elements are first discerned by the primary visual cortex (area V1) which includes the calcarine fissure and is called striate cortex because of distinct stripes in the gray matter associated with perception of color, shape, and motion. Secondary visual cortex refines these perceptions and integrates these basic elements into wholes, allowing association cortex to definitively identify the viewed objects or determining and guiding movement. For example, the stimuli of one straight line and two curved lines are initially processed by the primary visual cortex. This information is further processed with the portion of the three elements being noted and recognized as a familiar unitary stimulus. This is subsequently processed further by tertiary cortex and recognized as an upper

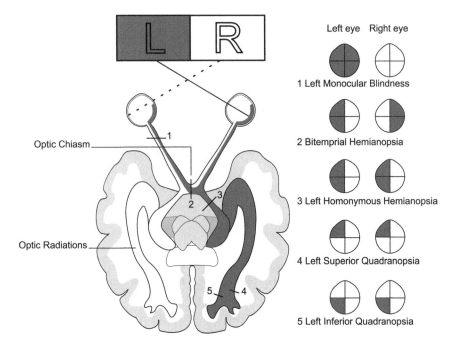

Fig. 9.2 Illustration of optic pathways from retina to primary visual cortex

case "B." While this is certainly a simplified example of the processing of the elements of a letter "B," the process of recognition of more complicated stimuli such as a face or landscape occurs much the same way. However, in the case of faces, there is a specialized area of the brain to recognize and process faces termed the fusiform face area (FFA) which lies in the fusiform gyrus of the occipito-temporal area. While termed the FFA, this area appears important for specialized visual object discrimination, such as for discriminating between birds and cars (Gauthier et al. 2000).

Visual Processing "Streams"

The visual processing system is traditionally divided into two general systems in humans: (1) a system for processing where stimuli are in space, the so-called "where" system (or Dorsal stream); and (2) a system for processing what a visual percept is, the so-called "what" system (or Ventral stream) (Fig. 9.3). The "Where" system begins in the occipital lobe involving the primary visual cortex (area V1) to V2 and V3 projecting to the middle temporal area (MT) and runs dorsally and superiorly to the medial superior area and parietal lobes. Alternatively, the "What" system also begins in primary visual cortex (V1), but with somewhat different pathways that project to V2 and V3 to V4 which then runs ventrally and inferiorly

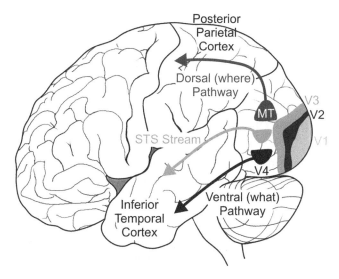

Fig. 9.3 Illustration of dorsal and ventral visual processing "streams" in human brain

to the posterior and inferior temporal lobes (including the fusiform gyrus). A third system, termed the superior temporal sulcus (STS) system, has been identified, and likely involves complex visuoconstructional and movement processing, running laterally from the primary occipital cortex (area V1) laterally along the superior temporal sulcus and includes regions of the superior temporal gyrus as well.

Rule of thumb: Visual processing "streams"

- "What" stream (visual processing pathway that recognizes objects) = Ventral pathway
- "Where" stream (visual processing where things are in space) = Dorsal pathway
- "Specialized movement" stream (visual analysis of movement of body parts and biological objects) = STS pathway

---

Visual and Visuospatial Deficits

Visual loss occurs with destruction or impairment of any point in the pathway from the retinas to the primary visual cortex. Lesions occurring before the optic chiasm result in monocular blindness (blindness in one eye). Lesions producing damage to the medial optic chiasm produces a bi-temporal hemianopsia resulting from the disruption of fibers from the medial retinas, which must cross at the optic chiasm. Post-chiasmic lesions produce contralateral visual field loss and are referred to as a homonymous hemianopsia. Lesions in the posterior geniculo striate radiations would produce a contralateral upper quadrant anopsia if in the inferior geniculo striate or a lower quadrant anopsia if in the superior geniculo striate. Figure 9.2 shows the lesion locations and visual deficits associated with each.

Visuoperceptual Distortions

A variety of visuoperceptual distortions have been identified. The visuoperceptual distortions are distinguished from visual agnosias in patients are able to identify objects, but their visual perception is altered in some fashion. Complaints may include perception of objects as too close (pelopsia), too far away (telopsia), larger than they really are (macropsia) or smaller than they really are (micropsia). A syndrome involving the distortion of visual perception and time has been described, the so-called *Alice in Wonderland* (or *Todd's*) syndrome (see Table 9.1 for summary of visual distortions).

Cortical Blindness or "Blind Sight"

Cortical blindness (Blind sight) is a rare condition occurring with damage to the primary visual cortex. Traditionally, this term is referred to bilateral occipital lobe damage, but is also present with unilateral occipital lobe destruction, which has been reported with vascular disease or traumatic brain injury. Individuals have no conscious awareness of vision in the damaged visual field(s), and will report being blind. However, these individuals are able to appreciate location or movement, without knowing the content. Individuals have been able to point to where a light was located in their "blind" visual field(s) and able to perceive orientation of lines without conscious perception. While a person with cortical blindness is unable to identify a face in their visual field, patients were able to "guess" the emotional expressions. Lastly, there is some processing of movement, but this perception is outside the clear awareness of patients.

Balint's Syndrome

First described in 1909 by Reszo Balint, but coined in 1954 by Hecaen and Ajuriaguerra, this is a disorder of visual perception and attention characteristically associated with three features: (1) *optic ataxia*, (2) *ocular apraxia*, and (3) a visual spatial inattention thought to reflect a *simultanagnosia*. *Optic ataxia* is the inability to coordinate visual guided reach for objects in space. The individual is unable to use his/her eyes to guide hand (or feet) movements to desired targets in space.

Table 9.1 Visuoperceptual deficits

Term	Description
Acromatopsia	Inability to distinguish colors
Alice in Wonderland (Todd's) syndrome	Alteration in the perception of time, generally for brief time periods. Perceptual alterations include macropsia, metamorphsia, micropsia, teleopsia, and pelopsia (collectively referred to as dysmetropsia). Objects may be perceived as too small (or far away) and/or too large (close). Associated with migraine headache, brain tumor, Epstein-Barr infection and use of psychoactive drugs. The syndrome has also been reported in association with epilepsy and ICP.
Anton's syndrome	Denial of cortical blindness
Balint's syndrome	Rare syndrome composing three classic features: (1) optic ataxia (unable to guide movements using visual information), (2) ocular apraxia (inability to voluntary move eyes), and (3) visual spatial inattention (features of simultanagnosia) Bilateral parieto-occipital damage.
Cortical Blindness (blind sight)	Blindness resulting from destruction of primary visual cortex. Patient's unable to identify or perceive colors, lines, shapes, or objects. Often associated with Anton's syndrome. Phenomena of "blind sight" occurs if patient with cortical blindness able to make better than chance identification of visual stimuli that are not consciously perceived. Blind sight thought to be possible due to intact parietal cortex and preserved visual pathway from superior colliculus.
Dysmetropsia	Term used to describe macropsia, micropsia, pelopsia, and teleopsia. Associated with retinopathy (swelling of the cornea), but also reported with Migraine headache, brain tumors, lesions of the occipital cortex, Epstein-Barr infection, epilepsy, psychoactive drug use, and psychiatric illnesses. Reported to occur at times in some otherwise healthy children and adolescents.
Figure-Ground Discrimination	Ability to distinguish overlapping objects. Impaired in simultanagnosia.
Macropsia (also known as megalopsia)	Visual distortion in which objects appear much bigger than the objects really are. Objects may also be perceived as closer than they really are (pelopsia), and objects may appear to move in towards the person. Perception may be like looking through a telescope.
Micropsia	Visual distortion in which objects appear much smaller than they really are. Objects are too small, and may be associated with teleopsia (perceived as being far off in the distance). The effect may be like looking through the wrong end of a telescope. Some have described objects as also appearing to "move away from them towards the distance." Strictly speaking, micropsia describes disruption of perception of size – not distance (teleopsia).
Metamorphsia	Visual distortion in which shapes and colors are distorted. Straight lines appear to bend.
Pelopsia	Visual distortion in which objects appear much closer (nearer) then the objects actually are.

(continued)

Table 9.1 (continued)

Term	Description
Teleopsia	Visual distortion in which objects appear further away than the objects actually are. Has been found in patients with parieto-temporal lesions as well, but most often associated with Migraine headache.
Ocular dysmetria	Deficit in the motor (ocular) movements of the eye, in which saccades are overshot or undershot. When trying to fixate on an object, the eye will appear to shake back and forth as the eye tries to adjust for over- and under-shooting the object in saccadic movements.
Visuo-Integration	Ability to mentally rotate or synthesize objects parts into whole
Visuo-Spatial Orientation	Ability to judge orientation of objects in space

Ocular apraxia is the inability to voluntarily shift eye gaze despite intact cranial nerves and functional ocular muscles. Should not be confused with ocular dysmetria (see Table 9.1). Individuals will exhibit a seemingly psychic stare and not be able to voluntarily "look away." Voluntary eye movements can occur if the patient closes his/her eyes. A visual spatial inattention occurs with the patient only being able to appreciate one aspect of a percept at a time. It has been described as almost a "tunnel" vision focusing on one percept. Minimizing the object for perception does not result in the whole image being seen, but a focus on the smaller detail aspects of the scene appreciated, and classically described as simultanagnosia, although some argue the features of the visual inattention of Balint's syndrome differs (subtly) from simultanagnosias. Balint's syndrome has traditionally been associated with bilateral occipito-parietal lesions, and often damage to the white matter underlying the angular gyrus for the dorsal "where" stream (e.g., Kolb and Whishaw 2009). Table 9.1 summarizes common visuoperceptual deficits.

Rule of thumb: Balint's syndrome

- Optic ataxia = loss of eye hand coordination
- Occular apraxia = loss of voluntary ability to shift gaze
- Simultanagnosia = cannot see anything but one aspect of an object at a time

---

Visual Agnosia

Agnosias develop when the meaning is striped from a percept, and there are problems associated with the cortical processing of stimuli which are *not* related to or explained by deficits in the sensory organ. Assuming the mechanisms of visual sensory perception are intact, patients may manifest several deficits in visual processing of stimuli. These deficits can be as basic as the perception of angular lines or as complex as an inability to synthesize or rotate visual images to make a recognizable object.

Deficits in visual processing can involve any aspect of the stimuli including color, texture and spatial orientation and integration.

Acromatopsia is an inability to distinguish among colors, typically in a range of color spectrum (i.e., blue-green, purple-red) and may be traumatically induced or congenital. Deficits may also be seen in inability to judge the spatial orientation of objects or lines in space. The type of visuospatial deficit typically involves deficits in distinguishing line orientation or curved and straight lines or the inability to separate figure and ground overlapping elements in a scene. Table 9.2 lists common visual agnosias.

Several visual agnosias have been delineated, which are associated with various parietal-occipital association cortices. While lesions to the occipital cortex tend to produce deficits in basic perceptual characteristics (i.e., color perception, orientation of stimuli), lesions to parieto-occipital cortex produces deficits in more complicated integrative and synthesizing visual functions. These deficits are included in visual object agnosia, of which two types have been identified, differentiated by clinical features and lesion locations.

Visual object agnosia is an inability to recognize (know) visually presented objects. This must not reflect a deficit in naming, so not only can the patient not name an object, but cannot demonstrate its use or point to the object when it is named by the examiner. Further, it is not a deficit of lack of familiarity or knowledge per se, with the patient being able to name and/or demonstrate use of objects when presented in other sensory domains (auditory, tactile, etc.). Often, real objects can be better perceived (known) than line drawings. The agnosia of visual objects will vary, such that some classes of objects are better known, while other classes of objects are not known (i.e., animals worse than trees or tools). Visual agnosias are further divided into Apperceptive and Associate subtypes.

1. *Apperceptive visual agnosia* is characterized by the inability to demonstrate accurate percept of objects. Patients are unable to draw the object on command, copy the object on paper, or match similar classes of objects together. The patient is unable to name the object and cannot sort groups appropriately (types of birds, four-legged mammals, etc.).
2. *Associative visual agnosia* is a deficit in perceiving an object with intact abilities to draw and match visual objects. It can be distinguished from the Apperceptive type by the ability of the patient to draw or match similar visual objects together, yet still be unable to name or demonstrate the use of the objects.

Rule of thumb: Visual agnosia

Inability to appreciate the meaning of a visual percept that is not due to loss of visual field or visual acuity or lack of familiarity with object/item. Demonstrate appropriate use of object if presented in another sensory modality (auditory, touch, etc.).

Table 9.2 Visual agnosias

Term	Description	Lesion location
Apperceptive Visual-Agnosia	Inability to perceive visual objects. Involves all visual objects. Patients unable to draw, copy or match (or sort) similar objects. Visual acuity is intact, and able to identify shades, colors, and light and dark lines.	Bilateral temporo-occipital-parietal. Often presents as recovery from cortical blindness
Associative Visual Agnosia	Inability to recognize visual objects. A visual percept "stripped of its meaning." Objects seen are not known, and can't be named or use demonstrated. However, objects can be drawn, copied, and matched (to a like visual object). Dollar bills can be matched together. May be associated with achromatopsia.	Bilateral posterior mesial temporo-occipital cortex (and underlying white matter).
Auto Prosopagnosia	Inability to identify one's own face	
Dorsal simultanagnosia	Unable to appreciate more than one feature of an object or scene at a time. Restriction in perceiving objects more pronounced than in ventral simultanagnosia. Individuals may bump into objects in their environment if several are placed close together (e.g., a couch and a coffee table).	Bilateral parieto-occipital
Prosopagnosia	Classically, the inability to identify familiar faces. However, deficit is the inability to identify specific members of a class. Generic recognition of objects (pen, person, cat) is intact, but patient unable to identify specific members within a class (distinguish types of pens or distinguish pet cat from stray, etc.).	Bilateral temporo-occiptial area, particularly the mesial and inferior lingual and/or parahippocampal gyri (or underlying white matter).
Simultaneous Visual Agnosia (Simultanagnosia)	Inability to perceive multiple aspects of a single object or multiple aspects of a scene	Bilateral parieto-occipital lesions or left inferior temporo-occipital.
Ventral simultanagnosia	Unable to appreciate multiple aspects of a scene. When trying to read, may read a word, but unable to read a sentence. Less complete restriction in visual perception than dorsal simultanagnosia.	Left inferior temporo-occipital

Simultaneous visual-agnosia (*Simultanagnosia*) is impairment in the ability to appreciate the multiple aspects of a single object or the relationship of multiple objects in a scene. The patient is unable to appreciate the totality of an object (e.g., picture of an elephant) but can identify discrete features of the object (e.g., eyes, tail, trunk, ears, etc.). Individuals with simultanagnosia are unable to read, as they can appreciate each letter but cannot see the words the letters spell out. Two types of simultanagnosia have been identified, dorsal and ventral types.

1. *Dorsal simultanagnosia* describes individuals unable to appreciate more than one feature of an object or scene at a time. Dorsal simultanagnosia is associated with bilateral occipitoparietal lesions
2. *Ventral simultanagnosia* is less "complete" with patients being able to identify some multiple features of an object or a scene, but unable to appreciate the entire scene. As an example, a patient with a ventral simultanagnosia may be able to identify two discrete people in a scene, but is unable to describe the scene as two people playing Frisbee. The patient may be able to read short words, but will have more difficulty with longer words and reading a printed sentence along a page. Ventral simultanagnosia has been reported with unilateral (left) inferior occipitoparietal (or is occipitotemporal) lobe lesion.

Prosopagnosia is a deficit in recognizing familiar faces. Patients can describe discrete aspects of a face, nose, mouth, eyes, but cannot recognize the face. Prosopagnosia is not limited to human faces; it has been reported for recognizing animals (e.g., pets). Both apperceptive and associative forms have been described, based on ability to match faces to categories (known and unknown faces). Individuals with the associative form of prosopagnosia can sort familiar faces from unfamiliar faces, but remain unable to name or point to familiar faces if the familiar face is named.

Apraxia

Apraxia refers to an inability to perform previously learned, sequential motor movements. Apraxia should not be confused with ataxia (see Chap. 2, this volume), which is the loss of ability to coordinate motor movements. This loss of ability to perform motor movements cannot be attributable to sensory or simple central or peripheral motor impairment or general condition such as dementia. While many classification schemas of apraxias have been proposed, the most pragmatic involve discrimination among Ideational and Ideomotor limb apraxias, and constructional apraxia. Ideational and Ideomotor apraxias may involve any number of functions such as buccofacial movement, feeding, grooming, dressing or tool usage. The discriminating characteristic between Ideomotor and Ideational Apraxias is the inability of patients with Ideomotor apraxia to pantomime motor skills either to imitation or command (demonstrate use of a hammer and nail, hair brush, scissors, etc.) and the failure of Ideational Apraxia patients to perform sequenced movements in complex motor behaviors despite often retaining the individual components of such behaviors (e.g., demonstrating how to write a letter, fold it, put it in an envelope, address it, and put a stamp on it).

Ideomotor apraxia patients have the greatest difficulty in performing tasks to command, but often improve when asked to imitate hand movements, and typically improve further when asked to perform behaviors with actual objects. This is most frequently assessed by asking patients to demonstrate a tool's use by command such as: show me how you would use a hammer, saw or screwdriver. Individuals with Ideomotor apraxia often use their hand as the tool rather than demonstrating a proper hand grip and subsequent hammer use movements. Similarly, these patients often have difficulty with daily tool use such as eating utensils, grooming tools (comb, toothbrush) or writing implements. Lesions are typically associated with left hemisphere in right-handed persons. These lesions typically involve the posterior parietal lobe and or the corpus callosum connecting the right and left parietal areas.

In contrast, Ideational apraxia involves the failure of sequential movements that make up a purposeful behavior while the constitutional parts remain intact. Patients with Ideational apraxia often appear to get lost in the steps involved in a task. For example, the steps in brushing your teeth might include grabbing your toothbrush, holding it in one hand, getting toothpaste, unscrewing the top, squeezing the toothpaste onto the brush, wetting the brush, screwing the top back on the toothpaste and then brushing, followed by rinsing your mouth and then rinsing your toothbrush. Individuals with ideational apraxia often fail at some point in the multi-step sequence. Ideational apraxias are often associated with lesion in the frontal lobes.

Constructional apraxia refers to a loss of ability to draw or make three-dimensional designs despite intact perceptional skills. Individuals with this type of deficit have difficulty with visuospatial relationships and often produce drawings or three-dimensional designs that have correct elements, but in which the elements do not correspond appropriately to each other (see Fig. 9.5 for an example). Individuals with right parietal lesions are most likely to manifest this type of apraxia. It should be noted that this type of apraxia can also be conceptualized as a visuo-agnosia. Table 9.3 lists the above noted apraxia and their associated lesion location and deficit.

Assessment of Visuospatial (Visual-Spatial) Functioning

Prior to assessing visuospatial skills, deficits in sensory functioning need to be ruled out as potential causes for abnormalities. These include assessment of visual acuity as well as occulo-motor movements and visual field deficits. As mentioned in previous chapters, occulo-motor deficits can be attributed to cranial nerve deficits in nerves III, IV or VI (see Chap. 4 for examination of cranial nerves). Visual acuity should be assessed by asking patients about their use of corrective lenses and their last optometrist/ophthalmologist examination, as well as performing a crude bedside examination using a Schnelling Chart. Visual fields should be tested laterally as well

Table 9.3 Apraxias

Type	Deficit	Lesion location
Ideomotor Limb Apraxia	Cannot perform motor movements to command. Difficulty exists with performance to imitation and with actual object	Left posterior Parietal lobe or corpus callosum connecting right and left posterior parietal regions
Ideational Limb Apraxia	Deficits in performing sequenced motor movements to complete a complex behavior, often despite preserved ability to perform individual components.	Typically frontal lobe lesions in supplemental motor cortex. Lesions are more severe with left frontal lesions, but occur with damage to either side.
Constructional Apraxia	Inability to copy a drawing or construct a three-dimensional design from a model.	Lesions are typically in the right parietal lobe.

as in vertical quadrants as it is possible that a patient may have a quadrant anopsis if lesions are restricted either to the area above the calcarine fissure (produces a lower contralateral quadrant anopsia) or below the calcarine fissure (produces an upper contralateral quadrant anopsia). Oculomotor (Ocular motor) movements can also be affected by frontal lobe lesions to the frontal eye fields and usually result in poor voluntary eye control in tasks requiring visual search and sustained gaze. To test, have the patient voluntarily look to the left, right, up and down.

Rule of thumb: Right versus left constructional apraxias

- Left Hemisphere (parietal lesions):
  - Drawings maintain gestalt but lack detail
  - Organization of spatial features appears piecemeal, but generally in appropriate area.
  - Block designs maintain general organization (2×2) but spatial detail (block) often rotated
  - Right sensory extinction, can be present Gerstmann's syndrome

- Right Hemisphere (parietal lesions):
  - Left visual inattention may be present

    Features of left side of drawing/figure omitted

  - Gestalt of figure often not maintained. Details may be present, but poorly organized.
  - Block designs "strung out" and basic organization (2×2) not maintained.
  - Left sensory extinction can be present.

Assessment and Interpretation of Visuoconstructional Functions

Traditionally, qualitative differences in visuoconstructional skills have been identified between patients with left hemisphere versus right hemisphere damage. The differences are thought to reflect the differences between hemisphere functions. For example, the left hemisphere is associated with analizing visual information into details, while the right hemisphere is associated with appreciating the overall gestalt of the visual percept. Damage to the left hemisphere impairs ability to form detailed percepts, and the constructional drawings tend to be overly simplistic, poorly organized and often lack attention to detail while maintaining the overall gestalt of the object. Performance on block design tests tend to reflect maintaining the gestalt but rotating a detail. Alternatively, patients with right hemisphere, particularly right parietal damage, tend to demonstrate constructional deficits in which the whole gestalt is lost and the drawing will be typified by poor spatial arrangement of many details in which the spatial gestalt may not be maintained. In addition, a visual inattention (or hemi-neglect) may be present such that features in the left hemi-field will be missing or incomplete. Right parietal damage results in block design performance in which the gestalt is not maintained, and the drawing may be "strung" out (such that a 2×2 format is not used). The detailed feature of various angles or spatial arrangements may be preserved but the gestalt is lost.

Bedside Assessment of Visuospatial (Visuoconstructional) Skills

Screening assessment of visuospatial skills can be done in interview at the bedside and give an indication of whether more formal, standardized assessment is necessary. Assuming that sensory deficits have been ruled out by assessing visual acuity, bedside assessment of visuospatial skills should progress from simple to more integrated skills. These skills should include assessment of perception, scanning, inattention/neglect, visual recognition, facial recognition, visual form discrimination, construction (drawing) and visual synthesis skills.

Figure 9.4 is an assessment sheet with procedures and examples of ways to assess these skills. It includes a brief assessment of perception of line orientation and form discrimination (Fig. 9.4 number 1) as well as basic color perception (number 2). Number 3 assesses visual scanning and cancellation. Number 4 is an example of a line bisection task in which the patient is instructed to draw a vertical line bisecting the horizontal lines on a page. The patient's performance is evaluated based on any systematic distortion of line bisection either right or left of center. Form recognition can be screened with number 5, while Fig. 9.4 number 6 assesses constructional ability and is useful in evaluating perceptual skills as well as organizational and synthesis skills. Patients need to integrate many elements into the reproduction of more complex drawing.

Assessment of perception at its basic level involves the ability of patients to appropriately perceive angles of straight and curved lines. Patients can be given a sheet with both curved and straight lines and be asked to match or point to the lines that are most similar. Patients should also be asked to name the color of objects in the environment across blue-green and red-purple spectrums to assure correct color perception.

Scanning and assessment of neglect should involve the use of both behavioral assessment and tasks which require cancellation. Behaviorally, patients can be simultaneously shown a different number of fingers on each hand of the examiner and asked to report the total number of fingers they were shown. With the patients gaze focused centrally (i.e., look at my nose), alternately flash multiple (2–3)

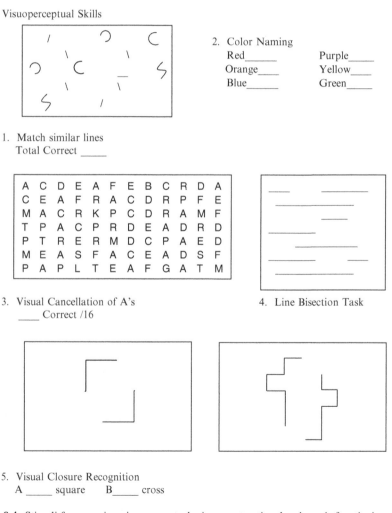

Fig. 9.4 Stimuli for assessing visuoperceptual, visuoconstructional and praxis functioning

Visuoconstructional skills

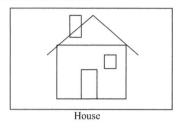

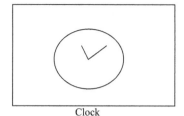

House   Clock

6. Figure Copying

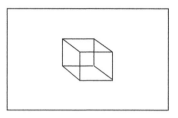

7. Drawing Cube and/or Clock (placing hands at 10 past 11).

Praxis skills

8. Ideomotor apraxia

Show me how to use a

	Command	Imitation	With object
Hammer			
Key			
Screwdriver			

9. Ideational Apraxia. Show me how to

	command	Imitation
Brush your teeth		
Strike a match and blow it out		

Fig. 9.4 (continued)

fingers with one hand and one finger with the other hand to each visual hemi-field and quadrant field. The patient should respond with the total number of fingers shown indicating appropriate perception in all tested visual fields. To confirm a request, fingers from both hands can be presented in the same visual field and should assure perceptual skills in a unilateral visual field. If neglect is present, similar further presentation can be done in the upper and lower visual field quadrants (both unilaterally and bilaterally) to discern a quadrant inattention or neglect. Visual scanning can be readily assessed by drawing letters at various orientations on a page in a random array. The patient is asked to cross off all of a specific letter and the examiner notes any items that are omitted and the side or quadrant in which these items are omitted. Similarly, patients can be shown horizontal lines in a random array on a sheet of paper and asked to draw a vertical line that bisects each horizontal line as close to the middle as possible. Patients should not distort or bias their responses consistently to the left or right.

Visual recognition and facial perception can be assessed quickly by asking patients to recognize and name objects and individuals in that environment. The examiner can carry pictures of common objects or famous people with them and ask for identifications to be made. Common objects may include phones, watches, cups, pens/pencils or books/magazines. Faces can include family members or well-known cultural figures, although identification of cultural figures varies considerably among individuals depending on age, gender and exposure to presented cultural icons.

Visual form recognition, drawing and visual synthesis skills can be assessed by showing patients common objects which have been drawn as separate parts and asking them to tell what that object would be if the parts were mentally rotated and assembled into a single object. Common objects may include cross or addition sign, square or circle. In addition, patients should be asked to copy and draw objects which require appropriate relational elements both in size, shape and elements within the object. For example, patients can be asked to copy a simple house and their copying should include a roof, chimney, walls, window and door in correct proportion and relation to each other. The patient can also be asked to draw an analog clock and put all the numbers in their correct positions. To assess further their ability to plan, they can be asked to place hands on the clock to represent a specific time. It is common for patients to be asked to set the hands so that the clock reads 11:10. Evaluation of patients performance can be judged not only on the correct position of the numbers, but the patient's understanding of the need to draw hands pointing at 11 and 2 in representing 11:10. The patient's ability to draw complex designs can be assessed by asking them to copy a three-dimensional drawing of a cube. Patients should be able to copy such a design if shown an example.

Laboratory (Outpatient) Neuropsychological Assessments

More thorough assessment of visual spatial and visual constructional tasks can (and should in many cases) be routinely completed. Common measures of visuoconstructional skills are the Wechsler Scales Block Design subtest and/or drawing a complex geometric figure such as the Rey-Osterrieth Complex figure, the Taylor complex figure or the Medical College of Georgia Complex Figures (see Lezak et al. 2004, for review). Figure 9.5 demonstrates a normal drawing of the Rey-Osterrieth Complex Figure along with drawings from patients with a left parietal lesion and a right parietal lesion, respectively. Note the patient with the left parietal lesion ability to preserve the overall design gestalt (the general features or shape is maintained), but the approach is simplistic and piecemeal approach to the task which has resulted in poor integration of sections and

Complex Figure Drawing

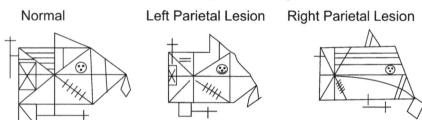

Normal   Left Parietal Lesion   Right Parietal Lesion

Fig. 9.5 Example of (**a**) normal drawing of Rey-Osterreith Complex Figure, and than copy by (**b**) a patient with left parietal lesion and by (**c**) a patient with a right parietal lesion

lack of details. Alternatively, the patient with the right parietal lesion exhibited left visual inattention (truncated left half of the figure) as well as an inability to synthesize and integrate the elements of the drawing suggesting perceptual deficits. These examples provide examples of post-acute left and right hemispheric constructional apraxic features. Namely, left hemisphere damage tends to result in maintained gestalt but simplistic designs, while patients with right hemisphere lesions tend to exhibit deficits in maintaining the gestalt of the figure (details without coherent organization).

References and Suggested Further Reading

Benton, A. L., Hannay, H. J., & Varney, N. R. (1975). Visual perception of line direction in patients with unilateral brain disease. *Neurology, 25*, 907–910. Reprinted in L. Costa & O. Spreen (Eds.) (1985). *Studies in neuropsychology*. Selected papers of Author Benton. New York: Oxford University Press.

Faustenau, P. S. (1996). Development and preliminary standardization of the "Extended Complex Figure Test" (ECFT). *Journal of Clinical and Experimental Neuropsychology, 18*, 63–76.

Gauthier, I., Skudlarski, P., Gore, J. C., & Anderson, A. W. (2000). Expertise for cars and birds recruits brain areas involved in face recognition. *Nature Neuroscience, 3*(2), 191–7.

Heilman, K., & Valenstein, E. (2003). *Clinical neuropsychology*. New York: Oxford University Press.

Hooper, H. E. (1983). *Hooper visual organization test manual*. Los Angeles: Western Psychological Services.

Hubley, A. M., & Tremlay, D. (2002). Comparability of total score performance on the Rey-Osterrieth Complex Figure and a modified Taylor Complex Figure. *Journal of Clinical and Experimental Neuropsychology, 24*, 370–382.

Kolb, B., & Whishaw, I. (2009). *Fundamentals of human neuropsychology* (5th ed.). New York: W.H. Freeman.

Lezak, M., Howieson, D., & Loring, D. (2004). *Neuropsychological Assessment,* (4th ed.) Oxford, New York.

Loring, D. W., & Meador, K. J. (2003). The Medical College of Georgia (MCG) Complex Figures: Four forms for follow-up. In J. Knight & E. Kaplan (Eds.), *Rey-Osterrieth handbook*. Odessa: Psychological Assessment Resources.

Taylor, L. B. (1979). Psychological assessment of neurosurgical patients. In T. Rasmussen & R. Marino (Eds.), *Functional neurosurgery*. New York: Raven.

Chapter 10
Frontal Lobe/Executive Functioning

James G. Scott and Mike R. Schoenberg

Abstract The frontal lobes represent a large area, consuming approximately one-third of the cortical surface of the brain. This area is involved directly and indirectly across a wide spectrum of human thought, behavior and emotions. The irony of the frontal lobes may best be described as the area of the brain we know the most about but understand the least. For example, frontal lobe functioning involves simple motor skills (both gross and fine), complex motor skills, sequenced motor skills, inhibition of motor skills and automatic motor skills, and these may be the simplest of the functions of the frontal lobes. The frontal lobes also subsume what is collectively referred to as executive skills. These functions include attention, reasoning, judgment, problem solving, creativity, emotional regulation, impulse control and awareness of aspects of one's and others' functioning. In this chapter, we will briefly discuss the anatomy of the frontal lobes, the basic and complex functions of the frontal lobes, and the informal assessment of frontal lobe functions.

> **Key Points and Chapter Summary**
>
> - Frontal lobes include a large area of the cortex and are involved directly or indirectly in most brain functions involving cognition, behavioral, and motor skills
> - Frontal lobe damage can have profound effects on attention, memory, language, problem solving/reasoning, and general comportment (personality/social behaviors, etc.)
> - Frontal lobe damage can be grouped into three syndromes determined by anatomical regions involved and associated with characteristic cognitive,

(continued)

J.G. Scott (✉)
Department of Psychiatry and Behavioral Sciences, University of Oklahoma
Health Sciences Center, Oklahoma City, OK, USA
e-mail: jim-scott@ouhsc.edu

M.R. Schoenberg and J.G. Scott (eds.), *The Little Black Book of Neuropsychology:*
A Syndrome-Based Approach, DOI 10.1007/978-0-387-76978-3_10,
© Springer Science+Business Media, LLC 2011

Key Points and Chapter Summary (continued)

> behavioral and/or mood symptoms: (1) Dorsolateral, (2) Orbitofrontal, and (3) Medial frontal syndromes
> - Behavioral and personality changes are often the most profound change seen in Frontal Lobe injuries and are not well measured by standardized tests
> - Cognition may be minimally impaired on standardized tests administered in controlled environments that minimize distraction and maximize motivation, particularly on tests which emphasize previously acquired knowledge

Anatomy of the Frontal Lobes

The frontal lobes represent the cerebral cortex anterior of the central sulcus, and accounts for 1/3 of the entire human neocortex, but represents more than a third of the cortical surface. The frontal lobe has been described in multitude of systems and areas, but we will review the frontal lobes in terms of basic functional organizations. The frontal lobes can be divided into three broad categories: (1) Primary motor cortex, (2) Premotor and supplementary motor cortex, and (3) Prefrontal cortex (see Figs. 10.1–10.3). The prefrontal cortex is often subdivided into three

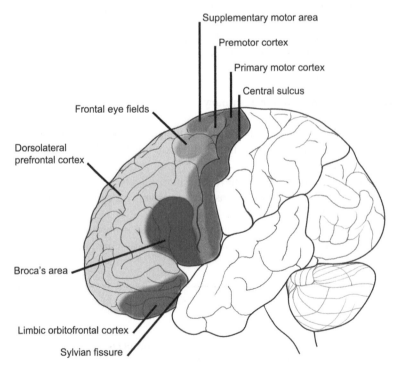

Fig. 10.1 Lateral view of the frontal lobe including primary motor, premotor, visual eye field, Broca's areas (Brodmann's area 44) and prefrontal region

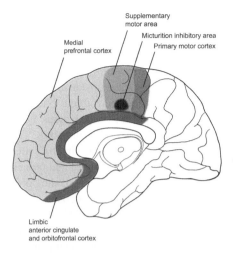

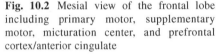

Fig. 10.2 Mesial view of the frontal lobe including primary motor, supplementary motor, micturation center, and prefrontal cortex/anterior cingulate

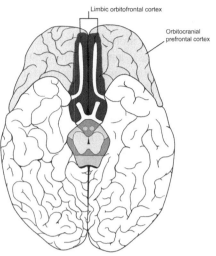

Fig. 10.3 Orbitofrontal (inferior frontal) view of the frontal lobe

functional domains, although some authors report two prefrontal functional domains. The three traditional prefrontal domains are: (a) dorsolateral prefrontal, (b) orbitofrontal (inferior or ventral frontal lobe), and (c) the medial frontal/anterior cingulate. The prefrontal cortex derived its name because this area of the frontal lobe received inputs (afferent fibers) from the dorsomedial nucleus of the thalamus. The prefrontal cortex also has extensive afferent and efferent connections to the temporal, parietal, and occipital lobes as well as reverberating (input and output) fibers to subcortical regions, including the basal ganglia, thalamus, hypothalamus, and tegmentum. The prefrontal projects to, but does not receive input from, the basal ganglia. Combined, the frontal lobe has classically been divided into six functional subdivisions (considering Broca's area, a separate subdivision of the premotor/supplementary area like the Frontal Eye Fields would yield seven subdivisions) (see Mesulam 2000; Salloway et al. 2001, for reviews):

1. Primary motor cortex
2. Premotor (supplementary) motor cortex
   (a) Broca's area
3. Frontal Eye Fields
4. Dorsolateral Frontal
5. Orbitofrontal (Inferior) Frontal
6. Medial frontal/anterior cingulate

Below, we will briefly review the functional neuroanatomy of each subdivision, and how lesions of the frontal lobes may present symptomatically within each functional area, and conclude with an overview of neuropsychological assessment for frontal lobe functions.

Primary Motor Cortex

The primary motor cortex is the most posterior aspect of the frontal lobes (pre-central gyrus), and contains a motor "humunuclus" representing a symatotopic representation of motor function for the contralateral body that is upside down (e.g., head towards the temporal lobe while the trunk is near the superior convexity and the legs are represented within the medial aspect of the pre-central gyrus lying within the interhemispheric fissure) (see Figs. 10.1, 10.2, 10.4, 10.5 and 10.6). The primary motor cortex is frequently termed the "motor strip" and is Brodmann's area 6. The primary motor cortex has efferent projections to the spinal cord and cranial nerve nuclei as well as the basal ganglia and red nuclei, forming part of the corticospinal or corticobulbar tracts, respectively. The initiation of the corticospinal and corticobulbar tracts is the premotor cortex (see below and Chap. 3). The primary motor cortex receives input from the premotor/supplementary motor cortex areas.

Lesions involving the primary motor cortex will result in contralateral motor weakness. Initially, the motor weakness may present as a flaccid hemiplegia (complete lack of motor strength), but strength will often recover to some extent, particularly if premotor and supplementary motor areas are preserved. Larger lesions may resolve into a spastic hemiparesis and smaller lesions may resolve into incoordination and mild hemiparesis which can be difficult to identify without careful examination.

Primary Facial Motor Cortex

The primary motor area involved in facial control (recall the upper part of the face is innervated bilaterally by the facial nerve) has some unique aspects summarized below. The primary motor cortex of the face is just superior to the perisylvian fissure and anterior to the central sulcus. Each hemisphere controls the contralateral half of the face (facial region above the eyes is controlled by both contralateral cortical and ipsilateral cranial nerve function). Focal damage to the language dominant (left) primary motor facial area is typically described as resulting in an expressive deficit (impaired receptive language but intact comprehension) thought to reflect an *oral apraxia*, along with contralateral hemiplegia of the lower face (Kolb and Whishaw 2009). The oral apraxia is the inability to coordinate the muscle movements necessary for speech production. Expressive speech deficits can also include agraphia (inability to write), thought to reflect damage to the closely situated supplementary area for fine motor movements of the hand. However, focal lesions can result in an initial global aphasia (impaired expressive and receptive speech). Patients with surgical removal of pre- and post-central gyrus involving the facial area have demonstrated recovery of facial expression usually within a month of surgery. However, recovery of speech is more gradual, and while speech production grossly recovers, more careful evaluation has revealed more profound residual impairments of generative verbal fluency, phonetic discrimination, spelling, and figural fluency. Remarkably, individuals with focal damage to the nondominant (right) primary facial motor cortex have exhibited chronic deficits in figural fluency to a greater extent than individuals with more extensive prefrontal nondominant (right) frontal damage. Deficits in verbal (and possibly figural) generative fluency might represent deficits in the motor preplanning needed for these tasks (Salloway et al. 2001).

Rule of thumb: Divisions of the frontal lobe

- Primary Motor
- Premotor/supplementary motor
  - Frontal Eye Fields
  - Broca's area
- Prefrontal
  - Dorsolateral
  - Orbitofrontal
  - Medial frontal/anterior cingulate

Premotor and Supplemental Motor

The premotor and supplemental motor cortex areas are involved in fine motor movements and sequenced motor movement such as writing or fastening buttons.

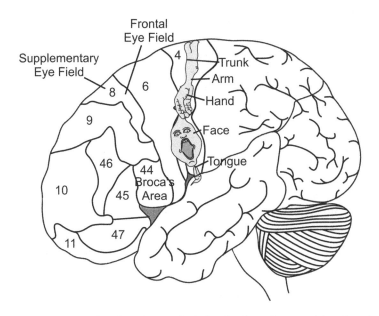

Fig. 10.4 Left dorsolateral prefrontal cortex including Brodmann's areas of dorsolateral cortex

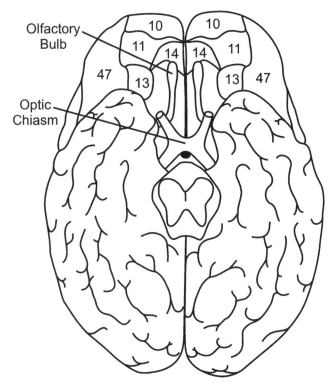

Fig. 10.5 Orbitofrontal/inferior frontal prefrontal cortex, including Brodmann's areas making up orbitofrontal areas

The premotor and supplementary motor cortices lie just anterior to the primary motor cortex, and includes Brodmann's areas 6 and 8. While many areas of the brain are involved in producing smooth, coordinated motor movements (i.e., the cerebellum and basal ganglia; see Chap. 3 for more details), the unique aspect of

---

Rule of thumb: Primary motor cortex

- Mediates contralateral Motor Movement
- Receives inputs from cerebellum, basal ganglia, supplemental motor cortex
- Projections form part of corticospinal and corticobulbar tracts
- Lesions produce contralateral motor weakness (hemiplegia or hemiparesis)
- Facial Primary Motor cortex is unique
  - Dominant hemisphere lesions cause expressive aphasia features (oral apraxia) with long-standing residual deficits in: generative verbal fluency, phonemic awareness, and spelling

the premotor/supplemental motor frontal cortex appears critical in two ways: (1) involved in acquiring novel motor skills which have not become overlearned, and (2) sequencing necessary motor movements. The premotor/supplementary area has projections directly to the cortico spinal and corticobulbar tracts, but *primarily* have connections to and from the basal ganglia. There are also projections to the primary motor cortex and thalamus. In addition to basal ganglia and thalamus, premotor and supplementary motor cortices receive input (afferent tracts) from the parietal and dorsolateral cortex. Thus, premotor and supplementary motor areas are able to execute complex motor actions and continually adjust and fine tune motor activity. Perhaps a simplistic example is the motor movement necessary for learning to ride a bicycle. Initially, it takes much more effort to focus on the conscious motor movements necessary for balance, propulsion and steering. This motor movement is not initially automatic, and the sequence of balance, pedal and steer is difficult to master and initially requires substantial prefrontal resources. With experience, these motor and sequencing aspects evolve into an automatic sequence of motor skills resulting in a complex behavior. As this occurs, the premotor cortex is less involved and other areas of the brain (cerebellum, parietal cortex) are more involved.

Lesions to the premotor and supplementary motor areas 6 (not involving the frontal eye fields, area 8) typically will result in motor apraxias of the contralateral body/limb, and not hemiparesis. Individuals will also have difficulty synthesizing sensory information into complex motor movements and complex motor sequencing will be incoordinated and may appear "choppy" or clumsy. However, simple motor movements remain fluid (not ataxic).

Broca's Area (Brodmann's Area 44 and 45)

Language production is also a function of the frontal lobes. For most individuals, the left lateral premotor area of the frontal lobe (i.e., Broca's area, Brodmann's area 44 and 45, see Chap. 3) controls expressive language. Lesions in this area can produce expressive aphasias or more subtle language impairment such as decreased verbal fluency and writing (see also Chaps. 7 and 16) or word-finding deficits (dysnomia). The right (nondominant) frontal lobe is less concerned with the actual production of speech, but rather contributes to expressive language *prosody* (see also Chaps. 7 and 16). Prosody refers to the vocal amplitude, tone and inflection that communicate nonsemantic meaning in vocal expressions such as emotion, questioning, confidence, lethargy, etc.

Lesions to Broca's area in the dominant hemisphere will result in loss of expressive speech. Depending upon the extent of damage, repetition may also be disrupted. Lesions to the nondominant hemisphere result in difficulties with expressive prosody (expressive aprosdy, see Chaps. 7 and 12 for details). Briefly, speech may sound monotone to others. Several different patterns of aphasia have been identified and extensively studied. These are reviewed in detail in Chap. 12, see also Chap. 7.

Rule of thumb: Pre-motor and supplementary cortex

- Anterior to primary motor cortex
- Beginning of the corticospinal and corticobulbar tracts
- Involved in production of complex movements and motor programming
- Connections with basal ganglia, parietal cortex, primary motor cortex, thalamus, and dorsolateral prefrontal cortex
- Lesions result in apraxias and discoordinated movement
- Broca's area, the expressive language center, in dominant hemisphere
- Frontal Eye fields involved in volitional eye movements and visual attention

---

Frontal Eye Fields

The premotor cortex also includes a region referred to as the frontal eye fields, which are involved in voluntary eye movements and fixation of gaze important for novel visually guided activities and visual attention. The frontal eye fields direct visual focus to central elements in an environment that allows us to successfully execute sequences of behaviors. The frontal eye fields (Brodmann's areas 8 and 8A) are anterior to the primary motor cortex. This area of supplementary motor cortex has afferent and efferent tracts to regions of the brain important for controlling eye movements, including the posterior parietal regions and the superior colliculus. As a simplistic act of dressing illustrates, one must first search out articles of clothing, locate each in space, plan motor movement to get each article, manipulate each article prior to putting it on and then successfully execute dressing, including fastening, buttoning and zipping. While many of these behaviors can become automatic through overlearning and repetition, the frontal eye fields must direct vision to each aspect for a successful behavior to be completed. Contrast this simple example with the visual demands in extracting or debulking a tumor located in the frontal lobe of a patient and you quickly become aware of the demands placed on the frontal eye fields every day.

Prefrontal Cortex (Dorsolateral, Orbitofrontal, and Medial Frontal/Cingulate Gyrus)

The Dorsolateral, Orbitofrontal (inferior or ventral frontal lobe) and Medial Frontal/Cingulate gyrus (anterior portion) areas compose the prefrontal cortex. The prefrontal cortex is comprised of Brodmann's areas 8, 9, 10, 44, 45, 46, and 47 on the lateral side, Brodmann's areas 10, 11, 12, 13, 14, and part of 45 on the ventral (inferior) side, and Brodmann's areas 8, 9, 10, 11, 13, and 32 on the mesial (medial) side (see Figs. 10.4–10.6, respectively). These areas have been

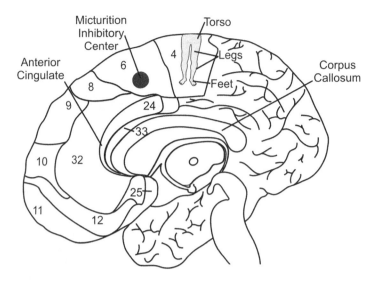

Fig. 10.6 Mesial frontal/anterior cingulate cortex including Brodmann's areas of the mesial frontal/anterior cingulate

subdivided into various regions, most commonly; the dorsolateral, orbitofrontal (inferior or ventral frontal lobe) and medial frontal/cingulate gyrus (anterior portion) areas. Another classification scheme involves the anterior prefrontal, medial prefrontal, and ventrolateral prefrontal regions. The roles and demarcations of these frontal lobe areas are less definitively agreed upon and more difficult to describe. Part of this difficulty arises from these functions being impaired or affected to differing degrees by injury to the frontal lobe cortex. These functions are often collectively referred to as "executive functions" and pertain to high level or complex aspects of cognitive, behavioral and emotional aspects of human behavior. These functions are necessarily complex and dependent on many regions of the brain. The proceeding description will necessarily be general and intended to give examples of the frontal lobe influences on these cognitive, behavioral and emotional aspects of frontal lobe functions. Table 10.1 summarizes the role of the frontal lobes.

Symptoms of Frontal Lobe Dysfunction: The "Frontal Lobe" Patient

It is not uncommon for a health care provider to mention "oh, that individual is pretty frontal" or "that individual has a frontal lobe syndrome". But what does that mean, and how is that determined? We will begin the behavioral syndrome review of frontal lobe disease with an overview of more generalized or diffuse prefrontal dysfunction

Table 10.1 Frontal lobe and executive functions

Domain	Region	Deficit
Motor	Left motor strip	Right gross, fine and coordination motor deficits
	Right motor strip	Left gross, fine and coordination deficits
	Left pre-motor	Poor contralateral sequencing and novel motor acquisition skills
	Right pre-motor	Poor contralateral sequencing and novel motor acquisition skills
	Frontal eye field	Contralateral voluntary eye movement/coordination
Cognitive	Diffuse frontal	Attentional deficits in sustained and voluntary alternation of attentional focus. Learning and retrieval.
	Posterior left frontal	Expressive language, naming, word finding, fluency
	Anterior left frontal	Verbal reasoning, verbal problem solving, sequencing, reduced generative verbal fluency
	Posterior right frontal	Expressive prosody
	Anterior right frontal	Visuospatial reasoning, visual problem solving, sequencing
Behavior/Emotional	Orbital frontal	Disinhibition, poor social skills, impulsivity, hyperactivity, emotional overreactivity.
	Dorsolateral frontal	Impaired problem solving, concrete, environmental dependency (stimulus bound behaviors), perseveration, poor sequencing, lack of self-monitoring for errors and self-correction. Impaired memory with reduced working memory, poor memory for temporal sequence of events, poor retrieval strategies with intact recognition.
	Medial frontal	Apathy, akinetic, mutism, leg weakness contralateral to lesion (may be bilateral). Abulia, apathy, socially disengaged, indifference, lack of initiation, emotionally underreactive with intermittent dysregulation.

and then turn to a description of selected "Frontal Lobe Syndromes." Table 10.1 summarizes the predominant roles of the frontal lobes and associated deficits.

Prefrontal Cortices (General/Diffuse Symptoms)

Many cognitive functions are mediated either directly or indirectly by the frontal lobes (dorsal lateral, medial, and orbital cortex) (see Kolb and Whishaw 2009; Lezak et al. 2004; Mesulam 2000; Salloway et al. 2001, for reviews). An overriding function involves many voluntary aspects of attention. Specifically, the ability to attend to relevant aspects of our environment and inhibit being distracted by incidental environmental stimuli is an important cognitive function of the frontal lobes. Failure of this function often has devastating results for individuals and usually is manifest as *tangentiality* or *circumloquaciousness* in language or distractibility in performing other tasks. The extent of the influence that voluntary attentional control can produce on other observed or measured skills should not be underestimated. In fact, voluntary attentional control is a prerequisite skill in everything from speaking to cooking and dressing. This function is frequently tested in terms of simple attention, sustained attention and voluntary rapid alternation of attention.

Environmental dependency (and *utilization behaviors*) can often be observed in patients with frontal lobe damage. Patients with environmental dependency respond in the usual way to a stimulus regardless of the appropriateness of the environmental situation. Environmentally bound behaviors can be initiated by an object, persons or situations. They may also be initiated by their own poorly inhibited thought processes. For example, patients may respond sexually to personnel who look at them and smile or respond angrily to personnel who make a request of them. Similarly, environmental cues such as the counter at a nursing station may solicit a patient to order auto parts because of its similarity to an auto parts store. Despite instruction not to shake an examiner's hand, this behavior can be elicited (hand shaking) by offering to shake the patient's hand. An internal trigger, such as a need to urinate, can elicit a patient to urinate in a potted plant. *Utilization behaviors* are a subtype of environmental dependency, and reflect the spontaneous use of an object without apparent need or desire. Examples of utilization behaviors can often be easily initiated by having a hairbrush, toothbrush, pen/pencil, comb, or cup/glass within reach of a patient with frontal lobe damage. Patients with utilization behaviors will, despite directions to not touch the items, reach out for the object(s) and begin using the object(s). For example, a patient may begin brushing his/her teeth without toothpaste or a sink or begin brushing his/her hair. Patients may "drink" from an empty cup or begin writing on a desk with a pen/pencil. These patients often demonstrate remorse for inappropriate behavior or verbal recognition of inappropriate behavior when their behavior is confronted, but will be unable to inhibit the behavior if the environmental trigger presents again.

Autonoetic awareness (Tulving 2002) is a term to describe self-awareness which has been defined as the autobiographical temporal continuum which is able to affect behavior through one's past personal experiences and goals. Patients with prefrontal damage in general, but particularly those with orbitofrontal damage, frequently exhibit deficits in autonoetic awareness (self-awareness) such that they have difficulty with self-regulation of behavior. Patients are unable to reference behaviors to past experiences or goals.

Memory functioning can be adversely affected by lesions of the prefrontal cortex. These are reviewed within each frontal lobe functional domain below. However, a hemispheric difference in memory functions involving frontal lobe regions has been identified and termed *Hemispheric Encoding and Retrieval Asymmetry* (HERA; see Tulving et al. 1994). This model posits the left prefrontal cortex is more involved during encoding of episodic and semantic memory material and less involved during retrieval. The right prefrontal cortex (and insula and parietal cortices) are thought to be more involved in retrieval of episodic memory material.

Paratonia (Gegenhalten) may be found with bilateral frontal lobe damage. Paratonia is presentation of increasing muscle tone to oppose efforts to passively move the limb by someone else. This can often be misinterpreted as purposeful noncompliance. Paratonia (gegenhalten) is load- and velocity-dependent resistance, and is outside the control of the patient. While it may be found following bilateral diffuse frontal lobe lesions, it can also be present following bilateral basal temporal lobe damage and more diffuse brain damage, including dementias and encephalopathies.

Several *neuropsychiatric syndromes* are associated with frontal lobe damage. *Personality changes* are commonly reported, particularly with orbitofrontal damage but also with dorsolateral or medial frontal damage (see below). Orbitofrontal personality changes are frequently described as overactive/manic, uncaring, narcissistic, and pleasure seeking. Commonly, these individuals are described as disinhibited and impulsive. Emotionally, patients generally have poor emotional regulation, but have a tendency to be overly reactive, in which their emotional response to a situation is often much greater than what might be anticipated or warranted. Individuals with orbito-frontal damage have also been labeled as *pseudopsychopathic* because of their personality changes noted above and apparent disregard for the feelings of others. Patients with dorsolateral or medial frontal damage may be perceived as indecisive, lazy, amotivated, apathetic, or passive. Some may be incorrectly described as "depressed." Indeed, the dorso-lateral syndrome has been referred to as *pseudo-depressive* or *apathetic* due to their appearance of indifference and abulia. Emotionally, patients with dorso-lateral damage tend to exhibit a propensity toward emotional underreactivity with variability or fluctuations when they do become emotionally engaged. Frequently, these individuals will exhibit emotional dysregulation that fluctuates from indifference to overreaction. Patients with mesial frontal damage also exhibit indifference, but exhibit more akinetic qualities, in which these patients may just sit motionless for hours and be potentially mute. These individuals have been incorrectly diagnosed as having catatonic schizophrenia. Other neuropsychiatric syndromes associated with frontal lobe damage include *reduplicative paramnesia* and *Capgras syn-*

drome. Reduplicative paramnesia is the delusion that a place or an object (clothes, furniture, house, food, etc.) has been exactly duplicated. Capgrass syndrome is the "imposter" delusion, such that the patient believes a person (or persons) has (have) been duplicated, and the person claiming to be the person is an imposter.

Finally, several frontal lobe reflexes (or release signs) normally present in infants are considered pathological in adult patients. While typically not present in adults, some of the reflexes may be present and the presence of one should not be interpreted as pathognomic of frontal lobe dysfunction. Among the reflexes, the grasp reflex is less often encountered in normal adults. If frontal release signs are present, there likely is frontal lobe dysfunction. The frontal release signs include: Glabbelar, Grasp, Palmomental, Root, Snout, and Suck reflexes which are briefly described:

- *Glabbelar reflex*. Failure to extinguish eye blink response to gentle tapping to the center of the forehead right above the nose.
- *Grasp reflex*. Perhaps the most helpful frontal release sign, as it is fairly specific of frontal lobe injury, and has localizing value to the contralateral supplementary motor area located in the medial frontal lobe. The grasp reflex occurs when the hand grasps onto an object (or examiner's finger). It is elicited by stroking the inside palm in a distal motion towards the base of the fingers. One may also stroke the proximal surface of the fingers (towards the palm). The grasp can be quite strong, allowing the person's torso to be lifted up from a lying position. Release may be voluntary or in some cases, takes considerable effort to release.
- *Palmomental reflex*. Ipsilateral contraction of the muscle of the chin (mentalis muscle) occurring to an unpleasant stimulus of the thenar eminence (body of the palm just proximal to the thumb). The ipsilateral corner of the mouth may also contract. The stimulus eliciting the reflex is started at the lower wrist and up the base of the thumb. The stimulus can be a tongue depressor or the handle of a reflex hammer.
- *Root reflex*. The turning of the patient's head ipsilateral to the side of the cheek that is lightly stroked. It is associated with the suck reflex in its adaptability for infants to breast feed.
- *Snout reflex*. The puckering of the lips to make a "snout" when the top lip is gently tapped (percussed). Typically, the Snout reflex can be elicited by gently tapping on the center of the upper lip when the lips are closed with your finger.

Rule of thumb: Frontal lobe reflexes

- Frontal Lobe Reflexes are normal in very young children and are suppressed through development
- Frontal Lobe reflexes are often seen in acute injuries or in severely impaired patients, but may not be seen in sub-acute populations or less severely impaired patients who continue to have cognitive, behavioral or motoric frontal lobe symptoms

- *Suck reflex.* Sucking movements of the lips when the lips are generally stroked or touched. The sucking movement can be elicited by stroking the upper or lower corners of the mouth.

Following a brief review of symptoms reflecting more generalized or diffuse dysfunction, we will review the traditional three prefrontal syndromes: (1) dorsolateral, (2) orbitofrontal, and (3) medial frontal. Another viewpoint that specifies two frontal lobe syndromes: (a) *syndrome of frontal abulia* and (b) *syndrome of frontal disinhibition* (e.g., Mesulam 2000) will be reviewed as well. The syndrome of frontal abulia has been associated with the dorsolateral frontal lobe syndrome while the syndrome of frontal disinhibition collapses the orbitofrontal and medial frontal syndromes together, as features of both are often observed in a patient (Mesulam 2000).

Rule of thumb: Frontal lobe syndromes

- Dorsolateral damage = dysexecutive syndrome also pseudodepressed syndrome
  - Poor problem solving, abulia/amotivational, perseverative, stimulus bound
- Orbitofrontal (inferior/ventral frontal) = Disinhibited/pseudopsychopathic syndrome
  - Disinhibited, emotional lability, impulsivity, lack of social graces, personality changes, poor smell discrimination
- Medial Frontal/Cingulate gyrus = akinetic/apathetic syndrome
  - Akinetic, amotivation, mute (if bilateral), leg weakness, urinary incontinence

---

Frontal Lobe Syndromes: Traditional Three (3) Syndrome Model

The three traditional frontal lobe regions have neuroanatomical connections to discrete areas of shared basal ganglia and thalamic nuclei structures. Each of the three systems have segregated tracts, but operate in parallel and have multiple areas where input and output of each region is directed to other parts of the prefrontal cortex and brain. The three systems are thought to process distinct cognitive and emotional information incorporating multiple sensory and motor information from other brain regions.

Dorsolateral Prefrontal (Dysexecutive or Frontal Convexity) Syndrome

Patients often appear distractible, apathetic and "depressed," but also have difficulty reasoning, problem solving, shifting attention, and maintaining a behavior for completion of a task (impersistence). Patients may exhibit environmental dependency and memory problems. The memory problems (detailed below) often reflect difficulty remembering the temporal sequence of when events occurred (as opposed to forgetting something occurred altogether). Learning rate is often slow, and the patient may not remember some things due to reduced working memory/attention but also reduced retrieval. Depending upon extent of lesion, motor weakness of the upper extremity contralateral to the lesion may be present.

Sequencing, problem solving and reasoning is impaired. The patient can have considerable difficulty with three-step motor sequencing along with sequencing figures or shapes (see Appendix). Problem solving and reasoning is concrete, but tends to be worse with divergent reasoning (reasoning that requires many possible solutions or answers) than convergent reasoning (drawing similarities or solutions from two or more things). For example, patients would have problems listing the uses for a brick. Besides the obvious use for construction, other uses might include a door stop, stepping stones, hammer, a paper weight, an exercise tool, etc. While many frontal lobe patients have difficulty with divergent reasoning, fewer problems may be found on the convergent reasoning tasks on many intelligence tests. Patients with dorsolateral damage have difficulty solving problems that require sequential steps for problem resolution. Failure reflects difficulty selecting the series of appropriate steps to reach a problem resolution. Their responses in such situations are often simplistic and fail to appreciate the complexities involved in the situation. For example, a patient discovering his/her refrigerator has quit working may recognize the need to have it repaired, but will not spontaneously appreciate the need to use, relocate or otherwise dispose of the contents. The patient will, however, answer correctly when prompted about the contents.

Insight and judgment is often poor. Individuals typically do not appreciate the depth or extent of their cognitive compromises. While patients are able to appreciate or recognize direct failure, they have a diminished capacity to appreciate the degree or extent of their deficits and anticipate the impact it is likely to have on their future performance despite previous failure. This often leads to an astonishing repetition of attempts and failures that are resistant to making adjustments to future attempts. They may exhibit perseveration or difficulty switching sets when they become engaged. Alternatively, persistence in completing a task (particularly one they are not interested in for themselves) can be reduced, especially when distracters are present in the environment. As an example, a patient spouse may say the patient will start a task if asked, but will get easily distracted and will not finish the task unless repeated requests and redirection to complete the task is given. Patients often exhibit environmental dependency. Verbal output is often reduced, and phrase length is typically shorter.

Memory can be worsened due to the disruption of several systems involved in learning and memory. First, working memory may be reduced and the patient more distractable. Working memory reflects two general processes, the maintenance of information in an attentional "store" and, the ability to manipulate this "online" material. Second, strategies for active learning and efficient encoding and retrieval may be disrupted. Third, memory for facts or events may be out of temporal sequence. Memory encoding of unrelated material is often poor, exhibiting a reduced learning curve. Spontaneous recall is often impaired, particularly for material not semantically (contextually) organized. Alternatively, encoding of material provided to the patient already semantically (contextually) organized that makes sense to the patient can improve encoding and retrieval. Recognition cues often improves recall. However, the temporal organization of memory is also frequently disrupted. Thus, patients may remember something happening a month ago as occurring yesterday. While the recall of events and situations may be perfectly reasonable, review of the patient's medical chart and/or report from a reliable collateral informant (spouse, adult child, friend, etc.) will quickly identify the poor temporal organization of memory.

Patients frequently appear to be emotionally blunted, apathetic, and abulic (hence the term "pseudodepressed"). However, when emotionally aroused, patients often exhibit difficulty regulating emotional expression, appearing to both over- and underreact to various situations. Patients will not be as behaviorally disinhibited as patients with orbito-frontal syndrome, they demonstrate attentional and initiation deficits that are no less impairing.

This presentation may reflect the dorsolateral (dysexecutive or frontal convexity) syndrome. Because of prominent deficits in problem solving, reasoning, and switching sets, this is known as the Dysexecutive syndrome. It has also been termed the pseudo-depressed syndrome due to patients often exhibiting apathy and abulia.

Anatomy: The dorsolateral cortex is anterior to the premotor and supplementary cortices and is also termed the frontal convexities, and includes Brodmann's areas 9 and 46 (see Fig. 10.4). Some also include the lateral aspects of Brodmann's area 10 (the anterior prefrontal or frontopolar region). This area of the cortex predominately has reciprocal projections from the posterior parietal and superior temporal sulcus. The dorsolateral prefrontal area also projects to the basal ganglia, thalamus, cingulate gyrus, and superior colliculus. The dorsolateral frontal region projects to the dorsolateral caudate nucleus which projects to the lateral and medial globus pallidus, which projects to the dorsomedial and ventral anterior thalamic nuclei and back to the prefrontal cortex. Note the dorsolateral cortex does not receive inputs from the striatum directly, but rather projections from the thalamus. The dorsolateral prefrontal areas are involved in complex human cognitive and behavioral func-

---

Rule of thumb: Dorsolateral frontal lobe damage = Dysexecutive syndrome

- Poor problem solving (concrete and rigid)
- Poor organizational strategies
- Impaired set-shifting, perseveration, and impersistence
- Memory may be disrupted
  - Reduced working memory, encoding/retrieval strategies, and temporal organization (order). Retrieval improved with recognition cues.
- Apathy and psychomotor slowing. Poor motivation/Abulia
- Decreased emotional range. May appear uncaring or emotionally unresponsive
- Contralateral upper extremity weakness

tions for making decisions, problem solving, sequencing and organizing behaviors. It is also associated with some attention and memory functions.

Causes of damage to the dorsolateral cortex are often the result of blunt trauma, occlusion of the anterior branch of the middle cerebral artery (or hemorrhage of ACA or MCA affecting the frontal convexities) and some neurodegenerative diseases (frontotemporal dementias). Frontal lobe tumors may also affect this area.

Orbitofrontal (Disinhibited/Pseudopsychopathy) Syndrome

Patients with lesions differentially affecting the orbitofrontal (the inferior or ventral surface of the frontal lobe) region will appear disorganized, behaviorally disinhibited, impulsive and overactive and often display emotional dysregulation. These individuals often demonstrate impulsivity and poor inhibition of behavior including inappropriate sexual behavior, inability to inhibit verbal outbursts and socially improper behavior. These individuals appear to have little empathy for others and will say and do things which may (at worst) appear purposeful efforts to hurt the feelings of others and (at best) appear uncaring. Patients may start new (or re-initiate) bad habits or addictive behaviors (e.g., start smoking, drinking, gambling) and may break social rules and norms to attain desired reinforcers. Work has found a functional distinction between the lateral and medial orbitofrontal areas. Lateral orbitofrontal regions are associated with the evaluation of punishment which leads to changes in behavior. Medial orbitofrontal regions are associated with the evaluation of reinforcers (primary or secondary) including the learning and memory for the reward value of reinforcers. In addition, a posterior and anterior distinction has also been made, such that the anterior orbitofrontal area is more involved in evaluation of more complex (secondary) reinforcers (such as money, social recognition, etc.) whereas the posterior orbitofrontal regions are more associated with primary reinforcers (e.g., gustatory).

Patients with orbitofrontal damage often exhibit poor judgment, and their behaviors are often governed by seeking reinforcers (often to extremes) and faulty reasoning initiated by environmental cues such as an object, person or situation. They may also be initiated by their own poorly inhibited thought processes. For example, patients may respond sexually to personnel who look at them and smile or respond angrily to personnel who make a request of them. Similarly, environmental cues such as the counter at a nursing station may solicit an orbitofrontal (disinhibited syndrome) patient to order auto parts because of its similarity to an auto parts store. These patients often demonstrate remorse for inappropriate behavior or verbal recognition of inappropriate behavior when their behavior is confronted. They tend to be hyperverbal and have difficulty with sustained attention. These individuals have little insight into how their behavior may affect others. These individuals may freely urinate in public or walk into other people's house to use the restroom, or to get desired things such as food, drugs, or money.

Memory functions are *not* consistently disrupted with lesions restricted to the orbitofrontal area. However, memory is often disrupted *if* damage includes the basal forebrain structures/septum, such that patients exhibit a classically described dense amnesia (Irle et al. 1992; Zola-Morgan and Squire 1993). Thus, damage restricted to the orbitofrontal region does *not* produce traditional memory impairment, which occurs when basal forebrain/septal structures are involved (Irle et al. 1992; Zola-Morgan and Squire 1993). The amnesia occurring with septal damage includes both antegrade as well as a temporally graded retrograde amnesia (see Chap. 9). Encoding is reduced due to poor attention. Learning rate is often deficient with a flat learning curve. Episodic memory is generally impaired, but recall of various events may appear (incorrectly) to be quite vivid reflecting confabulation. This confabulation does not appear to be a purposeful attempt to deceive, and is outside the person's awareness. That is, the examiner should not believe he/she has been purposely deceived by a patient with basal forebrain/septal damage.

Patients with lesions restricted to the orbitofrontal regions may perform normally on most traditional neuropsychological tests. Frequently, behavioral observation and report from reliable informants can provide needed information. However, patients do exhibit more risk-taking behaviors, are less likely to adjust their behavior to feedback, and perform poorly on tasks of behavioral disinhibition/emotional regulation (e.g., Frontal Systems Behavior Scale; FrSBe, Grace and Malloy 2001) and modulation of reward-related behaviors (i.e., Iowa Gambling test; Bechara et al. 2000).

The orbitofrontal area (and superior temporal sulcus) is important when individuals make judgments about others' personality characteristics based on their physical characteristics (Winston et al. 2002). Patients with ventral medial (orbitofrontal) lesions (right more than left) have difficulty appreciating deception (Stuss et al. 2001; Rowe et al. 2001).

Emotionally, patients with orbitofrontal dysfunction may exhibit difficulty regulating emotional expression when emotionally aroused and appear to overreact emotionally at various times. Individuals may present with a "hollow" jocularity termed *Witzelsucht*. This presents as an inappropriate humor and/or laughing, often with the patient making inappropriate jokes about self or others. Another common feature of the orbitofrontal syndrome is *anosmia* (or, more correctly, lack of smell discrimination). Because patients often exhibit disinhibition, impulsivity, hyperactivity, lack of insight or empathy for others, emotional lability, and distractability, predominant damage to the orbitofrontal cortex has been called the disinhibited or pseudopsychopathic syndrome.

Anatomy: The orbitofrontal lobe (i.e., the entire ventral or inferior surface of the frontal lobes) incorporates Brodmann's areas 10, 11, 12, 13, and 14, and has been further subdivided into several specific functional regions termed the lateral and medial orbitofrontal areas (see Fig. 10.5). The orbitofrontal area is very complex, and has connections with areas throughout the brain including all sensory modalities as well as limbic structures. The main connections are from the temporal lobe (superior temporal cortex, inferior temporal cortex, and amygdala) as well as parietal lobe (somatosensory cortex), insula (gustatory cortex), and pyriform (olfactory) cortex. There are also connections to the medial temporal lobe structures, cingulate gyrus, thalamus (medial dorsal and intralaminar nuclei), and hypothalamus. Projections of the orbitofrontal area to the hypothalamus and amygdala allow this area to influence the autonomic nervous system. The orbitofrontal area is implicated in a vast array of cognitive, emotional, and somatosensory functions, such as behavioral inhibition, emotional regulation, social cognition, memory, and smell discrimination (Frith and Frith 2003; Lezak et al. 2004; Mesulam 2000; Siegal and Varley 2002). Social cognition is an important aspect of behavior, allowing one to interact in complex social networks. An important aspect to social cognition is the ability to appreciate or attribute the mental perspectives to other people, termed *Theory of Mind* (ToM) (Frith and Frith 2003; Siegal and Varley 2002; Stuss et al. 2001). Neuroanatomic organization for ToM has been purported to involve amygdala, temporo-parietal junction, orbitofrontal, and medial frontal regions. While theory of mind (appreciate mental perspectives of others) was thought to be particularly mediated by medial frontal function (e.g., Frith and Frith 2003; Siegal and Varley 2002), other data argue the medial frontal lobes are not involved (Bird et al. 2004). We include social cognition and appreciation of others' mental function here, rather than medial frontal lobe (below), because some recent data do not support the involvement of the medial frontal lobe.

Lesions to the orbitofrontal area is often *not* limited to one focal area, but rather the typical causes of damage to the orbitofrontal area tends to result in diffuse damage to the inferior and ventral frontal lobe areas. The subcortical basal forebrain as well as the medial frontal lobe areas can also be affected. Thus, patients may also present with features of the medial frontal (akinetic-apathetic) syndrome detailed below. Damage is often caused by acceleration-deceleration closed head traumatic brain injuries (which often also affect the anterior temporal lobes as well), neurodegenerative diseases (frontotemporal dementias), brain tumor, and/or hemorrhagic stroke of an aneurysm of the ACoA (anterior communicating artery) or an ACA (anterior cerebral artery).

Rule of thumb: Orbitofrontal (inferior/ventral) Frontal lobe damage = Disinhibited or psycheduopsychopathic syndrome

- Disinhibited
  - Hyperactive, intrusive, pressured behavior
- Poor impulse control
  - Loss of social insight, poor situational awareness
- Distractible
  - Focus on single thing and unable to selectively guide attention away from competing stimuli
- Emotional lability/emotional dysregulation
  - Septal/basal forebrain damage can result in amnesia with confabulation

Medial Frontal (Akinetic/Apathetic) Syndrome

Patient symptoms of medial frontal lobe damage often include akinesia, lethargy, not spontaneously initiating behavior, and can appear indifferent to painful stimuli. Memory can be severely disrupted, with a dense antegrade amnesia. Bilateral lesions can result in an akinetic and mute state. Unilateral lesions often result in an incomplete akinetic state, with the patient regaining some self-initiated behaviors. Left medial frontal lesions affecting the anterior cingulate can present with features of a transcortical motor aphasia. Patients with medial frontal lesions often lack insight or awareness and frequently are described as having decreased arousal in general. These patients will often not initiate behavior or speech themselves. In some cases, these patients will be observed to remain in postures likely to be extremely uncomfortable for prolonged periods without complaint or attempt to change positions. Urinary and bowel incontinence can be present, and patients exhibit little concern about the incontinence, making little effort to clean themselves unless given prompt(s).

Memory functions can be severely disrupted (e.g., Bird et al. 2004), reflecting damage to septal region/basal forebrain structures sometimes affected by more extensive orbitofrontal lesions. Memory impairment associated with medial frontal (akinetic-apathetic) syndrome is an amnesia with antegrade as well as a temporally graded retrograde amnesia (see Chap. 8). Encoding is poor and the patient often exhibits a flat learning curve. Episodic memory is generally impaired. Some semantic and nondeclarative memory may be intact. Confabulation is frequently present. Like confabulation associated with more extensive orbitofrontal damage, confabulation is not purposeful, and lacks intent to purposefully deceive the examiner.

Patients with mesial frontal/anterior cingulated damage often demonstrate restricted emotional responses and appear disengaged from their environment. Individuals may exhibit little (no) interest in family or friends, exhibiting indifference and apparent lack of concern. Generally, patients will appear dull and unmotivated, but may respond if requested to perform specific behaviors. Patients may exhibit lower extremity weakness contralateral to the side of the lesion (bilateral leg weakness if damage was bilateral). If the corpus callosum is damaged, the patient may also exhibit the so-called alien hand syndrome if the dominant hemisphere is affected. The left extremities may not be under the volitional control of the patient, and the left hand may reach for objects and/or explore the immediate environment outside the apparent control of the patient.

Anatomy: The medial frontal cortex includes the cortex between the two frontal hemispheres, anterior to the primary motor strip, which includes the anterior portion of the cingulate gyrus and includes Brodmann's areas 24, 25, and 32 (see Fig. 10.6). This area of the cortex has connections with the temporal cortices, particularly the amygdala (anterior cingulate) and hippocampus (more posterior cingulated) along with the hypothalamus. Reciprocal connections are with lateral prefrontal cortex (Brodmann's areas 8,9,10, and 46), orbitofrontal cortex (Brodmann's area 47), parahippocampal gyrus, amygdala, insula, and claustrum. Afferent projects are from entorhinal and perirhinal cortex and hippocampus, thalamus, and tegmentum. Projections are also to substantia nigra pars compacta, subthalamic nucleus, hypothalamus, globus pallidus, and thalamus. This area of the brain is implicated in attention, behavioral inhibition, initiation and motivation, motor function (lower extremities), social cognition, including theory of mind, memory, mood, and autonomic (visceral) systems (e.g., Frith and Frith 2003; Lezak et al. 2004; Mesulam 2000: Siegal and Varley 2002; Stuss et al. 2001).

Rule of thumb: Medial frontal lobe damage = Akinetic/apathetic syndrome

- Akinetic and apathetic
- Little initiation of movement or speech
- Lack of interest and indifference
- Emotional blunting
- Memory can be impaired (amnesia with confabulation)
- Incontinence (bladder and sometimes bowel)
- Leg weakness

Prefrontal Syndromes: Two Syndromic Model

Below, we briefly review a two-syndromic model of prefrontal syndromes: (1) syndrome of frontal abulia and (2) syndrome of frontal disinhibition (e.g., Mesulam 2000).

(a) *Syndrome of Frontal Abulia.* This syndrome description is the same for that of the dorsolateral frontal lobe syndrome. Generally, patients exhibit poor problem solving, concrete reasoning, stimulus bound behaviors, lack of creativity, reduced (or no) initiative, apathy, and emotional blunting. Patients have difficulty planning and sequencing activities and exhibit deficits in strategic decision making in light of anticipated consequences for making various decisions.

(b) *Syndrome of Frontal Disinhibition.* This syndrome description reflects the fact that frontal lobe damage to the orbitofrontal area often also involves some aspects of the medial frontal lobe and basal forebrain, resulting in a general pattern of behavioral disinhibition, behavioral impulsivity, lack of judgment, reduced insight and foresight, and inability to delay gratification. Like orbitofrontal syndrome patients, the syndrome of frontal disinhibition may also include increased energy level and emotional reactivity. The individual's sleep–wake cycle can be disrupted, and they may not exhibit remorse for their behavior.

Bedside Assessment of Frontal Lobe Functions

General Assessment Issues

Frontal lobe damage can produce a range of deficits from subtle to grossly overt. The complexity of the frontal lobe involvement in many tasks both directly and indirectly means that their effect cannot only run the gamut from noticeable only to those who knew the patient well, to obvious to everyone in the environment but can also include functions which have an impact on other cognitive areas. For example, impairment in frontal lobes can produce simple, sustained and complex voluntary attention deficits which in turn have a discernable impact on seemingly unrelated tasks as object naming, copying a geometric figure or holding a conversation without becoming tangential or circumloquacious.

Assessment of frontal lobe functioning begins with good history taking and includes queries of both the patient and someone else who knows them well such as a parent, spouse, relative or friend. The content of this interview should include an assessment of changes in the cognitive, behavioral, and emotional functioning noted previously in this chapter. This discussion should inquire directly about change in these areas as there is considerable naturally occurring variability in behavior, cognition and emotional expressiveness across individuals. Table 10.2 outlines areas of inquiring for frontal lobe assessment. It is important to gain collateral information on these functions, as patient awareness of the existence or extent of the change in these areas of functioning is frequently diminished. If changes are noted, it is often helpful to try to establish an estimate of how much change has occurred and the frequency with which it occurs. It may be informative to ask both patients and collateral informants to give an estimate of current performance using 100% as a baseline and estimating the current level of functioning relative to that baseline. When using this table, we ask patients and a caregiver to rate how much change (percent) has occurred in the areas noted in Table 10.2, and this is written down in the column "Frequency/ Duration/Severity." This may also highlight the discrepancy between the patient's perception of change and the perceptions of others who know them well.

In addition to a history of change, many of the functions of frontal lobe deficits can be assessed bedside or informally in the outpatient clinic. While these techniques can yield important information, these functions can also be more precisely measured through formal, standardized, psychometrically evaluated means. The informal assessment of frontal lobe functions can often lead to the decision for referral or further formal assessment of frontal lobe functions identified or suspected to be impaired in the brief examination. Table 10.3 gives some examples of areas of assessment and assessment items.

Motor and Sequencing Skills

Patients with frontal lobe damage often have difficulty with fine motor skills and sequencing motor skills. They may exhibit difficulty both with tasks requiring

Table 10.2 Interview assessment of Frontal Lobe changes

Area	Change	Frequency/duration/severity[a]
Activity/energy	Hypoactive	
	Hyperactive	
Initiation	Hypo initiative (Abulic)	
	Disinhibited	
Social function	Decreased social skill	
	Social imperturbability	
	Social avoidance	
	Social disinhibition	
Emotional responsiveness	Overreactive	
	Underreactive	
	Rapidly variable	
Attention	Poor sustained attention	
	Difficulty switching attention	
	Perseveration	
Language	Disorganized	
	Unresponsive to questions asked	
	Lapses from attentional difficulty	
Memory	Increased variability/inconsistency	
	Poor detail recall	
	Difficulty with temporal order in recall	
Reasoning/sequencing	Difficulty sequencing tasks such as cooking, repair, or other frequent activities	
	Concrete understanding, inability to see from others perspective	
	Knows conceptually, but cannot problem-solve the solution, step or steps to resolve novel problem	

[a]Column can be used as part of a working guide to note (write down) extent of change in domains listed. We have used percentile change, ranging from no change (around zero%) to total change (100%) change in that function/behavior. In some situations, it may be appropriate to not ask percent change, but rather a qualitative description, such as "no, small, medium, or large" change in function has occurred

sustained rapid motor responses as well as sequenced, novel motor skills. Patients may also have difficulty with simple sequencing tasks, exhibiting perseveration. Patients can be asked to rapidly tap their thumb and index finger. They should be instructed to perform this after being shown the examiner performing the task. Observations should be made regarding their ability to sustain their fine motor speed for 15 seconds to ensure that there is no gross slowing or increasing rigidity as indicated by progressively smaller taps. A second task is to ask them to perform a novel three-step sequenced task (Luria's manual sequencing task) after being shown through modeling. In this case the examiner places his hand on a table first making a fist, then with palm flat (slap), then on the side (i.e., Karate chop). Figure 10.7 illustrates these movements. The patient is asked to mimic this "fist–palm–side" sequenced movement. After success or failure with one hand, the other hand should be tested. While it is not unusual for some patients (especially elderly) to require repeated modeling to acquire the appropriate sequence, if more than two trials are necessary, a sequencing deficit should be suspected. The patient should be able to complete three complete motor sequences without error.

Rapid motor sequencing can be assessed by asking patients to rapidly alternate hands from palm up to palm down. The examiner asks the patient to observe him (the examiner) doing the task and then requests that the patient mimic the task. The examiner places both hands down on a surface (typically a table or top of legs if seated) and then alternatingly lifts and rotates each hand to be palm up and then palm down. Each hand is rotated palm up and palm down and then the alternate hand is rotated. The alternate rotating is then increased in speed and should be sustained in rapid succession for 10–15 seconds. Patients should be expected to master the sequence of movements rapidly (one or two modeling trials) and be able to sustain the sequence for the duration of the task. If patients have difficulty, the examiner may try to teach the task by adding the verbal label, "all the way over, all the way back," to their demonstration to gauge if verbal cueing or prompting assists in acquiring or maintaining the task performance. If labeling the examiner's modeling of the behavior is unsuccessful, the examiner can take the patient's hands and rotate them and verbalize, "all the way over, all the way back," to see if kinetic cueing is effective in allowing them to master the task. In general, patients are expected to be able to rapidly master the task after being shown a demonstration. Failure to be able to perform rapid alternation or sustain rapid alternations over a 10- to 15-seconds timeframe should be considered an abnormal performance and reason for further psychometric investigation.

Rule of thumb: Bedside assessment

- Assess sustained attention with and without distraction
- Assess impulse control by conflicting verbal and behavioral gesture (i.e. say "Don't shake my hand" while simultaneously extending the hand)
- Assess perseveration by using repeating drawings such as loops or Ramparts
- Assess sequencing by asking patient to repeat three-step sequence or rapidly alternate hand movements

---

Perseveration and deficits in set-shifting may also be identified in having patients complete an alternating sequence such as ramparts (see Fig. 10.7) running half-way across the page. Frontal lobe patients often fail to alternate between rectangle and triangle (often with the patient perseverating making linked triangles or linked rectangles only). Similarly, an alternating pattern of cursive "m"s and "n"s can be used to elicit perseveration in frontal lobe patients (see Fig. 10.7). The patient is asked to complete the pattern, beginning where the examiner stopped. The task is evaluated based on the patient's ability to appropriately alternate and not repeat "m" or "n". A final task is for the examiner to draw (outside of the examinee's vision) a series of large figures with 3 loops each. The patient is asked to

Bedside Tests for Frontal Lobe Dysfunction

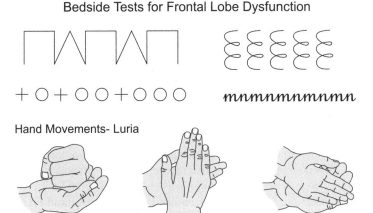

Hand Movements- Luria

Fig. 10.7 Luria's figures and sequencing tasks. Figures from left to right include ramparts, repeating loops, alternating +'s with increasing O's and alternating cursive M's and N's

complete making the looped figures until reaching the end of the page. Failure reflects having more or less than exactly three loops making up each of the figures. It is not unusual for patients with frontal lobe damage to make the figures with successively more loops (see Fig. 10.7).

Assessing Attention. Multiple aspects of attention can be impaired in frontal lobe patients (see also Chap. 6). They may have difficulty with simply attending to relevant stimuli in their environment without distraction, sustaining attention over time or in tasks which require them to switch voluntary attention rapidly. Simple attention can be evaluated by asking them to watch your finger as you move it slowly back and forth horizontally. They should be informed to keep their head still and track the examiner's finger with their eyes. This should be sustained for 15 seconds. The examiner can then add distraction to the task by prompting a discussion or purposefully diverting their gaze away from the patient. If the patient fails to maintain their voluntary gaze on the examiner's finger under either circumstance, the instructions can be repeated that the examiner wants them to maintain attention on the moving finger no matter what distractions are present. Patients with frontal lobe damage will often demonstrate difficulty with persistent voluntary attention and either lose attention to the task or have difficulty sustaining attention when confronted with verbal or visual competing stimuli in their environment.

Assessing Impulsivity/Disinhibition. The ability to initiate or inhibit a behavior is integrally linked to frontal lobe integrity. Patients with frontal lobe injuries often demonstrate changes in their ability to spontaneously initiate appropriate behavior or inhibit the enacting of overlearned or high frequency behavior. These deficits are most frequently observed early in the course of traumatic or acute injuries and progressively worsen in degenerative diseases involving the frontal lobes. These behaviors can be tested in examination of the patient in several ways. Perhaps the easiest way is to use contradictory verbal commands and physical gesture. In such a circumstance, the examiner would tell the patient not to take an object or shake a hand that is offered. This is typically done by offering an object to the patient such as a pen, cup, or paper while simultaneously telling them, "Don't take this." A patient who spontaneously takes the object should be asked to repeat what the instructions were and then given a second trial. Failure on a second trial would indicate difficulty with inhibiting the behavior. A second task which emphasizes a more subtle disinhibition is referred to as the *go–no-go* task. In this task, the examiner first instructs the patient to hold up one finger when the examiner holds up one finger and hold up two fingers when the examiner holds up two fingers (checking for cooperation and sufficient motor/sensory function). Complete a minimum of two trials in random order of holding up one and then two fingers. Once this is mastered, the examiner then instructs patients to hold up two fingers when the examiner holds up one finger, and to display one finger when the examiner displays two fingers. The examiner displays alternating one and two fingers increasingly rapidly. The patient is evaluated on accuracy of their responses, the consistency of accuracy (i.e., can they maintain response set), how quickly they respond (should be decreasing delay as task is learned), and their spontaneous recognition and correction of errors. Once their responses have stabilized with several correct responses, the examiner randomly alternates holding up one or two fingers and assesses the patient's ability to respond correctly. This sequence of trials should include at least one series in which the same number of fingers is held up repeatedly to allow a habitual response to be established from the patient, at which point the number of fingers displayed by the examiner is switched and the patient's ability to suppress what had become an overlearned response can be gauged. To establish this overlearned response, four to five trials with display of the same number of fingers by the examiner are typically required. Patients are typically expected to make some errors early in learning this task, but quick mastery is expected. Rapid recognition and correction of errors is expected.

Abstract Reasoning. Both verbal and nonverbal abstract reasoning can be impaired by frontal lobe injury. These patients tend to have greatest difficulty with divergent abstract reasoning tasks compared to relatively intact convergent reasoning. The conceptual difference between the two being the increased demand in divergent reasoning tasks to escape a single, sometimes concrete (right/wrong) answer of convergent reasoning and attempt to enact creative, multi-solution divergent solutions to a stated problem. Verbally, patients can be asked to list the similarities of a set of things and then be asked to list their differences. Both the similarities and differences should demonstrate an understanding of multiple ways the two are similar and different. The examiner can prompt for the other ways the objects are similar or different but should not provide answers. Examples that can be used may include a dog and a wolf, a shark and a whale, a house of representatives and a senate, a house and a hotel (see Table 10.3). The patient should be able to give 2–3 ways each pair is similar and different and be evaluated based on the quantity of responses, organization of responses and the quality of the explanation they can make for their answers.

Again, frontal lobe patients would be expected to have difficulty with switching from similarities to differences and providing adequate number of responses and/or organization of responses. Patients can also be asked to state what they might do in a situation such as their refrigerator quits working or they notice that their pet's behavior changes. Responses should include recognition that these may have multiple causes and that they can be systematically ruled out but may ultimately require seeking additional help (see Table 10.3).

Rule of thumb: Disrupted functions associated with frontal lobe

- Divergent reasoning more impaired than convergent reasoning
  - For example, test is to "tell me as many uses of a soda pop bottle
- Poor inhibition
  - Impulsive. Unable to perform "go–no-go" task.
- Set-shifting and perseveration
  - Unable to sequence simple squares and triangles on a page or put three, and only three loops in a series of three looped "3"-shaped figures on a page

---

Table 10.3 Verbal reasoning and cognitive flexability assessment

Object pairs	Similarities	Differences
Dog–wolf	Canine	Domesticated–wild
	Social	Geographically widespread–restricted
	Physical characteristics (legs, fur)	Size variable–typically large
	Carnivores	Seeks human contact–avoids human contact
	Mammals	
	Multiple pups	
Shark–whale	Live in water	Size
	Alive (breath oxygen)	Fish–mammal
	Swim	Bones–cartilage
	Widespread	Lungs–gills
	Similar physical characteristics (i.e., fins, skin, organs, teeth)	Horizontal swimming motion–vertical swimming motion
House of Representatives–Senate	Part of congress	Population proportioned–two per state
	Legislative branch	
	Elected	4-year term–6-year term
	Represent constituencies	Many more
	Work at capital	representatives–100 senators
	Pass bills	Rules and procedures differ

(continued)

Table 10.3 (continued)

Cognitive Flexability Problems	Potential Solutions
Refrigerator repair	Check power supply
	Secure alternate food storage
	Call repairman
	Check breaker box/circuit breaker
	Inspect power cord, electrical outlet
	Check with neighbors about power supply
Pet behavior	Check food supply
	Check for injuries
	Check temperature
	Recall past routine (diet, interactions, elimination)
	Inspect physically
	Call vet
	Call knowledgeable friend
	Offer desired object (treat, toy)

Object	Alternative Uses
Coat hanger	Hang clothes
	Probe
	Fastener
	Toothpick
	Guide wire
	Skewer
	TV antenna
	Open car door lock
	Holder, extender
	Sculpting
	Form for object (i.e., lamp shade)
	Made into tongs or a rod for reaching/grabbing objects
	Scraping tool
Brick	Building material
	Water saver device for commode tank
	Message delivery system
	Door stop
	Paper weight
	Hammer
	Stepping stone
	Landscaping
	Art object
	Motor vehicle chock
	Speed bumps
	Self-defense

Visual divergent reasoning can be assessed either by asking the patient to creatively list as many uses for a common object such as a coat hanger, knife or brick or asked to draw as many shapes/designs using four straight lines of similar length that touch as possible. In the first task, the patient should be able to generate at least 3–4 nontraditional uses for each object. Responses are not judged for the quality of the object as a substitute for another purpose or object, but rather for the presence of divergent abstraction and creativity. For example, a brick might be used as a paper weight, a door stop, a water-saving (displacement device) device in a commode tank, or an exercise device, etc (see Table 10.3). In the latter task, patients could draw a sequence, two Xs, a series of crosses, or a series of triangles with intersecting lines. Again, the quality of the designs should not be judged, but rather the diversity and number. Patients should be able to spontaneously draw 4–6 designs in less than a minute. Failures can be inquired as to what they found difficult about the task. Possible solution sets for a bedside figure fluency task is presented in Fig. 10.8.

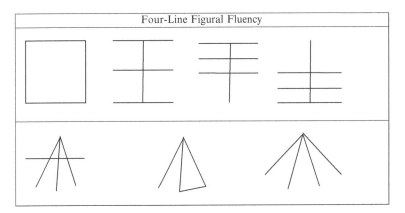

Fig. 10.8 Examples of solutions to a figural fluency task making at least six unique designs with four lines that touch

References and Suggested Further Reading

Bechara, A., Tranel, D., & Damasio, H. (2000). Characterization of the decision-making deficit of patients with ventromedial prefrontal cortex lesions. *Brain, 123*, 2189–2202.

Bird, C. M., Castelli, F., Malik, O., Frith, U., & Husain, M. (2004). The impact of extensive medial frontal lobe damage on "theory of mind" and cognition. *Brain, 127*, 914–928.

Frith, U., & Frith, C. D. (2003). Development and neurophysiology of mentalizing. *Philosophical Transactions of the Royal Society of London. Series B, Biological Sciences, 358*, 459–473.

Grace, J., & Malloy, P. F. (2001). *Frontal systems behavior scale (FrSBe): Professional manual.* Lutz: Psychological Assessment Resources.

Kolb, B., & Whishaw, I. (2009). *Fundamentals of human neuropsychology* (6th ed.). New York: W.H. Freeman.

Lezak, M. D., Howieson, D. B., & Loring, D. W. (2004). *Neuropsychological assessment* (4th ed.). New York: Oxford University Press.

Mesulam, M. (2000). *Principals of behavioral and cognitive neurology* (2nd ed.). New York: Oxford University Press.

Rowe, A. D., Bullock, P. R., Polkey, C. E., & Morris, R. G. (2001). "Theory of mind" impairments and their relationship to executive functioning following frontal lobe excisions. *Brain, 124*, 600–616.

Salloway, S. P., Malloy, P. F., & Duffy, J. D. (2001). *The frontal lobes and neuropsychiatric illness.* Arlington: American Psychiatric Publishing, Inc.

Stuss, D. T., Gallup, G. G., Jr., & Alexander, M. P. (2001). The frontal lobes are necessary for "theory of mind". *Brain, 124*, 279–286.

Stuss, D. T., & Knight, R. (2002). *Principles of frontal lobe function.* New York: Oxford University Press.

Tulving, E. (2002). Episodic memory: From mind to brain. *Annual Review of Psychology, 53*, 1–25.

Tulving, E., Kapur, S., Craik, F. I., Moscovitch, M., & Houle, S. (1994). Hemispheric encoding/retrieval asymmetry in episodic memory: Positron emission tomography findings. *Proceedings of the National Academy of Sciences of the United States of America, 91*, 2016–2020.

Winston, J. S., Strange, B. A., O'Doherty, J., & Dolan, R. J. (2002). Automatic and intentional brain responses during evaluation of trustworthiness of faces. *Nature Neuroscience, 5*, 277–283.

Chapter 11
Affect, Emotions and Mood

James G. Scott and Mike R. Schoenberg

Abstract Emotions and mood play a central role both in the outcome and the management of neurologic illness. The importance is magnified when faced with differentiating between a primary emotional etiology for presenting complaints or neurocognitive symptoms and the possibility of emotional symptoms being the result of a neurologic injury, or a process of dysfunction as a result of an attempt to adjust to changes produced from neurologic injury or neurodegenerative process. Differentiating among these three possibilities is not easy and depends as much on eliciting a detailed psychiatric history as it does on knowledge of the possible emotional sequelae of neurologic injury and anatomical correlates of emotional functioning.

This chapter outlines the currently used multi-axial system of the *Diagnostic and Statistical Manual of Mental Disorders*, 4th edition, Text Revised (DSM-IV-TR). This manual represents the currently accepted diagnostic criteria for mental disorders as outlined by the American Psychiatric Association and the American Psychological Association. While there is no shortage of controversy regarding the criteria for diagnosing mental illness, this system represents the best effort thus far to provide behavioral and objective criteria to a nosologically difficult area of medicine.

The DSM-IV-TR uses a multi-axial approach to diagnosis which incorporates the primary diagnosis (Axis I), personality disorders and mental retardation (Axis II), general medical conditions affecting or potentially affecting the mental disorder (Axis III), psychosocial and environmental deficits/difficulties (Axis IV), and a rating of global functioning on a likert-type scale with descriptive anchors (Axis V). Each of these axes will be reviewed with an emphasis on neurologic disease and commonly associated emotional sequelae. The interested reader is referred to the DSM-IV-TR referenced at the end of this chapter for a more detailed description of both the multi-axial system and specific mental disorders.

J.G. Scott (✉)
Department of Psychiatry and Behavioral Sciences,
University of Oklahoma Health Sciences Center, Oklahoma City, OK, USA
e-mail: jim-scott@ouhsc.edu

M.R. Schoenberg and J.G. Scott (eds.), *The Little Black Book of Neuropsychology:
A Syndrome-Based Approach*, DOI 10.1007/978-0-387-76978-3_11,
© Springer Science+Business Media, LLC 2011

Key Points and Chapter Summary

- Emotional disorders can be a direct or a secondary effect of neurologic disease.
- Diagnostic and Statistical Manual, 4th edition Text Revised (DSM-IV-TR) and International Classification of Disease, 10th edition (ICD-10) are used to classify emotional disorders.
- Many neurologic disorders produce symptoms which resemble psychiatric conditions.
- It is critical to differentiate behavioral changes associated with neurologic disease from those associated with psychiatric disease because both the appropriate treatment and the prognosis may be different.

Multiaxial Diagnostic System

Axis I

Axis I records the primary diagnosis of a mental disorder that is the focus of treatment. With the exception of personality disorders and mental retardation, all mental disorders are recorded on Axis I. This axis may contain as many primary diagnoses as are appropriate for the focus of treatment for the individual. For example, an elderly patient with Alzheimer's dementia may also suffer from depression and an anxiety disorder – all three of which may be listed on Axis I and be the focus of treatment. Table 11.1 lists the major classes of clinical disorders in DSM-IV-TR.

While this table is not exhaustive, it covers the major categories which are the primary Axis I diagnoses. In neuropsychology and neurology, the most common diagnoses are often in the categories of Delirium, Dementia and Cognitive Disorders Not Otherwise Specified (NOS). These diagnoses are often associated with general medical conditions listed under Axis III and result as a natural expression of the course of the neurologic illness or injury. The second most frequent categories seen in neurologically and medically compromised populations are mood disorders (particularly depression) and anxiety disorders (particularly post-traumatic stress disorder, acute stress disorder and generalized anxiety disorder). Alternatively, many neuropsychologists and non-psychiatrist physicians use the International Classification of Disease, 10th edition (ICD-10) to diagnose patients. This classification schema often has diagnoses which are more appropriate for patients with neurologic diseases for which emotional disorders are a direct result or secondary diagnosis.

Table 11.1 Primary diagnostic categories for DSM-IV-TR, Axis I

Category	Description
Disorders of infancy, childhood or adolescence	Includes learning disabilities, developmental delays, pervasive developmental disorders, attention deficit disorders, behavioral and conduct disorders
Delirium, dementia and amnestic and other cognitive disorders, NOS	Includes delirium associated with medical conditions and substance abuse, dementias including Alzheimer's, Vascular Dementia, Huntington's, Parkinson's, etc., and residual categories for Amnestic and other cognitive disorders not otherwise specified (NOS)
Mental disorder due to general medical condition	Includes personality and behavioral changes associated with known medical conditions which are recorded on Axis III
Substance-related disorders	Includes mental disorders that are related to intoxication, dependence or withdrawal of psychoactive substances such as alcohol, amphetamine, opioid or anxiolytics
Schizophrenia and other psychotic disorders	Includes a range of disorders marked by a loss of reality and associated with hallucinations, delusions or grossly disorganized thought processes. Examples include schizophrenia and psychoses associated with injury or illness
Mood disorders	Includes disorders like depression and bipolar disorders. These disorders are marked either by negative mood or by the fluctuation of mood from euphoric to dysphoric
Anxiety disorders	Includes generalized anxiety disorder, post-traumatic stress disorder, agoraphobia, obsessive-compulsive disorder, and simple phobias
Somatoform disorders	Includes disorders which are marked by an excessive concern of physical dysfunction for which physical explanations have been ruled out as the primary cause. These disorders include hypochondriasis, somatoform disorder, somatoform pain disorder, and conversion disorder.
Factitious disorders	Includes disorders in which the primary symptoms are produced consciously by the patient for secondary gain. The secondary gain may be monetary or may be to avoid responsibility, or gain or maintain sympathy and support from others
Sexual and gender identity disorders	Includes disorders of sexual arousal, sexual desire, sexual pain disorders, orgasmic disorders and sexual disorders associated with medical conditions
Paraphilias	Includes fetishes, sexual masochism, sexual sadism, pedophilia, exhibitionism
Eating disorders	Includes anorexia and bulimia
Impulse control disorders	Includes intermittent-explosive disorder, kleptomania, pyromania, pathological gambling and trichotillomania

Rule of thumb: Axis I

- Primary diagnosis of mental disorder that is the focus of treatment
- These disorders may be pre-existing or a result of neurologic disease

Axis II

Axis II includes personality disorders and mental retardation. While personality disorders can be a primary focus of treatment, they are not typically the focus of treatment for neuropsychologist or neurologists. Personality disorders are pervasive, long-standing and enduring personality traits which produce marked impairment for the individual in social, interpersonal, occupational or cultural functioning. Personality disorders are not of acute onset or associated with injury or neurologic compromise. If personality or behavioral changes are associated with a neurologic injury or etiology, these changes would be listed under Axis I in the category mental disorder due to general medical condition. These changes do, however, accompany injury to frontal lobe structures and are associated with many neurologic etiologies such as traumatic brain injury, stroke, and neurodegenerative disorders such as Alzheimer's, Huntington's disease or Fronto-Temporal Dementia. Table 11.2 lists the current DSM-IV-TR personality disorders.

Rule of thumb: Axis II
- Used to diagnose personality disorders and mental retardation
- Differentiation of longstanding personality disorders from acute behavioral changes associated with neurologic disease is critical as prognosis are often quite different
- Neurologic disease often results in exacerbation of pre-existing behavioral and personality characteristics which previously did not rise to the level of psychopathology

While many of the personality characteristics listed can be quite beneficial, the distinguishing characteristic remains in the excessive nature of the characteristic and in the presence of dysfunction caused by the characteristic in social, interpersonal or occupational functioning. While individuals with neurologic injuries can display dysfunction associated with personality, the changes in personality caused by an neurologic injuries are most commonly an exacerbation of a pre-existing characteristic which now begins to produce impairment in social, occupational of interpersonal functioning. For example, someone who premorbidly is cautious or distrustful of the motives of others, may exhibit frank paranoia or delusional paranoia after a brain injury or over the course of decline in a neurodegenerative disorder.

Axis III

Axis III records the presence of any general medical condition(s) which may cause, perpetuate or exacerbate any condition on Axis I. Conditions which influenced the condition listed on Axis I are noted on Axis III. Such conditions include acute as

Table 11.2 Personality disorders recorded on DSM-IV-TR, Axis II

Category	Description
Paranoid personality disorder	Marked by pervasive suspiciousness and distrust of others and ascribing malicious intent to the motives of others
Schizoid personality disorder	Marked by a lack of social relationships and restricted affective or emotional expressiveness
Schizotypal personality disorder	Marked by interpersonal discomfort around others, pattern of cognitive and perceptual distortions and eccentric behaviors
Antisocial personality disorder	Marked by behavior which disregards or violates the rights of others and by an absence or decrease in empathy
Borderline personality disorder	Marked by interpersonal volatility in relationships, impulsive behavior and erratic relationship instability
Histrionic personality disorder	Marked by excessive emotional volatility and attention seeking
Narcissistic personality disorder	Marked by self-aggrandizement, arrogance and belief that others are inferior, typically lacks empathy for others or insight into inflated sense of self
Avoidant personality disorder	Marked by social inhibition, avoidance of attention from others and negative self-evaluation
Dependent personality disorder	Marked by overdependence on others, idiosyncrasies, and avoidance of appropriate responsibility for themselves
Obsessive-compulsive personality disorder	Marked by preoccupation with perfectionism or maintaining appearance of perfection to others, overly concerned with orderliness and control

well as chronic medical conditions. For example, an acute eruption of acne vulgaris may be a contributing or exacerbating factor in a diagnosis of major depression listed in Axis I. Many conditions in neurology and neuropsychology pertain to this category and should be listed as contributing factors in the Axis I diagnosis. Differentiating between which is primary and which is secondary is often irrelevant for the treatment of both diagnoses. The decision as to primary diagnosis is often made clinically by history, assessing the temporal sequence of which presented first historically for the patient. For example, an individual who is diagnosed with Alzheimer's disease and develops depression is less likely to be diagnosed with primary depression, whereas persons with a history of depression and subsequent development of Alzheimer's disease are likely to have a primary of diagnosis of depression. While the sequence of development of the disorders (Alzheimer's and depression in our current example) does matter regarding expectations for outcome and patient management, it does not suggest that either of the disorders should go untreated. Rather, it emphasizes the need for multiple simultaneous treatments to prevent the potential exacerbation of one condition by the other. In many senses, the false dichotomy maintained by the separate diagnoses of physical (medical) conditions and "mental" conditions serves as a hindrance to recognition of the biopsychosocial interconnectedness and the often demonstrated superior treatment outcomes that accompany treating the whole person (biologically – psychologically and socially) rather than maintaining a false mind – body dualism.

Rule of thumb: Axis III

- Axis III often includes the neurologic diagnosis which brought the patient to the attention of the neuropsychologist or neurologist
- Other illnesses which contribute directly or indirectly to the emotional or behavioral symptoms identified on Axis I should be notes on Axis III

Axis IV

Axis IV pertains to psychosocial and environmental issues that impact the treatment and management of the primary diagnosis on Axis I. These issues are related to the individual's primary social, familial, educational, or occupational functioning and may pertain to changes in these areas of functioning due to or related to the primary diagnosis. These often are associated with current stressors experienced by the individual in their psychosocial functioning or environment. Any issue which is related to the cause, perpetuation or exacerbation of the primary diagnosis is listed and relevant to the treatment and management of the primary diagnosis. Table 11.3 lists major categories of psychosocial and environmental influences which impact treatment and treatment outcome.

Table 11.3 Psychosocial and environmental stress factors listed on Axis IV

Factor	Stressor
Family	Loss of family member, changes in living arrangements – separation, divorce, abuse within family, family conflicts
Social environment	Loss of friend, living alone, loss of social support/group, cultural estrangement
Education	Illiteracy, educational disruption, academic failure
Occupation	Loss of employment, work stress, change in occupation
Housing	Homelessness, discord with home owner/landlord
Economic	Financial hardship, poverty
Access to health care	Inadequate access to health care, transportation difficulties
Crime	Legal problems related to crime, incarceration, victim of crime

Axis V

Axis V relates to the individual's overall current global functioning. This takes into consideration the physical health and functional capacity of the person both currently and over the last 12 months. Two ratings are often employed – the first listing the highest level of functioning in the last 12 months and the second being a rating of current Global Assessment of Functioning (GAF). Table 11.4 lists the rating scale with verbal descriptions of each as described in DSM-IV-TR.

Table 11.4 Axis V global assessment of functioning (GAF)

GAF rating	Description
100–91	Superior functioning across social, occupational/education and interpersonal domains
90–81	Minimal symptoms, generally satisfied with life
80–71	Transient symptoms/dysfunction, related to temporary stresses
70–61	Mild symptoms, difficulty in one domain
60–51	Moderate symptoms difficulty in more than one domain or severe difficulty in one domain
50–41	Serious symptoms across domains
40–31	Serious symptoms with impairment in reality testing
30–21	Severe impairment, delusional or psychotic symptoms present affecting across all domains
20–11	Danger of hurting self or others. Impairment in ability to care for self or make decisions for self
10–1	Persistent danger of hurting self or others. Cannot make decisions for self

Mood/Emotions and Neurologic Illness

Increased rates of psychiatric symptoms/emotional problems are associated with any acute or chronic medical illness (see Hales and Yudofsky 2008; Lezak et al. 2004). This reflects at least two different, and often interacting, etiologies: (1) affective symptoms related to neurophysiologic changes in the CNS due to neurological disease or dysfunction and (2) the impact on emotional functioning resulting from psychosocial stressors. This biopsychosocial model is the predominate theoretical framework for understanding psychiatric symptoms/emotional problems at this time. Within this model, the psychosocial component reflects the process of adjustment to the changes produced with illness, frequently results in increased stress and elicits coping strategies which are not always adaptive to the patient within his/her environment and disease state. In examining the impact of an illness on mood, behavior and emotions, two factors are paramount. The first is an estimation of change in mood, behavior or emotions from premorbid functioning. The second issue involves examining the areas of the brain which are involved and analyzing the current and future anticipated changes in behavior and emotions.

The issue of change is critical in evaluating the impact of illness on emotional and behavioral functioning. It is important to get an accurate and reliable history of past emotional functioning from which to judge change in current emotional or behavioral functioning. This is crucial in differentiating a re-emergence or exacerbation of a pre-existing condition from a new manifestation of emotional symptoms or behaviors. While this may seem trivial at first glance, it is critical for determining the etiology for the psychiatric symptom/emotional problems as well as predicting the course and outcome of emotional and behavioral deficits associated with neurological dysfunction. As an example, the onset of visual hallucinations following a head injury of an adult patient is more likely to trigger a variety of questions and laboratory tests designed to assess for seizures or structural lesions than would be the onset of visual hallucinations in an elderly patient with a history of schizophrenia. The predictive value of obtaining a history is highlighted by consistent data establishing that individuals with extensive histories of recurrent emotional and behavioral deficits are both at much greater risk for subsequent development of such symptoms post injury or illness as well as at increased risk for poorer outcomes from treatment interventions than are individuals with no prior psychiatric history. Indeed, individuals with no psychiatric history are at lower risk for developing emotional and behavioral abnormalities following onset of neurological dysfunction or disease and have better remission rates with treatment.

In addition to obtaining a history of previously diagnosed emotional or behavioral disorders, it is important to obtain a reliable description of personality characteristics as these may be exacerbated to pathological levels following an injury or illness. These characteristics include past anger management, frustration tolerance, assertiveness – passivity, social interactions, suspiciousness, stubbornness, dependency, etc. An assessment of these characteristics will give indications of possible areas of concern in the development of current and future symptoms. It is also important to gain an understanding of the typical pre-injury coping skills/mechanisms of the individual, as these may be exacerbated following an injury and become a source of needed intervention or treatment. Table 11.5 provides a partial list of emotional and behavioral symptoms and coping skills/mechanisms history to be explored with the patient and a reliable collateral informant. These characteristics should be explored both in regard to the past and also as they pertain to any post-injury changes.

Table 11.5 Emotional history and coping skills history checklist

Emotional history	History	Current	Change
Depression			
Anxiety			
Bipolar disorder			
Post traumatic stress disorder			
Somatoform disorder			
Development delays			
Attention deficit disorder			
Substance abuse/dependency			
Schizophrenia/psychosis			
Factitious disorder			
Impulse control disorder			
Coping skills/mechanisms	History	Current	Change
Avoidance			
Hypo/hyper somnolence			
Eating (over/under)			
Substance use/abuse (including tobacco, alcohol and prescriptions)			
Obsessive behavior			
Compulsive behavior			
Agitation/irritability			
Aggression (verbal/physical)			

(continued)

Table 11.5 (continued)

Coping skills/mechanisms	History	Current	Change
Suspiciousness/distrust			
Over controlling			
Sexual behavior(hyper/hypo)			
Hyperactivity			
Emotional dysregulation (hyper/hypo)			
Inappropriate humor			
Hypervigilance/excessive worry			
Physical symptoms (headache, nausea, diarrhea, fatigue)			

The second issue regarding assessment of patients' emotional and behavioral symptoms is dependent on the type and location of an injury. Both acute and chronic neurologic injuries/illnesses can produce emotional/behavioral changes in patients. Particularly, injuries to the frontal lobes and those affecting the cortico-bulbar tracts bilaterally produce striking emotional and behavioral changes.

Injuries to the orbital-frontal region which involves the inferior medial and anterior frontal lobes produce behavioral changes, which have been termed the orbital-frontal personality syndrome (see Chapter 10 for elaboration). The emotional and behavioral symptoms involved include disinhibition, impulsivity, emotional volatility and socially inappropriate behavior. These individuals are often seen as disregarding the feelings or rights of others and are helpless in stopping or avoiding what they often readily verbalize as inappropriate behavior. This syndrome can be caused by anything that affects the orbital-frontal region, but is most frequently associated with traumatic brain injuries or ruptures of aneurysms involving the anterior communicating artery.

In addition, behavioral syndromes associated with dysfunction of the dorsal-lateral frontal cortex often results in producing decreased emotional responsiveness, poor awareness of deficits and decreased motivation or spontaneous behavior. These individuals are referred to as having a Dorso-Lateral-Frontal Lobe Syndrome (also termed Dysexecutive syndrome; see Chap. 10, this volume) and are often described as abulic, dull, emotionally unresponsive and appearing depressed. While these individuals are generally emotionally unresponsive, they are often capable of exaggerated emotional responses when they become emotionally stimulated and display difficulty in regulating or redirecting their emotional response. These changes can be seen with any etiology affecting the lateral and superior frontal convexities, but are most frequently associated with occlusive strokes involving the anterior branch of the middle cerebral artery or traumatic brain injuries. Interestingly, these behavioral/emotional syndromes often do not result in much change in cognitive functioning to the casual observer. Cognitive deficits are most frequently found in sustained attention, alternating attention, processing speed, and novel reasoning and problem-solving tasks requiring convergent or divergent reasoning. They do not often exhibit frank deficits in intelligence, language, visuo-spatial processing, or memory when attentional variability effects are considered.

A rare but interesting emotional phenomenon is pseudobulbar affect or affective incontinence (see also Chap. 10). This arises when there are bilateral lesions involving the cortico-bulbar tracts and results in the patient displaying an affective response (i.e., crying or laughter) but having no or minimal associated emotional feeling. These individuals often display inappropriate or grossly exaggerated emotional affective behaviors such as hysterical laughter or uncontrollable crying, but upon inquiry report no subjective appreciation of happiness or sadness. While this phenomenon is rarely seen in post-acute populations, there are several documented cases of persistent syndrome symptoms for years after injury. The phenomenon is rare and occurs most frequently in individuals with a history of neurologic injury to one cortico-bulbar tract and who then suffer an acute injury that involves the contralateral cortico-bulbar tract. Exaggerated negative dysphoria (crying) is seen much more frequently than euphoria (laughter). Again, this phenomenon is rare and typically remits or greatly improves in a few months following the injury. This is seen most frequently in individuals with a history of previous CVAs, transient ischemic attacks or multiple sclerosis, but can occur from any etiology affecting the bilateral cortico-bulbar tracts. Differentiation from depression or psychosis can often be made by both distracting the patient on to a neutral topic (What color are my shoes?) and asking them about the appreciation of the internal emotion when they have such an exaggerated/disproportional emotional display.

Finally, injuries to the right hemisphere can produce deficits in expressive and receptive prosody, which can have profound effects on emotional functioning. These individuals lack their previous social skill in understanding or communicating emotional states through the use of vocal tone and inflection or in readily grasping the subtle emotional variability in others' tone or inflection. The resulting behavioral and emotional changes are that these individuals are perceived as socially unskilled, concrete, emotionally unavailable and uncaring. While considerable variability exists among persons in social skill and emotional perception, these individuals represent changes from a previous level of emotional/social skill functioning which is obvious to others who previously knew them. It is, however, often associated or attributed to volitional behavior or negative personality characteristics and subsequently results in social and interpersonal difficulties and stresses. Table 11.6 summarizes the anatomical associations of behavioral and emotional changes.

Table 11.6 Emotional and behavioral symptoms associated with frontal lobe lesions

Lesion location	Behavioral/emotional symptoms
Orbital-medial-frontal lobe syndrome	Disinhibition, poor social control, emotional dysregulation, impulsivity, inappropriate social or sexual behavior, utilization behavior, distractibility
Dorsal-lateral-frontal lobe syndrome	Abulia, apathy, emotional restriction, emotional dysregulation when emotionally aroused, unmotivated, disregard for hygiene, decreased awareness of deficits, lack of spontaneity, decreased initiative

Below, we review some of the delusional misidentification syndromes. These are often associated with neurological disease, but may be associated with severe psychiatric syndromes as well (i.e., schizophrenia, bipolar disorder, etc.). The delusional misidentification syndromes include: Capgrass, Fregoli's, reduplicative paramnesia, and subjective doubles syndrome.

Capgrass syndrome: Delusional belief that a person (friend, spouse, or family member) has been replaced by an imposter. This imposter appears physically exactly like the person, and has the ability to provide memory for previous details about the person he/she is impersonating. Capgrass syndrome can also extend to the delusional belief that objects have been replaced by an duplicate, but not the original object (e.g., belief one's shoes have been replaced by duplicates). As an example, a patient may believe his/her clothes or shoes have been replaced by imposter garments, which look just like the patient's clothes and shoes, but are not theirs. Capgrass syndrome is associated with schizophrenia as a psychiatric illness, but also found among patients with dementia or brain injury. Patients with capgrass syndrome are able to identify faces (and do not have prosopagnosia); these individuals may have disruption of the autonomic processing aspect of facial recognition processing, such that viewing familiar faces (e.g., family members) does not result in an emotional autonomic response. Caprass syndrome has been reported among patients with dysfunction of the bifrontal lobes and/or diffuse non-dominant hemisphere lesions.

Fregoli syndrome (delusion): Belief that the same person known to the patient is able to disguise or change him/herself into other people the patient meets. While the people thought to be the same person may not look, sound, or behave at all alike, the patient is convinced that physiologically it is the same person who is able to disguise themselves "very well." The person able to disguise him/herself as other people the patient meets is usually identified as a persecutor of the patient. This syndrome is associated with schizophrenia as well as with damage to the right frontal or left temporoparietal areas.

Reduplicative paramnesia: Delusion that a place or location has been duplicated one more time. The place or location is either "relocated" or duplicated, but both must exist simultaneously. Reduplicative paramnesia can present with a patient believing that his/her home is not his/hers, but recognizes that the other house appears to be identical in detail, but is not the person's real place. Bensen et al. (1976) reported three cases, one of which believed there to be two identical hospitals, one of which was in his hometown. The syndrome has been reported to be often associated with bifrontal lesions, often with more diffuse right hemisphere damage. It is generally thought the disorder reflects a combination of impaired attention, memory, and visuoperceptual functions (Forstl et al. 1991).

Subjective doubles syndrome: Belief the patient has been duplicated, and the duplicate person is able to act independently of the patient. There may be more than one duplicate of the person, and the duplicates may have different characteristics or mannerisms. Reported for patients with neurological injury and psychiatric diseases (schizophrenia). Neurological injuries associated with subjective doubles syndrome tend to involve right hemisphere damage as well as frontal lesions. It can be comorbid with capgrass syndrome. Subjective doubles syndrome is not the belief that exact duplicates of the person exist, such that the duplicates are the same physiologically and psychologically/behaviorally. This delusion is also termed clonal pluralization of the self.

Visual Hallucinations

Visual hallucinations are more likely neurological than psychiatric, and the type of hallucination and associated phenomena can help identify etiology/neuroanatomical location. Individuals with visual hallucinations produced from neurologic disease often retain awareness that the experiences do not represent reality, often a distinguishing factor from schizophrenia. Simple shapes/figures reflect more posterior cortical involvement (occipital primary association cortex) while complex patterns more occipital-parietal. Hallucinations that occur for brief periods of time (e.g., <90 seconds), and are associated with loss of time, other associated somatosensory phenomena, motor dysfunction, or falling, are more likely to be associated with seizure activity. Visual hallucinations developing in older patients suggest encephalopathy, medication effects (e.g., excessive dopamine agonist), or neurodegenerative disorders (e.g., lewy body dementia).

Psychotic symptoms associated with depression are more typically auditory than visual and are often mood congruent (i.e., auditory perceptions are critical or negative in nature) and may be persistent, well formed and integrated into other delusional belief systems. In bipolar illness (previously called manic-depression), psychotic symptoms are associated primarily with the manic phase and are often dissociable from neurologic etiologies by history (occurring recurrently, with onset at an early age and no history of neurologic trauma or medical illness) as well as their mood congruent nature and lack of insight as to the irrationality of the experience.

Auditory Hallucinations

Auditory hallucinations may be neurologic or psychiatric. Quality of hallucination can provide clues as to likely etiology, but not always. Poorly formed auditory hallucinations (e.g., buzzing, ringing, etc.) are more likely related to neurologic or peripherial nerve problems (e.g., simple partial seizure, tinnitus, etc.). Running auditory commentary of an individual's actions or thoughts for extended periods of time (>several minutes) that is well articulated is more likely to be associated with psychiatric disease (e.g., schizophrenia). Auditory hallucinations of a repeated word/phrase may be neurologic or psychiatric. Auditory hallucinations of repeated words/phrases associated with other somatosensory phenomena, loss of awareness, or falls more likely represent neurological etiologies (i.e., seizure) than are auditory hallucinations of repeated words/phrases in isolation.

Olfactory and Gustatory Hallucinations

Olfactory and gustatory hallucinations more likely neurological. Table 11.7

Somatosensory Hallucinations

The perception of numbness, tingling, pain, bugs moving about the skin, or movement/ twitching may be either neurological or psychiatric. Determination of the origins are often very challenging. One helpful guide is the extent to which the somatosensory hallucination follows known dermatomes and/or myotomes (see Chap. 3).

Table 11.7 Differentiation of psychiatric and neuologic causes of emotional and behavioral symptoms

Emotion/behavior	Potential neurologic cause	Differentiation from psychiatric condition	Potential psychiatric cause	Differentiation from neurologic cause
Pseudobulbar affect/affective incontinence (uncontrollable crying or laughter)	Bilateral disruption of the corticobulbar tracts	No associated affect appreciated by patient (they do not feel happy or sad); redirection to neutral topic stops affective expression	Bipolar disorder; predominately manic	Confirm history of cyclical affective disorder of patient or family: no structural lesion identified on imaging or history of stroke, trauma or degenerative disorder
Impulsivity/ disinhibition	Frontal lobe disruption, particularly orbito-frontal	Significant change in social appropriateness following a neurologic injury or in the course of a degenerative disorder; minimal hyperactivity/sleep disturbance	Bipolar disorder: predominately Manic	History of bipolar disorder, associated insomnia, irritability, pressured speech, hyperactivity
Abulia/lack of initiation, motivation	Frontal lobe disruption, particularly dorso-lateral disruption; degenerative disorders in late stages	Little or no dysphoria associated with reduction in behavior; can frequently perform activities if directed and given structure	Major depressive disorder	Sadness, hopeless, helplessness associated with lack of motivation; recognizes need for behavior, but expresses no desire to perform(i.e., taking out trash)
Visual hallucinations	Temporal-parietal association cortices; often associated with lewy body disorder or trauma to temporal-parietal area in nondominant hemisphere (typically right); disruption may be transient as in seizures or transient ischemic attacks	No history of hallucinations before age 30, no excessive dopaminergic medications; insight into the factual nature of the hallucinations is often preserved	Schizophrenia; bipolar disorder manic phase; depression with psychotic features	Visual hallucinations are rare in psychiatric disorders; when present they are usually associated with acute exacerbations of long standing psychiatric conditions; usually mood congruent and insight into the factual nature of the hallucinations is usually lost

(continued)

Table 11.7 (continued)

Emotion/behavior	Potential neurologic cause	Differentiation from psychiatric condition	Potential psychiatric cause	Differentiation from neurologic cause
Auditory hallucinations	Temporal lobe lesions and transient disruption (e.g., Seizures)	Hallucinations are often sounds rather than intelligible voices; often are not mood congruent; are often transient rather than persistent	Schizophrenia, bipolar disorder in manic phase, major depressive disorder with psychotic features	Much more frequent than visual hallucinations, often mood congruent, often repetitive with command or negative content, associated with no physical trauma, but may be associated with stress or emotional trauma, history is often positive for previous occurrence of auditory hallucinations
Olfactory hallucinations	Frontal lobe seizures, less frequently frontal traumatic brain injury	Smells are typically unusual (i.e., metallic, acidic) and insight is often preserved as to the fact of the hallucination as not real	Schizophrenia	Rare, insight into the nonfactual nature of the olfactory sensation is often lost; may be incorporated into mood congruent delusion
Expressive aprosody	Lesions of the anterior dorsal right cortex (nondominant)	Retained awareness of what emotion should be expressed, but unable to modulate vocalizations to impart emotional meaning (i.e., cannot say "I'm going to the store" in contrasting happy, sad and angry tones)	Major depression	Prosody is usually retained, but patient may come across as monotone due to sadness and despair

Receptive aprosody	Lesions of the posterior right cortex (nondominant); can be associated with nonverbal learning disabilities and high level Autistic spectrum disorders (i.e., aspergers disorder)	Often retained awareness of emotions which should be understood, but failure to appropriately interpret and comprehend vocal tone and inflections which communicate emotional tone in language, patients are often surprised when others become frustrated after miscommunication, they often do not grasp sarcasm, innuendo, or detect frustration in others that lead to social awkwardness or rejection/avoidance	Major depression; schizophrenia, bipolar disorder	Not typically a major component of these disorders, but may appear as emotional nonresponsiveness/nonreciprocity. Differentiated from neurologic causes often by history and lack of relative change over time
Affective dis-modulation	Frontal lobe lesions; may be nonlocalizing and if so is typically associated with the severity of overall cognitive dysfunction or acuity of trauma (i.e., TBI)	Dysregulation occurs in the presence of environmental stimuli and is often disproportional to the evoking event (i.e., patient is over stimulated and reacts with hyperactivity/agitation and cannot self regulate back to stasis); when affective arousal is diminished, hypo arousal is often observed	Schizophrenia, bipolar	Arousal is often contextually driven in a desire to get something from the environment or avoid aversive stimuli in the environment, it is often precipitated by the demands of others in the environment and dissipates appropriately when the demand is reduced/removed
Perseveration	Frontal lobe or severe degenerative disorder	Perseveration is typically on some activity in the environment. Behavior is often non-seneschal and not mood congruent	Schizophrenia	Perseveration is often mood congruent and associated with self stimulation

(continued)

Table 11.7 (continued)

Emotion/behavior	Potential neurologic cause	Differentiation from psychiatric condition	Potential psychiatric cause	Differentiation from neurologic cause
Paranoia/suspiciousness	Nonlocalizing, associated with severity of impairment	Often is exacerbation of pre-existing non-pathological tendencies. Exacerbated by changes in patient that they do not have awareness of and attribute to the motives or behaviors of others (i.e., someone is stealing things they have misplaced, spouse is accused of infidelity because they do not know where they are at all times)	Schizophrenia	Often mood congruent and associated with a fixed pattern of delusions of persecution, grandiosity, or espionage. History is often associated with previous occurrences of paranoia/suspiciousness
Anxiety	Nonlocalizing, but may have preponderance for occurrence in right hemisphere lesions (nondominant)	Anxiety is associated with severity of compromise in cognition and often exacerbated by changes in environment or deviations from routine, often no identifiable attribution is made by the patient	Anxiety disorders	Anxiety is usually associated with a feared or dreaded stimuli. Attributions are made to impending disaster or worries about possible negative outcomes

References and Suggested Further Reading

American Psychiatric Association. (2000). *Diagnostic and statistical manual of mental disorders (DSM IV-TR)* (4th ed.). Washington, DC: American Psychiatric Press.

Bensen, A. L., Gardner, H., & Meadows, J. C. (1976). Reduplicative paramnesia. *Neurology, 26,* 147–151.

Fogel, B., Schiffer, R., & Rao, S. (1996). *Neuropsychiatry.* Baltimore: Williams & Wilkins.

Forstl, H., Almeida, O. P., Owen, A. M., Burns, A., & Howard, R. (1991). Psychiatric, neurological and medical aspects of misidentification syndromes: a review of 260 cases. *Psychological Medicine, 21,* 905–910.

Grant, I., & Adams, K. (1996). *Neuropsychological assessment of neuropsychiatric disorders* (2nd ed.). New York: Oxford University Press.

Hales, R. E., & Yudofsky, S. C. (2008). *Textbook of neuropsychiatry and behavioral neurosciences* (5th ed.). Washington, DC: American Psychiatric Press.

Lezak, M. D., Howieson, D. B., & Loring, D. W. (2004). *Neuropsychological assessment* (4th ed.). New York: Oxford University Press.

Chapter 12
Aphasia Syndromes

Mike R. Schoenberg and James G. Scott

Abstract The assessment of language is an essential component to neuropsychological evaluations. One that is often quickly summarized as "speech was fluent and articulate, with normal rate, rhythm, intonation, and prosody." While this may describe some aspects of speech, it by no means offers clinicians enough information to determine if language functions are impaired.

This chapter will approach the assessment of language from more of a diagnostic perspective. That is, we will approach language disorders based on well-described aphasia syndromes which are familiar to many. While this can be helpful, some readers uncertain of aphasia syndromes, but observing some disruption of language, are encouraged to review Chap. 7, which explores diagnosis of language disorders from a symptomatic (behavioral observation) perspective.

Aphasia syndromes denote an acquired language dysfunction due to neurological injury or disease. Aphasia syndromes are generally described by three language domains first detailed by Bensen and Geschwind: (1) fluent or nonfluent, (2) language comprehension, and (3) repetition. Additional components for assessing aphasia have been added, including naming, reading, and writing. Maintaining consistency with Chap. 7, reference to "dominant hemisphere" will refer to left hemisphere, since greater than 90% of people are left hemisphere dominant for language. Approximately 90–95% of the general population is right-handed.

Rule of thumb: Left hemisphere dominance for language

- Right handed – 90–95%
- Left handed – 60–70%

M.R. Schoenberg (✉)
University of South Florida College of Medicine, Departments of Psychiatry
and Neurosciences, Neurology, and Neurosurgery, Tampa, FL, USA
e-mail: mschoenb@health.usf.edu

M.R. Schoenberg and J.G. Scott (eds.), *The Little Black Book of Neuropsychology:*
A Syndrome-Based Approach, DOI 10.1007/978-0-387-76978-3_12,
© Springer Science+Business Media, LLC 2011

The clinical features of each aphasia syndrome are reviewed below along with neuroanatomical correlates. For rapid review, please see Tables 12.1 and 12.2 and Appendix. For more detailed discussion, please see Heilman and Valenstein (Clinical neuropsychology, 4th edn, Oxford University Press, New York, 2004), Kolb and Whishaw (Fundamentals of human neuropsychology, 6th edn, Worth, New York, 2008), Goodglass et al. (The assessment of aphasia and related disorders, 3rd edn, Pro-Ed, Austin, 2001), Lezak et al. (Neuropsychological assessment, 4th edn, Oxford University Press, New York, 2004), Mesulam (Principles of behavioral and cognitive neurology, 2nd edn, Oxford University Press, New York, 2000), and/or Victor and Ropper (Adams and Victor's principals of neurology, 7th edn, McGraw-Hill, New York, 2001) for reviews.

Key Points and Chapter Summary

- Most individuals (>90%) are left hemisphere dominant for language
  - Inferior frontal lobe associated with expressive speech (including writing).
  - Inferior temporo-parietal cortex associated with receptive language (including reading)
- The right hemisphere plays a significant role in prosodic aspects of language
  - Non-dominant frontal lobe associated with expressive prosody
  - Non-dominant temporo-parietal lobe associated with receptive prosody.
- Nonfluent aphasia syndromes have slow, effortful, halting speech that is difficult to understand.
- Fluent aphasia syndromes have speech that is fluent and effortless, but is difficult to understand due to lack of real words to convey meaning.
- Distinguish aphasia from psychosis, schizophrenia, other psychiatric illness, or delirium.
  - Aphasia: shorter sentences, paraphasias more common, and frequent dysnomia. Aphasias often have associated neurologic (motor/sensory) deficits.
  - Psychosis/schizophrenia "word salad" is marked by long, tangential responses to questions. Neologisms common while paraphasias rare. Rarely associated with focal neurologic symptoms

---

Clinical Classification of Aphasias

Nonfluent Aphasias

As a group, these aphasic syndromes share a common speech deficit in which verbal output is nonfluent. Speech output may be nonexistent or be slow and effortful.

Global Aphasia

> **Rule of thumb: Global aphasia**
>
> • Nonfluent aphasia with impaired comprehension and repetition.

Fluency: Patient may be entirely mute or have slow halting speech frequently only with incoherent grunts, single syllables, or single words (often neologisms) or short perseverative phrases (e.g., "I, I, I," or "doy, doy, doy" or "I go, I go, I go"). Patients may be able to utter single words or short phrases having an emotional context due to the spontaneous circumvention of typical voluntary language centers under emotional distress. Prosody and inflection may convey some apparent meaning to words, particularly anger or excitement.

Comprehension: Impaired. Comprehension of single words is often impaired, and markedly so for even simple sentences. Reading is similarly impaired. However, patients may follow gestural cues (i.e., hand gestures, facial cues, etc.) quite well. Some ability to comprehend prosodic cues such as vocal tone, volume and inflection is often retained.

Repetition: Impaired.

Naming: Impaired.

Writing: Impaired.

Frequent comorbid conditions: Right hemiparesis involving lower part of face (tongue may deviate to right) and both upper and lower extremities, right visual field defect, right hemianesthesia, Gerstmann's syndrome, visual agnosias, apraxias (including oral apraxia), and memory impairments.

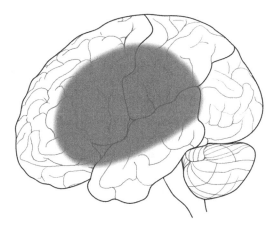

Fig. 12.1 Illustration of left hemisphere damage resulting in a global aphasia syndrome

Neuroanatomical correlates: Large lesions affecting both anterior and posterior areas of the left hemisphere regions involving both Broca's and Wernicke's areas.

Prognosis: Typically, evolve to Broca's (expressive) aphasia, with an improvement in comprehension (Fig. 12.1).

Mixed Transcortical Aphasia

Rule of thumb: Mixed transcortical aphasia

• Nonfluent aphasia with impaired comprehension, but intact repetition.

Fluency: Patient present with slow halting speech. Like global aphasia, speech may include only incoherent grunts, single syllables, or single words (often neologisms) or short perseverative phrases (e.g., "I, I, I," or "doy, doy, dog" or "I go, I go, I go"). Like global aphasia, patients may be able to utter single words or short phrases having an emotional context (e.g., profanity) when under emotional distress. Prosody and inflection may convey some apparent meaning to words, particularly anger or excitement.

Comprehension: Impaired. Like global aphasia, comprehension of single words and phrases is impaired. Reading is similarly impaired. Similarly, individuals may be able to respond appropriately to (nonverbal) gestures or facial expressions. Ability to comprehend prosodic cues such as vocal tone, volume and inflection can be intact.

Repetition: Intact. Single words and complete sentences can be repeated accurately. No comprehension of repeated words or phrases is apparent. Echolalia is common.

Naming: Impaired.

Writing: Impaired.

Frequent comorbid conditions: Right hemiparesis involving lower face and both extremities, right visual field defect, right hemianesthesia, Gerstmann's syndrome, visual agnosias, apraxias, memory impairments.

Neuroanatomical correlates: Isolation of the perisylvian fissure area by diffuse dominant hemisphere lesion. Lesion is large, affecting both anterior and posterior areas of the left hemisphere regions, sparing the arcuate fasciculus. Common etiology is an ischemic-based stroke.

Prognosis: Variable. Patients with vascular etiology may evolve to Broca's (expressive) aphasia or, in some cases, an anomic aphasia (Fig. 12.2).

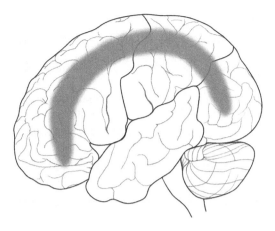

Fig. 12.2 Example of lesion resulting in Mixed transcortical aphasia syndrome

Broca's Aphasia

Rule of thumb: Broca's (expressive) aphasia

- Nonfluent aphasia with intact comprehension, but impaired repetition.

Fluency: Impaired. A range of nonfluent speech may be present, from almost complete lack of coherent speech as in global aphasia with single words and neologisms to slow halting speech with few content words and few verbs or adjectives. Verbal utterances are typically limited to less than four–five words in length (e.g., "I go, I go, I go" or "wife…down…hall."). Like global aphasia and mixed transcortical aphasia, patients can frequently utter words and phrases associated with an emotional context (e.g., profanity and obscenities), particularly when under emotional distress. In addition, patients can frequently exhibit much more fluent speech when asked to utter overlearned words (e.g., "no" or "hi") or sing familiar songs (e.g., "Happy Birthday" song). Prosody and inflection of words is typically impaired.

Comprehension: Intact. Comprehension of single words and short phrases are intact. Reading comprehension is also intact. Comprehension of more grammatically complex phrases, particularly syntactically-dependent sentences (e.g., "the cat was eaten by the mouse."), is often impaired. Ability to comprehend prosodic cues such as vocal tone, volume and inflection is intact.

Repetition: Impaired.

Naming: Impaired.

Writing: Impaired, effortful and very slow.

Frequent comorbid conditions: Right hemiparesis of lower part of face (and tongue) and upper extremity, apraxias (oral apraxia can be present), verbal memory can be impaired (Risse et al., 1984).

Neuroanatomical correlates: Lesion of dominant anterior hemisphere. May include left frontal and parietal lobes, including insula and white matter below these cortical areas. Less extensive lesions involving area anterior to central sulcus results in less severe (more transient) problems with, and better recovery of, language fluency. Posterior perisylvian fissure structures are preserved. Most typical etiology is infarct of superior division of middle superior artery (MCA).

Prognosis: Variable. Patients with vascular etiology frequently improve to an anomic aphasia with mild reduced fluency (Fig. 12.3).

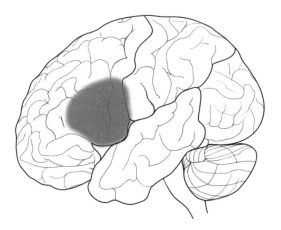

Fig. 12.3 Example of lesion resulting in Broca's aphasia

Transcortical Motor Aphasia

> **Rule of thumb: Transcortical motor aphasia**
> * Nonfluent aphasia with intact comprehension and repetition.

Fluency: Impaired, but less so than in Broca's or global aphasia. However, patients tend to be quite abulic, offering little speech spontaneously. A range of nonfluent speech may be present, varying from few single words and neologisms to slow halting speech consisting of mostly nouns and few verbs/adjectives, but devoid of conjunctives and prepositions. Verbal utterances are typically limited to less than four–five words in length (e.g., "I go, I go, I go" or "wife…down…hall."). Like the other nonfluent aphasias, patients can frequently utter words and phrases associated with an emotional context (e.g., profanity and obscenities), particularly when under emotional distress. Prosody and inflection of words is limited.

Comprehension: Intact. Comprehension of single words and short phrases is intact. Reading comprehension is also intact. Like Broca's aphasia, comprehension of syntactically-dependent phrases (e.g., "the cat was eaten by the mouse.") and multi-step instructions may be impaired. Ability to comprehend prosodic cues such as vocal tone, volume and inflection is intact.

Repetition: Intact, commonly for even long or complex sentences.

Naming: Impaired.

Writing: Impaired, effortful and very slow.

Frequent comorbid conditions: Depending upon location of lesion, can include either right upper extremity weakness (left frontal dorsolateral lesions) or right lower extremity weakness (medial frontal lesions). Apraxias and memory impairments may be present. Other executive dysfunction, perseveration and behavioral apathy may be present.

Neuroanatomical correlates: Lesion of dominant frontal lobe. Lesions may reflect dorsolateral damage anterior or superior to Broca's area. Lesion can involve mesial left frontal area associated with the anterior cingulated and supplementary motor area. Posterior perisylvian fissure structures are preserved. Alternatively, lesion can reflect damage of the dominant hemisphere basal ganglia or thalamus. Common etiology is infarct of left anterior cerebral artery (ACA) or anterior segment of the superior division of the middle superior artery (MCA).

Prognosis: Variable. Patients with vascular etiology can evolve to an anomic aphasia or symptoms may nearly resolve (Fig. 12.4).

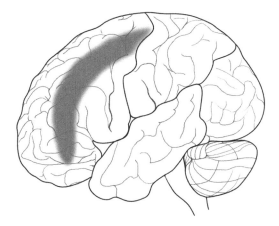

Fig. 12.4 Example of lesion resulting transcortical motor aphasia

Fluent Aphasias

Rule of thumb: Wernicke's (receptive) aphasia

- Fluent aphasia with impaired comprehension and repetition.

As a group, these aphasic syndromes all reflect intact verbal fluency. That is speech output is rapid and effortless. Speech content may be unintelligible, repetition impaired, or comprehension poor, but verbal utterances are effortless and fluent.

Wernicke's Aphasia

Fluency: Speech is fluent, but unintelligible. While speech output is effortless, rapid, and "sentence" length is normal, speech content is unintelligible due to paraphasias (phonemic and semantic) as well as frequent neologisms. Speech content is empty as there are few nouns or verbs, and mostly conjunctions and prepositions. Circumlocution is common, with the speaker frequently substituting "it or thing" for content words (e.g., "the thing whiffle sup it as tbe no...no be surk whe."). Speech can be rapid, particularly if the speaker is excited, which is sometimes referred to logorrhea or press of speech.

Comprehension: Impaired. Comprehension of single words and short phrases is often impaired, and patients have difficulty answering simple yes/no questions or following one-step commands. Reading comprehension is also impaired. Patients appear unaware speech is unintelligible. Ability to comprehend prosodic cues such as vocal tone, volume and inflection is often intact.

Repetition: Impaired. Patients may have difficulty repeating single words (often due to paraphasias), and clear impairment for short and longer sentences.

Naming: Impaired, with frequent paraphasias.

Writing: As with spoken speech, writing is often fluent with letters being identifiable, but the content of writing is unintelligible due to paraphasias and neologisms.

Frequent comorbid conditions: Frequently can present with *no* other obvious neurological signs. Anosagnosia of speech deficits is common. Right homonomyous visual field deficit, Gerstmann's syndrome, visuoconstructional apraxia, and/or memory impairments may be present depending on the extent of lesion and time since onset of disease.

Neuroanatomical correlates: Lesion of dominant inferior persylvian fissure (superior temporal lobe) and often extending superiorly to the parietal region affecting the supramarginal gyrus. Anterior perisylvian fissure structures are preserved. Common etiology is infarct of left inferior division of the middle cerebral artery (MCA).

Prognosis: Variable. Patients with vascular etiology will often exhibit improvement of comprehension, and can evolve to a transcortical sensory aphasia or sometimes conduction aphasia. Very good resolution would result in anomic aphasia (Fig. 12.5).

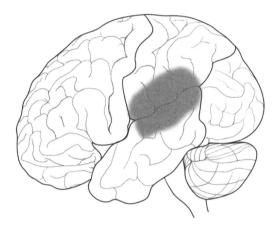

Fig. 12.5 Example of lesion resulting in Wernicke's aphasia

Transcortical Sensory Aphasia

Rule of thumb: Transcortical sensory aphasia

- Fluent aphasia with impaired comprehension, but intact repetition.

Fluency: Like Wernicke's aphasia, speech fluency is rapid and effortless, and speech content remains quite unintelligible due to paraphasias (phonemic and semantic) and neologisms. Speech content may be less devoid of nouns and verbs than Wernicke's aphasia. Circumlocution is common.

Comprehension: Impaired, but to less extreme than in classic Wernicke's aphasia. Comprehension of single words may be intact, and able to answer simple yes/no questions. However, comprehension of short phrases is often impaired, and patients are unable to follow two- or three-step instructions or understand syntacically-dependent phrases are impaired. Reading comprehension is similarly impaired. Like Wernicke's aphasia, patients are often unaware their speech is unintelligible, and ability to comprehend prosodic cues such as vocal tone, volume and inflection can be preserved.

Repetition: Intact. Patients are often able to repeat surprisingly complex sentences.

Naming: Impaired, with frequent paraphasias.

Writing: As with spoken speech, writing is often fluent with letters being identifiable, but the content of writing is similarly unintelligible due to paraphasias and neologisms.

Frequent comorbid conditions: Often right visual field loss. Right hemianasthesia is possible. Constructional apraxia may also be present.

Neuroanatomical correlates: Lesion of dominant temperoparietal-occipital area, or less often, the parieto-occipital area. The cerebral tissue affected is posterior (and often mesial) to Wernicke's area. Structures anterior to Wernicke's area are preserved. Common etiology is infarction of watershed zone between the inferior MCA territory and posterior cerebral artery (PCA) territory. Another common lesion is damage to the dominant hemisphere basal ganglia or thalamus. Neurodegenerative diseases, such as dementia of Alzheimer's type, can be associated with language impairment reflecting a transcortical sensory aphasia.

Prognosis: Variable. Patients with vascular etiology will often exhibit improvement of comprehension, and improve to an anomic aphasia or sometimes nearly resolve (Fig. 12.6).

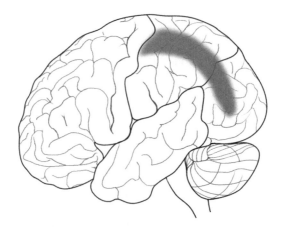

Fig. 12.6 Example of lesion resulting in Transcortical sensory aphasia

Conduction Aphasia

> **Rule of thumb: Conduction aphasia**
>
> • Fluent aphasia. Comprehension intact. Repetition impaired.

Fluency: Speech is generally fluent and rapid, but can be difficult to understand due to frequent phonemic paraphasias and pauses due to naming errors (dysnomia). While speech content is reduced by paraphasias and confrontation naming errors, speech is more meaningful and intelligible than produced with Wernicke's or transcortical sensory aphasias. Paraphasias are principally phonemic, and patients often engage in self-correction with increasingly close articulation of the desired word (circumlocution). Classically, some text books describe speech content as WNL/intact.

Comprehension: Grossly intact for conversational speech. Mild impairments may be evident with grammatically complex sentences (particularly syntacically-dependent phrases) and/or multi-step directions. Reading comprehension is grossly intact. Writing impaired with poor spelling (paraphasias). Prosodic cues such as vocal tone, volume and inflection are intact.

Repetition: Markedly impaired in light of preserved comprehension and somewhat fluent speech (frequent paraphasias). Patients are unable to repeat even simple phrases and often have difficulty with single words (e.g., "Massachusetts").

Naming: Impaired, with frequent phonemic paraphasias.

Writing: As with spoken speech, writing is fluent but can be difficult to understand due to misspelling (paraphasic errors).

Frequent comorbid conditions: Right hemianasthesia and apraxias are not uncommon. Some right facial weakness can be present. Acalculia can also be present. Right hemiparesis is rare.

Neuroanatomical correlates: Lesion of dominant temporoparietal area, particularly the supramarginal gyrus and underlying white matter such that the arcuate fasciculus is damaged. Wernicke's area and anterior structures are preserved. Common etiology is infarction of a limb of the inferior MCA territory.

Prognosis: Variable. Patients can recover and evolve to an anomic aphasia or almost completely resolve. Static lesions (head injury) will often result in retained deficit (Fig. 12.7).

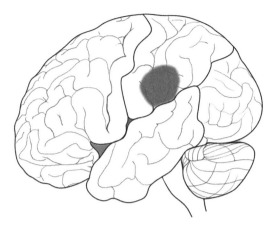

Fig. 12.7 Example of lesion resulting in Conduction aphasia

Anomic Aphasia

> **Rule of thumb: Anomic aphasia**
> - Expressive speech, comprehension, and repetition intact. Naming impaired.

Fluency: Intact, with speech content that is meaningful. While speech output is generally rapid and effortless, speech rate is interrupted by occasional pauses for apparent word finding problems. Circumlocution is present.

Comprehension: Intact. Comprehension of short and even complex sentences is often intact. Mild difficulty may be evident in complex multi-step directions and/or syntacically-dependent phrases. Reading comprehension is similarly intact.

Repetition: Intact, frequently even for complex sentences.

Naming: Impaired, with frequent circumlocution and/or paraphasias.

Writing: As with spoken speech, writing is fluent and content is intact. Some pauses in writing occur as with speech, suggesting word-finding difficulties.

Frequent comorbid conditions: Varies. Because anomic aphasia can present with a variety of neurological conditions (see below), may be associated with a variety of neurological and neuropsychological deficits. If limited to acute anomic aphasia, can be associated with Gerstmann's syndrome. Limb apraxia and acalculia can be present.

Neuroanatomical correlates: Except in the case of acute, isolated anomic aphasia, there is little localizing value. In acute isolated onset of anomic aphasia, lesion is often dominant (left) hemisphere outside the perisylvian language area in the inferior temporal area or angular gyrus of the parietal lobe area. Anomic aphasia is frequently identified in a variety of neurodegenerative conditions (e.g., dementia of Alzheimer's type), traumatic brain injuries, and conditions resulting in intracranial pressure (neoplasms, intraventricular hemorrhages, etc.). In addition, patients with anterior temporal lobectomy often present with an anomic aphasia. A semantic category organization has been proposed with famous faces/people more localized to anterior temporal tip, animals more localized to inferior temporal region, and tools more localized to left posterior lateral region (e.g., Damasio et al. 1996).

Prognosis: Variable. Anomic aphasia is the end phase of recovery from a broad range of mild to moderate aphasia syndromes, and remain quite static in these cases. Recovery from acute, isolated anomic aphasia from localized ischemic event can be nearly complete. Recovery from other etiologies, such as head injury and/or degenerative disorders may not occur, and in fact evolve to other aphasia syndromes (Fig. 12.8 and Table 12.1).

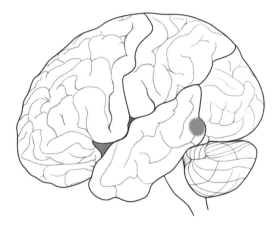

Fig. 12.8 Example of lesion resulting in Anomic aphasia

Alexia, Agraphia, and Aphemia

Rule of thumb: Alexia, agraphia, and aphemia
- Alexia is the inability to read not due to simple sensory (letter agnosia) or motor deficits (ocular apraxia).
- Agraphia is the inability to write not due to simple sensory or motor deficits.
- Aphemia refers to inability to speak not due to language deficit and is secondary to severe apraxia of musculature of mouth, larynx, and tongue needed for normal speech utterances. Distinguished from aphasia in that patients' ability to read and write is completely intact.

Alexia and *Agraphia* are frequently observed concurrently with aphasia syndromes identified above, and follow the pattern of deficits in comprehension (for alexia) or fluency (for writing) of the aphasia syndromes. However, both alexia and agraphia may be observed independently (and together), and should be individually assessed.

Table 12.1 Common aphasic syndromes

Aphasia syndrome	Expressive speech	Auditory comprehension	Repeat	Naming	Reading
Global	↓↓↓	↓↓↓	↓↓↓	↓↓↓	↓↓↓
Broca's	↓↓↓	↓/Normal	↓↓↓	↓↓/↓↓↓	↓/Normal
Trans motor	↓↓/↓↓↓	↓/Normal	Normal	↓/↓↓	Normal
Wernicke's	Fluent ↓↓↓	↓↓↓	↓↓↓	↓↓/↓↓↓	↓↓↓
Trans sensory	Fluent ↓↓↓	↓↓↓	Normal	↓↓↓	↓↓↓
Mixed trans	↓↓↓	↓↓↓	Normal	↓↓↓	↓↓↓
Conduction	Fluent ↓/↓↓	Normal	↓↓↓	↓/↓↓	Normal
Anomic	↓/Normal	Normal	Normal	↓↓↓	Normal
Aphemia/pure word mutism	Mute only Can write	Normal	Normal	Mute. Able to write	Normal
Alexia w/o agraphia (and pure word blindness)	Normal*	Normal	Normal	Normal	↓↓↓

Note: Trans motor=Transcortical motor aphasia; Trans sensory=transcortical sensory aphasia; Mixed trans=mixed transcortical aphasia; ↓=minimal impairment; ↓↓ moderate impairment; ↓↓↓=severe impairment

* Unable to read aloud

Alexia without agraphia is a classic syndrome in which a patient is able to write fluently with normal content, but who is unable to read, even their own writing. Other language functions, including fluency, comprehension, repetition, and naming are entirely intact.

> *Frequent comorbid conditions*: Right homonymous hemianopia and anomias, particularly color anomia.

> *Neuroanatomical correlates*: Alexia without agraphia is a classic disconnection syndrome, reflecting a lesion of the dominant (left) occipital lobe that involves the white matter of the posterior corpus collosum. This type of lesion may occur following an ischemic event of the posterior cerebral artery (PCA).

> *Prognosis*: Variable. Recovery from acute ischemic event can be nearly complete. Recovery from other etiologies, such as head injury, may not occur.

Alexia with agraphia reflects the inability to write or read, with other language functions preserved such that fluency, comprehension, repetition, and naming are intact. When alexia with agraphia predominate, mild dysnomia and/or paraphasias may be present.

> *Frequent comorbid conditions*: Components of Gerstmann's syndrome (agraphia, acalculia, finger agnosia, and right–left disorientation) are sometimes present.

> *Neuroanatomical correlates*: Discrete lesion of the dominant (left) angular gyrus in the inferior parietal lobe.

Prognosis: Variable. Recovery from acute ischemic event can be full.

Agraphia without aphasia reflects the inability to write in the absence of other language impairments, and is infrequently observed.

Frequent comorbid conditions: Components of Gerstmann's syndrome (agraphia, acalculia, finger agnosia, and right–left disorientation) are sometimes present.

Neuroanatomical correlates: Relatively small lesion of the dominant (left) angular gyrus in the inferior parietal lobe.

Prognosis: Variable. Recovery from acute ischemic event can be full.

Aphemia is an acquired inability to articulate speech, such that speech output is slow and very effortful. At its most severe, patients can present as being entirely mute. In milder forms, aphemia may sound as if the speaker was attempting to speak in an unusual accent. In all cases, writing is completely preserved as are the other language functions of comprehension, repetition, and naming.

Frequent comorbid conditions: None, on occasion paraphasias and mild dysnomia.

Neuroanatomical correlates: Discrete lesion of the dominant (left) frontal lobe affecting Broca's area.

Prognosis: Variable. Recovery from acute ischemic event can be full.

NOTE: when speech articulation problems are present since birth (e.g., developmental problem), the above speech disturbance is labeled *verbal apraxia* rather than aphemia.

Cortical Deafness, Nonverbal Auditory Agnosia, and Verbal Auditory Agnosia (Pure Word Deafness)

> **Rule of thumb: Cortical deafness, nonverbal auditory agnosia, and verbal auditory agnosia**
>
> - Cortical deafness – inability to respond to sounds (verbal auditory sounds or nonverbal sounds) not due to simple sensory or motor deficits.
> - Nonverbal auditory agnosia – inability to identify nonverbal sounds, but can accurately identify verbal sounds accurately (understand speech) not due to simple sensory or motor impairment.
> - Verbal auditory agnosia (pure word deafness) – inability to identify verbal sounds (speech sounds) but is able to identify nonverbal sounds and can read and write normally.

Cortical deafness is a rare, but classic acquired, syndrome in which a patient is unable to respond to either spoken language (verbal sounds) or nonverbal sounds (buzzer, dog bark, etc.). Despite being unable to "hear" sounds, patients can respond to written and gestural instructions. Repetition for writing is intact. Other language functions, including fluency and naming are entirely intact. Distinguish cortical deafness from cortical auditory disorder (both auditory agnosias) by the presence of patient complaining of deafness in the former. Acoustic reflexes are preserved, and patients will orient to sudden loud sounds.

Frequent comorbid conditions: Varies with extent of lesion. Acoustic errors in sound recognition. Paraphasias possible.

Neuroanatomical correlates: Bilateral lesions of Heschl's gyrus (primary auditory cortex). Also bilateral damage to white matter immediately ventral and lateral to the posterior portion of the putamen disrupting projections from medial geniculate bodies.

Prognosis: Variable. Some recovery frequent, but depends upon etiology and extent of lesions. Resolution to amusia, generalized auditory agnosia, and/or pure word deafness frequent.

Nonverbal auditory agnosia is the acquired inability to respond to nonverbal sounds (e.g., buzzer, dog bark) in light of preserved ability to respond accurately to speech sounds. Other language skills are entirely preserved.

Frequent premorbid conditions: Amusia.

Neuroanatomical correlates: Lesion of the nondominant (right) hemisphere of Heschl's gyrus and/or subcortical ascending auditory fibers from medial geniculate body.

Prognosis: Good. Typically recovers after several days to weeks.

Verbal auditory agnosia (*Pure word deafness*) reflects the acquired inability to understand spoken speech (verbal sounds) with intact ability to respond to nonverbal sounds. Other language functions, including fluency, comprehension (to written language), repetition (read material), and naming is entirely intact.

Frequent comorbid conditions: Paraphasias are sometimes present.

Neuroanatomical correlates: Discrete lesion of the dominant (left) Heschl's gyrus (primary auditory cortex) that also involves the underlying white matter thereby preventing input of the contralateral primary auditory area to left hemisphere language areas.

Prognosis: Good. Symptoms typically resolve over days to weeks.

Aprosodies

The right hemisphere also plays a significant role in language and communication (Heilman and Valenstein, 2003; Lezak et al., 2004). Impairment of the right hemisphere often leads to a group of impairments collectively referred to as Aprosodies (see Ross, 1997, 2000 for review). Prosody refers to the ability to express and interpret vocal tone, inflection and other nonlanguage auditory cues and extract meaning that facilitates communication. The quality of an increased tone at the end of the sentence, "Here he comes," relates that it was a question rather than an affirmative statement. Similar auditory cues are used in detecting sarcasm, irony, innuendo, and many other aspects of communication.

Prosodic functions are similarly represented as expressive and receptive language functions in the left hemisphere, with expressive prosody functions being associated with right anterior location and receptive prosody effects being associated with right posterior regions (Ross, 1997, 2000). The effect of prosody deficits in communication can be profound, leading to literal, inefficient communication, which has a significant impact on communication of emotional information. Individuals with expressive aprosody are often viewed by others as dull, emotionless, and lacking compassion and empathy. Their verbal output is frequently monotone, flat, and lacking the tone and inflection that correlates to the appropriate emotional state. When asked directly, they are often able to verbalize the presence of emotional states that they are not able to communicate in their verbal tone and inflection. Similarly, individuals with receptive aprosodies are often viewed as emotionally unavailable, lacking insight into others' emotional states or uncaring. They often miss verbal cues that would communicate the emotional states of others. This in turn leads to a decrease in appropriate emotional responsiveness and a generally literal interpretation of what is verbally said with little impact for the way it was verbalized or the context in which it occurred. Table 12.2 lists the major Aprosodies and their anatomical correlates.

Assessment

Please see Chap. 7 for a review of assessment of language disorders. Below, we provide an overview of a practical neuropsychological assessment of language disorders. There are many standardized assessment measures commercially available (see Lezak et al. 2004; Strauss et al. 2006, for reviews), and we discuss only some of the many currently available. However, our discussion below does *not* suggest a preference for one measure over another, but rather our familiarity with the measures discussed below. It is important to remember that neuropsychological (and neurological) syndromes are *not* an all or nothing phenomena. That is, a syndrome can be present in a range of severity, from subtle to severe. For example, a patient presenting with slow effortful speech consisting of short sentences (e.g., "I …go….home, I…..need….out."), who can repeat short sentences and has intact comprehension, but has difficulty repeating more complex sentences, would be considered to have Broca's aphasia in a mild to moderate form. Table 12.3 lists psychometric measures we commonly use in neuropsychological evaluations in the assessment of language functions.

Table 12.2 Types of aprosodies and associated deficits

Aprosodia syndrome	Anatomical location	Prosodic expression	Prosodic comprehension	Prosodic repetition	Gestural expressive	Gestural comprehend
Global	Right frontal, temporal and parietal	↓↓↓	↓↓↓	↓↓↓	↓↓↓	↓↓↓
Motor	Right lateral frontal, superior anterior temporal	↓↓↓	Normal	↓↓↓	↓↓/↓↓↓	↓/Normal
Trans motor	Right lateral frontal	↓↓	↓/Normal	Normal	↓↓	Normal
Sensory/ receptive	Right posterior/ inferior temporal lobe	Normal	↓↓↓	↓↓↓	Normal	↓↓↓
Trans sensory	Right inferior temporal/ parietal	Normal	↓↓↓	Normal	Normal	↓↓↓
Mixed trans	Right frontal and parietal	↓↓↓	↓↓↓	Normal	↓↓↓	↓↓↓
Conduction	Right superior temporal and inferior frontal lobes	Normal	Normal	↓↓↓	↓/Normal	Normal
Agestic	Variable right hemisphere	Normal	Normal	Normal	Normal	↓↓↓

Note: See Ross (1997, 2000) for reviews and more details

Assess for Fluency

This assessment is not simply administering a verbal fluency test e.g., Controlled Oral Word Association Test (COWAT; Benton and Hamsher 1989; Spreen and Struass, 1989) or confrontation naming tests (see Lezak et al. 2004, for review). Rather, the assessment must assess if the patient's speech output is effortless, articulate (well articulated), rapid, and understandable (intelligible). As reviewed above, several aphasia syndromes present with rapid, effortless speech that is not understandable. You will want to be able to assess what is the longest sentence the patient can speak accurately; typically, normal sentence length for native US English speakers is six–eight words. Are there word-finding problems (dysnomia)? Are there paraphasias? Semantic paraphasias include speaking (or writing) an incorrect word that is semantically related to the target word (i.e., "him" for "her" or "banana" for "apple"). Phonemic paraphasia involves speaking a word with an error in a letter sound (e.g., "carmel" for "camel" or "fump" for "dump"). Does the patient engage in circumlocution? Circumlocution can involve thematic circumlocution and provide a description of the term by general synonyms (e.g., "I want a …..thing, you know, the thing you use in your hand to say thank you with, you have one there [points to pen].") or much more vague (empty) circumlocution (e.g., "the two for…no…big damn...no…there is a one there….one…two..three..").

Assess for Comprehension

Comprehension is most easily assessed during the initial conversation. However, a careful step-by-step assessment will assure adequate evaluation of this domain. One might begin by asking open-ended questions (e.g., "What brought you in today?" or "Why are you here?"). Assessment should include asking the patient to respond to increasingly complex instructions/requests. The clinician may need to bring assistive devices (e.g., yes/no card or writing pad to assure other impairments will not limit evaluation of language comprehension). Comprehension can be assessed with single-step (point to the ceiling), two-step (point to the door and then the ceiling), and three-step (point to the door and then the floor, but first point to the ceiling) instructions. Comprehension can also follow with increasingly complex sentences. For example, a simple comprehension task can be asking a patient to state "what got hit?" given the following sentence: "the man hit the ball."; then "the man was hit by the ball." and finally more difficult still, with a passive negative statement "the man was not hit by the ball." Subtle comprehension deficits can also be ascertained by inquiring with serious sounding prosodic questions such as "Is my hair on fire?," followed with more difficult questions such as "Do kangaroos drive cars?" and "Do two pounds of candy weigh less than two pounds of rocks?"

Assess for Repetition

Have the patient begin by repeating simple sentences (The dog is big) to more complex sentences (The little man and the big dog ran around the tree). Finally, ask the patient to repeat grammatically dependent sentences (The cat was eaten by the mouse) and grammatically incorrect sentences (This pink circle heavier than red box).

Assess for Naming

Assess patients ability to name visual objects by pointing (what do you call this ____?) as well as auditory descriptions (what do we call a four legged animal that barks and is often a household pet?).

Assess for Reading and Writing

Have the patient write a sentence and have the patient read a sentence silently to his/herself and do what it says (e.g., "raise a hand above your head" or "stick out your tongue.") You may also assess for reading out loud, as often with nonfluent aphasias, reading comprehension will be intact while oral reading is impaired. One might have the patient read a sentence (s)he writes as well as a unique sentence (s) he has not had previous exposure to.

Have the most familiarity and clinical experience, but should not be construed to indicate the tests in Table 12.3 are superior to other measures of language functioning.

Ethnic, Age, Diversity and Psychiatric Considerations

The astute clinician will appreciate the need to be sensitive to, and appreciate the potential for, ethnic, age, and sociocultural impacts on the assessment of language. While a detailed analysis of these issues are beyond the scope of this text, we highlight some ethical and practical considerations below.

Cultural Considerations

First, and foremost, it is essential that assessment of language occur in the patient's primary language. If this is not possible due to some limiting factor, the clinician must weigh the relative merits of completing an evaluation that will underestimate language abilities and potentially result in an incorrect diagnosis or determination for the extent of language impairment. Clinical neuropsychologists are sensitive to cultural and ethnicity variables that may adversely affect the reliability and validity of assessment (see American Psychological Association 2002). It may be that the assessment of language functions occurs in the patient's second or third language that was acquired later in life and/or not as frequently used. Considerable work has identified that supplementary language areas can develop and/or the fluency or comprehension of the patient in the second or third language may have been reduced at baseline, thereby potentially leading the assessor to believe more language impairment exists than is actually present.

In addition to cultural/ethnicity variables of evaluating or treating an individual not having the same language as the assessor, one must also consider cultural factors with respect to the potential for differences in language dialects and customs for introducing the assessment and assessment procedures.

Pediatric Considerations

The assessment of language functions is particularly difficult in children to differentiate the presence of an acquired language deficit versus a developmental language

Table 12.3 Commonly used psychometric based tests of language

Language domain	Test	Author
Expressive	Boston diagnostic aphasia exam (BDAE)	Kaplan et al., (2001)
	Multilingual aphasia exam (MAE)	Benton and Hamsher (1989)
	Controlled oral word association test (COWAT)	Benton et al. (1994)
	Neuropsychological assessment battery (NAB)	Stern and White (2003)
	Semantic verbal fluency test (e.g., animals)	For review, see Straus et al. (2006)
	Woodcock-Johnson psychoeducational battery – 3rd Ed. (WJ-III)	Woodcock et al. (2001)
	Western aphasia battery (WAB)	Kertesz (1982)
• Writing/spelling	BDAE	
	NAB	
	Peabody individual achievement test – revised (PIAT-R)	Markwardt (1989, 1998).
	WAB	
	Wechsler Individual Achievement Test-2nd Ed. (WIAT-II)	Wechsler (2001)
	WJ-III	
	Wide Range Achievement Test-4th Ed. (WRAT-IV)	Wilkinson and Robertson (2006)
Receptive	BDAE	
	MAE	
	NAB	
	WAB	
	Token test (part of WAB)	
	WJ-III	
• Reading comprehension	BDAE	
	NAB	
	PIAT-R	
	WJ-III	
	WRAT-IV	
• Oral reading	Grey Oral Reading Test - 4th Ed. (GORT-4)	Wiederholt and Bryant (2001)
	WJ-III	
Repetition	BDAE	
	MAE	
	NAB	
	WAB	
Naming	Boston Naming test (part of BDAE)	Goodglass and Kaplan (2000)
	Columbia Auditory Naming test	Hamberger and Seidel (2003)
	MAE	
	NAB	
	WAB	

Note: The particular assessment instruments identified in this table are for convenience only, and authors have no preference for those listed or other measures which might also be available and not identified

problem, such as dyslexia or as a component of another neurodevelopmental process such as Autism or Asperger's disorder. It is essential to obtain a detailed history for the presence of developmental language problems prior to the onset of known or suspected neurological injury. In the case of early childhood trauma before onset of language functions, intra-hemispheric and/or inter-hemispheric language re-organization has been well documented (e.g., Kolb and Whishaw 2008)

Geriatric Considerations

Geriatric assessment of language disorders may, at first blush, appear more clear cut than in children or adults, but poses unique challenges. In particular, the assessment of language in older adults can be complicated by comorbid medical disorders that can adversely affect a patient's mental status, such as encephalopathies, sepsis, infections (e.g., acute urinary tract infection), cardiovascular insufficiency, pulmonary insufficiency, adverse effects from multiple medications, etc. The examiner should also not forget the potential impact of cultural differences in the doctor–patient relationship, in which the elderly may not wish to respond (functional mutism) during an assessment with a younger clinician.

Psychiatric Considerations

Distinguish aphasia from psychosis, schizophrenia, other psychiatric illness, or delirium may not seem important or difficult, but in clinical settings can be more difficult than is often readily appreciated. Perhaps this is the reason why articles and chapters reviewing the symptoms and signs of aphasia often do not include a discussion on differentiating psychiatric disorders from aphasias. It may also be the reason for some unfortunate patients with aphasia being diagnosed (and treated for) psychiatric disorders. We believe this is an important skill to develop and to provide an overview for distinguishing aphasia syndromes from psychiatric disorders.

Patients with schizophrenia, psychosis and thought disorders, bipolar disorders, primary mood disorders, and delirium can present with a variety of speech problems, including speech that is fluent but unintelligible. Patients with primary psychiatric disorders presenting with fluent but unintelligible speech may be mistaken for the language problems associated with a fluent aphasia (e.g., Wernicke's, transcortical sensory, or conduction aphasias). Similarly, patients with primary psychiatric disorder (or delirium) can also present with mutism or sparse verbal output that can be mistaken for the symptoms of a nonfluent aphasia (e.g., Broca's aphasia or, more often, transcortical motor or anomic aphasia).

Patients with aphasic syndromes can be misdiagnosed with a primary psychiatric disorder and not having a Wernicke's, conduction, and transcortical sensory aphasia may be misdiagnosed as having a psychiatric disorder, due to the appearance of bizarre speech output.

Patients with Broca's and transcortical motor, and mixed transcortical, are at risk of being mislabeled as having a primary psychiatric disorder. However, patients with an aphasia often present with symptoms of apathy and tearfulness.

Aphasia: shorter sentences, paraphasias more common, and frequent dysnomia. Aphasias often have associated neurologic (motor/sensory) deficits.

Patients with Broca's aphasia often present with tearfulness that is greater than observed for patients with more posterior dominant hemisphere lesions that result in fluent aphasias. Their affective expressions are exaggerated, reflecting damage to the frontal lobe (see Chaps. 3 and 10 for further review).

Psychosis/schizophrenia "word salad" is marked by long, tangential responses to questions. Neologisms common while paraphasias rare. Rarely associated with focal neurologic symptoms.

Appendix: Rapid Review Summary for Classic Aphasia Syndromes

	Neuroanatomical correlates	Figure
Aphasia syndrome		
Global	Lesion affecting anterior and posterior language areas (perisylvian or lateral fissure region)	
Expressive (Broca's)	Anterior language area, posterior left frontal region, including Brodmann's area 44	

(continued)

	Neuroanatomical correlates	Figure
Aphasia syndrome		
Transcortical Motor	Left anterior frontal sparing Broca's area (Brodmann's 44)	
Receptive (Wernicke's)	Temporoparietal damage affecting Wernicke's area (Brodmann's area 22, and often 39, 41, and 42)	
Transcortical Sensory	Posterior temporal and parietal dysfunction, sparing Wernicke's area	
Mixed Transcortical	Lesion damaging frontal and temporoparietal regions, but Broca's and Wernicke's areas spared	

(continued)

	Neuroanatomical correlates	Figure
Aphasia syndrome		
Conduction	Lesion of the supramarginal gyrus and arcuate fasiculus, but sparing both Broca's and Wernicke's areas.	
Anomic	Acute syndrome classically associated with a lesion posterior to Wernicke's area involving either the angular gyrus (not shown) or inferior temporal region (shown). However, other aphasia syndromes may clinically resolve to an anomic aphasia. Finally, diffuse head trauma and neurodegenerative diseases can present with an anomic aphasia.	

References

American Psychological Association. (2002). Ethical principles of psychologists and code of conduct. *American Psychologist, 57*, 1060–1073.

Benton, A. L., Hamsher, K., & de, S. (1989). *Multilingual Aphasia Examination*. Iowa City, IA: AJA Associates.

Benton, A. L., De Hamsher, S. K., & Sivan, A. B. (1994). *Multilingual aplasia examination* (3rd ed.). Iowa City, IA: AJA Associates.

Damasio, H., Grabowski, T. J., Tranel, D., Hichwa, R. D., & Damasio, A. R. (1996). A neural basis for lexical retrieval. *Nature, 380*, 499–505.

Kaplan, E., Goodglass, H., & Weintraub, S. (2001). *The Boston naming test*. Philadelphia: Lippincott Williams & Wilkins.

Goodglass, H., Kaplan, E., & Barresi, B. (2000). *The Boston diagnostic aphasia examination (BDAE-3)* (3rd ed.). Philadelphia: Lippincott Williams & Wilkins.

Goodglass, H., Kaplan, E., & Barresi, B. (2001). *The assessment of aphasia and related disorders* (3rd ed.). Austin, TX: Pro-Ed.

Hamberger, M., & Seidel, W. T. (2003). Auditory and visual naming tests: normative and patient data for accuracy, response time and tip-of-the-tongue. *Journal of the International Neuropsychological Society, 9*, 479–89.

Heilman, K. M., & Valenstein, E. (2003). *Clinical neuropsychology* (4th ed.). New York: Oxford University Press.

Kertexz, A. (1982). *Western Aphasia Battery*. San Antonio, TX: The Psychological Corporation.

Kolb, B., & Whishaw, I. Q. (2008). *Fundamentals of human neuropsychology* (6th ed.). New York: Worth Publishing Company.

Lezak, M. D., Howieson, D. B., & Loring, D. W. (2004). *Neuropsychological assessment* (4th ed.). New York: Oxford University Press.

Markwardt, F. C., Jr. (1989, 1998). *The peabody individual achievement test-revised*. Minneaplois, MN: NCS Pearson, Inc.

Mesulam, M. M. (2000). *Principles of behavioral and cognitive neurology* (2nd ed.). New York: Oxford University Press.

Risse, G. L., Rubens, A. B., & Jordan, L. S. (1984). Disturbances in long-term memory in aphasic patients: A comparison of anterior and posterior lesions. *Brain, 107*, 605–617.

Ross, E. D. (1997). The aprosodies. In T. E. Feinberg & M. J. Farah (Eds.), *Behavioral neurology and neuropsychology* (pp. 699–717). New York: McGraw-Hill.

Ross, E. D. (2000). Affective prosody and the aprosodias. In M. M. Mesulam (Ed.), *Principles of behavioral and cognitive neurology* (2nd ed., pp. 316–331). New York: Oxford University Press.

Spreen, O. & Strauss, E. (1998). *A Compendium of neuropsychological tests: Administration, norms, and commentary*. (2nd ed.). NY. Oxford University Press.

Stern, R. A., & White, T. (2003). *Neuropsychological assessment battery (NAB)*. Lutz, FL: Psychological Assessment Resources.

Strauss, E., Sherman, E. M. S., & Spreen, O. (2006). *A compendium of neuropsychological tests: administration, norms, and commentary* (3rd ed.). New York: Oxford University Press.

Victor, M., & Ropper, A. H. (2001). *Adams and Victor's principals of neurology* (7th ed.). New York: McGraw-Hill.

Wechsler, D. (2001). *Wechsler individual achievement test – 2nd Ed (WIAT-II)*. San Antonio, TX: The Psychological Corporation.

Wiederholt, J. L., & Bryant, B. R. (2001). *Gray oral reading test-fourth edition (GORT-4)*. Austin, TX: Pro-Ed.

Wilkinson, G. S., & Robertson, G. J. (2006). *Wide range achievement test-fourth edition*. Lutz, FL: Psychological Assessment Resources.

Woodcock, R. W., McGrew, K. W., & Mather, N. (2001). *Woodcock-Johnson III*. Itasca, IL: Riverside Publishing.

Chapter 13
Cerebrovascular Disease and Stroke

Cathy Sila and Mike R. Schoenberg

Abstract The term stroke encompasses a heterogeneous group of cerebrovascular diseases, each with distinctive clinical presentations, underlying causes and strategies for management. Stroke is the third leading cause of death in the USA and the most common cause of long-term disability in adults. Each year, approximately 750,000 strokes occur with 200,000 representing a recurrent stroke. There are approximately 5.5 million stroke survivors in the USA and it is estimated that about 13 million individuals have sustained a so-called "silent" stroke. Although stroke risk increases with age, all age groups are affected.

Key Points and Chapter Summary

- Stroke is the third leading cause of death in the USA
- Strokes are classified as ischemic or hemorrhagic
- Ische mic stroke results from an obstruction of blood flow by thrombosis or embolism to an artery supplying the brain and can be classified by their underlying cause as: Large Artery Atherosclerotic, Lacunar, Cardioembolic, Cryptogenic or Other.

(continued)

M.R. Schoenberg (✉)
Departments of Psychiatry and Neurosciences, Neurology, and Neurosurgery,
University of South Florida College of Medicine, Tampa, FL, USA
and
Case Western Reserve University School of Medicine
Department of Neurology
Cleveland, OH USA
e-mail: mschoenb@health.usf.edu

M.R. Schoenberg and J.G. Scott (eds.), *The Little Black Book of Neuropsychology:*
A Syndrome-Based Approach, DOI 10.1007/978-0-387-76978-3_13,
© Springer Science+Business Media, LLC 2011

Key Points and Chapter Summary (continued)

- A Transient Ischemic Attack is a temporary focal neurologic deficit of presumed vascular cause that does not result in neuroimaging evidence of infarction or resolving within 24 hours.
- Hemorrhagic stroke results from non-traumatic bleeding into the brain and is classified by the location: intracerebral (intraparenchymal), intra-ventricular, subarachnoid, subdural, or epidural
- Neuropsychological deficits are common after stroke and can be predicted based on the stroke subtype, vessel affected and location of the injury, but are influenced by underlying patient variables including comorbid health conditions.
- As with other sequelae of stroke, neuropsychological deficits improve over time and tend to recover over time. Mild deficits may only be detected with detailed neuropsychological assessment.
- Rehabilitation efforts focus on restoring function or compensatory strategies.

Section I: Stroke Pathophysiology, Neuroanatomy, and Clinical Features

Pathophysiology

A disruption of arterial flow results in rapid dysfunction of the underlying brain tissue due to two processes: (1) loss of oxygen and glucose necessary for cell processes, and (2) various alterations to cellular metabolism leading to loss of the cells integrity and cell death. Several changes occur acutely with ischemia: venous blood darkens with decreased oxygen saturation, blood becomes thicker (more viscous), the area of isch-emic tissue pales, and arteries narrow. At a molecular level, the normal cellular pro-cesses are disrupted (e.g., Krebs cycle) with ATP depletion, increased intracellular calcium and extracellular potassium. Ischemic cells release the excitatory neurotrans-mitters glutamate and aspartate, leading to an influx of sodium and calcium leading to disruption of the cell membrane and cellular swelling (edema) with cell death.

The core region of infarcted tissue is surrounded by a penumbra which represents a zone of hypoperfused tissue which is vulnerable but may remain viable. The extent of tissue injury is dependent upon the magnitude and duration of the drop in cerebral blood flow which is also dependent upon the support of collateral blood supply from other neighboring arteries. A reduction in cerebral blood flow is often first noted in the farthest territory supplied by that blood vessel. The region representing the boundary of blood flow from two neighboring vessels is termed the borderzone, or watershed. Although the core region is irreversibly damaged, the ischemic penumbra has a tem-porary potential for salvage before progressing to infarction. The focus of current acute ischemic stroke therapy is to restore cerebral blood flow and salvage the penumbra, and stroke research continues to look for a way to extend the timeframe for this to occur by stabilizing the neurochemical milieu or reducing metabolic requirements.

Rule of thumb: In the setting of an acute stroke, "time is brain"
- Irreversible neuronal damage can occur rapidly; early intervention can lead to improved outcomes.

Stroke Subtypes and Categorization

Strokes are categorized by pathophysiology (see Table 13.1 for summary). The major categorization of stroke is whether it is *Ischemic* or *Hemorrhagic*. The archaic term "cerebrovascular accident" should not be used. *Ischemic stroke* (IS) or *cerebral infarction* occurs when an arterial flow to the brain is obstructed and accounts for ~85% of all strokes. *Hemorrhagic stroke* occurs when an artery or vein ruptures causing intracranial bleeding and accounts for ~15% of all strokes. There are multiple subtypes of ischemic and hemorrhagic strokes, which we review below.

Rule of thumb: Stroke categorization
- Ischemic Stroke = obstruction in blood flow to brain (~85% of strokes)
- Hemorrhagic Stroke = bleeding into brain (~15% of strokes)

Ischemic Stroke or Infarction

Ischemic strokes can be classified in many ways: by clinical severity, by pathophysiologic process leading to the vascular occlusion, or by presumed underlying mechanism. The latter is the most clinically useful as the underlying mechanism will determine the optimum treatment plan for prevention of further vascular events. Most vessels become occluded through a process of *thrombosis* or *embolism*, or both. *Thrombotic* strokes describes strokes that occur when a vessel is occluded from clot formation at the site of a ruptured atherosclerotic plaque. *Embolic* strokes refer to a vascular occlusion from material originating from a more proximal source, such as a more proximal artery or the heart. The embolus is typically made up of fibrin, coagulated blood and/or a plaque; but may be some other material (e.g., tumor cells, air, etc.). While Transient Ischemic Attacks (TIAs) are an ischemic event, TIAs are discussed separately below.

The TOAST classification scheme is clinically useful and is the most often used in practice. Developed for prospective use in the Trial of Org 10172 in Acute Stroke Treatment (TOAST; Adams et al. 1993), it has limitations when used retrospectively, and employs the clinical presentation, results of neuroimaging studies and laboratory tests to

Table 13.1 Stroke subtypes

I. Ischemic stroke or infarction and transient ischemic attacks
   A. Large artery atherosclerosis
   B. Lacunar or small vessel arteriosclerosis
   C. Cardioembolism
   D. Cryptogenic
   E. Other known cause
      1. Cervicocephalic dissection
      2. Coagulopathy
      3. Non-atherosclerotic arteriopathy (e.g., CADASIL)
      4. Metabolic disorders (e.g., MELAS)
      5. Migraine
      6. Vasculitis
      7. Drug abuse
II. Hemorrhagic strokes
   A. Intracerebral hemorrhage
      1. Hypertension
      2. Amyloid angiopathy
      3. Arteriovenous Malformation (AVM)
      4. Hematologic disorder
      5. Hemorrhagic transformation of recent cerebral infarct
      6. Hemorrhage into tumor
   B. Subarachnoid hemorrhage
      1. Saccular aneurysm
      2. Arteriovenous malformation
      3. Hematologic disorder
      4. Mycotic (infectious) aneurysm
III. Cerebral venous thrombosis
   A. Dural sinus thrombosis
   B. Cortical venous thrombosis

determine an underlying mechanism with varying levels of certainty (definite, probable, and possible). The TOAST scheme classifies ischemic stroke into five subtypes: (1) large-artery atherosclerosis, (2) cardioembolism, (3) small-vessel occlusion, (4) stroke of other determined etiology, and (5) stroke of undetermined etiology (cryptogenic).

Large artery atherosclerosis involving the extracranial or intracranial vessels accounts for about 20% of ischemic strokes. Cardioembolism, which includes the heart and proximal sources of embolism, accounts for 15–20% of ischemic strokes. Lacunar infarcts, resulting from atherosclerotic occlusion of small perforating arteries from hypertension and diabetes, results in characteristic clinical syndromes and accounts for another 20–25% of ischemic strokes. Thus, forms of atherosclerotic disease and cardioembolism account for about two-thirds of all ischemic strokes. Rarer causes including cervicocephalic dissection, nonatherosclerotic arteriopathies, coagulopathies, metabolic disorders, migraine, vasculitis and drug abuse account for about 5% of ischemic strokes. The cause of the remaining 30% of ischemic strokes have been classified as *cryptogenic*, indicating the cause has not been established, either because an adequate diagnostic evaluation was not performed, an underlying condition was not documented at the time of the evaluation, or multiple potential causes were demonstrated. These proportions of the various subtypes vary by the age group under study with young adults having a higher percentage of "other" causes.

Transient Ischemic Attacks

Transient ischemic attacks (TIAs) are classically defined as a sudden, painless, focal neurologic deficit of presumed vascular origin that either results in no neuroimaging evidence of infarction or resolves within 24 hours (see also Chap. 15). The majority of TIAs last less than 1 hour, and only 15% of those persisting beyond 1 hour will resolve within 24 hours. Diffusion-weighted Magnetic Resonance Imaging (DWI MRI) has led to this revision in the TIA definition, as many events previously classified as a TIA by the <24 hours definition have evidence of infarction on brain imaging. The sensitivity of detecting cerebral injury on neuroimaging varies with the neuroimaging modality used (CT vs T2-weighted MRI vs DWI-MRI) and the duration of the symptoms in question such that no time interval is specific to distinguish between a TIA and an ischemic stroke. Neuroimaging evidence of a recent cerebral infarction is detected in 15–20% of brain CT scans and 50–71% of diffusion-weighted MRI (DWI) scans with symptoms persisting >6 hours but <24 hours (see Image A).

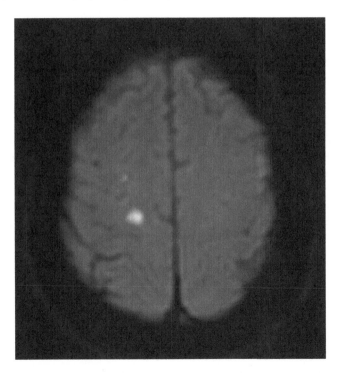

Image A. Diffusion-weighted MRI demonstrating a small infarct in the right parietal lobe (Shaded gray area; recall that on neuroimaging coronal and horizontal images are presented as if the patient is looking at you and thus right and left are reversed) in a patient with 6 hours of left arm paresthesias consistent with embolism to the right middle cerebral artery

The presumed mechanism is a transient occlusion of a cerebral vessel compromised by stenosis or from an embolus which undergoes spontaneous recanalization. TIAs are important warning symptoms of impending ischemic stroke and are considered a medical emergency warranting urgent medical attention. Within 3 months of a TIA, 8–10% of patients suffer a stroke with half of these occurring within the subsequent 48 hours (e.g., Johnston et al. 2000; Rothwell et al. 2005). The symptom features of TIA follow functional neuroanatomic association of the cerebral vasculature (see Tables 13.2, 13.3, 13.4, and 13.5 and Chap. 3, this volume for review).

An old term is *Reversible Ischemic Neurologic Deficit* (RIND), which represents a minor ischemic stroke lasting 24 hours but resolving within 7 days. This term is rarely used now, but the concept of specifying the extent of stroke recovery or residual disability is still useful. Clinical trials routinely add a functional outcome measure, such as the modified Rankin Scale (Bonita and Beaglehole 1988), to follow-up visits to assess the extent of stroke recovery.

Hemorrhagic Strokes

Hemorrhagic strokes are nontraumatic in origin, and result from the rupture of a vessel leading to blood within the brain. Hemorrhages may be *intracerebral* (*intraparenchymal*), *subarachnoid*, or *intraventricular*, alone or in combination, and account for ~15% of all strokes. Intracranial hemorrhages in the subdural space (subdural hemorrhage) or epidural space (epidural hemorrhage) are typically due to trauma, and are often excluded in the definition of stroke. Trauma may also result in intracerebral, subarachnoid, and/or intraventricular (see also Chaps. 3 and 21, this volume for a discussion of traumatic hemorrhages). *Intracerebral* or *intraparenchymal hemorrhage* (ICH) refers to bleeding within the brain tissue and accounts for ~10–12% of all strokes (and about 2/3 of all hemorrhagic strokes). *Subarachnoid hemorrhage* (SAH) involves bleeding within the subarachnoid space and accounts for about ~3–5% of all strokes (1/3 of all hemorrhagic strokes). Hemorrhagic stroke subtypes carry the highest mortality rates: 35–52% of patients die within the first 30 days (Carhuapoma and Hanley 2002). Below, we provide a more detailed discussion of hemorrhagic stroke classification and associated comorbidities.

Rule of thumb: Hemorrhagic stroke classification

- Intracerebral hemorrhage (~10–12%)
- Subarachnoid hemorrhage (~3–5%)
- Intraventricular hemorrhage

Intracerebral (Intraparenchymal) Hemorrhage (ICH)

Intracerebral (intraparenchymal) hemorrhages are nontraumatic by definition and can be further classified as *primary* or *spontaneous,* when the presumed underlying cause is rupture of small perforating vessels due to damage from chronic hypertension and degenerative changes in the arteries, or *secondary,* when associated with an identified precipitating cause such as a vascular malformation, aneurysm, tumor, complication of anticoagulant drugs, or an underlying bleeding disorder. Although survival has improved with early diagnosis and emergency care, early mortality remains high at 30–40% (e.g., Sturgeon and Folsom 2007), and most patients have residual motor, sensory, and/or neuropsychological deficits (see below for details). The location of the hemorrhage suggests the underlying cause. Hypertensive hemorrhages occur in locations supplied by small perforating vessels with 50% involving the deep nuclei (putamen, 35%; thalamus, 10%; caudate, 5%), 30% in the lobar white matter, and 20% occur in the posterior fossa (cerebellum, 15%; brain stem, 5%) (see Image B).

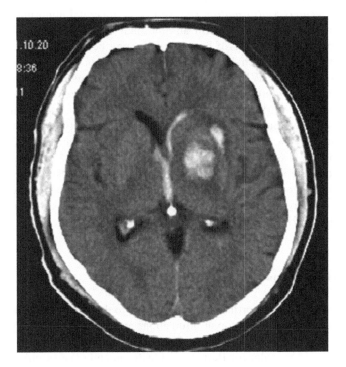

Image B. CT brain scan without contrast of a left basal ganglia intracerebral hemorrhage with extension into the intraventricular space in a patient with chronic hypertension

Nontraumatic intracerebral hemorrhages involving the cortex are more suggestive of an underlying structural abnormality such as an *arteriovenous malformation* (AVM) which is a congenital abnormality of blood vessels where the thin walls and increased blood flow predispose to bleeding. AVMs can be located in any region of the brain, but typically are inside the brain parenchyma. The incidence of hemorrhage for untreated AVMs is estimated to be 2–4% annually, with a mortality rate of 1–2% per year. Generally, patients are young and the hemorrhage is not large, so survival is better than other forms of hemorrhagic stroke. Scar tissue within the malformation often leads to seizures and may be the presenting feature of the lesion.

Amyloid angiopathy is the most common cause of ICH in the elderly, particularly when hypertension is not a factor. Cerebral amyloid angiopathy is the degeneration of vessel walls leading to multiple, recurrent hemorrhages, and is associated with progressive cognitive decline. The location of these hemorrhages is typically in the parieto-occipital or temporo-parietal lobar white matter and spare the locations typically favored by hypertensive hemorrhages. Although ICHs related to anticoagulant drug use and other bleeding etiologies are more frequently confluent, single, and lobar in location, there can be tremendous variability with multifocal involvement.

Arteriovenous Malformation (AVMs) is a congenital abnormality in which a network of blood vessels form an abnormal communication of arterial and venous blood. This tangle of blood vessels may be very small, such as a few millimeters, or a much larger network of vessels that requires increased cardiac output. The AVM is composed of an arterial vessel that branches, often many times, and connecting directly to the venous system. The blood vessels comprising the AVM are abnormal and have thin walls. Arteriovenous malformations can be located in any region of the brain, but typically are inside the brain parenchyma. The incidence of hemorrhage for untreated AVMs is estimated to be 2–4% annually, with a mortality rate of 1–2% per year. Generally, the hemorrhage is not large and most patients (about 90%) survive the initial bleed. The hemorrhage of an AVM may be limited to a small area of the parenchyma, or may involve hemorrhage into the ventricles (intraventricular), arachnoid (SAH), or dura (SDH).

Subarachnoid Hemorrhage (SAH)

Most subarachnoid hemorrhages (SAH) are due to the rupture of intracranial aneurysms that commonly develop at bifurcations and branch points within the Circle of Willis at the base of the brain (see Images C, D, and E). There are three types of aneurysms: (1) Saccular (or Berry), (2) Fusiform, and (3) dissecting. Most aneurysms are saccular (berry) aneurysms, which originate from a congenital weakness within the artery which enlarges to form a sac- or balloon-like structure protruding from the side of a vessel. In the elderly, atherosclerosis can lead to a fusiform enlargement (aneurysm) of intracranial vessels which are also classified as aneurysms. These rarely rupture but rather cause ischemic strokes by occluding thrombosis or act like an expanding mass and distort brain tissue. The third type of aneurysm is a dissecting aneurysm which is formed when the lumen of the vessel wall is torn, allowing blood to track between the layers of tissue making up the vessel wall; these have a variable prognosis.

The risk for rupture for incidental or asymptomatic saccular aneurysm overall is 1–2% per year. Factors that increase this risk include aneurysm size, multiplicity, location, and the patient's age. Although aneurysms of any size may rupture, many are between 5 and 10 mm in size. Most saccular aneurysms are idiopathic, but 15% are inherited and are associated with other vascular disorders such as polycystic kidney disease, co-arctation of the aorta, Ehlers-Danlos syndrome, neurofibromatosis, fibromuscular dysplasia, and arteriovenous malformations (AVMs).

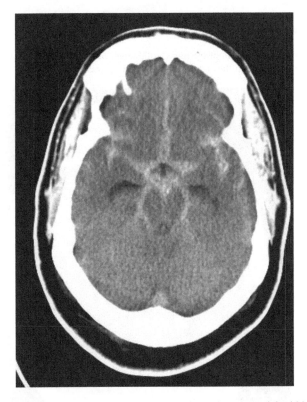

Image C. CT brain scan without contrast demonstrating hyperdense material within the sylvian fissures characteristic for an aneurysmal subarachnoid hemorrhage

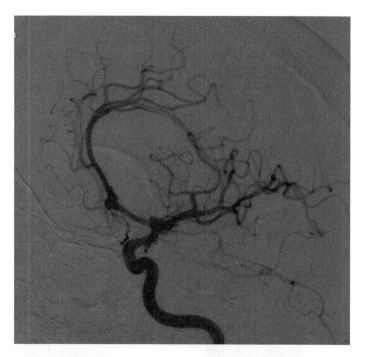

Image D. Cerebral angiogram of internal carotid artery demonstrating ACA and MCA distributions and berry aneurysm at the anterior communicating artery

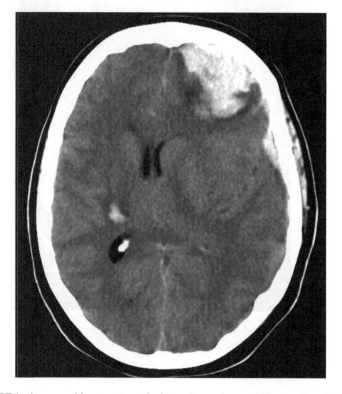

Image E. CT brain scan without contrast depicts a hemorrhage within a region of infarction located at the cortical surface characteristic for rupture of a mycotic aneurysm

Mortality rates are highest for SAH as the acute rupture of blood under arterial pressure produces an abrupt rise in intracranial pressure preventing cerebral blood flow. As of 2009, 10–20% of patients with SAH die prior to reaching the hospital, and 26–46% of surviving patients die within 6 months of the original SAH. The overall mortality rate for SAH has ranged from 32% to 67%. Neurological complications of SAH include rebleeding, vasospasm, and hydrocephalus.

Rebleeding is the re-occurrence of blood hemorrhaging after an initial bleed through a ruptured aneurysm, and has lead to mortality in up to 78% of patients. Rebleeding occurs in up to 50% of patients who are not surgically treated. Of these, about 20% of cases rebleed within 2 weeks of the original hemorrhage, and more than 30% rebleed within the first month. The incidence of rebleeding 6 months after the original SAH is about 2.2% per year in the first 10 years and then 0.9% per year in the following 10 years.

Vasospasm refers to the contraction of the intracerebral artery walls, resulting in lower flow and higher arterial pressure. Vasospasm may be diffuse; however, it occurs most often in arteries proximal to the subarachnoid blood, and is correlated with blood products in the subarachnoid space. Vasospasm typically occurs 2–12 days after the initial hemorrhage, and will present with a clinical presentation of worsening neurologic and/or neuropsychologic deficits. Up to 50% of patients with vasospasm will suffer an ischemic stroke (brain attack). The presentation is typically fluctuating neurologic and/or neuropsychologic symptoms associated with vascular territory (territories) of the artery(s) (see Clinical Symptoms and neuroanatomic correlates section, this chapter, below).

Hydrocephalus occurs in 15–60% of patients with SAH. Hydrocephalus presents acutely (within 3 days of SAH) in about 20% of patients, but may occur at any time (often within 4 weeks) after the hemorrhage. Hydrocephalus in these cases is due to blockage of CSF pathways. Clinical presentation is onset of confusion, cognitive deterioration (dementia), ataxic gait and incontinence. Treatment of acute or subacute hydrocephalus is typically ventriculostomy or lumbar puncture.

The Hunt and Hess scale (Hunt and Hess 1968) is often used to grade the severity of SAH, and is provided below:

Grade 1 = Headache, slight nuchal rigidity
Grade II = Severe headache, cranial nerve palsy, nuchal rigidity
Grade III = Lethergy, confusion, mild focal neurologic deficits
Grade IV = Stupor, decerebrate rigidity (posturing), hemiparesis
Grade V = Coma (no arousal with pain), decerebrate rigidity (posturing)

Clinical outcome can be predicted by the Hunt and Hess clinical scale. Patients with Grade I, II, and III SAH tend to have better outcomes than patients with Grade IV or V SAH. With appropriate treatment, 30% of patients with Grades I–III make good functional and neurologic outcomes, but even for survivors of lesser severity SAH, the effects of increased intracranial pressure and the delayed cerebral injury from vasospasm-induced cerebral infarction can result in significant long-term cognitive deficits (see Sect. Neuropsychological Assessment of Patients after Stroke, p. 338 below, for review of Neuropsychological deficits). Overall, about 66% of survivors of SAH and aneurysm clipping never return to the same quality of life.

Intraventricular Hemorrhage

Intraventricular hemorrhage (IVH) can occur in isolation but is more commonly seen as a complication of subarachnoid hemorrhage or intracerebral hemorrhage and has similar etiologies. In addition to the above-mentioned complications, IVH often results in hydrocephalus requiring ventricular drainage.

In summary, strokes are classified according to pathophysiology being either ischemic or hemorrhagic. While the hallmark clinical features of a stroke are the sudden onset of neurologic and/or neuropsychologic symptoms, the specific symptoms are determined by the location of the lesion and pathophysiology. As the arterial vascular supply is rather uniform and disease states tend to affect certain regions of the vasculature with regularity, the result is a series of recognizable patterns of neurologic deficit representing specific stroke subtypes. The pattern of signs and symptoms will not only suggest the specific vessel(s) affected but will also suggest the underlying mechanism. However, having an understanding of functional neuroanatomical organization of the nervous system and the vasculature of the brain is a prerequisite to understanding the signs and symptoms of strokes, and a brief review is provided here. Readers may also review Chap. 3, this volume.

Cerebral Vasculature

The vascular supply to the brain is provided by the carotid arteries (anterior circulation) and the vertebral-basilar arteries (posterior circulation) (Fig. 13.1 and Image F). Venous blood is returned to the heart via a complimentary network of veins both

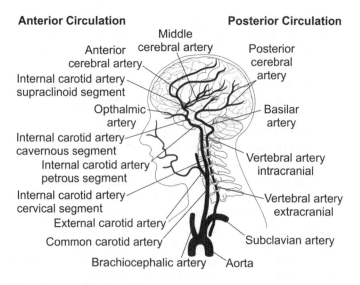

Anterior Circulation   **Posterior Circulation**

Fig. 13.1 Vasculature of head and brain

anterior and posterior which generally flow to the jugular vein (See Chap. 3, this volume, for review of the cerebral vasculature).

Anterior Circulation

The Common Carotid arteries arises from the Aorta (in some individuals, the Common Carotid arteries originate from the brachiocephalic arteries) and extend (one on the left side and one on the right side) up to the neck, where it branches into the *External Carotid* and *Internal Carotid* arteries (see Image F) . The External Carotid arteries provide blood to the face, scalp, and meninges. The Internal Carotid arteries extend nearly vertical until making a quick turn as it pierces the dura at the base of the brain. The Internal Carotid enters the Cavernous sinus (referred to as the Carotid Siphon (or cavernous segment), and then extends through subarachnoid space to branch (successively) into the Ophthalmic artery, Posterior Communicating artery (PComm or PCoA), Anterior Choroidal artery, Anterior Cerebral artery (ACA), and then Middle Cerebral artery (MCA) (OPAAM). See also Chap. 3 for review of cerebrovasculature anatomy.

Rule of thumb: OPAAM

To remember the arteries originating from the internal carotid artery:
  Ophthalmic artery
  Posterior communicating artery (PCoA)
  Anterior choroidal artery
  Anterior cerebral artery (ACA)
  Middle cerebral artery (MCA)

- *Ophthalmic artery* provides circulation to the optic nerve and retina.
- *Posterior Communicating (PComm or PCoA) arteries* form connections between the anterior and posterior circulations systems.
- *Anterior Choroidal arteries* provide circulation to a part of the Lenticular nucleus (i.e., globus pallidus and putamen), thalamus, and internal capsule (posterior limb).
- *Anterior Cerebral arteries* (ACAs) perfuse the anterior medial surface of the brain (area between the interhemispheric fissures dividing the two hemispheres of the brain), including the entire mesial frontal lobes, orbital frontal lobes, cingulate gyrus, corpus callosum, fornix (anterior segment), and may extend posteriorly to the mesial area of the parietal lobes.
- *Middle Cerebral arteries* (MC's) provide circulation to a large part of both hemispheres. The MCA runs horizontally along the base of the brain and before entering the Sylvian fissure, gives off a series of small perforating arteries, the

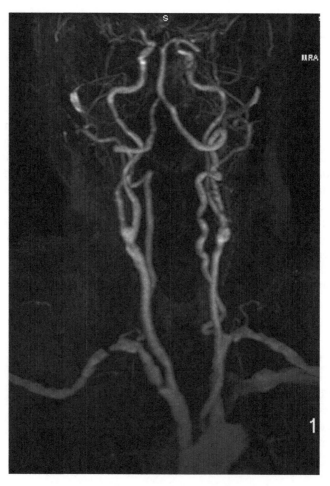

Image F. Magnetic Resonance Angiogram (MRA) beginning with the brachiocephalic artery at the bottom of the diagram showing the common carotid arteries and veterbral arteries. The vetebral arteries combine to the form the basilar artery at the top of the figure. Lateral to the basilar artery is the left and right internal carotid arteries. The MRA demonstrates multifocal areas of stenosis and irregularity consistent with atherosclerosis

Lenticulostriate arteries, and enter the brain through the anterior perforated substance providing blood to a large area of the basal ganglia and internal capsule. Once the MCA reaches the insula, it branches into the superior and inferior divisions. The superior division of the MCA provides circulation above the Sylvian fissure, including the lateral frontal and most of the lateral parietal lobes. The inferior division provides blood to the lateral temporal lobe and a posterior portion of the parietal lobes (see Image G).

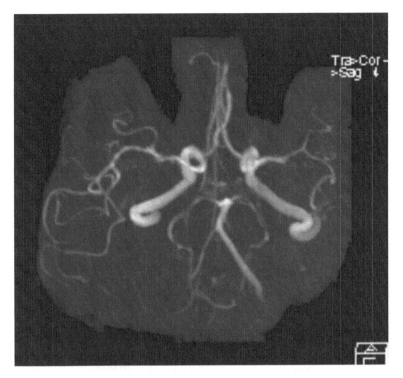

Image G. Magnetic Resonance Angiogram (MRA) of the Circle of Willis demonstrates an occlusion of the inferior division of the left middle cerebral artery in a patient presenting with a Wernicke's aphasia

Posterior Circulation

The posterior circulation includes the bilateral vertebral arteries, the basilar artery, and its branches. The vertebral arteries arise from the Subclavian arteries and are encased by the foramina transversaria of the cervical vertebrae to enter the skull via the foramen magnum. The vertebral arteries ascend along the ventral surface of the medulla, eventually joining together to form the *Basilar artery* usually at the pontomedullary junction. Along this course, the vertebral arteries give rise to *Anterior Spinal artery* and the *Posterior Inferior Cerebellar arteries* (PICA). Arising along with *Basilar artery* are the two *Anterior Inferior Cerebellar arteries* (AICAs). The Basilar artery then runs along the ventral surface of the pons and midbrain with branches that form the two *Superior Cerebellar arteries* (SCAs) and, at the distal end, terminating by dividing into the two *Posterior Cerebral arteries* (PCAs). *Posterior Cerebral arteries* perfuse the mesial and inferior temporal lobes (including the hippocampus) as well as the occipital lobes (both inferior, mesial, and lateral areas of the occipital lobes).

Circle of Willis

The anterior and posterior cerebral circulation systems are connected together by the Circle of Willis, which allows for collateral flow of the anterior and posterior systems as well as left to right (or right to left) (see Fig. 13.2). The anterior segment of the Circle of Willis include the Anterior Communicating artery (AComm or ACoA) which allows flow between the right and left ACAs. The ACAs form another aspect of the circle as they connect to the Internal Carotid Artery. The Internal Carotid arteries are connected to the posterior circulations via the bilateral PComms arteries (PCoA). The two PCAs branch off from the top of the Basilar artery. While a complete Circle of Willis is present in about 25% of normal adults, collateral flow is present to varying degrees. Having briefly reviewed functional neuroanatomy and cerebral vasculature, we now turn to clinical features and syndromes.

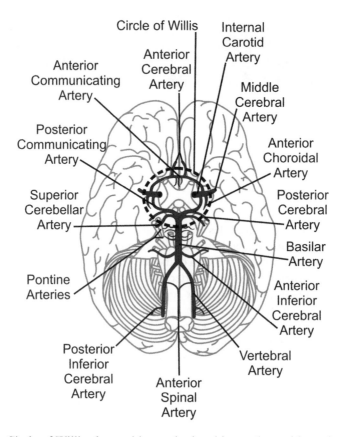

Fig. 13.2 Circle of Willis along with vertebral and internal carotid arteries

Clinical Symptoms and Neuroanatomic Correlates

The clinical presentation of a stroke is classically recognized as one of the most distinctive syndromes affecting the brain. The classic description of abrupt onset of nonconvulsive focal neurologic deficit is well known to health professionals and increasingly the public. Indeed, public education campaigns to improve recognition and reporting of stroke warning signs and symptoms have focused on the most common clinical presentations (National Stroke Association 2007) and include:

1. Sudden onset of weakness of the face, arm, and/or leg on one side of the body
2. Sudden onset of numbness/tingling of the face, arm, and/or leg on one side of the body
3. Sudden onset of confusion, trouble speaking, or understanding speech
4. Sudden trouble with vision in one or both eyes (diplopia, complaints of blurred or distorted vision)
5. Sudden onset of difficulty walking, loss of balance, discoordination, or vertigo
6. Sudden severe headache with no known cause

However, patients may also present with symptoms that are less acute or salutatory in onset, nonfocal (e.g., headache, loss of consciousness, etc.), or less commonly pure neuropsychological deficits (e.g., problems in memory, attention/executive, and/or pseudobulbar affect) that are not as readily recognized as symptoms of stroke. In addition, seizures are not uncommon, reported in about 8–9% of all ischemic strokes and 10–11% of all hemorrhagic strokes (Bladin et al. 2000). Below, we first review the general clinical features of ischemic and hemorrhagic strokes, followed by a discussion of specific cerebrovascular syndromes associated with different types of strokes.

Ischemic Strokes

The signs and symptoms of cerebral ischemia and infarction are determined by both the location and the extent of brain tissue injured. Focal neurologic and/or neuropsychologic deficits develop abruptly and are typically painless without depressed consciousness and evolve over the course of seconds to hours. Stroke progression can occur in 10–20% of patients usually in the setting of a thrombotic occlusion of a vessel with declining blood flow or repeated embolism. The neurologic and neuropsychologic deficits associated with stroke is linked to the areas of the brain perfused by the vessel(s) involved (see below and Table 13.3). Figures 13.3, 13.4, and 13.5 provide an overview of regions profused by cerebral vessels. Figure 13.6 shows vascular profusion of (1) the basal ganglia and (2) internal capsule. See Chap. 3 for overview of functional neuroanatomy of cerebral cortex and basal ganglia.

The treatment of acute ischemic stroke has advanced considerably over the years (see Table 13.7 in Treatment of Stroke and Rehabilitation section below for details) with the introduction of tissue plasminogen activators (t-PA) and other

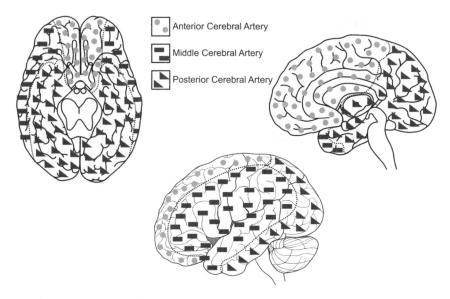

Fig. 13.3 Gross cerebral vascular profusion of cortex

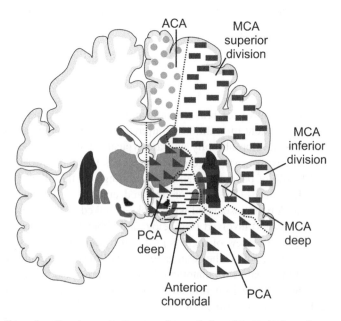

Fig. 13.4 Coronal section demonstrating vascular profusion of major brain regions

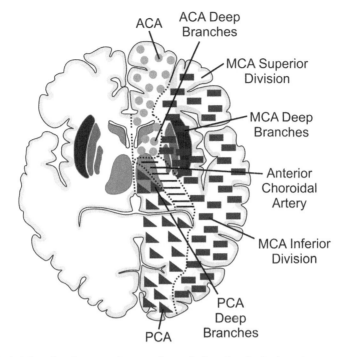

Fig. 13.5   Axial section demonstrating vascular profusion of major brain regions

revascularization therapies. t-PA converts plasminogen to the enzyme plasmin which is able to lyse fibrin within the recent thrombus thus restoring blood flow. Treatment with t-PA is not without risk, with hemorrhagic conversion being the primary morbidity of treatment. When tPA is given within an appropriate treatment protocol to 100 eligible patients within 3 hours of ischemic stroke symptom onset, 32 are substantially improved and 3 are harmed by the therapy. When tPA is given to a more select population at 3–4.5 hours of ischemic stroke symptom onset, 16 are substantially improved and 3 are harmed by the therapy. Studies have demonstrated 30% of patients treated with t-PA intravenously within 3 hours of symptom onset did not exhibit appreciable neurologic deficits 3 months or 12 months later (e.g., Kwiatkowski et al. 1999).

Hemorrhagic Strokes

The clinical presentation of hemorrhagic strokes will depend upon pressure within the bleeding vessel, anatomic location, size, extent of any mass effect, and occurrence of any secondary comorbid processes (edema, vasospasm, rebleeding, etc.). Symptoms may be focal (in the case of some ICH syndromes), generalized (in the case of some SAH) or

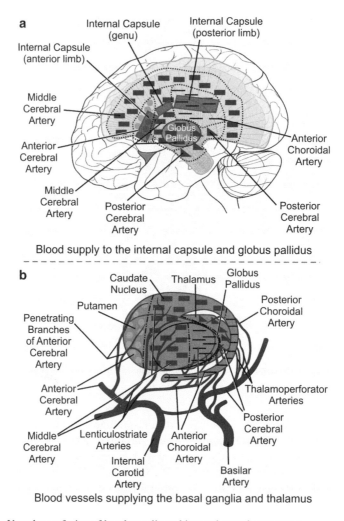

Fig. 13.6 Vascular profusion of basal ganglia and internal capsule structures

combinations of both. Prominent complaints of headache and altered consciousness or progressive obtundation are typical features of hemorrhagic strokes that help to distinguish them from ischemic strokes prior to obtaining neuroimaging. Seizures may also occur. The common clinical features of hemorrhagic strokes are reviewed below.

Intracerebral Hemorrhage (ICH)

In general, ICH presents as an acute, focal neurological deficit (e.g., hemiplegia), but as the hematoma expands, the deficit progresses with headache, emesis, and altered consciousness. Presence of headache and/or emesis is not universal, but is frequent.

Very small ICH in some parts of the brain (e.g., periventricular white matter) may not be associated with any clinical symptoms (i.e., "silent stroke"). Seizures have been reported in about 10% of all ICH within the first few days of the stroke, with rates ranging from 4% to 17%. Seizures are more common in lobar hemorrhages than hemorrhages involving deep white matter or brain stem. Onset of seizures after months or even years of the ICH may occur, but is less common (Bladin et al. 2000). Extension of the hemorrhage to ventricles or arachnoid space increases risk of developing hydrocephalus within days to weeks of the hemorrhage. The risk factor of ICH has not been shown to be directly linked to periods of high stress, with 90% of cases occurring when the patient was not stressed, but is more likely to occur during wakefulness than while sleeping (Caplan, 1993). Massive sized hemorrhages can present with abrupt onset of loss of consciousness and unsteady breathing, dilated and fixed pupils, and within several hours, death. However, the clinical presentation and course of ICH varies as a function of size of hemorrhage, location, and comorbid conditions. Symptoms worsen over minutes to at most several hours to days, followed by a period of gradually resolving symptoms over weeks to 2–3 months. This reflects the physiological processes of the brain and body with edema and subsequent breakdown of blood products in the parenchyma. Unlike ischemic strokes, the recovery of neurologic and/or neuropsychologic function can be much more complete, as ICH tends to displace brain parenchyma due to space occupying bleed as opposed to the direct damage to neurons and glia as a result of ischemia. As reviewed above, there are common locations of ICH, and the four most common ICH syndromes are reviewed below.

Putaminal hemorrhage. Hemorrhage involving the basal ganglia is the most common place of primary ICH. The hemorrhage often extends into the internal capsule. The typical clinical course is abrupt onset of headache followed over the course of several minutes (<30 minutes) of progressive deterioration with onset of facial paresis followed by hemiplegia contralateral to the side of the hemorrhage, homonymous hemianopsia (contralateral to side of lesion), slurred speech (nondominant hemisphere ICH) or aphasia (dominant hemisphere ICH), deviation of eyes towards the side of the lesion (pupils may remain normal), followed over the course of less than an hour by confusion and obtundation (loss of consciousness level). However, massive hemorrhages may present simply with abrupt onset of coma with hemiplegia contralateral to side of hemorrhage. Respirations become shallow, and as the brain stem becomes compressed, eyes become fixed and dilated, and decerebrate posturing occurs. Smaller hemorrhages confined to the putamen tend to produce either more motor or sensory deficits depending if the lesion is more anterior or posterior. Anterior putamen hemorrhages are associated with contralateral hemiparesis, Broca's aphasia (dominant hemisphere lesions only), abulia, and motor impersistence. Small hemorrhages restricted to the posterior putamen results in mild and more hemianesthesia, loss of visual pursuit to the contralateral hemispace, hemianopia, Wernicke's aphasia (dominant hemisphere lesions only) or anosagnosia (nondominant hemisphere lesions). Extension of these lesions to the lateral ventricle often results in change of mental status (drowsiness and stupor or agitation and confusion).

Thalamic hemorrhage. Symptoms vary depending upon the size of the hemorrhage, but the most common features are contralateral hemianesthesia, Wernicke's (fluent) aphasia (dominant hemisphere ICH) or contralateral neglect and anosagnosia (nondominant hemisphere ICH), and, frequently, various gaze and ocular abnormalities including vertical and lateral gaze palsies, pseudo-abducens palsies in which the eyes are deviated slightly inward and down, and asymmetrical skew deviation with the eye contralateral to the lesion being lower than the eye ipsilateral to the lesion. Ipsilateral Horner's syndrome and/or nystagmus may be present. Contralateral hemiparesis may also be present, but less pronounced than sensory deficits and due to impingement of the hemorrhage affecting the outlying internal capsule. Homonymous hemianopsia is also frequently reported, but is likely to remit after several days. Larger lesions can result in compression of the third ventricle which may result in hydrocephalus of the lateral ventricles, necessitating placement of a shunt. Extension of the hemorrhage to the third ventricle has been reported to result in less neurologic comorbidity, but frequently does result in hydrocephalus that requires surgical treatment.

Pontine hemorrhage. The clinical manifestations of pontine ICH tends to result in coma within minutes. Quadraplegia is often present due to disruption of both corticospinal and corticobulbar tracts. Decerebrate rigidity and small (so called "pin-point") pupils that are reactive to light frequently develop within minutes of the ICH. Lateral eye movements are absent. Mortality is common with pontine hemorrhages, with most (60 + %) dying within the first few hours. Small hemorrhages are less likely to result in coma or death. If the hemorrhage is small, symptoms include pinpoint pupils, lateral gaze palsies, hemianesthesia, quadraparesis, but retained consciousness. Recovery has been reported to be "functionally good" for a small number of patients with pontine ICH and retained consciousness.

Cerebellar hemorrhage. Common clinical signs include nausea and emesis, severe occipital headache, and truncal ataxia preventing the patient from walking, standing, and in some cases even sitting upright. Depending upon the size of the hemorrhage, symptom onset may be minutes to an hour or two. While consciousness is generally retained early in the symptom course, untreated ICH can lead to compression of the brain stem leading to rapid onset of coma, decerebrate posturing, and death within minutes. Ipsilateral conjugate lateral gaze palsy, ipsilateral sixth nerve palsy, or eye deviation to the contralateral side is often present. "Pin-point" pupils that are reactive to light may also be present. Other cerebellar signs, including dysarthria, dysphagia, limb ataxia or nystagmus may not be present. Vertical eye movements are retained. Sudden onset of these symptoms progressing over minutes should be considered a neurological emergency unless proven otherwise.

Lobar hemorrhages. The signs and symptoms of lobar hemorrhages vary substantially based on where the ICH occurs, but often include abrupt headache, drowsiness, and nausea with emesis. Seizures are reported in 15–24% of patients (electrographic in 31%), and among this group, a seizure was the first presenting symptom in about 10 % of the patients (Bladin et al. 2000). Lobar hemorrhages, when in the elderly, are frequently due to amyloid angiopathy.

Occipital hemorrhages tend to result in contralateral homonymous hemianopsia and pain around the ipsilateral eye. Temporal hemorrhages can result in a variety of symptoms including Wernicke's aphasia (dominant hemisphere lesions), memory impairment, pain involving the ipsilateral ear (or just anterior to it), and visual agnosias. Frontal lobe hemorrhages can result in a vast array of symptoms including contralateral hemiparesis, Broca's (nonfluent) aphasia (dominant hemisphere only), motor apraxias, dysexecutive (dorsolateral) syndrome, and frontal headache. Parietal lobe hemorrhages symptoms include anterior temporal region headache, contralateral hemianesthesia, aphasia symptoms (conduction aphasia), Gerstmann's syndrome (acalculia, dysgraphia, finger agnosia, and right/left confusion), and constructional apraxia.

Arteriovenous Malformation

As noted above, the clinical features of an AVM is typically completely silent, until the AVM hemorrhages. However, some neurologic symptoms have been associated with AVMs, including headache and seizure. Headache has been reported as the only symptom of AVM in 20% of patients while seizure was reported as the presenting symptom in 17–40% of patients. Seizures are not uncommon presenting symptom, reported in 17–40% (Hofmeister et al., 2000). Neurologic deficits that are progressive have been reported for large AVMs that either compress neighboring brain regions and/or through a phenomena called "intracerebral steal" in which large amounts of blood are shunted away from neighboring regions due the large vascular volume enabled by such AVMs. Finally, hemorrhage was the first clinical symptom in about half of patients with AVMs (42–50%). Although thought to be present since before birth, onset of clinical symptoms typically occurs between the ages of 10–30 years old, although clinical symptoms may not appear until one's 50s or even later. Neurologic and neuropsychologic deficits associated with hemorrhages of AVMs may involve SAH, subdural hemorrhage, intraventricular, and/or hemorrhage into brain parenchyma.

Subarachnoid Hemorrhage (SAH)

Subarachnoid hemorrhage clinical presentation has typically been described as one of the three patterns: (1) patient develops a sudden severe generalized headache with vomiting, (2) sudden severe generalized headache with vomiting and loss of consciousness, and (3) rapid onset of unconsciousness with no other complaints before the patient collapses to the ground (patient will suddenly topple to the floor). The most common is onset of sudden severe headache and initially retained consciousness. Because bleeding is predominantly around the brain, there are usually no early focal neurological findings (but see below). Most (90–95%) of saccular aneurysms arise from the Circle of Willis, with the four most common areas being: (1) anterior communicating artery (ACoA), (2) origin of the PComm from the internal carotid artery, (3) first large bifurcation of the MCA, and (4) arising from the bifurcation of the internal carotid artery to form the MCA and ACA. Below, we review the clinical features, etiology, and general prognosis for SAH arising from these four areas.

Rule of thumb: Top areas for saccular aneurysms at branch points within basal brain arteries

A. Internal carotid (anterior) vascular system (85–95% of all cerebral aneurysms)
  1. Anterior cerebral artery and Anterior communicating artery (ACA and ACoA) ~30–35%
  2. Terminal Internal Carotid Artery and Posterior communicating artery (tICA and PCoA) ~30–35%
  3. Middle cerebral artery (1st MCA bifurcation) ~20%
B. Vertebral-Basilar (posterior) vascular system (5–15% of all cerebral aneurysms)
  1. Basilar artery bifurcation (top of the basilar) ~5%
  2. Remaining posterior circulation arteries ~5%

The clinical syndrome of SAH shares many similarities in the acute phase. The common clinical picture is an abrupt onset severe headache followed by reduced arousal level, and sometimes coma. Sudden loss of consciousness occurs in about 20% of patients. Nuchal rigidity, seizures, papilledema, and/or retinal hemorrhage are common. Seizure as first presenting symptom occurred in 6–18% of patients with SAH (Pinto et al. 1996). Localizing features may not be present for one or more days, but cranial nerve palsies, particularly CN III, IV, and VI, are common. Lateralizing features, such as headache that primarily involves one hemisphere, monocular pain, or unilateral retinal hemorrhage may occur. While not common, some more localizing features may be present:

1. Paresis of one or both legs and/or presentation of retained consciousness with mutism and/or akinesia is suggestive of an ACoA aneurysm hemorrhage
2. A third nerve palsy can be indicative of a PComm aneurysm, but CN IV and VI palsies are often due to increased intracranial pressure.
3. Immediate hemiparesis and/or global aphasia is suggestive of an aneurysm of the first major bifurcation of the MCA.
4. Unilateral blindness with retained consciousness is suggestive of an ophthalmic artery or the branching of the internal carotid artery.

Outcome from SAH is difficult to predict, such as rebleeding, ischemic stroke due to vasospasm and/or hydrocephalus adversely affects outcome. In general, individuals with SAH that cannot be identified using angiography have a much better prognosis than patients in which the aneurysm is identifiable. Mortality and increased likelihood of poor outcome occurs with ventricular and/or intraparenchymal extension. Patients with extensions of the hemorrhage have increased likelihood of coma and development of hydrocephalus.

AComm (ACoA). Rupture of aneurysm of artery between the ACA arteries may result in damage to large or small area of the brain, but typically the inferior and mesial frontal lobes are damaged. Damage to the brain parenchyma can occur by a variety of causes, including blood products, ischemia due to decreased arterial blood volume and/or subsequent vasospasm, increased intracranial pressure and effects from craniotomy and/or infection. Damage may also affect the mesial thalamus and cingulate gyrus.

Up to 60% of patients who survive AComm aneurysms present with disabling neuropsychological deficits. Deficits frequently involve attention/concentration, executive skills, memory, and language functions as well as personality and mood changes related to bilateral frontal lobe dysfunction. Pseudobulbar affect may be present. Attention deficits typically include reduced sustained attention and increased distractibility. Executive impairments are common, and patients can present with a variety of cognitive and personality changes associated with mesial and/or orbitofrontal lobe syndromes including decreased initiation, behavioral apathy, reduced verbal output (mutism), or, alternatively, behavioral disinhibition, agitation, increased energy level, reduced personal hygiene, and difficulty learning from trial and error (see Chap. 10, this volume for detailed description of frontal lobe syndromes). Memory can be markedly impaired, particularly if basal forebrain areas are damaged. Memory impairment is of declarative (explicit) memory, and the patient can be densely amnestic. Confabulation is frequently found, and mood symptoms can include paranoia, delusions, and obsessive-compulsive behaviors.

Improvement in neuropsychological function after AcoA aneurysm rupture does occur, but most patients will exhibit residual impairments. Return to work and/or independence following ACoA aneurysm is typically poor. Of patients working full-time prior to AComm aneurysm rupture, about 50% do not return to the same level of work due to the long-term cognitive deficits frequently associated with ACoA aneurysms.

Cerebral Artery Syndromes

ACA, MCA, and PCA Cerebral Artery Syndromes

Table 13.2 reviews the neurologic and neuropsychologic symptoms associated with common cerebral arterial strokes. Importantly, the description below assumes normal neuroanatomical functional organization, with the patient being left hemisphere dominant for language.

Table 13.2 Cerebral arterial syndromes

Left ICA

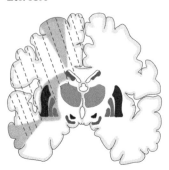

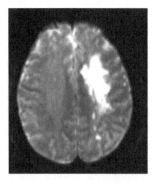

Image H. Transverse MRI DWI image of a left carotid thrombosis resulting in borderzone (watershed) infarct of left hemisphere

LEFT Internal Carotid Artery (ICA): "Silent" (having no symptoms) in 30–40% of cases due to collateral flow from posterior circulation and collateral flow from opposite internal carotid artery through the circle of Willis. Collateral flow to left ACA via ACoA from right ACA and posterior circulation (basilar artery) supplying flow to the left PCA usually results in sparing of medial frontal and the occipital and part of the parietal lobe. Thus ICA occlusion can result in limited borderzone (watershed) infarcts between the ACA-MCA and MCA-PCA regions (along with ischemia of deep MCA penetrating branches). However, if no collateral flow from circle of Willis, much more massive ischemic damage can occur, inclusive of left ACA and MCA areas.

"Incomplete ICA" (borderzone or watershed infarct): Mixed transcortical aphasia or transcortical motor aphasia is most common. Transcortical sensory aphasia possible. Right motor and sensory impairment of the trunk, hips, and proximal extremities. Gerstmann's syndrome. Agnosias. Memory deficits are possible. See Image H.

"Complete ICA": Right hemiparesis of contralateral body including lower face (primary and supplementary cortex). Right hemianesthesia, including pain, temperature, light touch, position, and vibration sense (primary sensory cortex). Global aphasia quite possible. Broca's aphasia also possible depending upon flow from posterior circulation and distribution of PCA territory. Agraphia, acalculia, finger agnosia, right/left confusion (Gerstmann's syndrome) may be present if flow from PCA is insufficient. Ideomotor apraxia, ideational apraxia, constructional apraxia (left frontal and parietal cortex). Acute ipsilateral monocular blindness (damage to optic nerve) and right homonymous hemianopsia, which tends to resolve (optic radiations). Frontal lobe behavioral problems (dorsolateral frontal lobe syndrome) including grasp, root, suck reflexes, impaired sequencing, poor problem solving. Memory may be impaired (particularly for verbal memory).

(continued)

Table 13.2 (continued)

LEFT ACA	LEFT ACA artery: Right leg motor and sensory loss (primary motor and sensory cortex, supplementary motor cortex). Frontal lobe behavioral problems (medial frontal syndrome) including akinesia, mutism, abulia (lack of initiative or drive). Patients may appear lazy or uncaring. While complete mutism is rare (except in the case of AComm aneurysms, with rupture causing damage to both right and left medial frontal areas), transcortical motor aphasia is more common. Memory deficits are possible, particularly with poor retrieval (see Image I).
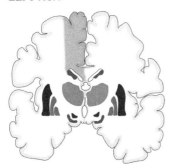 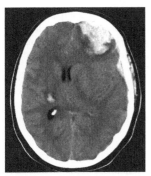 **Image I.** Left frontal hemorrhage into infarction resulting from a mycotic aneurysm	
Left MCA stem (Lateral view) 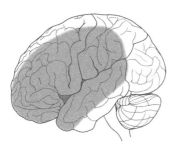	Move down to be parallel to figure. LEFT MCA stem: Right face, arm and leg motor and sensory loss (motor and sensory primary cortex, secondary motor cortex) resulting in a right hemiparesis and right hemianasthesia. Right homonymous hemianopsia is possible, left gaze preference (lesion of left frontal eye field that would drive eyes to right leading to left gaze). Global aphasia common (Most people are left hemisphere dominant for language). Motor apraxias and visuoconstructional deficits can be present. Acalculia and memory loss may occur. Mood changes are common (see Image D), frequently with depressive symptoms that can be quite prominent.

(continued)

Table 13.2 (continued)

Left MCA stem (Coronal view)

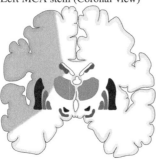

Left MCA deep territory 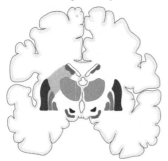	Left MCA deep territory: Right face, arm, and leg motor loss (aka. pure motor hemiparesis). Mild aphasia symptoms can be present in larger infarcts. The left basal ganglia involvement may produce deficits in movement. Mood changes with depression is common.
Left MCA inferior division 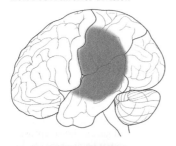	Left MCA inferior division: Fluent aphasia syndrome (Wernicke's or transcortical sensory) depending on extent of infarction. Right face and arm sensory loss (primary sensory cortex). Right visual field defect is common (particularly inferior quadrantanopsia). Right face and hand motor loss is possible, but will be mild. Gerstmann's syndrome is possible. Visuoconstructional/visuospatial deficits are possible. Mood changes, with symptoms of depression common (see Image J).

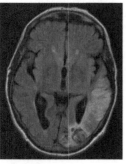

Image J. Left MCA inferior infarction

(continued)

Table 13.2 (continued)

Left MCA superior division	Left MCA superior division: Right face and arm motor loss (primary and secondary motor cortex). Some face and arm sensory loss may be present, depending on how posterior the vascular extended into the parietal lobe. Leg motor and sensory function unaffected. Nonfluent type of aphasia (Broca's or transcortical motor) depending upon extent of infarction. Mood changes, symptoms of depression common (see Image K).

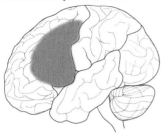

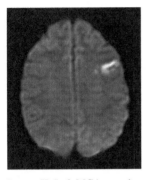

Image K. Left MCA superior
division infarct

Left PCA (Lateral view)	Left PCA: Right homonymous hemianopsia is common. Some kind of right visual field defect will be present. Visual agnosias are common. Alexia without Agraphia is possible. Transcortical Sensory Aphasia is possible with larger infarcts. Motor and sensory loss of the hand and face is possible if lesion is large and damages thalamus and internal capsule. Mood changes with depression can be present.

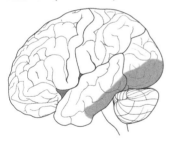

Left PCA (coronal section)

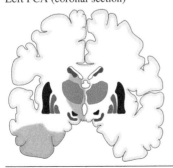

(continued)

Table 13.2 (continued)

Left ACA-MCA	Left ACA-MCA borderzone: Transcortical motor aphasia. Right motor and sensory impairment of the trunk, hips, and proximal extremities.

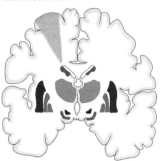

Left MCA-PCA	Left MCA-PCA borderzone: Transcortical sensory aphasia. Gerstmann's syndrome. Agnosias. Memory deficits are possible (verbal may be more impaired than "visual" memory, see Chap. 8).

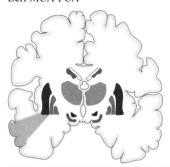

Right ICA

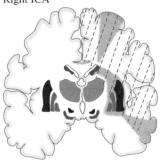

RIGHT Internal Carotid Artery (ICA): "Silent" (having no symptoms) in 30–40% of cases due to collateral flow from posterior circulation and collateral flow from opposite internal carotid artery through the Circle of Willis. Collateral flow to right ACA via ACoA from left ACA and posterior circulation (basilar artery) supplying flow to the right PCA usually results in sparing of medial frontal and the occipital and part of the parietal lobe. Thus, ICA occlusion can result in limited borderzone (watershed) infarcts between the ACA–MCA and MCA–PCA regions (along with ischemia of deep MCA penetrating branches). However, if no collateral flow from Circle of Willis, more massive ischemic damage can occur, inclusive of ACA and MCA areas.

"Incomplete ICA" (borderzone or watershed infarct): Aprosody (motor), but can be of a transcortical motor or mixed transcortical. Left motor and sensory impairment of the trunk, hips, and proximal extremities. Anosagnosia, left neglect, ideational apraxia, constructional apraxia (right frontal and parietal cortex). Memory deficits are possible, in particular visual/nonverbal memory.

(continued)

Table 13.2 (continued)

	"Complete ICA": Left hemiparesis of contralateral body including lower face (primary and supplementary cortex). Left hemianesthesia, including pain, temperature, light touch, position, and vibration sense (primary sensory cortex). Receptive and expressive aprosody quite possible. Expressive aprosody also possible depending upon flow from posterior circulation and distribution of PCA territory. Constructional apraxia (likely severe). Acute ipsilateral monocular blindness (prechiasmic damage to optic nerve) and left homonymous hemianopsia, but tends to resolve (optic radiations). Frontal lobe behavioral problems (dorsolateral frontal lobe syndrome) including grasp, root, suck reflexes, impaired sequencing, poor problem solving. Memory may be impaired (particularly for visual/nonverbal material).
Right ACA 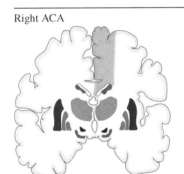	Right ACA: Left leg sensory and motor loss. Left arm weakness can occur in large infarcts. Frontal lobe behaviors (apathy, stimulus bound behaviors, jocularity, hypomania).
Right MCA (Lateral view) 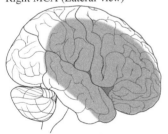 Right MCA (Coronal view) 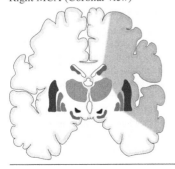	Right MCA stem: Left face, arm and leg motor and sensory loss (motor and sensory primary cortex, secondary motor cortex) resulting in a left hemiparesis and left hemianasthesia. Left homonymous hemianopsia possible, with right gaze preference (lesion of right frontal eye field which drives eyes to left). Profound hemi-neglect initially and may resolve to hemi-inattention. Speech intact. (Most people are left hemisphere dominant for language). Visuoconstructional deficits are prominent. Motor apraxia may sometimes occur. Memory impairments may be present. Anosagnosia common. Mood changes are common, with initial symptoms of hypomania and jocularity, but affective flattening may occur. Aprosody is common (see Image L and Chaps. 7 and 12, this volume).

Table 13.2 (continued)

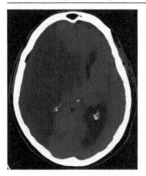

Image L. MRI ADC map showing right
MCA stem artery infarction

Right MCA deep territory	Right MCA deep territory: Left face, arm, and leg motor loss (aka. pure motor hemiparesis). Large infarcts may result in left hemineglect. Visuoconstructional deficits are possible.
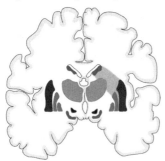	
Right MCA inferior division	Right MCA inferior division: Left face and arm sensory loss (primary sensory cortex). Left visual field defect is common (particularly inferior quadrantanopia). Left face and hand motor weakness is possible, but will be mild. Left hemineglect (that may gradually resolve to a left hemi-inattention). Initially, the left hemineglect can be pronounced, and limit the ability to evaluate for left visual field defects or any left motor weakness. Visuoconstructional/visuospatial deficits. Mood changes, with symptoms of hypomania or affective flattening is common. Receptive aprosody is likely (see Chap. 16, this volume, for review)
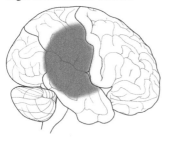	
Right MCA superior division	Right MCA superior division: Left face and arm motor weakness (primary and secondary motor cortex). Some face and arm sensory loss may be present, depending on how posterior the ischemic *penumbrae* extended into the parietal lobe. Leg motor and sensory function unaffected. Expressive aprosody may be present. Frontal lobe behaviors may be present, particularly dorsolateral syndrome behaviors of poor problem solving, impaired sequencing, perseveration, poor reasoning. Mood changes with hypomania and a hollow jocularity are common (see Image M).
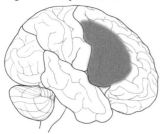	

(continued)

Table 13.2 (continued)

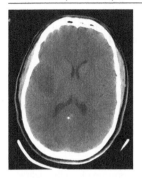

Image M. MRI showing right MCA
superior division infarction

Right PCA (Lateral view)	Right PCA: Left homonymous hemianopsia is common. Some kind of left visual field defect will be present. Visual agnosias are common. Aprosody (receptive) is possible. Motor and sensory loss of the hand and face is possible if lesion is large and damages thalamus and internal capsule. Mood changes with anxiety or depression can be present.

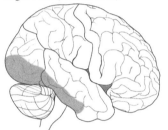

Coronal view

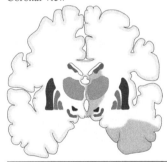

Right ACA-MCA borderzone (watershed)	Right ACA – MCA Borderzone(watershed): Left motor and sensory impairment of the trunk, hips, and proximal extremities. Visuoconstructional deficits are possible.

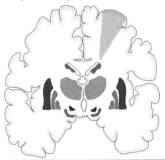

(continued)

Table 13.2 (continued)

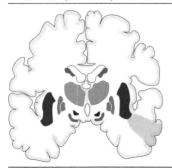

Right MCA – PCA borderzone (watershed):
Visuoconstructional and visuoperceptual deficits.
Visual agnosias possible. Memory deficits are
possible, particularly nonverbal material.

Note: MRI images are presented such that the left side of the image corresponds to the right side
of the brain.

The Lacunar Syndromes

Lacunes are small subcortical infarcts (generally considered to be < 1.5 cm in diameter) of small deep penetrating arteries. Classically, Fisher (1982) described five lacunar syndromes: pure motor hemiparesis, pure sensory stroke, sensorimotor stroke, ataxic hemiparesis, and clumsy-hand dysarthria. Other lacunar syndromes have been described (see Table 13.3 for list of common lacunar syndromes), but some lacunar infarcts may be asymptomatic. We discuss the lacunar syndromes of the thalamus in a subsection below, as these present with greater neuropsychological deficits.

Rule of thumb: Classic Lacunar Syndromes

- Pure Motor Hemiparesis
- Pure Sensory Syndrome
- Ataxic Hemiparesis
- Dysarthria-Clumsy Hand
- Sensorimotor Syndrome

Table 13.3 Lacunae syndromes

Syndrome	Clinical features	Vasculature	Localization
Pure sensory stroke	Taste may be impaired (olfaction intact) No vision loss No motor deficits No neuropsychological impairment Ipsilateral: None	Inferolateral (thalamogeniculate) artery	Ventral posterior lateral (VPL) nuclei of the thalamus. Taste impaired if larger lesion affecting ventral posteromedial (VPM) nuclei of thalamus
Pure sensorimotor stroke	Contralateral: hemisensory loss (light touch, proprioception, vibration sense, pain, and temperature) of the face, hand, leg. Taste may be impaired (olfaction intact). Hemiparesis of face, hand, leg. No neuropsychological impairment. Ipsilateral: None	Inferolateral (thalamogeniculate) artery Lenticulostriate arteries (or other perforating branches of the MCA).	Ventrolateral (VL) and VPL nuclei of the thalamus. Thalamic somatosensory projections, corticospinal and corticobulbar pathways (posterior limb of internal capsule) Loss of taste indicates VPM nuclei of thalamus
Pure motor hemiparesis (of face, arm, leg)	Contralateral: hemiparesis No sensory loss No neuropsychological impairment. Ipsilateral: None	Lenticulostriate arteries (or other perforating branches of the MCA). Perforating branches of PCA. Anterior choroidal artery	Posterior limb of internal capsule, Pons (anterior portion) Cerebral peduncle Corona radiata

(continued)

Table 13.3 (continued)

Syndrome	Clinical features	Vasculature	Localization
Pure motor hemiparesis with dysarthria. (dysarthria – clumsy hand)	Contralateral: hemiparesis of face and arm (and sometimes leg). (face>arm>leg). Dysarthric speech Dysphagia No sensory loss. No aphasia (receptive and expressive speech and repetition grossly intact). Assuming functional use of writing hand, the patient is able to write (and read) without difficulty. Ipsilateral: None	Penetrating branches of Basilar artery (paramedian). Lenticulostriate arteries (or other perforating branches of the MCA).	Medial pons damaging corticospinal and corticobulbar tracts. Cerebral peduncle genu of internal capsule
Pure motor hemiparesis with ataxia (Ataxic Hemiparesis)	Contralateral: hemiparesis and ataxia of face, arm, and leg. No sensory loss. No neuropsychological deficits. Important to distinguish clumsy hand movements due to hemiparesis (lesion of upper motor neurons) from apraxia Ipsilateral: None	Penetrating branches of Basilar artery (paramedian artery). Lenticulostriate arteries (or other perforating branches of the MCA).	medial pons damaging the corticospinal and corticobulbar tracts and pontine nuclei and the pontocerebellar tract. Less often due to internal capsule often including corona radiata.

Hemi-dystonic – putamen and globus pallidus	Contralateral: Variable presentation but may be asymptomatic. Presentation of movement disorders may occur, such as tremor or dystonia. Rarely associated with neuropsychologic deficits. Obsessive-compulsive symptoms reported. Ipsilateral: None	Lenticulostriate arteries (or other perforating branches of the MCA). Anterior choroidal artery (anterior putamen, globus pallidus) Recurrent artery of Heubner	Putamen and/or globus pallidus
Hemiballism/chorea – subthalamic nucleus	Contralateral: Classically associated hemiballismus of extremity [rapid flinging movement of the limb (see Chap. 21, this volume for details)]. Ipsilateral: None	Inferolateral (thalamogeniculate) artery	Subthalamic nucleus

Thalamic syndromes (Bogousslavsky et al. 1988; Graff-Radford et al. 1985)

Various thalamic syndromes have been described. Perhaps the best known are the pure sensory and the pure sensorimotor strokes, identified in Table 13.4. Table 13.5 reviews the clinical features and area of neuroanatomic damage resulting from occlusion of each arterial territory of the thalamus. Neuropsychological deficits can be pronounced in some thalamic syndromes (e.g., tuberothalamic artery) while entirely absent in others (e.g., inferolateral artery). Thalamic pain, a central pain disorder, can result from occlusion of the inferolateral (thalamogeniculate) artery and is contralateral to the lesion. Thalamic pain, if present, is usually associated with hemisensory loss, mild hemiparesis, choreoathetotic movements, and sometimes a mild hemiataxia and astereognosis. Outcome from occlusion to interolateral artery tends to be good. Alternatively, outcome from occlusion of the tuberothalamic or paramedian arteries tends to be poor, often with persistent neuropsychological deficits.

Rule of thumb: Thalamic syndromes

- Pure sensory syndrome or Sensorimotor syndrome
  OR
- Neuropsychological impairments
  - Memory, aphasia (dominant hemisphere), neglect (nondominant hemisphere), behavioral apathy

---

Rule of thumb: Thalamic pain (the Dejerine-Roussy syndrome)

- Central pain disorder (severe burning pain contralateral to lesion)
- Try to avoid touching patient on side contralateral to lesion
  - Pain is severe and burning contralateral to lesion with cutaneous hypersensitivity that limits rehabilitation and functional activities.
- Pain is not responsive to analgesics (e.g., morphine), and is variably responsive to antidepressants (tricyclics) or anticonvulsants (carbamazepine).

  - Medication can result in cognitive adverse effects.

Table 13.4 Thalamic vascular syndromes

Thalamic artery	Clinical features	Localization
Inferolateral (thalamogeniculate) artery	Contralateral hemisensory loss (light touch, position sense, vibratory sense, temperature, and pain), hemiataxia, and possible thalamic pain syndrome. Hemiparesis (usually mild) and loss of taste may also occur. No neuropsychological deficits. Two common subtypes: 1. Pure sensory stroke (see Table 13.3) 2. Pure sensorimotor stroke (see Table 13.3)	Ventral posterior (VPL) Ventral posterior medial (VPM) Ventral lateral (VL) Motor involvement affects corticospinal and corticobulbar pathways of internal capsule.
Paramedian arteries	Commonly includes a triad of deficits: 1. Impairment of declarative memory (anterograde amnesia). Deficit in memory tends to be retrieval deficits and inefficient consolidation. Bilateral lesion anterograde amnesia Unilateral less memory impairment Confabulation may be present. 2. Behavioral apathy with somnolescence (reduced level of alertness) Unilateral lesion less persistent apathy. Akinetic mutism can be present with bilateral lesion or dominant hemisphere lesion 3. Vertical gaze palsy Upward gaze more impaired than downward gaze. 4. Confabulation may be present	Intralaminar nuclei and Mediodorsal (MD) thalamic nuclei
Posterior choroidal artery	Contralateral homonymous quadrantanopia Larger lesion results in hemianopsia.	Lateral geniculate nuclei

(continued)

Table 13.4 (continued)

Thalamic artery	Clinical features	Localization
Tuberothalamic artery	Primarily neuropsychological deficits that are typically persistent and limit return to previous level of function.	Anterior thalamus
	Most common deficits are:	Anterior nucleus of thalamus
	Memory loss (e.g., anterograde amnesia). Impaired declarative (explicit) memory (autobiographical memory poor from time of lesion, and reduced ability to remember new facts).	Midline thalamic nuclei group
	Dominant hemisphere lesions more impairment in verbal memory	
	Nondominant hemisphere lesions more impaired "nonverbal" (visuospatial) memory.	
	Aphasia (dominant hemisphere lesions)	
	Executive dysfunction (e.g., disinhibition, apathy, lethargy, and abulia).	
	Dominant (left) hemisphere infarct deficits:	
	Aphasia symptoms including hypophonia, paraphasias, reduced spontaneous speech with short sentences, and some comprehension deficits. Repetition is intact.	
	Verbal memory can be particularly affected. Impaired encoding and consolidation.	
	Nondominant (right) hemisphere infarct deficits:	
	Nonverbal (visuospatial) memory may be more impaired than verbal memory.	
	Hemi-neglect and visuoconstructional and visual spatial deficits.	
	Bilateral infarcts present with pronounced apathy, lethargy, and dense anterograde amnesia.	
	Other neurologic deficits:	
	Contralateral facial paresis in which facial movement more impaired for facial movements to emotions (e.g., reduced involuntary smile to joke) than voluntary movement (e.g., request to show teeth) may be present.	

Brainstem Syndromes: Medulla, Pons, Midbrain

The clinical presentation of vertebral artery ischemia very considerably, largely dependent upon the vascular development of the individual and where the occlusion occurs. The anatomy of the vertebral arteries vary considerably from person to person, with almost 10% of individuals having only one functional vertebral artery supplying the basilar artery. In addition, the posterior inferior cerebellar artery (PICA) is traditionally depicted to arise from the vertebral artery; however, it is not uncommon for the PICA to arise from the basilar artery along with the anteroinferior cerebellar artery. These anatomic variations provide a host of variable clinical presentations typically taking on the form of various brain stem or lucanar syndromes described below. However, if the person has two patent and functional vertebral arteries, the occlusion of one may not result in any clinical deficits.

Basilar artery syndromes include the midbrain syndromes, paramedian thalamic and subthalamic syndromes (i.e., complete basilar and "top-of-the-basilar" syndromes as well as AICA and SCA syndromes). As the diameters of the vertebral arteries are often smaller than the Basilar artery, an embolus may not lodge until it reaches the top of the Basilar artery where it bifurcates into the smaller PCAs. In this setting, many perforator vessels are affected and the presentation is clearly more severe than one of the lacunar syndromes. Occlusion of the entire basilar artery (typically involving the lower third of the artery) is generally thrombotic from build-up of atherosclerotic plaque, and results in the so-called *complete basilar syndrome*. When perfusion is insufficient to spare the reticular activating, a rare, but devastating syndrome termed "locked-in" can occur. Table 13.5 provides the signs and symptoms, neuroanatomical localization, and syndrome name of common brain

---

Rule of thumb: Brain stem and Midbrain infarcts

- "crossed signs"

  – Contralateral hemiparesis and/or hemianesthesia
  – Ipsilateral facial weakness loss of sensation and/or ataxia of body

- Dysarthric speech (brain stem infarcts)
- Gaze palsies (brain stem and midbrain infarcts)

---

stem and midbrain vascular syndromes. Image N provides an example of radiographic image of medial medulla syndrome. While brain stem syndromes are not associated with neuropsychological deficits, patients with a "Top of the Basilar" syndrome exhibit memory impairment. In general, patients suffering brain stem or midbrain infarcts tend to exhibit persistent deficits with poor quality of life.

Table 13.5 Syndromes of midbrain and brain stem

Syndrome	Clinical features	Localization

"Top-of-the-Basilar" syndrome	Contralateral:
	  Ataxia (arm & leg)
	  Hemiparesis or tetraparesis (arm & leg)
	NOTE: motor features may not be present.
	  Visual field defects
	Ipsilateral:
	  CN III palsy
	Other neurologic deficits
	  Somnolence
	
	Neuropsychologic deficits
	  Visual hallucinations (poorly formed)
	  Memory impairment (poor encoding and consolidation reflecting anterograde amnesia)
	  Apathy and abulia. Akinetic mutism present in some cases.
		Basilar artery including paramedian arteries and midbrain
		
		CN III nucleus
		
		Rostral mesencephalic reticular formation.
		Primary visual cortex
		Dorsomedial thalamic nuclei (bilateral)
		Intralaminar thalamic nuclei

Midbrain tegmentum syndromes	Contralateral:
	  Hemiparesis (face, arm, leg)
	  Hemiataxia (face, arm, leg)
	  Tremor (resting)
	  Hyperkinesia (define) – (Benedikt's syndrome only)
	Ipsilateral:
	  CN III palsy
		Midbrain tegmentum, red nucleus, CN III, cerebral peduncle

Weber's syndrome	Contralateral:
	  Hemiparesis (face, arm, leg)
	Ipsilateral:
	  CN III palsy
	No neuropsychologic impairment
		Ventral midbrain, CN III, Cerebral peduncle.

Locked-In syndrome	Contralateral:
	  Hemiparesis (face, arm, leg)
	  Paralysis of tongue (mutism)
	Ipsilateral:
	  Hemiparesis (face, arm, leg)
	  Paralysis of tongue
	Other symptoms:
	  Often mute due to tongue paralysis
	  Lateral gaze palsy may be present
	  Bilateral bulbar involvement leading to dysphagia, and inability to protect airway requiring intubation.
	Note:
	  Patient is awake and alert due to sparing of midbrain and reticular formation.
	  Somatosensory pathways (touch, temperature, pain, proprioception, and vibration sense) often intact (intact medial lemniscus).
	  Vertical eye movements intact.
	  Patient often able to blink to command.
		Ventral pontine area (or cerebral peduncles) resulting in bilateral damage to corticospinal tracts

(continued)

Table 13.5 (continued)

Syndrome	Clinical features	Localization
Foville's syndrome	Contralateral: Hemiparesis (face, arm, leg) Hemianesthesia Internuclear ophthalmoplegia Ipsilateral: Facial hemiparesis Horizontal gaze palsy Other symptoms: Dysarthria No neuropsychological impairment	Medial pons and tegmentum damaging the corticospinal, corticobulbar tracts and facial colliculus.
Medial superior pontine syndrome	Contralateral: Hemiparesis (face, arm, leg) Can be hemianesthesia (touch, vibration, position sense) Ipsilateral: Cerebellar ataxia Internuclear ophthalmoplegia Myclonus of palate, pharynx, vocal cords No neuropsychological impairment	Occlusion of paramedian branches of upper basilar artery. Corticospinal tract Corticobulbar tract Medial lemniscus Cerebellar peduncle Central tegmentum
Lateral superior pontine syndrome (SCA syndrome)	Contralateral: Loss of pain and temperature (face, arm, leg) Loss of light touch, proprioception, and vibration sense (arm and leg). Ipsilateral: Cerebellar ataxia (face, arm, leg) falling to side of lesion Dizziness, vertigo, emesis Horizontal nystagmus Paresis of conjugate gaze Facial paresis Tremor of the upper extremity (static type) No neuropsychologic impairment	Occlusion of spinal cerebellar artery (SCA) Middle and superior peduncles Spinothalamic tract Medial lemniscus Corticobulbar tract Vestibular nuclei
Medial midpontine syndrome	Contralateral: Hemiparesis (face, arm, leg) Eye deviation Infrequently, loss of touch and proprioception (face, arm, legs) Ipsilateral: Cerebellar ataxia No neuropsychological impairment	Occlusion of paramedian branch of basilar artery Corticospinal (ipsilateral) Corticobulbar (ipsilateral) Cerebellar peduncle Posteriorly extending lesions affect medial lemniscus

(continued)

Table 13.5 (continued)

Syndrome	Clinical features	Localization

Lateral midpontine syndrome	Contralateral:
	  Can be hemianasthesia (light touch and proprioception) of arm and leg
	Ipsilateral:
	  Ataxia
	  CN V palsy (paresis of mastication muscles, positive jaw jerk reflex)
	  CN V sensory deficit (anesthesia of side of face)
	No neuropsychologic impairment
		Occlusion of short circumferential artery

Unilateral inferior pontine [Anterior inferior cerebellar artery (AICA)] syndrome	Contralateral:
	  hemiparesis (face, arm, leg)
	  hemianasthesia (light touch and proprioception) of arm and leg
	Ipsilateral:
	  Cerebellar ataxia
	  Facial hemiparesis
	  Horizontal gaze palsy
	  (Eyes look toward lesion and away from side of hemiparesis)
	  Facial hemianesthesia (light touch and proprioception)
	  Diplopia on lateral gaze
	  Loss of hearing and/or tinnitus
	Other symptoms
	  Dizziness, vertigo, emesis
	  Dysarthria
	No neuropsychologic impairment
		Occlusion of AICA artery
		Corticospinal tract
		Corticobulbar tract
		Middle cerebral peduncle
		
		Cerebellar hemisphere
		Medial lemniscus
		Abducens nucleus or paramedian pontine reticular formation (PPRF)
		Descending sensory tract of CN V
		
		Auditory nerve (CN VIII)
		Facial nerve (CN VII)

Medial inferior pontine (Pontine "wrong-way eyes") syndrome	Contralateral:
	  Hemiparesis (face, arm, leg)
	  Hemianasthesia (light touch and proprioception) of arm and leg
	Ipsilateral:
	  Horizontal gaze palsy (Eyes look away from lesion and toward side of hemiparesis)
	  Diplopia on lateral gaze
	  Cerebellar ataxia
	Other symptoms:
	  Dysarthria
	No neuropsychologic impairment
		Occlusion of paramedian branch of basilar artery
		Corticobulbar tract
		Medial lemniscus
		Abducens nucleus or paramedian pontine reticular formation (PPRF).

(continued)

Table 13.5 (continued)

Syndrome	Clinical features	Localization

Lateral inferior pontine syndrome	Contralateral:
	  Hemianasthesia (pain and temperature) of arm and leg
	Ipsilateral:
	  Facial hemiparesis
	  Horizontal gaze paralysis (eyes look away from lesion and toward side of hemiparesis)
	  Facial hemianesthesia (light touch and proprioception)
	  Cerebellar ataxia
	  Loss of hearing and/or tinnitus
	Other symptoms
	  Dizziness, vertigo, emesis
	  No neuropsychologic impairment
		Occlusion of AICA (incomplete).
		Spinothalamic tract
		Cerebellar peduncle
		Facial nerve (CN VII)
		Abducens nucleus or paramedian pontine reticular formation (PPRF).
		descending sensory tract of CN V
		
		Auditory nerve (CN VIII)

Medial medullary syndrome (see Image N).	Contralateral:
	  Loss of arm or leg motor function
	  Sensation of light touch, proprioception and vibration sense
	Ipsilateral:
	  Tongue weakness
	  No neuropsychological impairment
		Occlusion of small penetrating branches of Vertebral and Anterior Spinal arteries (paramedian branches)
		Infarct of medial medulla (damaging pyramidal tract, medial lamniscus, and hypoglossal nucleus)

Wallenberg's syndrome	Contralateral:
	  Loss of body sensation (arm and leg) to pain and temperature
	Ipsilateral:
	  Ataxia (arm and leg)
	  Loss of facial sensation to pain and temperature
	  Paralysis of soft palate, pharynx and vocal cord resulting in dysphagia and hoarseness
	  Horner's syndrome
	Other symptoms:
	  Nausea and vertigo often present
	  Nystagmus
	  No neuropsychological impairments
		Lesion to lateral medulla (damaging the inferior cerebellar peduncle, vestibular nuclei, trigeminal nucleus, spinothalamic tract, and sympathetic fibers)

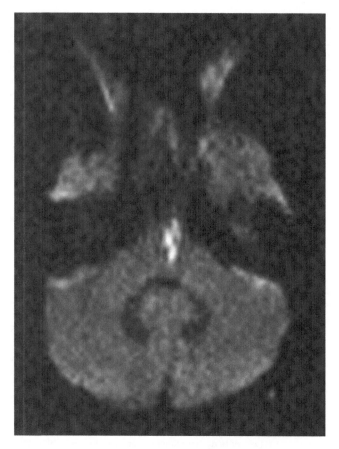

Image N. Diffusion-weighted MRI showing an acute medial medullary lacunar infarct presenting with dysarthria from an ipsilateral hypoglossal palsy and contralateral limb weakness and sensory loss

Leukoariosis

Periventricular and subcortical white matter gliosis and demyelination are a common consequence of medical conditions such as hypertension and diabetes. These changes, prominently demonstrated on MRI scans, are correlated with the cognitive changes of vascular dementia (see Image O). The differentia diagnosis of vascular dementia with

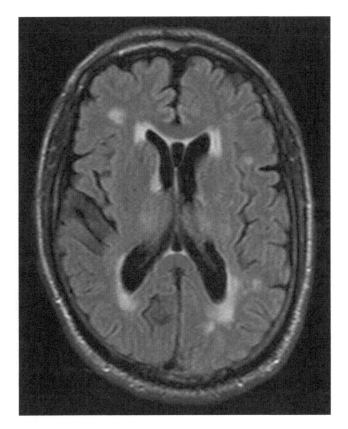

Image O. Magnetic Resonance Image (MRI) demonstrating periventricular and subcortical T2-weighted hyperintensities consistent with small vessel disease, or "leukoariosis"

multifocal white matter changes includes amyloid angiopathy and Cerebral Autosomal Dominant Arteriopathy with Subcortical Infarcts and Leukoencephalopathy (CADASIL). CADASIL results from mutations on the notch 3 gene on chromosome 19. As the MRI changes precede the clinical manifestations, neuroimaging should be considered when progressive cognitive decline is associated with a personal and family history of migraine headaches, seizures, TIAs and stroke, and particularly when affecting young individuals (see Chap. 28, this volume and Image P below).

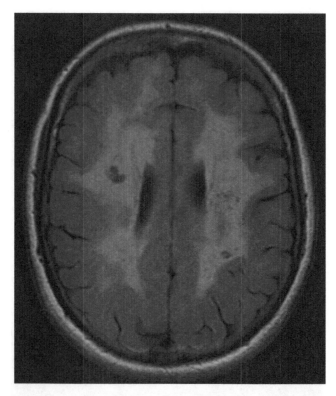

Image P. Profound white matter changes on MRI associated with cavitary changes in a patient with CADASIL

Section II: Neuropsychological Assessment of Patients after Stroke

Neuropsychological evaluation can help identify extent of cognitive and perceptual impairments, may assist in predicting outcome, and can be essential in guiding treatment and treatment progress. Treatment of stroke will likely include acute management of symptoms, rehabilitation and pharmaceutical intervention for medical risk factors (e.g., hypertension, hyperlipidemia, diabetes, etc.). Patients may also be prescribed medications with cognitive side effects, such as anticonvulsants (for seizure prophylaxis), antidepressants, anxiolytics and antipsychotics for concomitant mood and behavioral disorders. Rehabilitation after stroke commonly includes speech and language therapy, cognitive therapy, physical therapy, occupational therapy, and vocational therapy.

Deficits in neuropsychological function will depend upon size and location of lesion, time elapsed since the stroke, as well as the patient's age and co-morbid conditions. Assuming all other things being equal, the majority of functional recovery from stroke will occur over the first few (3–6) months, and additional, but less pronounced recovery occurs over the next 6–12 months. Improved functioning after 9–12 months is largely a function of compensation and adaptation to deficits rather than biological recovery, although younger patients may evidence some biological recovery of function years since injury (see Victor and Ropper 2001 for review). Although there is marked variability in the type and severity of neurologic/neuropsychologic comorbidities of cortical and subcortical strokes, recovery following damage to cortical structures and supratentorial white matter is more complete than recovery from deep pathways within the brain stem. While brain stem strokes are often more life threatening given the likelihood of affecting basic life support centers, they often produce profound physical impairment but may spare cortical areas and subsequently many cognitive processes (attention/executive, memory, language, vision, reasoning, personality, etc.). Cortical strokes in contrast produce the greatest risk for cognitive functioning deficits.

When to Conduct a Neuropsychological Evaluation

Neuropsychological assessment may be completed any time following a stroke. Common referral questions include requests to document the nature of the deficit, help develop rehabilitation interventions and/or placement decisions, assess for progression of neuropsychological functional recovery, and/or identify the development of complicating conditions (e.g., cerebral edema, hemorrhagic conversion, etc.). Neuropsychological assessment can be particularly helpful for patients with recovery that is mostly complete (and only subtle deficits are present), but continue to cause problems with work, school, or at home (see Victor and Ropper 2001 and Lezak et al. 2004 for review). In the acute and subacute stages, we recommend neuropsychological assessment be completed using brief bedside methods rather than administration of detailed or lengthy neuropsychological evaluation. Once a deficit is appreciated (e.g., hemi-neglect, hemiparesis, or aphasia syndrome), accommodation of the patient's recognized deficit in order to evaluate for other potential neuropsychological deficits is recommended. For example, in a sub-acute assessment of a right MCA infarct, it is unnecessary to continue to administer tests in a patient's left

---

Rule of thumb: Identifying cognitive strengths is often at least as important as identifying deficits

DON'T: repeatedly request that a patient attempt tasks where failure is likely (e.g., repeated motor testing of a patient with hemi-paresis).

DO: attempt to identify strengths and weakness. Accommodation and adaptation of neuropsychological tests is often necessary in acute and sub-acute stroke assessments. For example, presenting visual memory material in the right hemispace will better allow for assessment of visual memory function

visual field after a left hemi-neglect has been identified. Thus, stimuli to assess other neuropsychological domains (e.g., language, agnosias, memory, and executive functions) should be presented in the preserved visual hemi-space.

Neuropsychological evaluation may also be requested months to years after a stroke, and is particularly helpful in evaluating the extent and severity of residual neuropsychological deficits, identify strengths to assist with developing accommodation and adaptations along with speech/language and physical therapy (Lezak et al. 2004). Additionally, neuropsychological evaluation can also assist in determining the patient's competence to manage his/her personal affairs, make medical/legal/financial decisions, and/or capacity, and accommodations for the ability, to return to employment. In these cases, more detailed psychometric evaluation of the patient's neuropsychological functioning is often completed. Neuropsychological evaluation in patients suspected of multi-infarct and vascular dementia may be reassessed at 6- to 12-month intervals to assess for change in neuropsychological function with treatment.

Differences Between Ischemic and Hemorrhagic Strokes

The extent of neurological and/or neuropsychological deficits typically differ between ischemic and hemorrhagic strokes. As noted above, deficits resulting from ischemic strokes follow cerebral vascular neuroanatomic territory, while ICH can result in more diffuse dysfunction involving areas of several different cerebral vascular territories. Moreover, the ischemic process results in damage to the brain parenchyma, but if a patient survives a subdural hemorrhage, the neuropsychological deficits can be minimal as the brain parenchyma may not be damaged, but rather displaced by a volume of blood. Once the volume of blood is removed, the acute space occupying effect resolves, often with little of no residual deficit. Deficits resulting from ischemic stroke will also vary depending upon the completeness of occlusion, duration of the occlusion and the availability of anastomotic blood supply during the ischemic period (e.g., TIA versus completed stroke. For example, outcome from TIA can be complete, with detectable residual deficits apparent only from detailed neuropsychological evaluation (e.g., Lezak et al. 2004 for review). Alternatively, a MCA stroke can result in marked residual neuropsychological deficits in language, visuospatial, and executive deficits.

Neuropsychological (and neurological) outcome from hemorrhagic strokes vary more widely than ischemic strokes. While ischemic damage tends to result in damage to brain parenchyma itself within the vascular distribution territory, hemorrhagic strokes can damage brain tissue outside of the cerebral vascular distribution (e.g., intracerebral hemorrhages with intraventricular extension and/or due to herniation of tissue and subsequent ischemia). Alternatively, other hemorrhagic strokes (e.g., subdural) may not damage parenchyma, with the accumulating blood producing a space occupying lesion and subsequent displacement of brain parenchyma, but no long-term damage once the blood products are removed. Survivors of ICH can exhibit anything from marked neurological impairment (unable to live independently) to minimal neurological and/or neuropsychological deficits.

The next section reviews common neuropsychological and neurological presentations of strokes limited to certain vascular distributions. These descriptions assume the patient is left hemisphere dominant for language.

MCA Distribution Stroke

Typical physical deficits include contralateral motor weakness, particularly for tasks requiring fine manual dexterity, contralateral sensory deficits, and hemi-inattention evident by extinction to bilateral simultaneous stimulation. Hemi-inattention is much more common in right hemisphere strokes (producing left hemi-inattention) due to the right hemispheres unique role in processing and maintaining attention. Acutely, the patient often exhibits extinction to more than one sensory modality (or may even entirely ignore the left hemispace), which is termed hemi-neglect. Hemi-neglect often extends across tactile, auditory and visual stimuli acutely, but improves over days to several months to hemi-inattention (in one modality). The hemi-inattention may be subtle, such that the deficit is detectable only with formal testing procedures. Assessment of language, attention/concentration, memory (verbal and nonverbal) visuoconstructional/visuoperceptual, and executive functions along with personality and mood should be incorporated.

Rule of thumb: Strokes involving the MCA are the most common

Common Deficits include: Contralateral motor weakness, contralateral sensory deficits.
Left MCA: Aphasia and ideomotor apraxia
Right MCA: Constructional Apraxia, Aprosodia, dressing apraxia

Left MCA

Neuropsychological deficits often include language deficits (aphasia), visuoconstructional deficits, Gerstmann's syndrome (finger agnosia, acalculia, agraphia, and right-left confusion), and executive functions. Visuoconstructional deficits often reflect drawings that maintain the gestalt (general form) of the figure or design, but lack detail (see Chap. 9, this volume, for details). Memory impairments can be present, particularly in large "stem" MCA infarcts. Material-specific memory impairment for verbal material is likely. Nonverbal (visual) memory can be entirely normal. Dorsolateral frontal lobe impairments may also be present in large superior and/or stem MCA stroke. Acutely, aphasias are very frequently present. Language deficits may include poor verbal fluency (phonemic and/or semantic; Benton and Hamsher 1989; Spreen and Strauss 1998), confrontation naming (e.g., deficits on visual confrontation naming or auditory naming tasks; Kaplan, Goodglass and Weintraub 2001; Stern and White 2003), repetition, comprehension (e.g., Token Test; Boller and Vignolo 1966), reading, or writing. There are a number of Aphasia assessment batteries which are very helpful in detailed assessment of the type and severity of language deficits (Boston Diagnostic Aphasia Battery, Goodglass et al. 2000; Multilingual Aphasia Examination, Benton and Hamsher 1989; Neuropsychological Assessment Battery, Stern and White 2003; Western Aphasia Battery, Kertesz 1982). Please see Chap. 7: Language syndromes, and Chap. 16: Aphasias, for more details on language syndromes and features of aphasia. A "stem" MCA infarct will result in more neuropsychological deficits, reflecting dysfunction of both frontal as well as temporal and parietal cortex. A superior segment MCA infarct will typically not result in sensory deficits or comprehension language problems. An inferior segment MCA infarct will typically present with greater comprehension language deficits, sensory deficits, and ideomotor and ideational apraxias are common.

Right MCA

Neuropsychological deficits often include constructional apraxias (loss of gestalt of objects) and a left hemi-neglect or hemi-inattention. Recall that hemi-neglect is the "in-attention" to more than one sensory modality in hemi-space (e.g., not attending to visual stimuli or light touch). Hemi-inattention is the "in-attention" to one sensory modality in hemi-space (e.g., not paying attention to visual material in the left hemi-space). Dressing apraxia is common. Other deficits can include aprosodies (see Chaps. 7 and 16, this volume). Receptive aprosodies are common with "stem" or right inferior MCA stroke. Expressive aprosodies are common with "stem" or right superior MCA stroke. Executive dysfunction involving dorsolateral syndrome is also common. Memory impairments can be present, and material-specific memory impairment with poor visual (nonverbal) memory is likely.

ACA Distribution Stroke

Isolated ACA territory infarcts are uncommon as the path is circuitious for an embolus, but can be affected by occlusion from intracranial atherosclerosis or from vasospasm after rupture of an ACoA aneurysm.

Unilateral ACA strokes are associated with contralateral hemiparesis involving the leg more than the shoulder and sparing the hand, sensory deficit (in a similar distribution) and a variety of behavioral deficits. Abulia and emotional apathy are common and when severe, can manifest as akinetic mutism. Impairment of frontostriatal circuits can result in deficits in divided and focused attention as well as memory deficits. Delirium and agitation may alternate with apathy and mutism.

Neuropsychological Assessment of ACA stroke should include assessment of executive functions and attention/working memory, verbal and nonverbal (visual) memory, language, visuoconstructional and visual spatial, personality/behavior, and motor functions.

Rule of thumb: Deficits associated with ACA stroke

Contralateral weakness of feet/legs with falls, urinary incontinence, and apathy and abulia. Lack of spontaneous speech (mute with damage to both medial frontal lobes). Executive dysfunction.

Left ACA: Expressive language deficits.

Right ACA: Expressive aprosodies

ACoA aneurysm: Memory deficits, mutism, apathy, executive impairments.

Left ACA. Neuropsychological deficits commonly include executive dysfunction and expressive language deficits. Executive dysfunction can be more pronounced with dominant hemisphere lesions, and involve poor verbal reasoning, motor impersistence, abulia, and behavioral apathy. Patients may also present with features of a transcortical motor aphasia, and psychometric evaluation of phonemic verbal fluency may reveal deficits.

Right ACA. Neuropsychological deficits may present with executive dysfunction. Rather than language deficits, persons may reflect poor social insight and judgment. Impersistence, abulia, and apathy may also be present.

Bilateral ACA. The most common cause for damage to parenchyma of both ACA artery distributions is the result of a ruptured ACoA aneurysm (see above).

Neuropsychological deficits can involve mutism, memory impairments, behavioral apathy, lack of initiation, bilateral weakness (legs greater than arms) and cortical sensory loss involving feet/legs. Not all patients exhibit neuropsychological deficits following surgical repair of ACoA aneurysm (Bendel et al. 2009). Bendel et al. (2009) reported only 54% exhibited neuropsychological deficits following surgical repair. Memory may be affected to varying severity, with the patient exhibiting retrieval deficits and inefficient consolidation. Short-delay recall may be worse than long-delay recall (Lezak et al. 2004). Patients tend not to organize material for consolidation, and semantic clustering is often reduced (Lezak et al. 2004). Learning curve is flat or nearly flat and retrieval errors are common, with frequent false positive errors. False positive errors are often of semantically related distracters. Recognition memory is often impaired due to failure of release of proactive interference (improved memory for stimuli that differs from previously presented material), resulting in patients making false positive and false negative errors. Patients may also demonstrate impairment in prospective memory, the ability to "remember to remember" (Lezak et al. 2004).

Neuropsychological assessment may present with deficits on measures of complex and divided attention [e.g., Trails A & B (AITB 1944), Paced Auditory Serial Addition Test (PASAT; Gronwall 1977), Wechsler Memory Scale-3rd Ed. (WMS-III; Wechsler 2001a) Working Memory Index and memory e.g., Benton visual retention task (Benton 1974), complex figure immediate and delayed recall, Rey Auditory Verbal Learning test (Rey 1964), Wechsler Memory Scales (WMS; e.g., Wechsler 2001) tests, Wide Range Assessment of Memory and Learning, 2nd Ed. (WRAML-2, Sheslow and Adams 2003), etc. (see Lezak et al. 2004; Spreen et al. 2006 for reviews]. Varying expressive language deficits are often present, with the more severe cases exhibiting mutism. Executive function deficits reflect poor initiation, apathy, and reduced performance on Stroop tasks (Lezak et al. 2004). Behavioral and mood changes can be predominant.

PCA Distribution Strokes

Neurological deficits include contralateral homonymous hemianopsia (or quadrantanopsia), contralateral hemi-sensory loss. Neuropsychological deficits commonly include constructional apraxia, visuoperceptual deficits, color anomia, and memory loss. Memory loss often reflects poor encoding and an impaired learning curve. Material-specific memory impairment can be present, particularly for left PCA strokes. Short-delay and long-delay recall is often impaired.

Left PCA: Memory loss (verbal greater than nonverbal/visual), Transcortical sensory aphasia symptoms, alexia without agraphia, visuoconstructional deficits (mild loss of details but gestalt maintained. Drawings may appear "slavish" and block designs may be mildly reduced secondary to missing a detail).

Right PCA: Memory loss (nonverbal/visual greater than verbal), visuoconstructional and visuospatial deficits, agnosias (e.g., prosapagnosia), color anomia. Left hemi-sensory loss may be present. Hemi-neglect is common acutely and may resolve to more subtle hemi-neglect or hemi-inattention (often visual). Visuoconstructional deficits involve drawings that may be detailed but the gestalt of the object is often not maintained. Evidence of left hemi-neglect (or visual hemi-inattention) is common. Block design performance exhibits "stringing out" or other designs in which the gestalt is not maintained. Assessed with double simultaneous stimulation (hands and face), Line Bisection tests (Schenkenberg, Bradford and Ajax 1980), and/or Bell's test (Gauthier et al. 1989), Hooper Visual Organization test (Hooper 1983), Rey-Osterreith Complex Figure Test/Medical College of Georgia Complex Figures (Meador et al. 1993; Rey 1941), Test of Face Recognition (Benton, Sivan, Hamsher et al. 1994), Wechsler Intelligence Scales Block Design tests (e.g., Wechsler 2001b).

Behavioral deficits consisting of irritability, distractability, agitation and frank psychosis may occur, and when associated with visual hallucinations, can be mistaken for a toxic delirium and managed as a primary psychiatric disorder.

Neuropsychological Assessment of PCA stroke should include assessment of motor and sensory functions, language, verbal and nonverbal (visual) memory, visuoconstructional and visual spatial, executive functions and attention/working memory, personality/behavior, and motor functions.

Visual loss is typically recognized by the patient when the lesion is confined to the occipital lobe but when the parietal or temporal lobe is also involved, patients may not recognize their visual deficits and frankly deny that there is any problem at all (cortical blindness). This is more common when the right hemisphere is involved but also occurs with left hemisphere lesions and is particularly prominent when bilateral. Visual hallucinations of simple shapes or well-formed experiences, sometimes associated with other sensory experiences, are more noticeable during the evenings and nighttime and may be a source of significant distress. Specific syndromes include alexia without agraphia, alexia with agraphia, abnormal color naming, visual agnosia, constructional apraxia, visual amnesia, visual hypoemotionality, abnormalities of color perception and depth perception, and prosopagnosia. Balint's syndrome consists of asimultagnosia, optic ataxia and apraxia of gaze.

Rule of thumb: Deficits of PCA stroke

Contralateral sensory deficit of hands/arms (light touch, vibration, position). Contralateral visual field defect. Visuoconstructional/visuospatial deficits very common. Memory deficits may be present.

Left PCA: Receptive language deficits. Ideomotor apraxia. Gerstmann's syndrome. Visuoconstructional deficits (loss of details). Memory loss (often verbal).

Right PCA: Visuoconstructional/visuospatial deficits. Hemi-neglect or hemi-inattention. Receptive aprosodies. Memory loss (often nonverbal – visual).

Subcortical Strokes (Sparing Brain Stem Nuclei)

Due to the predictable anatomy of the small perforator vessels, occlusion of one of these arteries can result in recognizable "lacunar syndromes". The most common are the pure motor hemiparesis, ataxic hemiparesis, and pure sensory syndrome. For most patients, neuropsychological deficits are minimal or absent with a few, notable exceptions. Strokes involving the caudate nucleus have prominent behavioral abnormalities of a frontal-lobe nature, those involving the thalamus (particularly the dominant, mesial nuclei) results in confabulation, anterograde amnesia, and behavioral disruptions. Emotional incontinence or pseudobulbar affect can result with bilateral lesions or some brainstem lesions.

Multi-infarct states (leukoareosis) involving multiple and diffuse infarction of subcortical white matter and periventricular areas often produce neuropsychological deficits including bradyphrenia, psychomotor slowing, attention deficits, problems in efficient spontaneous recall and consolidation, visuoconstructional deficits, and executive dysfunction. Depression and apathy is common. The Hachinski Ischemia Scale (Hachinski et al. 1975) is a commonly used rating scale to help discern vascular dementia from other dementia etiologies. The Hachinski Ischemia Scale incorporates cognitive and behavioral symptoms common in vascular disease as well as risk factors for stroke (see Table 13.6). When applied to a patient with a dementia, scores less than 4 are indicative of AD while scores greater than 7 are associated with Vascular dementia (VaD).

Brain stem strokes. Deficits often involve motor and sensory deficits as well as dysarthria, dysphagia, and/or ataxia. Neuropsychological functions are generally entirely intact. Motor deficits can often be disabling. In addition, speech articulation and intelligibility may be severely impacted by dysarthria, limiting the patients ability to communicate via spoken language. Abilities to write (assuming dominant hand motor paresis is not present) and/or comprehension is entirely intact.

Table 13.6 Hachinski Ischemia Scale

Feature	Present	Absent
Abrupt Onset	2	0
Stepwise deterioration	1	1
		0
Fluctuating course	2	0
Nocturnal confusion	1	0
Relative preservation of personality	1	0
Depression	1	0
Somatic complaints	1	0
Emotional incontinence	1	0
History of hypertension	1	0
History of strokes (brain attacks)	2	0
Evidence of associated atherosclerosis	1	0
Focal neurological symptoms	2	0
Focal neurological signs	2	0
Total Score		
Scores<4 more likely AD		
Scores>7 more likely VaD		

Dysphagia (difficulty swallowing) may also be present, and can be life threatening. Patients with brain stem strokes are routinely evaluated for swallowing problems.

Emotional Regulation/Personality Changes

Emotional and personality changes frequently occur either as new onset emotional and/or personality disorder or as an exacerbation of a premorbid psychiatric disorder. The most common symptoms following stroke is depression and anxiety symptoms. Generally, patients with left hemisphere strokes initially present with symptoms of depression while patients with right hemisphere strokes are typically described as emotionally flat and indifferent to their motor and cognitive deficits. A meta-analysis found 52% of patients with stroke reported symptoms of clinical depression (see Lezak et al. 2004 for review). Hemispheric differences have been extensively studied, and a review is provided below.

Right Hemisphere

The most common affect change with right hemisphere strokes is indifference and affective flattening. Right hemisphere damage often results in reduced capacity to appreciate emotional based cues (both nonverbal and verbal). Patients can have marked difficulty appreciating the meaning of facial expressions and/or body posture and hand gestures. In addition, recall the right hemisphere is often involved in appreciating and expressing speech prosody (e.g., speech aprosodies). Thus, patients with right hemisphere damage may be unable (or very inefficient) at appreciating the meaning of changes in prosody and intonation to convey meaning. Due to expressive aprosodies, patient's speech is often described as flat and monotone, and may be interpreted as reflecting dysphoria to a casual observer. While speech prosody and intonation is blunted, speech is of often of normal rate and well articulated. It need not just be blunted monotone speech, but may also present with a sustained jocular type of speech. Indeed, the emotional meaning of speech with patients having right hemisphere damage may not reflect the patient's emotional state. Speech content may be about past events, which have little relevance to the listener, or may be repeated explanations for the patient's inability to do certain things. As an example, patients may offer repeated excuses for being in the hospital (which may not be accurate or reasonable), and often attempt to limit or avoid neuropsychological assessment, such as "I'm too tired." Finally, it is not uncommon for patients with right hemisphere dysfunction to present with paranoia and perseveration. Following acute emotional flattening, or indifference, patients with right hemisphere lesions develop increasing symptoms of depression and anxiety months and even years following the stroke. Among patients with right hemisphere lesions, symptoms of depression have been strongly related to posterior lesions 1–2 years post-stroke (e.g., Robinson and Starkstein 2002).

Left Hemisphere

Ischemic damage to the left hemisphere, particularly the caudate and left frontal lobe, are associated with symptoms of depression and the so-called "catastrophic reaction." Patients often appear tearful and/or anxious. Post-acute emotional changes are typically described as depressed. Rates of depression vary, but at least 50% of patients exhibit depressive symptoms following left hemisphere strokes (Lezak et al. 2004). Patients with left hemisphere stroke typically present acutely with symptoms of depression, and these symptoms gradually resolve over time (which is opposite of patients with right hemisphere stroke). Not all tearful patients are experiencing sadness, and may be reflecting pseudobulbar affect. As noted above, patients with stroke often exhibit reductions in socializing, and those patients with symptoms of depression tend to exhibit the greatest reduction in social activities years after stroke (Lezak et al. 2004).

Frontal and Subcortical

Frontal lobe damage caused by stroke can present with marked emotional and personality changes. Anterior Communicating Artery (ACoA) aneurysm patients may present with marked personality changes, particularly behavioral flattening, apathy, and abulia. Because orbital frontal damage may also occur, patients may also present with behavioral disinhibition, irritability, lack of concern for others, and reduced personal hygiene. Damage to the cortico-striato-thalamic-cortico circuitry often presents with symptoms of perseveration and compulsions that reflect an obsessive-compulsive disorder.

Damage to corticobulbar pathways (see Chap. 3, this volume) can release motor control of facial expressions from cortical control (pseudobulbar affective expression). Patients may have restricted spontaneous emotions yet experience sudden laughter or crying without an apparent emotional trigger. The extent of facial weakness does not correlate well with the presence of facial or bulbar motor weakness. The far more common pseudobulbar behavior is the appearance of crying. Asking the patient if (s)he is feeling sad/despondent and wants to cry can be very instructive in disentangling the potential presence of pseudobulbar affect from reactive responses to having a neurologic disease. The same line of question for apparent "forced" (pseudobulbar) laughing, asking the patient laughing if (s)he is feeling a sense of mirth (happiness/funny) is instructive in these cases. Pseudobulbar affect can be very troubling to family members and friends, as the initiation of crying or laughing behaviors can be, and are often in our experience, at very inappropriate social times. Knowing these behaviors are out of the patient's control and due to neurologic disease can be very reassuring to the patient and his/her family. Outbursts of Pseudobulbar affect (sometimes referred to as affective incontinence) can be redirected by directly asking the patient a neutral question such as "what color are your shoes" thus breaking the cycle of affective expression.

Treatment of Stroke and Rehabilitation

Stroke is a medical emergency. While a detailed review of the acute treatment of stroke is beyond the scope of this chapter, Table 13.7 provides an overview of stroke interventions. The acute treatment of ischemic stroke focuses on restoring blood flow, preventing reperfusion hemorrhage, and determining the cause to guide future pre-

---

Rule of thumb: Changes in personality and affect

Changes in mood/personality common in stroke.

Left hemisphere: "Catastrophic reaction." Most common is symptoms of depression and affective lability. Patient often extremely tearful.

Right hemisphere: Affective flattening and indifference. Patient speech may be monotone. Difficulty appreciating nonverbal cues in social settings.

Frontal/medial/subcortical: involvement of mesial frontal area or orbitofrontal areas often exhibit pronounced behavioral changes, including amotivation, pronounced apathy/abulia (akinetic) and agitation at times. Orbitofrontal involvement may result in behavioral changes of decreased inhibition, lack of regard for others and changes in sleep and libido. Pseudobulbar affect is associated with damage to the bulbar pathways. Pseudobulbar crying is most often but laughing also occurs. Terminate pseudobulbar affect is to ask neutral question "what color are your shoes?" while patient is crying/laughing.

Table 13.7 Treatments for stroke

Treatment	Treatment mechanism of action	Treatment indications
Tissue plasminogen activators (t-PA)	Metabolizes plasminogen to plasmin enzyme which hydrolyzes clotting proteins. Treatment window is generally regarded as 3 h of symptom onset.	Useful for thrombotic and thrombo-embolic (ischemic) strokes
	Intra-arterial tPA treatment window is up to 6 h of symptoms onset, but application requires angiographic evidence of vessel occlusion and direct arterial injection.	Increases risk for hemorrhagic conversion
Anticoagulant medication	Increases PT and/or PTT clotting time, and increases INR to 2–4.	Thrombotic stroke (particularly stenosis of large cerebral vessels) or occlusion due to carotid artery dissection.
Heparin, warfarin		Contraindicated in patients with endocarditis due to possible increased risk of bleeding with vasculitis or mycotic aneurysm, recent surgery, trauma or hemorrhagic stroke, and/or active or systemic bleeding.
Antiplatelet medication (aspirin, ticlopidine, clopidogrel, or dipyridamole)	Rather than reversing a stoke, antiplatelet medication has demonstrated effectiveness in reducing the risk of subsequent stroke (and myocardial infarction).	Embolic and/or thrombotic strokes
Surgical revascularization	Carotid endarterectomy for symptomatic or severe accessible carotid stenoses. Following a mild to moderate infarct, surgery recommended within 2 weeks to maximize the benefit of reducing a recurrent stroke.	Surgical benefit is greater for symptomatic (> 70% internal carotid stenoses) than symptomatic moderate (50–69% stenoses) or asymptomatic (> 60% stenoses).
Surgical treatment (angioplasty with/without stenting, balloon angioplasty)	Recanalization of vessel by angioplasty, stenting, and/or balloon angioplasty. Common surgical targets are internal carotid artery, common carotid artery, or subclavian arteries.	Carotid angioplasty and stenting is recommended over endarterectomy for surgically inaccessible lesions, and other anatomic high-risk conditions such as endarterectomy re-stenoses and radiation arteriopathy. Less evidence for effectiveness among patients with vertebral or basilar artery stenosis.

(continued)

Table 13.7 (continued)

Treatment	Treatment mechanism of action	Treatment indications
Treatment of edema	Hyperventilation and osmotic diuretic agents can provide temporary reduction in intracranial pressure, but may aggravate lateral tissue shifts causing a worsening of herniation.	Following a stroke by hours to days (typically about 2–3 days later), edema of the infarcted area generally occurs. In large strokes, edema can be fatal due to mass effect and brain herniation (particularly if brain stem affected).
	Surgical treatment, with hemicraniectomy can be lifesaving to these patients	Symptoms are typically worsening mental status hours to days after a stroke, and can progress to stupor and coma, often associated with signs of herniation such as ipsilateral IIIrd nerve palsy and bilateral lower extremity spasticity and Babinski signs.

ventive therapies. The acute treatment of hemorrhagic stroke focuses on controlling the bleeding and limiting the effects of increased intracranial pressure. Some patients may require surgical therapy to evacuate the clot, clip an aneurysm or remove an AVM. Nonsurgical, endovascular techniques of aneurysm coiling and AVM obliteration may spare a craniotomy for some patients. In all stroke patients, preventing medical complications such as pneumonia, sepsis, and deep venous thrombosis are important, as are maintaining adequate nutrition and restoring mobility. Once patients are medically stable to be discharged from the hospital, the longer term therapies of rehabilitation take center stage.

Neuropsychological Assessment and Rehabilitation

The role of neuropsychology within rehabilitation of stroke is a complex issue, and assessment of neuropsychological function in recovery from brain attack can play an important role in patient's return to independence. The neuropsychological evaluation provides an objective assessment of specific cognitive deficits and strengths as well as which behaviors and/or emotional functioning are present or disrupted. Such programs often will utilize a patient's neuropsychological strengths to help develop accommodation techniques for deficits. Without detailed neuropsychological assessment, many cognitive rehabilitation procedures cannot be undertaken and individuals can be provided unnecessary treatment (e.g., Engelberts et al. 2002).

The goal of rehabilitation is to improve a patient's ability to process and interpret information allowing the individual to function better in all aspects of life (adapted from NIH position statement for rehabilitation in TBI, 1999). Rehabilitation may be short-term or longer-term programs targeting specific motor, sensory, cognitive and/or behavioral/psychiatric functioning.

The two primary processes of rehabilitation are *restorative* or *compensatory*. Restorative therapy is designed to enhance a cognitive (or other) function to pre-injury levels or maximal residual function. Restorative therapy typically occurs in the acute phase of rehabilitation, and seeks to capitalize on the concurrence of biological recovery process. Ideally, restorative rehabilitation allows a patient's functioning to return to (or approximate) premorbid levels of mastery. For example, speech therapy may initiate a restorative treatment program to reacquire expressive language function. The second general process of rehabilitation is compensatory therapies. Rather than a goal to restore function, compensatory therapies focus on adapting the patient's function to a deficit (cognitive, motor, behavioral). Compensatory strategies may utilize either (or both) adaptations and/or accommodations to identified deficits. Adaptations often include teaching patients to complete a task or activity differently or modifying the environment to allow the patient to complete a task or activity with his/her current deficits. Compensatory methods often utilize assistive technologies or physical adaptations to accommodate the deficit(s). Examples of a compensatory strategies include the use of a memory notebook or Personal Data Assistant (PDA) in facilitating the patient with anterograde amnesia ability to live independently.

There are three principal types of accommodations: (1) Procedure accommodations, (2) Physical accommodations to environment, and (3) Utilization of assistive devices. Procedure accommodations are often easily implemented by developing sequenced set of steps to complete a more complex task (minimizing attention and memory demands). Physical accommodations adapt an environment (bedroom, kitchen, or work site) to allow a patient to complete tasks inclusive of the individual's identified neuropsychological deficits. Assistive devices have been increasingly used with progression of microelectronics, e.g., computer-based or electronic reminder alerts (alert may be auditory, tactile, or visual stimuli). Pagers, watches, and personal digital assistants (PDAs) have been increasingly used for reminder cues and/or enhance organizational skills. Physical assistive devices can be essential to a patient with severe physical limitations due to stroke.

Rehabilitation involves a step-like process in which gross (large-scale) behaviors/abilities must be present (or developed) before fine motor or specialty behaviors can occur. Recovery of motor function occurs first in proximal muscles prior to distal motor skills. Cognitive rehabilitation utilizes the same pattern, such that basic attention and sensory-perceptual functions must be retained (or developed) before higher level memory strategies or problem solving can be acquired.

Speech/Language Therapy: Neuropsychological assessment plays an important role in speech/language therapy. Assessment will identify cognitive strengths and weaknesses which are employed by the Speech/language therapist to develop a treatment plan.

Physical Therapy: Strengthening exercises are essential in recovering from motor deficits to resume safe ambulation and activities of daily living as well as addressing the deconditioning associated with bedrest.

Occupational Therapy: Functional exercises are essentially in recovering from perceptual and motor deficits to resume activities of daily living including functional activities and fine motor tasks. Driving specialists can also offer specialized assessments geared to determine the safety to resume independent driving.

Vocational Therapy: Results of the patient's neurological examination, rehabilitation assessment and neuropsychological testing are used by the Vocational counselor to advise the patient on suitability to return to the prior employment, ability to retrain for alternate employment, and types of alternate employment that would be possible given the residual deficits.

Rule of thumb: Neuropsychology in Rehabilitation from Stroke

Primary purposes of Rehabilitation:

1. Restorative – efforts to enhance cognitive or behavioral functions to return to pre-injury levels. Frequently programming initiated acutely to benefit from biological recovery processes.
2. Compensatory – effort to enhance performance of skills and/or activities by introducing adaptations and/or accommodations to a deficit in order for the patient to be able to perform or function a task that is functionally equivalent.
   (a) Adaptations – teaching patient different way to complete activity/skill or modifying environment to allow patient with deficits to perform a task/skill.
   (b) Accommodations – three primary types: (1) procedural, (2) physical, and (3) use of assistive devices.

Neuropsychological evaluations provide needed information to identify cognitive and behavioral deficits, quantify severity, and work with rehabilitation team to develop rehabilitation programming. Also enables monitoring of restorative rehabilitation programming over time.

References

Adams, H. P., Bendixen, B. H., Kappelle, L. J., Biller, J., Love, B. B., Gordon, D. L., et al. (1993). Classification of subtype of acute ischemic stroke. Definitions for use in a multicenter clinical trial. TOAST. Trial of Org 10172 in Acute Stroke Treatment. *Stroke, 24,* 35–41.

AITB (1944). *Army Individual Test Battery, Manual of directions and scoring,* War Department, Adjutant General's Office, Washington, DC (1944).

Bladin, C. F., Alexandrov, A. V., Bellavance, A., et al. (2000). Seizures after stroke: A prospective multicenter study. *Archives of Neurology, 57,* 1617–1622.

Bendel, P., Koivisto, T., Niskanen, E., Kononen, M., Aikia, M., Hanninen, T., et al. (2009). Brain atrophy and neuropsychological outcome after treatment of ruptured anterior cerebral artery aneurysms: A voxel-based morphometric study. *Neuroradiology, 51*(11), 711–722. ISN 0028-3940.

Benton, A. L. (1974). *Revised Visual retention Test (4th Ed.)*. New York: The Psychological Corporation.

Benton, A. L., & Hamsher, K. de S. (1989). *Multilingual aphasia examination*. Iowa City: AJA Associates.

Benton, A. L., Sivan, A.B., Hamsher, K. De S., et al. (1994). *Contributions to neuropsychological assessment. A clinical manual (2nd ed.)*. New York: Oxford University Press.

Bogousslavsky, J., Regli, F., & Uske, A. (1988). Thalamic infarcts: Clinical syndromes, etiology, and prognosis. *Neurology, 38*, 837–848.

Boller, F., & Vignolo, L. A. (1966). Latent sensory aphasia in hemisphere-damaged patients: An experimental study with the Token Test. *Brain, 89*, 815–831.

Bonita, R., & Beaglehole, R. (1988). Modification of Rankin Scale: Recovery of motor function after stroke. *Stroke, 19*, 1497–1500.

Caplan, L. R. (1993). Stroke: A clinical approach. Boston, MA: Butterworth-Heinemann.

Carhuapoma, J. R., & Hanley, D. F. (2002). Intracerebral Haemorrhage. In A. K. Asbury, G.M. McKhann, W. I. McDonald, P. J. Goadsby, & J. C. McArthur (Eds.) *Diseases of the Nervous System: Clinical Neuroscience and Therapeutic Principles. (3rd ed.)*. London: Cambridge University Press.

Fisher, C. M. (1982). Lacunar strokes and infarcts: A review. *Neurology, 32*, 871–876.

Gauthier, L., Dehaut, F., & Joanette, Y. (1989). The Bells Test: A quantitative and qualitative test for visual neglect. *International Journal of Clinical Neuropsychology, 11*, 49–54.

Goodglass, H., Kaplan, E., & Barresi, B. (2000). *The Boston Diagnostic Aphasia Examination (BDAE-3) (3rd ed.)*. Philadelphia: Lippincott Williams & Wilkins.

Graff-Radford, N. R., Damasio, H., Yamada, T., Eslinger, P. J., & Damasio, A. R. (1985). Nonhaemorrhagic thalamic infarction. *Brain, 108*, 485–516.

Gronwald, D. M. A. (1977). Paced Auditory Serial Addition Task: A measure of recovery from concussion. *Perceptual and Motor Skills, 44*, 367–373.

Hachinski, V. C., Iliff, L. D., Zilhka, E., Du Boulay, G. H., McAllister, V. L., Marshall, J., et al. (1975). Cerebral blood flow in dementia. *Archives of Neurology, 32*, 632–637.

Heilman, K. M., & Valenstein, E. (2003). *Clinical neuropsychology* (4th ed.). New York: Oxford University Press.

Hofmeister, C., Stapf, C., Hartmann, A., Sciacca, R. R., Mansmann, U., terBrugge, K., Lasjaunias, P., Mast, H., & Meisel, J. (2000). Demographic, morphological, and clinical characteristics of 1289 patients with brain arteriovenous malformations. *Stroke, 31*, 1307–1310.

Hooper, H. E. (1983). *Hooper Visual Organization Test Manual*. Los Angeles: Western Psychological Services.

Hunt, W. E., & Hess, R. M. (1968). Surgical risk as related to time of intervention in the repair of intracranial aneurysms. *Journal of Neurosurgery, 28*, 14–20.

Johnston, S. C., Gress, D. R., Browner, W. S., & Sidney, S. (2000). Short-term prognosis after Emergency Department diagnosis of TAI. *JAMA, 284*, 2901–2906.

Kaplan, E., Goodglass, H., & Weintraub, S. (2001). *The Boston naming test*. Philadelphia: Lippincott Williams & Wilkins.

Kertesz, A. (1982). *Western Aphasia Battery*. San Antonio: Psychological Corporation.

Kolb, B., & Whishaw, I. (2009). *Fundamentals of human neuropsychology* (6th ed.). New York: W.H. Freeman Press.

Kwiatkowski, T. G., Libman, R. B., Frankel, M., et al. (1999). Effects of tissue plasminogen activator for acute ischemic stroke at one year. *The New England Journal of Medicine, 340*, 1781.

Lezak, M. D., Howieson, D. B., & Loring, D. W. (2004). *Neuropsychological assessment* (4th ed.). New York: Oxford University Press.

Meador, K. J., Moore, E. E., Nichols, M. E., et al. (1993). The role of cholinergic systems in visuospatial processing and memory. *Journal of Clinical and Experimental neuropsychology, 15*, 832–842.

Mesulam, M. M. (2000). *Principles of behavioral and cognitive neurology* (2nd ed.). NY: Oxford University Press.

National Stroke Association. (2007). Stroke Symptoms. Available at: http://www.stroke.org/site/ PageServer?pagename=SYMP. *Accessed March 4*, 2007.

Pinto, A. N., Canhao, P., & Ferro, J. M. (1996). Seizures at the onset of subarachnoid haemorrhage. *Journal of Neurology, 243*, 161–164.

Rey, A. (1941). L'examen psychologique dans les cas d'encephalopathie traumatique. *Archives de psychologie, 28*, 286–340.

Rey, A. (1964). *L'examen clinique en psychologie. Paris*: Presses Universitaires de France.

Robinson, R. G., & Starkstein, S. E. (2002). Neuropsychiatric aspects of cerebrovascular disorders. In S. C. Yudofsky & R. E. Hales (Eds.), *Textbook of neuropsychiatry and clinical neurosciences* (2nd ed.). Washington, DC: American Psychiatric Press.

Ross, E. D. (1997). The aprosodies. In T. E. Feinberg & M. J. Farah (Eds.), *Behavioral neurology and neuropsychology* (pp. 699–717). New York: McGraw-Hill.

Rothwell, P. M., Giles, M. F., Flossmann, E., Lovelock, C. E., Redgrave, J. N. E., Warlow, C. P., et al. (2005). A simple score (ABCD) to identify individuals at high early risk of stroke after transient ischemic attack. *Lancet, 366*, 29–36.

Schenkenberg, T., Bradford, D. C., & Ajax, E. T. (1980). *Line bisection and unilateral visual neglect in patients with neurologic impairment. Neurology, 30*, 509–517.

Sheslow, D., & Adams, W. (2003). *Wide Range Assessment of Memory and Learning Second Edition administration and technical manual*. Lutz, FL: Psychological Assessment Resources.

Spreen, O., & Strauss, E. (1998). *A compendium of neuropsychological tests: Administration, norms, and commentary* (2nd Ed.). New York: Oxford University Press.

Strauss, E., Sherman, E. M. S., & Spreen, O. (2006). *A compendium of neuropsychological tests: Administration, norms, and commentary* (3rd ed.). New York: Oxford University Press.

Stern, R. A., & White, T. (2003). *Neuropsychological assessment battery*. Lutz: Psychological Assessment Resources.

Sturgeon, J. D., & Folsom, A. R. (2007). Trends in hospitalization rate, hospital case fatality, and mortality rate of stroke by subtype in Minneapolis-St. Paul, 1980–2002. *Neuroepidemiology, 28*, 39–45.

Victor, M., & Ropper, A. H. (2001). *Adam's and Victor's Principals of Neurology* – (7th ed.). New York: McGraw-Hill.

Wechsler, D. (2001a). *Wechsler Memory Scale-3rd Edition* (WMS-III). The San Antonio, TX: The Psychological Corporation.

Wechsler, D. (2001b). *Wechsler Adult Intelligence Scale-3rd Edition* (WAIS-III). The San Antonio, TX: The Psychological Corporation.

Chapter 14
Dementias and Mild Cognitive Impairment in Adults

Mike R. Schoenberg and Kevin Duff

Abstract Dementia does not describe a specific disease entity, but rather describes a clinical syndrome characterized by a loss of previously acquired cognitive functions that adversely affects an individual's ability to complete day to day activities. The decline in cognitive functioning is greater than what occurs during the normal aging process. This chapter will review prominent definitions of dementia and a number of the etiologies of this syndrome. The prodromal phase between dementia and normal aging, Mild Cognitive Impairment (MCI), is reviewed later in this chapter. Readers interested in a more detailed review of dementia syndromes and conditions presenting as dementia are referred to Mendez and Cummings (Dementia: a clinical approach, 3rd edn, Butterworth Heinemann, Philadelphia, 2003).

Key Points and Chapter Summary

- Normal aging is characterized by slight decrements in speed of processing, memory, and other cognitive abilities. Mild Cognitive Impairment is characterized by isolated impairments, usually in memory. Dementia, however, is characterized by severe impairments in two or more cognitive domains, as well as functional decline.
- The most common types of dementia are: Alzheimer's disease, vascular dementia, frontotemporal dementia, and Dementia with Lewy Bodies.
- A detailed history of symptom onset and the course of its progression can be very valuable in the differential diagnosis of dementia.

(continued)

M.R. Schoenberg (✉)
Departments of Psychiatry and Neurosciences, Neurology, and Neurological Surgery,
University of South Florida College of Medicine, Tampa, FL, USA
and
Case Western Reserve University School of Medicine, Cleveland, OH, USA
e-mail: mschoenb@health.usf.edu

M.R. Schoenberg and J.G. Scott (eds.), *The Little Black Book of Neuropsychology: A Syndrome-Based Approach*, DOI 10.1007/978-0-387-76978-3_14,
© Springer Science+Business Media, LLC 2011

Key Points and Chapter Summary (continued)

- Evidence-based neuropsychology can assist in the differential diagnosis of dementia through the identification of distinct cognitive and behavioral presentations.
- Neuropsychological batteries should be tailored to the suspected type of dementia, as well as the severity of the cognitive impairments. Broad coverage of cognitive domains is necessary to accurately evaluate the presence of dementia and its etiology.

Diagnostic Criteria and Definitions

There are several different sets of diagnostic criteria for dementia. Some are more clinically based, whereas others are pathologically based and primarily applied in research settings. Given notable differences between different types of dementia (e.g., Alzheimer's disease vs vascular dementia), specific diagnostic criteria have been developed to define clinical states that represent dementia. Below we review proposed diagnostic guidelines for the more common forms of dementia (see Mendez and Cummings (2003) for additional dementia diagnostic criteria).

Diagnostic and Statistical Manual – 4th Edition (*DSM*-IV; (American Psychiatric Association. Diagnostic and Statistical Manual of Mental Disorders & 4th ed., text revision ed. Washington DC: author 2000)) is a set of primarily clinical diagnostic criteria that define dementia, and then provide options to classify the cause of the dementia. Broadly, dementia within the *DSM*-IV requires a deficit in memory. Additionally, at least one other cognitive deficit must be present, including aphasia (i.e., language disturbance), apraxia (including constructional skills), agnosia (i.e., poor visual recognition with intact sensory function), or executive dysfunction (e.g., poor judgment, insight, abstract reasoning, etc.). These cognitive deficits must represent a decline from a previously higher level of functioning, and must be severe enough to interfere with work, school, activities of daily living, or other social activities. The diagnosis is excluded if the symptoms occur exclusively during an episode of encephalopathy (delirium) or if only a single cognitive impairment (e.g., aphasia) is present. Within the *DSM*-IV, there are several different etiological possibilities, some of which require additional conditions to be met for diagnosis. For example, the diagnosis of vascular dementia also requires focal neurological signs and symptoms or laboratory evidence of cerebrovascular disease. The different subtypes of dementia within the *DSM*-IV are listed in Table 14.1.

Alzheimer's Disease

National Institute of Neurological and Communicative Disorders and Stroke – Alzheimer's Disease and Related Disorders Association (NINCDS-ADRDA, (3))

Table 14.1 DSM-IV subtypes of dementia

Dementia of the Alzheimer's type
Vascular dementia
Dementia due to HIV disease
Dementia due to head trauma
Dementia due to Parkinson's disease
Dementia due to Huntington's disease
Dementia due to Pick's disease
Dementia due to Creutzfeldt-Jakob disease
Dementia due to general medical condition
Substance induced persisting dementia
Dementia due to multiple etiologies
Dementia not otherwise specified

developed a set of diagnostic criteria that have been widely utilized in research studies investigating Alzheimer's disease (AD). These criteria make the important distinction between *probable* and *possible* AD, with the former being more certain than the latter. Within these criteria, *definitive* AD can only occur with neuropathological confirmation (e.g., biopsy, autopsy).

1. Criteria for *probable* AD:
   (a) Dementia established by clinical examination and cognitive tests
   (b) Deficits in two or more areas of cognition
   (c) Progressive worsening of memory and other cognitive functions
   (d) No disturbance of consciousness
   (e) Onset between ages of 40 and 90, most often after age 65
   (f) Absence of systemic disorders or other diseases that could account for symptoms
   (g) Probable AD is further supported by:
       (i) Progressive deterioration of specific cognitive functions
       (ii) Impaired activities of daily living and altered patterns of behavior
       (iii) Neuropathologically confirmed family history of similar disorders
       (iv) Confirmatory laboratory results (lumbar puncture, EEG, CT, MRI)

2. Criteria for *possible* AD:
   (a) Dementia in the absence of other neurologic, psychiatric, or system disorders of sufficient severity to cause the dementia, and in the presence of variations in the onset, in the presentation, or in the clinical course.
   (b) May be made in the presence of a second systematic or brain disorder sufficient to produce dementia, which is not considered to be the cause of the dementia.
   (c) Should be used in research studies when a single, gradually progressive severe cognitive deficit is identified in the absence of other identifiable cause.

Vascular Dementia

National Institute of Neurological Disorders and Stroke – Association Internationale pour la Recherche et l'Enseignement en Neurosciences (NINDS-AIREN,

(Roman et al. 1993)) criteria are a collaborative effort to conceptualize and define vascular dementia (VaD) for research purposes. This group also noted that researchers could communicate their level of confidence in their diagnosis of VaD with the qualifiers of *probable* or *possible.*

1. Criteria for *probable* VaD:
   (a) Evidence of dementia (i.e., impairments of memory and other cognitive domains).
   (b) Evidence of cerebrovascular disease (e.g., focal neurological signs, brain imaging).
   (c) Relationship between dementia and cerebrovascular disease (e.g., dementia within 3 months post-stroke, fluctuating or stepwise course of cognitive deficits).
   (d) Other features that support the diagnosis: gait disturbance, falls, incontinence, pseudobulbar palsy, mood changes.

2. Criteria for *possible* VaD:
   (a) Dementia with focal neurological signs, but without neuroimaging evidence, or
   (b) Dementia with focal signs, but without temporal relationship between dementia and stroke, or
   (c) Dementia with focal signs, but with subtle onset and variable course.

Frontotemporal Dementia

Two sets of diagnostic criteria have been developed for frontotemporal dementias (FTD). The first (Neary et al. 1998) identifies both core features and supportive evidence:

1. Presence of core diagnostic features (i.e., insidious onset and gradual progression, early decline in social interpersonal functioning, early impairment in regulating personal conduct, early emotional blunting, early loss of insight).
2. Other features that support the diagnosis: behavioral disorder (e.g., decline in hygiene, mental rigidity, hyperorality, utilization behavior), speech/language disorder (e.g., altered output, echolalia, mutism), physical signs (e.g., primitive reflexes, incontinence, rigidity), diagnostic procedures (e.g., executive dysfunction on neuropsychological testing, anterior abnormalities on brain imaging).

The Lund and Manchester groups (Lund 1994) provide a more behavioral description of FTD, and these include:

1. Behavioral symptoms (e.g., loss of personal awareness, disinhibition, mental inflexibility, perseverations, impulsivity)
2. Affective symptoms (e.g., indifference, depression, aspontaneity), and
3. Speech symptoms (e.g., repetition of phrases, echolalia, mutism).

Dementia with Lewy Bodies

McKeith et al. (1996) proposed clinical diagnostic criteria for dementia with Lewy Bodies (DLB). The consensus criteria include a *central* feature (below), three *core* features associated with DLB, and six additional features (symptoms) that support a diagnosis of DLB. A diagnosis of *probable* DLB requires the central feature and at least two core features, whereas *possible* DLB requires the central feature and one core feature. Conformation of clinical diagnosis of DLB requires pathological study.

1. The *central* feature of DLB is a progressive decline of cognitive function that is sufficient to interfere with the individual's social or occupational functioning. Cognitive deficits often include attention, frontal-subcortical, visuospatial, and memory.
2. Core Features supporting a diagnosis of DLB include:
   (a) Fluctuating levels of consciousness/cognition with pronounced variations in arousal level/attention
   (b) Spontaneous parkinsonian motor features (extrapyramidal signs)
   (c) Visual hallucinations that are typically well formed and recurring
3. Features (symptoms) that support a diagnosis of DLB:
   (a) Repeated falls
   (b) Syncope
   (c) Transient loss of consciousness
   (d) Sensitivity to neuroleptic medications
   (e) Hallucinations in other modalities (i.e., auditory)
   (f) Systematized delusions
4. The following do *not* support a diagnosis of DLB:
   (a) Evidence of stroke – either with focal neurological exam or based on neuroimaging
   (b) Evidence of any physical illness or other brain disorder sufficient to account for clinical symptoms.

Recent evaluation of diagnostic criteria suggests that the presence of visual hallucinations is not consistently found in neuropathologically confirmed DLB. Fluctuation in mental status may also be a less useful diagnostic feature, but lack of consistent findings in pathologically confirmed DLB may also relate to variability in clinicians recognition of substantive fluctuation in mental status. Parkinsonism is found in most patients with DLB (minimum of 67% of pathologically confirmed DLB), and the co-occurrence of neuropsychological deficits within 12 months of extrapyramidal (parkinsonian) motor deficits has shown particularly reliable diagnostic utility.

Progressive Supranuclear Palsy

Clinical research diagnostic criteria were established by the National Institute of Neurological Disorders and Stroke (NINDS)/Society for PSP conference, identifying criteria for definite, probable, and possible Progressive Supranuclear Palsy (PSP). Within these criteria, *definite* PSP is made when patient has had a clinical history of probable or possible PSP and histopathological confirmation (e.g., biopsy, autopsy).

1. Criteria for *probable* PSP:
    (a) Vertical supranuclear gaze palsy
    (b) Prominent postural instability with falls within the first year of the disease
    (c) And other features of PSP as follows:
        (i)   Akinesia and/or rigidity that is symmetric and greater proximally than distally
        (ii) Abnormal stiffening and extension of the neck, particularly retrocollis
        (iii) Dysphagia and dysarthria early in the course of the disease
        (iv) Cognitive impairment early in the course of the disease including at least two of the following: apathy, impaired verbal fluency, frontal release signs, echopraxia or echolalia, impaired abstract reasoning.
    (d) Absence of systemic disorders or other diseases that could account for symptoms.

2. Criteria for *possible* PSP:
    (a) Gradually progressive disorder with onset when the individual is aged 40 years or older
    (b) Within the first year of disease onset, vertical supranuclear palsy or *both* slowed vertical saccades and prominent postural instability with unexplained falls
    (c) No evidence of other diseases that can explain the clinical features.

A diagnosis of PSP is less likely with any of the following: presence of dysautonomia or hallucinations in the absence of medication effects, prominent cerebellar signs, unilateral dysnomia, or early cortical dementia features (e.g., aphasia or agnosia).

HIV Associated Neurocognitive Disorders

Although initially described as AIDS dementia complex (Navia et al. 1986), the diagnostic criteria associated with cognitive impairment secondary to HIV and AIDS have evolved over the years. The earliest was HIV-dementia complex (Navia et al. 1986). In 1991, the American Academy Neurology proposed the HIV-Associated Dementia (HAD) and HIV-associated minor cognitive-motor disorder (MCMD). Most recently, Antinori et al. (2007) proposed a three subtype diagnostic model for HIV associated neurocognitive disorders (HAND) summarized below. All diagnoses below require confirmation of HIV infection, and objective neurocognitive testing can be used to empirically support the level of impairment.

- *HIV-associated dementia (HAD)*: Acquired neurocognitive deficits lasting at least 1 month in which either; (1) scores on neuropsychological tests in at least two neurocognitive domains (e.g., attention/working memory, information processing speed, executive functions, learning/memory, language/speech, visuo-perceptual/visuospatial, and/or motor skills) that are moderately to severely impaired (e.g., less than or equal to 2 standard deviations below demographically appropriate normative mean), *or* (2) scores of one neurocognitive domain are more severely impaired (<2.5 standard deviations below the mean) *and* at least one other neurocognitive domain is at least mildly impaired (i.e., ≤1 standard deviations below the mean). At least one of the impaired ability domains must be primarily cognitive.

  - The neurocognitive deficits are severe enough to cause major functional impairment in work or school or activities of daily living, and these neurocognitive and functional impairments may not be accounted for by confounding conditions (e.g., opportunistic CNS infections, systemic illness, medication effects, and/or substance abuse).

- *HIV-associated mild neurocognitive disorder (MND)*: Acquired neurocognitive deficits lasting at least 1 month in which scores on neuropsychological tests in at least two neurocognitive domains that are mildly impaired (i.e., 1 or more standard deviations below the mean). These deficits are severe enough to cause mild functional impairments in work or school or activities of daily living and these impairments are not better accounted for by comorbid conditions.
- *HIV-asymptomatic neurocognitive impairment (ANI)*: Acquired neurocognitive deficits lasting at least 1 month in which scores on neuropsychological tests in at least two neurocognitive domains that are mildly impaired (i.e., 1 or more standard deviations below the mean). However, the neurocognitive deficits do *not* cause any demonstrated or reported functional impairments.

  - In cases in which standardized neuropsychological assessment is not available, substitution with other assessment (e.g., MMSE or HIV Dementia Scale) can be used. In this case, an attempt should be made to approximate the criteria above (e.g., MND diagnosis requires mental status exam score to fall at least 1 standard deviations below demographically appropriate normative mean involving at least two neurocognitive domains and there is a mild functional deficit).

Before turning to etiologies for the dementias, it is noteworthy to point out some of the operational definitions for diagnosing dementia are more specific than others. For example, HAD specifies the number of standard deviations that cognitive test scores must fall below normative data to be considered impaired, whereas others are more general (e.g., "evidence of dementia" in VaD). Some diagnostic criteria are more cognitive-focused (e.g., AD), whereas others are more behaviorally focused (e.g., FTD). Many of these criteria sets allow for varying levels of certainty of the diagnosis (e.g., probable vs possible), but neuropsychological dysfunction is present in all dementias, and neuropsychological assessment assists in differential diagnosis and prognosis of dementia (Mendez and Cummings 2003; Kral 1962; Graham et al. 1997; Christensen et al. 1995; Petersen et al. 1999; Gutierrez et al. 1993; Morris and Cummings 2005; Petersen 2003; Petersen et al. 2001; Luis et al. 2004; Manly et al. 2008; Morris et al. 2001; Storandt et al. 2002; DeCarli et al. 2004; Griffith et al. 2006; Duff et al. 2007; Jack et al. 1999; Jack et al. 2000; de Leon et al. 2001; Tuokko et al. 2003; Chamberlain and Sahakian 2006; Rosenstein 1998; Wright and Persad 2007; Fleisher et al. 2007; Dubois et al. 2005; Carnahan et al. 2006; Peters 1989). The definitions of dementia have been revised as new research refines our understanding of the dementias and aging. Future changes will undoubtedly occur.

Etiologies of Dementia

Factors that can cause the syndrome of dementia can be divided into multiple classes. Some conditions are primarily degenerative and will slowly progress over time. At its broadest definition, dementia is anything resulting in a loss of previously acquired skill in multiple cognitive domains, and this potentially includes nearly every chronic disease. For this chapter, we will more narrowly focus on primary central nervous system diseases that have a neurodegenerative course for which the loss of cognitive (neuropsychological) function is a primary disease characteristic. Some of these degenerative conditions have hallmark neuropathological signs that differentiate them from other conditions (e.g., tau mutations in AD), while others are a secondary result of multiple illnesses that have a primary CNS deterioration (e.g., hypertension, diabetes, and hypercholesterolemia in VaD). Dementias can be caused by a variety of medical (e.g., cerebrovascular, metabolic, infectious, systemic) and psychiatric illnesses (e.g., substance abuse). Table 14.2 summarizes some of the etiologies for dementias. The table is not exhaustive, but includes both common and rare causes of dementia, and includes illnesses that can result in cognitive decline (dementia) in children and/or younger adults. For a review of conditions leading to cognitive decline in childhood through young adulthood, the readers may review Chap. 28, this volume.

Prevalence of Dementia

Dementia rates increase steadily with age (Launer et al. 1999). Cognitive impairment of this severity is rare in young and middle aged adults (e.g., 0.5%). Prevalence at age 60 is thought to be about 1 in 100. Prevalence at age 65 and older is 5–8%. Prevalence after age 74 years old is 15–20%. At age 85 years and older, prevalence is 30–50%.

Table 14.2 Etiologies of dementia

Degenerative dementias	Cerebrovascular disease
Alzheimer's disease	Subdural hematoma
Dementia with Lewy Bodies	Small vessel disease
Frontotemporal dementia/Pick's disease	Binswanger's disease
Huntington's disease	Multi-infarct dementia
Parkinson's disease	CADASIL
Corticobasal degeneration	Infections
Progressive supranuclear palsy	Syphilis
Multisystem atrophies	Chronic meningitis
Metabolic and deficiency conditions	Progressive multifocal leukoencephalopathy
Cushing syndrome	HIV infection/AIDS
Hepatic encephalopathy	Lyme disease
Hypothyroidism	Prion diseases
Porphyria	Creutzfeldt-Jakob disease
Wilson's disease	variant Creutzfeldt-Jakob disease
Vitamin deficiencies (B12, thiamine, folate)	Kuru
Hypoglycemia	Demyelinating disorders
Kidney disease (renal failure, dialysis)	Multiple Sclerosis
Head injury	Acute disseminated encephalomyelitis
Toxins and drugs	Systemic Disorders
Heavy metals	Systemic Lupus Erythematosus
Carbon monoxide	Sarcoidosis
Alcohol (Wernicke-Korsakoff Syndrome)	Neoplasms
Illegal drugs and prescription medications (e.g., anticholinergic)	Normal Pressure Hydrocephalus
Psychiatric syndromes	Epilepsy
Depression	

Clinical Descriptions of Common Dementia Conditions

A brief clinical description of common diseases presenting with dementia is presented below. These descriptions are summaries of multiple empirical studies, which can form a basis for evidence-based neuropsychology practice, and some relevant references are cited below each diagnostic condition. Readers are also encouraged to review Table 14.3, which provides a brief description of the historical, behavioral, neuropsychological, and psychological presentation of these conditions.

Alzheimer's Disease (AD)

Prevalence: AD is the most prevalent of dementia syndromes, accounting for about 35% of all cases of dementia. Another 15% of dementias include mixed pathologies of both AD and VaD. Therefore, 50% of all dementia are either pure or "mixed" AD.

Risk factors: Older age, female gender (but this might be an artifact of longevity differences in gender), lower levels of education, family history of dementia (especially with onset before age 65), homozygous for the apolipoprotein e4 allele (Apoe4), Down's syndrome, history of head injury, history of psychiatric illness, history of alcohol abuse.

Onset: The majority of cases of AD develop after age 65 (i.e., late onset AD). The number of cases significantly increases across the seventh, eighth, and ninth decades of life (2, 6, 50 + %, respectively). A minority of AD cases develop before age 65 (i.e., early onset AD), and these cases often demonstrate a stronger genetic etiology (familial).

Course: Late onset AD tends to have a slow and insidious course, lasting 10+ years. Early onset has a more rapid progression. Both types of AD are progressive, without remission. Several efforts have been made to scale the progression of AD. The Clinical Dementia Rating Scale (CDR, (Morris 1997)) is the most widely used such scale. CDR scores fall on a 5-point scale (0 = no impairment, 0.5 = questionable impairment/very mild dementia, 1 = mild deficit/dementia, 2 = moderate deficit/moderate dementia, 3 = severe deficit/severe dementia) based on six domains (memory, orientation, judgment/problem solving, community affairs, home/hobbies and personal care.

Behavioral Symptoms/Clinical Presentation: Early in the course of AD, subtle personality changes (e.g., less energy, socially withdrawn, greater dependence on others, indifference) may be evident. Symptoms of depression may be present, but often affect is dependent upon environmental stimuli (e.g., visiting grandchildren improves mood). Patients often will minimize cognitive problems, and may confabulate to cover memory deficits. As the disease progresses, agitation, confusion, wandering, apathy, decreased sleep and appetite, and emotional blunting become more common. Delusions and hallucinations can also occur later in AD.

Neuropsychological symptoms: Memory impairment and dysnomia are some of the earliest cognitive symptoms in AD. Memory loss reflects deficits in consolidation and recall with rapid forgetting of new information (e.g., retention rate <50%). Learning curve is impaired. Immediate memory may be less impaired than delayed recall, but is still below peers. Recognition memory is impaired, with frequent false positive or false negative errors. Confrontation naming is generally impaired, and markedly so as the disease progresses. Verbal fluency is often impaired, and semantic fluency may be worse than phonemic fluency. Constructional apraxia is common. Simple attention is intact until late in the disease. As AD progresses, global cognitive impairment is observed, with agnosia, apraxia, and aphasia defining the syndrome. Motor function is often preserved late into the disease, but eventually becomes impaired.

Neuropathology: Amyloid plaques and neurofibrillary tangles are the two most common markers of AD in the brain. These neuropathological conditions begin in the medial temporal lobes (entorhinal cortex, hippocampi), spread to the parietal and frontal cortices, and eventually consume most of the neocortex. These cellular changes lead to gross morphological changes in the brain, with MRI studies showing cortical atrophy that is more prominent in temporal and parietal areas. Enlargement of ventricles is an effect of this global cerebral atrophy.

Selected References: (Mendez and Cummings 2003; Launer et al. 1999; Salmon and Filoteo 2007; Kim et al. 2005; Yaari 2007)

Rule of thumb: Alzheimer's disease dementia

- Early onset of memory impairment (poor consolidation and recognition)
  - Learning curve flat, delayed recall impaired, false positive errors
- Dysnomia (poor confrontation naming)
- Visuoconstructional deficits
- No parkinsonism present early
- Social withdraw common
- Symptoms of depression can occur, but tend to vary with environment

---

Vascular Dementia (VaD)

Prevalence: Excluding "mixed" AD, VaD is the second most common cause of dementia. Approximately 10% of dementia cases are due to pure VaD, and another 15% are attributable to some combination of VaD and AD.

Risk factors: History of stroke, atherosclerosis, hypertension, diabetes, hyperc-holesterolemia, smoking cigarettes, obesity, male gender, and older age.

Onset: As individuals age, their risk for strokes and other vascular problems increase, and so does their risk for VaD. Onset of VaD typically occurs between 60 and 75 years of age.

Course: The course of VaD is quite variable due to the many different sizes and locations of ischemic events within the brain. Many cases progress in a "stepwise" manner, with periods of stability followed by rapid deterioration due to additional strokes. However, this "stepwise" course can be hard to identify and may appear more continuously progressive. Other cases can progress slowly and gradually, in which multiple remote ("old") ischemic events are identified by neuroimaging that were undetected by patients or their families.

Behavioral Symptoms/Clinical Presentation: The clinical presentation of VaD can vary widely, depending on the site of the stroke and penumbra. Neurological signs and symptoms can be minimal or severe (e.g., gait and balance problems, planter flexor response, increased deep tendon reflexes, spasticity, rigidity, visual field deficits, clonus, etc.). Symptoms of depression and anxiety are common. Apathy and social withdrawal are also common. Disinhibition can occur. Urinary incontinence may be present.

Neuropsychological symptoms: Psychomotor slowing, impaired attention/concentration, and visuoperceptual/constructional deficits could all be present. Memory is likely impaired on both immediate and delayed free recall tasks. This memory deficit, however, tends to reflect poor retrieval, as recognition cues improve recall. Language deficits can lead to aphasia syndromes depending upon lesion location. As additional strokes occur, more global cognitive and motor impairments will be observed.

Neuropathology: The neuroanatomical damage in VaD varies depending upon vascular etiology. Multi-infarct dementia typically reflects multiple small lesions throughout the white and grey matter of the cerebral cortex. Binswanger's disease reflects multiple small lesions throughout the white matter of the cerebral hemispheres, predominately affecting the internal capsule and periventricular white matter. Strategic vascular dementias can reflect focal lesions of the anterior thalamus or mediodorsal thalamus, or angular gyrus typically of the dominant hemisphere. In general, the lesion volume is not the best predictor of the severity of cognitive impairment, as strategic small infarcts in the thalamus can result in dense amnestic syndromes not usually observed until extensive diffuse periventricular microvascular disease is present.

Selected References: (Mendez and Cummings 2003; Roman et al. 1993; Zekry et al. 2002; Starkstein et al. 1996; Paul et al. 2001)

Rule of thumb: Vascular dementias (multi-infarct type)

- Neurologic signs (planter flexors, unilateral motor and/or sensory deficits) may be present
- Early deficits in processing speed, attention, executive functions, visuo-constructional skills are often seen
- Recognition memory may be intact early in the course of disease
- Poor rapid generative verbal fluency (phonemic may be more impaired than semantic)
- Psychomotor deficits including predominant slowing and fine motor co-odination deficits

---

Dementia with Lewy Bodies (DLB)

Prevalence: After AD, DLB is the second or third most prevalent of the neurodegenerative diseases, accounting for 12–27% of all diagnosed dementias.

Risk factors: Older age and other causes of dementia (e.g., patients with AD and Parkinson's disease (PD) often have Lewy bodies).

Onset: DLB usually develops earlier than AD and VaD, with onsets typically between 50 and 70 years of age.

Course: The course of DLB is slow and insidious, and it is often mistaken for other types of dementia (e.g., AD or PD) before correct diagnosis (note that some data suggest DLB and PD may reflect a continuum of disease pathology rather than two distinct diseases, see Chapter 19). Generally, the course is more rapid than AD, with a 5–7 year course from diagnosis. However, the clinical presentation is punctuated by periods (hours to days) of marked fluctuation in mental status/orientation, which gives it a more variable appearance. Patient families often remark on this variability when describing the deficits demonstrated by patients with DLB.

Behavioral Symptoms/Clinical Presentation: Dementia with fluctuating cognition/consciousness, parkinsonism, and recurrent visual hallucinations are the hallmark features of DLB, and all three features often present within a year or two of dementia (See also Chap. 21, this volume). Cognitive impairment alone, but more often cognitive impairment plus parkinsonism and/or visual hallucinations, are often the first symptoms to present in DLB. The fluctuation in mental status can be seen as temporary confusion and disoriented. In addition to visual hallucinations, depressive symptoms may be present (e.g., social withdrawal, dependence, irritability). The Parkinson-like motor impairments can include rigidity and decreased spontaneous movements. As the disease progresses, disability increases with worsening cognition, hallucinations and delusions, and parkinsonism. Treatments aimed at reducing hallucinations (e.g., neuroleptics) can actually worsen motor functioning in these patients. Unlike PD with dementia, DLB is diagnosed among individuals in whom neuropsychological deficits present concurrently with motor symptoms or within one year, while dementia associated with PD has been diagnosed among individuals whom present with prominent motor features without prominent neuropsychological deficits. often presents with neuropsychological deficits and parkinsonism or neuropsychological deficits prior to other symptoms, while dementia associated with PD develops after several years of parkinsonism. REM sleep behavioral disorder is also common in DLB. See also Chap. 19 for further discussion of associated features of DLB.

Neuropsychological symptoms: Frequently the most marked neuropsychological deficits involve attention/executive, particularly working memory, and visuoperceptual/visuoconstructional functions. Unlike AD, early in the course of DLB, memory (particularly delayed free recall) is not markedly affected, with memory often being mildly impaired due to poor encoding strategies. Recognition cues do not improve recall. Nonverbal (visual) memory may be more impaired than verbal memory, perhaps reflecting marked impairment in visuoperceptual/visuoconstructional skills. Early in disease, language functions may not be markedly affected, although deficits in verbal fluency (phonemic and semantic) and naming develop. Executive functions are often moderately to severely impaired. Disorientation to time and place is likely to occur as mental status fluctuates over hours to days. Later in the course of DLB, global cognitive impairment is notable, although mental status will continue to wax and wane.

Rule of thumb: Dementia with Lewy bodies (DLB)

- Onset of dementia within 12 months of parkinsonian motor deficits
  - (i.e., Co-occurrence of cognitive deficits and parkinsonian motor deficits)
- Fluctuating mental status/cognitive functioning over hours or days
- Early deficits in attention, executive, and visuoperceptual/constructional skills
  - Memory often not severely impaired early
- Visual hallucinations (well-formed)

Neuropathology: Gross pathology of the brain in patients with DLB might be absent (or quite minimal). It is the accumulation of Lewy bodies, alpha-synuclein protein, in the nuclei of neurons that differentiates this condition from other causes of dementia. Although Lewy bodies are present in PD and also in AD, it is their widespread (i.e., diffuse) distribution that separates DLB from these other conditions.

Selected References: (Mendez and Cummings 2003; McKeith et al. 1996; Ballard et al. 2001; Johnson et al. 2005; Zaccai et al. 2005)

Frontotemporal Dementia (FTD)

FTD has become an umbrella term to describe several clinical syndromes of dementia all sharing a pathology of frontotemporal lobar degeneration. There are several relatively clinically distinct FTDs. The FTDs include *frontal variant FTD* or *behavioral variant FTD* (of which *Pick's disease* is a subtype) and *primary progressive aphasia (PPA)*(Mendez and Cummings 2003). The terms either frontal variant FTD (fvFTD) or behavioral variant FTD (bvFTD) have been used to describe patients with changes in behavior and personality noted in Pick's disease (see below), but also include other forms of FTD, such as those that include onset of parkinsonian symptoms not typically associated with Pick's disease. Primary progressive aphasia (PPA) has traditionally been divided into *progressive nonfluent aphasia (PNFA)* and *semantic dementia (SD)*. However, a fluent form of PPA has been suggested (fPPA) as well as another subtype, termed *logopenic progressive aphasia* or *logopenic/phonological progressive aphasia.*

Prevalence: Representing the fourth most common form of dementia are FTDs, accounting for 5–9% of cases. Among persons under 60 years old, FTDs are the first or second most common type of dementia. Pick's disease, as a subtype of FTD, is thought to represent 20% of all FTDs.

Risk factors: Family history of dementia and older age (although cases after age 75 are rare). Majority of cases are not hereditary, but advances in genetics have identified autosomal dominant inheritance in 20–30% of cases. Various abnormalities of the tau protein gene on chromosome 17q21–22 have been identified.

Another histopathological risk factor recently identified is the presence of ubiquitin immunoreactive inclusions in cells or ubiquitin immunoreactive neuritis. More than 50% of FTD cases have ubiquitin, and have been termed frontotemporal lobar degeneration-ubiquitin (FTLD-U). A small group of FTDs have no consistent histopathological abnormality (e.g., not an FTLD-U) or identifiable genetic link.

Some cases of corticobasal ganglionic degeneration (CBGD) and PSP were found to share the tau pathology of some of the FTDs. Similarly, some of the ubiquitin-immunoreactive inclusions of FTDs have also been found in the upper and lower motor neurons of amyotrophic lateral sclerosis (ALS). The histological findings have led to a proposed FTD complex, which includes these clinically distinct diseases into a single nosology which have different clinical symptom presentation but shared histopathological features.

Onset: Developing earlier than most other common dementias, onset of FTDs is typically between 50 and 60 years of age (mean age of onset is 59). There are reports of FTDs onset in the early 20s.

Course: Gradually developing symptoms is the most common course in this type of dementia. However, once diagnosed, progression can be more rapid than AD, often evolving over 5–7 years. As FTDs progress, some patients present with parkinsonian features.

Behavioral Symptoms/Clinical Presentation: The clinical variants of FTD are typically described as having relatively distinct clinical presentations, but overlap in symptoms is often present.

1. *Frontal variant (fvFTD/bvFTD)* often presents with personality changes reflecting apathy, social withdrawal, loss of social awareness, decreased personal hygiene, affective flattening, and apathy. Less frequently, the behavioral disturbance might reflect social disinhibition, impulsivity, impersistence and perseveration. Language deficits (poor confrontation naming, reduced verbal fluency) are common. Other frequent frontal symptoms include utilization behaviors, perseveration, and stimulus-bound behaviors. Echolalia, echopraxia, and mutism may be present in rare, and/ or severe cases. Hoarding of unusual items and change in libido (increase or decrease) can occur. A fvFTD reflecting greater pathology of the right hemisphere has been reported [i.e., FTD-rv (right variant)], presenting with flat affect, socially aloof, and aprosodic speech. Greater left hemisphere (dominant hemisphere) involvement results in greater language impairment. As the disease progresses, more marked personality changes will occur, including emotional incontinence, stereotyped behaviors, and agitation or marked apathy and indifference. Frontal release signs (positive snout, grasp, and palmomental responses and/or glabellar sign) and/or oculomotor abnormalities may be present. Gait abnormalities with parkinsonian features are present in some cases, and can be pronounced in a minority of cases. These FTD with more prominent parkinsonian features may represent a unique subset type of FTDs that includes cortical basal ganglionic degeneration (CBGD) and some cases of PSP.

   i. *Pick's disease* is a subtype of fvFTD/bvFTD that is distinguished based on presentation of classic symptoms and the histological marker of Pick's bodies (see below). Classically, Pick's disease features include impulsivity, dysnomia, and Kluver–Bucy type syndrome of hyper-orality (excessive eating) and sensory stimulus seeking that has a compulsive quality.

2. *Primary progressive aphasias* [e.g., fluent primary progressive aphasia (fPPA), progressive nonfluent aphasia (PNFA), semantic dementia (SD)] collectively present with reductions in speech/language (see below) and/or verbal comprehension with social withdrawal and depression not uncommon. Traditionally, these disorders are not associated with changes in personality or behaviors (other than social withdrawal) and may also develop symptoms of anxiety and depression thought to be associated with loss of ability to speak. PNFA presents with speech articulation errors (dysarthria is common). Some patients with PNFA

develop motor features of CBGD and/or PSP such as oculomotor abnormalities and/or parkinsonian features. Semantic Dementia (SD) and logopenic forms do not present with motor speech deficits. No oculomotor abnormalities have been found in patients with SD.

Neuropsychological symptoms:

1. *fvFTD/bvFTD* (including Pick's disease) tends to present first with problematic changes in personality and social behaviors (e.g., poor social judgment, silliness/jocularity, impulsivity, disinhibition, decreased hygiene, and/or impersistence). The initial personality changes may present with increasing activity, disinhibition, impulsivity, lack of empathy and reduced regard for others. Alternatively, patients may present as "bored" or "depressed" and exhibit behavioral apathy, motor impersistence, amotivation, and emotionally blunting. Cognitive deficits of executive dysfunction reflected in impaired mental flexibility, distractibility, poor verbal fluency, and deficient problem solving (e.g., concrete verbal reasoning, poor design fluency/verbal fluency, and limited insight) will often follow personality changes. In contrast to patients with AD, patients with fvFTD exhibit greater executive impairment than memory impairment. Memory may be surprisingly intact, particularly in the first 2 years of the disease. However, memory impairments may become more apparent later in the course of the disease, particularly in difficulty accurately recalling the temporal sequence of events, proactive interference, and retrieval deficits. Language deficits (e.g., impaired confrontational naming, decreased phonemic verbal fluency, slower word reading and color naming) are present (see also PPAs below). Stimulus bound and utilization behaviors may be present, particularly in later stages of the disease. *Gagenhalten* or *paratonia* (involuntary resistance to efforts to passively move limbs) and *witzelsucht* (hollow and inappropriate humor/jokes) may be exhibited. Generally visuospatial skills, orientation, and arithmetic skills remain intact (but see SD below).
    (a) *Pick's Disease*, as a specific subtype of fvFTD/bvFTD, has a neuropsychological presentation that is similar to that described above. However, the features of hyper-orality and compulsive sensory stimulation seeking should be present.
2. *Primary Progressive Aphasia*
    (a) *Progressive nonfluent aphasia (PNFA)* presents with a largely circumscribed progressive decline in speech (and writing). Speech is non-fluent and effortful, and gradually presents with increasing phonological and grammatical errors. Comprehension of words and objects remain intact (as opposed to SD and logopenic types, below). Speech articulation is disturbed (i.e., dysarthria). Repetition is intact. Other cognitive domains remain largely unaffected for several years.
    (b) *Semantic dementia* (SD) is associated with loss of semantic knowledge, resulting in severe deficits in confrontation naming, poor verbal comprehension due to disrupted knowledge of word meanings, and visual agnosias (due to loss of knowledge of visual material). Conversational speech remains

quite fluent and is not dysarthric. While semantic memory is poor, performance on tests of episodic memory (e.g., word lists, stories, figures) are often intact, at least in the early stages. A diagnostic consensus statement (Neary et al. 1998) specifies a diagnosis of SD must include semantic knowledge impairments exhibited by impaired word knowledge and associate agnosia (difficulty recognizing/identifying objects) and/or prosopagnosia.

(c) *Logopenic (logopenic/phonologic) progressive aphasia* present with dysnomia, effortful speech, and impaired repetition and comprehension for sentences. However, single word repetition and comprehension is intact. Unlike SD, semantic knowledge of words and objects is intact. Memory, early in the disease, is intact.

Neuropathology: Given the multiple variants of FTD, there are various neuropathological etiologies. However, all are characterized by degeneration of some aspect of the frontal and/or temporal lobes. Degeneration tends to be asymmetric to match the clinical presentation.

1. *fvFTD/bvFTD:* Presents with atrophy, gliosis, and neuronal loss of frontal cortex. Predominant degeneration of frontal lobes with involvement of anterior temporal lobe cortices is typical.

   (a) *Pick's disease* (but not all fvFTD/bvFTD) is a tauopathy, with tau-positive inclusions, swollen (ballooned) neurons (Pick cells), and Pick bodies (i.e., argentophilic neuronal inclusions) in the frontotemporal regions of the cortex. Characteristic Kluver–Bucy symptoms are thought to reflect degeneration of the amygdala.

Rule of thumb: Fronto-temporal dementia

- Early onset of personality changes and executive dysfunction
- Deficits in language (confrontation naming and verbal fluency)
- Memory, visuoperceptual, and arithmetic skills can be intact (early stages)

Primary Progressive Aphasia characterized by

- Effortful speech (confrontation naming, verbal fluency, and/or comprehension)
- Mild arithmetic problems, attention deficits, ideomotor apraxia, and perseveration can be present with speech deficits during first two years, but this presentation cannot be the primary presentation.
- Memory and visuoperceptual skills intact and no apathy, disinhibition, or motor deficits the first 2 years of illness

Subtypes of PPA traditionally include:

- Progressive Nonfluent Aphasia – primarily disruption in articulation
- Semantic dementia – primarily disruption in semantic knowledge

2. *Progressive Nonfluent Aphasia* is commonly associated with greater degeneration of the left posterior frontal cortex, anterior insular, and basal ganglia. Many cases of PNFA are tauopathies, and do not to have AD pathology.
3. *Semantic Dementia* is often associated with polar and inferolateral temporal cortex atrophy (left greater than right). Many cases of SD are ubiquitin-positive, and represent a type of the FTLD-U dementias (see above).
4. *Logopenic* or *logopenic/phonological variant* has been reported with consistent reduction in metabolism of the posterior aspect of the left superior and middle temporal gyri and left parietal inferior lobule. Cases of logopenic type PPA were found to have AD pathology.

Selected References: (Mendez and Cummings 2003; Neary et al. 1998; Lund 1994; Bozeat et al. 2000; Forman et al. 2006)

Huntington's Disease (HD)

Prevalence: HD is a rare autosomal dominant neurodegenerative disorder that leads to motor dysfunction, psychiatric symptoms, and cognitive impairments. Not all patients with HD develop dementia, and HD probably accounts for 1–2% of dementias.

Risk factors: Earlier development of HD and greater genetic loading (i.e., longer CAG repeat lengths).

Onset: Although HD typically develops between the ages of 40 and 50 years old, juvenile cases can occur before the age of 20.

Course: Dementia slowly develops in individuals with HD.

Behavioral Symptoms/Clinical Presentation: Research suggests that behavioral and motor symptoms may develop at least 10 years before the diagnosis of HD. Depression and obsessive-compulsive traits are some of the earliest psychiatric symptoms. Subtle movement abnormalities are also present. As HD progresses, the motor and psychiatric symptoms worsen to include choreiform movements, personality changes, and delusions and hallucinations.

Neuropsychological symptoms: Early cognitive changes in HD include psychomotor slowing, executive dysfunction, and decreased working memory. Retrieval deficits probably explain most of the early "memory changes" in HD. Some of the cognitive declines might be an artifact of the loss f voluntary motor control. As with most other progressive dementias, the cognitive impairments in HD worsen across time, becoming more global and more profound.

Neuropathology: The subcortical striatum (caudate and putamen) is primarily affected in HD. However, extra-striatal changes have also been reported, and might better correlate with the different clinical presentations of HD.

Selected References: (Mendez and Cummings 2003; Paulsen and Conybeare 2005; Paulsen et al. 2008, 2001; Mendez 1994)

Rule of thumb: Huntington's disease (HD)

- Early onset of psychiatric changes may occur
- Movement disorder (voluntary and involuntary disturbances)
- Subcortical cognitive impairments can occur early in HD, with frank dementia occurring later

Parkinson's Disease with Dementia (PD-D)

Prevalence: Like with HD, Parkinson's disease (PD) is a neurodegenerative disease with motor, psychiatric, and cognitive dysfunction. Not all patients with PD will develop dementia (~30%), although rates ranging from 2% to 93% have been reported. PD-D probably accounts for 2% of all dementias.

Risk factors: Risk for dementia (and cognitive dysfunction in general) is higher for individuals with onset of PD after age 60.

Onset: Typically between 60 and 70 years of age.

Course: Insidious onset, slowly progressing over years. Cognitive deterioration is more rapid for patients with onset of PD later in life, particularly for those after age 70. Incidence of dementia in patients with onset of PD before age 45 is 10% of those with onset of PD after age 60.

Behavioral Symptoms/Clinical Presentation: Motor symptoms include resting tremor (typically), rigidity, bradykinesia/akinesia, and postural instability (See Chap. 21, this volume). Patients with PD are likely to suffer from apathy, symptoms of depression, anxiety, and sleep problems. Later in PD, marked gait impairment, dyskinesias, and urinary incontinence can develop. Falls can be a debilitating consequence of the motor dysfunction. Sleep problems, such as REM sleep disorder, and depression, may worsen. Visual hallucinations may develop, but are associated with doses of dopamine agonists. Patients often exhibit increasing "on–off" fluctuations, and derive less time with good motor control, and more quickly fluctuate between akinesia to dyskinesias.

Neuropsychological symptoms: Impairments in processing speed (bradyphrenia), attention/concentration, executive functions, and visuospatial and visuoconstructional abilities. Retrieval deficits likely explain early memory performances (e.g., poor immediate and delayed recall, but generally intact recognition). Language problems include hypophonia and micrographia. Confrontation naming and semantic and phonemic verbal fluency often impaired in PD-D. Patients with PD with greater impairment in digit span backwards, memory (reduced list learning and recognition memory), and more perseverative errors on the Wisconsin Card Sorting Test were at greater risk for developing dementia at 1 year follow-up (Woods and Troster 2003).

Neuropathology: Gross neuropathology associated with PD-D is in the substantia nigra, with depigmentation, neuronal loss, and Lewy bodies. Additionally, the characteristic brain changes of AD (plaques, tangles, hippocampal atrophy) are also seen in PD-D.

Selected References: (Mendez and Cummings 2003; Beatty et al. 2003; Emre et al. 2007; Jankovic 2008; Williams-Gray et al. 2006)

Rule of thumb: Parkinson's disease with dementia (PD-D)

- Parkinsonian motor deficits precede dementia by at least 1 year
- Bradyphrenia
- Micrographia, hypophonia, and masked facies (i.e., reduced facial expressions) are common
- Early executive function deficits with reduced flexibility, set-shifting
- Recognition memory is intact (cueing improves recall)
- Visuoconstructional/visuoperceptual impaired
- Apathy is not depression. Motor slowing may appear affective, but is neurological
- Visual hallucinations not prominent and if present are associated with dopamine agonist medication

---

Progressive Supranuclear Palsy (PSP) or Steele–Richardson–Olszewski Syndrome

Prevalence: Although PSP might be the third most common cause of parkinsonism (behind PD and DLB), it is quite rare as a cause of dementia, representing 1–2% of dementias.

Risk factors: Male gender, parkinsonism, older age, and lower education.

Onset: Typically between 40 and 70 years of age, with a mean age of onset of 63 years.

Course: Progressive decline. Rates of decline vary, but mortality was reported with a median disease duration of 9.7 years; however, disease course has ranged from 2 to 15+ years.

Behavioral Symptoms/Clinical Presentation: Prominent changes in gait with frequent falls, parkinsonism (bradykinesia, rigidity) without prominent resting tremor, and vertical gaze palsy are early clinical manifestations of PSP. Downward gaze palsy is more diagnostically useful, since upward gaze is normally reduced in healthy older adults. Horizontal gaze palsy often occurs later in the disease. Blink rate is slowed, and patients may appear to stare. Eyelid movements can be impaired, and development of involuntary closing of eyes (blepharospasm) or inability to open eyelids may occur. The upper eyelids are often retracted, and the unblinking, wide-eyed stare with raised eyebrows gives rise to a characteristic facial expression of surprise. The "applause sign" (can't clap hands together three times only, such that the patient often claps many more than three times) is likely present, and can be helpful to distinguish PSP from PD and FTD (Dubois et al. 2005). Pseudobulbar palsy, personality changes with apathy, and social withdrawal are also frequently present. Alternatively, affective instability may be present. As the disease progresses, these clinical manifestations worsen (e.g., inability to walk, more restricted gaze, urinary incontinence, more severe personality changes).

Neuropsychological symptoms: Psychomotor slowing (bradyphrenia) predominates. Executive dysfunction and impaired complex attention are common, but may not be pronounced early. Memory is not markedly impaired, but mild impairment is common. Memory is sensitive to interference. Speech is often dysarthric and may also be hypophonic. Confrontation naming is often mildly impaired. Visuoperceptual function may be nearly normal early in disease. With no time limits, patient responses can be remarkably accurate. Later in the course, cognitive impairments spread and worsen.

Neuropathology: Atrophy along with neurofibrillary tangles, and gliosis occur in the basal ganglia (globus pallidus, subthalamic nucleus, substantia nigra) and superior colliculus, substantia innominata, and pretectal area. PSP is considered a Tau protein disorder. Functional neuroimaging studies often demonstrate hypometabolism of fronto-subcortical regions, and PET labeling of dopamine has shown marked deficiency. Structural neuroimaging may demonstrate atrophy of the midbrain and hyperintensity of the red nucleus and/or globus pallidus.

Selected References: (Lubarsky and Juncos 2008; Esper et al. 2007)

Rule of thumb: Progressive supranuclear palsy (PSP)

- Early onset of supranuclear palsy (impaired vertical gaze, particularly downward gaze),
- Frequent falls (often backwards)
- Parkinsonism (axial rigidity),
- Bradyphrenia is pronounced. "Subcortical" dementia pattern with prominent executive dysfunction.
- No visual hallucinations.

Corticobasal Ganglionic Degeneration (CBGD)

Prevalence: Less than 1% of dementias.

Risk factors: Parkinsonism (onset is typically asymmetric rigidity unresponsive to levedopa and bradykinesia), positive family history, and older age.

Onset: Late 50s to 70 years of age is typical.

Course: Slowly progressive over 8+ years.

Behavioral Symptoms/Clinical Presentation: Early symptoms include: lateralized motor impairments (e.g., asymmetrical parkinsonism of rigidity or myoclonus) and bradykinesia. Tremor, if present, is typically present during action (postural) and may reduce or resolve at rest. Gait becomes ataxic and has a "shuffling" appearance. Symptoms of depression may be severe, whereas other neuropsychiatric symptoms are less common. Asymmetric cortical sensory loss (graphesthesia, astereoagnosis, and visual extinction) may be present.

Neuropsychological symptoms: Prominent ideomotor and ideational apraxia is often present. Alien limb (limb is "foreign" and moves seemingly on its own) is a hallmark, but present in only about 40% of cases. Dementia with particular deficits in executive function, complex attention, and verbal fluency is found. Early in the disease, memory is not markedly affected, and can be near normal. Recognition cues improve recall, reflecting a "subcortical" memory retrieval problem. Language functions are not prominently impaired, although reduced verbal fluency is common.

Neuropathology: Asymmetrical profiles are often identified on neuroimaging (structural and functional), especially in the frontoparietal regions. In addition to cortical loss, the substantia nigra is severely affected with intraneuronal inclusions. Inclusions are tau positive.

Selected References: (Murray et al. 2007; Boeve 2007)

Rule of thumb: Corticobasal ganglionic degeneration (CBGD)

- Prominent asymmetric motor deficits including parkinsonism (rigidity, bradykinesia), and limb dystonia
- Myoclonus and tremor (at action and rest) may be present
- Ideomotor and ideational apraxia (e.g., alien hand sign)
- Oculomotor function is often normal (as opposed to PSP)
- Dementia with early subcortical pattern (executive dysfunction)

Multisystem Atrophy (MSA)

Prevalence: MSA is a term to describe three previously identified causes of dementia (striatonigral disease, Shy–Drager syndrome, olivopontocerebellar atrophy) sharing parkinsonian features that are not improved with levodopa. The presentation includes components of parkinsonian movement disorders along with other neurologic, autonomic, cognitive and affective features. All three previously described syndromes have been combined into the term MSA since these three causes of dementia share a neuropathology of glial inclusions (see below).

Risk factors: Little is known about risk factors.

Onset: Typically between 50 and 60 years of age.

Course: Progression occurs over 8–10 years.

Behavioral Symptoms/Clinical Presentation: Patients present with different features of parkinsonism. Shy–Drager syndrome presents as having prominent signs of autonomic failure (postural hypotension, erectile dysfunction, anhidrosis, etc.). Olivopontocerebellar atrophy presents as having predominant cerebellar dysfunction reflecting ataxia. Striatonigrial degeneration presents as predominant symmetric parkinsonism (symmetric rigidity, bradykinesia, tremor, etc.) and is difficult to distinguish from PD. As opposed to PD, patients with MSA present with greater postural hypotension, erectile dysfunction, urinary and bowel incontinence, anhidrosis, constipation, and muscle rigidity. Little information is available on the behavioral/psychiatric manifestations of MSA.

Early: Parkinsonian features are typically symmetric with greater autonomic, and in the case of olivopontocerebellar atrophy, cerebellar features. Parkinsonian symptoms do not respond to levedopa. This can lead to the "wheel chair" sign, with patient's being limited to a wheel chair.

Late: Progressive autonomic and/or cerebellar failure. Fluctuating blood pressure, headaches, dysphagia, irregular heartbeat, and problems breathing.

Neuropsychological symptoms: Early cognitive impairments are often overshadowed by neurological and medical concerns (e.g., patients often quickly become wheel chair bound and suffer from autonomic failure). However, deficits in memory and attention/executive functions have been reported. Memory deficits are generally in slowed learning with reduced scores on immediate memory tasks while delayed memory scores may be normal or nearly normal. However, consistent with other "subcortical" dementia processes, patients with MSA often exhibit retrieval problems with intact recognition. Visuoconstructional deficits are also frequently present.

Neuropathology: All are characterized pathologically by glial inclusions (oligo-dendroglial cytoplasmic inclusions without Lewy bodies), most often in the putamen and basal ganglia.

Shy–Drager syndrome associated with degeneration of the basal ganglia and lateral horn neurons in the thoracic spinal cord.

Olivopontocerebellar atrophy associated with degeneration of basal ganglia and cerebellar nuclei in the midbrain and pons

Striatonigral disease associated with degeneration of striatum.

Selected References: (Kawai et al. 2008; Berent et al. 2002; Bhidayasiri and Ling 2008)

Rule of thumb: Multisystem atrophy (MSA)

- Parkinsonism features
- Autonomic dysfunction (greater than PD or CBGD or PSP)
- No response to dopamine agonists

Three clinically distinct MSA variants:

1. Olivopontocerebellar atrophy is characterized by prominent cerebellar dysfunction
2. Shy-Drager characterized by predominant autonomic failure
3. Striatonigral disease characterized by predominant symmetric parkinsonism

HIV Associated Neurocognitive Disorders (HAND)

The HIV virus enters the nervous system, and is found throughout the brain, particularly involving frontal and subcortical white and grey matter. HIV-related effects on the CNS (and PNS) are both direct and indirect and can include acute and protracted processes.

Prevalence: HIV-associated dementia (HAD) occurs in 6–66% of individuals with HIV, with current estimates for patients receiving highly active antiretroviral therapy (HAART) being 10% (although 37% has been reported). In the USA, prevalence in asymptomatic HIV patients is lower (<1%) and much higher for patients with advanced AIDS (10–20%). However, neurological involvement of HIV infection (HIV-associated neurocognitive disorders) are present in up to 65% of adults with HIV and the majority of children with HIV. Prevalence rates in countries without HAART is much higher, and may be the first or second most common cause of dementia after AD, with a recent study finding 31% of sub-Saharan HIV patients met criteria for HIV dementia and another 46% (77% in total) had some neuropsychological impairments. Incidence rate in the USA for 20–59 year-olds in 1990 is about 1.9:100,000.

Risk factors: HIV infection. HIV genes (DNA) present in CNS. Lower CD4 counts and/or higher CSF HIV viral load. Co-occurring Hepatitis C infection.

Onset: Variable. Can affect individuals of any age with HIV infection.

Course: Onset and progression varies, but generally thought to be slow with a long period (e.g., 2–20 years) of relative asymptomatic problems followed by increasing physical and neurocognitive morbidity as HIV infection evolves with AIDS, eventually leads to mortality. However, up to 44% of cases of asymptomatic HIV infection present with neurocognitive symptoms (10–30% is generally accepted). Course is usually progressive, but reduction in symptoms with antiretroviral therapy and protease inhibitors in un- or under-treated patients has been reported. Three subtypes identified among spectrum of extent of deficits (1) HIV-associated dementia, (2) HIV-associated mild neurocognitive disorder, and (3) HIV asymptomatic neurocognitive impairment (see above for diagnostic criteria)

Behavioral Symptoms/Clinical Presentation: Motor dysfunction often involves limb incoordination, weakness, corticospinal tract signs (hyperreflexia). Significant apathy and social withdrawal is common. Alternatively, onset of disinhibition, poor judgment, irritability, and emotional lability may also occur.

Neuropsychological symptoms: Early impairments can be mild, and typically involve attention/executive dysfunction, deficient verbal fluency and word finding problems, reduced memory, and/or psychomotor slowing (bradyphrenia). Deficits in fine manual speed and/or dexterity are common. Deficits in visuoperceptual/visuospatial functions develop along with worsening memory impairments. Memory deficits initially reflect inefficient encoding and poor retrieval (recognition cues improve recall), but worsen as disease progresses. Language functions remain grossly intact, although reductions in verbal fluency and word findings problems can be present early. As the dementia progresses, increasing global cognitive deterioration is present with onset of seizures, prominent motor deficits, mutism, incontinence, and, eventually, coma.

1. In addition, the HIV-related cognitive disorders, there are often complications associated with HIV infection that can lead to transitory or permanent neuropsychological deficits including: brain abscess (bacterial or fungal), cerebral taxoplasmosis, primary CNS lymphoma, progressive multifocal leukoencephalopathy, meningitis, encephalitis, meningoencephalitis, meningovasculitis, transverse myelitis, and vasculitis. Finally, about 4% of patients with HIV suffer a stroke (ischemic or hemorrhagic).

Neuropathology: Cerebral atrophy with prominent lesions of subcortical white matter and subcortical grey matter structures (e.g., basal ganglia and thalamus).

Selected References: (Mendez and Cummings 2003; Antinori et al. 2007; Dawes et al. 2008)

Rule of thumb: HIV associated neurocognitive disorders (HAND)

- HIV has direct and indirect effects on both CNS and PNS
- Neurocognitive deficits present in up to 65% of people with HIV, but neurological involvement may be very mild (i.e., HIV asymptomatic neurocognitive impairment)
- HIV dementia is rare in asymptomatic individuals with HIV
- Early neuropsychological deficits include:
  - Processing speed/psychomotor speed (bradyphrenia), attention/executive, verbal fluency, confrontation naming, visuoperceptual/visuoconstructional skills.
  - Memory deficits typically mild early in disease (inefficient encoding and retrieval)
  - Basic language functions remain intact early in disease

Normal Pressure Hydrocephalus (NPH)

Prevalence: NPH is a relatively infrequent cause of dementia, in which cerebrospinal fluid is not adequately absorbed. It is considered a form of communicating hydrocephalus in that there is no acute blockage of CSF circulation.

Risk factors: Little is known about risk factors.

Onset: Typically between 60 and 80 years in age.

Course: Onset and progression can be relatively rapid (e.g., months) compared to other causes of dementia. NPH is progressive if untreated, and surgical treatment with a shunting procedure has varying efficacy. Patients identified earlier in course of disease (within weeks to months) have better outcomes following placement of shunt for CSF removal than those patients whom suffered from NPH for years.

Behavioral Symptoms/Clinical Presentation: Classically described with 3 Ws (whacky, wobbly, and wet) reflecting dementia, ataxic gait, and urinary incontinence. Gait disturbances (e.g., ataxic, increasingly wide based, shuffling presentation) are often the earliest symptom of NPH, with falls occurring frequently. Early urinary urgency and/or incontinence are common. Significant apathy and social withdrawal are common. Patients with NPH remain aware of deficits until late in course.

Neuropsychological symptoms: Early impairments can be mild (or completely missed). Psychomotor slowing, mild memory problems, and executive dysfunction can fluctuate. Progression of NPH can lead to more significant cognitive impairments, including global dysfunction.

Neuropathology: Failure to reabsorb cerebrospinal fluid resulting in dialation of ventricles, particularly the lateral and third ventricles. The enlarged ventricles observed with structural neuroimaging is greater than what might occur due to changes in age and cortical atrophy, and not associated with the cortical atrophy typical of other progressive dementias. Frontal and temporal lobes may appear larger than normal. Functional imaging, however, is notable for generalized hypoperfusion.

Selected References: (Hellstrom et al. 2007; Graff-Radford 2007; Devito et al. 2005)

Rule of thumb: Normal pressure hydrocephalus (NPH) "Wet, whacky, and wobbly."

- Gait instability (shuffling apraxic gait).
- Urinary incontinence
- Psychomotor slowing (bradyphrenia)
- Confusion and disorientation is common. Awareness of deficits often retained
- Cognitive deficits mild early in course. Progressively worsen with untreated NPH
  - Impaired attention and executive functions often present early. Visuoconstructional deficits may also develop with dementia.
  - Early deficits in memory encoding. Recognition cues improve recall.
  - Language grossly intact (but scores poor due to bradyphrenia and confusion)
- Apathy and symptoms of depression. Hallucinations rare.

Table 14.3 Clinical presentation of Dementia syndromes (see end of chapter)

Cognitive Domain	AD	FTD	DLB	VaD	PD-D	PSP	CBGD	Depression
Behavioral Observation	Early –deny memory impairment, may appear depressed Late – irritable, paranoid, anosognosia Sundowning may be present.	Early – personality changes. Poor initiation, disinhibition, reflexive and stereotyped use of objects, poor mood modulation, poor judgment.	Early – fluctuation in mental status common. Mental status orientation fluctuates. Not sundowning. Visual hallucinations. Late – Pronounced mental status variation. Distractible. Psychiatric symptoms. Psychosis. Sensitivity to dopamine antagonists.	Apathy common, symptoms of depression, incontinence, psychomotor retardation. Neurologic signs (e.g., babinski, spasticity, abnormal reflexes). Gait instability, rigidity.	Early – slowed processing speed. Autonomic dysfunction not prominent. Apathy and/or depression symptoms common. Late – similar to DLD, BUT hallucinations not prominent and/or related to medication dosing. Depression common.	Early - Vertical gaze palsy. Upward gaze is first affected, but also reduced in normal aging. Downward gaze palsy more specific. Parkinsonism. Gait change with open eyed stare. Depression common.	Early – Apraxia (Alien hand sign present about 40%). Asymetric parkinsonian features (bradykinesia, rigidity and tremor). Tremor is course, also present with posture, and does not respond to levedopa. Gait abnormality.	Complain of cognitive problems, particularly forgetfulness. Progression of problems often rapid.
General Cognitive	Early – Verbal IQ WNL. Nonverbal IQ mildly impaired. Processing speed WNL. Late – IQ declines with slowed processing speed.	Early – verbal IQ WNL. Nonverbal IQ mildly impaired. Late – IQ declines.	Early – Vocabulary remains intact. Gross decline in attention. Verbal IQ WNL. Nonverbal IQ mildly impaired.	Early – May not be affected. Some deficit possible. Processing speed often impaired.	Early – Verbal IQ WNL. Nonverbal IQ mildly reduced due to poor motor speed and processing speed. Late –vocabulary often preserved.	Early –Generally considered WNL. Late - impaired.	Early – Verbal IQ WNL. Nonverbal IQ may be reduced due to motor impairments. Late – general deficits.	Early –IQ WNL. Psychomotor retardation common.

(continued)

Table 14.3 (continued)

Cognitive Domain	AD	FTD	DLB	VaD	PD-D	PSP	CBGD	Depression
					Disease			
Attention	Simple attention (e.g., digit span forward, Trails A) WNL. Complex attention (e.g., Letter #, Trails B) impaired.	Simple attention generally intact (e.g., digit span forwards, Trails A). Complex attention impaired (Trails B, digit symbol, arithmetic).	Early gross impairment. Working memory is particularly affected. Digit span, Trails A, etc. impaired. Poor ability to maintain vigilance.	Often impaired. Simple and complex attention impaired (Digit Span & Arithmetic. Trails A and B, vigilance often impaired).	Often impaired. Simple attention generally preserved (e.g., digit span). Complex attention (Trails B, digit symbol) impaired.	Varied. Simple attention intact (e.g., digit span). Complex attention (Trails B, digit symbol) impaired.	Early – mild to moderate deficits. Simple attention WNL. Complex attention impaired Visual inattention may be present. Late – moderate to severe deficits	Attention often variable. Some scores may be WNL other scores impaired. Depressed score less well than healthy controls but perform better than patients with dementia.
Learning/Memory	Early – Impaired encoding and retention (learning over trials, short and long-delay free recall and recognition). Retention <50%. High false+rate on recognition. Implicit memory intact. Remote memories (e.g., early adulthood) intact. Late – Immediate and delayed memory markedly impaired. Remote memories impaired. Semantic memory impaired.	Early - severe impairment in immediate free recall (CVLT or RAVLT). May not show much decline from immediate to delay recall.	Early – memory deficits may not be severe. Learning reduced due to poor encoding strategies. Visual memory may be more impaired than verbal memory. Memory more impaired than in similar staged patient with PD. Late – impairment in immediate and delayed memory. Recognition cues do not improve recall.	Memory impairment may be severe. Poor consolidation (e.g., semantic clustering CVLT, logical memory). Short and delayed free recall impaired. Recognition is often WNL.	Early – generally preserved, but learning may be slowed. Late – impairment in efficiency of encoding. Recognition improves recall and is WNL.	Early – generally preserved. Late – impairment common. Reflects reduced encoding. Recognition improves recall and is often WNL.	Early – mild to moderate impairment. Tend to reflect frontal/subcortical memory impairments (recognition cues improves recall)	Mixed. Immediate and delayed recall may be impaired. Patient often say "don't know." Good cued recall and recognition.

Language	Early – mild impairment in verbal fluency (semantic more impaired than phonemic). Confrontation naming mild impaired. Vocabulary not impaired. Late – impaired fluency (semantic and phonemic), naming, comprehension, reading.	Early – varied. Deficits in verbal fluency (phonemic more impaired than semantic). Confrontation naming impaired. Stereotyped output and/or reduced output common. Comprehension may be decreased (e.g., Token test).	Early – Varied. Deficits in semantic verbal fluency and confrontation naming. Hypophonia and micrographia may be present. Late – worsening symptoms as above.	Early - Mixed, depending upon lesions. Dysarthria may be present. Impaired verbal fluency (phonemic may be more impaired than semantic fluency), expressive aphasia with large lesions, may have impaired confrontation naming. Comprehension can be impaired.	Early - Impaired with dysarthria, hypophonia, and micrographia. Verbal fluency (phonemic and semantic) can be impaired. Confrontation naming impaired later in disease. Repetition and comprehension preserved.	Early -Slowed responses to questions Fluency impaired (phonemic worse than semantic)	Early – often WNL. Phonemic fluency may be impaired. Late – Fluency impaired (phonemic and semantic)	Early - Expressive and receptive language intact, often with cues. Verbal fluency, naming, comprehension, reading WNL (often improved with general encouragement).
Visuoperceptual/visuoconstructional	Early – May be impaired. Late – Impaired. Visuoperceptual and visuoconstructional deficits worsen as disease progresses.	Early – Often markedly impaired visuoperceptual skills and constructional apraxia. Late – Severe impairment	Early – Poor block design, planning in copy (drawing). Early - Simple figures drawn correctly. Late – generally impaired.	Early – Mixed. Can be mild to moderate impaired. Not all patients impaired. Late – Moderate to severe impairment common	Early – Impaired. Dysfunction beyond difficulty due to motor deficits.	Early – Mild to moderate impairment	Early – Mild to moderate impairment	Mixed, but visuoperceptual and visuoconstructional skills WNL.

(continued)

Table 14.3 (continued)

				Disease				
Cognitive Domain	AD	FTD	DLB	VaD	PD-D	PSP	CBGD	Depression
Executive functions	Early - mild impairments present. Poor problem solving, sequencing, abstract reasoning. Late – moderate to severe deficits. Utilization behaviors.	Severe perseveration. Utilization behaviors present. Poor reasoning, judgment, insight, sequencing, Cognitive inflexibility.	Early – moderate to severe dysfunction can be present. Reduced problem solving, sequencing, abstract reasoning. Late – severe impairment common.	Early – mild to moderate. Can be severe. Decreased problem solving, reasoning, initiation, and increase in perseverations.	Early – mild to moderate impairment (less than PSP). Reduced mental flexibility. Late – general impairment. Apathy, poor sequencing, abstract reasoning.	Early-prominent impairment. 'Applause' sign (Pts. unable to clap hands just 3 times). Impaired initiation/ perseveration.	Early- mild to moderate. Late – moderate.	Can be reduced, but often WNL. Set-shifting (Trails B) slightly reduced or WNL. Perseveration, utilization behaviors not present.
Sensory/Motor	Early – generally WNL. Olfaction may be impaired very early in AD. Late – dyspraxia common.	Poor motor programming (Luria alternating movements). Grasp, root, and snout reflexes may be present.	Parkinsonian motor dysfunction may be present, but after dementia presents. Dementia first	Mixed. Motor deficits common (i.e., paresis, poor fine motor skills). Sensory loss (i.e., extinction) often present. Deep tendon reflexes may be abnormal. Clonus possible.	Parkinsonian motor impairment presents before dementia. Dementia last. Akinesia and dyskinesias common. "On-Off" motor fluctuations.	Falls and gait problems. Falls are typically backward Parkinsonian features.	Asymetric motor/ sensory deficits.	Mixed, but grossly WNL. Deficits, if any, are inconsistent. Motor programming WNL. Deep tendon reflexes WNL.

History	Slow insidious onset, family history common, gradual decline. No neurological signs.	Early-Insidious onset (compared to AD). Mean age of onset = 54 years-old. Progression more rapid than AD. Personality changes prominent.	Slow insidious onset. Early – Mental status fluctuates and visual hallucinations. Gait abnormalities/ akinesia, tremor may occur after cognitive problems present.	Slow onset, may have stepwise progression. Hx of risk factors (i.e., stroke, diabetes, hyperlipidemia, hypertension). Other neurological signs (e.g., sensory extinction)	Dementia presents after movement disorder. Autonomic dysfunction not primary. Family history.	Slow insidious onset. Falls often present first, followed by neuropsychological deficits and psychological problems (anxiety and depression).	Early – asymetric onset of motor deficits. parkinsonian features (akinetic and rigid) followed by cognitive deterioration (often years after motor deficits).	Hx of depression, symptoms associated with increase stress. 2-26% of elderly depressed. Symptoms may decrease with enjoyable activities.
Task engagement	Early – generally good. Late – variable.	May be variable – often dependent on examiner cues.	Early – generally good. Late - may be reduced due to variable mental status.	Generally good until late in disease.	Generally good	Generally good	Generally good	Inconsistent performances may be present (e.g., digit forward worse than digit backward).
Cardinal Features	Social withdraw, poor memory with rapid forgetting, dysnomia, constructional apraxia.	Onset typically in 50s. Personality changes early with "Frontal" signs. PPA – language deficits	Variable mental status, parkinsonian motor symptoms (tremor not predominant), visual hallucinations.	Motor/sensory abnormalities, poor attention, Recognition cues improve recall. Apraxias common.	Slowed processing speed, attention deficits, constructional apraxia, learning slow, but retention can be normal. Parkinsonian motor features.	Vertical gaze palsy, falling backwards, "applause sign". Frontal/subcortical cognitive deficits	Ideomotor apraxia, asymmetric parkinsonian rigidity and bradykinesia. Alien Hand sign, later dementia	Complains of memory problems, good description of perceived difficulties, withdrawn, speech fluent and articulate. No apraxias.

Aging and Cognitive Impairment

Extensive empirical evidence indicates that some cognitive processes normally decline with age, while others remain more stable across the lifespan. (for reviews, see (Salthouse 2009; Baltes and Mayer 1999)). However, the identification of the transition from "normal aging" to a pathological process requiring treatment is an area of active research and debate. Numerous terms and diagnostic criterion have been proposed to distinguish normal aging from abnormal, including; (1) age-associated memory impairment (AAMI (Crook et al. 1986)), (2) aging-associated cognitive decline (Levy 1994), (3) benign senescent forgetfulness (Kral 1962), (4) cognitive impairment no dementia (CIND) (Graham et al. 1997), (5) mild cognitive disorder (Christensen et al. 1995), (6) mild cognitive impairment (MCI) (Petersen et al. 1999) (7) mild neurocognitive disorder (Gutierrez et al. 1993), and (8) questionable dementia (Morris and Cummings 2005). Further complicating the division between normal and abnormal aging processes is the variability in neuropathological and neuropsychological functions between and within samples. Prognostically, research studies have demonstrated that individuals who have suffered prior neurologic injuries or diseases are at increased risk for developing subsequent cognitive decline, which may contribute to the picture of dementia. For example, an individual whom suffered a moderate to severe head injury or ischemic stroke in middle adulthood is at increased risk for developing a dementia in older age. Although this information cannot yet be used on individual patient level to predict risk for dementia, this is a growing area of development in making the neuropsychology of dementia more evidence based. Below, we review MCI and CIND, which are commonly used concepts to describe the area between normal aging changes in cognition and dementia.

Mild Cognitive Impairment (MCI)

Petersen et al. (1999) proposed the term MCI to describe a select group of individuals from the Mayo Older Adult Normative Studies whom demonstrated cognitive decline, but did not meet diagnostic criteria for dementia. The initial criteria by the Mayo group for MCI were:

- Subjective memory complaint
- Objective memory deficit compared to age-matched peers (1.5 or more standard deviations below average)
- Otherwise cognitively intact
- Otherwise intact daily functioning
- Not demented

Subsequently, these criteria have been modified based on new findings (e.g., collateral information on subjective memory complaint is useful, memory deficit should be relative to age- and education-corrected normative data, some declines in other cognitive abilities are expected, mild deficits in activities of daily living might be present), but the concept has endured (Petersen 2003). Much like the criteria for

HIV-related cognitive dysfunction, the criteria for MCI has traditionally provided objective benchmarks (e.g., cognitive functioning falling 1.5 standard deviations below expectations) that allow for the diagnosis of this condition.

MCI has also evolved from a single condition to several different subtypes of MCI, including single domain impairment (either memory or non-memory) and multiple domain impairments (with or without memory impairment) (Petersen et al. 2001). Single domain memory impaired MCI (i.e., only memory score(s) ≤–1.5 SD) is termed amnestic MCI (aMCI). Single domain not memory impaired (i.e., other neuropsychological domain test score(s) ≤–1.5 SD) is termed nonamnestic MCI. Multi-domain MCI involving memory plus at least one other neuropsychological domain is termed multidomain amnestic MCI (aMCI+). It has been theorized that each subtype of MCI could progress to its own dementia outcome. For example, the single memory domain subtype of MCI is likely to progress to AD, whereas the single nonmemory domain subtype (e.g., executive dysfunction) might reflect a prodromal stage of FTD. Multiple domain MCI (e.g., deficits in memory and processing speed) might be indicative of eventual VaD. Although this theoretical framework has clear appeal and some studies have found support for the expected progression patterns (Luis et al. 2004), other studies have less consistently found that different clinical subtypes of MCI were associated with unique disease etiologies (Manly et al. 2008). Nevertheless, the identification of MCI, and increasingly the different MCI subtypes, has clear implications for initiating and evaluating treatments for neurodegenerative diseases, particularly in AD.

Although the Petersen et al. definition of MCI has been most widely referenced, a second view of MCI comes from Morris et al. at Washington University who argue that MCI is not a separate disease entity, but rather individuals with MCI are in a very early or mild, but definite, stage of AD (Morris and Cummings 2005; Morris et al. 2001). This is supported by the long-term prognosis of dementia diagnosis in many patients diagnosed with MCI (Storandt et al. 2002), as well as neuropathological findings that most patients with MCI have the hallmark signs of AD.

Regardless of the definition of MCI, it has attracted attention because of its practical and prognostic value. Whereas community-dwelling elders develop dementia at 1–2% per year, individuals with amnestic MCI developed dementia at 12–15% per year (Petersen et al. 1999). Although other studies have varied the definition of MCI and obtained different rates of progression, all indicate an increased risk of developing dementia in this "at-risk" sample. Other negative outcomes associated with MCI include: mortality, institutionalization, disability, and psychiatric symptoms.

Although MCI progresses to dementia at a higher-than-normal rate, not everyone with MCI will progress. Even over 6 years, 20–30% of the original Mayo sample of MCI participants did not develop dementia (Petersen et al. 1999), with similar rates reported for other studies. The search for variables to predict conversion from MCI to dementia is an active area of research, and neuropsychology is contributing to this evidence-based prognostic investigation. Demographically, increasing age and lower education have been linked to progression to dementia. Clinically, collateral reports of memory problems were more suggestive of dementia conversion. An important neuropsychological risk factor for converting to dementia from MCI is the presence of more severe memory deficits (DeCarli et al. 2004; Griffith et al. 2006) and/or executive dysfunction. Individuals with nonamnestic MCI are at less risk of converting to dementia than are patients with amnestic MCI. An absence of expected practice effects has also been linked to continued cognitive decline (Duff et al. 2007). Structural imaging has focused on medial temporal lobe volumes as indicators of potential progression. For example, Jack et al. (1999) found baseline hippocampal volumes on MRI were related to rates of progression from MCI to dementia. Similarly, rates of hippocampal volume change with sequential neuroimaging have shown utility in predicting progression to dementia (Jack et al. 2000). Structures outside the medial temporal lobe have also demonstrated significant changes in patients with MCI, but fewer of these structures have been linked with predicting conversion to dementia. Functional imaging (e.g., PET, fMRI) has been utilized, and patients who cognitively declined across 3 years had 18% lower resting metabolism in the entorhinal cortex compared to non-decliners (de Leon et al. 2001). Lastly, several biomarkers have been identified as potentially useful to identify disease progression, including APOE e4, increased cerebrospinal fluid levels of total tau protein and phosphorylated tau protein, and decreased levels of amyloid beta (Aβ) 40 and 42. However, no demographic, clinical, neuropsychological, imaging, or biomarker is a "gold standard" for identifying which patients will progress to dementia and whom will not. It is likely a combinations of markers (e.g., baseline hippocampal volume, executive dysfunction, inflamation markers, and/or APOE e4) will best predict progression.

Rule of thumb: Mild cognitive impairment (MCI)

Diagnosis:
- Complaints of cognitive impairment
- Objective deficit in neuropsychological function (i.e., 1.5 or more standard deviations below age- and education-matched normative data)
- Not demented and generally intact daily functioning

Subtypes:
- Amnestic-MCI = memory score
- Non-amnestic-MCI = one non-memory domain score
- Multi-domain MCI = two (or more) domain scores

Conversion:
- MCI → dementia 10–15% per year

Cognitive Impairment No Dementia (CIND)

The Canadian Study of Health and Aging sought to determine prevalence rates of dementia across Canada, which it reported at 8%. It also identified a condition that was not dementia, but had "the presence of various categories of [cognitive] impairment identified in the clinical examination and in a battery of neuropsychological tests" (Graham et al. 1997). This condition, CIND, was subtyped by likely causes of the cognitive impairment: delirium, substance abuse, depression, other psychiatric illness, circumscribed memory impairment, and mental retardation. The prevalence of CIND was reported as 16.8% of Canadian seniors, with the circumscribed memory subtype representing 5.3% of the sample. It is this latter group that most closely matched the definition of MCI. When followed across 5 years, individuals with CIND had two times the risk of death, two times the risk of being admitted to an institution, and five times the risk of being diagnosed with dementia (Tuokko et al. 2003). Although MCI and CIND do not completely overlap, the concept of CIND broadens the view of subsyndromal cognitive disorders and attempts to identify the underlying cause of the disorder. Like MCI, a diagnosis of CIND increases risk of dementia diagnosis.

Rule of thumb: Cognitive impairment no dementia (CIND)

Diagnosis:

- Objective deficit in neuropsychological function
- Not demented as determined by a clinical examination

Cognitive Decline in Childhood or Young Adulthood

Cognitive decline in childhood and young adulthood is rare, and difficult to identify. During childhood, any deterioration in cognitive and motor skills from a neurodegenerative condition or disease is affected by neurodevelopmental processes, making it difficult to ascertain the onset of cognitive and/or motor skill decline. In young adulthood, cognitive decline may occur with psychiatric symptoms, medication use/abuse, and/or illicit drug use/abuse. However, the importance of identifying the presence of conditions which present with cognitive deterioration in childhood and early adulthood is essential. Table 14.4 lists some diseases resulting in cognitive deterioration in childhood that may not have other predominant neurological or medical symptoms. Other causes having other neurologic manifestations include Rett's disorder in females as a childhood onset neurodegenerative disorder. In addition, various disorders affecting metabolic functions (e.g., Tay-Sachs disease, Neimenn-Pick disease, Batten/Kuf's disease, phenylketonurias (PKU), Wilson's disease, etc.) are frequently associated with cognitive deterioration. Sickle cell disease and cerebral autosomal dominant arteriopathy with subcortical infarcts and leukoencephalopathy (CADISIL) also cause neuropsychological decline due to cerebrovascular disease (e.g., ischemic stroke). Other etiologies for onset of dementia in childhood through early adulthood can include infection [e.g., AIDS infection or acute disseminated encephalomyelitis (ADEM)], dysfunction of cerebrospinal fluid (hydrocephalus or pseudotumor cerebri), lack of nutrition/metabolic (B12 deficiency) or disorder of endocrine/thyroid functions (Hashimoto's encephalopathy) or those associated with epilepsy encephalopathies (e.g., Landau-Kleffner syndrome). Please see Chap. 28 this volume for overview (see also (Griffith et al. 2006; Duff et al. 2007) for reviews).

Table 14.4 Disorders presenting in childhood or adolescence that have early predominant cognitive deterioration and/or personality/behavioral changes as primary feature without other neurological symptoms

Adrenoleukodystrophy
Adult GM2 Gangliosidosis
Gaucher disease (juvenile and adult form)
Hallervorden-Spatz disease
Kuf's disease (late onset NCL)
Lafora-body myoclonic episode
Metachromatic leukodystrophy
Mucolipidosis I

"Pseudodementia": Medication and Psychiatric Considerations for Cognitive Complaints

A vast array of conditions can cause cognitive deterioration. This chapter has reviewed features and etiologies of the more common neurological diseases giving rise to dementia. However, numerous other causes must be considered, and include infections [e.g., acute disseminated encephalomyelitis (ADEM)], strategic lesions resulting in cognitive impairment (e.g., anterior thalami infarct), medical disorders, medications, illicit drugs and alcohol abuse, psychiatric diseases, and poor testing effort/task engagement (with such poor effort, patient can appear "demented"). Delirium or encephalopathy is a common disorder encountered in the elderly, with prevalence rates ranging from 10% to 56% exhibited among elderly patients in hospitals. Etiology of encephalopathy or delirium can vary substantially (see Chap. 15, this volume), but is often related to infections (urinary tract infection), metabolic disturbances, medications, drugs/alcohol abuse/dependence, or combinations of the above. The evaluation for encephalopathy and delirium is reviewed in Chaps. 5 and 15, but in general onset of cognitive and behavioral abnormalities is relatively rapid (but may remain chronic for months or even years without treatment) that classically ebb and flow during the day and/or night. Typically, level of arousal varies with poor orientation along with fluctuating energy level (i.e., manic-like agitation to lethargic). Attention is often impaired and hallucinations (visual and/or tactile) are common. Medications with anticholinergic qualities, such as tricyclics, antihistamines, antiemetics, some cough suppressants, analgesics, etc., can adversely affect cognitive function. A relative rating system for anticholinergic effects has been developed (Carnahan et al. 2006) and rates medications from a low of 0 for no known effects to 3 for medications that are markedly anticholinergic (see Table 14.5). A mnemonic for symptoms associated with anticholinergic toxicity is: "Hot as a Hades, blind as a bat, dry as a bone, red as a beet, and mad as a hatter" (Peters 1989) for the hyperthermia, mydriasis, anhydrosis, vasodilation, and psychosis that is commonly observed. In addition to medications, various substances and drugs can result in

Table 14.5 Common medications with anticholinergic effects

Medication/class/use	Common examples
Narcotics	Morphine
	Hydrocodone
	Fentanyl
Benzodiazepines	Lorazepam
	Clonazepam
	Diazepam
Anti-depressants	Tricyclics (e.g., amitriptyline, imipramine, etc.)
	Selective Serotonin Reuptake Inhibitors (e.g., paroxetine, sertraline, etc.) – *Less effect than Tricyclics*
Antihistamines	Clemastine (Tavist)
	Diphenhydramine (Benadryl)
	Promethazine (Phenergan)
Cough and cold suppressants	Dextrophan/pseudoephedrine
Skeletal Muscle Relaxants	Cyclobenzaprine (Flexaril)
Antispasmodics	Atropine
	Oxybutnynin (Ditropan)
	Ranitidine (Zantac)
	Cimetidine (Tagamet)
Antidiarrhoeals	Diphenoxylate
Anti-Parkinsonian (some)	Trihexyphenldyl
	Benztropine
	Artane
Travel sickness medications	Meclizine
	Scopolamine
Anticonvulsants (some)	Oxycarbazine
	Carbamazepine
	Valproic acid
Sleep aids	Diphenhydramine

dementia. Alcohol remains a common cause of cognitive impairment, although debate continues whether the dementia related to alcohol abuse/dependence (Wernicke's or Korsokoff's syndrome) may be related to other conditions associated with alcohol abuse/dependence, such as hepatic encephalopathy, cerebrovascular disease, head injuries, and nutritional problems. Psychiatric disease is often found in the elderly, and patients with depression and/or anxiety may complain of, and perform poorly on, neuropsychological tests. In addition to patients with major depressive disorders, individuals with bipolar disease, schizophrenia, schizoaffective, and other mood disorders may perform poorly on neuropsychological tests. Participants with depression tend to perform poorly on neuropsychological tests and often respond to questions with "I don't know" or "I give up" or "I can't."

Rule of thumb: Conditions that can present as "pseudodementias"

- Infections (ADEM, urinary tract, etc.)
- Strategic lesions (vascular, infectious, space occupying)
- Traumatic head injury
- Medical disorders
- Metabolic dysfunction
- Toxins
- Medications (anticholinergics)
- Illicit drugs, alcohol abuse/dependence
- Psychiatric diseases

Rule of thumb: Anticholinergic toxicity

- Hot as a Hades, Blind as a bat, Dry as a bone, Red as a beet, and Mad as a hatter
    - Hot = patient has a fever (hyperthermia)
    - Blind = "blown" or dilated pupils (mydriasis)
    - Dry = skin dry and no perspiration (anhydrosis)
    - Red = patient will appear flush (vasodialation)
    - Mad = patient exhibits delirium (confusion/agitation/psychosis)

These patients may appear to be easily frustrated and tearful. Neuropsychological test performances vary across and within neuropsychological domains, and it is not uncommon for patients with depression to provide accurate examples to illustrate their memory problems. Spontaneous memory is poor, but cueing often improves recall, with "nay saying" response set (answering "no" to questions regardless of content). We provide an overview of the presentation of pseudodementia due to depression below. The neuropsychological features of severe and persistent mental illness are reviewed in Chap. 14. Finally, the possibility of somatoform, conversion, and malingering must also be considered in some cases. The potential for malingering is increased when there is clear secondary gains to being diagnosed with a dementia (e.g., in the case of criminal or civil litigation or applying for disability). Consideration to the above factors for etiology of a dementia has important implications for treatment and prognosis, as treatment can reverse cognitive deficits.

Depression or Pseudodementia (Psychiatric Related Reversible Dementia)

Prevalence: Depression and other psychiatric conditions account for about 4% of patients presenting with dementia symptoms. These are among the most common form of "reversible" conditions presenting as a dementia.

Risk factors: Prior depressive episodes with cognitive impairment, older age, lower education, and cerebrovascular lesions.

Onset: Can occur at any age, but chances of onset increases with age.

Course: Slowly develops and progresses over months, with waxing and waning of depressive and cognitive symptoms. Although cognitive impairments due to depression can significantly improve with the treatment of depression, some cases will progress to a "true" dementia.

Behavioral Symptoms/Clinical Presentation: Symptoms of depression will often appear early, including: depressed mood, anhedonia, social withdrawal, sleep and appetite disturbances, and irritability. Individuals commonly complain of "memory problems," which, on further examination, tend to reflect difficulties focusing and sustaining attention. Importantly, patients often provide accurate recent and remote histories, with discrete examples of their "memory problems." Fear of dementia is often present. During evaluation, patients often defer to family members to answer questions, "give-up" quickly on tasks, and give many "I don't know" responses to questions. As mood worsens or improves, cognitive complaints can worsen or improve, respectively.

Neuropsychological symptoms: Psychomotor retardation associated with depression often leads to impairments on measures requiring speed, effort, and attention. Symptom validity testing is often below criteria. Learning and memory scores often fall below expectations, while recognition memory is often normal or nearly normal (e.g., more "hits" than on delayed recall, although false negative errors can occur). Conversational speech is often fluent and articulate. Confrontation naming often normal or nearly normal. Fluency scores can be normal or impaired. Executive and visuoperceptual/visuoconstructional scores vary, but functions are grossly intact. Variable and inconsistent performances are usually present.

Rule of thumb: Depression-related pseudodementia

- Flat affect (tearfulness and affective feelings as opposed to apathy)
- Frequent "I don't know" responses to questions
- Conversational speech is typically fluid (and often articulate)
- Memory improves with recognition formats
- Tend to perform poorly on symptom validity testing
- History can be detailed and accurate with recent and remote events

Evaluate for potential of medication (anticholinergic) effects on cognition

Neuropathology: Minimal (or no) gross pathological changes. Aging related changes, such as mild cerebral atrophy and/or diffuse periventricular white matter changes is often present.

Selected References: (Chamberlain and Sahakian 2006; Rosenstein 1998; Wright and Persad 2007)

Evidence-Based Neuropsychology in Dementia

There is a growing literature providing empirical evidence for the unique contribution of neuropsychological assessment in the diagnosis and management of MCI and dementia. Neuropsychological scores can be crucial for making a diagnosis of MCI, and for identifying subtypes of MCI (Morris and Cummings 2005; Petersen 2003; Petersen et al. 2001; Luis et al. 2004; Manly et al. 2008; Morris et al. 2001; Storandt et al. 2002; DeCarli et al. 2004; Griffith et al. 2006). Although the importance of the differential diagnosis in MCI continues to be explored, different subtypes of MCI (i.e., different neuropsychological profiles) appear to have different rates of progression to dementia (or reversion to "normal" status) (Petersen et al. 2001; Luis et al. 2004; Manly et al. 2008; Morris et al. 2001; Storandt et al. 2002; DeCarli et al. 2004; Griffith et al. 2006; Tuokko et al. 2003; Fleisher et al. 2007; Chen et al. 2000; Busse et al. 2006). Neuropsychological deficits in multiple domains (amnestic MCI-multiple domain, nonamnestic MCI-multiple domain) and amnestic MCI-single domain increase the risk of progression to a diagnosis of dementia compared to individuals having MCI in one domain that is not memory (i.e., non-amnestic MCI) (Busse et al. 2006). Additionally, subjects with non-amnestic MCI multiple domain are more likely to progress to a dementia that is not of the Alzheimer's type than are patients diagnosed with amnestic MCI single or multiple domain. Specific neuropsychological measures have also been shown to predict future progression to dementia in patients with MCI. For example, in a large study of the progression of MCI to AD, Fleisher et al. (2007) found that the five best predictors of progression included four cognitive tests (Symbol Digit Modalities Test, delayed recall of a list of words, delayed recall of a paragraph, and global cognitive score) and one biomarker (APOE 4 status).

There is extensive empirical support for evidence-based neuropsychology practice in dementia. Indeed, the presence of neuropsychological deficits in older adults increases the risk for development of dementia and even death (Luis et al. 2004; Manly et al. 2008; Morris et al. 2001; Storandt et al. 2002; DeCarli et al. 2004; Griffith et al. 2006; Duff et al. 2007; Jack et al. 1999; Jack et al. 2000; de Leon et al. 2001; Tuokko et al. 2003; Fleisher et al. 2007; Chen et al. 2000; Busse et al. 2006; Barnes et al. 2009; MacDonald et al. 2008). Barnes et al. (2009) developed a Dementia Risk Index and found measures of neuropsychological function were independent predictors for the development of dementia 6 years later above and beyond demographic and other medical variables, including neuroimaging. The Dementia Risk Index (Barnes et al. 2009) found poor performance on the 3MS (Teng and Chui 1987) and digit symbol substitution test from the WAIS-R were independent predictive variables for development of dementia 6 years later. Similarly, Chen et al. (2000) found poor performance on delayed recall on a list learning task and Trails B were the best predictors of developing AD 1.5 years later. Development of dementia for patients with PD is also higher for patients exhibiting greater frontal/executive dysfunction (Woods and Troster 2003). Finally, neuropsychological data can provide unique data in the differential diagnosis of dementias, including AD, VaD, FTD (including FTD subtypes), DLB, PD-D, and dementia with cortical-basal ganglionic degeneration (CBGD) (see (Mendez and Cummings 2003) for review, (Diehl et al. 2005; Huey et al. 2009)). For example, Diehl et al. (2005) found performance on the Boston Naming Test and Animal fluency score correctly classified 90.5% of patients as either having AD, semantic dementia, or FTD. A correct classification rate between AD and semantic dementia was reported in 96.3% of patients using scores on the Boston Naming Test and MMSE total score (Diehl et al. 2005).

Assessment of Dementia

The diagnosis of dementia requires a thorough evaluation to identify its subtype and/or etiological cause. Many conditions must be ruled out to make even a "probable" diagnosis of dementia. Components of a comprehensive evaluation are listed in Table 14.6.

A neuropsychological evaluation is an important part of a comprehensive assessment for dementia. A clinical interview should inquire if there are problems with cognition, including memory, problem solving skills, and/or language. Evaluation of apraxias and agnosias are recommended. It is particularly helpful to identify the impact of any cognitive dysfunction on day-to-day functioning, since social or occupational impairment is necessary for the diagnosis of dementia in some criteria. The temporal onset and course of symptoms is absolutely essential, including motor dysfunction, urinary incontinence, cognitive complaints, and/or mood/personality changes. The evaluation of symptom onset is often *crucial* in the differential diagnosis of dementia syndromes, as well as distinguishing progressive neurodegenerative diseases from reversible causes of dementia. For example, a several-year history of progressive and insidious worsening memory with no motor impairment is more suggestive of AD than would the occurrence of gait problems, urinary urgency, and cognitive problems over several months (much more suggestive of NPH). Family history of, and risk factors for, dementia should also be ascertained. Ideally, information should be obtained from the patient and a reliable collateral source (e.g., spouse, adult child), as patient provided information can be compromised by dementia conditions.

An initial screening of cognitive functioning with a brief measure can be helpful to evaluate what extent of neuropsychological testing is needed. For example, scores of 20 or less on the Mini Mental Status Examination (MMSE) suggest that a brief neuropsychological assessment is all that is possible (or needed), although

Table 14.6 Components of a dementia evaluation

History and physical exam
Routine laboratory tests
  Chest x-ray
  Complete blood count
  Electrolyte and screening metabolic panel
  Thyroid function tests
  Syphilis serology
  Vitamin B12, folate
Neurological exam
CT or MRI
Psychiatric evaluation
Other tests for atypical presentation
  EEG
  Lumbar puncture
  HIV titer
  Lyme titer
  Serologic testing for vasculitis
  Heavy metal screening
  Angiography
  PET study
  Brain biopsy

a sensorimotor and cranial nerve exam can be helpful. However, the converse is not true: perfect scores on screening measures (MMSE = 30/30) does *not* mean neuropsychological functioning is normal.

Evidence-based neuropsychology practice is guided by extensive literature finding differential diagnosis of dementia and MCI should involve an evaluation of orientation, attention/executive, memory, language, and visuoperceptual/visuoconstructional skills. Orientation to person, place, time, and circumstances should be assessed. Simple and complex attention should be evaluated, as should visuospatial perception and visuoconstruction, along with praxis. Language assessment should include evaluation of naming, fluency, and comprehension. Prosody may be assessed in less impaired individuals. Memory testing should allow to test for learning, immediate free recall, delayed free recall, and recognition memory. Executive functions (e.g., planning, organizing, sequencing, set shifting, conceptual reasoning, response inhibition) should be assessed. Detailed assessment of all domains may not be necessary, but assessment of each domain has empirical support. We recommend an evaluation of motor function, if only basic motor speed. Finally, a brief evaluation of psychiatric functioning (e.g., depression, anxiety) is needed.

A vast number of neuropsychological measures may be employed, but the evaluation should be tailored to the extent of suspected neuropsychological impairment and should endeavor to assess the domains identified above. The battery of tests will need to be adapted to the patient skill level and patients with less severe deficits may require more extensive testing to accurately describe the presence and degree of deficit.

Tables 14.7 and 14.8 provide examples of neuropsychological batteries for patients with suspected mild and severe impairments, respectively. Although test selection should be guided by many factors, these are some examples of common measures used in the field for dementia evaluations.

Table 14.7 Examples of tests used in a memory disorders evaluation if mild impairments are suspected and/or rule-out pseudodementia due to depression

Clinical interview

North American Adult Reading Test or Wechsler Test of Adult Reading or Wide Range
  Achievement Test-4 Word Reading and/or Oklahoma Premorbid Intellectual Estimate-3

Wechsler Adult Intelligence Scale – 3rd Edition short form (*WAIS*-III) or *Wechsler Adult
  Intelligence Scale* – 4th Ed. (*WAIS*-IV; selected subtests for prorated PRI, VCI, and PSI) or
  Wechsler Abbreviated Scale of Intelligence (WASI)

Wechsler Memory Scale – 4th Edition or *California Verbal Learning Test* – 2nd Edition or *Rey
  Auditory Verbal Learning Test* or *Hopkins Verbal Learning Test-Revised* or *Brief Visuospatial
  Memory Test*-Revised

Boston Naming Test (60-item or 30-item)

Controlled Oral Word Association Test

Semantic verbal fluency test (e.g., Animals)

Language screening for repetition, comprehension, writing, and reading

Hooper Visual Organization Test and/or Benton Line Orientation Test

Rey-Osterreith Complex Figure Test

Praxis evaluation

Sensory-perceptual exam/screening

Finger Tapping Test

Wisconsin Card Sorting Test or Delis-Kaplan Executive Function Scale (selected subtests)

Trail Making Test Parts A and B

Geriatric Depression Scale (GDS) or Beck Depression Inventory – 2nd Edition (*BDI*-II)

Spielberger State-Trait Anxiety Inventory (STAI) or Beck Anxiety Inventory (BAI)

In very limited cases:Personality Assessment Inventory (PAI) or Minnesota Multiphasic
  Personality Inventory-2 (MMPI-2, short form). Note: If PAI or MMPI-2, GDS/BDI-II nor
  STAI/BAI administered

Table 14.8 Examples of tests used in a dementia evaluation if mild to moderate or moderate-severe impairments are suspected

Clinical Interview

Mini Mental Status Examination or Montreal Cognitive Assessment (MoCA) (Rosenstein 1998)[a]

Repeatable Battery for the Assessment of Neuropsychological Status (RBANS) or Dementia
  Rating Scale – 2nd Edition (DRS-2)[b]

Trail Making Test, Parts A and B

Controlled Oral Word Association Test

Semantic verbal fluency test (e.g., animals)

WAIS-III Similarities and Matrix Reasoning subtests[b]

Luria 3-step motor sequencing

Praxis evaluation

Sensory Perception exam/screening

Geriatric Depression Scale[b]

[a]MMSE or MOCA may not be administered if completed as part of earlier memory screen by physician or nurse

[b]May not be administered in patients exhibiting more severe dementia

References

American Psychiatric Association.(2000). *Diagnostic and statistical manual of mental disorders*, 4th ed., text revision ed. Washington DC: American Psychiatric Association.

Antinori, A., Arendt, G., Becker, J. T., et al. (2007). Updated research nosology for HIV-associated neurocognitive disorders. *Neurology, 69*, 1789–1799.

Ballard, C., O'Brien, J., Gray, A., et al. (2001). Attention and fluctuating attention in patients with dementia with Lewy bodies and Alzheimer disease. *Archives of Neurology, 58*, 977–982.

Baltes, P. B., & Mayer, K. U. (1999). *The Berlin aging study: Aging from 70 to 100*. Cambridge, England: Cambridge University Press.

Barnes, D. E., Covinsky, K. E., Whitmer, R. A., Kuller, L. H., Lopez, O. L., & Yaffe, K. (2009). Predicting risk of dementia in older adults. The late-life dementia risk index. *Neurology, 73*, 173–179.

Beatty, W. W., Ryder, K. A., Gontkovsky, S. T., Scott, J. G., McSwan, K. L., & Bharucha, K. J. (2003). Analyzing the subcortical dementia syndrome of Parkinson's disease using the RBANS. *Archives of Clinical Neuropsychology, 18*, 509–520.

Berent, S., Giordani, B., Gilman, S., et al. (2002). Patterns of neuropsychological performance in multiple system atrophy compared to sporadic and hereditary olivopontocerebellar atrophy. *Brain and Cognition, 50*, 194–206.

Bhidayasiri, R., & Ling, H. (2008). Multiple system atrophy. *The Neurologist, 14*, 224–237.

Boeve, B. F. (2007). Links between frontotemporal lobar degeneration, corticobasal degeneration, progressive supranuclear palsy, and amyotrophic lateral sclerosis. *Alzheimer Disease and Associated Disorders, 21*, S31–38.

Bozeat, S., Gregory, C. A., Ralph, M. A., & Hodges, J. R. (2000). Which neuropsychiatric and behavioural features distinguish frontal and temporal variants of frontotemporal dementia from Alzheimer's disease? *Journal of Neurology, Neurosurgery and Psychiatry, 69*, 178–186.

Busse, A., Hensel, A., Gühne, U., Angermeyer, M. C., & Riedel-Heller, S. G. (2006). Mild cognitive impairment: Long-term course of four clinical subtypes. *Neurology, 67*, 2176–2185.

Carnahan, R. M., Lund, B. C., Perry, P. J., Pollock, B. G., & Culp, K. R. (2006). The anticholinergic drug scale as a measure of drug-related anticholinergic burden: Associations with serum anticholinergic activity. *Journal of Clinical Pharmacology, 46*, 1481–1486.

Chamberlain, S. R., & Sahakian, B. J. (2006). The neuropsychology of mood disorders. *Current Psychiatry Reports, 8*, 458–463.

Chen, P., Ratcliff, G., Belle, S. H., Cauley, J. A., DeKosky, S. T., & Ganguli, M. (2000). Cognitive tests that best discriminate between presymptomatic AD and those who remain nondemented. *Neurology, 55*, 1847–1853.

Christensen, H., Henderson, A. S., Jorm, A. F., Mackinnon, A. J., Scott, R., & Korten, A. E. (1995). ICD-10 mild cognitive disorder: epidemiological evidence on its validity. *Psychological Medicine, 25*, 105–120.

Crook, T., Bartus, R. T., Ferris, S. H., Whitehouse, P., Cohen, G. D., & Gershon, S. (1986). Age-associated memory impairment: Proposed diagnostic criteria and measures of clinical change. Report of a National Institute of Mental Health Work Group. *Developmental Neuropsychology, 2*, 261–276.

Dawes, S., Suarez, P., Casey, C. Y., et al. (2008). Variable patterns of neuropsychological performance in HIV-1 infection. *Journal of Clinical and Experimental Neuropsychology, 30*, 613–626.

de Leon, M. J., Convit, A., Wolf, O. T., et al. (2001). Prediction of cognitive decline in normal elderly subjects with 2-[(18)F]fluoro-2-deoxy-D-glucose/positron-emission tomography (FDG/PET). *Proceedings of the National Academy of Sciences of the United States of America, 98*, 10966–10971.

DeCarli, C., Mungas, D., Harvey, D., et al. (2004). Memory impairment, but not cerebrovascular disease, predicts progression of MCI to dementia. *Neurology, 63*, 220–227.

Devito, E. E., Pickard, J. D., Salmond, C. H., Iddon, J. L., Loveday, C., & Sahakian, B. J. (2005). The neuropsychology of normal pressure hydrocephalus (NPH). *British Journal of Neurosurgery, 19*, 217–224.

Diehl, J., Monsch, A. U., Aebi, C., Wagenpfeil, S., Krapp, S., Grimmer, T., et al. (2005). Frontotemporal dementia, semantic dementia, and Alzheimer's disease: the contribution of standard neuropsychological tests to differential diagnosis. *Journal of Geriatric Psychiatry and Neurology, 18*, 39–44.

Dubois, B., Slachevsky, A., Pillon, B., Beato, R., Villalponda, J. M., & Litvan, I. (2005). "Applause sign" helps to discriminate PSP from FTD and PD. *Neurology, 64*, 2132–2133.

Duff, K., Beglinger, L. J., Schultz, S. K., et al. (2007). Practice effects in the prediction of long-term cognitive outcome in three patient samples: A novel prognostic index. *Archives of Clinical Neuropsychology, 22*, 15–24.

Emre, M., Aarsland, D., Brown, R., et al. (2007). Clinical diagnostic criteria for dementia associated with Parkinson's disease. *Movement Disorders, 22*, 1689–1707. quiz 1837.

Esper, C. D., Weiner, W. J., & Factor, S. A. (2007). Progressive supranuclear palsy. *Reviews in Neurological Diseases, 4*, 209–216.

Fleisher, A. S., Sowell, B. B., Taylor, C., Gamst, A. C., Petersen, R. C., & Thal, L. J. (2007). Clinical predictors of progression to Alzheimer disease in amnestic mild cognitive impairment. *Neurology, 68*, 1588–1595.

Forman, M. S., Farmer, J., Johnson, J. K., et al. (2006). Frontotemporal dementia: Clinicopathological correlations. *Annals of Neurology, 59*, 952–962.

Graff-Radford, N. R. (2007). Normal pressure hydrocephalus. *Neurologic Clinics, 25*, 809–832. vii–viii.

Graham, J. E., Rockwood, K., Beattie, B. L., et al. (1997). Prevalence and severity of cognitive impairment with and without dementia in an elderly population. *Lancet, 349*, 1793–1796.

Griffith, H. R., Netson, K. L., Harrell, L. E., Zamrini, E. Y., Brockington, J. C., & Marson, D. C. (2006). Amnestic mild cognitive impairment: Diagnostic outcomes and clinical prediction over a two-year time period. *Journal of the International Neuropsychological Society, 12*, 166–175.

Gutierrez, R., Atkinson, J. H., & Grant, I. (1993). Mild neurocognitive disorder: needed addition to the nosology of cognitive impairment (organic mental) disorders. *The Journal of Neuropsychiatry and Clinical Neurosciences, 5*, 161–177.

Hellstrom, P., Edsbagge, M., Archer, T., Tisell, M., Tullberg, M., & Wikkelso, C. (2007). The neuropsychology of patients with clinically diagnosed idiopathic normal pressure hydrocephalus. *Neurosurgery, 61*, 1219–1226. discussion 1227–1218.

Huey, E. D., Goveia, E. N., Paviol, S., Pardini, M., Krueger, F., Zamboni, G., et al. (2009). Executive dysfunction in frontotemporal dementia and corticobasal syndrome. *Neurology, 72*, 453–459.

Jack, C. R., Jr., Petersen, R. C., Xu, Y. C., et al. (1999). Prediction of AD with MRI-based hippocampal volume in mild cognitive impairment. *Neurology, 52*, 1397–1403.

Jack, C. R., Jr., Petersen, R. C., Xu, Y., et al. (2000). Rates of hippocampal atrophy correlate with change in clinical status in aging and AD. *Neurology, 55*, 484–489.

Jankovic, J. (2008). Parkinson's disease: clinical features and diagnosis. *Journal of Neurology, Neurosurgery and Psychiatry, 79*, 368–376.

Johnson, D. K., Morris, J. C., & Galvin, J. E. (2005). Verbal and visuospatial deficits in dementia with Lewy bodies. *Neurology, 65*, 1232–1238.

Kawai, Y., Suenaga, M., Takeda, A., et al. (2008). Cognitive impairments in multiple system atrophy: MSA-C vs MSA-P. *Neurology, 70*, 1390–1396.

Kim, K. Y., Wood, B. E., & Wilson, M. I. (2005). Risk factors for Alzheimer's disease: an overview for clinical practitioners. *The Consultant Pharmacist, 20*, 224–230.

Kral, V. A. (1962). Senescent forgetfulness: Benign and malignant. *Canadian Medical Association Journal, 86*, 257–260.

Launer, L. J., Andersen, K., Dewey, M. E., et al. (1999). Rates and risk factors for dementia and Alzheimer's disease: results from EURODEM pooled analyses. EURODEM Incidence Research Group and Work Groups. European Studies of Dementia. *Neurology, 52*, 78–84.

Levy, R. (1994). Aging-associated cognitive decline. *International Psychogeriatrics, 6*, 63–68.

Lubarsky, M., & Juncos, J. L. (2008). Progressive supranuclear palsy: a current review. *The Neurologist, 14*, 79–88.

Luis, C. A., Barker, W. W., Loewenstein, D. A., et al. (2004). Conversion to dementia among two groups with cognitive impairment: A preliminary report. *Dementia and Geriatric Cognitive Disorders, 18*, 307–313.

Lund, Manchester. (1994). Clinical and neuropathological criteria for frontotemporal dementia. The Lund and Manchester Groups. *Journal of Neurology, Neurosurgery and Psychiatry, 57*, 416–418.

MacDonald, S.W.S, Hultsch, D.F., & Dixon, R.A. (2008). Predicting impending death: Inconsistency in speed is a selective and early marker. *Psychology and Aging, 23*, 595–607.

Manly, J. J., Tang, M. X., Schupf, N., Stern, Y., Vonsattel, J. P., & Mayeux, R. (2008). Frequency and course of mild cognitive impairment in a multiethnic community. *Annals of Neurology, 63*, 494–506.

McKeith, I. G., Galasko, D., Kosaka, K., et al. (1996). Consensus guidelines for the clinical and pathologic diagnosis of dementia with Lewy bodies (DLB): report of the consortium on DLB international workshop. *Neurology, 47*, 1113–1124.

Mendez, M. F. (1994). Huntington's disease: update and review of neuropsychiatric aspects. *International Journal of Psychiatry in Medicine, 24*, 189–208.

Mendez, M. F., & Cummings, J. L. (2003). *Dementia: A Clinical Approach* (3rd ed.). Philadelphia: Butterworth Heinemann.

Morris, J. C. (1997). Clinical dementia rating: a reliable and valid diagnostic and staging measure for dementia of the Alzheimer type. *International Psychogeriatrics, 9*(Suppl 1), 173–176. discussion 177–178.

Morris, J. C., & Cummings, J. (2005). Mild cognitive impairment (MCI) represents early-stage Alzheimer's disease. *Journal of Alzheimer's Disease, 7*, 235–239. discussion 255–262.

Morris, J. C., Storandt, M., Miller, J. P., et al. (2001). Mild cognitive impairment represents early-stage Alzheimer disease. *Archives of Neurology, 58*, 397–405.

Murray, R., Neumann, M., Forman, M. S., et al. (2007). Cognitive and motor assessment in autopsy-proven corticobasal degeneration. *Neurology, 68*, 1274–1283.

Navia, B. A., Jordan, B. D., & Price, R. W. (1986). The AIDS dementia complex: I. Clinical features. *Annals of Neurology, 19*, 517–524.

Neary, D., Snowden, J. S., Gustafson, L., et al. (1998). Frontotemporal lobar degeneration: a consensus on clinical diagnostic criteria. *Neurology, 51*, 1546–1554.

Paul, R., Moser, D., Cohen, R., Browndyke, J., Zawacki, T., & Gordon, N. (2001). Dementia severity and pattern of cognitive performance in vascular dementia. *Applied Neuropsychology, 8*, 211–217.

Paulsen, J. S., & Conybeare, R. A. (2005). Cognitive changes in Huntington's disease. *Advances in Neurology, 96*, 209–225.

Paulsen, J. S., Ready, R. E., Hamilton, J. M., Mega, M. S., & Cummings, J. L. (2001). Neuropsychiatric aspects of Huntington's disease. *Journal of Neurology, Neurosurgery and Psychiatry, 71*, 310–314.

Paulsen, J. S., Langbehn, D. R., Stout, J. C., et al. (2008). Detection of Huntington's disease decades before diagnosis: the Predict-HD study. *Journal of Neurology, Neurosurgery and Psychiatry, 79*, 874–880.

Peters, N. L. (1989). Snipping the thread of life. Antimuscarinic side effects of medications in the elderly. *Archives of Internal Medicine, 149*, 2414–2420.

Petersen, R. C. (2003). *Mild Cognitive Impairment*. New York: Oxford Press.

Petersen, R. C., Smith, G. E., Waring, S. C., Ivnik, R. J., Tangalos, E. G., & Kokmen, E. (1999). Mild cognitive impairment: clinical characterization and outcome. *Archives of Neurology, 56*, 303–308.

Petersen, R. C., Doody, R., Kurz, A., et al. (2001). Current concepts in mild cognitive impairment. *Archives of Neurology, 58*, 1985–1992.

Roman GC, Tatemichi TK, Erkinjuntti T, et al. Vascular dementia: diagnostic criteria for research studies. Report of the NINDS-AIREN International Workshop. Neurology 1993;43: 250-260.

Rosenstein, L. D. (1998). Differential diagnosis of the major progressive dementias and depression in middle and late adulthood: a summary of the literature of the early 1990s. *Neuropsychology Review, 8*, 109–167.

Salmon, D. P., & Filoteo, J. V. (2007). Neuropsychology of cortical versus subcortical dementia syndromes. *Seminars in Neurology, 27*, 7–21.

Salthouse, T. A. (2009). When does age-related cognitive decline begin? *Neurobiology of Aging, 30*, 507–514.

Starkstein, S. E., Sabe, L., Vazquez, S., et al. (1996). Neuropsychological, psychiatric, and cerebral blood flow findings in vascular dementia and Alzheimer's disease. *Stroke, 27*, 408–414.

Storandt, M., Grant, E. A., Miller, J. P., & Morris, J. C. (2002). Rates of progression in mild cognitive impairment and early Alzheimer's disease. *Neurology, 59*, 1034–1041.

Teng, E. L., & Chui, H. C. (1987). The modified mini-mental state (3MS) examination. *The Journal of Clinical Psychiatry, 48*, 314–318.

Tuokko, H., Frerichs, R., Graham, J., et al. (2003). Five-year follow-up of cognitive impairment with no dementia. *Archives of Neurology, 60*, 577–582.

Williams-Gray, C. H., Foltynie, T., Lewis, S. J., & Barker, R. A. (2006). Cognitive deficits and psychosis in Parkinson's disease: a review of pathophysiology and therapeutic options. *CNS Drugs, 20*, 477–505.

Woods, S. P., & Troster, A. I. (2003). Prodromal frontal/executive dysfunction predicts incident dementia in Parkinson's disease. *Journal of the International Neuropsychological Society, 9*, 17–24.

Wright, S. L., & Persad, C. (2007). Distinguishing between depression and dementia in older persons: neuropsychological and neuropathological correlates. *Journal of Geriatric Psychiatry and Neurology, 20*, 189–198.

Yaari, R. (2007). Corey-Bloom J. Alzheimer's disease. *Seminars in Neurology, 27*, 32–41.

Zaccai, J., McCracken, C., & Brayne, C. (2005). A systematic review of prevalence and incidence studies of dementia with Lewy bodies. *Age and Ageing, 34*, 561–566.

Zekry, D., Hauw, J. J., & Gold, G. (2002). Mixed dementia: epidemiology, diagnosis, and treatment. *Journal of the American Geriatrics Society, 50*, 1431–1438.

Chapter 15
Episodic Neurologic Symptoms

Heber Varela and Selim R. Benbadis

Abstract Paroxysmal neurologic symptoms are common, and covering them extensively would almost amount to covering the entire field of neurology. Identifying their cause relies mostly on taking a good history. Despite advances in neuroimaging and adjunct diagnostic techniques, the clinical information remains the most important part of the diagnostic process. In particular, in regard to episodic neurologic symptoms, an accurate account of the time course is critical. How quickly symptoms develop or buildup, how long each "episode" lasts (seconds, minutes, hours), and how it resolves, for example, are very different among the entities described here. In short, while tests are briskly ordered, MRIs will never replace clinical judgment, and the importance of obtaining a good history cannot be overemphasized.

This chapter will cover the main and common cause of episodic neurologic symptoms. Based on the clinical presentation, we will divide entities into "global" symptoms and "focal" or localized symptoms.

Key Points and Chapter Summary

- Paroxysmal neurological symptoms are common and rely mostly on a good history for differential diagnosis.
- Global symptoms include seizures, syncope, encephalopathy and delirium and classically present with altered mental status and no focal or lateralizing signs.
- Focal symptoms can be negative (weakness, aphasia, visual loss or numbness) and/or positive (convulsions, dystonia, flashing lights and tingling). In general, mental status is preserved.

(continued)

H. Varela (✉)
Department of Neurology, University of South Florida College of Medicine
and James A. Haley Veterans Affairs Medical Center, Tampa, FL, USA
e-mail: heberluis@yahoo.com

M.R. Schoenberg and J.G. Scott (eds.), *The Little Black Book of Neuropsychology:*
A Syndrome-Based Approach, DOI 10.1007/978-0-387-76978-3_15,
© Springer Science+Business Media, LLC 2011

Key Points and Chapter Summary (continued)

- The physician should be familiar with the most common disorders causing each symptom in order to narrow the differential diagnosis and focus the testing needed to establish etiology/diagnosis and develop treatment plan.
- The neuropsychologist suspecting a previously unknown altered mental status in a patient (e.g., possible delirium, encephalopathy, seizure, TIA, etc.) should direct the patient to follow-up immediately with his/her referring physician and, if not possible, refer the patient to his/her treating primary care physician.

Global Symptoms

Loss of Consciousness and Convulsions

- Seizures:

   - Generalized tonic-clonic seizures, also known as "grand mal" seizures, are the most common and dramatic type of seizure. They are very stereotyped and consist of sudden loss of consciousness with onset of rigid muscle tone (tonic phase) followed by rhythmic jerky movements (clonic phase). The entire convulsion lasts 1–3 minutes. During the tonic phase the bladder may empty and patients may bite their tongue. Postictal somnolence lasts for minutes to a few hours. Some patients experience a brief prodromal vague sensation (e.g., depression, irritability) for a few hours before the event (Benbadis 2001).
   - *Other seizure types include* myoclonic seizures (brief and sporadic body jerk), tonic seizures (abrupt generalized tonic stiffening with LOC), and atonic (abrupt loss of muscle tone). The last two usually occur in severe childhood onset epilepsies with static encephalopathy (Benbadis 2001).

      See Chap. 16, this volume, for detailed review of seizures and epilepsy.

- *Psychogenic Nonepileptic Seizures (PNES)* also termed Psychogenic Nonepileptic Attacks (PNEA) are the main condition misdiagnosed as seizures, at least at epilepsy centers. They should be suspected in patients with a high frequency of seizures that is completely unaffected by medications. Specific triggers unusual for epilepsy, such as stress, getting upset or pain can be present. PNES tend to occur in the presence of an audience, and occurrence in the physician's office or waiting room is particularly suggestive (Benbadis 2005). Similarly, PNES tend not to occur in sleep. Some characteristics of the convulsions are associated with PNES. These include a very gradual onset or termination; pseudosleep; discontinuous (stop and go), irregular, or asynchronous (out of phase) activity; side-to-side head movements; pelvic thrusting; opisthotonic posturing; stuttering; weeping;

preserved awareness during bilateral motor activity; and persistent eye closure (Benbadis et al. 1996). The presence of likely psychogenic diagnoses, such as fibromyalgia, chronic pain or chronic fatigue syndrome, is strongly associated with PNES (Benbadis 2005). Similarly, a florid review of systems (especially written lists of symptoms or diagnoses, i.e., hypergraphia) suggests somatization (Benbadis 2006a). A premorbid psychiatric history should also raise the suspicion of PNES. EEG video monitoring is the "gold standard" for diagnosis of PNES (Benbadis 2006b). (See also Chap. 17 for detailed review of PNES/PNEA).

- *Syncope* is commonly known as fainting. In its most common etiology, vasovagal syncope, the episode occurs when the individuals are in the upright position (i.e., sitting or standing). A prodrome (i.e., presyncope) is typically present and is described as lightheadedness, giddiness or "feeling queasy." Patients become pale and diaphoretic and feel nauseated. This prodrome, which typically lasts for seconds or minutes, is followed by loss of consciousness, the patient falls (or slowly slumps) to the ground and lays motionless with eyes closed for several seconds, although not infrequently, brief myoclonic-like body jerks are seen, which are often mistaken for a seizure. The event terminates quickly once the patient is horizontal, in sharp contrast to the typical generalized tonic-clonic seizure duration of 30–90 seconds. Vasovagal syncope is typically triggered by clear precipitants (e.g., pain such as inflicted by medical procedures, emotions, cough, micturition, hot environment, prolonged standing, exercise). Tongue biting and urinary incontinence are typically absent. Cardiac diseases, such as arrhythmias and myocardial infarction as well as hypovolemia, are also known causes of syncope and should be investigated by EKG and blood pressure measuring in supine and upright positions. Syncope can usually be differentiated from seizures on the basis of history although at times this can be difficult.
- *Hypoglycemia* rarely causes complete LOC. When it does, it resembles syncope and is preceded by florid prodromes of hunger, weakness, tremulousness, malaise, and abnormal behaviors. Hypoglycemia typically occurs in reasonably obvious settings (e.g., diabetic patient on insulin or oral hypoglycemics). If prolonged and severe, hypoglycemia can also cause an epileptic seizure (Cryer 1999).
- *Narcolepsy* is characterized by frequent attacks of irresistible sleepiness, several times a day, usually after meals, while sitting in class or in unusual situations such as driving, talking or eating. The individual falls sleep usually for about 15 min, can be awaken easily, and feels somewhat refreshed afterwards. About 70% of narcoleptics report cataplexy, which consists of an abrupt loss of tone, typically triggered by emotions, most commonly laughter (Guilleminault and Gelb 1995). Other associated features include sleep paralysis and vivid and terrifying hallucinations (hypnagogic hallucinations). Sleep studies usually confirm the diagnosis by demonstrating a short sleep latency of less than 10 min and sleep-onset REM (appearing within 15 minutes after sleep onset).
- *Nonepileptic myoclonus* is defined as myoclonus that is not of cortical origin, i.e., not visible on EEG. Hiccups and hypnic jerks are examples of normal nonepileptic myoclonus, but abnormal nonepileptic myoclonus can be seen in metabolic or toxic encephalopathies and neurodegenerative diseases. *Hypnic*

jerks or sleep starts are benign myoclonic jerks that everyone has experienced on occasion. While they resemble the jerks of myoclonic seizures, their occurrence only upon falling asleep stamps them as benign nonepileptic phenomena. They occur at all ages and can lead to evaluations for seizures, especially when the jerks are unusually violent. They are easily identified on EEG-video by the fact that they occur in wake to stage 1 transition and have no EEG correlate associated with the jerks (Montagna et al. 1988).

• *Transient ischemic attacks (TIAs)* are brief, reversible, episodes of focal ischemic neurological disturbance. TIAs are important to be mentioned here due to the common misconception that they can cause global cerebral symptoms like LOC. TIAs in the carotid system do not present with transient LOC. In the case of attacks in the vertebrobasilar territory, an impairment of consciousness is a very rare manifestation and would almost always be in the context of focal signs of brain stem dysfunction (See also Chap. 13, this volume, for review of cerebrovascular disease and detailed review of TIAs).

Rule of thumb: LOC/Loss of awareness and convulsions

• Premonitory lightheadedness and rapid recovery of consciousness characterize syncope whereas convulsions and postictal confusion favor seizures
• Consider pseudoseizures if seizures are frequent and intractable, there is a psychiatric and chronic pain history, and the convulsions are non-clonic
• Check blood glucose especially in diabetic patients.
• TIAs typically do not cause loss of consciousness

• *Confusional states* (i.e., encephalopathies) manifest as impaired alertness, attention, recent memory and orientation. These abnormalities fluctuate in severity, being worse at night. Illusions (misinterpretation of reality) are common. In most advances stages of the illness, confusion gives way to stupor and finally to coma. The common etiologies of encephalopathy can be divided in three categories:

  – Systemic causes which include metabolic (e.g., uremia, liver disease, anoxia, hyponatremia, hypoglycemia, etc.), toxic (e.g., alcohol or drug intoxication/withdrawal), nutritional (B12 and Thiamine deficiencies) and infectious (e.g., sepsis, pneumonia). Asterixis ("flapping tremor") is common if the underlying cause is metabolic or toxic. Typically, there are no lateralizing neurologic sings and brain imaging studies and CSF examination are normal. EEG generally demonstrates diffuse slowing which is nonspecific. No clinical finding is pathognomonic of a specific etiology and the diagnosis is based on the history and laboratory tests. See Table 15.1 for some useful clinical features and laboratory findings that help orient the clinician to a specific etiology.
  – Structural brain lesions such as tumors, strokes, and abscesses can also present with acute confusion. However, in these instances the physical examination

Table 15.1 Clinical and laboratory features of common etiologies of encephalopathy

Disorder	Important clinical findings	Important laboratory findings
Liver failure	Asterixis, jaundice, ascites	Elevated blood ammonia, elevated liver enzymes
		EEG: Triphasic waves
Uremia	Hypertension, dry skin, uriniferous breath, myoclonic jerks, seizures	Elevated BUN and creatinine
		EEG: Triphasic waves
Anoxia	Rigidity, decerebrate posture	Hypoxemia
	Seizures, myoclonus	EEG: Periodic patterns
Hypoglycemia	Tremor, hunger, sweating, headache, palpitations	Low blood glucose (usually below 30 mg/dL)
Alcohol intoxication	Slurred speech, ataxia, alcohol breath	High alcohol levels
	Hypothermia, hypotenison	
Alcohol withdrawal	Tremors, seizures, delirium	Normal alcohol levels
Wernike's encephalopathy	Confusion, ataxia, ophtalmoplegia Aloholics	Low transketolase activity (index of thiamine deficiency)
B12 deficiency	Apathy, emotional instability Paresthesias, loss of vibratory sense, leg weakness, ataxia	Low blood B12 levels, low homocystheine and low methylmalonic acid

demonstrates focal signs (hemiparesis, Babinski sign, aphasia, etc.) and brain imaging studies are abnormal.

- Disorders that cause meningeal irritation such as meningoencephalitis and subarachnoid hemorrhage. The signs of meningeal irritation include headache, fever and nucal rigidity. Typically, there are no lateralizing neurologic signs and the CSF is abnormal demonstrating blood (subarachnoid hemorrhage) or pleiocytosis (meningitis).

- *Delirium* is a state of fluctuating confusion, marked by significant inattention, altered perception (illusions and hallucinations) and psychomotor overactivity (agitation, tremor, insomnia). Autonomic overactivity is a distinguishing feature and is manifested by tachycardia, profuse sweating, hypertension, and hyperthermia. After recovery, patients are typically amnestic to the episode. Delirium and encephalopathy are terms often used interchangeably since the diagnostic and therapeutic approach are similar. However, as described above, delirium has several distinguishing features, and recognizing them may help the clinician narrow the differential diagnosis since this condition is usually due to drug toxicity and withdrawal (most commonly alcohol) or systemic illness.

- It is of clinical importance to differentiate between delirium and dementia since the underlying pathologic process and prognosis are different. There are clear features that distinguish the two. Dementia develops slowly, has a chronic course, and is usually not reversible. In contrast, delirium generally develops acutely, has a fluctuating course (worse at night) and is frequently reversible if the underlying medical cause is removed. Dementia denotes intellectual deterioration, mainly in memory, with no disturbance of consciousness or perception whereas delirium manifests with prominent attention, consciousness is clouded and agitation and visual hallucinations are frequently present. A common situation encountered in everyday practice is that of an elderly patient with a pre-existing dementia (diagnosed or not) who enters the hospital displaying and acute confusional state or delirium. This condition, also known as "beclouded dementia," is usually triggered by an acute illness, more commonly intercurrent infections, electrolyte abnormalities, surgeries, or the administration of a new medication. All the clinical features that one observes in the acute confusional states can be present, and the manifestation of dementia might not be obvious before the onset of the complicated illness. Please see Chap. 14, this volume, for a detailed review of dementia and mild cognitive impairment (MCI).

- Review of Table 15.1 illustrates a summary of some common sources of encephalopathy and a summary of the clinical features and laboratory findings for each etiology. The EEG may be helpful to identify potential encephalopathies. For instance, periodic patterns are present in severe diffuse encephalopathies, more commonly anoxic and triphasic waves are typically seen in liver failure and uremia. Hypoglycemia is readily identified by low blood glucose and although there is some inter-individual variability in the blood glucose level resulting in encephalopathy, a common threshold are levels below 30 mg/dL. Wernicke's encephalopathy is characterized by the triad of confusion, ataxia and abnormal eye movements and is caused by thiamine (vitamin B1) deficiency, more commonly in alcoholics.

- *Seizures* can present as abnormal behaviors rather than convulsions and LOC (Benbadis 2001) (see also Chap. 16, this volume).

    - Complex partial seizures have a focal onset and impairment of awareness. They commonly originate in the temporal lobe. The episode may starts as a "simple" partial seizure (also called "aura"). The most common aura is some type of visceral sensation such as nausea, butterflies, or a rising epigastric sensation (French et al. 1993). This may be accompanied by fear, or fear may exist alone as the second most common aura. Other less common auras include olfactory and gustatory hallucinations, alteration of visual perceptions (micropsia, macropsia), and dyscognitive states (déjà vu, jamais vu). This initial event is followed by altered awareness where the individuals are out of contact with their surroundings and may demonstrate automatisms (lip smacking, chewing, swallowing, or picking on clothes). A postictal state is common and may last for minutes to hours. After the attack, the patient typically has no memory of the events.
    - *Absence seizures* are much briefer and present as arrest of activity with blank staring for only a few seconds. They almost always begin in childhood.

- *Transient global amnesia* consists of dramatic episodes of anterograde amnesia. Patients are alert and otherwise cognitively intact but cannot form new memories, and they ask repetitive questions about their environment. This lasts several hours and then resolves. The cause is not known, but transient global amnesia is not thought to represent a TIA or a seizure and usually does not recur (Quinette et al. 2006).

- *Dissociative fugue* is characterized by the sudden inability to remember pertinent information coupled with leaving home and taking on a different identity. The person is usually not aware that he/she has assumed a new identity.
- *Panic attacks* are paroxysmal manifestations of anxiety or panic disorder. Abrupt and intense fear is accompanied by at least four of the following symptoms: palpitations, diaphoresis, tremulousness or shaking, shortness of breath or sensation of choking, chest discomfort, nausea or abdominal discomfort, dizziness or lightheadedness, derealization or depersonalization, fear of losing control, fear of dying, paresthesias, and chills or hot flashes. The symptoms typically peak within 10 minutes. Panic disorder often coexists with other manifestations of anxiety such as agoraphobia and social phobia and also with depressive disorders. Panic attacks can be mistaken for seizures since fear is a relatively common (psychic) aura in patients with temporal lobe epilepsy. If the episode evolves into a clear seizure the diagnosis is easy but can be difficult in the absence of other seizure types (Biraben et al. 2001).

Parasomnias are short-lived paroxysmal behaviors that occur out of sleep. In particular, the non-REM parasomnias (night terrors, sleepwalking, and confusional arousals) can superficially resemble seizures since they include complex behaviors and some degree of unresponsiveness and amnesia for the event. The non-REM parasomnias are most common between ages 4 and 12 years, and night terrors are particularly common. They are often familial and may be worsened by stress, sleep deprivation, and intercurrent illnesses. Similarly, rhythmic movement disorder is a parasomnia typically seen at transition or stage 1 sleep, which can also resemble partial seizures. One common example is head banging (jactatio capitis). Among REM sleep parasomnias, nightmares rarely present a diagnostic challenge, but REM behavior disorder may with violent and injurious behaviors during REM sleep. The diagnosis of REM behavior disorder is usually easy as it affects older men and the description of acting out a dream is quite typical. However, EEG-video may be necessary to make the distinction, provided that the episodes are frequent enough. EEG-video will usually confirm the absence of an EEG seizure and usually shows that the behavior arises from a specific stage of sleep (Iranzo et al. 2005).

Rule of thumb: Confusion and mental status changes

- Encephalopathy presents with confusion, distractibility, memory loss, and decreased level of consciousness.
- Encephalopathy can be due to
  - Systemic (metabolic, infectious, toxic, etc.)
  - Structural
  - Irritation of meninges

(continued)

Rule of thumb: Confusion and mental status changes (continued)

- Delirium presents similar to encephalopathy, but differs with perceptual changes (hallucinations and/or illusions), psychomotor agitation, and autonomic dysfunction
- Parasomnias are paroxysmal behaviors occurring out of sleep (sleep walking, confusional awakening, night terrors).

Global Weakness

Generalized *fatigue* is not generally a symptom of neurologic disease, and is typically related to systemic factors. True *motor (muscular) weakness* (different from global fatigue) can be indicative of a neurologic process. When this is the case, mental status (sensorium, alertness, and attention) is normal.

- *Myasthenia Gravis* is an autoimmune disorder of the neuromuscular junction, which typically causes weakness of the ocular, facial, oropharyngeal, and limb muscles. Ptosis ("eye lid droop") and diplopia (i.e., double vision) are the most common presenting symptoms. Other symptoms include dysphagia, dysphonia and dysarthria due to weakness of the facial and bulbar muscles. Proximal limb and neck weakness is present in 20–30% of patients. The distinguishing feature in myasthenia is the fluctuation of the symptoms, worsening with activity or during the course of the day. This can be demonstrated on the physical examination by fatigable weakness. Deep tendon reflexes are spared. Weakness of the respiratory muscles can also be seen potentially leading to respiratory failure. The diagnosis is supported by a positive tensilon test, the presence acetylcholinesterase antibodies in the blood, and a detrimental response during EMG-NCS with repetitive nerve stimulation.
- *Lambert-Eaton myasthenic syndrome (LEMS)* is also a disorder of the neuromuscular junction caused by an autoimmune mechanism. It is clinically differentiated from myasthenia by the weakness predominantly affecting the proximal lower limb muscles and only mild involvement of the ocular and bulbar muscles. Deep tendon reflexes are typically decreased, but strength and reflexes can be improved by a brief period of contraction (facilitation). Autonomic symptoms, such as dry mouth are frequently part of the syndrome. The diagnosis is supported by the presence of facilitation during repetitive nerve stimulation and the detection in the blood of antibodies against presynaptic Voltage-gated calcium channels. LEMS can be associated with small cell lung cancer.
- *Periodic paralysis* can present with attacks of acute, severe limb weakness. Primary hyperkalemic periodic paralysis has its onset during childhood and manifests clinically with attacks of muscle weakness lasting less than a few hours and triggered by rest followed by strenuous exercise. Hypokalemic periodic paralysis is more common and also starts during childhood or adolescence with episodes of acute paralysis during the night or early morning and precipitated by meals rich in carbohydrates and sodium, stress or sleep following heavy

exercise. The ocular and bulbar muscles are typically spared. Reflexes are diminished or absent. The episodes last several hours.

- *Metabolic myopathies* are a group of disorders caused by abnormalities in muscle metabolism. It includes disorders of glycogen, lipid or mitochondria. Typical symptoms are exercise intolerance, muscle pain, stiffness, cramps, fatigue and sometimes weakness of proximal and distal muscles. Muscle biopsy provides a definite diagnosis.

Rule of thumb: Generalized weakness

- Weakness can reflect systemic illness or symptom of neurological process
- Neuromuscular diseases include:
  - Myastenia Gravis – predominately weakness of eye lids (eye lid droop), eyes, face, oropharyngeal, and limb muscles.
  - Lambert-Eaton myastenic syndrome - weakness of proximal lower extremities, mild weakness of eyes, eye lids or bulbar muscles, hyporreflexia and dry mouth.
- Metabolic myopathies often include muscle pain, stiffness, cramps, fatigue and weakness of proximal and distal muscles triggered by exercise.
- Episodic global weakness may indicate hyperkalemic periodic paralysis
- Somatic, conversion, factitious, or malingering disorders present with generalized weakness that is variable or inconsistent. Discontinuous resistance during testing of power ("give way weakness") is noted.

Dizziness and Vertigo

- *Benign Paroxysmal Positional vertigo* (*BPPV*) consists of brief (less than 1 min) episodes of vertigo prompted by change in head position, such as turning over in bed. Vertigo is described as an illusion of movement (usually spinning). Nausea can be present. Typically, BPPV manifests itself with symptomatic episodes lasting from a few days to several months, interspersed by asymptomatic intervals of several months to years in duration. The diagnosis is confirmed by the Dix–Hallpike maneuver which involves provocation of vertigo by positioning testing and observation of typical nystagmus (Lanska and Remler 1997).
- *Vertebrobasilar TIAs* are caused by transient focal ischemia in the territory supplied by the vertebrobasilar system, namely brain stem and cerebellum. They can also present with episodes of vertigo, but are almost always accompanied by other signs of brain stem dysfunction, such as diplopia, dysarthria, bifacial numbness, ataxia, and weakness or numbness of part or all of one or both sides of the body. Rarely, isolated vertigo can be a manifestation of vertebrobasilar insufficiency and should be suspected in patients with cerebrovascular risk factors (Gomez et al. 1996).

- *Basilar migraine* is a form of migraine with prominent brainstem symptoms. Patients are usually young women or children with a family history of migraine. The first symptoms of the attack involve visual phenomena affecting the whole of both visual fields, such as "flashing lights," scintillating scotomas and sometimes temporary blindness. The visual symptoms are often associated with vertigo, staggering, incoordination of the limbs, dysarthria and tingling in hands and feet. These symptoms last 10–30 minuntes, and are followed by a headache that is usually occipital. In some patients, the basilar-type aura at times occurs without a headache (Kirchmann et al. 2006).
- *Meniere disease and other labyrinthine diseases* is a constellation of diseases effecting the labyrinthines. Symptoms include recurrent, acute, recurring episodes of severe vertigo, often with nausea and vomiting as well as mild tinnitus and deafness. Other symptoms can include contralateral nystagmus (nystagmus to the side contralateral of the impaired labyrinthine). Falling or swaying while walking is often to the ipsilateral side of the labyrinthine impairment. In classic Meniere disease, vertigo attacks occur with rapid onset and last for minutes to 1–2 hours in duration.
- *Presyncope*, as described above, is the constellation of prodromal symptoms preceding a syncopal (i.e., fainting) episode. Patients complain of queasiness and lightheadeness. If the individual has enough time to lie down, LOC may be prevented. Patients frequently describe these symptoms as "dizziness" and can be confused with vertigo, which is an illusion of movement.
- *Vestibular Neuronitis (Labyrinthitis) (also known as acute unilateral peripheral vetibularopathy)* classically describes a paroxysmal, often single attack, of vertigo without tinnitus or deafness (as is found in Meniere disease) last several days in duration. Typical onset is in early to middle adulthood and may be preceded by upper respiratory infection. Vertigo onset is over hours to, at most, a few days of feeling "top heavy" or "off balance." During the period of severe vertigo, extreme nausea and vertigo are common. Symptoms subside in a number of days.

Rule of thumb: Dizziness and Vertigo

- Vertigo is NOT dizziness
  - Vertigo is a sensation of rotation, whirling or spinning (movement) and/ or perception of objects spinning around or moved rhythmically in one direction.
  - Dizziness as a complaint may include vertigo, but may also describe non-moving perception such as lightheadness, faintness (syncope), blurred vision, unsteadiness, etc.
- Causes of vertigo include:
  - Benign paroxysmal positional vertigo
  - TIAs (involving vertebral or basilar arteries)
  - Migraine (basilar)
  - Meniere disease and labyrinthine diseases
  - Vestibular neuronitis

Focal Symptoms

A focal neurologic deficit is a problem that affects a specific location, such as the left face or right face, one arm or leg or even just a small area such the tongue. Specific functions, such as speech, writing or calculation can also be involved as well as especial senses including vision, olfaction or taste. The problem typically occurs in the brain and rarely in the peripheral nervous system. It may result in negative symptoms (loss of movement or sensation, visual field cuts, etc.) or positive symptoms (abnormal movements, tingling or visualization of flashing lights). The type, location, and severity of the change can indicate the area of the brain or nervous system that is affected. The most common disorders causing transient focal neurologic symptoms are outlined in Table 15.2.

Table 15.2 Common disorders causing transient *focal* neurologic symptoms

	Clinical features	Time frame	Helpful tests
TIA	Negative symptoms (monocular visual loss, focal sensory loss or weakness)	Onset within a few seconds (<5 seconds), maximum deficit at onset	MRI-MRA Ultrasounds of neck vessels
		Duration: minutes	EKG, Echocardiogram
Seizure	Positive symptoms (twitching, tingling) Focal symptoms may evolve into generalized tonic clonic seizure	Onset or progressive march in several seconds	EEG MRI
Migraine	Mixed positive and negative symptoms Evolution into clear migraine	Onset or progressive march of symptoms over course of minutes	None

Abnormal Movements

- *Simple partial motor seizures* consist of simple motor movements, typically a single type of clonic or tonic contraction of a muscle or group of muscles. They are usually brief in duration (15 seconds to 2 minutes) and consciousness is not impaired. These seizures typically arise from motor regions of the frontal lobe. Interictal EEG may show focal epileptiform discharges localized to the affected area. Because the ictal discharge involves only a small area of the brain, ictal scalp EEG is only abnormal about 25% of the time (Devinsky et al. 1989) (see also Chap. 16, this volume, for review of seizures and epilepsy)/
- *Acute dystonic reactions* are caused by dopamine receptor blockers such as antipsychotics (neuroleptics, including atypical ones) and antiemetics, although other drugs can be involved (e.g., carbamazepine, lithium, trazodone, illicit drugs). They typically occur within 1–4 days of beginning the medication and are characterized

by torsion/twisting movements affecting the cranial, pharyngeal, and cervical muscles. The oculogyric crisis is a subtype characterized by acute conjugate eye deviation, usually in an upward direction. The typical attack lasts 1–2 hours, during which the abnormal movement occurs repetitively for seconds to minutes. These dystonic reactions respond very well and rapidly to anticholinergics (trihexyphenidyl, benztropine, diphenhydramine) and levodopa (Dressler and Benecke 2005).

- *Hemifacial spasm* (HFS) is a chronic progressive disorder that causes painless irregular clonic contractions of the facial muscles of one side. HFS typically affects the periorbital muscles first and then spreads to other (ipsilateral) facial muscles over a period of months to years. Over time or with exacerbations, the clonic movements can result in a sustained tonic contraction causing forceful (unilateral) eyelid closure. HFS can be idiopathic or symptomatic and may resemble a facial clonic seizure, but clear differences make the differentiation easy. By contrast, seizures are paroxysmal (not chronic progressive) and typically affect the perioral muscles (due to a large representation on the motor homunculus).
- *Tics* are characterized by involuntary, sudden, purposeless, repetitive, stereotyped, motor movements such as blinking, shoulder shrugging, mouth opening or vocalizations (sniffing, throat clearing, barking). Stereotypy and irresistibility are the main identifying features. The patient admits to making the movements and feels compelled to do so in order to relieve perceived tension. Such movements can be suppressed for a short time by an effort of will, but they reappear as soon as the subject's attention is diverted.

Rule of thumb: Focal abnormal movements

- Simple partial motor seizures
- Acute dystonic reactions
- Hemifacial spasm
- Motor tics

Weakness

- *Transient ischemic attacks (TIAs)* are by far the most common cause of focal weakness, especially in older individuals with cerebrovascular risk factors. Unlike the transient focal weakness in migraine which tend to spread from one part of the body to another within several minutes, symptoms in TIA are stroke-like, (i.e., maximal acutely and involving all affected parts simultaneously). Seizures do not manifest with ictal weakness. However, some confusion between TIA and seizures may occur when the seizure is not witnessed and the patient appears with a focal deficit (e.g., Todd's paralysis described below), especially since both will improve over time (minutes) (Benbadis 2007). In these cases, an accurate history of the event is essential to differentiate the two. Most TIA symptoms last 2–15 minutes, but may last from seconds up to 1 hour Episodes lasting more than an hour are more likely to leave permanent neurologic deficits. TIAs may result in a single episode of transient symptoms, but events recurring several times over days, weeks, or months also occur. It is important to separate a single transient episode from repeated ones that present with the same symptoms. The latter are more often a warning sign of impending vascular occlusion. See also Chap. 13 for details of cerebrovascular disease.

- *Todd's paralysis.* Following focal motor seizures there might be a transient paralysis of the affected limbs lasting for minutes to a few hours, usually in proportion to the duration of the seizure. Continued focal paralysis beyond this time usually indicates a focal brain lesion (stroke, tumor, etc.) as the cause of the seizure. A similar phenomenon can occur with seizures involving the language, sensory and visual areas.
- *Migraine auras* can cause transient focal neurologic symptoms, usually visual but sometimes include weakness. Migraine symptoms tend to evolve in minutes and "March" (spread from one involved part to the other). As the symptoms begin to recede, they are followed by a unilateral throbbing headache. In some patients, the weakness is prolonged and may outlast the headache. This condition is known as hemiplegic migraine and has a strong familial trait.
- *Spinal cord or plexus damage/impingement* can cause focal neurologic weakness that rarely may be transient or fluctuating.

Rule of thumb: Focal weakness/paralysis

- Transient ischemic attacks (TIAs) – symptoms tend to present acutely and resolve over minutes to an hour
- Migraine auras/headache – symptoms tend to present over minutes and can spread from one part to the other.
- Todd's paralysis – transient paralysis of the affected face and/or limb lasting minutes to hours following seizure
- Conversion/factitious/malingering disorder –weakness due to psychogenic etiology

Headaches and Facial Pain

- *Migraine* is characterized by periodic headaches beginning in childhood, adolescence or early adult life. Migraine with aura, termed *classic migraine*, presents with focal neurologic symptoms ("aura"), most often visual (flashing, flickering lights, scintillating scotomas) followed within several minutes by a unilateral, less often bilateral, throbbing headache accompanied by nausea, vomiting and sensitivity to light (photophobia) and sounds (phonophobia). More commonly the migraine headache appears without preceding neurologic symptoms (migraine without aura), and is termed *common migraine*. Migraine is a ubiquitous familial disorder. In about 60–80% of the classic migraine cases, several family members have migraine headache.

- *Cluster headaches* are characterized by severe, unilateral pain localized in the orbital, supraorbital and/or temporal area lasting from 15 to 180 minutes. The typical patient is a young adult man. The episodes occur from 1 every other day to 8 per day and nightly occurrence is characteristic. Autonomic symptoms are invariable present on the side of the pain and include rhinorrhea, lacrimation, conjunctival injection, ptosis and myosis. The headache tends to recur regularly for periods ("clusters") extending over 6–12 weeks followed by pain-free intervals of many months.
- *Paroxysmal hemicrania* is a unilateral headache that resembles cluster headaches in some respects including the short duration of the attacks (2–45 minutes), the location in the temporo-orbital region and the accompanying autonomic symptoms on the same side of the pain. Unlike cluster headaches, the episodes occur many times a day, are shorter (5–45 minutes) and recur daily for long periods that could extend to years (Goadsby 2001). This disorder affects more women than men and responds dramatically to Indomethacin.
- *Trigeminal neuralgia* presents with abrupt, paroxysmal, excruciating pain, described as stabbing or electric-like sensation, localized in the distribution of the trigeminal nerve (usually second and/or third divisions). The pain is of brief duration (from seconds to less than 2 minutes) and can be triggered by touching the face, brushing the teeth, talking or eating. The majority of the cases is idiopathic or due to compression of the nerve by a tortuous blood vessel and the physical exam is unremarkable. On the other hand, the finding of sensory loss in the face or abnormal corneal reflex should raise the suspicion of a structural brain lesion such as tumor, basilar artery aneurysm or multiple sclerosis.

Rule of thumb: Headache and facial pain

- Cluster headache is a severe unilateral pain localized in the orbital, supraorbital and/or temporal area lasting 15 minutes to 3 hours occurring typically at night, 1–8 times per day for weeks to 3 months followed by an interval of months with no headache (headaches occur in clusters).
- Migraine is typically a unilateral throbbing headache associated with nausea, phonophobia, and photophobia lasting minutes to hours
  - Common – no aura
  - Classic – headache preceded by aura
- Paroxysmal hemicrania is unilateral headache similar to cluster headaches but of shorter duration (2–45 minutes) occur more frequently per day and occur for longer periods of time (up to several years with daily headache). Respond to Indomethacin.
- Trigeminal neuralgia is abrupt paroxysmal excruciating pain of stabbing quality that last seconds to several minutes and localized to distribution of trigeminal nerve (typically 2nd and 3rd divisions). Onset can be triggered by touching the face, gums, eating, or talking. Compression of nerve due to blood vessel is most common.
- Conversion/Factitious/malingering disorder – headache with psychogenic etiology.

Limb Pain

- Episodic limb pain is usually caused by non-neurological conditions such as muscleskeletal disorders. However, the "shooting" character of the pain due to nerve root disease (radiculopathy) can be perceived as episodic or intermittent. Radiculopathies frequently cause paresthesias (numbness or tingling) and the physical examination typically reveals decreased sensation and, if severe, weakness and decreased deep tendon reflexes in the distribution of one or more roots. Painful dystonia (sustained, unnatural posture of a limb due to co-contraction of agonists and antagonists muscles) is not uncommon in patients with Parkinson's disease and occur frequently at night, particularly when the dopaminergic medications wear-off (Grandas and Iranzo 2004).

Aphasia

See also Chaps. 7 and 12 for detailed review of language problems and aphasia syndromes.
- *TIA* involving the cortical language areas are by far the most common cause of transient aphasia, fluent, non-fluent or both in which symptoms typically last several minutes. Commonly, the language disturbance is accompanied by negative symptoms, such as focal weakness and numbness, but it can present in isolation. In a patient with cardiovascular risk factors, a transient aphasia should be considered a TIA until proven otherwise.
- *Partial seizure* arising from the cortical language areas may give rise to a brief aphasic disturbance (ictal aphasia). In most cases, it is usually followed by other focal or generalized seizure activity, but may (rarely) occur in isolation. More commonly, aphasia is a component of a postictal state (postictal aphasia) which typically last minutes or a few hours.

Visual Loss

- *Transient monocular blindness or amaurosis fugax* is caused by atherosclerotic occlusive disease of the common or internal carotid artery. Transient ocular ischemia is the most common mechanism of transient visual loss (Biousse and Trobe 2005). Patients usually report negative symptoms usually described as a graying, blurring, darkening, fogging or dimming of vision in the eye. The visual loss can involve entirely or partially the field of vision in that eye. Some patients describe a curtain that descends quickly over the eye. The most important and common ophthalmoscopic finding in patients with transient monocular blindness is the presence of embolic cholesterol particles within retinal arteries.
- *Migraine.* Occasional patients with migraine have attacks of monocular visual loss. Descriptors of the visual loss are not different from those used by patients

with carotid artery occlusive disease. Most patients have complete loss of monocular vision rather than altitudinal symptoms (Winterkorn and Teman 1991). Some have had aching or discomfort in the eye during attacks. Attacks can be frequent and occur more than once a day. This diagnosis should be considered in patients with a personal history of migraine and after excluding other disorders such as carotid artery disease.

- *Increased intracranial pressure in patients with pseudotumor cerebri.* Patients with pseudotumor cerebri (benign intracranial hypertension) have transient visual obscuration (Merle et al. 1998). These are often monocular but can be binocular. The episodes are usually brief and often are precipitated by coughing, straining, or other maneuvers that elevate intracranial pressure. Prominent headaches are invariably associated (Digre 2002).

- *Optic Neuritis* typically begins with rapid (over hours), but not sudden, loss of vision, and is unilateral. Unlike transient ocular ischemia in which the symptoms last several minutes, the visual loss in optic neuritis progresses over hours or days (Glaser 1990). It is associated with pain (90%) in or behind the eye, particularly with eye movement. The involved pupil reacts poorly to light (afferent pupillary defect). This disorder most frequently affects young individuals and is frequently a manifestation of multiple sclerosis.

- *Giant Cell Arteritis* is probably the most frequent cause of ophthalmic artery disease. The disorder classically affects patients older than 65 and is frequently associated with headache, scalp tenderness, jaw claudication and systemic symptoms such as low-grade fever, malaise and weight loss. Most of these patients have persistent rather than transient monocular visual loss. Elevated ESR is nearly always present and the diagnosis is confirmed by a temporal artery biopsy.

Rule of thumb: Vision loss

- Transient monocular blindness (amaurosis faux) is loss of vision in one eye typically presenting as blurring or graying of vision due to transient ocular ischemia.
- Migraine auras/headache is typically described as monocular visual loss and can occur more than once per day.
- Pseudotumor cerebri (increased intracranial pressure) results in transient vision loss that is typically monocular but can be binocular. Vision loss of short duration (seconds to minutes) and associated with straining (coughing, laughing, sneezing, etc.).
- Optic neurotis is progressive loss of vision over several days and is associated with pain in or behind the affected eye and there is often an afferent pupillary defect (no pupil constriction)
- Conversion/factitious/malingering disorder – vision complaints due to psychogenic etiology

Sensory Symptoms ("Numbness, Tingling")

The main disorders that cause transient focal weakness, such as TIA, seizures and migraine can also present with focal sensory symptoms involving a limb, part of the face or the entire hemibody when the disease affects the somatosensory pathways (e.g., the parietal cortex). Focal seizures typically cause "positive" symptoms (e.g., tingling) that spread or "March" over seconds. In contrast, TIA produces negative symptoms ("dead numbness or sensory loss") involving all affected parts simultaneously. Migraine can produce both, negative and positive symptoms that typically "March" over minutes usually followed by the headache. Recurrent attacks of multiple sclerosis can manifest as focal numbness, tingling or pain, but the episodes classically evolve over days or weeks, not seconds or minutes.

Hallucinations

In general hallucinations that are of organic origin tend to be *unformed*, whereas hallucinations of psychiatric origin are *formed* and have a strong "content" (usually paranoid). The main causes for organic hallucinations are seizures and migraines.

- *Migraines* tend to cause visual hallucinations in the aura phase. They are usually unformed (fortification spectra), associated with a scotoma (negative symptom), and evolve or "March" slowly (over minutes). Of course they are usually followed by a typical headache, but "acephalgic" migraine does exist.
- *Hallucinations caused by seizures* can involve any of the five senses, are unformed, and evolve or "March" over seconds. Their epileptic nature can be impossible to prove or disprove when they occur with no other seizure types, since even ictal EEG does not help in "simple partial" seizures. Fortunately, when hallucinations are seizures, they usually will evolve into other (obvious) seizure types.

The most common disorders causing transient focal neurologic signs are illustrated in Table 15.2. Transient ischemic attacks (TIAs) typically produce negative symptoms, such as "dead numbness" and weakness reaching the maximal severity within seconds. The presence of carotid or vertebrobasilar artery disease on the MRI or a cardiac source of emboli identified by echocardiogram support the diagnosis. In contrast, focal seizures cause positive symptoms (twitching, tingling) that spread ("March") from one part of the body to another over a few seconds. The EEG confirms the diagnosis if an epileptic focus is identified.

References

Benbadis, S. R. (2001). Epileptic seizures and syndromes. *Neurologic Clinics, 19*, 251–270.

Benbadis, S. R. (2005). A spell in the epilepsy clinic and a history of "chronic pain" or "fibromyalgia" independently predict a diagnosis of psychogenic seizures. *Epilepsy & Behavior, 6*(2), 264–265.

Benbadis, S. R. (2006a). Hypergraphia and the diagnosis of psychogenic attacks. *Neurology,* *67*(5), 904.

Benbadis, S. R. (2006b). Psychogenic non-epileptic seizures. In E. Wyllie (Ed.), *The treatment of epilepsy: principles and practice* (4th ed., pp. 623–630). Philadelphia: Lippincott Williams & Wilkins.

Benbadis, S. R. (2007). Differential diagnosis of Epilepsy. *Continuum Lifelong Learning in Neurology,* *13*(4), 48–70.

Benbadis, S. R., & Chichkova, R. (2006). Psychogenic pseudosyncope: an underestimated and provable diagnosis. *Epilepsy & Behavior,* *9*(1), 106–110.

Benbadis, S. R., Lancman, M. E., King, L. M., & Swanson, S. J. (1996). Preictal pseudosleep: a new finding in psychogenic seizures. *Neurology,* *47*(1), 63–67.

Biousse, V., & Trobe, J. D. (2005). Transient monocular visual loss. *American Journal of Opthalmology,* *140,* 717–21.

Biraben, A., Taussig, D., Thomas, P., et al. (2001). Fear as the main feature of epileptic seizures. *Journal of Neurology, Neurosurgery and Psychiatry,* *70*(2), 186–191.

Cryer, P. E. (1999). Symptoms of hypoglycemia, thresholds for their occurrence, and hypoglycemia unawareness. *Endocrinology and Metabolism Clinics of North America,* *28*(3), 495–500. v–vi.

n, O., Sato, S., Kufta, C. V., et al. (1989). Electroencephalographic studies of simple partial seizures with subdural electrode recordings. *Neurology,* *39*(4), 527–533.

Digre, K. B. (2002). Idiopathic intracranial hypertension headache. *Current Pain and Headache Reports,* *6,* 217–25.

Dressler, D., & Benecke, R. (2005). Diagnosis and management of acute movement disorders. *Journal of Neurology,* *252*(11), 1299–1306.

French, J. A., Williamson, P. D., Thadani, V. M., et al. (1993). Characteristics of medial temporal lobe epilepsy: I. Results of history and physical examination. *Annals of Neurology,* *34,* 774–80.

Glaser, J. S. (1990). *Clinical neuro-ophthalmology* (2nd ed.). Philadelphia: Lippincott.

Goadsby, P. J. (2001, May 5–11) *Cluster and other short-lived headaches.* 53rd Annual Meeting of the American Academy of Neurology, Philadelphia, 2001.

Gomez, C., Cruz-Flores, S., Malkoff, C., Sauer, M., & Burch, C. (1996). Isolated vertigo as a manifestation of vertebrobasilar ischemia. *Neurology,* *47,* 94–97.

Grandas, F., & Iranzo, A. (2004). Nocturnal problems occurring in Parkinson's disease. *Neurology,* *63*(8), S8–S11.

Guilleminault, C., & Gelb, M. (1995). Clinical aspects and features of cataplexy. *Advances in Neurology,* *67,* 65–77.

Iranzo, A., Santamaria, J., Rye, D. B., et al. (2005). Characteristics of idiopathic REM sleep behavior disorder and that associated with MSA and PD. *Neurology,* *65*(2), 247–252.

Kirchmann, M., Lykke Thomsen, L., & Olesen, J. (2006). Basilar-type migraine, clinical, epidemiologic, and genetic features. *Neurology,* *66,* 880–886.

Lanska, D. J., & Remler, B. (1997). Benign paroxysmal positioning vertigo: classic descriptions, origins of the provocative positioning technique, and conceptual developments. *Neurology,* *48,* 1167–77.

Merle, H., Smadja, D., Ayeboua, L., et al. (1998). Benign intracranial hypertension. Retrospective study of 20 cases. *French Journal of Ophthalmology,* *21,* 42–50.

Montagna, P., Liguori, R., Zucconi, M., et al. (1988). Physiological hypnic myoclonus. *Electroencephalography and Clinical Neurophysiology,* *70*(2), 172–176.

Quinette, P., Guillery-Girard, B., Dayan, J., et al. (2006). What does transient global amnesia really mean? Review of the literature and thorough study of 142 cases. *Brain,* *129*(pt 7), 1640–1658.

Winterkorn, J. M., & Teman, A. J. (1991). Recurrent attacks of amaurosis fugax treated with calcium channel blockers. *Annals of Neurology,* *30,* 423–5.

Chapter 16
Epilepsy and Seizures

Mike R. Schoenberg, Mary Ann Werz, and Daniel L. Drane

Abstract Epilepsy represents an important area of clinical neuropsychological practice and research. Historically, clinical neuropsychology studies primarily involved patients with seizures that were not adequately controlled by anti-epileptic drugs, termed medically refractory or intractable epilepsy. However, the role of the neuropsychological evaluation and the clinical neuropsychologist has expanded well beyond a narrow focus on patients with medically intractable epilepsy. This chapter will provide an overview of the application of neuropsychology, psychology, and quality of life to patients with epilepsy, including a special section for the clinical neuropsychologist in the surgery team (see section "Neuropsychological (Cognitive and Behavioral) Comorbidity in Epilepsy"). Section "Neuropsychological Assessment Guide" provides an overview of assessment practices.

Key Points and Chapter Summary

- Epilepsy is a common neurological disorder often associated with neuropsychological and psychiatric comorbidity
- Neuropsychological deficits are greatest for patients with symptomatic epilepsies and catastrophic epilepsy syndromes, but idiopathic "benign" epilepsies have also been found to produce some mild neuropsychological deficits.
- Controlling seizures (seizure freedom) is strongly related to decreasing cognitive comorbidity
- 30 to 40% of patients with epilepsy are refractory to current medications

---

(continued)

M.R. Schoenberg (✉)
University of South Florida College of Medicine, Tampa, FL, USA
and
Adjunct Associate Professor, Case Western Reserve University
School of Medicine, Cleveland, OH, USA
e-mail: mschoenb@health.usf.edu

M.R. Schoenberg and J.G. Scott (eds.), *The Little Black Book of Neuropsychology:*   423
A Syndrome-Based Approach, DOI 10.1007/978-0-387-76978-3_16,
© Springer Science+Business Media, LLC 2011

Key Points and Chapter Summary (continued)

- Children with epilepsy commonly present with cognitive and psychiatric dysfunction
- Neuropsychological data have value in predicting surgical outcome among adults with no currently identifiable lesion on structural neuroimaging and temporal lobe seizure onset

---

The neuropsychologist providing services to individuals with epilepsy may involve a variety of roles (e.g., Baxendale and Thompson 2010), which are based on evidence-based neuropsychology (e.g., Chelune 2008). These roles can include any one or a combination of the six highlighted below:

1. *Predicting cognitive and psychiatric outcome.* Neuropsychological data have been shown to be independent predictors of cognitive outcome following neurological surgery for treatment of medication refractory epilepsy (e.g., Baxendale and Thompson 2010; Chelune 1995; Chelune and Najm 2001; Rausch 2006; Stroup et al. 2003; Seidenberg et al. 1998). An emphasis is to identify patients at high risk for meaningful decline in cognitive and behavioral functioning (generally regarded as decline sufficient to result in functional change in social, occupational or self care).

   (a) More generally, neuropsychological baseline data may be used, along with other variables, to identify children and adults at increased risk for the development of neuropsychological, cognitive, academic, and psychiatric problems from time of first recognized seizure (Byars et al. 2008; Fastenau et al. 2009).

   (b) *Predicting seizure freedom.* Although limited to select cases, emerging studies have shown neuropsychological data can add unique variance in predicting likelihood a patient will be seizure-free after surgical treatment (e.g., Helmstaedter and Kockelmann 2006; Keary et al. 2007; Potter et al. 2009; Sawrie et al. 1998; Seidenberg et al. 1998). Often the additive predictive value is demonstrated for individuals with normal neuroimaging (i.e., nonlesional) or incongruent ictal and inter-ictal EEG findings, and generally have not included multiple non-invasive studies in addition to neuropsychological data (e.g., MEG/MSI, fMRI, PET, SISCOM studies). A recent study combining multiple predictors did not find that neuropsychological data added unique variance (Bell et al. 2009).

2. *Assessing post-surgical cognitive and behavioral function.* Post-surgical neuropsychological evaluation can help guide post-surgical: (1) medical treatment and rehabilitation, (2) educational/vocational planning, (3) assist in determining competency, and/or (4) assist in making placement decisions (e.g., Baxendale and Thompson 2010; Fastenau et al. 2004; Hermann et al. 2008).

3. *Assisting to lateralize and/or localize the presence of brain dysfunction.* Within surgical contexts, neuropsychological data have limited utility at this time (Baxendale and Thompson 2010), although support for lateralizing value is present

(Akunama et al. 2003; Helmstaeder 2004; Hennessy et al. 2001; Keary et al. 2007; Potter et al. 2009; Rausch 2006; Sawrie et al. 1998). Alternatively, neuropsychological data have clear utility to evaluate the functional adequacy of mesial temporal lobes and other cerebral areas (e.g., Baxendale and Thompson 2010; Chelune 1995; Hermann et al. 2008; Seidenberg et al. 1998; Stroup et al. 2003).

4. *Providing a baseline assessment of cognitive function.* Neuropsychological data provide an objective method to monitor for changes in patients' cognitive and behavioral functioning over time (i.e., longitudinal assessment of cognitive function for patients with focal or generalized epilepsies) (Hermann et al. 2008; Helmstaedter et al. 2003).

   (a) As above, neuropsychological assessment at the time of first recognized seizure can identify those children at increased risk for onset of academic deficits, and assist in formulating interventions to offset potential for further neuropsychological and academic deficits (Fastenau et al. 2009; Austin et al. 2010).

5. *Assessing the effects of anti-epileptic medications (AEDs) on cognition/psychological function* (e.g., Aldenkamp et al. 2003; Drane and Meador 2002; Kluger and Meador 2008; Loring et al. 2007) (see Table 16.8).

6. *Identify and formulate treatment plans for patients with psychogenic nonepileptic seizures* (also termed psychogenic nonepileptic attacks) (See Chap. 17, this volume).

The clinical care of epilepsy has reflected an area of medicine having a strong multidisciplinary model, particularly with respect to neuropsychology (see section "Neuropsychological (Cognitive and Behavioral) Comorbidity in Epilepsy"). Neurological surgery is often successful at eliminating seizures in selected patients (e.g., Ojemann and Valiante 2006). However, resection of brain tissue presents with a variety of risks extending beyond more traditional surgical morbidity (i.e., hemorrhage, infection) and mortality (i.e., death) such as post-operative neurological (e.g., somatosensory loss or hemiparesis), cognitive, and/or psychiatric morbidity (e.g., Baxendale and Thompson 2010; Ojemann and Valiante 2006). The cognitive risks to neurological surgery were highlighted by the report of Scoville and Milner (1957) of patient HM, who underwent bilateral temporal lobectomy in 1953 for treatment of refractory epilepsy that resulted in a profound amnestic syndrome. Thus, the clinician and patient must balance the potential of being seizure-free following surgical treatment against the possible neurological, neuropsychological, psychiatric, and psychosocial risks to the patient's outcome (Ojemann and Jung 2006). The pre-surgical neuropsychological evaluation continues to provide important data to inform this clinical decision process (e.g., Hermann et al. 2007; Stroup et al. 2003). From a research standpoint, data from patients who underwent elective neurological surgery have helped to formulate our current understanding of the functional neuroanatomy of memory and language (e.g., Hermann et al. 1999; Lezak et al. 2004; Ojemann et al. 1989). Indeed, the understanding of human neuropsychology owes a debt to patients who have provided data over many years.

This chapter is meant as a targeted review of the neuropsychological aspects of epilepsy and its treatment. However, we will also endeavor to provide a review of the diagnosis of epilepsy, seizure classification, seizure semiology, and the

Table 16.1 Diagnostic tools in epilepsy

Study	Description	Purpose
Neurological Exam	Cursory mental status exam along with cranial nerve, motor, coordination and sensory exams.	Lateralize and/or localize neurologic dysfunction
EEG interictal	Regional slowing, sharp waves, spikes and polyspikes	Support a diagnosis of epilepsy and help determine epilepsy syndrome
Ictal Video-EEG	Provides seizure semiology and EEG changes during a seizure	Diagnose epilepsy and determine epilepsy syndrome
MRI	High resolution imaging. Studies at Epilepsy Centers include specific high resolution imaging sequences with increased sensitivity	Identify lesions that are associated with epilepsy such as tumors, vascular malformations, and cortical malformations
Interictal PET	Measures regional blood flow and glucose metabolism in the brain.	These are often decreased at the seizure focus consistent with impaired brain function. The area of hypometabolism (dysfunction) is usually larger than the seizure focus, and may be bilateral. The area of hypometabolism can decrease (improved regional blood flow) after successful epilepsy surgery.
Ictal SPECT	Short half-life radioligands serving as indirect measures of neuronal activity based on regional blood flow changes in the brain.	Blood flow markedly increases during a seizure. The radioligand must be injected immediately at seizure onset to identify the seizure onset zone and not seizure propagation pathways
Wada's test (Intra-carotid amobarbital, methohexital, or ethosuxomide test)	Amobarbital, methohexital, or ethosuxomide is injected into an internal carotid artery resulting in a short duration of brain anesthesia to areas of the brain affected (usually the middle cerebral, anterior cerebral, and, less often, posterior cerebral artery areas). During the period of anesthesia (often measured by EEG) and typically lasting 3–5 min with amobarbital, language and memory function are evaluated. The patient is asked to follow commands, repeat, and name words/pictures. Memory is assessed after drug effects has worn off with recall and recognition of words and/or objects previously presented.	Lateralize language functions (comprehension, repetition, naming, fluency, reading) to a hemisphere as well as lateralize memory function. Generally considered to measure the functional adequacy of each hemisphere to support language and memory function.

(continued)

Table 16.1 (continued)

Study	Description	Purpose
MEG/MSI	Record magnetic fields produced by currents from cortical neurons. Sharp waves corresponding to those seen on surface EEG can be identified. During Magnetic Source Imaging (MSI), functional mapping of language, motor and sensory cortex is done.	Localize inter-ictal activity from the seizure focus. MEG can detect sharp waves from deep cortical sulci that may not be detectable by surface EEG. MSI may provide alternative to Wada's test and fMRI to identify functional areas of cognitive functions (language and memory).
fMRI	Measures cerebral blood flow, known as BOLD MRI sequences. Areas of brain involved in performing tasks theorized to have increased blood flow.	Functional mapping of eloquent cortex. That is cortex involved in activities such as language and hand movement. Also been applied to memory function.

prevalence and incidence of seizures and epilepsy. Because neuropsychologists are integral members of epilepsy centers, it is important for the neuropsychologist to be aware of factors affecting the treatment and variables affecting surgical outcome, both in terms of neuropsychological outcome and of seizure freedom. We then summarize the treatment of seizures and components of a pre-surgical evaluation for medication refractory (intractable) epilepsy. Finally, we summarize decades of research attempting to delineate risk factors for post-surgical neuropsychological impairment following neurological surgery for the treatment of medically refractory epilepsy. Table 16.1 lists some common terms in epilepsy and epilepsy treatment.

Making a Diagnosis

Seizures are paroxysmal (abrupt) events due to abnormal hypersynchronous discharge of neurons associated with behavioral change. Seizures may be provoked due to a variety of conditions or unprovoked. Anyone can have a seizure that is provoked. Common etiology for a provoked seizure include: (1) hyponatremia (low sodium in the blood), (2) hypoglycemia (low blood sugar), (3) injury to the brain parenchyma (stroke, open head injury, infection of CNS), (4) sudden cessation of drinking alcohol in a person physically addicted to alcohol, and (5) overdose of some medications and/or drugs.

Epilepsy is traditionally defined as the occurrence of more than one unprovoked seizure (e.g., seizures not provoked by illness or brain injury). However, diagnosing epilepsy is a complicated process and involves both identifying the *type* of seizure (generalized or focal) as well as the presumed etiology of the epilepsy (or epilepsy syndrome). Epilepsy syndromes include seizures with similar semiology and epidemiologic characteristics. For example, juvenile myoclonic epilepsy is genetic in etiology and includes absence, myoclonic, and generalized tonic-clonic seizures often upon awakening that typically has an onset in adolescence. A classification scheme for epilepsy is evolving, but the most commonly used is the International League Against Epilepsy (Epilepsy 1989) and includes approximately 30 distinct syndromes (see Appendix 1). This classification system is being revised, and a proposed revision was published in 2001 (see Appendix 2) (Engel and Epilepsy 2001). Another classification scheme combining EEG, etiology and syndrome features has also been proposed (Hamer and Luders 2001). In summary, remember that patients with epilepsy have seizures, but not all patients who have had a seizure meet diagnostic criteria for epilepsy.

Diagnosing seizures is ideally made by measuring the neuronal activity of the brain by placement of electrodes on the scalp, termed an electroencephalogram (EEG), as well as semiology. Electrode placement has been standardized. Figure 16.1 displays the placement of EEG electrodes with the older 10–20 standard international system for electrode placement which consists of 21 electrodes. Figure 16.2 displays the newer 10–10 standard international system for electrode placement consisting of 64 electrodes. (Society 1986). The semiology of a seizure reflects the evaluation of the behavioral features associated with the period immediately before a seizure (pre-ictal period), during a seizure (ictus or ictal period), and immediately following a seizure (post-ictal period). The time between seizures is termed the inter-ictal period. Seizure semiology (i.e., clinical expression of a seizure) varies depending upon the localization of seizure onset, duration, and propagation pathways of discharging neurons. These are reviewed in detail below (see also Tables 16.6 and 16.7).

Fig. 16.1 The 10–20 International electrode placement system. Electrodes on left are odd numbered, electrodes on right are even numbered

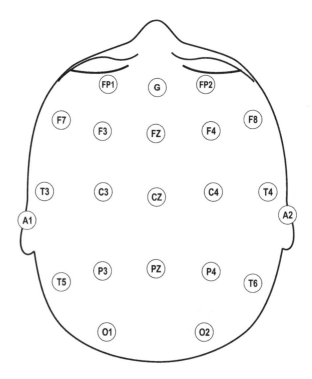

Fig. 16.2 The 10–10 international system for electrode placement. Electrodes on left are odd numbered, electrodes on right are even numbered

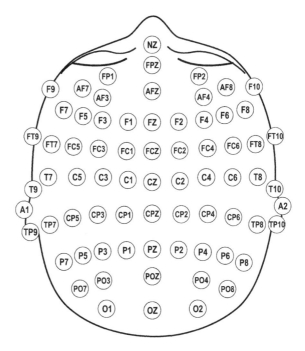

Seizures must be distinguished from other conditions that can mimic features of a seizure. Common conditions that may present with symptoms suggestive of a seizure include:

1. Cardiac conditions

    (a) Structural (i.e., hypertrophic cardiomyopathy, aortic stenosis, etc.)
    (b) Rhythm (i.e., sick sinus syndrome, ventricular tachycardia, etc.)

2. Migraine headache
3. Metabolic conditions (hypoglycemia, hyponatremia, etc.)
4. Parasomnias
5. Paroxysmal movement disorders
6. Psychogenic nonepileptic seizures/attacks (PNES/PNEA)
7. Reflex neurogenic syncope (autonomic neuropathy, vasovagal, post-exertional, cough induced, micturition induced, medication related, etc.)
8. Transient ischemic attack(s)/stroke

Incidence/Prevalence

Seizures/epilepsy is the third most common neurological disorder after headache and dementia (see Table 16.2). In general, the prevalence of epilepsy is thought to be about 1%. The lifetime prevalence rate of epilepsy is thought to be about 3%. The lifetime prevalence rate of seizures is about 9–10%.

Table 16.2 Prevalence of seizures/epilepsy

	Seizures (%)	Epilepsy (%)
Life time prevalence	9–10	3
Point prevalence	0.6	1

Table 16.3 Prevalence of posttraumatic epilepsy

	Epilepsy (%)
Closed head injury	0.7–7.3
Normal Imaging – mild TBI	0.7–1
Normal imaging – moderate to severe TBI	1.2–5
Imaging abnormal	10–25
Open head injury	35–80
Korean and Vietnam Veterans	53

The annual incidence rate of seizures ranges 44–88 per 100,000. It is thought about 300,000 people in the USA have a seizure each year. The incidence rate for seizures is highest for individuals under the age of 2 years old and older than 65 years old.

Injury or infection to the brain increases the risk for developing seizures and epilepsy. A seizure due to injury is termed post-traumatic seizure (PTS), and experiencing two or more seizures after a head injury is termed post-traumatic epilepsy (PTE). While the terminology and definition of PTS and PTE are evolving, it is now considered a seizure is provoked if occurring within 7 days of the traumatic brain injury (TBI). Seizures after the first 7 days are defined as unprovoked. Another differential is for "early" and "late" seizures. Early seizures are those occurring after 24 hours of TBI but within 7 days of TBI. Late seizures are defined as onset of seizures 7 days after injury. The risk of post-traumatic seizures and epilepsy is lowest for closed head injuries and highest for penetrating head injuries. Seizure risk also varies by injury severity, such that individuals with mild closed head brain injury have a risk of seizure that is less than 1% (0.7%), increasing to 1.2% for moderate TBI, and 10% with severe TBI. The risk of PTE is highest for penetrating injuries, and is generally considered to be about 53%. The risk of having an unprovoked seizure *after* a first unprovoked seizure is about 86%. Most post-traumatic epilepsy develops within the first year of injury, but post-traumatic seizures may develop years after the injury. Table 16.3 summarizes prevalence for TBI. Risk factors for developing PTE are depressed skull fracture, brain contusion, intracranial hemorrhage, longer coma duration, lower Glasgow Coma Scale score, and older age at time of TBI.

Seizure Classification

Seizures (as opposed to epilepsy) are classified as being *focal* or *generalized* in onset (see Table 16.4). There is a third classification, unclassified epileptic seizures, which is not reviewed here (see Appendix). *Focal seizures* begin in a focal area of the cerebral cortex and are usually associated with an underlying structural abnormality. Structural abnormalities may include focal developmental malformations (e.g., cortical dys-

Table 16.4 Seizure types

Focal seizures	Generalized seizures
Simple partial (aura)	Absence
Complex partial	Myoclonic
Secondarily generalized	Tonic
	Atonic
	Clonic
	Tonic-clonic

genesis that can be gross or microscopic), vascular malformations, traumatic scarring, or neoplasms. Importantly, focal does not necessarily mean a small circumscribed lesion, as focal seizures often arise from an epileptogenic region that involves a broad area of cerebral dysfunction. *Generalized seizures* have an onset on ictal scalp EEG that occurs simultaneous in both cerebral hemispheres. Diagnosis is currently made by clinical history, seizure semiology, EEG, and often neuroimaging correlation (International League Against Epilepsy 1989).

Focal Seizures

Focal seizures have been divided into simple partial, complex partial, and secondarily generalized seizures. However, the newly emerging diagnostic scheme for epilepsy and seizures has proposed avoiding the terms "simple partial" and "complex partial" to describe seizures. Instead, it is preferred to describe seizures on the basis of whether or not (1) the onset is focal or generalized in origin and (2) if consciousness is lost during the ictal phase of the seizure. However, the new classification scheme remains to be finalized, and we provide the traditional classification of focal seizures below.

1. *Simple Partial*
Simple partial seizures involve at least one focal area of the brain, and do *not* impair consciousness. Clinical characteristics of simple partial seizures can involve sensory, motor, autonomic, or psychic phenomena (e.g., deja-vu, jamais-vu, or dreamy state). Indeed, a simple partial seizure may present clinically as any discrete human experience. A simple partial seizure typically lasts a few seconds, although they can last for a few minutes. Historically, non-motor simple partial seizures were referred to as auras. See Tables 16.6 and 16.7 for localizing details.

2. *Complex Partial*
Complex partial seizures involve at least one focal area of the brain, and impair awareness. Typically, a complex partial seizure starts as a simple partial seizure or aura which evolves to a complex partial seizure with impaired consciousness. During a complex partial seizure, an individual will demonstrate impaired responses to environmental stimuli. Alternatively, individuals may begin with a complex partial seizure without a preceding simple partial seizure or the aura may be forgotten during the complex partial seizure. Complex partial seizure duration varies from a few seconds to a few minutes (average is 83 seconds). This is the most common

type of seizure with 50–60% of all patients with epilepsy having complex partial seizures. The seizure semiology (behaviors during a seizure) often provides major clues as to where seizures start in the brain.

3. *Secondarily generalized seizures*
Focal seizures may evolve from simple partial to complex partial to secondarily generalized seizures. Generalized tonic-clonic seizures have been termed "grand mal" seizures. These characteristic seizures first involve an epileptic cry (air forced out against a closed glottis) followed by generalized stiffening and then bilateral jerking of extremities. The generalized tonic-clonic seizure almost always lasts less than 3 min.

Generalized Seizures

Generalized seizures are currently thought to involve both hemispheres at onset and are classified into six major categories reviewed below. We also discuss febrile seizures separately below, as these may represent either a generalized and/or focal seizure(s):

1. *Absence Seizures*
Brief episodes of impairment of consciousness with no warning and short duration (typically less than 20 s). There are several epilepsy syndromes that include absence seizures including childhood absence, juvenile absence and juvenile myoclonic epilepsy (JME). Childhood absence epilepsy is associated with a 3-Hz spike and wave complexes on EEG. Children can have dozens or hundreds of seizures per day. Onset occurs in childhood or adolescence, and may persist to adulthood. Generally associated with little clinical symptoms other than a brief "blank stare" can be appreciated. These seizures need to be distinguished from attention deficit hyperactivity disorder and complex partial seizures as certain anti-epileptic drugs may be of no benefit or even worsen absence seizures.

2. *Atonic seizures*
Brief loss of muscle tone of the postural muscles. The seizures may consist of a simple head drop or, if proximal leg muscles are involved, a crumple to the floor which can result in injuries. It is often impossible to determine from the clinical history if seizure related falls are due to myoclonic, atonic, or tonic seizures. The term Astatic seizure is often used as an umbrella for "falling seizures." Ictal EEG is similar to tonic seizures, frequently with high-frequency electrographic beta or attenuation.

3. *Clonic seizures*
Brief rhythmic jerking movements of muscles frequently affecting both upper and lower extremities during which consciousness is impaired. Ictal EEG often shows bilateral epileptiform discharges.

4. *Tonic seizures*
Sudden onset of bilateral tonic extension or flexion of the head, trunk, or extremities for several seconds. If standing, patients' may fall to the ground. Seizures typically

occur during drowsiness or just after falling asleep or waking up. EEG correlate of ictal tonic presentation is often high frequency (beta) electrographic discharge with low amplitude.

5. *Myoclonic seizures*
Present as lightning fast-like jerks usually involving symmetric movements of the head, distal limbs or axial musculature. Involvement of the pelvic girdle can result in falls. Myoclonic seizures typically cluster over a period of several minutes with no loss of awareness. These may evolve to a generalized tonic-clonic seizure. Myoclonic seizures may occur as part of epilepsy syndromes with benign prognosis, such as JME, or severe neurodegenerative disorders (e.g., Jacob-Creuzfeldt disease).

6. *Primary generalized tonic-clonic seizures*
Colloquially termed "grand-mal" seizures that present as: (1) tonic extension of extremities (and trunk) for about 20 s followed by (2) clonic synchronous rhythmic muscle movements generally lasting about 45 s. Generalized tonic-clonic seizures are generally associated with a period of post-ictal confusion. This type of seizure does not present with a "warning" compared to a secondarily generalized tonic-clonic seizure which may be preceded by a simple partial seizure. EEG ictal presentation is bilateral spike or polyspikes and slow wave complexes.

Febrile Seizures

Defined as seizure(s) associated with fever, but without evidence of intracranial infectious process or defined cause. For the seizure(s) to be termed febrile, the seizure must occur in children aged 1 month to 5 years of age, and the child must not have a history of neonatal seizure or other unprovoked seizure, and the seizure must not meet criteria for another acute systematic seizure (Guidelines for epidemiologic studies on epilepsy 1993). A febrile seizure is commonly understood as a generalized convulsive seizure, but a febrile seizure may also be focal.

Febrile seizures are common, with an incidence rate of 2–5% of children in the USA. Incidence rates vary worldwide, ranging from a low of 0.35% in Hong Kong to a high of 14% in Guam.

There are two types of febrile seizures, simple and complex. A simple febrile seizure is a generalized seizure lasting less than 15 minutes in duration that is non-focal and do not recur within 24 hours. A complex febrile seizure is a febrile seizure that is focal in onset and/or may be of extended duration (more than 15 minutes in duration), or when a seizure recurs within 24 hours of a another febrile seizure. There is evidence for a genetic predisposition for febrile seizures, and febrile seizures tend to run in families. The genetic basis as not been established for most individuals having a febrile seizure. A history of a simple febrile seizure does not increase the risk for having an unprovoked seizure later in life over the risk for the general population. However, the risk for developing epilepsy is increased with a history of complex febrile seizure, family history of epilepsy, developmental delays, and/or neurological abnormality. A study found 27% of patients having a complex febrile seizure with normal MRI and EEG developed epilepsy. Treatment of febrile seizure has been controversial, and no treatment for seizure (AED medication) is indicated for individuals with simple febrile seizure. Those with increased risk for development of epilepsy (complex febrile seizure, developmental delay, and/or family history of epilepsy) has also not shown clear benefit (reduced risk for onset of epilepsy) from treatment by AEDs.

Seizure Semiology

The importance of seizure semiology is increasingly recognized in the classification and diagnostic categorization of epilepsies (Lachhwani and Kotagal 2006). Moreover, close attention to the behavioral presentation of a seizure, along with an aura/simple partial seizure (if present) can provide useful localization information. A summary of common behaviors during seizures with associated anatomical correlates is provided in Table 16.5. Behaviors that may have lateralizing value are presented in Table 16.6.

Table 16.5 Summary of seizure localization based on behavioral presentation

Location	Behavioral presentation
Frontal lobe	
Dorsolateral	Forced head and eye deviation (termed version) is common. Seizures are typically tonic, but may also be clonic. Disruption of speech common for dominant hemisphere seizures.
Opercular	Swallowing, salivation, speech arrest, facial clonic activity
Orbitofrontal, cingulate, and mesial frontal	Motor agitation, emotional feelings and complex gestural automatisms. The movements can be bizarre and include bicycle pedaling and pelvic thrusting in which awareness is retained and there can be little post-ictal confusion. The vigorous movements combined with emotional expression can lead to a misdiagnosis of psychogenic origin (psychogenic nonepileptic seizures). Clues that argue for epilepsy include the stereotypy and brief duration.
Supplementary motor area (mesial and anterior to primary motor strip)	Asymmetric tonic posturing of bilateral limbs, monotonous vocalization, and variably preserved consciousness.
Motor strip (precentral gyrus)	Focal motor seizures that can evolve to sequential areas of motor strip (Jacksonian March).
Insular Cortex	Rising epigastric sensation, nausea, autonomic changes such as changes in heart rate or piloerection. Gustatory (taste) hallucinations may also be associated with insular cortex seizures.
Left perisylvian fissure	Peri-ictal aphasia.
Temporal lobe	Typical includes wide-eyed stare with behavioral arrest → oro-alimentary automatismsisms → manual autisms (hand washing, picking at clothes).
Mesial	Rising epigastric sensation, fear, deja-vu, jamais-vu, and dreamy states. Olfactory (smell) hallucinations related to anterior mesial (amygdala) involvement. Rising epigastric sensation associated with insular cortex and superior bank of sylvian fissure.

(continued)

Table 16.5 (continued)

Location	Behavioral presentation
Lateral	Posterior lateral temporal onset can present as visual hallucinations. These hallucinations are generally well formed and include people and/or objects. Some lateral temporal seizures can also present with auditory hallucinations. Poorly formed sounds (buzzing) reflects involvement of Heschls gyrus. If sounds are lateralizable (left or right), onset is generally contralateral to where sound is heard.
Anterior/amygdala	Sense of fear or panic is common. Olfactory (smell) hallucinations classically associated with amygdala/uncinate cortex seizures. Smells are usually unpleasant (burning rubber, etc.).
Parietal lobe	In general, parietal lobe seizures can present with somatosensory (tingling or burning) and/or sense of movement. Seizures may propagate frontally or temporally, producing semiology that leads to false localization.
Dominant parietal lobe	Loss of language functions can occur, frequently receptive and/or conductive aphasia features.
Nondominant	Loss of orientation/neglect and metamorphopsia (visual phenomena) and/or asomatognosia (lack of awareness of body)
Anterior	Somatosensory sensation. Somatosensory phenomena may be positive or negative. Positive symptoms reflect tingling, electrical "shock" feeling, sensation that body part(s) is being moved, and/or pain, etc. Negative phenomena include loss of sensation, such as numbness, feeling body part(s) is/are missing, or neglect. Loss of muscle tone is also possible.
Posterior	Immobility and/or visual phenomena. Alteration of vision perception (metamophopsia) and/or complex visual hallucination is common. Can experience perception that objects are closer or farther away or other complex visual distortions. Visual hallucinations are well-formed objects and/or people/animals. Differs from visual hallucinations in that visual phenomena will be of short duration and, commonly, same image(s). Rarely associated with auditory hallucinations at onset.
Inferior	Disorientation and vertigo may be present. Involvement of superior bank of the Sylvian fissure (and/or insular cortex – see mesial temporal lobe) associated with abdominal sensations, including sensation of rising epigastric sensation.
Occipital lobe	Positive or negative visual phenomena most common. Positive visual features are hallucinations of elementary visual phenomena. Typically, these are not well formed and include perception of colors, shapes, and/or lights. Negative phenomena is loss of vision, including scotomas, hemianopsia, or general graying/blacking out of vision (amaurosis). The visual phenomena are contralateral to side of seizure. Post-ictal phenomena can last for hours. Other features include eye movements that may be either tonic or clonic, sensation of eye movements, nystagmus, or eye blinking.
Other Locations	
Hypothalamus (hypothalamic hamarotoma)	Gelastic seizure (e.g., laughing without feeling of mirth) is common. May also present similar to temporal lobe seizures.

Table 16.6 Lateralizing signs during seizures

Behavioral presentation	Localization
Aphasia (expressive or receptive). Post-ictal paraphasias	Dominant (typically left) hemisphere
Auditory phenomena (unformed) such as buzzing, humming, or other nondescript hearing change.	Primary auditory association cortex and Heschl's gyrus
Auditory phenomena (well formed) such as intelligible sounds (song) or voice.	Secondary auditory association cortex
Automatism (unilateral) such as picking at clothes and other nonpurposeful extremity movements.	Ipsilateral to extremity
Dystonic arm posturing (unilateral)	Contralateral to extremity
Eye/head deviation especially immediately preceding secondary generalization	Contralateral to direction of version
Figure four (4) sign (as secondary generalization develops, one arm becomes the extended long stroke of "4" while the other arm is abducted proximally and flexed at elbow completing the "hook of the 4").	Contralateral to extended arm
Lip smacking/chewing movements	Insular cortex
Nose wiping after a seizure (post-ictal)	Ipsilateral to hand used to wipe nose
Talking throughout the seizure/ictal speech	Nondominant (typically right) hemisphere
Urinary urgency sensation before seizure (peri-ictal)	Nondominant hemisphere
Visual phenomena (unformed) sometimes in visual hemifield	Contralateral occipital cortex
Visual phenomena (formed) that includes objects, animals, people, etc.	Contralateral occipitotemporal lobe
Vomiting during a seizure (ictal vomiting)	Nondominant (typically right) hemisphere

Post-ictal Behaviors

After a complex partial or generalized tonic-clonic seizure a patient is typically confused (post-ictal confusion). Individuals have experienced a loss of awareness and suddenly or gradually "return to reality." Individuals may exhibit a range of behaviors and/or emotions. The observation of post-ictal behaviors can assist in identifying the type and localization of seizures (Privitera, Morris, and Gillam 1991). Post-ictal confusion and/or aphasia can last for a few minutes to an hour. Post-ictal aphasia is largely related to extent and duration of seizure. However, seizures presenting with short duration and post-ictal aphasia are often localized to the language dominant perisylvian or lateral frontal area. Post-ictal mood disorders may also occur. These can include symptoms of dysphoria and anxiety. Post-ictal psychosis is a rare, but serious condition. Post-ictal psychosis had been associated with right temporal lobe seizures, but emerging data suggest patients with either right or left hemisphere seizures can develop post-ictal psychosis.

Epilepsy Etiology and Syndromes

Epilepsy is classified according to presumed etiologies and epileptic syndromes, and includes: (1) idiopathic, (2) symptomatic (and probably symptomatic), and (3) familial. In addition, three special epilepsy categories have also been proposed: epileptic encephalopathies, reflex epilepsies, and progressive myoclonic epilepsies (see Table 16.7). Idiopathic epilepsies have no underlying structural brain pathology that can currently be identified nor have any neurologic signs or symptoms. These epilepsies likely have a genetic component. Symptomatic epilepsies are the result of one or more known structural brain lesion(s) that may be developmental (e.g., cortical dysgenesis) or acquired (e.g., traumatic injury). Probably, symptomatic epilepsy syndrome replaces the previous term "cryptogenic" and refers to epilepsies with presumed structural brain lesion that has not yet been identified. Familial epilepsies have a clear genetic component.

In general, the classification system identifies epilepsies according to localization, semiology, and understood etiology. Some selected syndromes are included below, but the focus for the rest of the chapter will be on focal seizures.

Table 16.7 Presumed etiology for epilepsy

Name	Etiology
Idiopathic	Presumed genetic. Etiology is thought to reflect molecular dysfunction such as a channelopathy (disruption of neuronal activity due to dysfunction of
Symptomatic	Related to known structural abnormality.
Probably symptomatic (previously cryptogenic)	Related to a structural abnormality that is not identifiable with current available methods.
Familial	Demonstrated to be genetic. Typically autosomal dominant
Special epilepsy categories	
Epilepsy encephal opathies	Reflects syndromes in which the epileptic abnormalities may contribute to progressive neurologic/neuropsychological dysfunction (e.g., Dravet syndrome, Landau–Kleffner syndrome, Lennox–Gastaut syndrome, West syndrome, etc.)
Reflex epilepsies	Epilepsies associated with specific sensory stimuli (e.g., Idiopathic photosensitive occipital lobe epilepsy, primary reading epilepsy, startle epilepsy, etc.)
Progressive myoclonus epilepsies	Refers to a series of rare epilepsy syndromes all having myoclonic seizures as part of the disease presentation. Includes severe myoclonic epilepsy of infancy (Dravet syndrome), Lafora disease, mitochondrial encephalopathies, etc.

Selected Epilepsy Syndromes

Idiopathic Syndromes

Benign Childhood Epilepsy with Centrotemporal Spikes

Benign childhood epilepsy with centrotemporal spikes (BECTS), also known as benign rolandic epilepsy, typically presents between the ages of 3 and 13 years of age. It is common, accounting for about 24% of all epilepsies in children. The EEG inter-ictally shows very high amplitude sharp waves with a field centrotemporally, involving the precentral and postcentral gyri of the perisylvian region (see Chap. 3 for neuroanatomic reference). Seizures predominately occur during sleep or shortly after awakening. The epileptiform discharges markedly increase in frequency during non-REM sleep. Seizures are focal (simple partial) with onset in the centrotemporal region and spread to adjacent areas and may secondarily generalize. Seizures onset may shift from one hemisphere to the other. Rarely, atypical EEG patterns may present, including continuous spike-and-wave during slow sleep or focal motor facial status epilepticus. Seizure frequency is generally low; although significant variation occurs (about 10% may have only one recognized seizure while about 20% can have multiple seizures in a 24-hours period). Ictal features classically present with motor, sensory, and autonomic symptoms (hypersalivation), generally involving one side of the mouth, face, and throat. Patients may present with drooling, guttural noises, involuntary clonic retraction of one side of the face, tonic contraction of mouth and/or tongue, numbness and/or tingling of hemi-face, lips, and/or gums, and speech arrest. Sensory and/or motor activity of the hand, trunk, and/or leg as well as abdominal pain has been reported. This syndrome as well as *benign partial epilepsy of childhood with occipital paroxysms* is a dominantly inherited condition with normal MRI despite the "focal" EEG findings. Prognosis is generally considered excellent, and BECTS is considered an age-related syndrome, in which almost all patients exhibit seizure remission (so-called "growing out of seizures") by adulthood, often by age 16 years. Treatment may not require medication, and the initiation of AEDs is typically not made until the patient has a second unprovoked seizure. Because seizures almost always disappear by adulthood, medical treatment beyond this point is not needed.

Neuropsychological morbidity was traditionally not associated with BECTS. However, compared to controls, child aged patients have exhibited significantly lower scores on tests of general cognitive function (IQ), attention, memory (short- and long-term), language (e.g., phonemic verbal fluency, comprehension), visuo-perceptual/visuospatial skills, and behavioral problems (e.g., impulsivity, mood lability) (e.g., Elger et al. 2004). Academic problems requiring accommodations is not uncommon. In general, neuropsychologic deficits have been more related to frequency of EEG abnormalities than the number of clinical seizures. Neuropsychological function of adolescents and young adults with remission of BECTS has generally not differed from healthy controls.

Rule of thumb: Benign childhood epilepsy with centrotemporal spikes (aka benign rolandic epilepsy)

- Onset typically 3–13 years of age
- Seizures arise from centrotemporal region (often switching sides)
- Seizures commonly occur during sleep or when walking up
- Considered an age-limited epilepsy syndrome (seizures often remit by 16 years old)
- Neuropsychological deficits: Generally mild in childhood, and include attention/working memory, delayed and immediate memory, phonemic verbal fluency, comprehension, visuospatial, and behavioral problems. Persistent deficits into adulthood *not* generally present, and no long-term cognitive morbidity

Childhood Absence Epilepsy

Childhood absence epilepsy (CAE) is common, accounting for 2–10% of all epilepsies (10–15% of all epilepsies in childhood). The seizures reflect the classic 3-Hz spike and wave complexes on EEG that are often induced by hyperventilation. Clinically, these seizures often present as a brief (few seconds) "blank" stare, although longer seizures up to 20–30 seconds in duration can be associated with automatisms such as blinking or mouth movements. There is loss of awareness, and children have no memory of events during a seizure. There are no post-ictal sensory, motor, or cognitive changes. Onset typically occurs between ages 4–8 years (peak period is 6–7 years old). Children can have dozens or hundreds of seizures per day. These seizures need to be distinguished from Attention Deficit Hyperactivity Disorder (ADHD) and complex partial seizures, as certain AEDs may be of no benefit or even worsen absence seizures. A helpful clinical distinction between absence seizures and complex partial (focal) seizures is the lack of post-ictal manifestations after absence seizures. Prognosis is generally considered quite good (but see below for vocational and psychosocial function in adulthood), with about 80% responding to medication treatment. Complete remission rates are highly variable, but majority of patients with typical CAE remit in late teens to early adulthood. Those patients with generalized tonic clonic seizures are at increased risk for persistent seizures. First line AEDs include ethosuximide and valproic acid as well as lamotrigine and topiramate. Alternatively, carbamazepine and oxcarbazepine exacerbate absence seizures, and gabapentin is ineffective at reducing absence seizures. Exacerbation of absence (and myoclonic) seizures has also been reported for some patients treated with tiagabine and vigabatrin.

Neuropsychological dysfunction has traditionally not been associated with CAE, save for higher rates of diagnosed learning disorders and ADHD. Indeed, as a group, children with CAE have demonstrated overall intelligence quotients (IQ) scores that are slightly above average. However, Fastenau et al. (2009) found that

children with CAE exhibited, as a group, significant deficits in attention/executive/
constructional, language, and learning/memory domains when compared to healthy
siblings within 6 months of the first seizure being recognized. Deficits in children
with idiopathic generalized seizures included attention/executive/constructional,
language, and learning/memory deficits. There were no significant deficits in measures of academic achievement. Similarly, other work has found mild neuropsychologial deficits among children with CAE in attention, memory (visual/nonverbal),
and visuospatial functions. Deficits in language function (verbal fluency, naming,
comprehension) and verbal memory are less consistently found, but both language
and verbal memory deficits have been reported (e.g., Henkin et al. 2005; Pavone
et al. 2001). Psychiatric diagnoses (e.g., Attention Deficit Hyperactivity Disorders
and anxiety disorders) have been reported for over half of patients with CAE.
Duration of seizures, seizure frequency, and AED treatment were associated with
more neuropsychological and psychological problems. While prognosis is generally considered good, long-term outcome studies found patients with CAE at risk
for lower vocational attainment, poor social adjustment, and increased rates of
psychiatric diagnoses in adulthood compared to healthy peers or to patients with
juvenile rheumatoid arthritis (e.g., Wirrell et al. 1997).

Rule of thumb: Childhood absence epilepsy

- Onset typically 4–8 years of age
- Seizures have characteristic generalized 3-Hz spike and wave complexes
- Seizures brief (several seconds) staring spells with loss of awareness
- May remit in adulthood, but some patients continue to seizures into
  adulthood.
- Neuropsychological deficits: Traditionally considered mild to none, but
  new data suggest mild deficits in attention/executive, delayed and immediate memory (visual/nonverbal), visuospatial, and increased rates of learning disorders, ADHD, and anxiety disorders. With seizure remission,
  deficits do not persist into adulthood. However, patients with absence
  seizures in adulthood exhibit neuropsychological deficits.

Juvenile Myoclonic Epilepsy (JME)

Juvenile myoclonic epilepsy onset is usually in adolescence, although occasionally
diagnosis is not made until after the fourth decade. JME is considered an inherited
epileptic syndrome, with six abnormal genes mapped to chromosomes 6 and 15.
It is assumed to be an autosomal dominant disorder with incomplete penetrance.
A relatively common epilepsy syndrome, JME accounts for about 3–12% of all
epilepsies (higher rates reported from hospital records, lower rates from population
studies). Affected individuals usually have three types of seizures: myoclonus,
generalized tonic clonic, and absence. Myoclonic seizures (jerks) with preserved

consciousness is a cardinal feature of JME, and the only seizure type for about 17% of patients with JME. The myoclonic jerks are generally bilateral and involve the shoulders and/or arms, although involvement of the lower extremities, head, or trunk has been reported. Lateralized myoclonus does occur. The majority (about 80%) of patients with JME will present with generalized tonic clonic seizures in addition to myoclonic seizures. While absence seizures are less often found in patients with JME (about 28% of patients), when present, absence seizures are typically the first clinical manifestation of JME. Classically, the seizures are markedly exacerbated by sleep deprivation and occur shortly after awakening. The EEG shows more irregular 3–7-Hz generalized discharges. Brain imaging is normal in patients with JME, although neuropathologic studies have reported microscopic abnormalities (increased partially dystopic neurons, indistinct boundary between lamina 1 and 2 of the cerebral cortex, and irregular columnar arrangement of some cortical neurons termed microdysgenesis). Prognosis is generally considered good, although JME is considered a lifelong condition. Treatment with AEDs (e.g., levetiracetam, lamotrigine, topiramate, zonisamide, valproic acid) is often efficacious in controlling seizures. Vagus nerve stimulation (VNS) implantation has been offered to select patients with medication refractory JME. Surgical resection is *not* indicated for JME.

Cognitive function in patients with JME has traditionally been viewed as unaffected, and IQ is often in the average ranges. However, more detailed neuropsychological studies have demonstrated that patients with JME can exhibit mild deficits in processing speed, attention/working memory, language (confrontation naming and verbal fluency), memory (verbal immediate and verbal and visual delayed), visuospatial, and executive functions (i.e., abstract reasoning, mental flexibility, behavioral inhibition) when compared to matched healthy peers. Patients with JME have more pronounced deficits in executive function than matched patients diagnosed with temporal lobe epilepsy (see below for neuropsychological deficits of temporal lobe epilepsy). An association between neuropsychological deficits and duration of epilepsy has been observed, although this trend disappears for patients with more education (12 years or more), particularly those with college education.

Rule of thumb: Juvenile myoclonic epilepsy (JME)

- Onset typically in adolescence, but diagnosis delayed past 4th decade reported.
- Triad of seizure types: myoclonus, generalized tonic clonic, and absence
- Myoclonus with preserved awareness is the cardinal feature of JME
- Seizures exacerbated by sleep deprivation and 20–30% with photic stimulation.
- Neuropsychological deficits: Generally mild, but deficits in processing speed, attention/working memory, language (verbal fluency, naming), memory (verbal immediate and delayed), visuospatial, and executive functions reported. Most consistent deficits are in executive function, which can be more pronounced than patients with temporal lobe epilepsy. Deficits typically *not* present in adulthood.

Epileptic Encephalopathies (Previously Generalized, Symptomatic Epilepsies)

These epilepsy syndromes have been described as being multifocal or "pseudogeneralized" epilepsies since the EEG have inter-ictal and ictal features of epilepsies with MRI-detectable diffuse or multifocal lesions of variable etiology.

West's Syndrome

West's syndrome accounts for about 2% of all epilepsies, but 25% of epilepsies in the first year of life. Associated with a high mortality rate (5–31%), it is a classic epilepsy syndrome presenting with a characteristic triad of infantile spasms, developmental arrest, and inter-ictal EEG pattern that is distinctively "chaotic" (called hypsarhthmia). The EEG consists of high voltage multifocal spikes, sharp waves, and slow waves in a random distribution usually presenting between the ages of 6–18 months. Diagnosis can be made if two of the three characteristic features are present. "Infantile spasms" has been used to describe the seizure type, and the term infantile spasm has also been used to describe the epilepsy syndrome.

Treatment is usually a course of adrenocorticotropic hormone (ACTH) or prednisone. Second line medication includes several AEDs. However, there is no one treatment that yields satisfactory control, and in some cases, patients with identified focal lesions can obtain reduction in seizures from surgical treatment. Prognosis is generally poor, with a variety of neurologic, neuropsychological, academic, and psychiatric problems. Psychomotor slowing, autistic features, and up to 70% of patients will present with moderate to severe mental retardation. Patients with West's syndrome can develop other types of seizures, and 18–50% develop Lennox – Gastaut syndrome.

Rule of thumb: West's syndrome (aka infantile spasms)

- Onset typically between 6 and 18 months of age.
- Clinical triad of infantile spasms, developmental arrest and hypsarhthmia EEG pattern
- Mental retardation, autistic features, and behavioral problems common.

Lennox–Gastaut Syndrome

Lennox–Gastaut syndrome is rare, accounting for 0.5–4% of all epilepsies, but accounts for about 10% of epilepsy in children with onset of seizures before 5 years of age. A classic epilepsy syndrome often following West's syndrome with a mean age of onset around 27 months of age, with the majority presenting by 6 years of age.

This severe epilepsy syndrome is difficult to medically control, and is characterized by a mix of seizure types (Gastaut et al. 1966; Markand 2003). Seizure types include atonic, atypical absences, and tonic seizures that occur frequently throughout the day. Children may appear clumsy (due to falls) and also present with episodes of eyelid retraction, staring, and apnea. The inter-ictal EEG has a classic generalized 1.5–2.5-Hz slow spike and wave discharge pattern in childhood. In adulthood, EEG abnormalities show multifocal independent epileptic discharges. About 75% of patients with Lennox–Gastaut syndrome have symptomatic epilepsy (identifiable underlying pathologies) including encephalitis/meningitis, brain malformations (cortical dysplasias), tuberous sclerosis, hypoxic/ischemic injuries, other brain lesions (particularly frontal lobe), and/or birth/early infant trauma. Prognosis is considered poor (but is somewhat variable), and patients typically manifest developmental delays, psychomotor slowing, mental retardation, and behavioral problems including autistic features (Oguni et al. 1996). Corpus callosotomy can be helpful in minimizing drop attacks (atonic seizures) (Maehara and Shimizu 2001), and vagus nerve stimulation is considered as a palliative option (Majoie et al. 2001).

Rule of thumb: Lennox-Gastaut syndrome

- Onset typically between 26 and 28 months of age (most by age 6 years old).
- Triad of seizure types: Atonic, atypical absence, and tonic seizures.
- Interictal EEG has classic 1.5–2.5-Hz slow spike and wave discharges
- Mental retardation, autistic features, and behavioral problems common.

Landau–Kleffner Syndrome

Also called Acquired Epileptic Aphasia, it is a rare (less than 1% of epilepsies), but unique, epilepsy syndrome associated with acquired aphasia (receptive and expressive speech) and epileptic discharges of the temporoparietal regions beginning in the first decade of life (Landau and Kleffner 1957; Robinson et al. 2001). Symptoms present after a period of normal motor and language development. Seizure onset is associated with onset of language problems, but deterioration in language can precede the presentation of seizures. Inattention to auditory stimuli and receptive language dysfunction are often the first symptoms of language dysfunction (although initial loss of expressive speech has been reported). In addition to an acquired aphasia, children will often present with a myriad of other psychomotor and behavioral problems and may appear on the autistic spectrum. Prognosis is variable, and some patients do experience an improvement in aphasic symptoms while others do not. Patients with younger age of onset (5 years and younger) tend to exhibit less improvement in language than older patients (6 years old and older). Resolution of language deficits are not strongly associated with resolution of EEG abnormalities, which may decrease with age. Neurological surgery, multiple subpial transection of the epileptic cortex (eloquent language cortex), has shown to improve language function in up to 79% of patients who had been unable to speak for a minimum of 2 years.

Rule of thumb: Landau–Kleffner syndrome (aka Acquired Epileptic Aphasia)

- Onset typically between 3 and 10 years of age (occurs after a period of normal language development).
- Seizures: Clinical seizures may not be present, but epileptic abnormalities on EEG in temporoparietal area required.
- Language decline may precede presentation of seizures.
- Recovery of language function strongly related to age of onset:
- Less than 6 years of age have worse outcome than older patients

Symptomatic or Probably Symptomatic Partial (Focal) Epilepsies

These are epilepsies with focal onset of seizures, and may be amenable to resection of the epileptogenic zone (minimal area of brain tissue needed to be removed for seizure freedom). These include temporal lobe epilepsies, but also other neocortical epilepsies (frontal, parietal, and occipital) as well as Rasmussen syndrome, hemi-convulsion-hemiplegia syndrome, and migrating partial seizures of early infancy. Etiology may be dysplastic tissue, mesial temporal sclerosis, tumor, hemorrhage, or other focal abnormality. Focal epilepsies can present with a simple partial seizure (aura) and/or other semiology (behavioral presentation of the seizure, including aura, and post-ictal phenomena) that provide clues as to localization or hemisphere lateralization of seizure onset (see Tables 16.5 and 16.6).

Temporal Lobe Epilepsy (TLE)

TLE is the most common type of epilepsy, thought to affect 25% of children and 50% of adults with epilepsy. Among patients diagnosed with complex-partial (focal) seizures, 70–90% of patients have seizures arising from the temporal lobe. Patients with mesial temporal sclerosis (MTS), which is neuronal loss and gliotic scarring of the hippocampal formation/mesial temporal lobe structures, are typically medication refractory. Individuals with TLE are often ideal candidates for surgical treatment to achieve seizure control (see section "Neuropsychological (Cognitive and Behavioral) Comorbidity in Epilepsy") (Wiebe et al. 2001). In general, about 60–80% of carefully selected patients are seizure-free at 1 year, although some variability does exist.

Temporal lobe seizures typically involve an aura (Gupta et al. 1983). Although variable, classically, the aura of temporal lobe epilepsy typically involves wide eyed stare followed by oro-alimentary automatisms (lip smacking, swallowing and chewing) and/or automatisms of the upper extremities (pill rolling or picking movements of the hands). Auras typical of mesial temporal onset include rising epigastric sensation, fear, deja-vu, jamais-vu, and dreamy states. Auditory and complex visual auras suggest lateral temporal neocortical onset. Patients with lateral TLE more often report unformed auditory hallucinations (e.g., buzzing or ringing) or sound distortion (e.g., perceive sounds are farther away or differ in pitch or tone). The auditory hallucination may also be a formed sound (e.g., voices of others and/or songs). Other lateralizing features include unilateral automatisms, unilateral dystonic posturing, and post-ictal paraphasias (Chee et al. 1993). Patients with lateral TLE less often exhibit characteristic automatisms (e.g., oro-alimentary) and contralateral dystonia than do patients with mesial temporal lobe onset (Gil-Nagel and Risinger 1997).

Neuropsychological impairment is frequently identified among patients with TLE, and may include deficits in general cognitive ability (IQ), academic achievement, language (i.e., naming and verbal fluency), memory, attention/executive, motor skills, and visuospatial/constructional skills (see section "Neuropsychological (Cognitive and Behavioral) Comorbidity in Epilepsy" for more detail) (e.g., Elger et al. 2004; Fastenau et al. 2009; Hermann et al. 1997; Hermann et al. 2008).

Risk Factors for TLE. Patients suffering from a complicated febrile seizure (characterized by long duration or focal features) are at greater risk (5–20 times) for the development of TLE than patients having no history of complicated febrile seizure (Tarkka et al. 2003). However, individuals with a history of uncomplicated febrile seizure do *not* have an increased risk of TLE over that of the general population. Among patients with identified TLE and hippocampal sclerosis, 40–60% have a history of a childhood complicated febrile seizure.

Pathology Associated with TLE. About 70% of TLE patients have evidence of hippocampal sclerosis. Others may have developmental misgrowth of cortical structures (cortical dysgenesis, cortical malformation), benign growths such as DNET (dyembroplastic neuroepithelial tumor) or gangliogliomas, malignant tumors, or vascular malformations. Some patients have mesial temporal sclerosis plus an additional pathology (dual pathology).

Rule of thumb: Temporal lobe epilepsy (TLE)

Term for epilepsy with seizures arising from temporal lobe. TLE is divided into two types:
1. Mesial temporal lobe seizure onset (MTLE) (account for ~80% of patients)
2. Lateral temporal lobe seizure onset.

Features of MTLE
1. Seizures present with an aura (simple partial seizure before losing awareness).

(continued)

Rule of thumb: Temporal lobe epilepsy (TLE) (continued)

  (a) Most frequent auras associated with MTLE are:
    i. Rising epigastric sensation
    ii. Fear
    iii. déjà-vu
    iv. Pilorection (goose pimples)
    v. Memory flashbacks
    vi. Olfactory hallucinations (uncinate fits)
    vii. Dreamy states
Features of lateral TLE
1. Presentation similar to MTLE, but auras can differ:
  (a) Auditory hallucinations – unformed (e.g., buzzing, muffled sound or ringing).
  (b) Visual hallucinations (unformed figures, objects, rarely faces)
TLE often refractory to medication – about 33% medication refractory in 2009
Seizure freedom in about 70% of selected patients after temporal lobectomy.

Frontal Lobe Epilepsy

Frontal lobe epilepsy (FLE) is less well researched than TLE, but has increased interest. It is estimated that 20% of patients with refractory partial (focal) seizures have frontal lobe epilepsy. Of those patients with FLE, most patients have seizure onset involving the dorsolateral prefrontal cortex. Outcome for patients having surgical treatment is less well known, but recent studies suggest seizure-free rates vary from less than 30–100% of patients. Seizure-free rates are highest for those individuals with a lesion demonstrated by MRI. Seizure-free rates at 1 year for individuals with a demonstratable lesion is about 70%.

Typical features of seizures in frontal lobe epilepsy are seizures of a relative short duration that may occur in clusters which result in no clear loss of awareness. Inter-ictal EEG can be normal, or demonstrate unilateral or bilateral abnormalities that can include the temporal leads. Compared to seizures from the temporal lobe, frontal lobe seizures are often briefer, and involve more motor activity. The behavioral features of frontal lobe epilepsy vary widely depending on localization of onset and propagation (Williamson et al. 1985), and some have behavioral features that may be misidentified as nonepileptic events (i.e., pelvic thrusting and wild random limb movements) (Savqi et al. 1992). The more common seizure types in frontal lobe epilepsy are summarized below:

(a) *Dorsolateral*: Several more typical presentations are described below:

  1. *Focal motor seizures.* Seizures begin with unilateral clonic motor jerks corresponding to the region of the motor strip (precentral gyrus) with epileptic

discharges. The seizure may spread to sequential areas of the motor strip resulting in clonic motor activity as dictated by the motor functional organization of the precentral gyrus (Jacksonian March). Consciousness (awareness) is maintained unless the seizure propogates outside the motor (and supplementary motor) areas of the frontal lobe.

2. *Supplementary motor area (anterior to the primary motor strip) seizures*: Semiology is sudden asymmetric tonic posturing of both limbs, forced head and eye deviation (termed version) away from the seizure focus, monotonous vocalization (or speech arrest), and variably preserved consciousness.

3. *Frontal lobe complex partial seizures.* Seizures present behaviorally as sudden onset of vigorous bilateral motor automatisms of extremities that can appear as nonpurposeful movements or organized purposeful activity (e.g., swimming like arm motions, bicycling, laughing, shouting, etc.). Termed "hypermotor seizures," these are the seizure semiology classically associated with frontal lobe epilepsy. Hypermotor seizures can exhibit aggressive or sexually related behaviors. Most patients (50–90%) have an aura of tightness or tingling of body parts, a vague psychic feeling, or fear. Awareness is lost during these seizures, and the patient is amnestic for the event. These seizures can arise from the frontopolar, opercular-insular, cingulate gyrus (anterior portion), and orbtiofrontal areas (see also below).

4. *Frontal lobe absence seizures (dialeptic seizures).* These seizures, which frequently occur in clusters, involve a sudden arrest in motor/speech activity that lasts several seconds in duration. Awareness is lost during the ictal period, but there is no post-ictal confusion. Subtle automatisms may be present with frontal lobe absence seizures. Can be associated with mesial frontal or orbitofrontal seizure onset.

5. Aphasic seizures. Seizures with speech arrest.

(b) *Opercular:* Seizures behaviorally characterized by swallowing, salivation, speech arrest, and sometimes clonic activity of the face.

(c) *Orbitofrontal, cingulate, and mesial frontal*: Semiology can include motor agitation, emotional feelings and complex gestural automatisms, that are also associated with frontal complex partial seizures (see above and Table 16.6). The behavioral/neurologic features of seizures involving these regions can be bizarre and include "bicycle pedaling" and pelvic thrusting. Consciousness can be retained and there may be little post-ictal confusion. The vigorous movements along with the emotional content can lead to a misdiagnosis of psychogenic origin [see Chap. 17 for coverage of psychogenic nonepileptic seizures (aka psychogenic nonepileptic attacks)]. Clues that argue for epilepsy include the stereotypy and brief duration.

Neuropsychological deficits in FLE have been highly variable, ranging from deficits in attention to gross deficits in attention/executive functions (e.g., planning, initiation, maintaining or altering behavior, and/or anticipating outcomes), language, and motor functions (Risse 2006). Less researched than patients with TLE, patients with frontal lobe epilepsy can exhibit diffuse as well as focal deficits (Risse 2006) (see section "Neuropsychological (Cognitive and Behavioral) Comorbidity in Epilepsy," for more details).

Rule of thumb: Frontal lobe epilepsy (FLE)

Term for epilepsy with seizures arising from the frontal lobes. Patients with FLE often have short seizures, which can present in a myriad of ways, and the behavioral features can easily be ascribed to PNES (i.e., pelvic thrusting).

Seizure freedom is less known, but varies from 30% to 100% of selected patients after frontal resections. Best seizure-free rates among patients with lesional findings on MRI (tumor, focal dysgenesis, etc.).

Parietal Lobe Epilepsy

Like frontal lobe epilepsies, parietal lobe epilepsies are less well researched, but there is increasing interest (Kim et al. 2004b). Focal onset in parietal lobe is relatively rare (6–8% of partial/focal epilepsies). Seizure semiology can present with elemental sensory (tingling, numbness, visual), motor (asymmetric simple motor or automotor), vertigo, psychic/mood, or little semiology (dialeptic) before loss of awareness. Parietal lobe epilepsies can spread to the frontal lobe, and present with clinical features consistent with frontal lobe epilepsy or to the temporal lobe mimicking features of temporal lobe epilepsy. Seizure freedom is reported to vary considerably, and like other focal epilepsies, is higher for those individuals in which a lesion is identified. Seizure freedom (Engle Class I) has been reported to vary from 53% to 88% of patients (Cascino et al. 2005; Kim et al. 2004b).

Neuropsychological dysfunction may involve impairment in language and/or praxis, but there is little neuropsychological data on selected cohorts of patients with parietal lobe focal onset epilepsies.

Rule of thumb: Parietal lobe epilepsy (PLE)

Term for epilepsy with seizures arising from the parietal lobes. Patients with PLE can have seizures that present with features of frontal or temporal lobe epilepsy patients.

Early reports suggest 55–88% of selected patients are seizure free after resections. Best seizure-free rates among patients with lesional findings on MRI (tumor, focal dysgenesis, etc.).

Occipital Lobe Epilepsy

Occipital lobe epilepsy is uncommon (Salanova et al. 1992). Localization is usually suggested by a visual aura. Visual auras include elementary hallucinations such as flashing lights or colors with or without movement. Some may have ictal blindness. Spread to adjacent visual association areas may produce more complex hallucinations of formed objects such as people or illusions such as distortion of proportion, size or contours. Other manifestations may include contralateral eye deviation, blinking, a sensation of eye movement, or nystagmus. Subsequent seizure spread may be to the frontal or temporal lobes just as described for parietal lobe epilepsy.

Rule of thumb: Occipital lobe epilepsy (OLE)

Term for epilepsy with seizures arising from the Occipital lobes. The most common clinical onset is visual aura (about 60%). Visual aura may be simple or complex, and may be positive (shape, animal, face, etc.) or negative (blind spot).

Seizure freedom for selected patients is not well established, and varies from 45% to 85%, with about 60–65% being generally accepted. Patients with developmental lesions (e.g., cortical dysplasia) are less likely to be seizure free (45%) than patients with tumors (e.g., gliomas) (85%).

Neurologic/neuropsychological risks generally include visual field defects and visuoperceptual deficits.

Treatment of Seizures

It is important to note that not all seizure presentations require pharmacological treatment. If, after a first seizure, a neurologic evaluation, EEG and MRI are normal, AEDs are not prescribed and a diagnosis of epilepsy is not made as most will not go on to have a second seizure. As noted previously, as many as 10% of the general population will have a seizure, but only 10% of this population will develop subsequent seizures necessary for the diagnosis of Epilepsy. For our purposes, we will focus on patients diagnosed with epilepsy. Front line treatment is medication. Additional therapies for those patients having seizures despite medication include: (1) diet and behavioral therapies and (2) surgery [including surgical resection and implantation of medical devices including vagus nerve stimulator (VNS) and forms of deep brain stimulator (DBS)].

Medication Treatment

Initiation of AEDs is the front line treatment for patients with epilepsy. Only four frontline AEDs were available prior to 1995. Currently, over a dozen are available, and more are in development. Some AEDs are "broad spectrum" and treat both partial and generalized epilepsies. Others are "narrow spectrum" and may not treat partial epilepsies (i.e., ethosuccimide) or may worsen myoclonic epilepsies (i.e., gabapentin). The recently developed AEDs have not significantly increased the percent of patients who are seizure-free, but do offer different side effect profiles, which are often less pronounced than the older AEDs (see Table 16.8). Side effects can be either positive or negative. For example, topiramate may help with weight loss but can have an adverse effect on cognition in some individuals. Most investigators have found 60–70% of patients with epilepsy are successfully treated with AEDs (e.g., Kwan and Brodie 2000). Alternatively, 30–40% of patients with epilepsy continue to have seizures despite medications.

Table 16.8 Cognitive and behavioral/mood effects of antiepileptic drugs (AEDs)

	Behavior/mood	Cognitive function
Carbamazepine	↓	↓↕
Clonazepam	↓↓↓	↓↓↓
Gabapentin	↓	↓
Lamotrigine	↑[b]	↕?↑
Levetiracetam	↓	? ↓
Lucosamide	?↓	?↓ (dizziness ↓↓)
Oxcarbazepine	↓	↓↕
Phenytoin	↓	↓↓↓
Phenobarbital	↓↓↓	↓↓↓
Pregabilin	↓↑	?↓ (dizziness ↓↓)
Sodium valproate	↓[b]	↓
Tiagabine	↓	?↕
Topiramate	↓↑[b]	↓↓↓[a]
Zonisamide	?↓	?↓↓↓

Note: ↓ = negative impact; ↕ = no meaningful impact; ↑ = positive impact; ? limited or inconsistent data
[a]Some participants exhibit more deficits than others in dose dependent fashion
[b]Reports of positive impact on mood and/or mood stabilization

After failing more than three AEDs, the likelihood of achieving seizure control with another AED trial was found to be around 3 % in one study (Kwan and Brodie 2000) around 3% (Kwan and Brodie 2000). Typically, individuals failing two to three adequate AED trials are labeled as medication refractory (intractable) and considered for surgical intervention. Those who are not surgical candidates can be treated with other therapies (see below).

Refractory Epilepsies

The majority of patients with medication refractory epilepsy have complex partial (focal) seizures of a symptomatic (or probably symptomatic) origin. Patients with focal epilepsy involving the temporal lobes, particularly those with mesial temporal sclerosis (MTS), are typically intractable to medication. Patients with intractable epilepsy are at risk (1 per 200 patient years) for death secondary to a seizure, termed sudden unexplained death in epilepsy or SUDEP (Tomson et al. 2008). In addition, patients with refractory epilepsies are at risk for progressive neuropsychological

Rule of thumb: Refractory epilepsy

- 30 to 40% of patients with epilepsy are currently refractory to medication
- Majority of refractory epilepsies have focal seizures that arise from the temporal lobe
- Seizure freedom with surgical resection occurs in about 70% of patients versus a small minority of patients (< 10%) 3% with subsequent trials of medication, making surgery a highly effective treatment for refractory epilepsy

deficits (e.g., Hermann et al. 2008; Helmstaedter and Kockelmann 2006), psychiatric dysfunction (e.g., Hermann et al. 2000, 2003; Hermann et al. 2008), poor academic achievement (Austin et al. 1998), reduced occupational success, and lower quality of life (e.g., Poochikian-Sarkissian et al. 2007). Alternatively, a landmark randomized study (Wiebe et al. 2001) confirmed the efficacy of seizure surgery for treatment of refractory temporal lobe epilepsy with ~60% becoming seizure-free with temporal lobectomy, but only ~8% becoming seizure-free with continued medication management. While temporal lobectomy carries an approximate 5–10% risk of complications such as death, stroke or infection, the only death in the clinical trial occurred in the medically managed group. Seizure-free rates for selected patients with temporal lobe epilepsies vary, but 60–80% after 1 year is generally accepted, and patients presenting with MTS are typically ideal candidates for surgical treatment to achieve seizure control (seizure-free rates after 1 year above 90% have been reported). Patients with clear TLE, but no MTS can also be good surgical candidates (Ojemann 2006). Thus, seizure control after surgical treatment may decrease the risk of seizure related complications, including death, and can improve quality of life and independence.

The purpose of elective neurosurgical treatment is complete resolution of seizures. However, the determination of "seizure freedom" has varied in the literature, with some experts considering lack of "debiliating" seizures as a good outcome, while other experts argue the term "seizure-free" should equate to having no seizures of any kind. Several classification schemes have been developed, with perhaps the most common being that by Engel et al. (1993) (see Table 16.9). We now summarize the surgical and nonsurgical treatments for refractory epilepsies.

Table 16.9 Engel et al. (1993) classification scale for outcome from surgery for treatment of epilepsy (Adapted from Engel et al. 1993)

Engel class	Seizure outcome
Ia	Seizure-free without auras
Ib	No disabling seizures (e.g., complex partial), but patient may have simple partial seizures (auras).
II	Rare (several per year) disabling (complex partial or complex partial seizures that secondarily generalize) seizures
III	Greater than 50% reduction in frequency of disabling seizures
IV	Less than 50% reduction in frequency of disabling seizures

Surgical Treatments

Surgical interventions for medication refractory epilepsy currently include: (1) surgical resection of brain parenchyma thought to be necessary for cessation of seizures (the epileptogenic zone), (2) hemispherectomy, (3) corpus callosotomy, (4) multiple subpial resection, (5) implantation of vagus nerve stimulator (VNS), and (6) implantation of a deep brain stimulator (DBS). Stereotaxic gamma-knife radiation, in which focused radiation is directed at a specific target intracranially, has also been used, and is briefly described below.

1. *Anterior Temporal Lobectomy (ATL)*
   Surgical resection in which the anterior temporal lobe is resected en bloc. There are multiple ATL procedures, and resections vary from 3 to 8 cm measured from the anterior tip of the temporal lobe. Left (language dominant) temporal resections often include the anterior 3–5 cm of the temporal lobe, while right (nondominant) temporal resections typically involve the anterior 4–8 cm. Extent of resection has traditionally been determined in one of two ways. The first approach tailors the extent of the resection to the patient's pathophysiological findings obtained either extraoperatively or intraoperatively (Ojemann and Valiante 2006). Extraoperative techniques to tailor a resection include placing subdural grid, strip, or depth electrodes in the region of the suspected epileptogenic zone, and typically obtaining ictal onset data. Intraoperatively, surgeons typically rely on inter-ictal epileptic activity to determine the extent of resection. With the tailored approaches, functional mapping is often used to determine eloquent cortex (e.g., language and motor) (Ojemann et al. 1989). The second approach bases the extent of the temporal resection on anatomical standards (Falconer et al. 1955). Resections typically include most of the medial and lateral temporal structures, while much of the superior temporal gyrus is retained in the dominant hemisphere.

(a) *Amygadalohippocampectomy*: In an effort to minimize cognitive/psychological post-surgical deficits associated with standard temporal lobectomy, anatomically standardized operations resecting primarily the medial temporal lobe structures have been developed and gaining popularity (Hori et al. 2003; Neimever 1958; Wieser and Yasargil 1982). These procedures are typically referred to as amygadalohippocampectomy (Neimeyer 1958). There are three more commonly employed routes used to access the medial temporal structures, i.e., transcortical (going through the superior temporal gyrus), subtemporal (going through the basal temporal cortex), or trans-sylvian (going through the middle temporal gyrus) (Olivier 2000; Shimizu et al. 1989). There are also differences in opinion regarding the extent of resection of medial temporal structures (Feindel and Rasmussen 1991), although most contemporary series of patients include a resection of some or all of the hippocampal formation. Whether or not the selected amygadalohippocampectomies actually convey an advantage in terms of either seizure outcome or post-operative neuropsychological functioning remains controversial (Burchiel and Christiano 2006). When the epileptic focus involves eloquent cortex, e.g., primary motor or sensory cortex, Wernicke's or Broca's area(s), resection can be combined with multiple subpial transection (see below). This latter technique utilizes small cuts perpendicular to the cortical surface to disrupt horizontal connections needed for seizure spread, but allow the columnar processing necessary for normal cognitive functioning.

2. *Hemispherectomy*

The removal of all (or most of) an entire hemisphere. There are two common procedures of hemispherectomy, functional hemispherectomy and anatomical hemispherectomy (Schramm 2002). The procedure is generally limited to those patients with functional hemiparesis and severe seizures (e.g., Rasmussen's encephalitis or Sturge–Weber syndrome). While seemingly dramatic, these procedures can offer patients a favorable outcome from a typically crippling epilepsy syndrome, and up to 75% of patients can have a good outcome, defined as no additional significant deteriation of function beyond the neurological and neuropsychological deficits present at time of surgery. Surgical complications do occur, and may include motor, sensory, cognitive, and psychological deficits. A recent study of Rasmussen encephalitis found post-surgical changes in motor (hemiparesis) and sensory (hemianopsy) in all patients. Beyond worsening in motor and sensory function with surgery, neuropsychological functioning remained stable in 52% of patients, worsened in 38% of patients, and improved in about 10% of patients. Language function did not change after surgery in all patients not having pre-surgical language impairment, regardless of side of surgery. Of those with language impairments before surgery, 33% of patients had improved language, 25% worsened, and about 42% of patients did not exhibit meaningful change (Terra-Bustamante et al. 2009).

3. *Corpus callosotomy*

A procedure in which the corpus collusum is transected in order to minimize the spread of seizures from one hemisphere to another. Typically, this procedure is limited to patients with unknown seizure focus or multiple seizure foci with debilitating seizures that are frequently atonic and/or tonic in nature (e.g., "drop attacks"), which can result in injury. Outcome is variable, but the outcome of the procedure is not to decrease seizure frequency per se, but rather to alter the "spread" of the seizures to spare one hemisphere and hopefully limit the behavioral effect of seizures (i.e., preventing drop attacks). Following callosotomy, various disconnection syndromes are present initially, particularly when stimuli are presented to one hemisphere alone (Van Wagenen and Herren 1940). Classic neuropsychologic syndromes of agnosias, apraxias (e.g., alien hand phenomena), alexia, and agraphia have been reported (Gazzaniga 1984; Sass et al. 1988). The severity of disconnection syndrome generally decreases over a period of months such that the deficit is often not appreciable in everyday activities.

4. *Multiple subpial transection*

A surgical procedure in which horizontal axonal fiber tracts in the brain are transected while preserving the vertical oriented axonal fiber tracts (Morrell et al. 1989). The surgery is currently offered to patients with seizure focus in eloquent cortex (i.e., cortex with vital functions such as motor, sensory, or language functions and is increasingly employed with memory functions) (Wyler 2006). This procedure arose from observations that seizures typically propagate along horizontal axonal fiber tracts while cortical functions (motor, language) typically propagate along vertical axonal fiber tracts. Surgical transection limits the spread of seizures. Preliminary studies of multiple subpial resection found benefit of greater than 95% seizure reduction in 71% of patients with generalized seizures, 62% of patients with complex partial seizures, and 62% of patients with simple partial seizures (Spencer et al. 2002). However, data are limited at this time, and concerns remain regarding the long-term outcome for seizure freedom with this procedure.

5. *Vagus Nerve Stimulator implantation*

Vagus nerve stimulation (VNS) is the chronic stimulation of the left vagal nerve by implantation of an electrode attached to the left vagus nerve and a programmable signal generator placed subdermally under the clavicle. Vagus nerve stimulation is approved by the US Food and Drug Administration (FDA) as adjunctive treatment of adult and adolescent patients with refractory complex partial seizures. In general, VNS is thought to benefit about 33% of patients with a 50% or greater reduction in the frequency and severity of seizures. The other 67% of patients obtained no significant benefit. Studies have shown about 10% of patients can become seizure-free. Recent data indicates the benefits of VNS increase after 1 year of treatment, with 12 year follow-up data now available (e.g., Uthman et al., 2004). VNS treatment is typically reserved for patients who are not surgical candidates and/or have had unsuccessful surgical resection procedures. Benefits of VNS have also been observed among a limited number of patients with auras (simple-partial seizures) of relatively long duration. These patients can sometimes turn on the VNS during their auras, which reportedly can lead to the avoidance of the seizure progressing to a complex partial or secondarily generalized tonic-clonic event. The mechanism underlying the benefit of VNS remains unknown, but is thought to reflect alteration of the vagus nerve afferents to the brainstem. This is thought to alter the reticular activating, autonomic, and limbic systems, including the noradrenergic neurotransmitter system. Common adverse effects of VNS include cough, dyspnea, voice alteration (hoarseness), parethesias, and throat pain. Less common adverse effects include left vocal cord paralysis and left lower facial nerve (CN VII) paralysis. There is evidence VNS has a positive effect on depression, and VNS was recently approved for treatment of patients with refractory major depressive disorder.

6. *Deep Brain Stimulator (DBS) implantation*

Deep brain stimulator (DBS) implantation has revolutionized the treatment of movement disorders (see Chap. 19, this volume). DBS is increasingly being applied to medication refractory epilepsy (e.g., Boon et al. 2007; Fisher 2008). DBS surgery involves implantation of very thin electrodes to apply chronic electrical stimulation to brain structures, commonly the thalamus, basal ganglia, or cingulate gyrus. There are two DBS systems, an "open loop" system and a "closed loop" system. The open loop system maintains a static electrical stimulation parameter based on external programming. The "closed loop" system allows for the monitoring and alteration of the electrical stimulation settings by the function of the brain by an implanted recorder and dynamic computer system. Both methods are currently being investigated as adjunctive therapy for refractory epilepsy. Clinical trials continue to determine ideal brain targets and stimulation parameters. Adverse effects of DBS can include infection, hemorrhage, and depending upon stimulation location, aphasia, dysarthria, weakness, as well as cognitive and mood/behavioral effects.

Several studies have reported promising results of long-term high frequency DBS in reducing, and in some cases, eliminating medical refractory epilepsy (Boon et al. 2007; Fisher 2008). Boon et al. (2007) reported outcome of a prospective open label trial of DBS of mesial temporal structures for 10 carefully selected patients. Following at least 1 year of DBS, 1 patient was seizure-free and an additional 6 patients exhibited a greater than 50% reduction in seizures. An additional 2 patients had a 30–49% reduction in seizures. Only 1 patient (10%) failed to respond to DBS. Recently, initial results of a prospective, randomized, double-blind clinical trial of DBS targeting the anterior thalamus in refractory epilepsy known as the Stimulation of the Anterior Nucleus of the Thalamus in Epilepsy (SANTE) were presented (Fisher 2008). At the end of the blinded phase of the study (4 months post-op), 37% of patients receiving DBS exhibited a significant reduction in the median frequency of seizures compared to 14.5% of patients receiving no stimulation. Through the open label period (13 months after DBS surgery), the entire sample (both those in the experimental and control arms) exhibited a 40% reduction in seizure frequency. These results are promising for individuals who have refractory epilepsy and are not candidates for other neurosurgical treatments. Neuropsychological outcome from DBS for medication refractory epilepsy is unknown.

7. Stereotaxic gamma-knife radiation treatment

Gamma-knife radiation treatment uses focused radiation in several beams to target an area of tissue. Each beam alone does not result in brain damage, but the focused concentration of where all the beams converge results in radiation doses sufficient to cause cell death in a pre-planned discrete area. This procedure is particularly well suited to treatment of brain tumors that would otherwise be inoperable. Gamma-knife radiation has also been applied to vascular malformations with favorable outcomes. Recently, sterotaxic gamma-knife radiation has been applied to patients with temporal lobe epilepsy (Regis et al. 1999). A recent multi-center trial reported seizure freedom rates at 36 months post-gamma-knife radiosurgery of 76% in a high dose group (receiving 24 Gy) and 59% in the low dose group (receiving 20 Gy), which approached the seizure freedom rates of standard ATL without the potential surgical risks of infection (Barbaro et al. 2009). The benefits to seizure reduction related to gamma-knife radiation are not immediately appreciated, with the average time to seizure freedom reported to be about 12 months after the procedure (Bartolomei et al. 2008). Interestingly, patients often experience an increase in simple-partial seizures at the onset of seizure reduction (Regis et al. 1999). This coincides with the onset of structural neuroimaging changes 9–12 months after surgery. A long-term (6–10 years) seizure freedom rate (Engle I) is reported to be ~60% (Bartolomei et al. 2008). Neuropsychological outcome from gamma-knife surgery may be better than standard temporal lobectomy, with pilot data finding that a significant decline in verbal memory occurred in 15% of subjects, while 12% of participants exhibited a significant improvement (Barbaro et al. 2009). Another study found a significant decline in verbal memory among 100% of patients ($n = 3$), while no decline in visual memory, IQ, or language/speech measures was evident (McDonald et al. 2004).

Diet and Behavioral Therapies (Ketogenic and Other Diets)

Dietary changes to initiate ketosis represent a first line treatment for epilepsies associated with deficiency in glucose transporter protein and pyruvate dehydrogenase. The ketogenic diet has also demonstrated efficacy for patients with Lennox–Gastaut syndrome. Efficacy for treating symptomatic (or probably symptomatic) epilepsies with complex partial (focal) seizures is unknown. Ketosis occurs when the brain shifts from primary glucose metabolism to ketone body metabolism due to a diet that is high in fats and low in carbohydrates and protein. The fat to carbohydrate and protein ratio is ideally 4:1. While often effective, it is often difficult to maintain this diet over long periods of time and there is a potential long-term health risk from the high lipid diet.

Other therapies for medication refractory epilepsy can include behavioral treatment and hormone treatment. Neither intervention has good support and will not be discussed here.

Presurgical Evaluation

Once a patient has failed to respond to adequate medication trials, surgical evaluation should proceed. The pre-surgical evaluation will typically include a comprehensive neurological evaluation that includes a detailed history, high quality MRI, and video-EEG study (Velis et al. 2007). Neuropsychological evaluation is often ordered, and increasingly considered a core study in the evaluation of surgical candidacy (Baxendale and Thompson 2010; Rausch 2006). Other procedures to identify the seizure focus/epileptic region and/or areas of eloquent cortex include functional neuroimaging studies such as functional MRI (fMRI), SPECT, PET, and/or MEG/MSI studies (e.g., Baxendale and Thompson 2010; Juhasz and Chaugani 2003; Van Passchen et al. 2007; Ryvlin et al. 1998). The Wada's test may also be utilized in surgical planning. SPECT studies, particularly an ictal SPECT can be helpful in localizing the seizure focus (Van Passchen et al. 2007). PET studies can also prove useful in identifying areas of dysfunction not presenting on structural MRI studies (Ryvlin et al. 1998). Often the hypometabolic region is larger than the area generating seizures, even involving the contralateral lobe, which may improve after successful seizure surgery. Finally, MEG and MSI is increasingly used in epilepsy centers to identify inter-ictal activity suggesting the seizure focus (Pataraia et al. 2005). Increasingly, fMRI and MEG/MSI are being used to localize brain functions including language and memory and used to map the area of surgical resection (Baxendale and Thompson 2010; Tovar-Spinoza et al. 2008). Based on these studies, determination as to surgical candidacy is made, and treatment options provided to the patient. We now provide a brief review of the neuropsychological aspects of the presurgical evaluation and then turn our attention to the neuropsychological aspects of epilepsy more generally.

Pre-surgical Neuropsychological Evaluation: Basic Concepts

Pre-surgical neuropsychological evaluations assist in predicting cognitive/psychological risks to surgery (post-surgical cognitive decline), can help to confirm seizure localization in some cases, and can aid in determining probability of seizure-free outcome (e.g., Loring et al. 2009).

In most comprehensive epilepsy centers providing surgery (Level III and IV centers), clinical neuropsychologists are considered core members of the treatment team. One role of the clinical neuropsychologist is to provide consultation to the team and the patient with respect to likely cognitive and psychological risks to undergoing elective neurosurgical treatment. Data a neuropsychologist uses include a pre-surgical neuropsychological evaluation, medical history, results from EEG studies, structural and functional neuroimaging results and/or Wada's test results. Data obtained from various neuroimaging techniques (e.g., structural and functional MRI) and intra- or extraoperative cortical stimulation mapping of language and other cognitive functions can be very helpful in refining prediction for outcome and/or developing rehabilitation/treatment programing (e.g., Baxendale and Thompson 2010). The clinical neuropsychologist should also be aware of the medical aspects of epilepsy which can impact the patient's neuropsychological outcome, as well as the potential impact of AEDs and other medications. Equally important, is providing information about the patient's neuropsychological risks to NOT having surgery (see section "Neuropsychological (Cognitive and Behavioral) Comorbidity in Epilepsy").

Neuropsychological (Cognitive and Behavioral) Comorbidity in Epilepsy

Neuropsychological Prognosis for Patients Diagnosed with Epilepsy

For many epilepsies, particularly idiopathic epilepsies, cognitive and behavioral/mood function had been thought to be generally unaffected. However, more recent data have raised questions about the long-term cognitive functioning and quality of life of patients with epilepsies successfully managed with medication and/or the so-called "benign" epilepsies (e.g., Camfield et al. 1993; Dodrill 2004; Helmstaedter 2004; Hermann et al. 2008; Sillanpaa et al. 1998). Patients with epilepsy have consistently reported higher unemployment, less occupational success, lower educational achievement, and are less likely to marry and have children than are healthy peers in the general population (see Hermann et al. 2008 for review). The etiology for the increased risk of neuropsychological (cognitive and behavioral/mood) dysfunction is multifactorial (e.g., Helmstaedter 2004; Hermann et al. 2008). Variables implicated in the neuropsychological dysfunction among patients with epilepsy include: (1) underlying pathology giving rise to seizures, (2) the epileptic electroneurophysiological dysfunction – particularly frequency and severity of seizures, (3) antiepileptic medications, (4) medical complications (multiple episodes of status epilepticus, falls resulting in head injuries, etc.), and (5) other factors (e.g., psychosocial variables, neurodevelopmental and aging effects) (see Fig. 16.3).

Reviewing this figure highlights the interactive, non-independent inter-relationships of these factors on neuropsychological function, the epilepsy syndrome/underlying pathology, and psychosocial functioning. Neurodevelopmental forces can have positive and negative impacts on neuropsychological function. For example, seizures from the language dominant hemisphere are known to result in inter- and/or intra-hemispheric reorganization of neuropsychological functions, allowing for normal or near normal neuropsychological functioning (e.g., Liegeois et al. 2004; Muller et al. 1999; Satz et al. 1988). In addition, aging processes of the brain also impact patients with epilepsy, in which patients with refractory epilepsy appear to be at higher risk for development of dementia than the general population. Anti-epileptic medication has increasingly been recognized as having adverse neuropsychological effects on the patient, although the magnitude of adverse cognitive effect is generally considered to be small (e.g., Aldenkamp et al. 2003; Gomer et al. 2007; Loring et al. 2007). However, data indicate some AEDs (e.g., benzodiazapines, sodium valproate) can adversely impact neurodevelopmental processes (Olney 2002), and initial data sug-

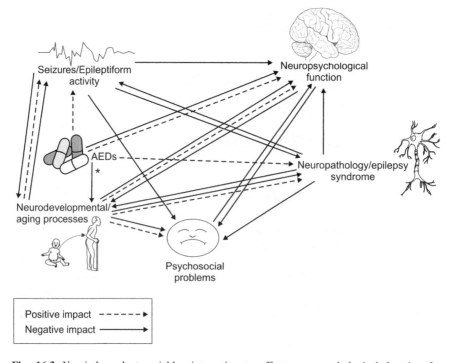

Fig. 16.3 Non-independent variables interacting to affect neuropsychological function for patients with epilepsy.*Note*: * Adverse effect shown only for neurodevelopmental processes and is limited some medications and not all individuals exposed have demonstrated adverse effect (Adapted from Baker and Taylor 2008)

gest the adverse impact of AEDs on neurodevelopmental processes do occur in children prenatally exposed to at least some AEDs (e.g., sodium valproate) (Meador 2008; Meador et al. 2009). The potential for negative impact on neurodevelopmental processes in a child with seizure onset not previously exposed remains to be determined. Clearly, the relative contributions of these variables to neuropsychological dysfunction vary. For example, the impact of underlying neuropathology and seizures in some idiopathic epilepsies is reduced given the lack of structural lesion and often well-controlled seizures, thus leaving the factors largely affecting neuropsychological function to be the epilepsy syndrome itself, effect of AEDs, and potentially, medical complications (Elger et al. 2004).

In the remainder of this section, we review what is known about the neuropsychological functioning of patients with epilepsy, including emerging data suggesting aspects of behavioral and cognitive function are compromised in at least some individuals at seizure onset (Fastenau et al. 2009) or even before the first recognized seizure (Jones et al. 2007). Further, some patients with epilepsy experience a progressive decline in cognitive functioning over time (e.g., Helmstaedter et al. 2003; Seidenberg et al. 2007). We also summarize cognitive differences between the generalized epilepsies and patients with focal seizures, and then review the impact of surgical intervention on cognition.

Cognitive and Behavioral Dysfunction Before Seizure onset?

There is recent evidence to argue the presence of cognitive and behavioral problems are present prior to the first recognized seizure in at least some individuals (Hermann et al. 2008; Jones et al. 2007). For example, Jones et al. (2007) found about one-quarter of children diagnosed with new onset epilepsy exhibited academic problems prior to first recognized seizure. Additionally, nearly half of children with new onset epilepsy exhibited psychiatric and behavioral problems prior to first recognized seizure than age-matched peers (primarily depressive disorders, anxiety disorders, and ADHD). Taken together, these data suggest some epilepsy syndromes manifest with cognitive and psychiatric dysfunction prior to seizure onset.

Cognitive Status at Seizure Onset

In patients with symptomatic epilepsy, the etiology of seizure onset (i.e., brain tumor, cortical dysgenesis, head trauma, encephalitis, developmental disorder) typically produces brain dysfunction independent of the epilepsy syndrome. However, epidemiological studies have found children and adults with new onset epilepsy, including those with idiopathic onset (i.e., unknown etiology for seizures), exhibit some deficits in cognitive functioning, higher rates of academic problems, and increased rates of psychiatric syndromes (e.g., Elger et al. 2004; Davies and Goodman 2003; Fastenau et al. 2009; Noeker et al. 2005; Rutter et al. 1970).

Children. Neuropsychological deficits in attention/executive, memory, processing speed, visuoconstructional/visuospatial skills along with academic achievement problems and psychiatric disorders have been observed for children at seizure onset. Children with idiopathic focal (localized) epilepsies (e.g., benign epilepsy with cen-trotemporal spikes) tend to exhibit the least neuropsychological deficits, with some studies observing no neuropsychological deficits (Fastenau et al. 2009). Patients with symptomatic focal and patients with idiopathic generalized epilepsies tend to exhibit neuropsychological deficits. While academic problems have previously been reported among children with first onset epilepsy, Fastenau et al. (2009) did not find deficits in academic achievement in a well-controlled study of children with a variety of epilepsy syndromes. Indeed, the authors argued that neuropsychological evaluation in children with one or more identified risk factors for cognitive deficits may provide an avenue to arrest or reduce the adverse affects of epilepsy and neuropsychological deficits on academic development. The risk factors for neuropsychological dysfunc-tion in children with a first recognized seizure were: (1) multiple unprovoked sei-zures [odds ratio (OR) = 1.97], (2) use of antiepileptic medications (OR = 2.27), (3) symptomatic/cryptomgenic etiology of seizures (OR = 2.15), and (4) epileptiform discharges on the EEG at first recognized seizure (OR = 1.90). The presence of all four risk factors increased the risk of neuropsychological deficits within 6 months of first recognized seizures to three times that of their healthy siblings. The adverse effect of seizures (electroneurophysiological dysfunction) on neuropsychological function is clear for both children and adults, and in children can serve as a biomarker for deficits in processing speed and other neuropsychological functions. Interestingly, research has found children with first recognized seizure do not consistently exhibit MRI structural abnormalities (Fastenau et al. 2009; Hermann et al. 2008).

Adults. Neuropsychological deficits in memory, attention/executive, reaction time, and visuomotor tasks have been observed in at least some patients at the time of first recognized seizure.

Taken together, greater neuropsychological and behavioral/psychiatric problems are observed among patients with epilepsy around the time of first recognized sei-zure, arguing against the possibility neuropsychological deficits merely reflect a progression of disease based on the adverse impact of recurrent seizures and/or AEDs. However, decades of research with patients having medication refractory epilepsy has established greater neuropsychological dysfunction with earlier age of onset and longer duration of seizures, raising the clear possibility that at least some epilepsy syndromes are a progressive disease.

Epilepsy as a Potentially Progressive Disorder

There has been interest for many years in determining whether epilepsy syndromes contribute to declines in physiological and neuropsychological status over time (e.g., Hermann et al. 2006, 2008; Seidenberg et al. 2007; Strauss et al. 1995). While the majority of these studies have used a cross-sectional design, several longitudinal studies have reported data more recently. Longitudinal data provide actuarial data for change in cognitive, behavioral, and brain neurophysiology over time among patients with epilepsy (Seidenberg et al. 2007; Hermann et al. 2008). Further, Seidenberg et al. (2007) argued for including a healthy control group in order to recognize change in neurocognitive functioning. Longitudinal studies without control groups failed to recognize decline, as this can be obscured by practice effects related to repeat testing (e.g., Helmstaedter et al. 2003; Holmes et al. 1998). More specifically, recent studies have demonstrated that patients with epilepsy often fail to show normal improvements in scores with repeat testing (practice effects) exhibited by healthy controls (e.g., Seidenberg et al. 2007; Thompson and Duncan 2005). While evidence for frank deterioration in neuropsychological function over time has varied, more robust findings for decline in memory is evident (Hermann et al. 2006; Seidenberg et al. 2007).

In general, duration of epilepsy, age of seizure onset, as well as seizure frequency play a role in the occurrence of progressive cognitive decline (Dodrill 1986; Jokeit and Ebner 2002; Jokeit and Ebner 1999; Oyegbile et al. 2004), although not all studies have found this relationship (Holmes et al. 1998). While it has been suggested the impact of duration of epilepsy on cognitive decline may also reflect the impact of chronic AED use and inter-ictal epileptiform activity (Thompson and Duncan 2005), research with children and adults with first onset seizure and naive to AEDs exhibited neuropsychological dysfunction, arguing that neuropsychological dysfunction is not due to AED use (although clearly can be further adversely affected by AEDs) (Fastenau et al. 2009). At least one study has also suggested that experiencing two or more different seizure types correlates strongly with poor outcome over time (Dodrill et al. 1984). Seidenberg et al. (2007) suggested a 3- to 4-year follow-up period is sufficient to detect change over time, but argued changes in cognition may be more apparent with longer test–retest time intervals.

Cognitive deterioration across epilepsy syndrome types is quite variable, although certain syndromes are more associated with cognitive dysfunction (e.g., temporal lobe epilepsy) than others (benign epilepsy syndromes). For example, patients with temporal lobe epilepsy are generally considered to be at high risk for cognitive morbidity, with data suggesting at least 20–25% experience a progressive decline in cognitive function over time, defined as 3–7 years (Hermann et al. 2008; Seidenberg et al. 2007). Moreover, patients with Lennox–Gastaut and Landau–Kleffner syndromes often exhibit catastrophic cognitive impairments, including mental retardation in the former and acquired global aphasia in the latter. In contrast, patients with JME tend not to exhibit neuropsychological impairment in adulthood, arguing against long-term adverse cognitive effects. Similarly, long-term cognitive outcome for patients with benign childhood epilepsy with centrotemporal spikes (rolandic epilepsy) is thought to be good, although mild neuropsychological dysfunction is found in childhood. Thus, cognitive dysfunction is often present across epilepsy syndromes, but evidence for cognitive deterioration is limited to a subset of epilepsy syndromes (e.g., temporal lobe epilepsy).

Neuroimaging has also found structural and functional brain abnormalities which support the hypothesis that uncontrolled (medication refractory) epilepsy is a progressive disease. Most of these studies have been conducted in patients with

TLE, and indicate patients often exhibit significant abnormalities that extend outside of the epileptogenic temporal lobe (Hermann et al. 2003). Using volumetric MRI analysis, TLE patients exhibited significant reductions in (1) total cerebral tissue, (2) white matter volumes, (3) neocortical thickness, (4) parietal and frontal lobes, and (5) thalamic volumes as compared to normal controls (Bernasconi et al. 2004; Bernasconi et al. 2005; Gong et al. 2008; Hermann et al. 2003; Keller and Roberts 2008). While some data suggest extra-temporal atrophy may represent early cerebral damage, increasing evidence suggests such abnormalities are progressive in nature and likely due to structural brain changes associated with ongoing seizure activity (e.g., deafferentation of white matter following chronic seizure occurrence). A recent diffusion tensor imaging (DTI) study found that fronto-temporal white matter integrity is disrupted by seizure activity in TLE patients in the hemisphere ipsilateral to seizure onset (Lin et al. in press). In addition, studies have demonstrated prefrontal metabolic abnormalities among patients with TLE using both PET (Jokeit et al. 1997) and magnetic resonance spectroscopy (MRS) (Mueller et al. 2004). The metabolic abnormalities can normalize following treatment resulting in seizure freedom (Cendes et al. 1997). The forces affecting the extent and progression of impairment appears to reflect a combination of noxious and beneficial factors impacting the brain (e.g., underlying disease pathology, duration and type of seizures, chronic AED exposure, seizure freedom, psychosocial variables, neurodevelopmental/aging forces).

Neuropsychological Profiles

Below, we summarize the neuropsychological findings for patients with both generalized epilepsy syndromes and focal epilepsies.

Generalized Epilepsy Syndromes

In general, generalized seizures are more likely to impair cognitive functions than are partial seizures, particularly for patients with multiple episodes of status-epilepticus (Dodrill 1986; Hennric Jokeit and Schacher 2004). While there are a number of different primary generalized epilepsy syndromes, the onset of seizures in all these syndromes is defined as involving electrical discharges that appear simultaneous throughout the brain on scalp EEG. In actuality, there is debate over whether seizures originate in the thalamus or the cortex (Holmes et al. 2004; McCormick 2002; Slaght et al. 2002). It also known that frontal lobe structures play a significant role in generalized epilepsies (Pavone and Niedermeyer 2000). Accordingly, patients with generalized epilepsies have exhibited impairment in functions associated with the frontal lobes (executive functions), such as mental flexibility, working memory, and task shifting. Concordantly, MRI morphometry has revealed frontal lobe abnormalities in patients with primary generalized epilepsy (Savic et al. 1998).

Neurocognitive Profiles in Focal Epilepsy and the Impact of Surgical Intervention

There is a vast literature examining the cognitive and emotional/psychiatric functioning in patients with focal epilepsy, particularly for TLE. This emphasis reflects TLE being the most common focal epilepsy syndrome, and the predominant subset of patients referred to epilepsy surgery programs. The surgical evaluation process has allowed extensive data to be collected across electroneurophysiological, neuroanatomical (gross to molecular level), neurophysiological, neurological, neuropsychological, psychiatric, psychological, quality of life, as well as a variety of psychosocial/cultural variables. The goal for the collection and analysis of data has been to establish seizure focus and propagation as well as predict surgical outcome (seizure freedom, cognitive, psychiatric) to improve quality of life and reduce morbidity/mortality.

Neuropsychological outcome is increasingly considered an important marker of successful seizure surgery outcome (e.g., Baxendale et al. 2006; Hermann and Loring 2008; Lineweaver et al. 2006), and several variables have consistently shown to reduce risk for cognitive morbidity following seizure surgery (longer duration of seizures, mesial temporal sclerosis, impaired pre-surgical memory scores, Wada's test failure when testing the ipsilateral side, etc.) (e.g., Glosser et al., 1995). Detailed below, prototypical neuropsychological profiles that have lateralizing/localizing value (e.g., material-specific memory deficits in TLE) have been identified. In this section, we will also discuss other schemas for conceptualizing or predicting the deficits associated with TLE that go beyond the prototypical models. We also summarize the more limited research on the various extratemporal epilepsies. Finally, the major findings related to predicting surgical outcome is detailed for patients with TLE.

Findings in Temporal Lobe Epilepsy

Preoperative: For many years, the prototypical pattern of deficit in presurgical TLE patients has been described as a material-specific pattern of memory dysfunction (Milner 1958). The lateralization of dysfunction has been used to predict the side of seizure onset (see predicting side of seizure, below). In particular, greater auditory memory deficits are often observed in patients in language-dominant TLE, while visual memory deficits have been more associated with nondominant TLE (Blakemore and Falconer 1967; Jones-Gotman 1986; Loring et al. 1988; McDonald et al. 2001; Milner 1968b; Pillon et al. 1999; Wilde et al. 2001). This finding has also been bolstered by neuroimaging studies that have found that auditory/verbal and nonverbal/visual stimuli can preferentially activate the left or right MTL, respectively (Golby et al. 2001; Powell et al. 2005). However, the "text-book" profile for temporal lobe epilepsy has not been found consistently (Barr et al. 1997; Pigott and Milner 1993; Wilde et al. 2001). Indeed, nonverbal/visual memory deficits associated with nondominant hemisphere dysfunction have been particularly difficult to establish. Overall, material-specific memory dysfunction can be observed in presurgical TLE patients, and individuals with TLE can exhibit a range

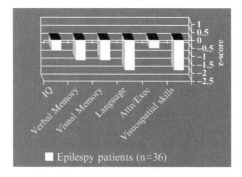

Fig. 16.4 Pre-surgical neuropsychological deficits for adults with temporal lobe epilepsy

---

Rule of thumb: Neuropsychological domains impaired in TLE

- Memory (may be material specific, or generally impaired verbal/visual memory)
- Attention/executive
- Language (confrontation naming, word reading, semantic verbal fluency)
- Visuospatial/constructional
- IQ and/or achievement
- Fine motor (grooved pegboard)

---

of other deficits, including impaired speech (particularly visual or auditory naming and verbal fluency), attention/executive, and visuospatial/constructional functions. Finally, it is not uncommon for patients with TLE to exhibit reduced overall IQ as well as academic achievement. For example, Fig. 16.4 graphs the average performance of adult patients with TLE ($n=36$) who underwent pre-surgical evaluation at the University of South Florida Epilepsy Center (Fig. 16.4). Our data are similar to other pre-surgical findings.

Language deficits and seizure lateralization: Seizure lateralization has been predicted by naming deficits (Busch et al. 2005). Busch et al. provided a regression equation using the Boston Naming Test (BNT) to aid in preoperative seizure localization. Hamberger and colleagues have also introduced an auditory naming task that may also have value in predicting preoperative seizure lateralization (i.e., Columbia Auditory Naming Test) (Hamberger and Seidel 2003; Hamberger and Tamny 1999). However, these data are limited, and there are no consistent findings with respect to auditory naming failure and seizure lateralization (Hermann et al. 1988b). While the predictive value for seizure lateralization of naming tasks remains to be determined, extensive research finds that patients with TLE, particularly those with dominant seizure onset, are more likely to experience deficits in naming ability (e.g., confrontational naming, naming to description) than healthy controls and patients with extratemporal seizure onset (e.g., Hamberger and Tamny 1999; Mayeux et al. 1980). Left TLE groups tend to perform worse than right TLE groups on visual confrontational naming tasks (Hamberger et al. 2010; Hermann et al. 1988a, b; Langfit and Rausch 1996), although the right TLE groups often perform worse than healthy controls (Langfit and Rausch 1996).

The confrontation naming deficits among patients with TLE can be extensive. Patients with left (dominant) TLE are impaired at naming famous faces (Drane et al. 2008; Glosser et al. 2003; Seidenberg et al. 2002), and at least two of these studies suggested these deficits may be worse following ATL resection. Drane et al. (Drane et al. 2008; Drane et al. 2004) have recently extended these findings to include other visually complex item categories (e.g., famous landmarks, nonunique animals) even when performance is normal on a standard naming test [i.e., Boston Naming Test (BNT)]. The broader naming deficits in TLE are supported by functional imaging that highlight a critical role for the anterior temporal lobes in naming certain object categories (Damasio et al. 1996; Griffith et al. 2006).

Deficits in verbal fluency (i.e., generating items from categories and/or letter fluency) are commonly found among patients with TLE (Troster et al. 1995). However, pre-operative deficits in semantic fluency (category fluency) have not shown consistent value in seizure lateralization, since impaired scores are observed for patients with either dominant or nondominant temporal lobe epilepsy (Bartha et al. 2005; Joanette and Goulet 1986; Martin et al. 1990), and frontal lobe epilepsy (Drane et al. 2006). Semantic fluency requires both an executive component mediated by frontal lobe regions (i.e., organization/retrieval from semantic memory stores as well as initiation of action and self-monitoring) (Sylvester and Shimamura 2002) and a semantic memory component thought to be mediated by the temporal lobes (Martin and Fedio 1983). Patients with frontal lobe seizure onset can be distinguished preoperatively from patients with TLE using a semantic fluency paradigm that contrasts cued and uncued performance (Drane et al. 2006). Similarly, performance on letter fluency tasks can be impaired preoperatively due to both frontal lobe and temporal lobe dysfunction (Helmstaedter et al. 1996; Martin et al. 2000). Thus, simply having a poor score on a semantic or phonemic verbal fluency task may not be of localizing or lateralizing value, but may be helpful for localizing (temporal vs frontal) if the component parts of the tests are examined.

Visuospatial and visuoperceptual deficits are frequently found among patients with TLE. These deficits may be more pronounced in patients with nondominant (right) TLE, but the lateralizing aspect of visuoconstructional deficits are not consistent, with both left and right TLE patients performing poorly (see Lezak et al. 2004).

Adults and children with TLE may demonstrate deficits in executive functioning tasks (Hermann and Seidenberg 1995; Keary et al. 2007; Kim et al. 2007; Martin et al. 2000; Rzezak et al. 2007). The "nociferous cortex hypothesis" of Wilder Penfield is sometimes invoked to explain this phenomenon (Penfield and Jasper 1954), in which epilepsy disrupts widespread neural networks. Functional neuroimaging data have demonstrated patients with TLE often show hypometabolism of the frontal lobes that correlates with executive dysfunction (Jokeit et al. 1997; Takaya et al. 2006).

With the exception of interest in visual memory functioning, less work has been focused on the nondominant TL in the context of epilepsy. While current visual memory test scores and memory complaints are not strongly associated, most neuropsychological studies do not adequately assess function of the right (nondominant) temporal lobe (see Chap. 3 this volume). For example, route learning/way finding is rarely clinically assessed, yet several experimental studies suggest performance on these tasks is compromised by right anterior TL damage (Spiers et al. 2001). Similarly, patients with right (nondominant) TLE often exhibit object recognition deficits, and deficits in identifying famous faces and some animals has been found among patients status post-right ATL (Drane et al. 2004, 2008; Seidenberg et al. 2002). Clinically, patients with these deficits have greater difficulty recognizing familiar individuals, which seems to contribute to compromised social functioning.

Taxonomic description of neuropsychological function in epilepsy. A new approach to studying the neuropsychologic aspects of epilepsy has been to assess if distinct patient groups could be empirically derived based on similarities and differences in presurgical neuropsychological function (Hermann et al. 2007). Among patients with TLE, three distinct cognitive phenotype patient groups emerged; (1) minimally impaired, (2) predominately memory impaired, and (3) memory, executive, and speed impaired. The minimally impaired group accounted for 47% of the total sample. This group did not differ from healthy controls in regards to IQ or perception. While scores on measures of immediate and delayed memory, confrontation naming, executive control processes (e.g., generative fluency), and psychomotor speed were significantly below the mean of healthy control group, the difference in scores was no more than one (1) standard deviation (SD). Thus, these lower scores are probably not clinically meaningful. Structural neuroimaging found the minimally impaired group exhibited hippocampal volume atrophy, but no other significant differences from the control group. The predominately memory impaired group included about 27% of the TLE sample. As a group, immediate and delayed memory scores were more than 2 SDs below the mean of the healthy control group, and also displayed mild deficits in all remaining cognitive domains (IQ, perception, language, executive, and psychomotor speed). This patient cluster exhibited greater structural brain abnormalities, with more atrophy of the hippocampus along with significantly less total cerebral brain volume and CSF volume. The memory, executive, and speed impaired group included about 29% of the TLE patients. As a group, this patient taxonomy exhibited the greatest neuropsychological impairment, scoring 2 or more SDs below controls on measures of IQ, immediate and delayed memory, language, executive, and psychomotor speed. In contrast to the primarily memory impaired group, the most pronounced deficits were in executive and psychomotor speed. The third cluster tended to be the oldest sample, having the longest duration of epilepsy, taking the most antiepileptic medications, and showing the greatest volumetric brain abnormalities. Volumetric brain abnormalities included marked hippocampal atrophy and significant changes in total cerebral tissue, reduced gray and white matter, and greater CSF volume. This group also exhibited the worst cognitive course of the three samples.

The material-specific pattern of memory dysfunction model may be impacted by other task parameters and disease-related variables. For example, material-specific findings may be easier to detect when examining both learning and recall patterns rather than only examining one trial learning (Jones-Gotman et al. 1997; Majdan et al. 1996). Further, material-specific findings may be altered by side of seizure onset (Vannest et al. 2008; Weber et al. 2007), and both temporal lobes may eventually be impacted by a chronic duration of unilateral TLE (Cheung et al. 2006). While this review highlights considerable variability in the pre-surgical neuropsychological presentation of patients with epilepsy, patients experience *better* seizure control and *better* functional outcome when the prototypical neurocognitive profiles line up with other diagnostic findings (e.g., EEG, MRI) (Holmes et al. 2003; Lineweaver et al. 2006). We now turn to post-operative neuropsychological findings.

Post-operative findings. While it is increasingly appreciated that meaningful post-operative neuropsychological deficits should mark a clear adverse comorbidity to neurosurgical treatment to be avoided (e.g., Hori et al. 2003; Loring et al. 2009), patients can exhibit post-operative declines in neurological and neuropsychological function. A common neurologic deficit of a standard ATL is a visual field defect due to resection of some optic radiations of Meyers loop resulting in a superior quadrantopsia. Decline in memory, particularly among patients having dominant (left) ATL, can occur (e.g., Chelune et al. 1993; Lineweaver et al. 2006). Indeed, 10–50% of patients having had an ATL will exhibit a decline in memory (Lineweaver et al. 2006; Martin et al. 1998) that is greater than expected for practice and error effects (e.g., reliable change). While the rate of decline in memory may seem excessive, keep in mind that 20–25% of patients with medication refractory epilepsy have exhibited declines in memory over a period of several years, and that there is also a risk for death due to SUDEP in medication refractory epilepsy.

Language/naming decline after ATL is also not uncommon. Patients having dominant TL resections may exhibit significant declines in naming (~40), while those undergoing nondominant TL resection typically do not (Davies et al. 1998; Hamberger et al. 2010; Hermann et al 1999; Martin et al. 1998; Saykin et al. 1995). The role of the hippocampus versus extramesial temporal involvement for naming was recently demonstrated by Hamberger et al. (2010), in which visual naming was affected by hippocampal resection while auditory naming was not. This pattern highlights the differential involvement of the dominant TL in naming abilities, with the hippocampus being implicated in visual, but not auditory, naming. While the BNT is clearly affected by ATL (e.g., Hamberger et al. 2010), Drane et al. (2006) suggest the BNT may lack sensitivity to some language problems experienced by patients following ATL, since the BNT does not include specific item categories most impacted by ATL surgery.

Standard anterior TL resection typically does *not* lead to declines in basic language function (comprehension, repetition, and expression) (Saykin et al. 1995). While classic aphasia is not present following ATL, decline in semantic (category) fluency following dominant ATL resection does occur. While a decline in semantic verbal fluency following nondominant TL resection can occur (Martin et al. 1990), but more pronounced adverse affects on semantic verbal fluency generally occurs for patients with dominant ATLs (Jokeit et al. 1998). Post-operative decline is typically *not* observed on letter fluency tasks. Rather, patients whom are seizure-free can exhibit a post-operative improvement in performance. The improved performance is thought to reflect the pre-surgical widespread disruption of neural networks by epilepsy (see Nociferous Cortex hypothesis below) (Helmstaedter et al. 1998).

Improved neuropsychological function following ATL has been reported for patients who are seizure-free. Patients who underwent a nondominant (right) TL can exhibit an improvement in verbal memory post-operatively (e.g., Martin et al. 1998).

Resolution of seizures can result in significant improvement on neuropsychological tasks associated with frontal lobe function (Hermann et al. 1988; Martin et al. 2000), suggesting the distributed networks are functioning better in the absence of electrophysiological disruption. Indeed, functional neuroimaging studies have found frontal lobe activation "normalizes" for some patients who are seizure-free after ATL (Maccotta et al. 2007).

Frontal Lobe Epilepsy

Research examining the neuropsychological functioning of patients with frontal lobe epilepsy (FLE) is less extensive than for TLE (e.g., Helmstaedter 2004; Jobst et al. 2000). Patients with FLE (children and adults) often exhibit deficits in attention/executive functions (working memory, response inhibition, complex problem solving, verbal fluency, design fluency) and motor functions (psychomotor speed, coordination, motor sequencing and bimanual hand movements) when compared to controls and patients with TLE (Helmstaedter et al. 1996; Hernandez et al. 2002; McDonald et al. 2005; Milner 1968a; Upton and Thompson 1996; but see also Cocoran and Upton 1993). Fluency, both verbal and design, is often impaired among patients with FLE. Deficits in semantic and phonemic verbal fluency can occur. Action (verb) fluency is also decreased in FLE patients (Drane et al. 2006). Design fluency can be impaired in FLE patients relative to other epilepsy patients or healthy controls, with some studies suggesting lateralization to the nondominant hemisphere (Helmstaedter et al. 1996; Jones-Gotman and Milner 1977; Suchy et al. 2003), but not consistently (McDonald et al. 2005). Other areas of impairment include: (1) cost estimation (Upton and Thompson 1996), (2) reasoning (Upton and Thompson 1999), determining temporal order (McAndrews and Milner 1991), and social cognition (e.g., humor appreciation, recognition of facial emotion, perception of eye gaze expression) (Farrant et al. 2005). Helmstaedter (2001) reported patients with FLE had more behavioral problems than patients with TLE and healthy controls. Alternatively, patients with FLE had less behavioral problems than patients with frontal lobe structural lesions.

Memory impairment among people with FLE can be similar to patients with TLE. However, the type and severity of memory deficits can differ from that observed in TLE. For example, worse performance may be found on memory tasks requiring efficient encoding and/or retrieval (list learning tests). Patients with FLE also exhibit greater deficits in release of proactive interference, such that earlier memory interfere with learning new information (Pigott and Milner 1993). Patients with FLE also have difficulty recalling the temporal order of when events/information occurred/learned (Milner et al. 1985; Milner et al. 1991).

In summary, patients with FLE present with a variety of deficits involving motor functioning, executive control processes, attention, speed of processing, aspects of memory, and possible behavioral abnormalities. While overlap in neuropsychological deficits exist between patients with TLE and FLE, there also appear to be some distinct neuropsychological differences between patients with FLE and TLE, that may yet be useful for confirming the region of seizure onset (i.e., differences in reasons for memory deficits, complex motor programming, etc.).

Post-operative decline in motor and neuropsychological functions can occur with unilateral frontal lobe resections (Helmstaedter et al. 1996; Jobst et al. 2000). McDonald et al. (2001) also reported post-operative patients with FLE did not display release from proactive interference, and there was no difference between the TLE and FLE groups in terms of consolidation of stimuli (i.e., they showed similar rates of retention over trials).

Posterior Cortical Epilepsy

Posterior cortical epilepsies (PCEs) is a term to describe patients with seizures arising from the parietal, occipital, or occipital border of the temporal lobe (Dalmagro et al. 2005). Referrals for surgical evaluation to epilepsy centers is rare, accounting for less than 10% of surgical patients, but do respond favorably to surgical treatment for carefully selected patients (Binder et al. 2008; Blume et al. 1991).

Neuropsychological studies of PCE are emerging (Binder et al. 2008; Blume et al. 2005; Luerding et al. 2004). Defects in visual processing are common, and vary from visual field cuts to deficits in facial processing, color perception, object localization, object recognition (including letters/words), and other visuospatial/visuoconstructional skills (Kiper et al. 2002). Deficits in sensory discrimination, arithmetic, and language functioning (spelling, reading, etc.) have also been reported. Patients with seizure onset involving the mesial occipital lobe exhibited more visual-field defects (e.g., 40–50%) than patients with lateral occipital lobe seizure onset (e.g., 0–18%). Patients with seizure onset involving the parietal lobes tend to exhibit deficits in visuoperceptual/ visuospatial and/or visuoconstructional deficits (Siegel and Williamson 2000). Children with occipital lobe seizure onset exhibited academic problems, psychiatric disorders (i.e., primarily depression), and visuospatial deficits (including problems with face processing) (Chilosi et al. 2006).

Post-operative data are generally lacking, but surgical resections risk visual field defects (42% of occipital lobe epilepsy experienced new or increased field cuts), Following resections for PCE, an index of nonverbal general cognitive function (WAIS-R Performance IQ) mildly declined, while verbal IQ remained stable and some performances on measures of executive functions improved.

Factors That May Obscure Neuropsychological Profiles in Presurgical Epilepsy Patients

A variety of factors can obscure neuropsychological deficits attributable to the underlying epilepsy syndrome/pathology. These variables reflect effects from treatment (effect of AED medications), comorbid medical and psychiatric conditions, acute ictal/inter-ictal epileptiform activity, test selection, emotional/mood, task engagement/effort and/or unrelated disease variables (sleep deficits) (see Fig. 16.3). As potential sources of error, these variables can obfuscate dysfunction due to underlying disease and/or effect from seizures, and lead to error in studying neuropsychological functioning of patients with epilepsy.

As noted earlier, many AEDs can have both positive and negative impacts on neuropsychological function (Loring et al. 2007). While AEDs might improve function by reducing or eliminating seizures, AEDs effect of lowering neuronal excitability can lead to cognitive deficits. For example, topiramate may adversely affect attention, verbal fluency, and processing speed, which is entirely separate from the effects of the underlying neuropathology (Kockelmann et al. 2003). The effects of AEDs can be quite pronounced in some individuals, thereby confounding the ability to identify any lateralizing or localizing neuropsychological deficits. Adverse effects from medication could also lead to underestimating the patient's level of cognitive function. Knowledge of the impact of AEDs is critical to interpreting neuropsychological test results. In general, we do *not* advocate a patient withdrawing AEDs prior to a neuropsychological evaluation, as this increases risk for seizures and related medical morbidity/mortality. Discontinuation of AEDs should only be done with supervision of the patients treating physician.

Medical and psychiatric conditions comorbid with epilepsy can also introduce measurement error into neuropsychological assessment (Lezak et al. 2004). Seizures may develop following a head injury or be the presenting symptom of brain tumor(s), stroke, or encephalitis. The primary disease or injury contributes uniquely to the patient's pattern of dysfunction, and there may be multifocal dysfunction related to brain tumor(s) as well as the cerebral dysfunction of epilepsy. For example, patients with focal TL seizure onset resulting from post-traumatic epilepsy may exhibit significant executive dysfunction due to the head trauma. Psychiatric comorbidities, particularly depression and anxiety symptoms, are higher for patients with epilepsy than the general public (Blumer et al. 1995; Manchanda 2002). Scores on neuropsychological tests can be adversely affected by depression and anxiety (Lezak et al. 2004).

Finally, there is growing awareness that acute ictal or inter-ictal epileptiform discharges can alter neuropsychological functioning. While the impact of epileptiform activity can accentuate lateralized dysfunction in the case of focal seizure onset (Privitera et al. 1991), it can also obscure this pattern when there is secondary generalization or non-focal inter-ictal discharges (Aarts et al. 1984; Aldenkamp and Arends 2004; Binnie 2003; Kasteleijn-Nolst Trenite and Vermeiren 2005).

Problems with features of test design and selection can also muddle the interpretation of neurocognitive data. For example, it is frequently argued that neuropsychological tests are not particularly sensitive to nondominant mesial temporal functions, thought to reflect "visual" memory functions (Jones-Gottman 1996). For example, the Family Pictures subtest of the Wechsler Memory Scale, 3rd edition (Wechsler 1997) contributes to the Visual Memory index from this battery, yet variance of the test loads on a verbal factor (Dulay et al. 2002). Thus, patients whom have had a dominant (left) TL resection can exhibit a decline on Family Pictures, as well as the Visual Memory index to which it contributes (Chapin et al. 2009). Thus far, it has been extremely difficult to develop a visual memory test that does not allow for verbal processing/mediation of information. Similarly, more complex list learning tasks place greater demands on executive systems than do less complex contextual memory tasks (e.g., story recall) (Tremont et al. 2000), and list learning can be impaired due to lesions in many brain regions (Umeda et al. 2006).

Overall, prototypical neuropsychological profiles can be identified in some cases of epilepsy, but have not been identified in others. There are many potentially confounding factors that can make it challenging to obtain an accurate baseline measure of neuropsychological function in patients with epilepsy. We believe it is increasingly possible to recognize and control for variables that can potentially adversely affect neuropsychological function. In this manner, one may be able to better assess neuropsychological deficits and predict surgical outcome.

Predicting Seizure Freedom, Side of Seizure Onset, and Cognitive Outcome Following Epilepsy Surgery

Predicting Seizure Freedom from Epilepsy Surgery

Seizure-free Rates

With selected patients with TLE, up to 90% of patients have been reported to be seizure-free at 1 year, but vary from study to study (Wiebe et al. 2001). Reasons for the variability are not entirely clear, but include center differences in patient selection, surgical techniques and outcome classification system used (Ojemann and Jung 2006). It is generally accepted that 1-year seizure-free rates for patients with TLE undergoing an ATL is ~70%. Recent long-term longitudinal data report 10-year seizure-free rates ranging from 37% to 80%. Overall, patients with mesial temporal sclerosis as the sole pathology is associated with the highest seizure freedom at 1 year (90+%), and are most likely to remain seizure-free at 10+ years after surgery. Also, many patients are not "cured" of their epilepsy and remain on AEDs (Andermann et al. 1993). It can be viewed that epilepsy surgery has taken an intractable patient and made them responsive to medication. Thus far, laterality of epileptic zone (right versus left) TLE is not a predictor of being seizure-free.

Variables Predicting Seizure Remission

Factors that predict seizure remission have been an area of aggressive research. Recent data suggest neurological and demographic variables provide the best predictors of being seizure-free (unilateral EEG abnormalities, single pathology of mesial temporal sclerosis, duration of seizures, age of seizure onset). Neuropsychological variables have shown less predictive value, but significant variance to lateralizing seizure onset or predict seizure outcome has been demonstrated in some cases (e.g., Hennessy et al. 2001; Helmstaedter and Kockelmann 2006; Keary et al. 2007; Sawrie et al. 1998; Seidenberg et al. 1998). In addition, it is important for the neuropsychologist to provide input to the epilepsy surgery program regarding the potential neuropsychological risks with surgery. It can be the case in which a patient may present with neurological findings supportive of having a good seizure-free outcome, but at the risk of pronounced neuropsychological deficits could out weight the potential benefits of a patient becoming seizure-free (Hermann and Loring 2008). The variables found to predict being seizure-free is presented below. A more detailed review of evidence-based neuropsychology for predicting neuropsychological outcome follows.

Importance of brain pathology in predicting seizure freedom. The brain pathology underlying epilepsy can be the best predictor of seizure freedom. Meta-analysis (Tellez-Zenteno et al. 2010) found patients (with either TLE or extratemporal epilepsy) exhibiting a lesion by MRI or histopathology were 2.5 times (95% CI 2.1, 3.0, $p < 0.001$) more likely to be seizure-free than patients without a lesion. Patients with TLE were 2.7 times more likely to be seizure-free. Among patients with extratemporal lobe epilepsy, patients with a lesion were 2.9 times more likely to be seizure-free.

Mesial temporal sclerosis (MTS) is the most common pathology found in patients with TLE. MTS is defined as gliosis and loss of neurons within the hippocampal formation. Hippocampal sclerosis is associated with loss of neuron density in the CA1, hillar regions, and CA3 of the hippocampus. The CA2 area is often spared. MRI findings of MTS include decreased volume associated with increased fluid attenuated inversion recovery (FLAIR) and T2 signal of the hippocampas. MTS is the sole pathology in about 65% of adult cases. Isolated MTS is associated with an especially good surgical outcome, with about 90% of patients remaining seizure-free at 1 year, and 80% seizure-free at 10 years (Cohen-Gadol et al. 2006) (see Table 16.10).

When the MRI is negative in temporal lobe epilepsy, pathology after en bloc resection often shows "microscopic" abnormalities deviating from the normal cortical structure. A panel of neurologists and neuropathologists in 2004 described and categorized these abnormalities (Palmini et al. 2004), which include architectural abnormalities of laminar or columnar organization or dysmorphic neurons.

Table 16.10 Impact of presurgical structural abnormality on seizure freedom after anterior temporal lobectomy

Years seizure-free	Percent of patients seizure-free	
	Structural abnormality (%)	No structural abnormality (%)
2	89 ± 5	77 ± 18
3	83 ± 6	64 ± 20
5	72 ± 7	58 ± 21
10	56 ± 9	40 ± 2

Surgical outcome for temporal lobectomies with pathology showing dysplasia has ranged from 60% to 70% free of disabling seizures (Engel class I) with a mean follow-up duration of 2.8–4.4 years. Seizure-free outcome is less positive than for isolated MTS, presumably because the microdysgenesis is more diffuse and less circumscribed than MTS.

Neurological and Demographic Variables Predicting Seizure Remission

The most important variables predicting seizure freedom includes results from EEG, structural MRI, age at time of surgery, and duration of epilepsy. A summary of the effects of these variables on seizure remission is below.

1. Unilateral inter-ictal EEG with seizure focus restricted to unilateral hemisphere.
2. Presence of exclusively ipsilateral temporal inter-ictal epileptiform discharges.
3. Presence of structural abnormalities, including focal cortical dysgenesis, cyst, or mesial temporal sclerosis (MTS).
4. Younger patients are more likely to be seizure-free.

   (a) Younger patients (<30 years of age) at time of surgery are more likely to be seizure-free
      i. $94\% \pm 5\%$ were seizure-free at 2 years
      ii. $89\% \pm 6\%$ were seizure-free at 3 years
      iii. $78\% \pm 8\%$ were seizure-free at 5 years
      iv. $66\% \pm 10\%$ were seizure-free at 10 years
   (b) Middle aged patients (30 ± 59) recently found to have comparable likelihood of being seizure-free (Grivas et al. 2006).
5. Shorter duration of pre-operative epilepsy increases likelihood patient will be seizure-free (less likely to relapse) (see Table 16.11)

Risk Factors for Surgery Failure (Continued Uncontrolled Seizures)

1. Presence of bilateral EEG abnormalities.
2. Presence of secondarily generalized tonic-clonic seizures with TLE.
3. No structural pathology with high resolution MRI (imaging negative).
4. Contralateral memory function intact on Wada's test (TLE only).

Table 16.11 Duration of epilepsy as predictor of seizure freedom after anterior temporal lobectomy

Years seizure-free	Percent of patients with refractory epilepsy seizure-free after anterior temporal lobectomy	
	<20 years of epilepsy (%)	20+ years of epilepsy (%)
2	92 ± 5	82 ± 10
3	86 ± 7	77 ± 10
5	80 ± 8	60 ± 12
10	69 ± 10	37 ± 15

Neuropsychological variables predicting seizure remission: Evidence-based Neuropsychology: In general, neuropsychological data are not helpful in predicting seizure outcome. However, some studies have shown neuropsychological data incrementally improves prediction of seizure freedom (Hennessy et al. 2001; Potter et al. 2009; Sawrie et al. 1998). Hennessy et al. (2001) found impaired verbal memory was associated with better seizure-free outcome for patients having a left temporal lobectomy. Potter et al. (2009) observed that an index of language function that included confrontation naming along with nonverbal memory added unique variance to predicting seizure freedom beyond that provided by demographic variables (side of surgery, age of epilepsy onset) and MRI findings of hippocampal sclerosis. Overall, the multivariate prediction model provided accurate classification of 93% of the patients whom were seizure-free and not seizure-free.

Predicting Side of Seizure Onset

In general, electroneurophysiological and structural neuroimaging are the most powerful predictors of side of seizure onset. Ictal EEG remains the gold standard for assessing side of seizure onset. Additional data, including MRI structural imaging to identify structural pathology as well. In cases in which the seizure onset cannot be well lateralized and localized, PET studies, SISCOM and MEG/MSI are increasingly being employed to identify the epileptogenic and/or seizure onset zone.

Neuropsychology Variables Predicting Side of Seizure Onset: Evidence-based Neuropsychology

While neuropsychologial deficits have long been associated with side of surgery, only more recently has the incremental variance of neuropsychological data to determining side of surgery (side of seizure onset) been explored. Neuropsychological data do provide significant prediction to lateralizing side of seizure onset (e.g., Akanuma et al. 2003; Busch et al. 2005; Drane et al. 2008; Hamberget et al. 2010; Helmstaedter and Kockelmann 2006; Jones-Gottman et al. 1993; Keary et al. 2007; Kim et al. 2004a; Kneebone et al. 1997; Moser et al. 2000; Rausch and Babb 1993; Sass et al. 1992; Seidenberg et al. 1998). Indeed, Sawrie et al. (2001) found logical memory scores to significantly improve prediction of seizure lateralization among patients with bilateral hippocampal atrophy. While memory scores are generally found to be predictive of side of seizure onset, other neuropsychological measures of language [confrontation naming (BNT) and WRAT-III word reading], and executive functions (Wisconsin Card Sorting Test) have also shown predictive value. Keary et al. (2007) found that a multivariate model provided the correct lateralization of seizure onset in 69% of mixed left and right TLE cases. It should also be noted that Wada test results also have predictive value (and may be more predictive) to lateralize side of seizure onset (Perrine et al. 1995).

Predicting Memory Impairment following ATL: Evidence-based Neuropsychology

Defining post-surgical outcome as a marker of surgical success (Hermann and Loring 2008), much attention has been focused on predicting the relative risk of decline for patients with TLE and represents an area of evidence-based neuropsychology. A constellation of variables have consistently shown to be predictive of neuropsychological outcome (see below). Among these, particularly strong predictors are the neuropsychological presurgical test scores, which provide unique variance to predicting memory outcome, and form a cornerstone for evidence-based neuropsychology practice and research (e.g., Baxendale et al. 2006; Chelune 1995; Chelune and Najm 2001; Helmstaedter 2004; Hermann and Loring 2008; Lineweaver et al. 2006; Martin et al. 1998). As an example, Chelune and Najm (2001) report a relative risk for a post-surgical memory deficit that is 4.9 times greater for individuals with memory scores above 90 (mean 100 and standard deviation 15) compared to those with memory scores below 90.

Hippocampal Adequacy versus Hippocampal Functional Reserve

Chelune (1995) detailed two perspectives for predicting post-surgical cognitive outcome from epilepsy surgery. One hypothesis was the *functional reserve of the contralateral hippocampus* predicted post-surgical memory outcome (functional reserve hypothesis). The second hypothesis, known as the *functional adequacy* model, predicted the functional adequacy of the ipsilateral hippocampus tissue resected would determine the risk for material specific memory decline.

The *functional reserve* hypothesis was based primarily on studies documenting severe amnestic disorders of patients with bilateral mesial temporal lobe dysfunction and in several cases, bilateral temporal lobe resection (Scoville and Milner 1957). Additional support was provided by data from Wada's testing, as patients with poor memory when the contralateral (e.g., remaining) temporal lobe was tested (injecting the ipsilateral side) exhibited more memory deficits post-surgically. However, the presence of a functionally intact contralateral hippocampal structure has not predicted material specific memory impairment following unilateral ATL.

The *functional adequacy* model has been supported by data that the functional adequacy of the ipsilateral hippocampus (memory functioning of the temporal lobe structures to be resected) better predicts material specific memory declines after ATL. From this model, it is predicted that individuals with left (dominant) TLE with intact memory function, are likely to experience more pronounced decline in verbal memory than patients with left TLE whose left hippocampal memory functioning is impaired. This has generally been supported, particularly the observation that patients with high pre-surgical memory functioning are at greater risk for significant declines in memory (both verbal and visual) than those patients with low average or poor pre-surgical memory functioning.

Cognitive Outcome from Anterior Temporal Lobectomy

Overall, $10\% \pm 0.6\%$ of TLE patients undergoing ATL experience a significant decline (defined by change in scores that is statistically significant in group studies) in memory. When controlling for practice effects and error, $18\% \pm 50\%$ of patients exhibited declines on at least one memory test (Baxendale et al. 2006; Dikmen et al. 1999; Lineweaver et al. 2006; Martin et al. 1998). Individuals with MTS and lower presurgical memory scores are significantly less likely to exhibit a decline in memory than individuals with average or better memory scores. Fewer patients with nondominant (right) TLE whom undergo a right ATL will exhibit a significant decline in visual memory (or verbal memory) and some may have an improvement in verbal memory test scores. Indeed, Martin et al. (1998) found 31% of patients having a right ATL scored better on a measure of verbal delayed memory. This same study also found 16% of patients having a left ATL also scored significantly better on this verbal memory test. Lange et al. (2003) completed a cluster analysis and found several common memory outcomes. Following left ATL, about 53% of patients exhibited impaired verbal and visual memory scores. The other 47% of patients exhibited impaired verbal memory (immediate and delayed), but average visual memory scores. Following right ATL, a small majority (59%) of patients exhibited poor performance on visual memory tests but performed normally (if not somewhat better than pre-surgical performances) on verbal delayed memory tasks. The other 42% of patients having had a right ATL performed poorly on both verbal and visual memory tests. Other changes with right ATL may also include reductions in an individual's ability to appreciate the nonverbal cues to interpersonal interactions. For example, appreciation of facial emotional recognition is associated with nondominant (right) amygdala function, and impaired appreciation of fearful expressions has been found in patients following right ATL (McClelland et al. 2006). Interestingly, only patients with early onset epilepsy (less than 6 years of age) exhibited a deficit in appreciating fearful facial expression.

Long-term neuropsychological outcome data suggest individuals undergoing left temporal lobectomy may exhibit decline in verbal memory for up to 2 years after surgery (Alpherts et al. 2006). Individuals having a right temporal lobectomy had an overall increase in verbal memory scores at 6 months after surgery, but these gains were lost at 2 years after surgery. Relatively little memory change has been observed in memory from 2 to 6 years after surgery. The best predictors of post-operative memory scores 6 years after surgery were side of seizure (left TLE had lower scores than right TLE), pre-operative verbal memory scores (higher scores more predictive of decline), and age at surgery (older patients at increased risk for memory decline).

Evidence-based Neuropsychology: Variables Important in Predicting Post-surgical Neuropsychological Outcome

1. *Presence of hippocampal/mesial temporal lobe sclerosis*
   Memory decline. In general, the risk for material specific memory decline *decreases* in patients with hippocampal sclerosis. Decreased neuronal density (scelrosis) of the CA1, CA3, and hillar regions is associated with worse verbal memory (e.g., story passage, verbal-paired associates, word lists) (Sass et al. 1990).
   Language/naming decline. The risk of significant dysnomia following ATL is decreased when MTS is present (Davies et al. 1998).

   - 19% of patients with MTS exhibited decline in BNT scores
   - 80% of patients without MTS exhibited a decline in BNT scores

2. *Pre-surgical neuropsychological immediate and delayed memory scores.*
   In general, the better (more intact) a patient's neuropsychological memory is prior to surgery, the greater the person's risk will be for memory decline. This is particularly true for left TLE patients with verbal memory functioning that is average or better when compared to peers (Baxendale et al. 2006; Chelune 1995; Chelune et al. 1998; Chelune and Najm 2001; Lineweaver et al. 2006; Sawrie et al. 1998).

   (a) Chelune (1995) reported patients undergoing left TL, about half (45.7%) of patients with WMS-R Verbal memory index scores 90 or greater exhibited a 10 or more points decline in verbal memory upon post-surgical evaluation. About 1/3 (36.7%) of patients with verbal memory index scores between 80 and 89 exhibited a 10 point or more decline after surgery. Among patients with verbal memory index scores of 79 or below, only 5% exhibited a decline of 10 or more points.

       i. Patients with Memory Index scores greater than 90 (mean of 100 and standard deviation of 15) at baseline have a 4.9 times greater likelihood of exhibiting a memory deficit post-operatively than patients with baseline memory scores that are less than 90.

   (b) Material-specific memory decline with right ATL is less consistent, but most experts agree decline in visual memory tasks is likely among patients with average or better visual memory test scores that undergo a right ATL, particularly if there is no right hippocampal sclerosis or other structural lesion.

   (c) *Pre-surgical Wada's test results.*
       Evidence-based practice for Wada's test has become increasingly complex. The relative incremental validity of Wada's test results over neuroimaging and neuropsychological data continue to be debated (e.g., Andelman et al. 2006; Baxendale et al. 2008; Elshorst et al. 2009; Loring et al. 2009). Memory decline is less likely among patients in which memory recall is

impaired when the contralateral temporal lobe is injected (testing of the ipsilateral temporal lobe), but memory is intact when the temporal lobe to be resected is injected (testing the contralateral temporal lobe function) (e.g., Andelman et al. 2006).

Pre-surgical neuropsychological memory scores and Wada's test scores may not be redundant. Naugle et al. (1993) found Wada's test scores and neuropsychological test scores were independent predictors of post-surgical WMS-R memory index scores. However, others (Baxendale 2009; Lineweaver et al. 2006) have argued that Wada's test scores do not add meaningfully to predicting post-operative memory outcome.

(d) *Presurgical IQ*

Patients with higher cognitive functioning (better cognitive "reserve") typically have a better outcome from surgery overall. Patients presenting with impaired memory scores, but IQ scores in the average ranges, are at less risk for substantial declines in memory than those patients with neuropsychological memory scores being in the average ranges.

3. *Duration of epilepsy*

Patients with a longer duration of epilepsy are at less risk for post-surgical cognitive decline (but likely have poorer neuropsychological function prior to surgery).

4. *Age at onset of seizures*

Patients with early age of onset epilepsy are at decreased risk for significant decline in confrontation naming following left ATL.

5. *Type of surgery*

(a) Post-surgical memory decline (decrease in verbal memory test scores) may be less with more focused resections (amygdalohippocampectomies) as compared to standard ATL (Elger et al. 2004; Lacruz et al. 2004), although this is disputed. Change in language functioning (e.g., scores on confrontation naming and verbal fluency tasks) are not significantly affected by extent of resection, but often decline among patients who are left hemisphere language dominant and undergo a left ATL.

(b) Extent of superior temporal gyrus resection correlated with decline in BNT scores among patients undergoing left ATL. Most patients undergoing left ATL will exhibit a decline in BNT scores; however, 24% of one series did not exhibit a significant decline.

Other Points/Factoids for Predicting Neuropsychological Outcome from Epilepsy Surgery

1. There is evidence for extra-temporal lobe dysfunction in TLE, particularly for frontal lobe dysfunction associated with reduced PET activity in the ipsilateral frontal lobe of patients with medically refractory TLE. With good post-surgical outcome (e.g., remission of seizures), PET activity in the ipsilateral frontal lobe (as well as neuropsychological test scores) often improve (but see above regard-

ing 6-year neuropsychological outcome) (e.g., Jobst et al. 2000). This may reflect the effect of the epileptic focus negative effect on ipsilateral brain function, and the so-called "nociferous cortex" hypothesis (Penfield and Jasper 1954).

2. Many patients experience a transitory period of more diffuse cognitive dysfunction following ATL, which generally resolves within days to several months. More chronic cognitive dysfunction with ATL at 6 months is usually limited to material specific memory loss and sometimes a decrease in language (e.g., confrontation naming and verbal fluency).

3. Post-surgical decline in memory, and also non-memory functions, occurs in a proportion of dominant hemisphere ATL patients when evaluated several (5–10) years after surgery (Helmstaedter et al. 2003). Likewise, Alpherts et al. (2006) found a decline in verbal memory scores from 6 months post-operative evaluation to 2 years post-operative evaluation among individuals having left or right temporal lobectomies. Individuals exhibited no significant change in memory scores from 2 years to 6 years post-operative follow-up evaluations.

4. Cognitive outcome is better for patients whom are seizure-free versus those patients who do not become seizure-free. However, Alpherts et al. (2006) report memory outcome assessed 6 years after surgery was not related to being or remaining seizure-free.

Impact of Wada's (Intracarotid Amobarbital/Methohexital) Procedure for Predicting Outcome

Wada's test is, arguably, the gold standard for evaluating the lateralized functional neuroanatomical organization of language and memory (Baxendale 2009). Predicting neuropsychological outcome from Wada's test remains an important variable for neuropsychologists to consider (Loring et al. 2009). Some comprehensive epilepsy centers have replaced Wada's test with fMRI and/or MEG; however, predicting neuropsychological outcome from these procedures remain less well understood than Wada's test, and research suggest data obtained from Wada's test are, to some extent, independent from those of fMRI or MEG. This may well be related to the behavioral affect of the procedure. Wada's test assesses behavior with inactivation, while fMRI and MSI assess behavior with activation (Loring & Meador 2008). Predicting outcome from Wada's test will be discussed in terms of language dominance and side of anticipated surgery (see Table 16.12 for summary). Glosser et al. 1995 prediction estimates below assumes a valid Wada's test (good behavioral response to anesthesia with contralateral hemiparesis, hemianesthesia, angiogram demonstrating normal cerebral vasculature, adequate patient cooperation, and the examiner administered Wada's test correctly). If EEG is used, EEG should demonstrate adequate ipsilateral hemisphere slowing during the administration of the to-be remembered items)).

Table 16.12 Relative risk for decline in memory and language function after ATL

	Ipsilateral language	Contralateral language	Bilateral language
IAP Memory			
Ipsilateral +/contralateral +	↓↓	↓↓	↓↓
Ipsilateral +/Contralateral −	↓	↓	↓
Ipsilateral −/Contralateral +	↓↓↓↓	↓↓↓	↓↓↓
Ipsilateral −/Contralateral −	↓↓↓	↓↓↓	↓↓↓
IAP Language			
Language loss	↓↓↓	↓	↓↓

Language Dominant to Ipsilateral Side of Surgery

Memory adequate with ipsilateral injection but poor for contralateral injection. This test result is favorable. Decreased risk of memory decline following surgical resection.

Memory adequate with ipsilateral and contralateral injection. This test result is somewhat favorable, but there is considerable risk for verbal memory decline. Extent of risk largely dependent upon neuropsychological verbal memory test scores (average or better scores at high risk) and structural MRI. Some risk also for "visual" memory decline.

Memory poor with ipsilateral injection and adequate with contralateral injection. This test result is a "failure." High risk for memory decline. See "Wrong-way" Wada section.

Memory poor with ipsilateral injection and contralateral injection. This test result is a "failure." However, relative risk must be weighed against pre-operative neuropsychological memory test scores. Poor memory pre-operatively reduces relative risk of pronounced memory decline following surgical resection, and raises concern Wada's test was invalid. The relative potential benefit of seizure freedom and outcome must be balanced upon the functional level of the patient. Among patients with poor memory on neuropsychological functioning, but functioning independently, surgical resection could worsen the amnestic syndrome, decreasing the patient's functional independence.

Language Dominant to Contralateral Side of Surgery

Memory adequate with ipsilateral injection but poor for contralateral injection. This test result is favorable. Decreases risk of memory decline following surgical resection.

Memory adequate with ipsilateral and contralateral injection. This test result is also somewhat favorable, but there is risk for memory ("visual" and verbal) decline. Extent of risk largely dependent upon neuropsychological memory test scores (average or better scores at higher risk) and structural MRI.

Memory poor with ipsilateral injection and adequate with contralateral injection. This test result is a "failure." High risk for memory decline. See "Wrong-way" Wada section.

Memory poor with ipsilateral injection and contralateral injection. See bilateral memory test failure above.

The "wrong-way"/"Reversed" Wada's test. This describes a test result in which the ipsilateral injection to the side of the proposed surgical resection (testing the contralateral hemisphere language and memory function) results in poor memory functioning. Alternatively, injection of the contralateral hemisphere to the proposed resection (testing ipsilateral hemisphere language and memory function) results in adequate memory. Traditionally, this test finding (so-called "failing" Wada's test) is generally considered to pose considerable neuropsychological risk to the patient with an amnestic syndrome following surgery being the worst case outcome (Loring et al. 2009). While decades of research establish patients with "wrong way" Wada's test results are at increased risk for memory decline, data suggest the risk of memory decline may be similar to those patients without structural pathology (Lacruz et al. 2004). The astute reader will recall that patients without structural pathology are at increased risk for memory decline. Thus, while having a "wrong way" Wada test result does not absolutely preclude surgical treatment, the risk of memory decline is greater. Indeed, patients with average or near average pre-operative neuropsychological memory scores will almost certainly exhibit a meaningful decline in memory following a standard ATL.

Rule of thumb: Predicting neuropsychological outcome: How to avoid the "double looser" (not seizure free and memory/language loss)

Good Prognostic Features (decreased likelihood of reliable decline in memory/language)

- Presence of lesion (e.g., mesial temporal sclerosis) ipsilateral to seizure focus
- Unilateral EEG abnormalities
- Presurgical lateralizing neuropsychological data in which memory impaired for ipsilateral temporal lobe (e.g., patient with left TLE exhibiting poor verbal memory, but good visual memory)
- Presurgical memory scores below 90 are 4.9 times at lower risk for reliable memory decline postoperatively than patients with memory scores above 90
- Longer duration of epilepsy
- Higher presurgical general cognitive ability (IQ)
- Asymmetric functional neuroimaging findings (PET hypometabolism ipsilateral to seizure focus)
- Asymmetric Wada's test results with ipsilateral injection memory is good while controlateral injection memory is impaired

Predicting confrontation naming outcomes

- Reliable decline in confrontation naming more likely for patients with resection of language dominant temporal lobe and intact naming score and/or shorter duration of epilepsy
- Reliable decline less likely with presurgical naming deficits and with longer duration of epilepsy

Psychiatric Status and Quality-of-life in Epilepsy

Reviewing Fig. 16.3 highlights the inter-related affect of psychosocial factors in epilepsy. Patients with epilepsy (both adults and children) are diagnosed with psychiatric disorders at a greater frequency than in the general population (Gaitatzis et al. 2004), and report a poor quality of life than healthy peers (Jacoby and Baker 2008). Treatment of epilepsy, including epilepsy surgery, can have a positive impact on mood and adjustment. In addition to understanding that certain psychiatric diseases commonly occur in patients with epilepsy, it is also important to recognize that some patients also experience acute psychiatric symptoms that are ictal, peri-ictal, or inter-ictal manifestations of their seizures, many of which may not fit the standard diagnostic rubrics of the Diagnostic and Statistical Manuel of Mental Disorders IV (DSM-IV). It appears psychiatric symptomatology (depression and/or anxiety symptoms) have been found *before* the onset of epilepsy (Austin et al. 2001), and there has been a growing debate about whether each disease may uniquely contribute to the development of the other in some cases. Neuropsychologists need to recognize behavioral deficits and psychiatric issues when they occur, both to identify and address these problems, as well as to consider their concomitant impact upon neuropsychologic status. Thus, the neuropsychological evaluation of patients with epilepsy should include an assessment of emotional/psychiatric functioning as well as quality-of-life. It should be noted that a neuropsychological evaluation is not equivalent to a psychiatric evaluation, and the patient with epilepsy will benefit from both.

Common psychiatric disorders occurring in epilepsy include mood disorders (major depressive disorders, bipolar disorder symptoms), anxiety disorders, psychosis, personality disorders, and substance abuse (Hermann et al. 2000; LaFrance et al. 2008). A variety of factors can contribute to psychiatric or behavioral disturbance in ES patients, including the ictal seizure discharge, the peri- or post-ictal state, CNS pathology, effects of AEDs, adverse psychosocial consequences of having epilepsy (reactive), and cognitive and temperamental (personality) attributes. Prevalence estimates of psychiatric disturbance in epilepsy tend to range from 20% to 50%, with higher estimates arising in specialty clinics and lower estimates coming from community-based samples. Similar prevalence rates have been observed in children and adults (Davies and Goodman 2003; Rutter et al. 1970). Studies examining prevalence rates of psychiatric comorbidity in epilepsy have been limited by a lack of large community-based surveys (Manchanda 2002), and a frequent failure to employ reliable standardized measures of psychopathology (Swinkels et al. 2005). However, study methodology and measures have improved over the past decade, particularly for symptoms of depression.

Depression in Epilepsy

The association between epilepsy and depression has been recognized for recorded medical history. Hippocrates noted in about 400 BC that: "Melancholics ordinarily become epileptics, and epileptics melancholics: What determines the preference is the direction the malady takes; if it bears upon the body, epilepsy, if upon the intelligence, melancholy (Lewis 1934)."

Prevalence rates of depression in epilepsy range from 10% to 60% among patients with recurrent seizures and from 3% to 9% in patients with controlled epilepsy (Ettinger et al. 2004; Fuller-Thomson and Brennenstuhl 2009; Gilliam and Kanner 2002; Kanner and Palac 2000). Variability across studies has been attributed to genuine differences across samples (e.g., Canadian vs USA), methods of sampling and statistical analysis, and differences in assessment instruments. Increased risk of depression among patients with epilepsy is associated with female gender, minority status, older age, being unmarried, unemployment, lower levels of education, and lower socioeconomic status (Ettinger et al. 2004; Fuller-Thomson and Brennenstuhl 2009; Jacoby et al. 1996; Mensah et al. 2006). However, epilepsy is an powerful risk factor for depression. For example, Fuller-Thomson and Brennenstuhl (2009) found epilepsy resulted increased odds of depression by 43% after adjusting for demographic factors.

Patients with epilepsy also experience higher rates of suicidal ideation and suicidal behavior than the general population. The lifetime prevalence rate of suicide and suicide attempts is between 5% and 14.3% in people with epilepsy, which is 6–25 times higher than in the general population (Robertson 1997).

Despite the increased risk for depression and suicide in epilepsy, mood disorders in this population often go unrecognized and/or untreated by practitioners. For example, Fuller-Thomson and Brennenstuhl (2009) found nearly 40% of patients with depression had not received mental health treatment, suggesting that better screening for psychiatric conditions is needed in this population. The reasons for not recognizing depression in this population appear to be multi-factorial and include: (1) patients may minimize their psychiatric symptoms for fear of being further stigmatized, (2) clinical manifestations of certain types of depressive disorders in epilepsy differ from depressive disorders in patients without epilepsy, and (3) clinicians frequently fail to inquire about psychiatric symptoms (Gilliam and Kanner 2002; Hermann et al. 2000). Both patients and clinicians can minimize symptoms of depression because they consider depression to be a "normal adaptation process" to having epilepsy (Kanner and Palac 2000). The concern that antidepressant drugs may lower the seizure threshold has also resulted in reluctance among some clinicians to use psychotropic drugs to treat patients with epilepsy (Gilliam and Kanner 2002).

Although there is general agreement that prevalence rates of psychiatric co-morbidity is higher among patients with epilepsy than the general population, the relationship between seizure type, seizure focus, and psychiatric status remains uncertain. Depression is more common among patients with TLE, as these groups have been shown to have lifetime prevalence rates for major depression of up to 50% (Gaitatzis et al. 2004). Patients with multiple seizure types also appear to experience greater emotional maladjustment than those without (Dodrill 1984; Hermann et al. 1982). Comorbid depression in epilepsy has been associated with a greater likelihood of adverse events to AEDs, more frequent visits to physicians, and higher costs of medical care related to seizures and not to the cost of psychiatric treatment (Cramer et al. 2004). Depression is also associated with a poor outcome following ATL to control seizures (Anhoury et al. 2000; Kanner et al. 2009).

Intriguing findings involve evidence that depression often antedates seizure onset, and that epilepsy and depression may be bidirectional in terms of causality. For example, behavioral abnormalities have been observed more than 6 months prior to seizure onset in children with new onset seizures as compared to sibling controls (Austin et al. 2001; Dunn et al. 2002). Jones et al. (2007) demonstrated that approximately 45% of children with new onset seizures exhibited a DSM-IV Axis I disorder that antedated their seizure onset. Academic problems were thought to precede initial seizure onset in children (Berg et al. 2005), but this was not confirmed in a large prospective study of first onset seizure (Fastenau et al. 2009). Taken together, these data argue an underlying neurobiological influence (that is not appreciated in current structural neuroimaging technologies) apart from seizures and AED treatment is leading to both seizures and psychopathology (Hermann et al. 2006).

Treatment of Depression in Epilepsy. There are limited data regarding the efficacy of standard treatment interventions (pharmacological or psychothera-peutic) for depression in patients with epilepsy (Kanner and Schacter 2008). However, patients with epilepsy respond favorably to pharmacological treatment, and some data suggest antidepressant medication may have some anticonvulsant properties at therapeutic doses (e.g., Alper 2008). The effectiveness of psycho-logical treatment at reducing depressive symptoms has also been demonstrated for patients with epilepsy. Gilliam (1990) reported that patients involved in psycho-therapy not only showed significant improvement in rating scales of depression and anxiety, but also showed a decline in seizure frequency. Emerging research suggest the presence of a psychiatric disorder increases the risk for seizures (lowers the seizure threshold), while antidepressant medications may reduce the risk for seizures among patients with epilepsy (Alper 2008).

Rule of thumb: Depression in epilepsy

- 10–60% of patients with active epilepsy meet criteria for depressive disorder
- 3–9% of patients with controlled epilepsy meet criteria for depressive disorder
- Risk of suicide 6–25 times the general population
- Treatment of depressive symptoms undertreated/under-recognized
- Treatment for depressive symptoms is efficacious
- Depressive symptoms can antedate seizure onset

Anxiety in Epilepsy

Anxiety disorders are the second most common psychiatric disorder among patients with epilepsy, with prevalence rates reported to vary from 10% to 50% (see Mensah et al. 2007). Rates of anxiety in community based samples are generally lower, ranging from 14% to 25%. Hospital based studies report prevalence of anxiety disorders range from 25% to 50%, and studies among patients whom are candidates for epilepsy surgery due to refractory TLE report prevalence rates of 10–31%. Anxiety symptoms are frequently comorbid with symptoms of depression, and there is an increased association of anxiety symptoms with female gender, unemployment, perceived side-effects of AEDs and chronic ill health, as well as lower educational attainment. Anxiety symptoms were not strongly associated with epilepsy variables, including side of seizures or if seizures were focal or generalized (e.g., Kanner and Schacter 2008; Mensah et al. 2007).

Treatment of anxiety disorders in epilepsy. Like the treatment of depression, psychopharmacological and psychological treatment have demonstrated some success, although both are less well researched than treatment for depression in epilepsy.

Rule of thumb: Anxiety in epilepsy

- 10 to 50% of patients with active epilepsy meet criteria for anxiety disorder
- Anxiety symptoms/disorders often comorbid with depressive symptoms/ disorders
- Treatment of depressive symptoms undertreated/under-recognized
- Anxiety symptoms not associated with side of seizure
- Treatment for anxiety symptoms is efficacious

Broader Psychopathology in Epilepsy

We have chosen to focus on depression in epilepsy, as it appears to be the most commonly occurring psychiatric comorbidity. Nevertheless, anxiety disorders, substance abuse, personality disorders, and psychosis also occur with significant frequency in this population.

Role of Neuropsychology in Managing the Psychiatric Aspects of Epilepsy. Clinical neuropsychologists represent a core group of clinicians that can obtain objective data on the presence of psychiatric disorders in patients, which is necessary to track disease prevalence and to recognize the need for intervention. Neuropsychological evaluations frequently include a psychometric based instrument of mood/psychiatric functioning, and many epilepsy centers also include a measure of quality-of-life. Measure of mood are useful for monitoring levels of distress, tracking change over time, and picking up on critical issues in need of intervention (e.g., active suicidal ideation). Personality profiles can also provide greater insight into the presence of disease, and the underlying personality traits that may contribute to their development and recalcitrance. Measures of mood do not typically allow for making psychiatric diagnoses, and do not provide any information with regard to lifetime prevalence rates. Kanner and colleagues have demonstrated that knowledge of psychiatric syndrome and personal and familial psychiatric history can be of benefit in predicting adverse responses to AEDs, and in determining the optimal treatment regimen for patients with such comorbid conditions (Kanner 2009; Kanner et al. 2003).

Quality of Life and Psychosocial Consequences

Patients with epilepsy experience higher rates of unemployment, lower income, lower education, and remain unmarried at rates that exceed the general population (Kobau et al. 2006; Strine et al. 2005). The worst functioning tends to be observed in patients with active epilepsy, and those with comorbid psychiatric conditions. A review found quality of life (QOL) is lower for patients with epilepsy than the general population and lower than among patients with other chronic medical conditions (e.g., asthma) (Jacoby and Baker 2008; Jacoby et al. 2009). Factors that have particular salience in affecting quality of life include epilepsy/medical (seizure frequency, side-effects of AEDs) and psychosocial (psychiatric symptoms of anxiety/depression, psychological resilience, family/social stigma, and discrimination) variables. A particularly powerful affect on QOL is from perceived seizure frequency followed by perceived adverse effects of AEDs. Nonepilepsy variables (psychosocial) appear to have less impact, but several variables, including family/parent variables can significantly impact children with epilepsy. In general, psychosocial variables negatively affecting QOL include presence of psychiatric disorders and/or perception of stigma. Interestingly, an aspect of cognitive function, the so-called "cognitive reserve" phenomena finds that individuals with higher educational and/or occupational attainment and/or increased involvement in tasks that involved cognitive activity appears to moderate QOL by modifying cognitive morbidity in epilepsy. In general, patients with higher cognitive reserve report better QOL than those individuals with less cognitive reserve/activities.

In general, patients experiencing one or few seizures, and then are seizure-free, report an initial acute dip in QOL after the seizure(s), and then gradual return to normal (or near normal) QOL 1–2 years after the seizure (last seizure) as compared to healthy peers without a seizure. For patients with active epilepsy (defined as having had a seizure in the last 12 months), QOL is lower than individuals with one or several unprovoked seizures, and no additional seizures. There is a clear relationship between frequency of seizures (particularly the patients' *perceived* seizure frequency), with seizures occurring monthly or more had the lowest quality of life, while QOL was better (but not normal) for individuals having a seizure once a year. For those individuals with active epilepsy, treatment variables have a large impact. In general, individuals having successful surgery (Engle Class Ia or 1b) after 1 or 2 years, have better QOL than individuals with continued epilepsy. QOL can profoundly improve for patients whom are seizure-free shortly after successful surgery, and the majority of patients' QOL was normal (or near normal) compared to healthy peers without epilepsy 2–3 years after being seizure-free. For patients not having successful surgery, QOL is generally poor, and may decline beyond baseline pre-surgical levels. Decline in QOL from presurgical baseline particularly likely for patients with ongoing seizures and experiencing a neuropsychological decline (memory loss) after surgerical treatment. Modifiable variables that can improve QOL include reducing seizure frequency, reducing AEDs, promote cognitive activity/reserve, reduce psychopathology (eliminate or minimize anxiety and/or depression symptoms), and try to reduce negative social/cultural variables of stigma and discrimination (Jacoby and Baker 2008).

Rule of thumb: Quality of life in epilepsy

– Epilepsy associated with lower quality of life
– Patients less likely to be employed, have less education, have less income, and more likely to be single.
– Quality of life related to epilepsy/medical and psychosical variables
  • Epilepsy/medical – most important predictors of quality of life
    ○ Perceived seizure frequency (lower QOL with more frequent seizures)
    ○ Perceived adverse effects from AEDs
    ○ Perceived cognitive problems due to epilepsy and/or AEDs
    ○ Limitations in independence due to seizures/not driving/unemployment
  • Psychosocial variables decrease QOL
    ○ Psychiatric comorbidity
      Presence of social stigma of epilepsy
– QOL improves to near normal levels with seizure freedom
    • Surgical patients QOL increased to near healthy peers within 2–3 years of being seizure-free
– Variables improving QOL
– Reducing seizure frequency
– Reducing AEDs
– Promote cognitive reserve/activity
– Decrease psychiatric symptomatology
– Reduce family/social/cultural stigma/discrimination of epilepsy

---

Neuropsychological Assessment Guide

Neuropsychological evaluations for patients with epilepsy are generally broad and we believe should incorporate sensory and motor testing along with symptom validity tests (SVTs) (see Table 16.13 for a recommended neuropsychological assessment battery).

Table 16.13 Summary of basic neuropsychological assessment battery

Neuropsychological domain	Recommended assessment procedure	
General cognitive	Wechsler intelligence scales	
Attention/executive	Wechsler intelligence scales attention subtests (i.e., digit span, digit symbol, letter-number sequencing)	
	Trail making test	
	Wisconsin card sorting test	
	Figural fluency test (D-KEFS or Ruff)	
Psychomotor speed/reaction time	Reaction time test	
	Finger tapping test	
	Grooved pegboard test	
Language	Boston naming test	Children add:
	Columbia auditory naming test	Achievement screen of word knowledge, receptive vocabulary, sentence reading, spelling, arithmetic skills
	Controlled oral word association test (COWAT)	
	Semantic verbal fluency	
Memory/learning	Rey auditory verbal learning test (RAVLT)	
	Wechsler memory scales	
Visuoperceptual/visuoconstructional	Rey-Osterrieth complex figure test (or Taylor figure)	
	Wechsler block design	
Emotion/mood/quality of life	Beck Depression Inventory – 2nd Ed.	
	Beck Anxiety Inventory	
	QOLIE-10 or QOLIE-31	
Task engagement	At least one SVT (Symptom Validity Test)	
Sensory-perceptual	Light touch (hand and face)	
	Visual fields	
	Apraxia	
	Auditory extinction to finger rub	

Review of medical records: This is absolutely crucial for a proper neuropsychological evaluation. Important records for review include EEG report identifying the suspected seizure focus and/or seizure types. Often, a report of the MRI study of the brain will identify any structural abnormalities, particularly involving the temporal lobe. The presence of mesial temporal sclerosis greatly aides in predicting neuropsychological outcome. Report for language dominance based on either or combination of Wada's (intracarotid amytal/brevital) test, fMRI, and/or MEG/MSI is helpful to predict memory and language outcome. Knowledge of age of seizure onset and duration of epilepsy can be helpful. Review of the medication regimen is recommended to identify AEDs or other medications that may negatively affect neuropsychological function (see Table 16.8).

Clinical Interview: Carefully listen for dysnomias, paraphasias, or slurring. Also, carefully watch for abnormal eye movements or episodes in which the patient appears to briefly pause while talking or "space off." These brief episodes when you think the patient may be thinking may actually reflect a seizure. Ask the patient if (s)he has experienced a loss of time or if they recall what they were thinking about. You might also carefully evaluate the patient's orientation. Look also for facial asymmetries (Tinuper et al. 1992), which can occur among patients with epilepsy.

Sensory-perceptual examination: The clinical neuropsychologist can evaluate for gross visual field cuts, tactile sensory function (extinction task), simple audition functions, and apraxias. We recommend evaluating for hemi-inattention to visual, auditory, and tactile sensation. Inattention can be rapidly assessed by using a brief bedside bilateral simultaneous stimulation test. One may also assess for finger agnosia, astereognosis, Right/Left orientation, and apraxia. Cranial nerve exam and evaluation of deep tendon reflexes may also assist the neuropsychologist complete the evaluation.

Motor examination: Evaluation of grip strength and manual dexterity of both upper extremities is recommended.

Neuropsychological psychometric instruments: The selection of instruments should (1) have demonstrated validity (evidence-based) and (2) assist the neuropsychologist to make some statement about the relative risk for neuropsychological impairment following surgery. Ideally, this will include a statement about the type and extent of neuropsychological and psychological impairments that may occur from the proposed surgical procedure (e.g., right anterior temporal lobectomy). Secondarily, the neuropsychologist may assist with confirming the lateralization or localization of the seizure focus, keeping in mind that this information will be misleading in some patients and assumes normal functional neuroanatomic organization (i.e., left hemisphere dominant for language). While the selection of specific assessment instruments can certainly differ (e.g., assessing verbal memory), the assessment should assess domains likely to be adversely affected by the epilepsy syndrome and/or proposed neurological surgery procedure. The neuropsychological measures specified below are guides, and as new tests are developed, neuropsychologists should evaluate the evidence-based research of older and newer instruments, and how new tests may better serve the needs of the patient (Loring and Bauer 2010).

General Cognitive

The assessment of general cognitive functioning can be helpful in epilepsy surgery evaluations, but differences in Verbal IQ and Performance (nonverbal) IQ should *not* be used to discriminate left TLE from right TLE. Borderline to impaired general cognitive functioning prior to elective surgery could raise concerns about poorer general outcome short-term, and place the patient at increased risk for decline in neuropsychological function over the long term, perhaps reflecting magnified age-related changes. Poor general cognitive functioning may also raise questions about the patient's ability to cope with psychosocial stressors, independently manage medications, and understand the benefits and potential risks of elective neurological surgery. Patients with early onset of refractory epilepsy, long duration of epilepsy, and history of multiple episodes of generalized tonic-clonic status epilepticus typically exhibit significantly worse IQ scores than patients with shorter duration of seizures, later onset of seizures, and no history of generalized tonic-clonic status epilepticus.

Recommended measures: Wechsler Intelligence Scales have an extensive literature. Abbreviated administration or short-form versions are often used. The processing speed and working memory indices can be useful for examining the effects of medications, acute seizures, and other transient, acute factors.

Academic achievement measures: Including a measure of academic functioning can be helpful, and is often important in academic placement issues for children and adolescents. For children, we recommend a screening of word reading, reading comprehension, spelling and arithmetic skills. In adults, an assessment of reading ability can be useful in TLE cases, while arithmetic may be more important in extratemporal resections (i.e., parietal).

Recommended measures: Wide Range Achievement Test – 4th Edition (WRAT-IV), Peabody Individual Achievement Test – Revised (PIAT-R), Woodcock-Johnson Test of Psychoeducational Achievement – 3rd Edition.

Attention/Concentration and "Executive Functions"

We recommend an evaluation of simple, focused, and divided attention.

Recommended measures (Attention): Commonly used measures include digit span forwards and backwards as well as letter number sequencing from the Wechsler Intelligence Scales, digit symbol/symbol digit/coding subtests of the Wechsler Intelligence Scales, Trail Making Test, parts A and B, Symbol Digit Modalities Test (SDMT), etc. A measure of reaction time is often helpful as well.

"Executive functions" refers to a range of complex cognitive and behavioral adaptive functions often associated with frontal lobe function, but also involve other brain regions (see Chap. 10, this volume for details).

Recommended measures (executive functions): Commonly included measures include the Wisconsin Card Sorting Test, Category Test of the Halstead–Reitan battery, Figural fluency task (e.g., DKEFS Figural Fluency, Ruff Figural Fluency Test), verbal fluency (Controlled Oral Word Association Test; COWAT), Stroop Color-word task, competing programs/serial motor programming tasks, Go/No-Go tasks. Other tests include the Iowa Gambling task. In addition, assessment for motor impersistence, motor weakness, and personality changes including apathy, social disinhibition, and/or irritability is suggested.

Language and Speech: Psychometric evaluation of naming and generative fluency is critical in the evaluation of epilepsy surgery patients. These domains are frequently impaired among patients with epilepsy, and can also be negatively impacted by neurological surgery. Reading and spelling functions may also be assessed, and can also be impacted by some surgical interventions. Inter-ictally, patients with epilepsy rarely exhibit gross aphasia symptoms, but aphasic symptoms post-ictally can predict seizure laterality and seizure outcome (Privetera et al. 1991).

Recommended measures: Boston Naming Test, Columbia Auditory Naming Test, COWAT, semantic verbal fluency task. Assessment of reading and spelling may include the PIAT-R, WRAT-4, or W-J III. Measures of vocabulary both receptive and expressive can be helpful in the assessment of children with epilepsy (Peabody Picture Vocabulary Test – 3rd Edition and Vocabulary subtest of the WAIS-III or WISC-IV).

Learning/Memory: Neuropsychological assessment of declarative memory functions has predictive value of post-surgical memory outcome. Moreover, in cases in which structural neuroimaging fails to identify a lesion, assessment of memory has been shown to be predictive of surgical outcome and side of seizure onset (e.g., Hennessy et al. 2001; Sawrie et al. 1998, 2001). Deficient short-term spontaneous recall of verbal material (paragraphs, list of words, and word-pairs), with normal verbal intellectual functioning is indicative of focal language dominant (left) mesial temporal lobe dysfunction. Poor recall of verbal material, particularly list learning tasks, as well as word-pairs or short paragraphs is consistently associated with mesial temporal sclerosis and histopathological evidence of CA1 and CA3 hippocampal gliosis. The predictive value of "visual" memory tests on outcome is not consistent. While nondominant (right) hemisphere seizure onset can present with specific deficits in recall of complex geometric shapes and human faces, patients with right TLE can also exhibit deficits in verbal and nonverbal (visual) memory. It is thought the major shortcoming of current "visual" memory tasks is that the stimuli can be verbally encoded.

Recommended measures: Verbal memory tests include the Rey Auditory Verbal Learning Test (RAVLT) or California Verbal Learning Test (CVLT). The RAVLT has more predictive value identifying left TLE than the CVLT (Loring et al. 2008). As of 2010, we are unaware of any visual memory measure that consistently discriminates patients with right TLE from left TLE. Visual memory tasks we recommend include the Rey-Osterrieth Complex Figure (or Taylor Complex figure). The WMS-IV visual memory tests may prove valuable, but data are too limited at this time. Other commonly used "visual" memory tests (Benton Brief Visual Retention Test, Hospital Facial Memory Test, Medical College Georgia Complex Figure (MCG-CF) test, or the WMS-III) has also not consistently distinguished right TLE from left TLE.

Visuoperceptual/Visuoconstructional skills: Deficits are common, but scores on measures of visuoconstructional tests has *not* consistently discriminated patients with left TLE from right TLE. Although rarely present, visual inattention has clear indications for the lateralization of brain dysfunction (see Lezak et al. 2004).

Recommended measures: Frequently used measures of visuoconstructional and visuoperceptual function include the Rey–Osterreith Complex Figure (or Taylor complex figure test) and the Block Design subtest of the Wechsler Intelligence scales. The Benton Tests [e.g., Judgment of Line Orientation, Facial Recognition Test (FRT)] are also widely used. Patients with TLE have exhibited post-operatively decline on the FRT in one study. A newer measure, the Visual Object Space Perception Battery, may hold promise to improve lateralization, and includes four subtests that load on a perceptual factor and four that load on a spatial processing factor (Rapport et al. 1998). Bedside assessments of visuoconstructional skills can also be used in lower functioning patients such as drawing a clock face, cube, or the Halstead–Reitan aphasia screening instrument.

Psychological/Emotional Functioning

Evaluation for symptoms of depression and anxiety is important in evaluating patients with refractory epilepsy given the high comorbidity of psychiatric symptoms in this population (Kanner 2003). It should be recognized that patients may present with symptoms of anxiety and depression secondary to the neurophysiological dysfunction associated with the epilepsy syndrome. There is currently no conclusive data regarding hemispheric laterality for symptoms of depression or anxiety symptoms. Furthermore, the so-called "temporal lobe personality" associated with interpersonal "stickiness" and religiosity is *not* consistent among patients with TLE. A rare, but disabling, psychiatric feature associated with TLE is psychosis. Psychosis can result from post-ictal psychosis or may appear as part of a rare schizophrenic-like presentation. Even more rare is the onset of psychosis following ATL. In addition, the patient's expectations for surgery outcome, and ways to cope with both good and poor surgical outcome, need to be assessed. A component of this should include an evaluation to the extent that the individual exhibits somatic pre-occupation and/or a history of psychogenic nonepileptic seizures (PNES, or pseudoseizure) and/or panic attacks. The presence of PNES along with refractory epilepsy would *not*, in our view, prohibit a patient from undergoing surgical treatment for the refractory epilepsy, but the presence of PNES should alert the team to increased risk for poor surgical outcome from a psychiatric and quality of life standpoint. Lastly, assessment of the patients social support network is recommended.

Recommended measures: Screening for symptoms of depression and anxiety can include the Beck Depression Inventory – 2nd Edition (BDI-2) and Speilberger State-Trait Anxiety Inventory (STAI). More detailed assessment of may include the Minnesota Multiphasic Personality Inventory – 2nd Edition (MMPI-2) or the Personality Assessment Inventory (PAI).

Quality of life: Assessment of quality of life with epilepsy can be obtained from the Quality of Life in Epilepsy Inventories, of which there are long and short versions. We use the 10-item version (QOLIE-10).

Analysis of Change in Neuropsychology Test Scores

Repeat neuropsychological evaluations are common in epilepsy, with the goal being to evaluate for change in neuropsychological function following surgical or medical interventions. In addition to monitoring for change following surgical intervention, increasing attention is being given to monitoring for the cognitive effects of AEDs. Another common referral is to evaluate for change in cognitive functioning for individuals with refractory epilepsy to monitor their progress. Traditional approaches have included evaluation of change in neuropsychology test scores by change in raw scores and some in standard scores. Beginning in the 1990s, two much more sophisticated measures of change were developed: (1) the Reliable Change Indices (RCI's) and (2) standard regression-based (SRB) change score norms (Heaton et al. 2001; Hermann et al. 1996; Sawrie et al. 1996). The statistical approaches vary, but a common theme is to statistical control for test-retest effects and measurement error (Temkin et al. 1999). Measurement of change is typically based on well-selected clinical samples of patients whom are typically medically managed to determine the extent of change (if any) that might occur with the disease and medical treatment alone. Once change over time due to progression of disease has been determined, comparison to change associated with a new treatment (surgery, etc.) allows clinicians to empirically answer if a change from time one to time two is greater than what might have occurred due to disease and measurement error. However, the change is based on a clinical population, in this case patients with epilepsy, so using particular RCI values to other patient populations or healthy controls should not be done.

We provide RCI and SRB change scores below (see Tables 16.14, 16.15, 16.16, and 16.17). These tables summarize available RCI and/or SRB data we were aware of as of 12/2009. While RCI/SRB are available for some commonly used measures in epilepsy, by no means are there plentiful data at this time. One might attempt to develop RCI at the 80% and 90 % confidence intervals for neuropsychological measures using the test manual using the following algorithm: $Sdiff = (SEM1^2 + SEM2^2)^{1/2}$. However, keep in mind this is the least accurate measures of reliable change, as it is based on healthy controls.

Table 16.14 Reliable change of common neuropsychological tests for adult epilepsy patients after anterior temporal lobectomy

Test or neuropsychological domain	Practice correct	80% RCI CI	90% RCI CI	Metric	Source
Intellectual Functioning					
Wechsler Adult Intelligence Test – 3rd edn. (WAIS-III)					Martin et al. (2002)
Full scale IQ	+1	$\leq -5, \geq +7$	$\leq -6, \geq +8$	Standard score	
Verbal IQ	0	$\leq -6, \geq +6$	$\leq -8, \geq +8$	Standard score	
Performance IQ	+3	$\leq -5, \geq +11$	$\leq -7, \geq +13$	Standard score	
Verbal comprehension Index	+1	$\leq -5, \geq +7$	$\leq -7, \geq +9$	Standard score	
Perceptual organization index	+3	$\leq -5, \geq +11$	$\leq -8, \geq +14$	Standard score	
Working memory index	−2	$\leq -15, \geq +9$	$\leq -17, \geq +13$	Standard score	
Wechsler Adult Intelligence Test – Revised (WAIS-R)					Hermann et. al. (1996)
Full scale IQ	+1	$\leq -4, \geq +8$	$\leq -6, \geq +10$	Standard score	
Verbal IQ	+3	$\leq -4, \geq +6$	$\leq -5, \geq +7$	Standard score	
Performance IQ	+2	$\leq -4, \geq +8$	$\leq -6, \geq +10$	Standard score	
Information	0	$\leq -3, \geq +3$	$\leq -4, \geq +4$	Scaled score	
Digit span	0	$\leq -3, \geq +3$	$\leq -4, \geq +4$	Scaled score	
Vocabulary	0	$\leq -2, \geq +2$	$\leq -3, \geq +3$	Scaled score	
Arithmetic	0	$\leq -3, \geq +3$	$\leq -4, \geq +4$	Scaled score	
Comprehension	0	$\leq -3, \geq +3$	$\leq -4, \geq +4$	Scaled score	
Similarities	0	$\leq -4, \geq +4$	$\leq -5, \geq +5$	Scaled score	
Picture completion	+1	$\leq -3, \geq +5$	$\leq -4, \geq +6$	Scaled score	
Picture arrangement	0	$\leq -4, \geq +4$	$\leq -5, \geq +5$	Scaled score	
Block design	0	$\leq -3, \geq +3$	$\leq -3, \geq +3$	Scaled score	
Object assembly	0	$\leq -3, \geq +3$	$\leq 4, \geq +4$	Scaled score	
Digit symbol	0	$\leq -3, \geq +3$	$\leq -3, \geq +3$	Scaled score	

Academic achievement

Wide Range Achievement Test-Revised (WRAT-R)					Hermann et. al. (1996)
Reading	+2	≤ −5, ≥ +9	≤ −7, ≥ +11	Standard score	
Spelling	+2	≤ −5, ≥ +9	≤ −6, ≥ +10	Standard score	
Arithmetic	+1	≤ −7, ≥ +9	≤ −9, ≥ +11	Standard score	

Processing speed

Adult Memory and Information Processing Battery (AMIPB)[a]					Baxendale and Thompson (2005)[b]
Information processing A total		< −11.3, > +11.3	< −14.7, > +14.7		
Information processing A speed		< −8.7, > +8.7	< −11.3, > +11.3		
Information processing B total		< −8.4, > +8.4	< −10.8, > +10.8		
Information processing B speed		< −8.0, > +8.0	< −10.3, > +10.3		
Trail making test – A	−2	≤ −17, ≥ +13	≤ −21, ≥ +17	Raw (seconds)	Hermann et. al. (1996)

Executive functions

Wisconsin card sorting test					Hermann et. al. (1996)
Categories	0	≤ −3, ≥ +3	≤ −4, ≥ +4	Raw	
Preservative responses	−1	≤ −18, ≥ +16	≤ −21, ≥ +21	Raw	
Trail making test-B	+3	≤ −47, ≥ +53	≤ −61, ≥ +67	Raw (seconds)	

Memory

AMIPB[a]					Baxendale and Thompson (2005)[b]
Story recall – immediate		< −10, > +10	< −12.9, > +12.9		
Story recall – delayed		< −9.4, > +9.4	< −12.1, > +12.1		
List learning total 1–5		< −9.6, > +9.6	< −12.4, > +12.4		
List learning delay		< −2.9, > +2.9	< −3.8, > +3.8		
List B		< −3.0, > +3.0	< −3.9, > +3.9		
Figure immediate recall		< −17.5, > +17.5	< −22.5, > +22.5		
Figure delayed recall		< −24.9, > +24.9	< −32.0, > +32.0		

(continued)

Table 16.14 (continued)

Test or neuropsychological domain	Practice correct	80% RCI CI	90% RCI CI	Metric	Source
Design learning total 1–5		< −10.0, > +10.0	< −12.8, > +12.8		Martin et al. (2002)
Design learning delay		< −3.9, > +3.9	< −5.1, > +5.1		
Wechsler Memory Scale – 3rd edn. (WMS-III)					
Auditory immediate index	+1	≤ −11, ≥ +13	≤ −14, ≥ +16	Standard score	
Visual immediate index	+3	≤ −11, ≥ +17	≤ −15, ≥ +21	Standard score	
General immediate memory	+2	≤ −9, ≥ +13	≤ −12, ≥ +16	Standard score	
Auditory delayed index	−2	≤ −15, ≥ +11	≤ −19, ≥ +15	Standard score	
Visual delayed index	+5	≤ −9, ≥ +19	≤ −13, ≥ +23	Standard score	
Auditory recog. delayed index	−1	≤ −18, ≥ +16	≤ −22, ≥ +20	Standard score	
General memory index	+1	≤ −13, ≥ +15	≤ −16, ≥ +18	Standard score	
Working memory index	−2	≤ −18, ≥ +14	≤ −22, ≥ +18	Standard score	
Logical memory I	0	≤ −3, ≥ +3	≤ −3, ≥ +3	Scaled score	
Logical memory II	0	≤ −3, ≥ +3	≤ −4, ≥ +4	Scaled score	
Faces I	+1	≤ −2, ≥ +4	≤ −3, ≥ +5	Scaled score	
Faces II	+1	≤ −2, ≥ +4	≤ −3, ≥ +5	Scaled score	
Verbal paired associates I	0	≤ −3, ≥ +3	≤ −3, ≥ +3	Scaled score	
Verbal paired associates II	0	≤ −3, ≥ +3	≤ −4, ≥ +4	Scaled score	
Family pictures I	0	≤ −3, ≥ +3	≤ −3, ≥ +3	Scaled score	
Family pictures II	0	≤ −3, ≥ +3	≤ −4, ≥ +4	Scaled score	
Letter/number sequencing	0	≤ −3, ≥ +3	≤ −4, ≥ +4	Scaled score	
Spatial span	+1	≤ −3, ≥ +5	≤ −4, ≥ +6	Scaled score	
Wechsler Memory Scale					
Logical memory I	+2	≤ −4, ≥ +8	≤ −5, ≥ +9	Raw score	Hermann et. al. (1996)

Logical memory II	+1	≤ −5, ≥ +7	≤ −7, ≥ +9	Raw score	Hermann et. al. (1996)
Logical memory% retention	+2	≤ −30, ≥ +32	≤ −39, ≥ +43	Raw score	
Associate learning-easy	0	≤ −3, ≥ +3	≤ −4, ≥ +4	Raw score	
Associate learning-hard	+1	≤ −3, ≥ +5	≤ −4, ≥ +6	Raw score	
Visual reproduction I	+1	≤ −3, ≥ +5	≤ −3, ≥ +5	Raw score	
Visual reproduction II	+1	≤ −3, ≥ +5	≤ −4, ≥ +6	Raw score	
Visual reproduction% retention	−1	≤ −29, ≥ +27	≤ −37, ≥ +35	Raw score	
California Verbal Learning Test					
Total words	+2	≤ −8, ≥ +12	≤ −11, ≥ +15	Raw score	
Trial 1	+1	≤ −3, ≥ +5	≤ −3, ≥ +5	Raw score	
Trial 2	+1	≤ −3, ≥ +5	≤ −4, ≥ +6	Raw score	
Trial 3	+1	≤ −4, ≥ +4	≤ −4, ≥ +4	Raw score	
Trial 4	0	≤ −4, ≥ +6	≤ −5, ≥ +7	Raw score	
Trial 5	+1	≤ −3, ≥ +5	≤ −3, ≥ +5	Raw score	
Short delay free recall	+1	≤ −6, ≥ +8	≤ −8, ≥ +10	Raw score	
Long delay free recall	+2	≤ −2, ≥ +6	≤ −3, ≥ +7	Raw score	
Discriminability	+3	≤ −13, ≥ +19	≤ −17, ≥ +23	Raw score	
False positives	−1	≤ −7, ≥ +5	≤ −8, ≥ +6	Raw score	
Recognition hits	+1	≤ −3, ≥ +5	≤ −4, ≥ +6	Raw score	

Language

Multilingual Aphasia Examination (MAE)					Hermann et. al. (1996)
Visual naming	0	≤ −7, ≥ +7	≤ −8, ≥ +8	Raw score	
Sentence repetition	0	≤ −4, ≥ +4	≤ −4, ≥ +4	Raw score	
Oral fluency	−1	≤ −12, ≥ +10	≤ −14, ≥ +12	Raw score	
Oral spelling	0	≤ −3, ≥ +3	≤ −4, ≥ +4	Raw score	
Token test	0	≤ −4, ≥ +4	≤ −5, ≥ +5	Raw score	
Aural comprehension	0	≤ −2, ≥ +2	≤ −2, ≥ +2	Raw score	
Reading comprehension	0	≤ −2, ≥ +2	≤ −2, ≥ +2	Raw score	

(continued)

Table 16.14 (continued)

Test or neuropsychological domain	Practice correct	80% RCI CI	90% RCI CI	Metric	Source
Visuospatial				Raw score	
Form Discrimination Test	0	≤ −5, ≥ +5	≤ −6, ≥ +6	Raw score	Hermann et. al. (1996)
Hooper Visual Organization Test	+1	≤ −2, ≥ +4	≤ −3, ≥ +5	Raw score	
Line Orientation Test	+2	≤ −2, ≥ +6	≤ −3, ≥ +7	Raw score	
Facial Recognition Test	0	≤ −5, ≥ +5	≤ −6, ≥ +6	Raw score	

[a]AK Coughlan and SE Hollows. Adult memory and information processing battery. UK, Leeds: St. James Hospital; 1985
[b]RCI data from personal communication. Assistance with Table by Eric Rinehardt, PhD, Department of Psychiatry and Neurosciences, University of South Florida College of Medicine, Tampa, FL, USA

Table 16.15 Summary of proportion (%) of adults with epilepsy exhibiting change on selected neuropsychological measures after anterior temporal lobectomy

Test or neuropsychological domain	Decline	Stable	Improve
Memory			
California verbal learning test			
Long delay free recall – Dominant ATL	46	54	0
Long delay free recall – Nondominant ATL	11	89	0
Wechsler memory scale – Revised			
Logical memory II – Dominant ATL	37	60	3
Logical memory II – Nondominant ATL	11	82	7

(From Stroup et al. 2003) RCI's were used to assess change

Table 16.16 Reliable change of common neuropsychological tests for pediatric epilepsy patients based on healthy standardization samples

Test or neuropsychological domain	Practice correct	90% RCI CI	Metric
Wechsler Intelligence Scale for			
Children – 3rd edn. (WISC-III)			
Full Scale IQ	7.72	≤ –0, ≥ +16	Standard score
Verbal IQ	2.32	≤ –6, ≥ +11	Standard score
Performance IQ	12.35	≤ 1, ≥ +23	Standard score
Verbal comprehension index	2.26	≤ –7, ≥ +12	Standard score
Perceptual organization index	10.99	≤ 0, ≥ +2	Standard score
Freedom from distractibility index	2.96	≤ –10, ≥ +16	Standard score
Processing speed index	9.09	≤ –5, ≥ +23	Standard score
Information	0.47	≤ –3, ≥ +4	Scaled score
Similarities	0.81	≤ –3, ≥ +4	Scaled score
Arithmetic	0.31	≤ –3, ≥ +4	Scaled score
Vocabulary	0.14	≤ –3, ≥ +3	Scaled score
Comprehension	0.26	≤ –4, ≥ +4	Scaled score
Digit Span	0.74	≤ –2, ≥ +4	Scaled score
Picture completion	1.78	≤ –2, ≥ +6	Scaled score
Coding	1.97	≤ –2, ≥ +6	Scaled score
Picture arrangement	2.96	≤ –1, ≥ +7	Scaled score
Block design	1.04	≤ –2, ≥ +4	Scaled score
Object assembly	1.57	≤ –3, ≥ +6	Scaled score
Symbol search	1.53	≤ –2, ≥ +3	Scaled score
Child Memory Scale (CMS)			
Visual immediate index	11.06	≤ –7, ≥ +29	Standard score
Visual delayed index	8.50	≤ –9, ≥ +26	Standard score
Verbal immediate index	12.13	≤ –1, ≥ +26	Standard score
Verbal delayed index	11.35	≤ –4, ≥ +26	Standard score
General memory index	16.42	≤ 5, ≥ +27	Standard score
Attention/concentration index	3.95	≤ –9, ≥ +17	Standard score
Learning index	9.43	≤ –5, ≥ +24	Standard score
Auditory delayed recognition	3.88	≤ –12, ≥ +20	Scaled score
Dot learning	0.75	≤ –3, ≥ +5	Scaled score
Dot total	0.98	≤ –3, ≥ +5	Scaled score

(continued)

Table 16.16 (continued)

Test or neuropsychological domain	Practice correct	90% RCI CI	Metric
Dot short delay	0.78	≤ −4, ≥ +6	Scaled score
Dot long delay	0.56	≤ −3, ≥ +5	Scaled score
Stories immediate	1.68	≤ −2, ≥ +6	Scaled score
Stories delayed	1.97	≤ −2, ≥ +6	Scaled score
Stories delayed recognition	1.11	≤ −3, ≥ +5	Scaled score
Faces immediate	2.60	≤ −2, ≥ +7	Scaled score
Faces delayed	2.25	≤ −2, ≥ +6	Scaled score
Word pair learning	2.07	≤ −1, ≥ +5	Scaled score
Word pair total	2.32	≤ −1, ≥ +5	Scaled score
Word pair immediate	0.87	≤ −3, ≥ +5	Scaled score
Word pair long delay	1.78	≤ −2, ≥ +5	Scaled score
Word pair delayed recognition	0.17	≤ −4, ≥ +4	Scaled score
Numbers	0.73	≤ −3, ≥ +4	Scaled score
Sequences	0.53	≤ −3, ≥ +4	Scaled score
Family pictures immediate	1.23	≤ −4, ≥ +6	Scaled score
Family pictures delayed	1.39	≤ −3, ≥ +6	Scaled score
Word list learning	1.72	≤ −2, ≥ +5	Scaled score
Word list delayed	1.33	≤ −3, ≥ +6	Scaled score
Word list delayed recognition	0.68	≤ −3, ≥ +4	Scaled score

Note: Data obtained from Haut et al. (2006). Reliable Change Indices developed from data published for the Wechsler Child Intelligence Scale-3rd Ed. (WISC-III; Wechsler, 1991) and Child Memory Scale (CMS; Cohen, 1997). Assistance with Table by Eric Rinehardt, PhD, Department of Psychiatry and Neurosciences, University of South Florida College of Medicine

Table 16.17 Summary of proportion (%) of pediatric patients with epilepsy exhibiting change on selected neuropsychological measures with and without surgery (From ML Smith et al. 2004)

Test or neuropsychological domain	Surgical (*n* = 30)			Nonsurgical (*n* = 21)		
	Decline	Stable	Improve	Decline	Stable	Improve
Intelligence						
WISC-III & WAIS-III						
Verbal comprehension index	10.3	86.3	3.4	15.8	84.2	0.0
Perceptual organization index	6.9	89.7	3.4	5.3	84.2	10.5
Freedom from distractibility index	21.4	75.0	3.6	15.8	78.9	5.3
Processing speed index	7.1	85.8	7.1	10.5	84.2	5.3
Memory						
Children's Memory Scale and Denman Neuropsychology Memory Scale						
Recall of story	34.5	44.8	20.7	33.3	47.7	19.0
Children's auditory verbal learning Test-2						
Recall of word list	39.3	50.0	10.7	15.0	75.0	10.0
Rey-Osterrieth Complex Figure; Children's Memory Scale; Denman Neuropsychology Memory Scale						
Recall of geometric design	29.6	51.9	18.5	18.8	49.9	31.3
Recognition of faces	12.0	52.0	36.0	10.5	73.7	15.8

(continued)

Table 16.17 (continued)

Test or neuropsychological domain	Surgical (*n* = 30)			Nonsurgical (*n* = 21)		
	Decline	Stable	Improve	Decline	Stable	Improve
Academic achievement						
Wechsler Individual Achievement Test						
Reading decoding	3.4	96.6	0.0	0.0	100	0.0
Reading comprehension	23.1	73.1	3.8	5.3	84.2	10.5
Spelling	6.9	93.1	0.0	10.0	85.0	5.0
Arithmetic	20.7	69.0	10.3	5.0	90.0	5.0
Visual sustained attention						
Vigilance and distractibility tasks from Gordon Diagnostic System						
Vigilance						
Correct	42.3	26.9	30.8	21.1	36.8	42.1
Errors of commission	34.6	50.0	15.4	10.5	42.1	47.4
Distractibility						
Correct	30.4	34.8	34.8	14.3	42.8	42.9
Errors of commission	17.4	34.8	47.8	0.0	35.7	64.3

Note: Mean age is 13. Data reflects various seizure foci and severity pre surgery. Change reflects ≥ or ≤ 1 SD 1 year post surgery; WISC-III = Wechsler Intelligence Scale for Children – 3rd Edition; WAIS-III = Wechsler Adult Intelligence Scale – 3rd Edition. Assistance with Table by Eric Rinehardt, PhD, Department of Psychiatry and Neurosciences, University of South Florida College of Medicine, Tampa, FL USA.

Summary

Epilepsy is a disease associated with more than one unprovoked seizure, and is a common neurological disorder. In general, the prognosis for most epilepsies are good. Neuropsychological deficits are observed in focal epilepsies as well as some idiopathic generalized epilepsies. Moreover, neuropsychological studies of the "benign epilepsy" syndromes, which have identified subtle deficits in some cases, has begun to change our understanding of epilepsy and seizures themselves.

Neuropsychologists are integral members of the epilepsy surgical team, and neuropsychological data provide important data to the diagnosis and management of patients with epilepsy. Within the frame of neuropsychological science and practice, epilepsy provides data for guiding an evidence-based neuropsychology practice. Neuropsychological data have clear implications for predicting post-surgical memory and language outcome following anterior temporal lobectomy for medication refractory epilepsy. Moreover, there are data establishing that neuropsychological data are helpful in predicting the side of seizure onset (lateralized dysfunction in focal epilepsy), and there are limited contexts in which neuropsychological data can assist in predicting seizure outcome (seizure freedom). These limited settings tend to involve cases in which there is no clear lesion or for which EEG findings for lateralization are mixed. However, these data are preliminary and largely do not integrate other non-invasive neuroimaging techniques that have recently been developed (e.g., MEG/MSI, functional neuroimaging, or PET studies), although Potter et al. 2009 did find limited support for neuropsychological variables in a multivariate model including MRI data. However, another recent study combining multiple non-invasive studies (MRI, SISCOM) to predict seizure outcome did not find neuropsychological data added to the prediction of seizure freedom (Bell et al. 2009).

Neuropsychological study is providing a longitudinal perspective for epilepsy, in which the presence of neuropsychological dysfunction appears to be present at the time of first recognized seizure (e.g., Fastenau et al. 2009), and this data are not consistently associated with structural brain changes. Moreover, data are developing that establish neuropsychological dysfunction may be progressive over time, and when present at first onset seizure appear to increase the risk for further cognitive and academic deficits. The long-term course of epilepsy remains to be detailed, but initial data suggest neuropsychological function may be quite stable for years (up to 10 years) for some patients, but appears to decline in 20–25% of patients. The long-term impact of seizure surgery on cognitive dysfunction remains to be delineated, but initial deficits may resolve at 1 or 2 years after surgery, although initial data for long-term follow-up in older patients suggest there may be decline, particularly for verbal memory and left temporal resections.

The impact of epilepsy on neuropsychological function and quality of life is beginning to emerge. While a detailed review of QOL was beyond the scope of this chapter, the literature clearly indicate epilepsy/medical variables of perceived seizure frequency and adverse effects of AEDs have a negative effect on QOL, and treatment resulting in seizure freedom improves quality of life. In addition to these epilepsy related variables, reducing psychiatric symptoms of anxiety and/or depression, increasing cognitive activity, and improving resilience variables of the patient along with reducing negative stigma and discrimination of epilepsy can improve QOL. The role of the neuropsychologist cannot only provide consultation for assessing, monitoring over time, and predicting cognitive outcome but can also improve patients QOL.

Appendix 1. International Classification of Epilepsies, Epileptic Syndromes, and Related Seizure Disorders

I. Localization-related (focal, partial, local)
   A. Idiopathic (primary)
      1. Benign childhood epilepsy with centrotemporal spikes (benign rolandic epilepsy).
      2. Childhood epilepsy with occipital paroxysms.
      3. primary reading epilepsy
   B. Symptomatic (secondary)
      1. Temporal lobe epilepsies
      2. Frontal lobe epilepsies

      3. Parietal lobe epilepsies

      4. Occipital lobe epilepsies

      5. Chronic progressive epilepsia partialis continua of childhood (Kojewnikoff's syndrome).

      6. Syndromes characterized by seizures with specific modes of precipitation (e.g., reflex epilepsies and startle epilepsies).

    C. Probably symptomatic (formally cryptogenic), defined by:

      1. Seizure type

      2. Clinical features

      3. Etiology

      4. Anatomical localization

b. Generalized

    A. Primary Idiopathic, in order of age of onset.

      1. Benign neonatal familial convulsions

      2. Benign neonatal convulsions

      3. Benign myoclonic epilepsy in infancy

      4. Childhood absence epilepsy (pyknolepsy).

      5. Juvenile absence epilepsy

      6. Juvenile myoclonic epilepsy (of Janz).

      7. Epilepsy with generalized tonic-clonic convulsions on awakening

      8. Other generalized idiopathic epilepsies

      9. Epilepsies with seizure precipitated by specific modes of activation.

    B. Probably symptomatic (formally cryptogenic), in order of age of onset

      1. West's syndrome

      2. Lennox-Gastaut syndrome

      3. Epilepsy with myoclonic-astatic seizures

      4. Epilepsy with myoclonic absences

    C. Symptomatic (secondary)

      1. Nonspecific etiology

        a. Early myoclonic encephalopathy

        b. Early infantile epileptic encephalopathy with suppression bursts

        c. Other symptomatic generalized epilepsies

      2. Specific syndromes

        a. Neurological diseases with seizures as a prominent feature.

c. Epilepsies undetermined whether focal or generalized

    A. With both focal and generalized seizures

      1. Neonatal seizures

      2. Severe myoclonic epilepsy of infancy

      3. Epilepsy with continuous spike waves during slow-wave sleep

      4. Acquired epileptic aphasia (Landau-Kleffner syndrome)

      5. Other undetermined epilepsies

d. Special syndromes

    A. Situation-related seizures

      1. Febrile convulsions

2. Isolated seizures or isolated status epilepticus

3. Seizures occurring only with acute metabolic or toxic events due to factors such as alcohol, drugs, eclampsia, and nonketotic hyperglycemia.

Appendix 2. Example of Newly Proposed Classification of Epilepsy Syndromes (2001)

I. Localization-related (focal, partial, local)
  A. Idiopathic (primary) epilepsies of infancy and childhood
    1. Benign infantile seizures
    2. Benign childhood epilepsy with centrotemporal spikes (benign rolandic epilepsy).
    3. Childhood epilepsy with occipital paroxysms.
  B. Familial (autosomal dominant)
    1. Benign familial neonatal seizures
    2. Benign familial infantile seizures
    3. Autosomal dominant nocturnal frontal lobe epilepsy
    4. familial temporal lobe epilepsy
    5. familial focal epilepsy with variable foci
  C. Symptomatic (or probably symptomatic) epilepsies
    1. Limbic epilepsies
      a. Messial temporal lobe epilepsy with hippocampal sclerosis
      b. Mesial temporal lobe epilepsy defined by specific etiologies
      c. Other types defined by location and etiology
    2. Neocortical epilepsies
      a. Rasmussen syndrome
      b. Hemiconvulsion-hemiplegia syndrome
      c. Other types defined by location and etiology (frontal, parietal, and occipital lobe epilepsies)
    3. Migrating partial seizures of early infancy
II. Generalized
  A. Idiopathic, in order of age of onset.
    1. Benign myoclonic epilepsy in infancy
    2. Epilepsy with myoclonic astatic seizures
    3. Childhood absence epilepsy (pyknolepsy).
    4. Epilepsy with myoclonic absences
    5. Idiopathic generalized epilepsies with variable phenotypes
      a. Juvenile absence epilepsy
      b. Juvenile myoclonic epilepsy (of Janz).
      c. Epilepsy with generalized tonic-clonic seizures only
    6. Other generalized idiopathic epilepsies
  B. Familial
    7. Benign neonatal familial convulsions

III. Epileptic encephalopathies (epileptiform abnormalities may contribute to progressive dysfunction).
  A. Early myoclonic encephalopathy
  B. Ostahara syndrome
  C. West's syndrome
  D. Dravet syndrome (also known as severe myoclonic epilepsy in infancy).
  D. Myoclonic status in nonprogressive encephalopathies
  E. Lennox-Gastaut syndrome
  F. Landau-Kleffner syndrome (acquired epileptic aphasia)
  G. Epilepsy with continuous spike-waves during slow-wave sleep.
IV. Reflex epilepsies
  A. Idiopathic photosensitive occipital lobe epilepsy
  B. Other visual sensitive epilepsy
  C. Primary reading epilepsy
  D. Startle epilepsy
  e. Progressive myoclonus epilepsies
  A. Various specific diseases
  f. Seizures not necessarily requiring a diagnosis of epilepsy
  A. Benign neonatal seizures
  B. Febrile seizures
  C. Reflex seizures
  D. Alcohol or other drug induced seizures
  E. Immediate and early post-traumatic seizures
  F. Single seizures or isolated clusters of seizures
  G. Rarely repeated seizures (oligoepilepsy)

References

Aarts, J. H., Binnie, C. D., Smit, A. M., & Wilkins, A. J. (1984). Selective cognitive impairment during focal and generalized epileptiform EEG activity. *Brain, 107*(1), 239–308.

Akanuma, N., Alarcon, G., Lum, F., et al. (2003). Lateralising value of neuropsychological protocols for presurgical assessment of temporal lobe epilepsy. *Epilepsia, 44*, 408–418.

Aldenkamp, A. P., & Arends, J. (2004). The relative influence of elileptic EEG discharges, short nonconvulsive seizures, and type of epilepsy on cognitive function. *Epilepsia, 45*(1), 54–63.

Aldenkamp, A. P., De Krom, M., & Reijs, R. (2003). Newer antiepileptic drugs and cognitive issues. *Epilepsia, 44*(Suppl 4), 21–29.

Alper, A. (2008). Do antidepressants improve or worsen seizures in patients with epilepsy? In A. M. Kanner & S. Schacter (Eds.), *Psychiatric controversies in epilepsy* (pp. 255–268). London: Elsevier Inc.

Alpherts, W. C., Vermeulen, J., van Rijen, P. C., da Silva, F. H., & van Veelen, C. W. (2006). Dutch Collaborative Epilepsy Surgery Program. Verbal memory decline after temporal epilepsy surgery? A 6 year multiple assessments follow-up schedule. *Neurology, 67*, 626–631.

Andelman, F., Kipervasser, S., Neufeld, M. Y., Kramer, U., & Fried, I. (2006). Predictive value of Wada memory scores on postoperative learning and memory abilities in patients with intractable epilepsy. *Journal of Neurosurgery, 105*, 20–26.

Andermann, F., Bourgeois, B., Leppik, I. E., Ojemann, L., & Sherwin, A. L. (1993). Postoperative pharmacotherapy and discontinuation of antiepileptic drugs. In J. J. Engel (Ed.), *Surgical treatment of the epilepsies* (2nd ed., pp. 679–684). New York: Raven Press.

Anhoury, S., Brown, R. J., Krishnamoorthy, E. S., & Trimble, M. R. (2000). Psychiatric outcome after temporal lobectomy: A predictive study. *Epilepsia, 41,* 1608–1615.

Austin, J. K., Huberty, T. J., Huster, G. A., & Dunn, D. W. (1998). Academic achievement in children with epilepsy or asthma. *Developmental Medicine and Child Neurology, 40*(4), 248–255.

Austin, J. K., Harezlak, J., Dunn, D. W., Huster, G. A., Rose, D. F., & Ambrosius, W. T. (2001). Behavior problems in children before first recognized seizures. *Pediatrics, 107,* 115–122.

Austin, J. K., Perkins, S. M., Johnson, C. S., Fastenau, P. S., Byars, A. W., Degrauw, T. J., & Dunn, D. W. (2010). Self-esteem and symptoms of depression in children with seizures: Relationships with neuropsychological function and family variables over time. Epilepsia, (epub ahead of print).

Baker, G. A., & Taylor, J. (2008). Neuropsychological effects of seizures. In S. C. Schachter, G. I. Holmes, & D. Kasteleijn-Nolst Trenite (Eds.), *Behavioural aspects of epilepsy: Principles and practice* (pp. 93–98). New York: Demos.

Barbaro, N. M., Quigg, M., Broshek, D. K., Ward, M. M., Lamborn, K. R., Laxer, K. D., et al. (2009). A multicenter, prospective pilot study of gamma knife radiosurgery for mesial temporal lobe epilepsy: Seizure response, adverse events, and verbal memory. *Annals of Neurology, 65,* 167–175.

Barr, W. B., Chelune, G. J., Hermann, B. P., Loring, D. W., Perrine, K., Strauss, E., et al. (1997). The use of figural reproduction tests as measures of nonverbal memory in epilepsy surgery candidates. *Journal of the International Neuropsychological Society, 3,* 435–443.

Bartha, L., Benke, T., Bauer, G., & Trinka, E. (2005). Interictal language functions in temporal lobe epilepsy. *Journal of Neurology, Neurosurgery and Psychiatry, 76,* 808–814.

Bartolomei, F., Hayashi, M., Tamura, M., Rey, M., Fischer, C., Chauvel, P., et al. (2008). Long-term efficacy of gamma knife radiosurgery in mesial temporal epilepsy. *Neurology, 70,* 1658–1663.

Baxendale, S. A. (2009). The Wada test. *Current Opinion in Neurology, 22,* 185–189.

Baxendale S., & Thompson P. (2005). Defining meaningful postoperative change in epilepsy surgery patients: measuring the unmeasurable? *Epilepsy and Behavior, 6,* 207–211.

Baxendale, S., & Thompson, P. (2010). Beyond localization: The role of traditional neuropsychological tests in an age of imaging. *Epilepsia, 51,* 2225–2230.

Baxendale, S. A., Thompson, P. J., Harkness, W., & Duncan, J. S. (2006). Predicting memory decline following epilepsy surgery: A multivariate approach. *Epilepsia, 47,* 1887–1894.

Baxendale, S. A., Thompson, P. J., & Duncan, J. S. (2008). Evidence-based practice: A reevaluation of the intracarotid amobarbital procedure (Wada test). *Archives of Neurology, 65,* 841–845.

Bell, M. L., Rao, S., So, E. L., Trenerry, M., Kazemi, N., Stead, S. M., et al. (2009). Epilepsy surgery outcomes in temporal lobe epilepsy with normal MRI. *Epilepsia, 50,* 2053–2060.

Berg, A. T., Smith, S. N., & Frobish, D. (2005). Special education needs of children with newly diagnosed epilepsy. *Developmental Medicine and Child Neurology, 47,* 749–753.

Bernasconi, N., Duchesne, S., Janke, A., Lerch, J., Collins, D. L., & Bernasconi, A. (2004). Whole-brain voxel-based statistical analysis of gray matter and white matter in temporal lobe epilepsy. *Neuroimage, 23,* 717–723.

Bernasconi, N., Natsume, J., & Bernasconi, A. (2005). Progression in temporal lobe epilepsy: Differential atrophy in mesial temporal structures. *Neurology, 65*(2), 223–228.

Binder, D. K., Lehe, M. V., Kral, T., Bien, C. G., Urbach, H., Schramm, J., et al. (2008). Surgical treatment of occipital lobe epilepsy. *Journal of Neurosurgery, 109,* 57–69.

Binnie, C. D. (2003). Cognitive impairment during epileptiform discharges: Is it ever justifiable to treat the EEG? *Lancet Neurology, 2*(12), 725–730.

Blakemore, C. B., & Falconer, M. A. (1967). Long-term effects of anterior temporal lobectomy on certain cognitive functions. *Journal of Neurology, Neurosurgery and Psychiatry, 30,* 364–367.

Blume, W. T., Whiting, S. E., & Girvin, J. P. (1991). Epilepsy surgery in the posterior cortex. *Annals of Neurology, 29,* 638–645.

Blume, W. T., Wiebe, S., & Tapsell, L. M. (2005). Occipital epilepsy: Lateral versus mesial. *Brain, 128,* 1209–1225.

Blumer, D., Montouris, G., & Hermann, B. (1995). Psychiatric morbidity in seizure patients on a neurodiagnostic monitoring unit. *The Journal of Neuropsychiatry & Clinical Neuroscience, 7,* 445–456.

Boon, P., Vonck, K., De Herdt, V., Van Dycke, A., Goethals, M., Goossens, L., et al. (2007). Deep brain stimulation in patients with refractory temporal lobe epilepsy. *Epilepsia, 48,* 1551–1560.

Burchiel, K. J., & Christiano, J. A. (2006). Review of selective amygdalophippocampectomy techniques. In J. W. Miller & D. L. Silbergeld (Eds.), *Epilepsy surgery: Principles and controversies* (pp. 451–463). New York: Taylor & Francis.

Busch, R. M., Frazier, T. W., Haggerty, K. A., & Kubu, C. S. (2005). Utility of the Boston Naming Test in predicting ultimate side of surgery in patients with medically intractable temporal lobe epilepsy. *Epilepsia, 46*(11), 1773–1779.

Byars, A. W., Byars, K. C., Johnson, C. S., DeGrauw, T. J., Fastenau, P. S., Perkins, S., Austin, J. K., & Dunn, D. W. (2008). The relationship between sleep problems and neuropsychological functioning in children with first recognized seizures. *Epilepsy and Behavior, 13,* 607–613.

Camfield, C., Camfield, P., Smith, B., Gordon, K., & Dooley, J. (1993). Biologic factors as predictors of social outcome of epilepsy in intellectually normal children: A population-based study. *The Journal of Pediatrics, 122,* 869–873.

Cascino, G. D., Hulihan, J. F., Sharbrough, F. W., & Kelly, P. J. (2005). Parietal lobe lesional epilepsy: Electroclinical correlation and operative outcome. *Epilepsia, 34,* 522–527.

Cendes, F., Andermann, F., Dubeau, F., Matthews, P., & Arnold, D. (1997). Normalization of neuronal metabolic dysfunction after surgery for temporal lobe epilepsy: Evidence from proton MR spectroscopic imaging. *Neurology, 49*(6), 1525–1533.

Chapin, J. S., Busch, R. M., Naugle, R. I., & Najm, I. M. (2009). The family pictures subtest of the WMS-III: Relationship to verbal and visual memory following temporal lobectomy for intractable epilepsy. *Journal of Clinical and Experimental Neuropsychology, 31,* 498–504.

Chee, M. W., Kotagal, P., Van Ness, P. C., Gragg, L., Murphy, D., & Luders, H. O. (1993). Lateralizing signs in intractable partial epilepsy: Blinded multiple-observer analysis. *Neurology, 43,* 2519–2525.

Chelune, G. J. (1995). Hippocampal adequacy versus functional reserve: Predicting memory functions following temporal lobectomy. *Archives of Clinical Neuropsychology, 10*(5), 413–432.

Chelune, G. J. (2008). Evidence-based research and practice in clinical neuropsychology. *The Clinical Neuropsychologist, 24,* 454–467.

Chelune, G. J., & Najm, I. (2001). Risk factors associated with postsurgical decrements in memory. In H. O. Lüders & Y. Comair (Eds.), *Epilepsy surgery* (2nd ed., pp. 497–504). New York: Lippincott: Williams & Wilkins.

Chelune, G. J., Naugle, R. I., Luders, H., Sedlak, J., & Awad, I. A. (1993). Individual change after epilepsy surgery: Practice effects and base-rate information. *Neuropsychology, 7,* 41–52.

Cheung, M. C., Chan, A. S., Chan, Y. L., Lam, J. M., & Lam, W. (2006). Effects of illness duration on memory processing of patients with temporal lobe epilepsy. *Epilepsia, 47*(8), 1320–1328.

Chilosi, A. M., Brovedani, P., Moscatelli, M., Bonanni, P., & Guerrini, R. (2006). Neuropsychological findings in idiopathic occipital lobe epilepsies. *Epilepsia, 47*(Suppl. 2), 76–78.

Cocoran, R., & Upton, D. (1993). A role for the hippocampus in card sorting? *Cortex, 29,* 293–304.

Cohen, M. (1997). *Child Memory Scale (CMS).* San Antonio, TX: The Psychological Corporation.

Cohen-Gadol, A. A., Wilhelmi, B. G., Collignon, F., White, J. B., Britton, J. W., Cambier, D. M., et al. (2006). Long-term outcome of epilepsy surgery among 399 patients with nonlesional seizure foci including mesial temporal lobe sclerosis. *Journal of Neurosurgery, 104*(4), 513–524.

Cramer, J. A., Blum, D., Fanning, K., Reed, M., & Group, t. E. I. P. (2004). The impact of comorbid depression on health resource utilization in a community sample of people with epilepsy. *Epilepsy & Behavior, 5,* 337–342.

Dalmagro, C. L., Bianchin, M. M., Velasco, T. R., Alexandre, J. V., Walz, R., Terra-Bustamonte, V. C., et al. (2005). Clinical features of patients with posterior cortical epilepsies and predictors of surgical outcome. *Epilepsia, 46*(9), 1442–1449.

Damasio, H., Grabowski, T. J., Tranel, D., Hichwa, R. D., & Damasio, A. (1996). A neural basis for lexical retrieval. *Nature, 380,* 499–505.

Davies, S. H. I., & Goodman, R. (2003). A population survey of mental health problems in children with epilepsy. *Developmental Medicine and Child Neurology, 45,* 292–295.

Davies, K. G., Bell, B. D., Bush, A., Hermann, B. P., Dohan, F. C. J., & Jaap, A. S. (1998). Naming decline after left anterior temporal lobectomy correlates with pathological status of resected hippocampus. *Epilepsia, 39*(4), 407–419.

Dikmen, S. S., Heaton, R. K., Grant, I., & Temkin, N. R. (1999). Test – retest reliability and practice effects of Expanded Halstead – Reitan Neuropsychological Test Battery. *Journal of the International Neuropsychological Society, 5*(4), 346–356.

Dodrill, C. (1984). Number of seizure types in relation to emotional and psychosocial adjustment in epilepsy. In R. J. Porter et al. (Eds.), *Advances in epileptology: XVth Epilepsy international symposium* (pp. 541–544). NY: Raven Press.

Dodrill, C. (1986). Correlates of generalized tonic-clonic seizures with intellectual, neuropsychological, emotional, and social function in patients with epilepsy. *Epilepsia, 27*(4), 399–411.

Dodrill, C. (2004). Neuropsychological effects of seizures. *Epilepsy & Behavior, 5*(suppl 1), S21–S24.

Dodrill, C., et al. (1984). Number of Seizure Types in relation to emotional and psychosocial adjustment in epilepsy. In R. J. porter (Ed.), *Advances in epileptology: XVth epilepsy international symposium* (pp. 541–544). New York: Raven Press.

Drane, D. L., & Meador, K. J. (Eds.). (2002). *Cognitive toxicity of antiepileptic drugs.* Boston: Butterworth-Heinemann.

Drane, D. L., Ojemann, G. A., Tranel, D., Ojemann, J. G., & Miller, J. W. (2004). Category-specific naming and recognition deficits in patients with temporal lobe epilepsy. *Journal of the International Neuropsychological Society, 10*(Suppl. 1), 202.

Drane, D. L., Lee, G. P., Cech, H., Huthwaite, J. S., Ojemann, G. A., Ojemann, J. G., et al. (2006). Structured cueing on a semantic fluency task differentiates patients with temporal versus frontal lobe seizure onset. *Epilepsy & Behavior, 9*(2), 339–344.

Drane, D., Ojemann, G., Aylward, E., Ojemann, J., Johnson, L., Silbergeld, D., et al. (2008). Category-specific naming and recognition deficits in temporal lobe epilepsy. *Neuropsychologia, 46*(5), 1242–1255.

Dulay, M. F., Schefft, B. K., Marc Testa, S., Fargo, J. D., Privitera, M., & Yeh, H. S. (2002). What does the family picture subtest of the Wechsler Memory Scale-III measure? Insight gained from patients evaluated for epilepsy surgery. *The Clinical Neuropsychologist, 16*(4), 452–462.

Dunn, D. W., Harezlak, J., Ambrosius, W. T., Austin, J. K., & Hale, B. (2002). Teacher assessment of behaviour in children with new-onset seizures. *Seizure, 11,* 169–175.

Elger, C. E., Helmstaedter, C., & Martin, K. (2004). Chronic epilepsy and cognition. *Lancet Neurology, 3,* 663–672.

Elshorst, N., Pohlmann-Eden, B., Horstmann, S., Schulz, R., Woermann, F., & McAndrews, M. P. (2009). Postoperative memory prediction in left temporal lobe epilepsy: The Wada test is of no added value to preoperative neuropsychological assessment and MRI. *Epilepsy & Behavior, 16,* 335–340.

Engel, J. J., & Epilepsy, I. L. A. (2001). A proposed diagnostic scheme for people with epileptic seizures and with epilepsy: Report of the ILAE Task Force on Classification and Terminology. *Epilepsia, 42*(6), 796–803.

Engel, J. J., Van Ness, P. C., Rasmussen, T. B., & Ojemann, L. M. (1993). Outcome with respect to epileptic seizures. In J. J. Engel (Ed.), *Surgical treatment of the epilepsies* (pp. 609–621). New York: Raven Press.

Epilepsy, I. L. A. (1989). Proposal for revised classification of epilepsies and epileptic syndromes: Commission on classification and terminology of the international league against epilepsy. *Epilepsia, 30*(4), 389–399.

Ettinger, A., Reed, M., & Cramer, J. (2004). Depression and comorbidity in community-based patients with epilepsy or asthma. *Neurology, 63*(6), 1008–1014.

Falconer, M. A., Meyer, A., Hill, D., Mitchell, W., & Pond, D. A. (1955). Treatment of temporal-lobe epilepsy by temporal lobectomy: A survey of findings and results. *Lancet, 268*, 827–835.

Farrant, A., Morris, R. G., Russell, T., Elwes, R., Akanuma, N., Alarcon, G., et al. (2005). Social cognition in frontal lobe epilepsy. *Epilepsy & Behavior, 7*(3), 506–516.

Fastenau, P. S., Johnson, C. S., Perkins, S. M., Byars, A. W., DeGrauw, T. J., Austin, J. K., et al. (2009). Neuropsychology status at seizure onset in children: Risk factors for early cognitive deficits. *Neurology, 73*, 526–534.

Fastenau, P. S., Shen, J., Dunn, D. W., Perkins, S. M., Hermann, B. P., & Austin, J. K. (2004). Neuropsychological predictors of academic underachievement in pediatric epilepsy: Moderating roles of demographic, seizure, and psychosocial variables. *Epilepsia, 45*, 1261–1272.

Feindel, W., & Rasmussen, T. (1991). Temporal lobectomy with amygdalectomy and minimal hippocampal resection: Review of 100 cases. *Canadian Journal of Neurological Science, 18*, 603–605.

Fisher, R. S. (2008). Non-pharmacological approach: Release of the "Stimulation of the Anterior Nucleus of the Thalamus in Epilepsy (SANTE)" trial results. Program presentation at *the 62nd annual meeting of the American Epilepsy Society*, Seattle, December, 6, 2008.

Fuller-Thomson, E., & Brennenstuhl, S. (2009). The association between depression and epilepsy in a nationally representative sample. *Epilepsia, 50*(5), 1051–1058.

Gaitatzis, A., Trimble, M. R., & Sander, J. W. (2004). The psychiatric comorbidity of epilepsy. *Acta Neurologica Scandinavica, 110*, 207–220.

Gastaut, H., Roger, J., Soulayrol, R., Tassinari, C. A., Regis, H., Dravet, C., et al. (1966). Childhood epileptic encephalopathy of children with diffuse slow spike-waves (otherwise known as "petit mal variant") or Lennox syndrome. *Epilepsia, 7*, 139–179.

Gazzaniga, M. S. (1985). Some contributions of split-brain studies to the study of human cognition. In A. G. Reeves (Ed.), *Epilepsy and the corpus callosum* (pp. 341–348). New York: Plenum Press.

Gilliam, R. A. (1990). Refractory epilepsy: An evaluation of psychological methods in outpatient management. *Epilepsia, 31*, 427–443.

Gilliam, F., & Kanner, A. M. (2002). Treatment of depressive disorders in epilepsy patients. *Epilepsy & Behavior, 3*(5, Supplement 1), 2–9.

Gil-Nagel, A., & Risinger, M. W. (1997). Ictal semiology in hippocampal versus extrahippocampal temporal lobe epilepsy. *Brain, 120*, 183–192.

Glosser, G., Salvucci, A. E., & Chiaravalloti, N. D. (2003). Naming and recognizing famous faces in temporal lobe epilepsy. *Neurology, 61*, 81–86.

Glosser, G., Saykin, A. J., Deutsch, G. K., O'Connor, M. J., & Sperling, M. R. (1995). Neural organization of material-specific memory functions in temporal lobe epilepsy patients as assessed by the intracarotid amobarbital test. *Neuropsychology, 9*(4), 449–456.

Golby, A. J., Poldrack, R. A., Brewer, J. B., Spencer, D., Desmond, J. E., Aron, A. P., et al. (2001). Material-specific lateralization in the mesial temporal lobe and prefrontal crotex during memory encoding. *Brain, 124*, 1841–1854.

Gomer, B., Wagner, K., Frings, L., Saar, J., Carius, A., Härle, M., et al. (2007). The influence of antiepileptic drugs on cognition: A comparison of levetiracetam with topiramate. *Epilepsy & Behavior, 103*, 486–494.

Gong, G., Concha, L., Beaulieu, C., & Gross, D. W. (2008). Thalamic diffusion and volumetry in temporal lobe epilepsy with and without mesial temporal sclerosis. *Epilepsy Research, 80*(2 – 3), 184–193.

Griffith, H. R., Richardson, E., Pyzalski, R. W., Bell, B., Dow, C., Hermann, B. P., et al. (2006). Memory for famous faces and the temporal pole: Functional imaging findings in temporal lobe epilepsy. *Epilepsy & Behavior, 9*(1), 173–180.

Grivas, A., Schramm, J., Kral, R., von Lehe, M., Helmstaedter, C., Elger, C. E., et al. (2006). Surgical treatment for refractory temporal lobe epilepsy in the elderly: Seizure outcome and neuropsychological sequels compared with a younger cohort. *Epilepsia, 47*(8), 1364–1372.

Guidelines for epidemiologic studies on epilepsy (1993). Commission on epidemiology and prognosis, International league against epilepsy. *Epilepsia*, 34, 592–596.

Gupta, A. K., Jeavons, P. M., Hughes, R. C., & Covanis, A. (1983). Aura in temporal lobe epilepsy: Clinical and electroencephalographic correlation. *Journal of Neurology, Neurosurgery and Psychiatry, 46*(12), 1079–1083.

Hamberger, M. J., & Seidel, W. T. (2003). Auditory and visual naming tests: Normative and patient data for accuracy, response time, and tip-of-the-tongue. *Journal of the International Neuropsychological Society, 9*(3), 479–489.

Hamberger, M. J., & Tamny, T. R. (1999). Auditory naming and temporal lobe epilepsy. *Epilepsy Research, 35*, 229–243.

Hamberger, M. J., Seidel, W. T., McKhann, G. M., & Goodman, R. R. (2010). Hippocampal removal affects visual but not auditory naming. *Neurology, 74*, 1488–1493.

Hamer, H. M., & Luders, H. O. (2001). A new approach for classification of epileptic syndromes and epileptic seizures. In H. O. Luders (Ed.), *Epilepsy surgery* (2nd ed.). New York: Lippincott, Williams & Wilkins.

Haut, J. S., Busch, R. M., Klaas, P. A., Lineweaver, T. T., Naugle, R. I., Kotagal, P., & Bingaman, W. (2006). Reliable change index scores for memory (CMS) and IQ (WISC-III) among children with medically-refractory epilepsy. *Epilepsia*, 47(s4), 111.

Heaton, R. K., Temkin, N., Dikmen, S., Avitable, N., Taylor, M. J., Marcotte, T. D., et al. (2001). Detecting change: a comparison of three neuropsychological methods, using normal and clinical samples. *Archives of Clinical Neuropsychology, 16*(1), 75–91.

Helmstaedter, C. (2001). Behavioral aspects of frontal lobe epilepsy. *Epilepsy & Behavior, 2*, 384–395.

Helmstaedter, C. (2004). Neuropsychological aspects of epilepsy surgery. *Epilepsy & Behavior, 5*(Suppl. 1), S45–S55.

Helmstaedter, C., & Kockelmann, E. (2006). Cognitive outcomes in patients with chronic temporal lobe epilepsy. *Epilepsia, 47*(Suppl. 2), 96–98.

Helmstaedter, C., Kemper, B., & Elger, C. E. (1996). Neuropsychological aspects of frontal lobe epilepsy. *Neuropsychologia, 34*(5), 399–406.

Helmstaedter, C., Gleissner, U., Zentner, J., & Elger, C. E. (1998). Neuropsychological conse-quences of epilepsy surgery in frontal lobe epilepsy. *Neuropsychologia, 36*, 681–689.

Helmstaedter, C., Kurthen, M., Lux, S., Reuber, M., & Elger, C. E. (2003). Chronic epilepsy and cognition: A longitudinal study in temporal lobe epilepsy. *Annals of Neurology, 54*(4), 425–432.

Helmstaedter, C., Van Roost, D., Clusmann, H., Urbach, H., Elger, C. E., & Schramm, J. (2004). Collateral brain damage, a potential source of cognitive impairment after selective surgery for control of mesial temporal lobe epilepsy. *Journal of Neurology, Neurosurgery and Psychiatry, 75*(2), 323–326.

Henkin, Y., Sadeh, M., Kivity, S., Shabtai, E., Kishon-Rabin, L., & Gadoth, N. (2005). Cognitive function in idiopathic generalized epilepsy of childhood. *Developmental Medicine and Child Neurology, 47*, 126–132.

Hennessy, M. J., Elwes, R. D. C., Honavar, M., Rabe-Hesketh, S., Binnie, C. D., & Polkey, C. E. (2001). Predictors of outcome and pathological considerations in the surgical treatment of intractable epilepsy associated with temporal lobe lesions. *Journal of Neurology, Neurosurgery and Psychiatry, 70*, 450–458.

Hermann, B., Seidenberg, M., & Jones, J. (2008). The neurobehavioral comorbidities of epilepsy: Can a natural history be developed? *Lancet Neurology, 7*, 151–160.

Hermann, B., & Loring, D. W. (2008). Improving neuropsychological outcomes from epilepsy surgery. *Epilepsy & Behavior, 13*, 5–6.

Hermann, B., & Seidenberg, M. (1995). Executive system dysfunction in temporal lobe epilepsy: Effects of nociferous cortex versus hippocampal pathology. *Journal of Clinical and Experimental Neuropsychology, 17*(6), 809–819.

Hermann, B. P., Dikmen, S. S., & Wilensky, A. J. (1982). Increased psychopathology associated with multiple seizure types: Fact or artifact? *Epilepsia, 23*, 587–596.

Hermann, B. P., Wyler, A. R., & Richey, E. T. (1988a). Wisconsin Card Sorting Test performance in patients with complex partial seizures of temporal-lobe origin. *Journal of Clinical and Experimental Neuropsychology, 10*, 467–476.

Hermann, B. P., Wyler, A. R., Steenman, H., & Richey, E. T. (1988b). The interrelationship between language function and verbal learning/memory performance in patients with complex partial seizures. *Cortex, 24*(2), 245–253.

Hermann, B. P., Seidenberg, M., Schoenfeld, J., Peterson, J., Leveroni, C., & Wyler, A. R. (1996). Empirical techniques for determining the reliability, magnitude, and pattern of neuropsychological change after epilepsy surgery. *Epilepsia, 37*(10), 942–950.

Hermann, B. P., Seidenberg, M., Schoenfeld, J., & Davies, K. (1997). Neuropsychological characteristics of the syndrome of mesial temporal lobe epilepsy. *Archives of Neurology, 54*, 369–376.

Hermann, B., Davies, K., Foley, K., & Bell, B. (1999). Visual confrontation naming outcome after standard left anterior temporal lobectomy with sparing versus resection of the superior temporal gyrus: A randomized prospective clinical trial. *Epilepsia, 40*(8), 1070–1076.

Hermann, B., Seidenberg, M., & Bell, B. (2000). Psychiatric comorbidity in chronic epilepsy: Indentification, consequences, and treatment of major depression. *Epilepsia, 41*(Suppl 2), S31–S41.

Hermann, B., Seidenberg, M., Bell, B., Rutecki, P., Sheth, R. D., Wendt, G., et al. (2003). Extratemporal quantitative MR volumetrics and neuropsychological status in temporal lobe epilepsy. *Journal of the International Neuropsychological Society, 9*(3), 353–362.

Hermann, B., Jones, J., Sheth, R., Dow, C., Koehn, M., & Seidenberg, M. (2006). Children with new-onset epilepsy: Neuropsychological status and brain structure. *Brain, 129*, 2609–2619.

Hermann, B., Seidenberg, M., Lee, E. J., Chan, F., & Rutecki, P. (2007). Cognitive phenotypes in temporal lobe epilepsy. *Journal of the International Neuropsychological Society, 13*, 12–20.

Hernandez, M. T., Sauerwein, H. C., Jambaque, I., De Guise, E., Lussier, F., Lortie, A., et al. (2002). Deficits in executive function and motor coordination in children with frontal lobe epilepsy. *Neuropsychologia, 40*(4), 384–400.

Holmes, M. D., Dodrill, C. B., Wilkus, R. J., Ojemann, L. M., & Ojemann, G. A. (1998). Is partial epilepsy progressive? Ten-year follow-up of EEG and neuropsychological changes in adults with partial seizures. *Epilepsia, 39*, 1189–1193.

Holmes, M. D., Miles, A. N., Dodrill, C. B., Ojemann, G. A., & Wilensky, A. J. (2003). Identifying potential surgical candidates in patients with evidence of bitemporal epilepsy. *Epilepsia, 44*(8), 1075–1079.

Holmes, M. D., Brown, M., & Tucker, D. M. (2004). Are "generalized" seizures truly generalized? Evidence of localized mesial frontal and frontopolar discharges in absence. *Epilepsia, 45*(12), 1568–1579.

Hori, T., Yamane, F., Ochiai, T., Hayashi, M., & Taira, T. (2003). Subtemporal amygdalohippocampectomy prevents verbal memory impairment in the language-dominant hemisphere. *Stereotactic and Functional Neurosurgery, 80*, 18–21.

International League Against Epilepsy (1989). Proposal for the revised classification of epilepsies and epileptic syndromes. *Epilepsia, 30*, 389–399.

Jacoby, A., & Baker, G. A. (2008). Auality-of-life trajectories in epilepsy: A review of the literature. *Epilepsy & Behavior, 12*, 557–571.

Jacoby, A., Baker, G. A., Steen, N., Potts, P., & Chadwick, D. W. (1996). The clincial couse of epilepsy and its psychosocial correlates: Findings from a UK community study. *Epilepsia, 32*(2), 148–161.

Jacoby, A., Snape, D., & Bakere, G. (2009). Determinants of quality of life in people with epilepsy. *Neurologic Clinics, 27*, 843–863.

Joanette, Y., & Goulet, P. (1986). Criterion-specific reduction of verbal fluency in right brain-damaged right-handers. *Neuropsychologia, 24*, 875–879.

Jobst, B. C., Siegel, A. M., Thadani, V. M., Roberts, D. W., Rhodes, H. C., & Williamson, P. D. (2000). Intractable seizures of frontal lobe origin: Clinical characteristrics localizing signs and results of surgery. *Epilepsia, 41*, 1139–1152.

Jokeit, H., & Ebner, A. (1999). Long term effects of refractory temporal lobe epilepsy on cognitive abilities: A cross sectional study. *Journal of Neurology, Neurosurgery and Psychiatry, 67*, 44–50.

Jokeit, H., & Ebner, A. (2002). Effects of chronic epilepsy on intellectual functioning. *Progress in Brain Research, 135*, 455–463.

Jokeit, H., & Schacher, M. (2004). Neuropsychological aspects of type of epilepsy and etiological factors in adults. *Epilepsy & Behavior, 5*(Supplement 1), 14–20.

Jokeit, H., Seitz, R. J., Markowitsch, H. J., Neumann, N., Witte, O. W., & Ebner, A. (1997). Prefrontal asymmetric interictal glucose hypometabolism and cognitive impairment in patients with temporal lobe epilepsy. *Brain, 120*, 2283–2294.

Jokeit, H., Heger, R., Ebner, A., & Markowitsch, H. J. (1998). Hemispheric asymetries in category-specific word retrieval. *NeuroReport, 9*, 2371–2373.

Jones, J. E., Watson, R., Sheth, R., Caplan, R., Koehn, M., Seidenberg, M., et al. (2007). Psychiatric comorbidity in children with new onset epilepsy. *Developmental Medicine and Child Neurology, 49*(7), 493–497.

Jones-Gotman, M. (1986). Right hippocampal excision impairs learning and recall of a list of abstract designs. *Neuropsychologia, 24*, 659–670.

Jones-Gotman, M. (1996). Psychological evaluation for epilepsy surgery. In J. Engel Jr. (Ed.), *Surgical treatment of the epilepsies*. Raven Press: New York.

Jones-Gotman, M., & Milner, B. (1977). Design fluency: The invention of nonsense drawings after focal cortical lesions. *Neuropsychologia, 15*, 653–674.

Jones-Gotman, M., Smith, M. L., & Zatorre, R. J. (1993). Neuropsychological testing for localizing and lateralizing the epileptogenic region. In J. Engel Jr. (Ed.), *Surgical treatment of the epilepsies* (pp. 263–271). New York: Raven Press.

Jones-Gotman, M., Zatorre, R. J., Olivier, A., Andermann, F., Cendes, F., Staunton, H., et al. (1997). Learning and retention of words and designs following excision from medial or lateral temporal-lobe structures. *Neuropsychologia, 35*, 963–973.

Juhasz, C., & Chugani, H. T. (2003). Imaging the epileptic brain with positron emission tomography. *Neuroimaging Clinics of North America, 13*, 705–716.

Kanner, A. M. (2009). Can antiepileptic drugs unmask a susceptibility to psychiatric disorders? *Nature Clinical Practice Neurology, 5*, 132–133.

Kanner, A. M., & Palac, S. (2000). Depression in epilepsy: A common but often unrecognized comorbid malady. *Epilepsy & Behavior, 1*(1), 37–51.

Kanner, A. M., & Schacter, S. (2008). *Psychiatric controversies in epilepsy*. London: Elsevier Inc.

Kanner, A. M., Wuu, J., Faught, E., Tatum, W. O., 4th, Fix, A., French, J. A., et al. (2003). A past psychiatric history may be a risk factor for topiramate-related psychiatric and cognitive adverse events. *Epilepsy & Behavior, 4*(5), 548–552.

Kanner, A. M., Byrne, R. W., Chicharro, A. V., Wuu, J., & Frey, M. (2009). Is a lifetime psychiatric history predictive of a worse postsurgical seizure outcome following a temporal lobectomy? *Neurology, 72*, 793–799.

Kasteleijn-Nolst Trenite, D. G., & Vermeiren, R. (2005). The impact of subclinical epileptiform discharges on complex tasks and cognition: Relevance for aircrew and air traffic controllers. *Epilepsy & Behavior, 6*, 31–34.

Keary, T. A., Frazier, T. W., Busch, R. M., Kubu, C. S., & Iampietro, M. (2007). Multivariate neuropsychological prediction of seizure lateralization in temporal epilepsy surgical cases. *Epilepsia, 48*(8), 1438–1446.

Keller, S. S., & Roberts, N. (2008). Voxel-based morphometry of temporal lobe epilepsy: An introduction and review of the literature. *Epilepsia, 49*(5), 741–757.

Kim, H., Yi, S., Son, E., & Kim, J. (2004a). Lateralization of epileptic foci by neuropsychological testing in mesial temporal lobe epilepsy. *Neuropsychology, 18*, 141–151.

Kim, C. H., Lee, S. A., Yoo, H. J., Kang, J. K., & Lee, J. K. (2007). Executive performance on the Wisconsin Card Sorting Test in mesial temporal lobe epilepsy. *European Neurology, 57*, 39–46.

Kim, D. W., Lee, S. K., Yun, C. H., Kim, K. K., Lee, D. S., Chung, C. K., et al. (2004b). Parietal lobe epilepsy: The semiology, yield of diagnostic workup, and surgical outcome. *Epilepsia, 45*, 641–649.

Kiper, D. C., Zesiger, P., Maeder, P., Deonna, T., & Innocenti, G. M. (2002). Vision after early-onset lesions of the occipital cortex: I. Neuropsychological and psychophysiological studies. *Neural Plasticity, 9*, 1–25.

Kluger, B. M., & Meador, K. J. (2008). Teratogenicity of antiepileptic medications. *Seminars in Neurology, 28*(3), 328–335.

Kneebone, A. C., Chelune, G. J., & Luders, H. O. (1997). Individual patient prediction of seizure lateralization in temporal lobe epilepsy: A comparison between neuropsychological memory measures and the intracarotid amobarbital procedure. *Journal of the International Neuropsychological Society, 3*, 159–168.

Kobau, R., Gilliam, F., & Thurman, D. J. (2006). Prevalence of self-reported epilepsy or seizure disorder and its association with self-reported depression and anxiety: results from the 2004 HealthStyles Survey. *Epilepsia, 45*, 1915–1921.

Kockelmann, E., Elger, C. E., & Helmstaedter, C. (2003). Significant improvement in frontal lobe associated neuropsychological functions after withdrawal of topiramate in epilepsy patients. *Epilepsy Research, 54*, 171–178.

Kwan, P., & Brodie, M. J. (2000). Epilepsy after the first drug fails: Substitution or add-on. *Seizure, 9*(7), 464–468.

Lachhwani, D. K., & Kotagal, P. (2006). Ictal semiology and the presurgical workup. In J. W. Miller & D. L. Silbergeld (Eds.), *Epilepsy surgery: Principles and controversies* (pp. 296–302). New York: Taylor & Francis.

Lacruz, M. E., Alarcón, G., Akanuma, N., Lum, F. C., Kissani, N., Koutroumanidis, M., Adachi, N., Binnie, C. D., Polkey, C. E., & Morris, R. G. (2004). Neuropsychological effects associated with temporal lobectomy and amygdalohippocampectomy depending on Wada test failure. *Journal of Neurology, Neurosurgery, and Psychiatry, 75*, 600–607.

LaFrance, W. C., Jr., Kanner, A. M., & Hermann, B. (2008). Psychiatric comorbidities in epilepsy. *International Review of Neurobiology, 83*, 347–383.

Landau, W. M., & Kleffner, F. R. (1957). Syndrome of acquired aphasia with convulsive disorder in children. *Neurology, 7*, 523–530.

Lange, R. T., Hopp, G., & Chelune, G. (2003). Profile Analysis of WAIS-III and WMS-III Performance Following Temporal Lobe Lobectomy. *Journal of the International Neuropsychological Society, 9*, 278.

Langfit, J. T., & Rausch, R. (1996). Word-finding deficits persist after left anterotemporal lobectomy. *Archives of Neurology, 53*(1), 72–76.

Lewis, A. J. (1934). Melancholia: A historical review. *The Journal of Mental Science, 80*, 1–42.

Lezak, M. D., Howieson, D. B., & Loring, D. W. (2004). *Neuropsychological assessment* (4th ed.). New York: Oxford University Press.

Liegeois, F., Connelly, A., Cross, H. J., Boyd, S. G., Gadian, D. G., Vargha-Khadem, F., et al. (2004). *Brain, 127*, 1229–1236.

Lin, J. J., Riley, J. D., Juranek, J., & Cramer, S. C. (2008). Vulnerability of the fronto-temporal connections in temporal lobe epilepsy. *Epilepsy Research, 82*, 162–170.

Lineweaver, T. T., Morris, H. H., Naugle, R. I., Najm, I. M., Diehl, B., & Bingaman, W. (2006). Evaluating the contributions of state-of-the-art assessment techniques to predicting memory outcome after unilateral anterior temporal lobectomy. *Epilepsia, 47*, 1895–1903.

LoGalbo, A., Sawrie, S., Roth, D. L., Kuzniecky, R., Knowlton, R., Faught, E., & Martin, R. (2005). Verbal memory outcome in patients with normal preoperative verbal memory and left mesial temporal sclerosis. *Epilepsy and Behavior, 6*, 337–341.

Loring, D. W., & Meador, K. J. (2008) . Wada and fMRI testing. In B. Fisch (Ed.). *Principles and practices of electrophysiological and video monitoring in epilepsy and intensive care*. Demos Medical Publishing, New York.

Loring, D. W., & Bauer, R. M. (2010). Testing the limits: Cautions and concerns regarding the new Wechsler IQ and Memory scales. *Neurology, 74*, 684–690.

Loring, D. W., Lee, G. P., Martin, R. C., & Meador, K. J. (1988). Material-specific learning in patients with partial complex seizures of temporal lobe origin: Convergent validation of memory constructs. *Journal of Epilepsy, 1*, 53–59.

Loring, D. W., Marino, S., & Meador, K. J. (2007a). Neuropsychological and behavioral effects of antiepilepsy drugs. *Neuropsychology Review, 17*(4), 413–425.

Loring, D. W., Meador, K. J., Williamson, D. J., Wiegand, F., & Hulihan, J. (2007b). Topiramate dose effects on neuropsychological function: Analysis from a randomized double-blind placebo-controlled study. *AES Abstracts, 2*, 234.

Loring, D. W., Strauss, E., Hermann, B. P., Barr, W. B., Perrine, K., Trenerry, M. R., et al. (2008). Differential neuropsychological test sensitivity to left temporal lobe epilepsy. *Journal of the International Neuropsychological Society, 14*, 394–400.

Loring, D. W., Bowden, S. C., Lee, G. P., & Meador, K. J. (2009). Diagnostic utility of Wada memory asymmetries: Sensitivity, specificity, and likelihood ratio characterization. *Neuropsychology, 23*, 687–693.

Luerding, R., Boesebeck, F., & Ebner, A. (2004). Cogntive changes after epilepsy surgery in the posterior cortex. *Journal of Neurology, Neurosurgery and Psychiatry, 75*, 583–587.

Maccotta, L., Buckner, R. L., Gilliam, F. G., & Ojemann, J. G. (2007). Changing frontal contributions to memory before and after medial temporal lobectomy. *Cerebral Cortex, 17*(2), 443–456.

Maehara, T., & Shimizu, H. (2001). Surgical outcome of corpus callosotomy in patients with drop attacks. *Epilepsia, 42*, 67–71.

Majdan, A., Sziklas, V., & Jones-Gotman, M. (1996). Performance of healthy subjects and patients with resection from the anterior temporal lobe on matched tests of verbal and visuoperceptual learning. *Journal of Clinical and Experimental Neuropsychology, 18*, 416–430.

Majoie, H. J., Berfelo, M. W., Aldenkamp, A. P., Evers, S. M., Kessels, A. G., & Renier, W. O. (2001). Vagus nerve stimulation in children with therapy-resistant epilepsy diagnosed as Lennox-Gastaut syndrome: Clinical results, neuropsychological effects, and cost-effectiveness. *Journal of Clinical Neurophysiology, 18*, 419–428.

Manchanda, R. (2002). Psychiatric disorders in epilepsy: Clinical aspects. *Epilepsy & Behavior, 3*, 39–45.

Markand, O. N. (2003). Lennox-Gastaut syndrome (Childhood epileptic encephalopathy). *Journal of Clinical Neurophysiology, 20*, 426–441.

Martin, A., & Fedio, P. (1983). Word production and comprehension in Alzheimer's disease: The breakdown of semantic knowledge. *Brain and Language, 19*, 124–141.

Martin, R. C., Loring, D. W., Meador, K. J., & Lee, G. P. (1990). The effects of lateralized temporal lobe dysfunction on formal and semantic word fluency. *Neuropsychologia, 28*, 823–829.

Martin, R. C., Sawrie, S. M., Roth, D. L., Gilliam, F. G., Faught, E., Morawetz, R. B., et al. (1998). Individual memory change after anterior temporal lobectomy: A base rate analysis using regression-based outcome metholodolgy. *Epilepsia, 39*, 1075–1081.

Martin, R. C., Sawrie, S. M., Edwards, R., Roth, D. L., Faught, E., Kuzniecky, R. I., et al. (2000). Investigation of executive function change following anterior temporal lobectomy: Selective normalization of verbal fluency. *Neuropsychology, 14*(2), 501–508.

Martin, R., Sawrie, S., Gilliam, F., Mackey, M., Faught, E., Knowlton, R., et al. (2002). Determining reliable cognitive change after epilepsy surgery: Development of reliable change indices and standardized regression-based change norms for the WMS-III and WAIS-III. *Epilepsia, 43*(12), 1551–1558.

Mayeux, R., Brandt, J., Rosen, J., & Benson, D. F. (1980). Interictal memory and language imparment in temporal lobe epliepsy. *Neurology, 30*, 120–125.

McAndrews, M. P., & Milner, B. (1991). The frontal cortex and memory for temporal order. *Neuropsychologia, 29*(9), 849–859.

McClelland, r S, Garcia, R. E., Paraza, D. M., Shih, T. T., Hirsch, L. J., Hirsch, J., et al. (2006). Facial emotion recognition after curative nondominant temporal lobectomy in patients with mesial temporal sclerosis. *Epilepsia, 47*(8), 1337–1342.

McCormick, D. (2002). Cortical and subcortical generators or normal and abnormal rhythmicity. *International Review of Neurobiology, 49*, 99–114.

McDonald, C. R., Bauer, R. M., Grande, L., Gilmore, R., & Roper, S. (2001). The role of the frontal lobes in memory: Evidence from unilateral frontal resections for relief of intractable epilepsy. *Archives of Clinical Neuropsychology, 16*, 571–585.

McDonald, C. R., Delis, D. C., Norman, M. A., Tecoma, E. S., & Iragui, V. J. (2005). Discriminating patients with frontal-lobe epilepsy and temporal-lobe epilepsy: Utility of a multilevel design fluency test. *Neurpsychology, 19*, 806–813.

McDonald, C. R., Delis, D. C., Norman, M. A., Wetter, S. R., Tecoma, E. S., & Iragui, V. J. (2005). Response inhibition and set shifting in patients with frontal lobe epilepsy or temporal lobe epilepsy. *Epilepsy and Behavior, 7*, 438–446.

McDonald, C. R., Norman, M. A., Tecoma, E., Alksne, J., & Iragui, V. (2004). Neuropsychological change following gamma knife surgery in patients with left temporal lobe epilepsy: A review of three cases. *Epilepsy & Behavior, 5*, 949–957.

McDonald, C. R., Delis, D. C., Norman, M. A., Tecoma, E. S., & Iragui, V. J. (2005a). Discriminating patients with frontal-lobe epilepsy and temporal-lobe epilepsy: Utility of a multilevel design fluency test. *Neurpsychology, 19*(6), 806–813.

McDonald, C. R., Delis, D. C., Norman, M. A., Wetter, S. R., Tecoma, E. S., & Iragui, V. J. (2005b). Response inhibition and set shifting in patients with frontal lobe epilepsy or temporal lobe epilepsy. *Epilepsy & Behavior, 7*, 438–446.

McLachlan, R. S. (1993). Suppression of interictal spikes and seizures by stimulation of the vagus nerve. *Epilepsia, 34*, 918–923.

Meador, K. J. (2008). Effects of in utero antiepileptic drug exposure. *Epilepsy Currents, 8*, 143–147.

Meador, K. J., Baker, G. A., Browning, N., Clayton-Smith, J., Combs-Cantrell, D. T., Cohen, M., et al. (2009). Cognitive function at 3 years of age after fetal explosure to antiepileptic drugs. *The New England Journal of Medicine, 360*, 1597–1605.

Mensah, S. A., Beavis, J. M., Thapar, A. K., & Kerr, M. (2006). The presence and clinical implications of depression in a community population of adults with epilepsy. *Epilepsy & Behavior, 8*, 213–219.

Mensah, S. A., Beavis, J. M., Thapar, A. K., & Kerr, M. P. (2007). A community study of the presence of anxiety disorder in people with epilepsy. *Epilepsy & Behavior, 11*, 118–124.

Milner, B. (1958). Psychological deficits produced by temporal lobe excision. In H. C. Solomon, S. Cobb, & W. Penfield (Eds.), *The brain and human behavior: Proceedings of the Association for Research in Nervous and Mental Disease*. Baltimore: The Williams and Wilkins Company.

Milner, B. (1968a). Effects of different brain lesions on card sorting. *Archives of Neurology, 9*, 90–100.

Milner, B. (1968b). Visual recognition and recall after right temporal-lobe excision in man. *Neuropsychologia, 6*(3), 191–209.

Milner, B., Petrides, M., & Smith, M. L. (1985). Frontal lobes and the temporal organization of memory. *Human Neurobiology, 4*, 137–142.

Milner, B., Corsi, P., & Leonard, G. (1991). Frontal-lobe contribution to recency judgments. *Neuropsychologia, 29*(6), 601–618.

Morrell, F., Whisler, W. W., & Bleck, T. P. (1989). Multiple subpial transection: A new approach to the surgical treatment of focal epilepsy. *Journal of Neurosurgery, 70*, 231–239.

Moser, D. J., Bauer, R. M., Gilmore, R. L., Dede, D. E., Fennell, E. G., Algina, J. J., et al. (2000). *Archives of Neurology, 57*, 707–712.

Mueller, S. G., Laxer, K. D., Cashdollar, N., Flenniken, D. L., Matson, G. B., & Weiner, M. W. (2004). Identification of abnormal neuronal metabolism outside the seizure focus in temporal lobe epilepsy. *Epilepsia, 45*(4), 355–366.

Muller, R.-A., Rothermel, R. D., Behen, M. E., Muzik, O., Chakraborty, P. K., & Chugani, H. T. (1999). Language organization in patients with early and late left-hemisphere lesion: A PET study. *Neuropsychologia, 37*, 545–557.

Naugle, R. I., Chelune, G. J., Cheek, R., Luders, H., & Awad, I. A. (1993). Detection of changes in material-specific memory following temporal lobectomy using the Wechsler Memory Scale-revised. *Archives of Clinical Neuropsychology, 8*(5), 381–395.

Neimeyer, P. (1958). The transventricular Amygdalohippocampectomy in temporal lobe epilepsy. In M. Baldwin & P. Bailey (Eds.), *Temporal lobe epilepsy* (pp. 461–482). Springfield: CC Thomas.

Noeker, M., Haverkamp-Krois, A., & Haverkamp, F. (2005). Development of mental health dysfunction in childhood epilepsy. *Brain & Development, 27*, 5–16.

Oguni, H., Hayashi, K., & Osawa, M. (1996). Long-term prognosis of Lennox-Gastaut syndrome. *Epilepsia, 37*(Suppl. 3), 44–47.

Ojemann, G. A. (2006). MRI-normal mesial temporal epilepsy is a common, surgically remedial condition. In J. W. Miller & D. L. Silbergeld (Eds.), *Epilepsy surgery: Principles and controversies* (pp. 98–99). New York: Taylor & Francis.

Ojemann, L. M., & Jung, M. E. (2006). Outcomes of temporal lobe epilepsy surgery. In J. W. Miller & D. L. Silbergeld (Eds.), *Epilepsy surgery: Principle and controversies* (pp. 661–689). New York: Taylor & Francis.

Ojemann, G. A., & Valiante, T. (2006). Resective surgery for temporal lobe epilepsy. In J. W. Miller & D. L. Silbergeld (Eds.), *Epilepsy surgery: Principles and controversy* (pp. 403–413). New York: Taylor and Francis.

Ojemann, G., Ojemann, J., Lettich, E., & Berger, M. (1989). Cortical language localization in left, dominant hemisphere. An electrical stimulation mapping investigation in 117 patients. *Journal of Neurosurgery, 71*(3), 316–326.

Olivier, A. (2000). Transcortical selective amygdalohippocampectomy in temporal lobe epilepsy. *Canadian Journal of Neurological Science, 27*, S68–S76. discussion S92.

Olney, J. W. (2002). New insights and new issues in developmental neurotoxicity. *NeuroToxcology, 23*, 659–668.

Oyegbile, T. O., Dow, D., Jones, J., Rutecki, P., Sheth, R., Seidenberg, M., et al. (2004). The nature and course of neuropsychological morbidity in chronic temporal lobe epilepsy. *Neurology, 62*, 1736–1742.

Palmini, A., Najm, I., Avanzini, G., Babb, T., Guerrini, R., Foldvary-Schaefer, N., et al. (2004). Terminology and classification of the cortical dysplasias. *Neurology, 62*(6 Suppl. 3), S2–S8.

Pataraia, E., Lindinger, G., Deecke, L., Mayer, D., & Baumgartner, C. (2005). Combined MEG/EEG analysis of the interictal spike complex in mesial temporal lobe epilepsy. *Neuroimage, 24*(3), 607–614.

Pavone, A., & Niedermeyer, E. (2000). Absence seizures and the frontal lobe. *Clinical Electroencephalography, 31*, 153–160.

Pavone, P., Bianchini, R., Trifiletti, R. R., Incorpora, G., Pavone, A., & Parano, E. (2001). Neuropsychological assessment in children with absence epilepsy. *Neurology, 56*, 1047–1051.

Penfield, W., & Jasper, H. H. (1954). *Epilepsy and the functional anatomy of the human brain.* Boston: Little, Brown.

Perrine, K., Westerveld, M., Sass, K. J., Spencer, D. D., Devinsky, O., Dogali, M., et al. (1995). *Epilepsia, 36*, 851–856.

Pigott, S., & Milner, B. (1993). Memory for different aspects of complex visual scenes after unilateral temporal- or frontal-lobe resection. *Neuropsychologia, 31*(1), 1–15.

Pillon, B., Bazin, B., Deweer, B., Ehrlé, N., Baulac, M., & Dubois, B. (1999). Specificity of memory deficits after right or left temporal lobectomy. *Cortex, 35*(4), 561–571.

Poochikian-Sarkissian, S., Wennberg, R. A., Sidani, S., & Devins, G. M. (2007). Quality of life in epilepsy. *Canadian Journal of Neuroscience Nursing, 29*(1), 20–25.

Potter, J. L., Schefft, B. K., Beebe, D. W., Howe, S. R., Yeh, H. S., & Privitera, M. D. (2009). Presurgical neuropsychological testing predicts cognitive and seizure outcomes after anterior temporal lobectomy. *Epilepsy & Behavior, 16*, 246–253.

Powell, H. W., Koepp, M. J., Symms, M. R., Boulby, P. A., Salak-Haddadi, A., Thompson, P. J., et al. (2005). Material-specific lateralization of memory encoding in the medial temporal lobe: Blocked versus event-related design. *Neuroimage, 27*, 231–239.

Privitera, M. D., Morris, G. L., & Gillam, F. (1991). Postictal language assessment and lateralization of complex partial seizures. *Annals of Neurology, 30*, 391–396.

Rapport, L. J., Millis, S. R., & Bonello, P. J. (1998). Validation of the Warrington theory of visual processing and the visual object and space perception battery. *Journal of Clinical and Experimental Neuropsychology, 20*, 211–220.

Rausch, R. (2006). Integrative neuropsychology in the preoperative workup of the epilepsy surgery patient. In J. W. Miller & D. L. Silbergeld (Eds.), *Epilepsy surgery: Principles and controversies* (pp. 183–199). New York: Taylor & Francis.

Rausch, R., & Babb, T. L. (1993). Hippocampal neuron loss and memory scores before and after temporal lobe surgery for epilepsy. *Archives of Neurology, 50*, 812–817.

Regis, J., Bartolomei, F., Rey, M., Genton, P., Dravet, C., Semah, F., et al. (1999). Gamma knife surgery for mesial temporal lobe epilepsy. *Epilepsia, 40*, 1551–1556.

Risse, G. L. (2006). Cognitive outcomes in patients with frontal lobe epilepsy. *Epilepsia, 47* (Suppl. 2), 87–89.

Robertson, M. M. (1997). Suicide, parasuicide, and epilepsy. In J. Engel & T. A. Pedley (Eds.), *Epilepsy: A comprehensive textbook* (pp. 2141–2151). Philadelphia: Lippicott-Raven.

Robinson, R. O., Baird, G., Robinson, G., & Simonoff, E. (2001). Landau-Kleffner syndrome: Course and correlates with outcome. *Developmental Medicine and Child Neurology, 43*(4), 243–247.

Rutter, M., Graham, P., & Yule, W. (1970). *A neuropsychiatric study in childhood. Clinics in developmental medicine Nos. 35/36*. London: S.I.M.P./William Heineman Medical Books.

Rzezak, P., Fuentes, D., Guimaraes, C. A., Thome-Souza, S., Kuczynski, E., Li, L. M., et al. (2007). Frontal lobe dysfunction in children with temporal lobe epilepsy. *Pediatric Neurology, 37*(3), 176–185.

Salanova, V., Andermann, F., Olivier, A., Rasmussen, T., & Quesney, L. F. (1992). Occipital lobe epilepsy: Electroclinical manifestations, electrocorticography, cortical stimulation and outcome in 42 patients treated between 1930 and 1991. Surgery of occipital lobe epilepsy. *Brain, 115*, 1655–1680.

Sass, K. J., Spencer, D. D., Spencer, S. S., Novelly, R. A., Williamson, P. D., & Mattson, R. H. (1988). Corpus callosotomy for epilepsy. II. Neurologic and neuropsychological outcome. *Neurology, 38*(1), 24–28.

Sass, K. J., Spencer, D. D., Kim, J. H., Westerveld, M., Novelly, R. A., & Lencz, T. (1990). Verbal memory impairment correlates with hippocampal pyramidal cell density. *Neurology, 40*(11), 1694–1697.

Sass, K. J., Sass, A., Westerveld, M., Lencz, T., Novelly, R. A., Kim, J. H., et al. (1992). Specificity in the correlation of verbal memory and hippocampal neuron loss: Dissociation of memory, language, and verbal intellectual ability. *Journal of Clinical and Experimental Neuropsychology, 14*, 662–672.

Satz, P., Strauss, E., Wada, J., & Orsini, D. L. (1988). Some correlates of intra- and interhemispheric speech organization after left focal brain injury. *Neuropsychologia, 26*, 345–350.

Savic, I., Seitz, R. J., & Pauli, S. (1998). Brain distortions in patients iwth primarily generalized tonic-clonic seizures. *Epilepsia, 39*, 364–370.

Savqi, S., Katz, A., Marks, D. A., & Spencer, S. S. (1992). Frontal lobe partial seizures and psychogenic seizures: Comparison of clinical and ictal characteristics. *Neurology, 42*(7), 1274–1277.

Sawrie, S. M., Chelune, G. J., Naugles, R. I., & Luders, H. O. (1996). Empirical methods for assessing meaningful neuropsychological change following epilepsy surgery. *Journal of the International Neuropsychological Society, 2*, 556–564.

Sawrie, S. M., Martin, R. C., Gilliam, F. G., Roth, D. L., Faught, E., & Kuzniecky, R. (1998). Contribution of neuropsychological data to the prediction of temporal lobe epilepsy surgery outcome. *Epilepsia, 39*, 319–325.

Sawrie, S. M., Martin, R. C., Gilliam, F. G., Knowlton, R., Faught, E., & Kuzniecky, R. (2001). Verbal retention lateralizes patients with unilateral temporal lobe epilepsy and bilateral hippocampal atrophy. *Epilepsia, 42*, 651–659.

Saykin, A. J., Stafiniak, P., Robinson, L. J., Flannery, K. A., Gur, R. C., O'Connor, M. J., et al. (1995). Language before and after temporal lobectomy: Specificity of acute changes and relation to early risk factors. *Epilepsia, 33*(11), 1071–1077.

Schramm, J. (2002). Hemispherectomy techniques. *Neurosurgery Clinics of North America, 13*(1), 113–134.

Scoville, W. B., & Milner, B. (1957). Loss of recent memory after bilateral hippocampal lesions. *Journal of Neuropsychiatry and Clinical Neuroscience, 12*(1), 103–113.

Seidenberg, M., Hermann, B., Wyler, A. R., et al. (1998). Neuropsychological outcome following anterior temporal lobectomy in patients with and without the syndrome of mesial temporal lobe epilepsy. *Neuropsychology, 12*, 303–316.

Seidenberg, M., Griffith, R., Sabsevitz, D., Moran, M., Haltiner, A., Bell, B., et al. (2002). Recognition and identification of famous faces in patients with unilateral temporal lobe epilepsy. *Neuropsychologia, 40*, 446–456.

Seidenberg, M., Pulsipher, D. T., & Hermann, B. (2007). Cognitive progression in epilepsy. *Neuropsychology Review, 17*(4), 445–454.

Shimizu, H., Suzuki, I., & Ishijima, B. (1989). Zygomatic approach for resection of mesial temporal epileptic focus. *Neurosurgery, 25*, 798–801.

Siegel, A. M., & Williamson, P. D. (2000). Parietal lobe epilepsy. *Advances in Neurology, 84*, 189–199.

Sillanpaa, M., Jalava, M., Kaleva, O., & Shinnar, S. (1998). Long-term prognosis of seizures with onset in childhood. *The New England Journal of Medicine, 338*, 1715–1722.

Slaght, S. J., Leresche, N., Deniau, J. M., Crunelli, V., & Charpier, S. (2002). Activity of thalamic reticular neurons during spontaneous genetically determined spike and wave discharges. *The Journal of Neuroscience, 22*(6), 2323–2334.

Smith, M.L., Elliott, I.M., and Lach L. (2004). Cognitive, psychosocial and family function one year after pediatric epilepsy surgery. *Epilepsia, 45*, 650–60.

Society, A. E. (1986). Guidelines in EEG, 1-7 (revised 1985). *Journal of Clinical Neurophysiology, 3*, 131–168.

Spencer, S. S., Schramm, J., Wyler, A., O'Connor, M. O. D., Krauss, G., Sperling, M., et al. (2002). Multiple subpial transection for intractable parital epilepsy: An international meta-analysis. *Epilepsia, 43*, 141–145.

Spiers, H. J., Burgess, N., Maguire, E. A., Baxendale, S. A., Hartley, T., Thompson, P. J., et al. (2001). Unilateral temporal lobectomy patients show lateralized topographical and episodic memory deficits in a virtual town. *Brain, 124*, 2476–2489.

Strauss, E., Hunter, M., & Wada, J. (1995). Risk factors for cognitive impairment in epilepsy. *Neuropsychology, 9*(4), 457–463.

Strine, T. W., Kobau, R., Chapman, D. P., Thurman, J., Price, P., & Balluz, L. S. (2005). Psychological distress, comorbidities, and health behaviors among US adults with seizures: Results from the 2002 National Health Interview Survey. *Epilepsia, 46*(7), 1133–1139.

Stroup, E., Langfitt, J., Berg, M., et al. (2003). Predicting verbal memory decline following anterior temporal lobectomy (ATL). *Neurology, 60*, 1266–1273.

Swinkels, W. A. M., Kuyk, J., van Dyck, R., & Spinhoven, P. (2005). Psychiatric comorbidity in epilepsy. *Epilepsy & Behavior, 7*(1), 37–50.

Sylvester, C.-Y. C., & Shimamura, A. P. (2002). Evidence for intact semantic representations in patients with frontal lobe lesions. *Neuropsychology, 16*(2), 197–207.

Takaya, S., Hanakawa, T., Hashikawa, K., Ikeda, A., Sawamoto, N., Nagamine, T., et al. (2006). Prefrontal hypofunction in patients with mesial temporal lobe epilepsy. *Neurology, 67*(9), 1674–1676.

Tarkka, R., Paakko, E., Pyhtinene, J., Uhari, M., & Rantala, H. (2003). Febrile seizures and mesial temporal sclerosis: No association in a long-term follow-up study. *Neurology, 60*, 215–218.

Tellez-Zenteno, J. F., Hernandez-Ronquillo, L., Moien-Afshari, F., & Wiebe, S. (2010). Surgical outcomes in lesional and non-lesional epilepsy: A systematic review and meta-analysis. *Epilepsy Research, 89*, 310–318.

Temkin, N. R., Heaton, R. K., Grant, I., & Dikmen, S. S. (1999). Detecting significant change in neuropsychological test performance: A comparison of four models. *Journal of the International Neuropsychological Society, 5*(4), 357–369.

Terra-Bustamante, V. C., Machado, H. R., Santos-Oliveira, R. D., Escorsi-Rosset, S., Yacubian, E. M. T., Naffah-Mazzacoratti, M. D. G., et al. (2009). Rasumussen encephalitis: Long-term outcome after surgery. *Child Nervous System, 25*, 583–589.

Thompson, P. J., & Duncan, J. S. (2005). Cognitive decline in severe intractable epilepsy. *Epilepsia, 46*(11), 1780–1787.

Tinuper, P., Plazzi, G. P. F., Cerullo, A., Leonardi, M., Agati, R., Righini, A., et al. (1992). Facial asymmetry in partial epilepsies. *Epilepsia, 33*(6), 1097–1100.

Tomson, T., Nashef, L., & Ryvlin, P. (2008). Sudden unexpected death in epilepsy: Current knowledge and future directions. *Lancet Neurology, 7*(11), 1021–1031.

Tovar-Spinoza, Z. S., Ochi, A., Rutka, J. T., Go, C., & Otsubo, H. (2008). The role of magnetoencephalography in epilepsy surgery. *Neurosurgical Focus, 25*(3), 1–6.

Tremont, G., Halpert, S., Javorsky, D. J., & Stern, R. A. (2000). Differential impact of executive dysfunction on verbal list learning and story recall. *The Clinical Neuropsychologist, 14*(3), 295–302.

Troster, A. I., Warmflash, V., Osorio, I., Paolo, A. M., Alexander, L. J., & Barr, W. B. (1995). The roles of semantic networks and search efficiency in verbal fluency performance in intractable temporal lobe epilepsy. *Epilepsy Research, 21*(1), 19–26.

Umeda, S., Nagumo, Y., & Kato, M. (2006). Dissociative contributions of medial temporal and frontal regions to prospective remembering. *Review of Neuroscience, 17*, 267–278.

Upton, D., & Thompson, P. J. (1996). General neuropsychological characteristics of frontal lobe epilepsy. *Epilepsy Research, 23*, 169–177.

Upton, D., & Thompson, P. J. (1999). Twenty questions task and frontal lobe dysfunction. *Archives of Clinical Neuropsychology, 14*(2), 203–216.

Uthman, B. M., Reichl, A. M., Dean, J. C., Eisenschenk, S., Gilmore, R., Reid, S., et al. (2004). Effectiveness of vagus nerve stimulation in epilepsy patients: A 12-year observation. *Neurology, 63*(6), 1124–1126.

Van Passschen, W., Dupont, P., Sunaert, S., Goffin, K., & Van Laere, K. (2007). The use of SPECT and PET in routine clinical practice in epilepsy. *Current Opinion in Neurology, 20*(2), 194–202.

Van Wagenen, W. P., & Herren, R. Y. (1940). Surgical division of commissural pathways in the corpus callosum. *Archives of Neurology and Psychiatry, 44*, 740–759.

Vannest, J., Szaflarski, J. P., Privitera, M. D., Schefft, B. K., & Holland, S. K. (2008). Medical temporal fMRI activation reflects memory lateralization and memory performance in patients with epilepsy. *Epilepsy & Behavior, 12*(3), 410–418.

Velis, D., Plouin, P., Gotman, J., da Silva, F. L., & Neurophysiology, I. D. S. o. (2007). Recommendations regarding the requirements and applications for long-term recordings in epilepsy. *Epilepsia, 48*(2), 379–384.

Weber, B., Fliessbach, K., Lange, N., Kugler, F., & Elger, C. E. (2007). Material-specific memory processing is related to language dominance. *Neuroimage, 37*, 611–617.

Wechsler, D. (1991). *The Wechsler Intelligence Scale for Children – Third Edition (WISC-III)*. San Antonio, TX: The Psychological Corporation.

Wechsler, D. (1997). *Wechsler Memory Scale* (3rd ed.). San Antonio: The Psychological Corporation.

Wiebe, S., Blume, W. T., Girvin, J. P., & Eliasziw, M. (2001). Effectiveness and efficiency of surgery for temporal lobe epilepsy group. A randomized, controlled trial of surgery for temporal-lobe epilepsy. *The New England Journal of Medicine, 345*(5), 311–318.

Wieser, H. G., & Yasargil, M. G. (1982). Selective amygdalohippocampectomy as a surgical treatment of mesiobasal limbic epilepsy. *Surgical Neurology, 17*, 445–457.

Wilde, N., Strauss, E., Chelune, G. J., Loring, D. W., Martin, R. C., Hermann, B. P., et al. (2001). WMS-III performance in patients with temporal lobe epilepsy: Group differences and individual classification. *Journal of the International Neuropsychological Society, 7*, 881–891.

Williamson, P., Spencer, D. D., Spencer, S. S., Novelly, R. A., & Mattson, R. H. (1985). Complex partial seizures of frontal lobe origin. *Annals of Neurology, 18*, 497–504.

Wirrell, E. C., Camfield, C. S., Camfield, P. R., Dooley, J. M., Gordon, K. E., & Smith, B. (1997). Long-term psychosocial outcome of typical absence epilepsy: Sometimes a wolf in sheeps' clothing. *Archives of Pediatric Adolescent Medicine, 151*, 152–158.

Wyler, A. R. (2006). Multiple subpial transections: A review and arguments for use. In J. W. Miller & D. L. Silbergeld (Eds.), *Epilepsy surgery: Principles and controversies* (pp. 524–529). New York: Taylor & Francis.

Chapter 17
Neuropsychology of Psychogenic Nonepileptic Seizures

Daniel L. Drane, Erica L. Coady, David J. Williamson, John W. Miller, and Selim Benbadis

Abstract Nonepileptic seizures (NES) are operationally defined as episodes of involuntary movement, altered responsiveness, or subjective experience that resemble epileptic seizures (ES), but are not accompanied by the abnormal electrical discharges in the brain that is a seizure. (Lesser, 1996; Reuber and Elger, 2003). When these episodes are caused by psychological processes, they are termed psychogenic nonepileptic seizures (PNES). Other terms, such as psychogenic nonepileptic attacks (PNEA) (Duncan and Oto, 2008a) or episodes, have been suggested more recently. The reasoning behind replacing the term "seizure" in PNES is twofold: (1) decrease the confusion among physician and other healthcare providers that the events are not electroneurophysiological (and do not require antiepileptic medication or acute emergent medical intervention when presenting to an emergency department/emergency room), and (2) decrease confusion among patients and their families that the events are not "seizures" and are not due to neurologic disease. Because PNES is currently the most prevalent term, we will use it throughout the rest of this chapter. However, it is likely that further changes in terminology will be made over the next decade in an effort to minimize pejorative connotations and improve descriptive accuracy.

Patients with PNES utilize considerable medical resources via emergency departments, hospitalizations, physician visits, and unnecessary pharmaceutical treatment. The lifetime cost of treating undiagnosed PNES may be equivalent to that of epilepsy, estimated to be $231,432 per patient in 1995 (Begley et al., 2000). Overall, psychogenic symptoms (inclusive of PNES as well as other conversion and factitious disorders) account for 10% of all medical visits. Patients with PNES are often treated similarly to patients with epilepsy and receive antiepileptic drugs (AEDs) that are unnecessary for many years before an accurate diagnosis is achieved (Abubakr et al., 2003;

D.L. Drane (✉)
Emory University School of Medicine
Atlanta, GA, USA
and
University of Washington, School of Medicine
Seattle, WA, USA
e-mail: ddrane@emory.edu

M.R. Schoenberg and J.G. Scott (eds.), *The Little Black Book of Neuropsychology: A Syndrome-Based Approach*, DOI 10.1007/978-0-387-76978-3_17,
© Springer Science+Business Media, LLC 2011

Reuber et al., 2002). The exposure of patients to AEDs is not inconsequential (see Chap. 16, this volume for review of AED medication side-effects). Prevalence of PNES varies by setting, with rates as high as 44% in tertiary epilepsy centers (Szaflarski et al., 2000). Thus, for the neuropsychologist who interacts regularly with an epilepsy team, patients with PNES are likely to be part of clinical practice.

Obtaining a better understanding of the etiology of PNES and its clinical features is important for several reasons. Foremost, this diagnosis is typically associated with genuine suffering that in many cases can be alleviated. Improved diagnosis of PNES events is critical to developing appropriate treatments for this disorder. Some clinicians have suggested that 75–95% of patient with PNES show improvement in their condition if an accurate diagnosis can be established, with 19–52% of these patients seeing their PNES events resolve (Ettinger et al., 1999; Ettinger et al., 1999; Walczak et al., 1995). The likelihood of improvement is particularly good for those patients whose PNES began relatively recently and who have few comorbid psychiatric diagnoses (Kanner et al., 1999; Lempert and Schmidt, 1990).

Another benefit of understanding patients with PNES is the unique perspective they provide in the development, diagnosis, and treatment of medically-unexplained symptom presentations. Within neuropsychology, such presentations are often seen in the context of litigation or other forms of compensation seeking. This is far less often the case in patients with PNES. Furthermore, there exists a "gold standard" diagnostic technology for PNES that simply does not exist for other such disorders. Thus, we are able to gain insight and understanding into the cause and course of PNES unobscured by confounds related to compensation-seeking or ambiguous diagnoses.

This chapter provides an overview of PNES, including diagnosis, semiology, prevalence, etiology, neuropsychological features, associated psychopathology, and treatment. We encourage healthcare providers to approach these patients with care and respect. While PNES poses many challenges, neuropsychology is uniquely suited to help patients, their families, and their healthcare providers.

Key Points and Chapter Summary

- Video EEG is the gold standard for diagnosing psychogenic nonepileptic seizures (PNES); however, neuropsychological assessment can provide data helpful for diagnosis and planning treatment by assessing emotional and cognitive functioning and assisting in treatment planning and implementation.
- Contrary to clinical lore, epileptic seizures and PNES co-occur relatively infrequently (less than 15% of the time).
- There is no single psychological profile associated with PNES, and some of these patients are at higher risk for poor psychological and social adjustment.
- Psychogenic status epilepticus and reported histories of abuse are particularly poor prognostic signs.

(continued)

> **Key Points and Chapter Summary** (continued)
>
> • Symptom validity testing can provide valuable guidance when drawing conclusions about the presence and severity of neuropsychological impairment, particularly in the absence of obvious neurodevelopmental delay or an objectively-documented seizure within the 24 hours preceding testing.
> • An integrated treatment team with clear communication between neurology and mental health professionals is most likely to meet with success, and some progress is beginning to be made in describing the types of medical and psychological treatment that are most likely to be successful.

Definition and Diagnosis

Epilepsy has always been with us, appearing in Egyptian hieroglyphics earlier than 700 BC (Fisch and Olejniczak 2001). Descriptions of psychogenic events also date back several centuries, with reports that Hippocrates and Aretaeus distinguished between epileptic and "hysterical" seizures (Gates and Erdahl 1993; Massey 1982). Since that time, descriptions of psychogenic-based spells have been commonplace, and much effort has been made to distinguish PNES from epilepsy. For example, during the late 1800s, Gowers wrote about "hysteroid seizures," Charcot described "epileptiform hysteria" (Krumholz 1999), and Freud described hysterical seizures (Freud 1966). The term *pseudoseizure*, reportedly first coined by Liske and Forster (Liske and Forster 1964) has been one of the more frequently used terms for PNES. The term PNES has come to replace pseudoseizures, since the term *pseudo* is often accompanied by negative connotations, and PNES is both more specific and less pejorative. More recently, some have used labels for these events that dropped the word "seizure" in order to prevent diagnostic and etiological confusion, replacing it with attack, spell, or episode.

While the gold standard for the diagnosis of PNES is continuous long-term video-EEG (vEEG) that captures the patient's typical spell, clinicians and researchers still disagree over the behavioral component needed to diagnose an event as PNES, as well as the criteria used to rule out seizure activity (e.g., some clinicians will capture a PNES event during monitoring, yet assume the patient also had epilepsy based on self-report alone). Video-EEG monitoring involves obtaining continuous EEG data synchronized with video recording of the patient's behavior for a span of 1–7 days in the hospital. There are numerous specialty epilepsy centers throughout the world that perform vEEG monitoring, and more centers are being established. Patients are often taken off of AEDs during monitoring, or the doses are reduced to increase the chance a patient will experience a clinical event in this controlled environment. If certain activities or stimuli are associated with eliciting a patient's typical event, an effort is sometimes made to recreate these conditions (e.g., exercise, sleep deprivation, photic stimulation).

Some groups, such as the Regional Epilepsy Center at the University of Washington (UW), have established conservative diagnostic criteria for PNES, such that events are not classified solely on the basis of subjective report (see Appendix for the UW diagnostic classification scheme) (Martin et al. 2003; Syed et al. 2008). The UW diagnostic criteria for PNES require: (1) a definitive motor component (e.g., shaking or writhing of the torso or limbs, convulsive or rocking movements, head shaking), and (2) a discrete episode of unresponsiveness in the absence of epileptiform activity on EEG or another known physiological cause (e.g., syncope). An *indeterminant* spell, in contrast, is one in which the motor component was restricted to minor motor movements (e.g., myoclonic jerks) in a fully responsive individual, or the spell is evident only by the subjective patient report about his or her internal state (e.g., patient reports feeling "funny" or hot). The absence of epileptiform EEG activity in events of this type does not definitively demonstrate the event was a PNES. Frontal lobe seizures and simple partial seizures, for example, can result in both types of behavioral and subjective phenomena in the absence of epileptiform EEG abnormality on standard scalp monitoring (French 1995) (see also Chap. 16 this volume). However, other epileptologists may disagree, and may classify these same events as PNES. The diagnostic decision in these less definitive spells should be influenced by the perceived risk of a misclassification error (e.g., potentially discontinuing AEDs in a patient with epilepsy misdiagnosed as having PNES or prescribing AEDs to a patient not having seizures).

Diagnosis of spells based purely on patient self-report or even clinical observation of an actual event leaves room for error, but still occurs in both clinical and research settings. While there are behavioral features of spells more commonly observed with either PNES or epileptic seizures (ES) events (see Table 17.1 for a list), there are usually exceptions for both types of paroxysmal events. Deacon et al. (2003) found epileptologists were accurate at identifying seizures, but tended to overdiagnose PNES as epileptic seizures when relying on clinical history alone rather than the results of vEEG monitoring in patients with suspected temporal lobe epilepsy. Likewise, while a few behaviors (e.g., ictal stuttering; Vossler et al. 2004) may be highly specific to PNES, they often do not occur with great frequency, and thus provide good specificity but lack diagnostic sensitivity (Cuthill and Espie 2005; Hoerth et al. 2008).

A common practice in diagnosing PNES is to obtain a single EEG recording on an outpatient basis. This practice often fails to produce definitive results in diagnosing either patients with epilepsy or PNES. These studies are useful only if the typical event is captured and/or clearly epileptic seizure activity is recorded. The absence of evidence does not preclude the presence of either PNES or ES. While long-term vEEG monitoring increases the likelihood of capturing a patient's typical event over ambulatory EEG, both ambulatory and long-term EEG suffers from the same weakness, namely needing to capture the typical patient event(s). For diagnostic and financial reasons, experts have derived various "induction techniques" to increase the chance of recording the patient's usual event. Induction techniques have included the use of hyperventilation, photic stimulation, saline injection,

Table 17.1 Usefulness of behavioral semiology to distinguish between psychogenic nonepileptic seizures (PNES) and epileptic seizures (ES)

Semiology/behavior	PNES	ES	Research studies (representative)
Tongue biting	Low frequency/uncommon (self-report is much higher)	Common	Peguero et al. (1995)
Urinary incontinence	Rare (self-report is much higher)	Common	Benbadis et al. (1995) and Oliva et al. (2008)
Weeping	Occasional	Very Rare	Bergen and Ristanovic (1993)
Ictal stuttering	Uncommon	Absent	Vossler et al. (2004)
Ictal eye closure	Common (eyes closed for longer periods)	Low frequency (often brief when it occurs)	Chung et al. (2006) and Syed et al. (2008)
"Teddy bear sign"	Uncommon	Rare	Burneo et al. (2003)
Pelvic thrusting	Low frequency	Uncommon (but occurs in frontal lobe seizures)	Devinsky et al. (1996) and Geyer et al. (2000)
Self-injury	Low frequency to common	Common	Peguero et al. (1995)
Post-ictal drowsiness or confusion	Uncommon	Frequent	Ettinger et al. (1999)
Long spell duration	Common	Rare	Devinsky et al. (1996) and Sagyi et al. (1992)
Situational onset	Common	Rare	Cragar et al. (2002)
Purposeful movements	Occasional	Very Rare	Cragar et al. (2002)
Self-reported sleep events	Low Frequency	Common	Duncan et al. (2004)
Sleep event during vEEG	Uncommon	Common	Bazil and Walczak (1997)

PNES = psychogenic nonepileptic seizures, *ES* epileptic seizures, *vEEG* video-EEG monitoring

hypnosis or simple suggestion (Benbadis 2001). However, a weakness of induction techniques is that the patient's typical spell may not occur (be monitored), and thus not provide an answer regarding PNES versus ES. Indeed, atypical spells occurred in 15% of patients with epilepsy and 8% of patients with PNES when a saline injection induction technique was used (Walczak et al. 1994). For diagnosis, it is important to capture the patient's typical event.

Rule of thumb: Continuous vEEG of typical episode is the gold standard to diagnosis PNES

- Neuropsychological assessment, behavioral features of the ictal event, demographic variables, and the presence of comorbid psychiatric features can play an adjunctive diagnostic role (particularly helpful when a typical event is not captured during vEEG monitoring).
- Inducing PNES may be useful for diagnosis, but the typicality of the observed spell should always be ascertained before drawing diagnostic conclusions.

There are a number of paroxysmal events, some of which have been termed nonepileptic seizure of other physiological origin, that can appear like a seizure or PNES and involve a physiological rather than psychogenic etiology (see Chap. 15 for review). Briefly, etiologies for paroxysmal spells not due to seizure include cardiovascular disorders, metabolic disturbances, and movement disorders. These other paroxysmal events typically make up only a very small proportion of the referrals seen in specialty epilepsy centers.

The use of the term *seizure* for all of these spells regardless of etiology (i.e., epileptic seizure versus psychogenic nonepileptic seizure/attack versus nonepileptic seizure of other physiological origin) has led to diagnostic confusion and is often misunderstood by patients and healthcare providers alike. Patients will often go away from a feedback session still thinking they have some form of epileptic seizure. Similarly, healthcare providers with less direct experience with epilepsy are often reluctant to discontinue antiepileptic drugs due to their persisting concern that psychogenic "seizures" represent epilepsy. Due to such confusion, some clinicians refer to these events as "nonepileptic episodes" in discussions with patients.

Prevalence and Incidence

Variability in diagnostic decision rules for PNES events and epileptic seizures used by different medical providers throughout the world has contributed to confusion regarding the *incidence* (the rate of newly identified cases of a given condition over a specified time span), *prevalence* (the proportion of a population with it at a given time) and co-existence of these disorders. In addition, selection biases as well as small study samples have contributed to wide variations in estimates of prevalence rates of PNES.

The easiest information to obtain regarding rates of PNES occurrence involves the number of patients with PNES identified by long-term vEEG monitoring. Based on all referrals to epilepsy centers, 10–50% of patients receive a diagnosis of PNES (with or without comorbid epilepsy). The higher estimates have occurred in more recent years, as rates of 10–20 % of patients referred for vEEG are found in reviews from the 1980s and 1990s (Gates et al. 1985; Scoot 1982). Potential reasons for the variability in the prevalence include differences in referral patterns, different diagnostic criteria used, increased monitoring of patients with paroxysmal events, and/or increased rates of this condition (Table 17.2).

Studies of PNES incidence have typically been made using estimates based on data obtained at specialty epilepsy centers. Szaflarski et al. (2000) estimated the 4-year incidence of PNES for one county in Ohio, USA based on vEEG monitoring. Almost 44% of the patients referred for vEEG monitoring experienced a PNES event, with 34.5% of patients diagnosed with PNES only. The average annual PNES incidence was reported as 3.03/100,000, but increased to 4.6/100,000 the last year of the study. In contrast, a European trial reported a 1.4/100,000 incidence rate (Sigurdardottir and Olafsson 1998). The Centers for Disease Control suggest 300,000 to 400,000 people may experience PNES in the USA. However, no definitive epidemiological study has been conducted.

Benbadis and Hauser (2000) estimated the prevalence of PNES based on calculations from data regarding the prevalence of epilepsy (0.5–1% of the general population), the proportion of patients with epilepsy diagnosed with intractable epilepsy (20–30%; Engel and Shewmon 1993; Mattson 1980), the proportion of patients with intractable epilepsy referred to epilepsy centers (20–55% of intractable patients are thought to be referred; Engel and Shewmon 1993; Engel 1996), and the proportion of such patients found to have PNES (10–20% of all referrals; Gates et al. 1985; Scoot 1982). In turn, they calculated prevalence rates for of PNES using the lower and higher estimates for these ranges; which resulted in estimated prevalence rates ranging from 1/50,000 to 1/3,000, or 2–33 per 100,000 persons.

Rule of thumb: PNES Prevalence trends and comorbidity

- As many as 50% of patients presenting to tertiary epilepsy centers in the US experience PNES
- 10–34% of patients referred for vEEG diagnosed as having PNES exclusively.
- The prevalence of PNES has increased over the past decade.

Table 17.2 Prevalence of PNES, epilepsy, a single seizure, and patients with both PNES and epilepsy

	PNES only	Epilepsy	Seizure (single)
Life time prevalence	Unknown	3%	9–10%
Point Prevalence	0.0002–0.0003%	1%	0.6%
Incidence (per 100,000)	4.6	30	55

PNES = psychogenic nonepileptic seizures

Prevalence of PNES/Epilepsy Co-Occurrence (CO)

Determining the prevalence rate of PNES among individuals diagnosed with epilepsy has proven challenging. Prevalence rates vary based on diagnostic criteria and on whether one considers how many patients *with epilepsy* have PNES or how many patients *with PNES* have epilepsy. The latter is probably the more useful statistic, as arguably the more medically dangerous situation is not diagnosing epileptic seizures in someone already diagnosed with PNES. O'Sullivan and colleagues (2007) reported as many as 50% of patients with PNES will also have comorbid epilepsy; however, studies using more explicit and conservative diagnostic criteria place this figure far lower, typically less than 10% (Benbadis et al. 2001; Lesser et al. 1983; Martin et al. 2003).

> **Rule of thumb: Prevalence of epileptic seizures and PNES**
>
> Only 5–10 % of patients diagnosed with PNES using vEEG also have seizures when using well-defined diagnostic criteria and vEEG.

Etiology

Despite decades of study, we still do not "know" what causes or maintains PNES. However, a variety of correlates have been identified: demographic variables, medical, social, and psychiatric history as well as psychological test results.

Demographic Correlates

The most common demographic presentation of the patient with PNES is the same as that seen with other functional somatic syndromes: females with somatic complaints beginning in young adulthood (LaFrance and Devinsky 2004; Neumann and Buskila 2003; Reuber and Elger 2003; Tojek et al. 2000). See Table 17.3 for a listing of some of the characteristic studies demonstrating the higher incidence of PNES events among women.

Similarly, data concerning the typical age of onset of PNES are strikingly consistent. PNES events tend to begin in early adulthood, often between 20 and 30 years of age (Reuber and Elger 2003). There is some suggestion that age of onset may vary by phenomenology of PNES, in which PNES associated with epilepsy and developmental delay has an earlier onset while PNES associated with health-related trauma is later in onset (Duncan and Oto 2008a, b; Reuber 2008). It is not uncommon for children as young as 8 years old to have PNES events, although it is believed the onset of PNES in middle or older adult age is less common (Kellinghaus et al. 2004). As the onset of PNES moves later into adulthood, the ratio of women to men appears to decrease (Duncan et al. 2006).

Table 17.3 Demographic features that have been commonly associated with PNES events

Demographic feature	Characteristic studies	Findings
Higher incidence of PNES among women	Reuber et al. (2004)	Of 85 patients diagnosed with PNES, 82.3% were female.
	Reuber and Elger (2003)	Review article indicating approximately three-quarters of all patients with PNES are female.
	Fiszman et al. (2004)	In a meta-analysis of 17 studies of patients with PNES taken from neuropsychological literature between 1945 and 2004, found women comprised 64–100% of the samples.
Age of onset is most typically during young adult years	Reuber et al. (2003b)	Mean age of onset = 20.3 years
	Reuber et al. (2002a)	Mean age of onset = 25.5 years
	Reuber et al. (2002a)	Mean age of onset = 26.1 years

PNES = psychogenic nonepileptic seizures

Rule of thumb: Demographic characteristics of patients with PNES

- PNES more common in women than men
- PNES often begins between 20 and 30 years old

Medical Histories

In addition to its potential relationship with epilepsy, PNES has been reported after brain injury, neurosurgery (Fiszman et al. 2004), and in patients with mental retardation (Reuber et al. 2003). Patients with PNES frequently report more neurological injury or disease than patients with epilepsy (e.g., head trauma, CNS infection, possible birth traumas) (Dodrill and Holmes 2000; Drake 1993; Wilkus and Dodrill 1984, 1989). However, such histories are typically based upon self-report, and may not be valid (Schrag et al. 2004).

Again mirroring the tendency demonstrated in other groups with functional somatic syndromes, patients with PNES report higher rates of fibromyalgia, chronic pain syndromes, and other medically unexplained illnesses than age-matched controls. Benbadis (2005b) found 75% of patients evaluated in an epilepsy clinic during a 5-year period who had been previously diagnosed with fibromyalgia or a chronic pain syndrome were later diagnosed with PNES. Also, 75% of the patients who had a spell while waiting in the lobby or examination room were diagnosed with PNES. Benbadis hypothesized that PNES may be a product of coping with fibromyalgia/chronic pain. However, he also noted that fibromyalgia and chronic pain are broad diagnoses that are often considered psychogenic themselves.

Body mass index (BMI) may also differ in patients with PNES. Patients with PNES tend to have higher BMIs than patients with epilepsy (30.5 vs 26.1) (Marquez et al. 2004).

Rule of thumb: Medical history of patients with PNES

- More neurological trauma/dysfunction reported (in addition to epilepsy)
- More common with diagnosis of fibromyalgia, chronic pain, chronic fatigue syndrome, multiple chemical sensitivity, etc.
- Higher body mass index (BMI)

Social Histories

A factor frequently mentioned in discussions of PNES etiology is a history of long-term psychological conflict. Some authors have described unresolved conflict as evidenced by chronic use of poor coping techniques. These poor coping techniques are often accompanied by patient reported histories of abuse during childhood, head trauma, psychiatric disturbance, and socially reinforced behaviors that mimic epilepsy symptoms. Histories of physical, sexual, or emotional abuse, in particular, are commonly reported. Bowman and Markand (1996) found 84% of patients with PNES had a history of abuse including; sexual (67%), physical (67%), and other trauma (74%). Other studies (Alper et al. 1993; Duncan and Oto 2008a; Fiszman et al. 2004; Selkirk et al. 2008) report lower but still substantial rates of abuse that exceed controls. A meta-analysis examining the frequency of traumatic events and post-traumatic stress disorder (PTSD) in PNES populations found 44–100% reported a history of general trauma, whereas 23–77% reported histories of physical and/or sexual abuse (Fiszman et al. 2004). Selkirk et al. (2008) provide data suggesting patients experiencing PNES within the context of a reported history of abuse tend to have worse social and psychological adjustment than patients with PNES whom do not have an abuse history. Thus, abuse history may be relevant in better understanding etiology, but also the relative likelihood of poor adjustment.

LaFrance and Devinsky (2004) proposed a conceptual model that incorporated the prevalent themes of chronic maladjustment and abuse, and divided PNES into two categories: posttraumatic and developmental. *Posttraumatic* PNES result from an individual's maladaptive response to chronic contact with traumatic experiences. Patients with posttraumatic PNES have often been exposed to physical, sexual or psychological trauma. *Developmental* PNES, in contrast, is thought to arise from an individual's difficulties in coping with the psychosocial tasks encountered along the developmental spectrum. For example, it is common for PNES to occur in the midst of trauma or social or family conflict (Berkhoff et al. 1998). Psychogenic events are common in patients with personal conflict over anger, expression of anger, dependency, sexuality, and extensive patterns of avoiding one's awareness of these frustrations (Abubakr et al. 2003). Patients with a history of poor adjustment after troublesome interactions with others, and those with difficulties in managing anger may manifest their poor psychosocial adjustment in the form of PNES (Lesser 2003). Additionally, patients with PNES perceive their families as being less supportive of each other, exhibit less commitment, and also place less of an emphasis on ethical values when compared to healthy controls and patients with epilepsy (Szaflarski et al. 2003).

> **Rule of thumb: Social history of patients with PNES**
> - More likely to have history of abuse (sexual, physical, etc.)–84% of patients
> - More common for PNES to occur in times of trauma or family/interpersonal conflict
> - More likely with individuals having poor coping skills and/or poor psychosocial adjustment

Psychiatric Comorbidities

In addition to a history of aversive childhood events and poor psychosocial development, patients with PNES tend to report more psychiatric symptoms than the general population as well as patients with epilepsy. Anywhere from 43% to 100% of patients with PNES meet criteria for a psychiatric disorder (Bowman 2001; Drane et al. 2006; Stroup et al. 2004). This is almost twice the rate reported for patients with epilepsy (Szaflarski et al. 2003), who themselves have a higher rate of psychiatric comorbidities than the general population. Common psychiatric co-morbidities in patients with PNES include PTSD, panic disorder with or without agoraphobia and other anxiety disorders, depressive disorders, personality disorders, prior conversion disorders, somatization disorders and dissociative disorders (Bowman 1993, 2006; Reuber and Elger 2003; Reuber et al. 2003).

Somatization, conversion, and dissociation. Using DSM-IV criteria, patients with a diagnosis of PNES will most often receive a diagnosis of conversion disorder, though other diagnoses (e.g., factitious disorder) can certainly present in the epilepsy clinic as well. Perhaps the most obvious traits characterizing patients with PNES are higher levels of somatization, suggestibility, and dissociation (Bowman 2006; Goldstein et al. 2000). These processes, by definition, are core components of the disorder. Conversion disorder, a specific type of somatoform disorder, is the current classification for a disorder Sigmund Freud originally termed *hysteria*. The phrase *conversion* extended from the hypothesis that the patient's somatic symptom represented "a symbolic resolution of an unconscious psychological conflict, reducing anxiety and serving to keep the conflict out of awareness" (American Psychiatric Association 2000). PNES are frequently seen in conversion disorders, with 15% of conversion disordered patients exhibiting PNES events (Devinsky et al. 2001). This relationship works in the other direction as well, as Devinsky et al. (2001) found that 9 out of 79 patients with PNES had other conversion symptoms, such as paralysis and nonanatomic sensory loss.

Goldstein et al. (2000) found that patients with PNES scored significantly higher than healthy controls on a measure of dissociative experiences. In this study, patients with PNES specifically used escape–avoidance behaviors and tended to use more emotionally-based coping strategies. In contrast, the control group used significantly more problem-focused coping techniques. Thus, escape avoidance and emotion-based coping may be coping mechanisms that increase risk for the development of PNES.

Anxiety. Given the rates of abuse and trauma described earlier, the prevalence of PTSD in this population comes as no surprise. Fiszman and colleagues (2004) found higher rates of PTSD in patients with PNES than those seen in the general population, which the Department of Veteran's Affairs estimates to be at approximately 8%(United States Department of Veterans Affairs, n.d.). PTSD symptoms are reported in patients with epilepsy as well, however, but in and of themselves are not sufficient to diagnose PNES (Dikel et al. 2003).

Patients with PNES report higher levels of anxiety more generally, some displaying chronic anxiety as a heightened trait (van Merode et al. 2004). Mokleby and colleagues (2002) found that patients with PNES have significantly higher levels of self-reported anxiety, anger, hostility, and depression when compared to healthy controls. This is consistent with the idea that hostility is often manifested as a coping style in individuals with anger and mistrust in others (Lesser 2003).

Depression. Of significant clinical concern is the high rate of depression in patients with PNES, as this conveys a higher risk for suicide. Further, it is not unusual for patients with PNES to have a history of parasuicidal behavior. Reuber et al. (2000) noted this was particularly true of patients who have a history of psychogenic status epilepticus (with features resembling epileptic status epilepticus, in that the patient has repeated PNES events without recovery in between). In a case series of five patients who originally presented with postoperative status epilepticus but whose episodes were later diagnosed as psychogenic in origin, nearly two-thirds of the patients had a history of suicide attempts (Reuber et al. 2000)

Eating disorders. Although investigated less frequently, there is some indication that bulimia may also be more frequent among patients presenting with psychogenic status epilepticus (Rechlin et al. 1997). Rechlin and colleagues found that one-third of a PNES sample hospitalized for PNES "status epilepticus" was bulimic. Consistent with Reuber and colleagues (2000), this PNES group was also characterized by higher than expected rates of personality disorder and suicide attempts.

Personality disorders. Estimates of the prevalence of personality disorder among patients with PNES vary widely, ranging from 30 to 80% (Harden et al. 2009; Lacey et al. 2007. The most carefully diagnosed sample to date (via the Structured Clinical Interview for the DSM-IV, Axis II version, or SCID-II) yields one of the highest prevalence rates, though the sample size ($n = 16$) was quite small (Harden et al. 2009). Notably, estimates of personality pathology among patients with epilepsy are also higher than those seen in the general population, ranging from 18% to 75%. Again, the study of Harden and colleagues (also with 16 patients with epilepsy) yielded the estimate on the high end of this range. There is a clear distinction between the personality pathology seen most commonly in PNES versus patients with epilepsy, as patients with epilepsy tend to be avoidant and dependent (cluster C), whereas patients with PNES more frequently demonstrate pathological emotional lability or idiosyncratic perceptions of their social environment (clusters A & B). Common personality disorder diagnoses in the PNES population are borderline, histrionic, and antisocial personality disorder. This is relevant clinically, as personality disorder among patients with PNES is associated with intractability and diminished access to appropriate treatment (Harden et al. 2003; Kanner et al. 1999).

Rule of thumb: Psychiatric history of patients with PNES

- Psychiatric comorbidity is higher in PNES than for patients with epilepsy
- PNES is a conversion disorder
- Patients with PNS have high rates of depression and at risk for suicidal gestures

---

Psychological Testing and Evidence-Based Psychology Practice

Patients with PNES tend to have distinctive profiles on personality testing, often reflecting aspects of somatization (Cragar et al. 2005; Cragar et al. 2003; Locke et al. 2010; Wagner et al. 2005; Wilkus and Dodrill 1989). Patients with PNES often show significant clinical elevations on Scales 1, 2, 3, 6, 7, and 8 of the MMPI/MMPI-2, with the most common profile configuration being the 1-3/3-1 profile (scale 1: Hypochondriasis; scale 3: Hysteria) (Cragar et al. 2005). On the MMPI-2-RF, elevations are seen on validity scales Fs and FBS-r, restructured clinical scales RC1 and RC3, and somatic scales MLS, GIC, HPC, and NUC (Locke et al. 2010). On the NEO-PI-R, patients with PNES tend to score higher on the Neuroticism scale, particularly facets of anxiety, angry hostility, and depression, but lower on the Extraversion and Agreeableness scales, potentially reflecting a facet of modesty (Cragar et al. 2005).

A number of studies have been conducted to determine how well such characteristics distinguish patients with PNES from patients with epilepsy. Wilkus and Dodrill (1984) suggested that PNES should be suspected when one of three MMPI configural patterns is present: (1) scale 1 or 3 exceeds 69 and is one of the two most elevated scales, disregarding scales 5 and 0, (2) scale 1 or 3 exceeds 79 regardless of whether either is a high point, or (3) both 1 and 3 exceed 59, and both are at least 10 points higher than scale 2. These rules have been generalized to the MMPI-2 (Warner et al. 1996). Other configural patterns have been suggested (Derry and McLachlan 1996). Dodrill and Holmes (2000) reviewed nine studies examining the sensitivity of the MMPI/MMPI-2 to PNES, and found an overall accuracy of 71% for these configural patterns. An evidence-based neuropsychology/psychology practice finding is that, if a patient with seizures of uncertain etiology meets these criteria, they are approximately *five times more likely* to be diagnosed with PNES than with epilepsy (Williamson et al. 2007). Storzbach et al. (2000) developed an algorithm by which diagnostic accuracy can be improved to approximately 80% by also taking duration of spells and results of routine EEG's into account (Schramke et al. 2007; Storzbach et al. 2000), establishing an evidence-based neuropsychology practice when using the MMPI-2.

Approximately 30% of patients with epilepsy produce this same profile on the MMPI/MMPI-2. It has been assumed that such elevations in patients with epilepsy are related to endorsement of symptoms associated with their seizures (e.g., loss of consciousness, lapses in awareness, bizarre sensory experiences). However, patients with epilepsy actually endorse these and other items that directly indicate ictal symptoms only infrequently (Nelson et al. 2004). In addition, the majority of patients with epilepsy (~70%) do not produce significant elevations on Scales 1 and 3 despite this apparent overlap of symptoms.

Although the MMPI/MMPI-2 clearly has the most extensive evidence-based support for use with this population, data have recently been published with other scales as well. Wagner et al., (2005) developed an algorithm to discriminate patients with epilepsy from patients with PNES using the Personality Assessment Inventory (PAI). An evidence-based neuropsychology/psychology finding was that PNES was approximately 15 times more likely when the T-score from the Health Concerns subscale was less than the T-score from the Conversion subscale.

Cragar et al. (2005) have explored personality characteristics of patients with PNES as well as using the NEO-PI-R to supplement the information gained from the MMPI-2. Cluster analysis of the data derived from the two measures combined revealed three distinct clusters of patients with PNES (Cragar et al. 2005). The first group was characterized as experiencing negative affect, low levels of energy and sociability, and clinical symptoms of depression via the MMPI-2 Scale 2. This cluster was termed the "depressed neurotics" and had MMPI-2 elevations on Scales 2 and 3. The second group clustered around a profile that was characterized by somatic tendencies when dealing with psychosocial stress factors. This group was called the "somatic defender" and had MMPI-2 elevations on Scales 1 and 3, with a lower score on Scale 2 (i.e., conversion V pattern). The third group, the "activated neurotic" group, was characterized by negative affect similar to that of the "depressed neurotics" but were more actively, socially engaged, thus exhibiting anxiety as a symptom of distress where elevations were highest on Scales 1 and 8.

Rule of thumb: Evidence-based practice for psychological assessment of patients with PNES

- 5 times more likely to be diagnosed with PNES than epilepsy if:
  - MMPI-2 Scale 1 or 3 exceeds Tscore of 64 and is one of the two most elevated scales

  Or
  - MMPI-2 Scale 1 or 3 exceeds T-score of 74 regardless of whether either is a high point

  Or
  - Both MMPI-2 Scales 1 and 3 exceed Tscore of 54, and both are at least 10 points higher than scale 2.
- 5 times more likely to be PNES when the T-score from the PAI Health Concerns subscale was less than the PAI T-score from the Conversion subscale

---

Neuropsychological Testing

In contrast to the psychological and emotional differences consistently found when comparing patients with epilepsy to patients with PNES, such differences are not evident when comparing the performances of the two groups on neuropsychological tests. No focal patterns of cognitive abnormalities have been found among patients with PNES. However, studies have reported that patients with PNES score as poorly as, or often worse than, patients with epilepsy (Dodrill and Holmes 2000; Drake et al. 1993; Hermann 2000; Wilkus and Dodrill 1984, 1989), although not consistently (Sackellares et al. 1985) (Table 17.4).

The question then becomes "why would a group without significant, objectively-verifiable neuropathology (PNES) perform as badly as patients with epilepsy?" There have been three proposed reasons for worse neuropsychological scores in PNES as compared to patients with epilepsy:

1. Patients with PNES have actual neuropathological insults that current neuroimaging technology cannot detect (Dodrill 2008; Dodrill and Holmes 2000; Drake 1993; Wilkus and Dodrill 1984, 1989). This hypothesis is based on the finding that patients with PNES frequently report more neurological injury or disease (e.g., head injury, CNS infection) than patients with epilepsy.
2. Patients with PNES perform worse than patients with epilepsy due to intervening variables such as the detrimental effects of medication, pain, physical fatigue, and forms of emotional distress that have been variably linked to impaired cognitive performance (e.g., depression, anxiety, post-traumatic stress disorder).

Table 17.4 Summary of representative studies comparing neurocognitive function in patients with PNES to patients with ES

Study reference	Specific findings	Neurocognitive deficits
Wilkus and Dodrill (1984, 1989)	Both groups perform outside of normal limits on approximately half of the measures in the Neuropsychological Battery for Epilepsy	PNES = ES or
Dodrill and Holmes (2000)		PNES <= ES
Drake et al. (1993)	4 of 20 individuals with PNES performed in the mentally retarded range, while an additional 13 exhibited cognitive impairment on the Halstead-Reitan Battery	PNES impaired relative to normative data
Hermann (2000)	No difference in neurocognitive performance between small groups of patients with either PNES or ES	PNES = ES
Sackellares et al. (1985)	Patients with PNES performed better than patients with generalized ES or those with co-occurring ES and PNES	ES < PNES
Prigatano and Kirlin (2009)	Patients with ES performed worse than patients with PNES on a few variables (e.g., naming). Memory performance correlated with anxiety levels for the PNES sample only	ES < PNES
Drane et al. (2006)	Both groups perform outside of normal limits on approximately half of the measures in the Neuropsychological Battery for Epilepsy. However, the patients with PNES failed SVT measures at a much higher rate, and this accounted for their decreased performance	ES < PNES

PNES = psychogenic nonepileptic seizures, *ES* epileptic seizures

3. Patients with PNES perform worse than patients with epilepsy due to inconsistent task engagement, as evidenced by much higher rates of symptom validity test failure in patients with PNES than seen in patients with epilepsy (Drane et al. 2006). Mechanisms for poor task engagement could subsume hypothesis #2, although these researchers have expanded the range of these latent variables to include psychological processes (e.g., dissociative tendencies, and motivation issues).

Research examining the relative merits of these explanations continues. From our perspective, we have noted SVT failure rate for selected patients with epilepsy who have not had a seizure in the past 24 h and do not have pronounced neurodevelopmental delay is 8%, the same as reported in general medical populations (Mittenberg et al. 2002; Williamson et al. 2005). In contrast, despite the lack of identifiable seizure activity or lifelong cognitive disability, the SVT failure rate of patients with PNES remains at or above 28%. There is a growing evidence-base neuropsychology research that the most likely reason patients with PNES perform poorly on neuropsychological tests is poor task engagement (explanation #3 above), the cause of which is more difficult to ascertain and probably varies between patients.

It is important to note what can, and cannot, be interpreted from SVT failure in this patient group (see also Chap. 18, this volume). SVT performance rarely tells one *why* a patient performs in such a manner as to compromise the interpretability of test results. While patients with PNES as a group put forth less effort than patients with epilepsy, malingering (conscious effort to perform poorly) does *not* appear to be a major contributor to the SVT failures seen in the PNES population (Orbach et al. 2003). A number of other factors which could be proposed to negatively impact SVT performance include (1) fatigue, (2) depression or psychiatric symptomatology, (3) pain, and (4) side effects of medications. We know pain and depression do not necessarily lead to poorer SVT performance (Gervais et al. 2004; Gervais et al. 2001; Rohling et al. 2002), and there is no evidence that AEDs impair cognitive performance to such an extent as to cause SVT failure. However, careful examination of the impact of specific AEDs on performance on specific SVTs has yet to be reported. Likewise, patients with epilepsy sometimes experience epileptiform discharges that do not manifest themselves in visible behavioral changes but may have effects upon cognition (Aldenkamp and Arends 2004); the extent to which such discharges may affect SVT performance has yet to be examined. It may well be that some patients with PNES perform poorly on neuropsychological tests for reasons other than poor motivation.

Rule of thumb: Neuropsychological Assessment and SVTs in patients with PNES

- Patients with PNES often exhibit equivalent or greater neurocognitive dysfunction as patients with ES.
- SVT failure rate of patients with PNES 28+% (8% for patients with epilepsy)
- SVT failure of patients with PNES may partially reflect invalid performances resulting from psychological factors or other possible variables (e.g., effects of medications, pain).

Counting Elephants: Are There Meaningful PNES Subtypes?

We are all familiar with the story of the four blind children, each of whom excitedly describe to their teacher their respective finds of (1) a rough but warm and pliable tree, (2) a curved bone, (3) a rough and pliable tube-like object, and (4) a large, flat leathery pad of some sort, and how surprised these children are when their teacher that they have just described the leg, tusk, trunk, and ear of a single animal. Without the presence of an overriding, unifying principle that can bring together the morass of correlates of PNES that have been described, we remain unsure about the extent to which we are playing the part of the blind children or the teacher. A number of groups have attempted to bring some sense of order to the disparate findings for PNES phenomenology, although each group has organized the data from different perspectives (Cragar et al. 2005; Drane et al. 2006; Duncan and Oto 2008a; Holmes et al. 2001; Kuyk et al. 2003; LaFrance and Devinsky 2004; Selkirk et al. 2008). LaFrance and Devinsky (2004) proposed post-traumatic versus developmental PNES. Cragar et al. (2005) divided PNES patients into subtypes based on personality characteristics derived from psychological testing. The Glasgow group has demonstrated subgroup differences if one categorizes according to the presence of developmental delay (Duncan and Oto 2008a), age of onset (Duncan et al. 2006), or report of sexual abuse (Selkirk et al. 2008). We have viewed these patients from the perspective of performance on symptom validity testing (SVTs) (Drane et al. 2006) or behavioral presentation of the PNES events (Benbadis 2005a, b). Each of these perspectives provides a starting point for further questions, many of which have yet to be explored, e.g., to what extent do the proposed subtypes predict response to treatment? Are different types of treatment indicated for different subtypes? Does the level of emotional suffering and disability vary according to subtype? Answers to these questions will provide information critical for treatment planning.

At a broader level, one cannot help but be struck by the similarities between the histories and presentations of patients with PNES and patients with other disorders in which emotional processes are felt to play an important role. Some of these have long been characterized variably as functional somatic syndromes or varying manifestations of somatoform, somatization, or conversion disorders. As evident in Table 17.5, these disorders share a number of similarities in the manner and extent to which affected patients differ from the general population. Are these similarities merely coincidence, or do they speak to a common primary neurological, psychological, metabolic, environmental, and genetic contribution to these problems that can bolster our understanding of these disorders and thereby help to alleviate the suffering of those affected? Or, alternatively, do they speak to a common final pathway depicting the manner in which certain individuals react to disparate primary problems? These questions have certainly been taken up by others (Binder and Campbell 2004; Brown 2004), but remain critical to understanding the extent to which we are dealing with varying manifestations of the same underlying problem or similar manifestations of fundamentally different problems.

Table 17.5 Comparison of syndromes with prominent emotional features

	Gender Ratio	Age of onset	History of Trauma	Association With Higher BMI	Educational Attainment & SES	Comorbid Psychiatric Condition
PNES	F>M (3:1)	Most common in young adulthood	Frequent (>70%)	Yes	Higher Rates Among Low Education and Low SES	Frequent
Fibromyalgia	F>M (7–9:1)	Most common in 40s to 60s	Common[a]	Yes	Some evidence of higher rates among low SES	Common
Chronic Fatigue Syndrome	F>M (4:1)	Most common in 40s to 50s	Common to Frequent	No (due to diagnostic criteria)[b]	Higher Rates Among Low Education and Low SES	Frequent
Chronic Daily Headache	F>M (1.7–2:1)	Most common in 20s to 30s	Common	Yes	Higher Rates Among Low Education and Low SES	Frequent
IBS	F>M (2–3:1)	Most common in young adulthood	Common	Yes	Higher Rates Among Individual from Higher SES	Common

PNES=psychogenic nonepileptic seizures, *IBS* irritable bowel syndrome, *BMI* body mass index, *F>M* female greater prevalence than male, *SES* socioeconomic status. Ratios represent rough approximations based on available data

[a]Trauma in the fibromyalgia group often appears to include physical injury (e.g., onset following a car accident), whereas the other groups in this table are more likely to report childhood abuse (e.g., physical, sexual, emotional)

[b]High BMI is typically included among exclusionary criteria for CFS, as this condition is believed to be independently associated with fatigue

Treatment

The first step of any treatment of PNES is helping the patient to understand the nature of the problem. Clear communication between clinician and patient can be challenging under optimal circumstances, but is even more so when the patient is motivated to maintain a neurological explanation for their difficulties rather than to acknowledge the potential contribution of emotional issues, as is often the case in those with PNES. This crucial interaction has received more attention of late (LaFrance et al. 2006; Shen et al. 1990; Thompson et al. 2005; Thompson et al. 2009); however, the "correct" way to go about it remains a matter of debate (see also Chap. 29 this volume). As pointed out by LaFrance and colleagues (2006), disagreement persists on such issues as (1) the terms "nonepileptic" versus "psychogenic" versus "functional," (2) the word "seizure," (3) providing the diagnosis with the aid of a videotape of the patient's spell versus a standardized verbal explanation, and (4) use of written information versus the clinician's standard verbal explanation. Potential algorithms to provide this information have been provided and to some extent reviewed in terms of their performance (Shen et al. 1990; Thompson et al. 2005); however, the variations on the theme identified by LaFrance and colleagues (2006) have yet to be investigated. The available protocols (e.g., Shen et al. 1990; Thompson et al. 2005) we view as starting points that await further validation.

Unfortunately, even if the clinician is able to effectively engage the patient in an understanding of the problem, an evidence-based practice treatment protocol has not been agreed upon. The literature on the treatment of PNES is far less impressive than the work done on diagnosis and characterization (LaFrance et al. 2006; LaFrance et al. 2008; Lesser 2003; Reuber et al. 2005; Rusch et al. 2001; Wood et al. 2004). There are few randomized controlled trials (but see Ataoglu et al. 2003; Brooks et al. 2007), however even the are difficult to interpret or generalize to other treatment settings. For instance, in one of the randomized controlled trials (Ataoglu et al. 2003), how the diagnosis of PNES was made is unclear, and patients with comorbid Axis I or Axis II disorders were excluded. Given the high rates of psychiatric comorbidity discussed above, it is hard to imagine how the resulting sample would be representative of many of the patients with PNES needing treatment. Other common limitations include (1) a preponderance of unblinded, uncontrolled trials, (2) inconsistent description and definition of PNES diagnosis, (3) small numbers of subjects, (4) inconsistent outcome variables, and (5) characterization of "psychotherapy" as an undifferentiated treatment strategy.

The relative dearth of evidence-based treatment protocols for PNES likely reflects several reasons for services in the USA:

1. *Structure of the USA health care system serving these patients.* Much of this work takes place in tertiary epilepsy centers, as this is where the gold standard diagnostic technique (vEEG) is most likely to available. By definition, many of the patients seen at these centers are there for diagnostic consultation rather than as patients for whom the epileptologists have primary responsibility. Thus, ongoing coordination of patient care by the neurologist after making the diagnosis is often not possible.

In addition, the staffing and finances of such centers are often not designed to accommodate ongoing treatment such as psychotherapy but instead are designed around the practice of consultation followed by referral for treatment.

2. *Reticence to assume responsibility of care.* Similar to other somatoform disorders, patients with PNES live in a gray diagnostic world between medical specialties, in this case, between neurology and psychiatry. Often, particularly in the absence of a functioning multidisciplinary team (arguably the typical treatment setting in the USA), the treating neurologist believes the psychiatric underpinnings of the patient's disorder mandates that a mental health professional assumes primary responsibility for care. Alternatively, the mental health professional, sometimes spooked by the possibility there may in fact be "something neurological going on" that has yet to be detected, feels the neurologist should continue to play a prominent role in the ongoing care of the patient. Benbadis has pointed out the lack of attention to somatization in the psychiatric literature and at psychiatric conferences is striking, given its inherent psychological basis and its base rate relative to other forms of psychiatric illness (Benbadis 2005a). The patient often senses these different perspectives and is left without knowing whom to rely upon as the primary professional coordinating care.

3. *Challenge of the patients.* Simply stated, patients with Cluster B personality disorders and patients who fundamentally disagree with the treating professional's conceptualization of the underlying problem are more challenging to treat. Such issues are more prevalent among patients with PNES (and somatization more broadly). Thus, while the systemic issues described above complicate decisions about who should assume responsibility, the fact of the matter is that the number of professionals actively trying to solve these systemic issues remains relatively small because of the inordinate amount of resources (e.g., physician time and energy) that these patients often consume.

None of these issues are likely to be resolved soon, so we are left with trying to sort out the available data. Unfortunately, the limited data available from well-designed studies preclude meta-analysis, so the reader is encouraged to examine the recent reviews (Brooks et al. 2007; LaFrance and Barry 2005; Reuber and Elger 2003; Rusch et al. 2001), and examine the original studies to implement a protocol with evidence-based support and that matches with the clinician's style and resources The treatments that are most likely to work for given subgroups of patients (perhaps defined by some of the subtype classifications noted earlier) have yet to be determined. Thus, we offer the following observations on the current trends in this literature:

1. A more focused effort to prospectively evaluate promising therapies targeted specifically at the issues viewed as problematic for patients with PNES (LaFrance et al. 2006; LaFrance and Barry 2005)
2. Rather than treating psychotherapy as an undifferentiated intervention, acknowledgment of the varied types of psychotherapeutic intervention available and employing different types of intervention for different putative etiologies (Rusch et al. 2001)
3. Emphasis on the need for continued involvement of the neurologist in the care of the patient with PNES, preferably as part of a multidisciplinary team (Kanner 2008).

Research has identified several treatment prognostic indicators. The duration a patient is diagnosed with having PNES versus seizures or epilepsy is a powerful predictor of treatment outcome. Patients with a history of longer duration of incorrect diagnosis tend to have worse outcomes in which there is maintenance of PNES symptoms. In addition, the duration a patient with PNES is treated with AEDs is also a prognostic indicator. Patients treated with AEDs for longer periods of time demonstrate worse outcomes, maintaining PNES symptoms for longer periods of time. As noted above, the social consequences of PNES are not inconsequential, and more than half of patients having PNES symptoms for more than 10 years in duration remain on disability for income. Because data indicate patients with PNES incorrectly diagnosed and/or treated with AEDs have worse outcomes, Benbadis has argued that the assessment for PNES may not be sufficiently sensitive. A recent study found that the average delay from onset of symptoms to diagnosis of PNES is 7 years.

PNES in Children and Adolescents

The astute reader will have noticed the lack of any reference to children in our discussion. This is not because PNES occur only in adulthood; on the contrary, psychogenic nonepileptic events have been noted in children as young as 6 years of age (Kotagal et al. 2002; Lancman et al. 1994; Vincentiis et al. 2006). The few empirical investigations available have suggested a few general trends among pediatric patients with PNES: (1) as patients get younger, the gender ratio moves closer to 1:1, (2) as patients get younger, the rate of the epilepsy co-occurrence increases, and (3) family dysfunction is common, though not necessarily physical, emotional, or sexual abuse (Kotagal et al. 2002; Patel et al. 2007; Vincentiis et al. 2006). Family histories of epilepsy also appear to be more common, as are comorbid psychiatric disorders, depression in particular (Vincentiis et al. 2006). Children have a better prognosis for recovery (i.e., resolution of PNES symptoms) following diagnosis of PNES than do adults (Wyllie et al. 2002; Wyllie et al. 1990; Wyllie et al. 1999). Unfortunately, there have been no controlled trials for the treatment of PNES in children, with some authors suggesting that until we have established more firmly the rates of comorbid developmental and psychiatric issues (e.g., ADHD, depression, anxiety, PTSD), such trials are premature (LaFrance et al. 2006).

Neuropsychological Assessment Strategies with PNES

In our opinion, an adequate neuropsychological evaluation of patients with PNES should include obtaining a thorough history, having the patients complete appropriate measures of mood/personality (evidenced-based practice supports MMPI-2 or PAI) and quality of life, and performing at least a core collection of neurocognitive measures [evidence-based neuropsychology practice suggests including a symptom validity task(s)].) A careful history will identify potential risk factors for either PNES (e.g., sexual abuse or trauma, history of fibromyalgia or chronic pain) or epilepsy (e.g., neurological injury or disease) and can be useful for understanding the development and maintenance of PNES (and subsequently for guiding treatment). The MMPI/MMPI-2 and the PAI provide evidence-based formulas for predicting the likelihood a given patient experiences PNES (see section "Psychological Testing/Evidence-Based Psychology Practice"). Finally, the use of neuropsychological tests helps to establish the functional capacity of the patient, and possibly point to a cognitive impact of medication regimens. For example, it is not uncommon for patients with PNES to experience comorbid chronic pain issues, and it is possible a patient is being treated with medications that dull/slow their cognitive processes. Establishing functional and intellectual capacity can be valuable for determining appropriate treatment. Of note, symptom validity testing has empirical support for establishing the interpretability of any neuropsychological assessment regardless of potential reasons for invalidity. Many researchers failing to use SVT measures have concluded patients with PNES have profound cognitive impairment and are unable to benefit from standard psychotherapeutic interventions. Table 17.6 includes some suggestions for specific tests that we have found useful as part of neuropsychological assessments with this patient population.

Table 17.6 Examples of possible neuropsychological tests and measures to use with a PNES population

Mood and personality measures:
    Minnesota multiphasic personality inventory (MMPI)/(MMPI2)
    Personality assessment inventory (PAI)
Quality of life measures:
    Quality of Life in Epilepsy (QOLIE-89)
Symptom validity measures:
    Word Memory Test
    Victoria Symptom Validity Test
Neurocogntive measures – general intelligence:
    Wechsler adult intelligence scales
Estimates of Premorbid Function:
    American national adult reading test (AMNART)
    Wechsler test of adult reading (WTAR)
Language:
    Boston naming test
    Letter and semantic fluency tests
Attention:
    Trailmaking test
    Working memory index from some version of the WAIS
Visuo-perception/visual-spatial:
    Visual object and space perception (VOSP) battery
Memory and learning:
    Wechsler memory scales (select subtests)
    List learning paradigm (e.g., Rey Auditory Verbal Learning Test)
Executive control processes:
    Stroop color-word interference test
    Wisconsin card sorting test

PNES = psychogenic nonepileptic seizures

Future Directions for Research, Detection, and Treatment of PNES

To make optimal progress in PNES, researchers and clinicians need to carefully define this condition and make the diagnostic classification rules clear. While vEEG represents the gold standard for diagnosis, working towards a consensus definition of the behavioral component of PNES would be helpful. In addition, we may find that combining diagnostic tools allows us to bolster our confidence in decisions where vEEG has failed to capture any typical spells. For example, it is likely the presence of demographic and medical variables (e.g., history of sexual abuse, co-morbid fibromyalgia), specific personality profiles, and performance on symptom validity testing can be combined with EEG data to provide a more accurate decision about "indeterminate" cases than clinical judgment alone. Research should continue developing classification algorithms, assessment of subtypes of patients with PNES, and potential etiological factors that may contribute to the onset of PNES. Improving diagnostic abilities could both cut down on the costs associated with this condition and what is often a lengthy time span between its onset and identification. Understanding the subtypes and their etiologies has the potential to increase sensitivity or specificity for treatment decisions and to lead to strategies to prevent the onset of this condition in potentially vulnerable populations. Efforts to determine why neuropsychological/psychological test scores can be so variable and often invalid (demonstrate lack of adequate task engagement in testing) among patients with PNES also need to be further explored (e.g., potential impact of comorbid conditions such as chronic pain and its treatment with analgesics or dissociation associated with chronic abuse histories). Finally, development and evaluation of specific treatment strategies for patients with PNES remains in its infancy, and represents a very important area of outcomes research that has been sorely missing. There is clearly a newfound interest in this large patient population, exhibited both by the USA National Institutes of Health and many USA national organizations devoting to the care of epilepsy, and this interest bodes well for the future care of individuals suffering from this malady.

Appendix

Diagnostic Nomenclature Used at the University of Washington Regional Epilepsy Center

Epileptic Seizures (ES) – Evidence of definite EEG abnormalities during video-EEG monitoring. This includes both ictal and interictal epileptiform activity.

Psychogenic Nonepileptic Seizures (PNES) – Episodes of unresponsiveness or behavioral abnormality in the absence of EEG changes. Subjective episodes (e.g., "funny" feeling) or minor motor movements (e.g., myoclonic jerks) are not felt to be definitive enough to warrant this diagnosis.

Physiological Nonepileptic Seizures (PhyNES) – Episodes of unresponsiveness or behavioral abnormality in the absence of EEG changes, but due to another specific physiological cause (e.g., movement disorders, sleep disturbance, syncopal episodes).

Indeterminate Spells (IS) – Diagnosis given to patients who either have no spells during vEEG monitoring or those that only experience subjective episodes (e.g., patient indicates that are experiencing a feeling of fear or disgust) or minor motor movements (e.g., myoclonic jerks) in the absence of EEG change.

Co-Occurrence (CO) – Both ES and PNES events have been established using the above criteria during a single or across multiple vEEG admissions.

References

Abubakr, A., Kablinger, A., & Caldito, G. (2003). Psychogenic seizures: Clinical features and psychological analysis. *Epilepsy & Behavior, 4*(3), 241–245.

Aldenkamp, A., & Arends, J. (2004). The relative influence of epileptic EEG discharges, short nonconvulsive seizures, and type of epilepsy on cognitive function. *Epilepsia, 45*(1), 54–63.

Alper, K., Devinsky, O., Perrine, K., Vazquez, B., et al. (1993). Nonepileptic seizures and childhood sexual and physical abuse. *Neurology, 43*(10), 1950.

American Psychiatric Association. (2000). *Diagnostic and statistical manual of mental disorders (DSM-IV-TR)* (4th ed.). Arlington: American Psychiatric Publishing.

Ataoglu, A., Ozcetin, A., Icmeli, C., & Ozbulut, O. (2003). Paradoxical therapy in conversion reaction. *Journal of Korean Medical Science, 18*(4), 581–584.

Bazil, C. W., & Walczak, T. S. (1997). Effects of sleep and sleep-stage on epileptic and nonepileptic seizures. *Epilepsia, 38*, 56–62.

Begley, C. E., Famulari, M., Annegers, J. F., Lairson, D. R., Reynolds, T. F., Coan, S., et al. (2000). The cost of epilepsy in the United States: an estimate from population-based clinical and survey data. *Epilepsia, 41*(3), 342–351.

Benbadis, S. R. (2001). Provocative techniques should be used for the diagnosis of psychogenic nonepileptic seizures. *Archives of Neurology, 58*(12), 2063.

Benbadis, S. R. (2005a). The problem of psychogenic symptoms: Is the psychiatric community in denial? *Epilepsy & Behavior, 6*, 9–14.

Benbadis, S. R. (2005b). A spell in the epilepsy clinic and a history of "chronic pain" or "fibromyalgia" independently predict a diagnosis of psychogenic seizures. *Epilepsy & Behavior, 6*(2), 264–265.

Benbadis, S. R., & Hauser, W. A. (2000). An estimate of the prevalence of psychogenic nonepileptic seizures. *Seizure, 9*, 280–281.

Benbadis, S. R., Wolgamuth, B. R., Goren, H., Brener, S., & Fouad-Tarazi, F. (1995). Value of tongue biting in the diagnosis of seizures. *Archives of Internal Medicine, 155*(21), 2346–2349.

Benbadis, S. R., Agrawal, V., & Tatum, W. O. (2001). How many patients with psychogenic nonepileptic seizures also have epilepsy? *Neurology, 57*, 915–917.

Bergen, D., & Ristanovic, R. (1993). Weeping as a common element of pseudoseizures. *Archives of Neurology, 50*, 1059–1060.

Berkhoff, M., Briellmann, R. S., Radanov, B. P., Donati, F., & Hess, C. W. (1998). Developmental background and outcome in patients with nonepileptic versus epileptic seizures: a controlled study. *Epilepsia, 39*(5), 463–469.

Binder, L. M., & Campbell, K. A. (2004). Medically unexplained symptoms and neuropsychological assessment. *Journal of Clinical and Experimental Neuropsychology, 26*(3), 369–392.

Bowman, E. S. (1993). Etiology and clinical course of pseudoseizures: Relationship to trauma, depression, and dissociation. *Psychosomatics, 34*(4), 333–342.

Bowman, E. S. (2001). Psychopathology and outcome in pseudoseizures. In A. B. Ettinger & A. M. Kanner (Eds.), *Psychiatric issues in epilepsy* (pp. 355–377). Philadelphia: Lippincott, Williams, and Wilkins.

Bowman, E. S. (2006). Why conversion seizures should be classified as a dissociative disorder. *The Psychiatric Clinics of North America, 29*(1), 185–211.

Bowman, E. S., & Markand, O. N. (1996). Psychodynamics and psychiatric diagnoses of pseudo-seizure subjects. *The American Journal of Psychiatry, 153*(1), 57–63.

Brooks, J. L., Goodfellow, L., Bodde, N. M., Aldenkamp, A., & Baker, G. A. (2007). Nondrug treatments for psychogenic nonepileptic seizures: What's the evidence? *Epilepsy & Behavior, 11*(3), 367–377.

Brown, R. J. (2004). Psychological mechanisms of medically unexplained symptoms: An integrative conceptual model. *Psychological Bulletin, 130*(5), 793–812.

Burneo, J. G., Martin, R., Powell, T., Greenlee, S., Knowlton, R. C., Faught, R. E., et al. (2003). Teddy bears: An observational finding in patients with non-epileptic events. *Neurology, 61*(5), 714–715.

Chung, S. S., Gerber, P., & Kirlin, K. A. (2006). Ictal eye closure is a reliable indicator for psychogenic nonepileptic seizures. *Neurology, 66*(11), 1730–1731.

Cragar, D. E., Berry, D. T. R., Fakhoury, T. A., Cibula, J. E., & Schmitt, F. A. (2002). A review of diagnostic techniques in the differential diagnosis of epileptic and nonepileptic seizures. *Neuropsychology Review, 12*(1), 31–64.

Cragar, D. E., Schmitt, F. A., Berry, D. T. R., Cibula, J. E., Dearth, C. M. S., & Fakhoury, T. A. (2003). A comparison of MMPI-2 decision rules in the diagnosis of nonepileptic seizures. *Journal of Clinical and Experimental Neuropsychology, 25*(6), 793.

Cragar, D. E., Berry, D. T., Schmitt, F. A., & Fakhoury, T. A. (2005). Cluster analysis of normal personality traits in patients with psychogenic nonepileptic seizures. *Epilepsy & Behavior, 6*(4), 593–600.

Cuthill, F. M., & Espie, C. A. (2005). Sensitivity and specificity of procedures for the differential diagnosis of epileptic and non-epileptic seizures: a systematic review. *Seizure, 14*(5), 293–303.

Deacon, C., Wiebe, S., Blume, W. T., McLachlan, R. S., Young, G. B., & Matijevic, S. (2003). Seizure identification by clinical description in temporal lobe epilepsy: How accurate are we? *Neurology, 61*(12), 1686–1689.

Dean, A. C., Victor, T. L., Boone, K. B., & Arnold, G. (2008). The relationship of IQ to effort test performance. *The Clinical Neuropsychologist, 22*(4), 705–722.

Derry, P. A., & McLachlan, R. S. (1996). The MMPI-2 as an adjunct to the diagnosis of pseudo-seizures. *Seizure, 5*, 35–40.

Devinsky, O., Sanchez-Villasenor, F., Vazquez, B., Kothari, M., Alper, K., & Luciano, D. (1996). Clinical profile of patients with epileptic and nonepileptic seizures. *Neurology, 46*, 1530–1533.

Devinsky, O., Mesad, S., & Alper, K. (2001). Nondominant hemisphere lesions and conversion nonepileptic seizures. *Journal of Neuropsychiatry and Clinical Neuroscience, 13*(3), 367–373.

Dikel, T. N., Fennell, E. B., & Gilmore, R. L. (2003). Posttraumatic stress disorder, dissociation, and sexual abuse history in epileptic and nonepileptic seizure patients. *Epilepsy & Behavior, 4*(6), 644.

Dodrill, C. B. (2008). Do patients with psychogenic nonepileptic seizures produce trustworthy findings on neuropsychological tests? *Epilepsia, 49*(4), 691–695.

Dodrill, C. B., & Holmes, M. D. (2000). Psychological and neuropsychological evaluation of the patient with non-epileptic seizures. In J. R. Gates & A. J. Rowan (Eds.), *Non-epileptic seizures* (2nd ed.). Boston: Butterworth-Heinemann.

Drake, M. E. (1993). Conversion hysteria and dominant hemisphere lesions. *Psychosomatics: Journal of Consultation Liaison Psychiatry, 34*(6), 524.

Drake, M. E., Huber, S. J., Pakalnis, A., & Phillips, B. B. (1993). Neuropsychological and event-related potential correlates of nonepileptic seizures. *The Journal of Neuropsychiatry and Clinical Neurosciences, 5*(1), 102.

Drane, D. L., Williamson, D. J., Stroup, E. S., Holmes, M. D., Jung, M., Koerner, E., et al. (2006). Cognitive impairment is not equal in patients with epileptic and psychogenic nonepileptic seizures. *Epilepsia, 47*(11), 1879–1886.

Duncan, R., & Oto, M. (2008a). Predictors of antecedent factors in psychogenic nonepileptic attacks: multivariate analysis. *Neurology, 71*(13), 1000–1005.

Duncan, R., & Oto, M. (2008b). Psychogenic nonepileptic seizures in patients with learning disability: comparison with patients with no learning disability. *Epilepsy & Behavior, 12*(1), 183–186.

Duncan, R., Oto, M., Russell, A., & Conway, P. (2004). Pseudosleep events in patients with psychogenic non-epileptic seizures: prevalence and associations. *Journal of Neurology, Neurosurgery and Psychiatry, 75*(7), 1009–1012.

Duncan, R., Oto, M., Martin, E., & Pelosi, A. (2006). Late onset psychogenic nonepileptic attacks. *Neurology, 66*(11), 1644–1647.

Engel, J. J. (1996). Surgery for seizures. *The New England Journal of Medicine, 334*, 647–652.

Engel, J., Jr., & Shewmon, D. A. (1993). Overview: Who should be considered a surgical candidate? In J. Engel Jr. (Ed.), *Surgical treatment of epilepsies* (Vol. 2, pp. 23–34). New York: Raven Press.

Ettinger, A. B., Devinksy, O., Weisbrot, D. M., Ramakrishna, R. K., & Goyal, A. (1999a). A comprehensive profile of clinical, psychiatric, and psychosocial characteristics of patients with psychogenic nonepileptic seizures. *Epilepsia, 40*, 1292–1298.

Ettinger, A. B., Dhoon, A., Weisbrot, D. M., & Devinksy, O. (1999b). Predictive factors for outcome of nonepileptic seizures after diagnosis. *Journal of Psychiatry and Clinical Neuroscience, 11*(4), 458–463.

Fisch, B. J., & Olejniczak, D. W. (2001). Generalized tonic-clonic seizures. In E. Wyllie (Ed.), *The treatment of epilepsy* (pp. 369–393). Philadelphia: Lippincott, Williams, and Wilkins.

Fiszman, A., Alves-Leon, S. V., Nunes, R. G., D'Andrea, I., & Figueira, I. (2004). Traumatic events and posttraumatic stress disorder in patients with psychogenic nonepileptic seizures: a critical review. *Epilepsy & Behavior, 5*(6), 818–825.

Francis, P., & Baker, G. A. (1999). Non-epileptic attack disorder (NEAD): A comprehensive review. *Seizure, 8*, 53–61.

French, J. (1995). Pseudoseizures in the era of video-electroencephalogram monitoring. *Current Opinion in Neurology, 8*(2), 117–120.

Freud, S. (1966). Hysteria. In J. Strachey (Ed. & Trans.), *The standard edition of the complete psychological works of Sigmund Freud* (Vol. 1, pp. 41–59). London: Hogarth Press.

Gates, J. R., & Erdahl, P. (1993). Classification of non-epileptic events. In A. J. Rowan & J. R. Gates (Eds.), *Non-epileptic seizures* (pp. 21–30). Boston: Butterworth-Heinemann.

Gates, J. R., Ramani, V., Whalen, S., & Lowenson, R. N. (1985). Ictal characteristics of pseudoseizures. *Archives of Neurology, 42*, 1183–1187.

Gervais, R. O., Russell, A. S., Green, P., Allen, L. M., Ferrari, R., & Pieschl, S. D. (2001). Effort testing in patients with fibromyalgia and disability incentives. *The Journal of Rheumatology, 28*, 1892–1899.

Gervais, R. O., Rohling, M. L., Green, P., & Ford, W. (2004). A comparison of WMT, CARB, and TOMM failure rates in non-head injury disability claimants. *Archives of Clinical Neuropsychology, 19*(4), 475.

Geyer, J. D., Payne, T. A., & Drury, I. (2000). The value of pelvic thrusting in the diagnosis of seizures and pseudoseizures. *Neurology, 54*, 227–229.

Goldstein, L. H., Drew, C., Mellers, J., Mitchell-O'Malley, S., & Oakley, D. A. (2000). Dissociation, hypnotizability, coping styles and health locus of control: characteristics of pseudoseizure patients. *Seizure, 9*(5), 314–322.

Green, P., Iverson, G. L., & Allen, L. (1999). Detecting malingering in head injury litigation with the Word Memory Test. *Brain Injury, 13*(10), 813.

Green, P., Rohling, M. L., Lees-Haley, P. R., & Allen, L. M. (2001). Effort has a greater effect on test scores than severe brain injury in compensation claimants. *Brain Injury, 15*(12), 1045.

Harden, C. L., Burgut, F. T., & Kanner, A. M. (2003). The diagnostic significance of video-EEG monitoring findings on pseudoseizure patients differs between neurologists and psychiatrists. *Epilepsia, 44*(3), 453–456.

Harden, C. L., Jovine, L., Burgut, F. T., Carey, B. T., Nikolov, B. G., & Ferrando, S. J. (2009). A comparison of personality disorder characteristics of patients with nonepileptic psychogenic pseudoseizures with those of patients with epilepsy. *Epilepsy & Behavior, 14*(3), 481–483.

Hermann, B. P. (2000). Neuropsychological assessment in the diagnosis of non-epileptic seizures. In J. R. Gates & A. J. Rowan (Eds.), *Non-epileptic seizures*. Boston: Butterworth-Heinemann.

Hoerth, M. T., Wellik, K. E., Demaerschalk, B. M., Drazkowski, J. F., Noe, K. H., Sirvin, J. I., et al. (2008). Clinical predictors of psychogenic nonepileptic seizures. *The Neurologist, 14*, 266–270.

Holmes, M. D., Dodrill, C. B., Bachtler, S., Wilensky, A. J., Ojemann, L. M., & Miller, J. W. (2001). Evidence that emotional maladjustment is worse in men than in women with psychogenic nonepileptic seizures. *Epilepsy & Behavior, 2*(6,Part1), 568.

Howe, L. L., & Loring, D. W. (2009). Classification accuracy and predictive ability of the medical symptom validity test's dementia profile and general memory impairment profile. *The Clinical Neuropsychologist, 23*(2), 329–342.

Kanner, A. M. (2008). Is the neurologist's role over once the diagnosis of psychogenic nonepileptic seizures is made? No! *Epilepsy & Behavior, 12*(1), 1–2.

Kanner, A. M., Parra, J., Frey, M., Stebbins, G., Pierre-Louis, S., & Iriarte, J. (1999). Psychiatric and neurologic predictors of psychogenic pseudoseizure outcome. *Neurology, 53*(5), 933–938.

Kellinghaus, C., Loddenkemper, T., Dinner, D. S., Lachwani, D., & Luders, H. O. (2004). Nonepileptic seizures of the elderly. *Journal of Neurology, 251*(6), 704–709.

Kotagal, P., Costa, M., Wyllie, E., & Wolgamuth, B. (2002). Paroxysmal nonepileptic events in children and adolescents. *Pediatrics, 110*(4), e46.

Krumholz, A. (1999). Nonepileptic seizures: Diagnosis and management. *Neurology, 53*(5 Suppl. 2), S76–S83.

Kuyk, J., Swinkels, W. A. M., & Spinhoven, P. (2003). Psychopathologies in patients with nonepileptic seizures with and without comorbid epilepsy: How different are they? *Epilepsy & Behavior, 4*(1), 13.

Lacey, C., Cook, M., & Salzberg, M. (2007). The neurologist, psychogenic nonepileptic seizures, and borderline personality disorder. *Epilepsy & Behavior, 11*(4), 492–498.

LaFrance, W. C., Jr., & Barry, J. J. (2005). Update on treatments of psychological nonepileptic seizures. *Epilepsy & Behavior, 7*(3), 364–374.

LaFrance, W. C., Jr., & Devinsky, O. (2004). The treatment of nonepileptic seizures: historical perspectives and future directions. *Epilepsia, 45*(Suppl 2), 15–21.

LaFrance, W. C., Jr., Alper, K., Babcock, D., Barry, J. J., Benbadis, S., Caplan, R., et al. (2006). Nonepileptic seizures treatment workshop summary. *Epilepsy & Behavior, 8*(3), 451–461.

LaFrance, W. C., Jr., Rusch, M. D., & Machan, J. T. (2008). What is "treatment as usual" for nonepileptic seizures? *Epilepsy & Behavior, 12*(3), 388–394.

Lancman, M. E., Asconape, J. J., Graves, S., & Gibson, P. A. (1994). Psychogenic seizures in children: long-term analysis of 43 cases. *Journal of Child Neurology, 9*(4), 404–407.

Lempert, T., & Schmidt, D. (1990). Natural history and outcome of psychogenic seizures: a clinical study in 50 patients. *Journal of Neurology, 237*(1), 35–38.

Lesser, R. P. (1996). Psychogenic seizures. *Neurology, 46*, 1499–1507.

Lesser, R. P. (2003). Treatment and outcome of psychogenic nonepileptic seizures. *Epilepsy Currents, 3*(6), 198–200.

Lesser, R. P., Leuders, H., & Dinner, D. S. (1983). Evidence for epilepsy is rare in patients with psychogenic nonepileptic seizures. *Neurology, 33*, 502–504.

Liske, E., & Forster, F. M. (1964). Pseudoseizures: Problems in diagnosis and management of epileptic patients. *Neurology, 14*, 41–49.

Locke, D. E. C., Kirlin, K. A., Thomas, M. L., Osborne, D., Hurst, D. F., Drazkowski, J. F., et al. (2010). The Minnesota multiphasic personality inventory-2-restructured form in the epilepsy unit. *Epilepsy & Behavior, 17*(2), 252–258.

Loring, D. W., Lee, G. P., & Meador, K. J. (2005). Victoria symptom validity test performance in non-litigating epilepsy surgery candidates. *Journal of Clinical and Experimental Neuropsychology, 27*(5), 610.

Marquez, A. V., Farias, S. T., Apperson, M., Koopmans, S., Jorgensen, J., Shatzel, A., et al. (2004). Psychogenic nonepileptic seizures are associated with an increased risk of obesity. *Epilepsy & Behavior, 5*(1), 88–93.

Marshall, P., & Happe, M. (2007). The performance of individuals with mental retardation on cognitive tests assessing effort and motivation. *The Clinical Neuropsychologist, 21*(5), 826–840.

Martin, R., Burneo, J. G., Prasad, A., Powell, T., Faught, E., Knowlton, R., et al. (2003). Frequency of epilepsy in patients with psychogenic nonepileptic seizures monitored by video-EEG. *Neurology, 61*(12), 1791–1792.

Massey, W. E. (1982). History of epilepsy and hysteria. In T. R. Riley & A. Roy (Eds.), *Pseudoseizures* (pp. 1–20). Baltimore: Williams and Wilkins.

Mattson, R. H. (1980). Value of intensive monitoring. In J. A. Wada & J. K. Penry (Eds.), *Advances in epileptology* (pp. 43–51). New York: Raven Press.

Mittenberg, W., Patton, C., Canyock, E. M., & Condit, D. C. (2002). Base rates of malingering and symptom exaggeration. *Journal of Clinical and Experimental Neuropsychology, 24*(8), 1094.

Mokleby, K., Blomhoff, S., Malt, U. F., Dahlstrom, A., Tauboll, E., & Gierstad, L. (2002). Psychiatric comorbidity and hostility in patients with psychogenic nonepileptic seizures compared with somatoform disorders and healthy controls. *Epilepsia, 43*(2), 193–198.

Nelson, L. D., Elder, J. T., Groot, J., Tehrani, P., & Grant, A. C. (2004). Personality testing and epilepsy: comparison of two MMPI-2 correction procedures. *Epilepsy & Behavior, 5*(6), 911–918.

Neumann, L., & Buskila, D. (2003). Epidemiology of fibromyalgia. *Current Pain and Headache Reports, 7*(5), 362–368.

O'Sullivan, S. S., Spillane, J. E., McMahon, E. M., Sweeney, B. J., Galvin, R. J., McNamara, B., et al. (2007). Clinical characteristics and outcome of patients diagnosed with psychogenic nonepileptic seizures: A 5-year review. *Epilepsy & Behavior, 11*, 77–84.

Oliva, M., Pattison, C., Carino, J., Roten, A., Matkovic, Z., & O'Brien, T. J. (2008). The diagnostic value of oral lacerations and incontinence during convulsive "seizures". *Epilepsia, 49*(6), 962–967.

Orbach, D., Ritaccio, A., & Devinsky, O. (2003). Psychogenic, nonepileptic seizures associated with video-EEG-verified sleep. *Epilepsia, 44*(1), 64.

Patel, H., Scott, E., Dunn, D., & Garg, B. (2007). Nonepileptic seizures in children. *Epilepsia, 48*(11), 2086–2092.

Peguero, E., Abou-Khalil, B., Fakhoury, T., & Matthews, G. (1995). Self-injury and incontinence in psychogenic seizures. *Epilepsia, 36*, 586–591.

Prigatano, G. P., & Kirlin, K. A. (2009). Self-appraisal and objective assessment of cognitive and affective functioning in persons with epileptic and nonepileptic seizures. *Epilepsy & Behavior, 14*(2), 387–392.

Rechlin, T., Loew, T. H., & Joraschky, P. (1997). Pseudoseizure "status". *Journal of Psychosomatic Research, 42*(5), 495–498.

Reuber, M. (2008). Psychogenic nonepileptic seizures: answers and questions. *Epilepsy & Behavior, 12*(4), 622–635.

Reuber, M., & Elger, C. E. (2003). Psychogenic nonepileptic seizures: Review and update. *Epilepsy & Behavior, 4*(3), 205–216.

Reuber, M., Enright, S. M., & Goulding, P. J. (2000). Postoperative pseudostatus: Not everything that shakes is epilepsy. *Anaesthesia, 55*(1), 74–78.

Reuber, M., Fernandez, G., Bauer, J., Helmstaedter, C., & Elger, C. E. (2002a). Diagnostic delay in psychogenic nonepileptic seizures. *Neurology, 58*(3), 493–495.

Reuber, M., Fernandez, G., Bauer, J., Singhh, D. D., & Elger, C. E. (2002b). Interictal EEG abnormalities in patients with psychogenic nonepileptic seizures. *Epilepsia, 43*(9), 1013–1020.

Reuber, M., House, A. O., Pukrop, R., Bauer, J., & Elger, C. E. (2003a). Somatization, dissociation and general psychopathology in patients with psychogenic non-epileptic seizures. *Epilepsy Research, 57*(2–3), 159–167.

Reuber, M., Pukrop, R., Mitchell, A. J., Bauer, J., & Elger, C. E. (2003b). Clinical significance of recurrent psychogenic nonepileptic seizure status. *Journal of Neurology, 250*(11), 1355–1362.

Reuber, M., Qurishi, A., Bauer, J., Helmstaedter, C., Fernandez, G., Widman, G., et al. (2003c). Are there physical risk factors for psychogenic non-epileptic seizures in patients with epilepsy. *Seizure, 12*(8), 561–567.

Reuber, M., Pukrop, R., Bauer, J., Derfuss, R., & Elger, C. E. (2004). Multidimensional assessment of personality in patients with psychogenic non-epileptic seizures. *Journal of Neurology, Neurosurgery and Psychiatry, 75*(5), 743–748.

Reuber, M., Howlett, S., & Kemp, S. (2005). Psychologic treatment of patients with psychogenic nonepileptic seizures. *Expert Review of Neurotherapeutics, 5*(6), 737–752.

Rohling, M. L., Green, P., Allen, L. M., & Iverson, G. L. (2002). Depressive symptoms and neurocognitive test scores in patients passing symptom validity tests. *Archives of Clinical Neuropsychology, 17*(3), 205.

Rusch, M. D., Morris, G. L., Allen, L., & Lathrop, L. (2001). Psychological treatment of nonepileptic events. *Epilepsy & Behavior, 2*(3), 277–283.

Sackellares, J., Giordani, B., Berent, S., Seidenberg, M., Dreifuss, F., Vanderzant, C., et al. (1985). Patients with pseudoseizures: Intellectual and cognitive performance. *Neurology, 35*, 116–119.

Sagyi, S., Katz, A., Marks, D. A., & Spencer, S. S. (1992). Frontal lobe partial seizures and psychogenic seizures: Comparison of clinical and ictal characteristics. *Neurology, 42*, 1274–1277.

Schrag, A., Brown, R. J., & Trimble, M. R. (2004). Reliability of self-reported diagnoses in patients with neurologically unexplained symptoms. *Journal of Neurology, Neurosurgery and Psychiatry, 75*, 608–611.

Schramke, C. J., Valeri, A., Valeriano, J. P., & Kelly, K. M. (2007). Using the Minnesota multiphasic inventory 2, EEGs, and clinical data to predict nonepileptic events. *Epilepsy & Behavior, 11*(3), 343–346.

Scoot, D. F. (1982). Recognition and diagnostic aspects of non-epileptic seizures. In T. L. Riley & A. Roy (Eds.), *Pseudoseizures* (pp. 21–34). Baltimore: Williams & Wilkins.

Selkirk, M., Duncan, R., Oto, M., & Pelosi, A. (2008). Clinical differences between patients with nonepileptic seizures who report antecedent sexual abuse and those who do not. *Epilepsia, 49*(8), 1446–1450.

Shen, W., Bowman, E. S., & Markand, O. N. (1990). Presenting the diagnosis of pseudoseizure. *Neurology, 40*(5), 756–759.

Sigurdardottir, K. R., & Olafsson, E. (1998). Incidence of psychogenic seizures in adults: a population-based study in Iceland. *Epilepsia, 39*(7), 749–752.

Storzbach, D., Binder, L. M., Salinsky, M. C., Campbell, B. R., & Mueller, R. M. (2000). Improved prediction of nonepileptic seizures with combined MMPI and EEG measures. *Epilepsia, 41*(3), 332–337.

Stroup, E. S., Drane, D. L., Wilson, K. S., Miller, J. W., Holmes, M. D., & Wilensky, A. J. (2004). Utility of the personality assessment inventory (PAI) in the evaluation of patients on a long-term monitoring unit. *Epilepsia, 45*(Suppl. 7), 239–240.

Syed, T. U., Arozullah, A. M., Suciu, G. P., Toub, J., Kim, H., Dougherty, M. L., et al. (2008). Do observer and self-reports of ictal eye closure predict psychogenic nonepileptic seizures? *Epilepsia, 49*(5), 898–904.

Szaflarski, J. P., Ficker, D. M., Cahill, W. T., & Privatera, M. D. (2000a). Four-year incidence of psychogenic nonepileptic seizures in adults in Hamilton County, OH. *Neurology, 55*, 1561–1563.

Szaflarski, J. P., Ficker, D. M., Cahill, W. T., & Privitera, M. D. (2000b). Four-year incidence of psychogenic nonepileptic seizures in adults in Hamilton County, OH. *Neurology, 55*(10), 1561.

Szaflarski, J. P., Szaflarski, M., Hughes, C., Ficker, D. M., Cahill, W. T., & Privitera, M. D. (2003). Psychopathology and quality of life: psychogenic non-epileptic seizures versus epilepsy. *Medical Science Monitor, 9*(4), 113–118.

Thompson, N. C., Osorio, I., & Hunter, E. E. (2005). Nonepileptic seizures: reframing the diagnosis. *Perspectives in Psychiatric Care, 41*(2), 71–78.

Thompson, R., Isaac, C. L., Rowse, G., Tooth, C. L., & Reuber, M. (2009). What is it like to receive a diagnosis of nonepileptic seizures? *Epilepsy & Behavior, 14*(3), 508–515.

Tojek, T. M., Lumley, M., Barkley, G., Mahr, G., & Thomas, A. (2000). Stress and other psychosocial characteristics of patients with psychogenic nonepileptic seizures. *Psychosomatics: Journal of Consultation Liaison Psychiatry, 41*(3), 221.

van Merode, T., Twellaar, M., Kotsopoulos, I. A., Kessels, A. G., Merckelbach, H., de Krom, M. C., et al. (2004). Psychological characteristics of patients with newly developed psychogenic seizures. *Journal of Neurology, Neurosurgery and Psychiatry, 75*(8), 1175–1177.

Vincentiis, S., Valente, K. D., Thome-Souza, S., Kuczinsky, E., Fiore, L. A., & Negrao, N. (2006). Risk factors for psychogenic nonepileptic seizures in children and adolescents with epilepsy. *Epilepsy & Behavior, 8*(1), 294–298.

Vossler, D. G., Haltiner, A. M., Schepp, S. K., Friel, P. A., Caylor, L. M., Morgan, J. D., et al. (2004). Ictal stuttering: A sign suggestive of psychogenic nonepileptic seizures. *Neurology, 63*, 516–519.

Wagner, M. T., Wymer, J. H., Topping, K. B., & Pritchard, P. B. (2005). Use of the personality assessment inventory as an efficacious and cost-effective diagnostic tool for nonepileptic seizures. *Epilepsy & Behavior, 7*(2), 301–304.

Walczak, T. S., Williams, D. T., & Berten, W. (1994). Utility and reliability of placebo infusion in the evaluation of patients with seizures. *Neurology, 44*, 394–399.

Walczak, T. S., Papacostas, S., Williams, D. T., Scheuer, M. L., Lebowitz, N., & Notarfrancesco, A. (1995). Outcome after diagnosis of psychogenic nonepileptic seizures. *Epilepsia, 36*(11), 1131–1137.

Warner, M. H., Wilkus, R. J., Vossler, D. G., & Dodrill, C. B. (1996). MMPI-2 profiles in differential diagnosis of epilepsy vs. psychogenic seizures. *Epilepsia, 37*(Suppl 5), 19.

Wilkus, R. J., & Dodrill, C. B. (1984). Intensive EEG monitoring and psychological studies of patients with pseudoepileptic seizures. *Epilepsia, 25*, 100–107.

Wilkus, R. J., & Dodrill, C. B. (1989). Factors affecting the outcome of MMPI and neuropsychological assessments of psychogenic and epileptic seizure patients. *Epilepsia, 30*, 339–347.

Williamson, D. J., Drane, D. L., Stroup, E. S., Wilensky, A. J., Holmes, M. D., & Miller, J. W. (2005). Recent seizures may distort the validity of neurocognitive test scores in patients with epilepsy. *Epilepsia, 46*(8), 74.

Williamson, D. J., Drane, D. L., & Stroup, E. S. (2007). Symptom validity tests in the epilepsy clinic. In K. B. Boone (Ed.), *Assessment of feigned cognitive impairment: A neuropsychological perspective* (pp. 346–365). New York: Guilford.

Wood, B. L., Haque, S., Weinstock, A., & Miller, B. D. (2004). Pediatric stress-related seizures: Conceptualization, evaluation, and treatment of nonepileptic seizures in children and adolescents. *Current Opinion in Pediatrics, 16*(5), 523–531.

Wyllie, E., Friedman, D., Rothner, A. D., Luders, H., Dinner, D., Morris, H., 3rd, et al. (1990). Psychogenic seizures in children and adolescents: outcome after diagnosis by ictal video and electroencephalographic recording. *Pediatrics, 85*(4), 480–484.

Wyllie, E., Glazer, J. P., Benbadis, S. R., Kotagl, P., & Wolgamuth, B. (1999). Psychiatric features in children and adolescents with pseudoseizures. *Archives of Pediatric and Adolescent Medicine, 153*(3), 244–248.

Wyllie, E., Benbadis, S. R., & Kotagal, P. (2002). Psychogenic seizures and other nonepileptic paroxysmal events in children. *Epilepsy & Behavior, 3*, 46–50.

Chapter 18
Somatoform Disorders, Factitious Disorder, and Malingering

Kyle Boone

Abstract Somatoform Disorders, Factitious Disorders and Malingering are among the most difficult issues for clinical neuropsychologists to differentiate. This chapter reviews diagnostic criteria for these disorders and emphasizes the differentiating characteristics among these disorders. The chapter reviews the current literature relating to applying Neuropsychological evaluation to assist in differential diagnosis of these disorders. The chapter also discuss the course, treatment and outcome of these disorders.

Key Points and Chapter Summary

- Somatoform disorders are relatively rare in the general population (1–3%); however, estimates of their prevalence in medical populations are much higher and have been reported to approach 20–30% in some neurologic practices.
- Differentiation of Somatoform Disorders, Factitious Disorder and Malingering requires a detailed understanding of the patients medical history, awareness of the production of symptoms and the motivations for producing the symptoms.
- In assessing cognitive complaints in Somatoform Disorders, Factitious Disorder and Malingering, multiple clinical and statistical procedures should be used.

Definition/Terminology

Broadly, somatoform disorders are characterized by somatization, a process in which an individual becomes preoccupied and over identified with, and even creates, on a nonconscious basis, physical symptoms that are not found to have a

K. Boone (✉)
Center for Forensic Studies, Alliant International University, Alhambra, CA, USA
e-mail: kboone@alliant.edu

M.R. Schoenberg and J.G. Scott (eds.), *The Little Black Book of Neuropsychology: A Syndrome-Based Approach*, DOI 10.1007/978-0-387-76978-3_18,
© Springer Science+Business Media, LLC 2011

medical cause or that are out of proportion to any objective medical findings. The DSM-IV describes the following putative subtypes of somatoform disorder:

- Somatization Disorder: combination of unexplained pain, gastrointestinal, sexual, and peudoneurological symptoms which present before age 30,
- Conversion Disorder: unexplained sensory and/motor symptoms which mimic a neurological or general medical condition
- Pain Disorder: unexplained pain symptoms thought to be causally related to psychological factors
- Hypochondriasis: chronic fear and/or fixed belief, that one has a serious disease despite the absence of confirming medical laboratory findings and which is due to misperception of benign bodily symptoms.
- Body Dysmorphic Disorder: preoccupation with imagined or inflated defect in physical appearance.
- Undifferentiated Somatoform Disorder: unexplained physical symptoms lasting at least 6 months but below the threshold for a somatization disorder
- Somatoform Disorder Not Otherwise Specified: somatoform symptoms not meeting criteria for any of the other disorders.

Although the DMS-IV is silent regarding the occurrence of nonphysiologic cognitive symptoms in the somatoform disorders, available literature and clinical observation indicate that they are commonly present. Examination of Freud's original writings on conversion disorder describe reversible amnesia and clouding of consciousness accompanying hysterical attacks and neuralgias (Mace 1994), and more recently, nonphysiological cognitive symptoms have been described in the context of nonepileptic seizures (Williamson et al. 2007). In addition, nonplausible cognitive complaints have been reported in such probable somatization disorders as toxic mold exposure (McCaffrey and Yantz 2007), multiple chemical sensitivity (McCaffrey and Yantz 2007), and chronic fatigue syndrome (Suhr and Spickard 2007), as well as in chronic pain/ fibromyalgia (Suhr and Spickard 2007). Further, presentations in which individuals claim significant cognitive dysfunction but on cognitive exam are found to be cognitively normal would suggest hypochondriasis (Boone, 2009a and Boone, 2009b).

Concerns have been raised regarding the diagnostic criteria for somatoform conditions, given evidence that large samples of patients may meet only partial criteria yet show substantial disruption in quality of life (Kroenke et al. 1997). In addition, the discrete somatoform diagnostic categories appear to be arbitrarily defined, with patients falling into various categories at differing points in time and/ or within several categories at once. Some have suggested that illness preoccupation would be better conceptualized as an overarching construct (Liu et al. 1997) identified through the generic terms of somatization, health anxiety, and/or medically unexplained symptoms. Alternatively, other researchers have noted the considerable overlap between somatization and anxiety/depressive conditions (e.g., 80%; Henningsen et al. 2005), with some suggesting that the somatoform subcategories would be better captured by other psychiatric diagnoses (e.g., hypochondriasis/health anxiety in the anxiety disorders, conversion disorder under dissociative disorder, and somatization with personality disorders; Mayou et al. 2005).

Prevalence

According to the DSM-IV, prevalence of the somatoform disorders is relatively low, for example, <1–3% for Somatization Disorder and Conversion Disorder in the general population, and 4–9% for Hypochondriasis in general medical practice. However, "abridged" somatization disorder (requiring fewer criteria than the full condition) was noted to be present in over 4% of the general population (Escobar et al. 1987), with consistent findings of full or partial somatization disorders in 20% of patients in a general medical care settings, and full criteria for somatoform disorder in 30% of patients in neurology clinic settings (Lamberty 2007).

Etiology

Originally, somatoform disorders (especially conversion disorders) were conceptualized within psychoanalytic theory as representing psychological conflict that was "converted" and displaced into dysfunction of a body part or system. More modern theories have viewed somatoform symptoms as being created by psychological distress that is not properly identified as such in nonpsychologically minded individuals; the resulting stress "has to go somewhere" and appears in the form of physical complaints that these patients are more comfortable facing than the underlying emotional pain. Recent empirical studies point to several factors as contributing to the development of somatization: (1) longstanding elevated fears and concerns regarding bodily functions including hypervigilance to physical symptoms and perceptions that one is particularly fragile and vulnerable (Kellner et al. 1987; Rief et al. 1998), (2) social factors such as problematic early attachment (Waller et al. 2004), sexual abuse (Samelius et al. 2007; Spitzer et al. 2008), family history/modeling of functional symptoms (Taylor and Asmundson 2004), and lowered levels of social support (Nakao et al. 2005), as well as the possibility that somatization is adaptive from an evolutionary perspective in terms of securing resources (Mealy 1995), and (3) psychiatric disorders including depression (Lieb et al. 2007), anxiety/panic attacks (Demopulos et al. 1996), and histrionic personality disorders (Demopulos et al. 1996). However, these variables are generally static/trait characteristics and would

Rule of thumb: Conceptualizing intent

- Nonconscious Processes:
  - Somatization, conversion, and pain disorders – creation of nonphysiologic symptoms
  - Hypochondriasis – *belief in* symptoms despite normal laboratory, imaging, and other test results
- Conscious Processes:
  - Malingering – deliberating feigning of symptoms for external goals
  - Factitious – deliberate feigning of symptoms *for psychological reasons*

not explain acute onset or fluctuating course of somatoform symptoms. In fact, somatoform symptoms likely develop in predisposed individuals when illness is particularly advantageous to the individual (e.g., in allowing one to be excused from stressful work responsibilities, in securing support and attention from others, in providing one with a special identity and unique life role, etc).

Malingering and Factitious Disorder

Definition/Terminology

According to the DSM-IV, malingering refers to conscious, deliberate feigning of symptoms for an obvious external incentive (i.e., for monetary compensation in the context of a lawsuit or disability benefits, to avoid military duty or criminal responsibility, to obtain drugs, etc.). As such, it is viewed as a volitional act which emerges in relation to external contingencies and is not a static condition.

In contrast, in factitious disorder, the symptom feigning is also thought to be conscious and deliberate, but the goal of the symptom fabrication is obscure and idiosyncratic to the individual. For example, in factitious disorder, the individual often appears to crave the notoriety and attention from medical personnel that accompany unusual symptoms, and to derive fulfillment from believing that one has "out-smarted" the typically better-educated medical personnel.

In both malingering and factitious disorders, symptom feigning can appear in discrete cognitive skills such as memory (verbal and/or visual), processing speed, motor function, visual perceptual/spatial skills, math calculation ability, basic attention, language skills including reading and spelling, executive/problem-solving, and remote memory. Alternatively, subjects may feign global cognitive impairment such as that observed in dementia or mental retardation. The choice of which symptoms to fabricate is driven by beliefs held by the individual as to what cognitive deficits accompany the disorder that is being feigned (i.e., brain injury, toxic exposure, anoxia, stroke, dementia, etc.), and is likely based on the type of cognitive symptoms that have been observed in persons with those disorders, and also how the disorders have been depicted on TV and in movies.

Prevalence

Malingering is found in those situations in which there is external incentive to be symptomatic. Mittenberg et al. (2002) reported survey results showing that experienced neuropsychologists estimate that in the presence of motive to feign symptoms (litigating or disability seeking), 41% of mild traumatic brain injury, 39% of fibromyalgia/chronic fatigue, 34% of chronic pain, 30% of neurotoxic, 26% of electrical injury, 16% of depressive disorders, 14% of anxiety disorders, 11% of dissociative disorders, 9% of seizure disorders, and 9% of moderate/severe head injury patients were judged to be fabricating cognitive deficits. Within a workers' compensation stress claim sample, 15–17% have been found to be feigning deficits in cognitive function (Boone et al. 1995; Sumanti et al. 2006). The base rate for malingered neurocognitive dysfunction in pretrial inpatient criminal defendants referred for neuropsychological evaluation likely ranges from 63% to 73% (Denney 2007). Thus, malingering of cognitive symptoms is not rare, which has precipitated admonitions within the field of neuropsychology that measures of response bias be routinely administered, particularly in contexts in which there is motive to be symptomatic (AACN 2007; Bush et al. 2005).

Rates of factitious disorder are much lower, with estimates ranging from 0.3% in neurological inpatients (Bauer and Boegner 1996), 0.6% of psychiatric consults (Kapfhammer et al. 1998), 0.8% of referrals to hospital-based psychiatric consultation and liaison services (Sutherland and Rodin 1990), to 1.3% of surgery, neurology, internal medicine, and dermatology patients (Fliege et al. 2007); no data are available regarding specific prevalence of factitious-related cognitive symptom fabrication.

Etiology

Malingering is a volitional act in the service of a tangible goal, and thus, traditional concepts of "etiology" do not apply. In contrast, the deliberate feigning of symptoms in the absence of such obvious goals as monetary compensation or avoidance of criminal or work responsibility typically only occurs in conjunction with significant psychiatric disturbance, and in particular, borderline personality disorder (Sutherland and Rodin 1990). The goal of such factitious behavior is to adopt the sick role, and while the acts themselves are conscious, the motivations behind the behaviors are considered to be nonconscious (Wang et al. 2005). Common associated characteristics include employment within the healthcare system and particularly maladaptive coping skills (Wang et al. 2005).

Differential Diagnosis: Distinguishing Somatoform Disorder from Malingering/Factitious Conditions and Genuine Illness

The DMS-IV is of limited use in conceptualizing and diagnosing feigned cognitive symptoms; it was published in 1994, prior to the appearance of the large majority of the current literature on cognitive symptom validity tests. Further, some of its assertions regarding malingering have been found not to be accurate. For example, the listed diagnostic criteria for malingering include anti-social personality disorder and lack of cooperation in evaluation and treatment. However, available research shows no link between antisocial personality traits and failure on symptom validity tests, at least within workers' compensation and civil litigation settings (Boone et al. 1995; Greiffenstein et al. 1995; Sumanti et al. 2006). Similarly, individuals feigning in these contexts tend to be overtly cooperative and solicitous during the examination, likely because they do not wish to antagonize the examiner into rendering a report unfavorable to their case.

The diagnosis of a somatoform disorder versus malingering or factitious disorder as expressed in cognitive symptoms involves first determining whether the patient exhibits credible cognitive performance, as assessed through the administration of indicators of response bias. Current recommended practice is to utilize several effort indicators interspersed throughout the cognitive exam (AACN 2007; Bush et al. 2005) to continuously sample effort (Boone 2009a, b). Response bias is not static and typically fluctuates across an evaluation depending on individual patient beliefs as to what skill deficits constitute brain dysfunction (e.g., if the person believes that motor dysfunction is a prominent finding in brain injury, evidence of response bias is likely to occur on measures of motor function). Failure on two or more effort indicators has been found to best discriminate between credible and noncredible populations (Larrabee 2003; Meyers and Volbrecht 2003; Suhr et al. 1997; Victor et al. 2009), although the more failed indicators the more confidence in conclusions. For example, failure on four or more tests approaches perfect specificity in that this number of failures is rare in truly symptomatic clinic populations (Victor et al. 2009). However, careful consideration should be given to the possibility of false positive effort test failures in populations particularly at risk for performing poorly on measures of response bias despite applying adequate effort, such as dementia (Dean et al. 2009), mental retardation (Dean et al. 2009), psychosis (Goldberg et al. 2007), and illiteracy and/or math disability (Victor and Boone 2007; Ziegler et al. 2008a; b).

The goal of a neuropsychological evaluation is to document level of cognitive function. However, if a patient fails numerous effort indicators, this objective is no longer attainable (because test scores are not valid), and instead the goal becomes to document level of effort. In the situation in which a patient fails one or two preliminary measures of response bias, it can be argued that there is no purpose in continuing with standard cognitive tests until adequacy of effort is assured. Should the patient continue to fail effort indices, the case can be made for defaulting to an "effort" battery (see Table 18.1 for a list of selected free-standing effort tests as well as embedded indices derived from standard cognitive tests). Once incontrovertible documentation of response bias is obtained (e.g., in many cases, patients will fail five or more indicators, performances that are 100% predictive of symptom feigning), the exam may be discontinued. The embedded effort indicators are contained in measures of verbal memory and visual memory, attention, processing speed, and motor function, and standard scores from these tests can be used to show that performances are markedly below those expected for the condition at issue (i.e., mild TBI). Additionally, it can at times be useful to administer standard cognitive tests that do not include effort indicators to illustrate performances on identical tests on sequential exams have "ping ponged" around in a nonsensical manner.

- If a patient is documented to fail numerous measures of response bias, the next step is to attempt to determine if the symptom fabrication is conscious, nonconscious, or both. Unfortunately, available exam techniques do not distinguish between conscious and nonconscious cognitive symptom fabrication. For example,

Table 18.1 Sensitivity rates for common measures of response bias/effort with a minimum specificity of 88% for "real world" noncredible subjects

FREE-standing effort indices	Sensitivity	References
TOMM		Greve et al. (2008)
Trial 2		
Cut-off ≤ 48 (for TBI)	70%	
Cut-off ≤ 49 (for pain)	55%	
Retention		
Cut-off ≤ 48 (for TBI)	70%	
Cut-off ≤ 48 (for pain)	50%	
Word memory test		Greve et al. (2008)
IR		
Cut-off ≤ 75 (for TBI)	59%	
Cut-off ≤ 87.5 (for pain)	60%	
DR		
Cut-off ≤ 77.5 (for TBI)	63%	
Cut-off ≤ 87.5 (for pain)	57%	
Con 1		
Cut-off ≤ 72.5 (for TBI)	63%	
Cut-off ≤ 82.5 (for pain)	55%	
Warrington Recognition Memory Test – Words		Kim et al. (2008)
Cut-off ≤ 42 (for mixed sample)	90%	
Rey Word Recognition Test		Nitch et al. (2006)
Cut-off for combination score ≤ 9 (for TBI)	82%	
Cut-off ≤ 5 (for male mixed sample)	63%	
Cut-off ≤ 7 (for female mixed Sample)	81%	
Portland Digit Recognition Test		Greve et al. (2008)
Easy		
Cut-off ≤ 24 (for TBI)	74%	
Cut-off ≤ 26 (for pain)	47%	
Hard		
Cut-off ≤ 19 (for TBI)	56%	
Cut-off ≤ 20 (for pain)	47%	
Total		
Cut-off ≤ 44 (for TBI)	70%	
Cut-off ≤ 46 (for pain)	41%	
Dot counting test		Boone et al. (2002a);
E-score cut-off ≥ 17 (for mixed sample)	73–79%	Boone and Lu (2007)
E-score cut-off ≥ (for TBI)	72%	
B test		Boone et al. (2002b)
E-score cut-off ≥ 150 (for mixed sample)	64%	
E-score cut-off ≥ 90 (for TBI)	77%	
Validity indicator profile		Ross and Adams (1999)
Verbal invalid	27%	
Nonverbal invalid	45%	

(continued)

Table 18.1 (continued)

FREE-standing effort indices	Sensitivity	References
Rey 15-item		Boone et al.
Standard administration		(2002c);
Cut-off < 9 (mixed sample)	46%	Boone and Lu
With Recognition trial		(2007)
Cut-off < 20 (mixed sample)	56–71%	
Embedded effort indices		
CVLT forced choice recognition		Root et al. (2006)
Cut-off ≤ 14 (mixed sample)	44%	
RAVLT		Boone et al.
Recognition		(2005)
Cut-off ≤ 9 (mixed sample)	67%	
Equation	74%	
Cut-off ≤ 12 (mixed sample)		
Rey complex figure equation		Lu et al. (2003);
Cut-off ≤ 45 (mixed sample)	64–74%	Boone and Lu
		(2007)
RAVLT/RO Discriminant Function		Sherman et al.
Cut-off ≤ –0.40 (mixed sample)	61–71%	(2002); Boone
		and Lu (2007)
Digit span		Babikian et al.
ACSS		(2006);
Cut-off ≤ 5 (mixed sample)	36–47%	Babikian and
RDS		Boone (2007)
Cut-off ≤ 6 (mixed sample)	38–57%	
Vocabulary minus Digit Span		
Cut-off ≥ 5 (mixed sample)	5% (IQ ≤ 85) – 50% (IQ >85)	
Finger tapping (dominant – mean of 3 trials)		Arnold et al.
Men		(2005)
Cut-off ≤ 35 (mixed sample)	50%	
Women		
Cut-off ≤ 28 (mixed sample)	61%	

Specificity of all indices and measures ≥ 88%

significantly below chance performance on forced choice symptom validity tests has been argued to be a "gold standard" for identifying malingered symptoms, yet 25% of hypnotized individuals, whose behavior is thought not to be under conscious control, when instructed to display memory impairment, obtain scores at this level (Spanos et al. 1990). The MMPI-2 has been traditionally used to identify somatization as evidenced by a "conversion V" (i.e., particular elevations on the hypochondriasis and hysteria scales), although more recent studies have shown that individuals thought to be deliberately faking physical symptoms also show this pattern (Larrabee 1998). Interestingly, preliminary functional neuroimaging studies appear to demonstrate comparable areas of brain activation in both deliberate lying and conversion disorder (right frontal and anterior cingulate areas; Ganis et al. 2003; Halligan et al. 2000; Kozel et al. 2004a; Kozel et al. 2004b; Langleben et al. 2002; Marshall et al. 1997; Tiihonen et al. 1995).

- These findings raises the obvious question as to whether "nonconscious" symptom production in fact exists since it cannot be distinguished from conscious feigning on psychometric and imaging parameters. However, the wealth of clinical experience argues that that there is a distinction between patients who only don their symptoms for medical evaluations conducted during the course of a lawsuit or disability exam versus patients who adopt an invalid lifestyle in which their symptoms become a prominent part of their identity. Malingerers and individuals with factitious disorder "know" their symptoms are false; they are engaging in "other" deception but not self-deception. In contrast, somatoform patients are not consciously aware of their symptom creation and thus are, on some level, primarily deceiving themselves.

  - The determination of malingering/factitious versus somatoform currently is one of "art" and requires obtaining qualitative information regarding the degree to which a patient "believes" in his/her symptoms. This can be gauged by obtaining information as to whether the symptoms are present continuously versus just in a medical evaluation context (e.g., through surveillance tapes, by querying individuals who know the patient regarding the extent to which the patient displays symptoms in nonmedical settings, etc.). In addition, possible conscious components to a symptom presentation can be inferred when a patient is found to "censor" information harmful to his/her litigated case (e.g., denying history of pre-accident symptoms which are, in fact, documented in medical records). However, complicating the picture is that conscious and nonconscious symptom fabrication may not be mutually exclusive, but may instead lie on a continuum of other deception versus self deception, or lie on two separate continua, one reflecting other deception and the other measuring self deception. Further, a patient's placement on the trajectories may not necessarily be static. Thus, determination of nonconscious versus conscious bases for symptom fabrication is problematic and often not possible.

- If the patient passes measures of response bias, the next step is to determine if any cognitive abnormalities are identified on formal neuropsychological measures.

  - If the patient scores essentially within normal limits despite complaints of prominent cognitive impairment, this would raise the possibility of hypochondriasis, which is characterized by fixed belief in the presence of illness in the absence of any objective evidence of dysfunction. Evidence of somatization on the MMPI-2 [elevation on somatic complaints (RC1) as well as low score on cynicism (RC3) or 1–3 codetype on traditional clinical scales; moderately elevated FBS] or other personality inventories would further buttress a diagnosis of hypochondriasis.

  - If the patient shows significant cognitive abnormalities on formal testing, the next step would be to determine what condition(s) in the patient's medical and psychiatric history could be etiological, such as moderate to severe brain injury and other neurologic conditions, learning disability and attention deficit

disorder, depression, psychosis, chronic medical illnesses, substance abuse and/
or medication overuse, etc. However, somatization often co-occurs with actual
medical disorders, and would be illustrated by personality test findings showing
elevations on scales measuring somatic complaints. Unfortunately, there is a
common misperception within neuropsychology that personality inventories
were developed on, and for, psychiatric populations, and that findings do not
translate well to neurologic populations. In fact, the MMPI hypochondriasis
scale was developed on normal controls, psychiatric patients, medical patients, and
patients diagnosed with hypochondriasis (Greene 1991). Observed elevations on
hypochondriasis scales are often attributed to expected and realistic concern
over actual physical illness. However, reference sources for the MMPI-2 note
that actual medical patients show only minor, nonsignificant elevations on the
hypochondriasis scale, and indicate that "if a client with actual physical illness
obtained a T score of 65 or higher on Scale 1, there are likely to be hypochondriacal features in addition to the physical condition, and the client is probably
trying to manipulate or control significant others in the environment with the
hypochondriacal complaints" (Greene 1991, p. 137) (Fig. 18.1).

Course and Treatment Outcomes

Studies show that approximately 50% of young adults diagnosed with a somatoform
condition were still symptomatic 4 years later (Lieb et al. 2002), while 2/3 of indi-

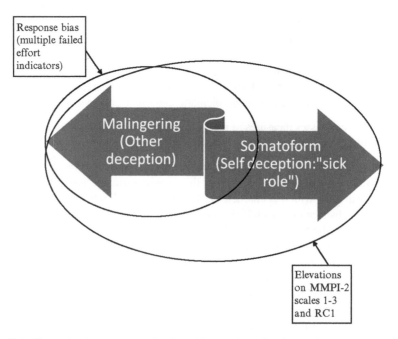

Fig. 18.1 Illustration for a conceptualization of Somatoform disorders and malingering

viduals diagnosed with hypochondriasis still met criteria for the disorder 4–5 years later (Barksy et al. 1998). In primary care, patients fulfilling criteria for abridged somatization disorder, 18% were still symptomatic 12 months later, and 16% were rated as showing residual hypochondriacal worries (Simon et al. 2001); depression and anxiety were predictors of both onset and persistence of somatization. Cognitive behavioral therapy has received the most empirical support for treatment of somatoform disorders. Intensive cognitive behavioral treatment has been associated with positive response in over 60% of patients, with nonresponse predicted by greater pre-treatment hypochondriasis, more somatization symptoms and psychopathology, more inaccurate cognitions regarding body functions, more psychosocial dysfunction, and more utilization of healthcare services (Hiller et al. 2002)

Unfortunately, factitious disorder appears to be even less treatable than somatoform disorders. Available research shows no difference in outcomes between confrontational versus nonconfrontational approaches, and between psychotherapy or medication versus no treatment (Eastwood and Bisson 2008).

Rule of thumb: Testing for response bias

Do the following:
- Employ multiple effort indices to provide greater confidence in conclusions
- Utilize effort indices with adequate sensitivity (see Table 18.1)
- Select measures of response bias/cut-offs appropriate for the differential diagnosis (e.g., actual versus feigned mild traumatic brain injury, psychosis, depression) and demographic and other characteristics of the test-taker (low IQ, learning disability, ethnicity/language, gender, etc.)
- Choose a range of effort indices that encompass various cognitive domains (e.g., memory, attention, processing speed, visual spatial skills), and in particular those which overlap with claimed symptoms (e.g., decreased memory, math skills, thinking speed, etc.)
- Provide results of effort indices in your report but in a manner that does not compromise test security (e.g., do not describe test stimuli or format)

References

American Board of Clinical Neuropsychology. (2007). American Academy of Clinical Neuropsychology (AACN) practice guidelines for neuropsychological assessment and consultation. *The Clinical Neuropsychologist, 21*, 209–231.

American Psychiatric Association. (1994). *Diagnostic and statistical manual of mental disorders* (4th ed.). Washington: American Psychiatric Association.

Arnold, G., Boone, K. B., Lu, P., Dean, A., Wen, J., Nitch, S., et al. (2005). Sensitivity and specificity of Finger Tapping Tset scores for the detection fo suspect effort. *The Clinical Neuropsychologist, 19*, 105–120.

Babikian, T., & Boone, K. (2007). Intelligence tests as measures of effort. In K. B. Boone (Ed.), *Assessment of feigned cognitive impairment: A neuropsychological perspective*. New York: Guilford Press.

Babikian, T., Boone, K. B., Lu, P., & Arnold, B. (2006). Sensitivity and specificity of various Digit Span scores in the detection of suspect effort. *The Clinical Neuropsychologist, 20*, 145–159.

Barksy, A. J., Fama, J. M., Bailey, E. D., & Ahern, D. K. (1998). A prospective 4- to 5- year study of DSM-III-R hypochondriasis. *Archives of General Psychiatry, 55*, 737–744.

Barsky, A. J., Bailey, E. D., Fama, J. M., & Aher, D. K. (2000). Predictors of remission in DSM hypochondriasis. *Comprehensive Psychiatry, 41*, 179–183.

Bauer, M., & Boegner, F. (1996). Neurological syndromes in factitious disorder. *The Journal of Nervous and Mental Disease, 184*, 281–188.

Boone, K. B. (2009a). Fixed belief in cognitive dysfunction despite normal neuropsychological scores: Neurocognitive hypochondriasis? *The Clinical Neuropsychologist, 23*(6), 1016–36.

Boone, K. (2009b). The need for continuous and comprehensive sampling of effort/response bias during neuropsychological examinations. *The Clinical Neuropsychologist, 23*(4), 729–41.

Boone, K. B., & Lu, P. (2007). Non-forced Choice Effort Measures. In G. Larrabee (Ed.), *Assessment of malingered neuropsychological deficits*. New York: Oxford University Press.

Boone, K. B., Savodnik, I., Ghaffarian, S., Lee, A., Freeman, D., & Berman, N. (1995). Rey 15-item Memorization and Dot Counting scores in a 'Stress' claim worker's compensation population: Relationship to personality (MCMI) scores. *Journal of Clinical Psychology, 51*, 457–463.

Boone, K. B., Lu, P., & Herzberg, D. (2002a). *Rey dot counting test*. Los Angeles: Western Psychological Services.

Boone, K. B., Lu, P., & Herzberg, D. (2002b). *The b test*. Los Angeles: Western Psychological Services.

Boone, K. B., Salazar, X., Lu, P., Warner-Chacon, K., & Razani, J. (2002c). The rey 15-item recognition trial: A technique to enhance sensitivity of the Rey 15-item Memorization Test. *Journal of Clinical and Experimental Neuropsychology, 24*, 561–573.

Boone, K. B., Lu, P., & Wen, J. (2005). Comparison of various RAVLT scores in the detection of noncredible memory performance. *Archives of Clinical Neuropsychology, 20*, 301–319.

Bush, S. S., Ruff, R. M., Troster, A. I., Barth, J. T., Koffler, S. P., Pliskin, N. H., et al. (2005). Symptom validity assessment: Practice issues and medical necessity (NAN Policy and Planning Committee). *Archives of Clinical Neuropsychology, 20*, 419–426.

Dean, A. C., Victor, T. L., Boone, K. B., & Arnold, G. (2008). The relationship of IQ to effort test performance. *The Clinical Neuropsychologist, 22*(4), 705–22.

Dean, A. C., Victor, T. L., Boone, K. B., Philpott, L. M., & Hess, R. A. (2009). Dementia and effort test performance. *The Clinical Neuropsychologist, 23*(1), 133–52.

Demopulos, C., Fava, M., McLean, N. E., Alpert, J. E., Nierenberg, A. A., & Rosenbaum, J. F. (1996). Hypochondriacal concerns in depressed outpatients. *Psychosomatic Medicine, 58*, 314–320.

Denney, R.L., Houston, C.M. (2007). Base rates of response bias and malingering neurocognitive dysfunction among criminal defendants referred for neuropsychological evaluation, *The Clinical Neuropsychologist, 21*, 899–916.

Eastwood, S., & Bisson, J. I. (2008). Management of factitious disorders: A systematic review. *Psychotherapy and Psychosomatics, 77*, 209–218.

Escobar, J. I., Burnam, M. A., Karno, M., Forsythe, A., & Golding, J. M. (1987). Somatization in the community. *Archives of General Psychiatry, 44*, 713–718.

Fliege, H., Grimm, A., Eckhardt-Henn, A., Gieler, U., Martin, K., & Klapp, B. F. (2007). Frequency of ICD-10 factitious disorder: Survey of senior hospital consultants and physicians in private practice. *Psychosomatics, 48*(1), 60–64.

Ganis, G., Kosslyn, S. M., Stose, S., Thompson, W. L., & Yurgelun-Todd, D. A. (2003). Neural correlates of different types of deception: An fMRI investigation. *Cerebral Cortex, 13*, 830–836.

Goldberg, H. E., Back-Madruga, C., & Boone, K. B. (2007). The impact of psychiatric disorders on cognitive symptom validity test scores. In K. B. Boone (Ed.), *Assessment of feigned cognitive impairment: A neuropsychological perspective*. New York: Guilford Press.

Greene, R. L. (1991). *The MMPI-2/MMPI: An interpretive manual*. Needham Heights: Allyn and Bacon.

Greiffenstein, M. F., Gola, T., & Baker, J. W. (1995). MMPI-2 validity scales versus domain specific measures in detection no factitious traumatic brain injury. *The Clinical Neuropsychologist, 9*, 230–240.

Greve, K. W., Ord, J., Curtis, K. L., Bianchini, K. J., & Brennan, A. (2008). Detecting malingering in traumatic brain injury in chronic pain: A comparison of three forced-choice symptom validity tests. *The Clinical Neuropsychologist, 22*, 896–918.

Halligan, P. W., Athwal, B. S., Oakley, D. A., & Frackowiak, R. S. (2000). Imaging hypnotic paralysis: Implications for conversion hysteria. *Lancet, 355*, 986–987.

Henningsen, P., Jakobsen, T., Schiltenwolf, M., & Weiss, M. G. (2005). Somatization revisited: Diagnosis and perceived causes of common mental disorders. *The Journal of Nervous and Mental Disease, 193*, 85–92.

Hiller, W., Weibbrand, R., Rief, W., & Fichter, M. M. (2002). Predictors of course and outcome in hypochondriasis after cognitive-behavioral treatment. *Psychotherapy and Psychosomatics, 71*, 318–325.

Kapfhammer, H. P., Rothenhausler, H. B., Dietrich, E., Dobmeier, P., & Mayer, C. (1998). Artifactual disorders-between deception and self-mutilation. Experiences in consultation psychiatry at a university clinic. *Der Nervenarzt, 69*, 401–409.

Kellner, R., Abbott, P., Winslow, W. W., & Pathak, D. (1987). Fears, beliefs, and attitudes in DSM-III hypochondriasis. *The Journal of Nervous and Mental Disease, 175*, 20–25.

Kozel, F. A., Padgett, T. M., & George, M. S. (2004a). A replication study of the neural correlates of deception. *Behavioral Neuroscience, 118*, 852–856.

Kozel, F. A., Revell, L. J., Lorberbaum, J. P., Shawstri, A., Elhia, J. D., Horner, M. D., et al. (2004b). A pilot study of functional magnetic resonance imaging brain correlates of deception in healthy young men. *The Journal of Neuropsychiatry and Clinical Neurosciences, 16*, 295–305.

Kroenke, K., Spitzer, R. L., de Gruy, F. V., Hahn, S. R., 3rd, Linzer, M., Williams, J. B., et al. (1997). Multisomatoform disorder: An alternative to undifferentiated somatoform disorder for the somatizing patient in primary care. *Archives of General Psychiatry, 54*, 352–358.

Lamberty, G. J. (2007). *Understanding somatization in the practice of clinical neuropsychology.* New York: Oxford University Press.

Langleben, D. D., Schroeder, L., Maldjian, J. A., Gur, R. C., McDonald, S., Ragland, J. D., et al. (2002). Brain activity during simulated deception: An event-related functional magnetic resonance study. *Neuroimage, 15*, 727–732.

Larrabee, G. (1998). Somatic malingering on the MMPI and MMPI-2 in personal injury litigants. *The Clinical Neuropsychologist, 12*, 179–188.

Larrabee, G. J. (2003). Detection of malingering using atypical performance patterns on standard neuropsychological tests. *The Clinical Neuropsychologist, 17*, 410–425.

Lieb, R., Zimmermann, P., Friis, R. H., Hofler, M., Tholen, S., & Wittchen, H. U. (2002). The natural course of DMS-IV somatoform disorders and syndromes among adolescents and young adults: A prospective-longitudinal community study. *European Psychiatry, 17*, 321–331.

Lieb, R., Meinlschmidt, G., & Araya, R. (2007). Epidemiology of the association between somatoform disorders and anxiety and depressive disorders: An update. *Psychosomatic Medicine, 69*, 860–863.

Liu, G., Clark, M. R., & Eaton, W. W. (1997). Structural factor analyses for medically unexplained somatic symptoms of somatization disorder in the epidemiologic catchment area study. *Psychological Medicine, 27*, 617–626.

Lu, P., Boone, K. B., Cozolino, L., & Mitchell, C. (2003). Effectiveness of the Rey-Osterrieth complex figure test and the Meyers and Meyers recognition trial in the detection of suspect effort. *The Clinical Neuropsychologist, 17*, 424–440.

Mace, C. J. (1994). Reversible cognitive impairment related to conversion disorder. *The Journal of Nervous and Mental Disease, 182*, 186–187.

Marshall, J. C., Halligan, P. W., Fink, G. R., Wade, D. T., & Frackowiak, R. S. (1997). The functional anatomy of a hysterical paralysis. *Cognition, 64*, B1–B8.

Mayou, R., Kirmayer, L. J., Simon, G., Kroenke, K., & Sharpe, M. (2005). Somatoform disorders: Time for a new approach in DSM-V. *The American Journal of Psychiatry, 162*, 847–855.

McCaffrey, R. J., & Yantz, C. (2007). Cognitive complaints in multiple chemical sensitivity and toxic mold syndrome. In K. B. Boone (Ed.), *Assessment of feigned cognitive impairment: A neuropsychological perspective*. New York: Guilford Press.

Mealy, L. (1995). The sociobiology of sociopathy: An integrated evolutionary model. *Behavior and Brain Sciences, 18*, 523–599.

Meyers, J. E., & Volbrecht, M. E. (2003). A validation of multiple malingering detection methods in a large clinical sample. *Archives of Clinical Neuropsychology, 18*, 261–276.

Mittenberg, W., Patton, C., Canyock, E. M., & Condit, D. (2002). Bases rates of malingering and symptom exaggeration. *Journal of Clinical and Experimental Neuropsychology, 24*, 1094–1102.

Nakao, M., Tamiya, N., & Yano, E. (2005). Gender and somatosensory amplification in relation to perceived work stress and social support in Japanese workers. *Women & Health, 42*, 41–54.

Nitch, S., Boone, K. B., Wen, J., Arnold, G., & Warner-Chacon, K. (2006). The utility Rey Word Recognition Test in the detection of suspect effort. *The Clinical Neuropsychologist, 20*, 873–887.

Rief, W., Hiller, W., & Margraf, J. (1998). Cognitive aspects of hypochondriasis and the somatization syndrome. *Journal of Abnormal Psychology, 107*, 587–595.

Root, J. C., Robbins, R. N., Chang, L., & van Gorp, W. (2006). Detection of inadequate effort on the California Verbal Learning Test (2nd ed): Forced choice recognition and critical item analysis. *Journal of the International Neuropsychological Society, 12*, 688–696.

Ross, S. R., & Adams, K. M. (1999). One more test of malingering. *The Clinical Neuropsychologist, 13*, 112–116.

Samelius, L., Wijma, B., Wingren, G., & Wigma, K. (2007). Somatization in abused women. *Journal of Women's Health (Larchmt), 16*, 909–918.

Sherman, D. S., Boone, K. B., Lu, P., & Razani, J. (2002). Re-examination of a Rey Auditory Verbal Learning Test/Rey Complex Figure discriminant function to detect suboptimal effort. *The Clinical Neuropsychologist, 16*, 242–250.

Simon, G. E., Guereje, O., & Fullerton, C. (2001). Course of hypochondriasis in an international primary care study. *General Hospital Psychiatry, 23*, 51–55.

Spanos, N., James, B., & de Groot, H. (1990). Detection of simulated hypnotic amnesia. *Journal of Abnormal Psychology, 99*, 179–182.

Spitzer, C., Barnow, S., Gau, K., Freyberger, H. J., & Grabe, H. J. (2008). Childhood maltreatment in patients with somatization disorder. *Australian and New Zealand Journal of Psychiatry, 42*, 335–341.

Stone, D., Boone, K. B., Back-Madruga, C., & Lesser, I. (2006). Has the rolling uterus finally gathered moss? Somatization and malingering of cognitive deficit in six cases of 'toxic mold' exposure. *The Clinical Neuropsychologist, 20*, 766–785.

Suhr, J., & Spickard, B. (2007). Including measures of effort in neuropsychological assessment of pain-and fatigue-related medical disorders: Clinical and research implications. In K. B. Boone (Ed.), *Assessment of feigned cognitive impairment: A neuropsychological perspective.* New York: Guilford Press.

Suhr, J., Tranel, D., Wefel, J., & Barrash, J. (1997). Memory performance after head injury: Contributions of malingering, litigation status, psychological factors, and medication use. *Journal of Clinical and Experimental Neuropsychology, 19*, 500–514.

Sumanti, M., Boone, K. B., Savodnik, I., & Gorsuch, R. (2006). Noncredible psychiatric and cognitive symptoms in a Worker's Compensation 'Stress' claim sample. *The Clinical Neuropsychologist, 20*, 754–765.

Sutherland, A. J., & Rodin, G. M. (1990). Factitious disorders in a general hospital setting: Clinical features and a review of the literature. *Psychosomatics, 31*, 392–399.

Taylor, S., & Asmundson, G. J. G. (2004). *Treating health anxiety: A cognitive-behavioral approach.* New York: Guilford Press.

Tiihonen, J., Kuikka, J., Viinamaki, H., Lehtonen, J., & Partanen, J. (1995). Altered cerebral blood flow during hysterical paresthesia. *Biological Psychiatry, 37*, 134–135.

Victor, T., & Boone, K. (2007). The false positive rate for common effort tests in individuals diagnosed with learning disabilities. Poster presented at the annual International Neuropsychological Society meeting, Baltimore.

Victor, T. L., Boone, K. B., Serpa, J. G., & Buehler, J. (2009). Interpreting the meaning of multiple effort test failure. *The Clinical Neuropsycholoigst, 23*, 297–313.

Waller, E., Scheidt, C. E., & Hartman, A. (2004). Attachment representation and illness behavior in somatoform disorder. *The Journal of Nervous and Mental Disease, 192,* 200–209.

Wang, D., Nadiga, D. N., & Jenson, J. J. (2005). Factitious disorders. In B. J. Sadock & V. A. Sadock (Eds.), *Kaplan & Sadock's comprehensive textbook of psychiatry* (8th ed.). Philadelphia: Lippincott, Williams, & Wilkins.

Williamson, D. J., Drane, D. L., & Stroup, E. S. (2007). Symptom validity tests in the epilepsy clinic. In K. B. Boone (Ed.), *Assessment of feigned cognitive impairment: A neuropsychological perspective.* New York: Guilford Press.

Ziegler, E. A., Boone, K. B., Victor, T. L., & Zeller, M. (2008). The specificity of digit span effort indicators in patients with poor math abilities. Poster presented at the Sixth Annual American Academy of Clinical Neuropsychology conference, Boston.

Ziegler, E. A., Boone, K. B., Victor, T. L., & Zeller, M. (2008). The specificity of the dot counting test in patients with poor math abilities. Poster presented at the Sixth Annual American Academy of Clinical Neuropsychology conference, Boston.

Chapter 19
Parkinson's Disease and Other Movement Disorders

Steven A. Gunzler, Mike R. Schoenberg, David E. Riley, Benjamin Walter, and Robert J. Maciunas

Abstract This chapter reviews the anatomy, physiology, treatment and cognitive/neuropsychological aspects of movement disorders, of which Parkinson's disease (PD) and parkinsonism are common manifestations. The neurologic, cognitive and behavioral aspects of movement disorders are covered in detail as are contemporary treatments and treatment outcomes. This chapter starts with an overview of the functional neuroanatomy of movement and discusses normal motor movement and disordered motor movement. We review the role of the basal ganglia and other anatomical areas implicated in movement disorders including Parkinson's disease and parkinsonism and the role of dopamine and other neurotransmitters in disorders of movement. The next section reviews the clinical presentation of the movement disorders, inclusive of a description of each disorders cardinal symptoms and the differentiating characteristics among movement disorders. The cognitive and emotional symptoms associated with movement disorders are also discussed in detail. The later part of this chapter discusses the available treatment for movement disorders such as pharmacotherapy and surgical options and the motor and cognitive outcomes from such treatments. Next, the chapter provides a detailed analysis for the pre-surgical evaluation of patients being considered for surgical treatment, including a review of the pre- and post-operative neuropsychological assessment of patients with movement disorders. We discuss the changes in neuropsychological function that may be predicted post-surgically. Finally, we propose directions for future research in the course and treatment outcomes in motor, cognitive and behavioral symptoms associated with movement disorders.

S.A. Gunzler (✉)
Department of Neurology, The Neurological Institute, University Hospitals Case Medical Center and Case Western Reserve University School of Medicine, Cleveland, OH, USA
e-mail: Steven.Gunzler@UHhospitals.org

M.R. Schoenberg and J.G. Scott (eds.), *The Little Black Book of Neuropsychology: A Syndrome-Based Approach*, DOI 10.1007/978-0-387-76978-3_19, © Springer Science+Business Media, LLC 2011

Key Points and Chapter Summary

- Movement disorders are many and varied, each exhibiting anatomical and physiological characteristics that present with distinct cognitive and behavioral symptoms.
- Movement disorders have many etiologies, including genetic, traumatic or idiopathic and involve anatomical, physiological or neurotransmitter abnormalities that affect the motor system at many points along pathways governing motor movement.
- Parkinson's disease and other types of parkinsonism are common movement disorders that share motor, cognitive and behavioral symptoms, but which must be distinguished due to different prognoses and responses to treatment.
- Parkinson's disease is associated with classic symptoms of tremor, rigidity, akinesia, and postural instability as well as non-motor features including neuropsychological dysfunction.
- Parkinson's plus syndromes often exhibit subtle differences in symptom onset and/or severity that assist in differential diagnosis.
- Essential tremor is associated with action tremor, often without significant neuropsychological dysfunction.
- Cortical-basal ganglionic degeneration is a movement disorder characterized by asymmetric parkinsonism, apraxia, and neuropsychological deficits
- Neuropsychological impairment is associated with multiple movement disorders and may present as either an early symptom or later in the course of the neurodegenerative process.
- Surgical treatments for movement disorder are generally considered cognitively safe resulting in improved motor function, but some individuals experience adverse neuropsychological and behavioral changes. Adverse outcomes can be reduced or mitigated with pre- and post-surgical neuropsychological evaluations.

Section I: Common Movement Disorders: Neurological and Neuropsychological Features

Parkinsonism

Parkinsonism is a syndrome comprising four cardinal physical features: resting tremor, rigidity, akinesia (or bradykinesia), and postural instability. The resting tremor is typically a slow tremor that occurs, as the label suggests, mainly when the involved body part is inactive. Rigidity is increased muscle tone, causing a stiffness of the trunk and limbs. "Akinesia" describes a lack of movement, while "bradykinesia" means slowness of movement. Postural instability is an inability to maintain one's self in a stable or balanced position and a form of disequilibrium that often predisposes parkinsonian patients to falls. A common definition used in clinical

Rule of thumb: Parkinson's disease symptoms = TRAP

- Tremor, Rigidity, Akinesia/Bradykinesia, and Postural instability.

Table 19.1 Common etiologies for parkinsonism

Disorders that can cause parkinsonism	
Cortical-basal ganglionic degeneration	Pantothenate kinase-associated neurodegeneration
Creutzfeld-Jakob disease	Parkinson's disease
Drug-induced parkinsonism	Progressive supranuclear palsy
Hereditary forms of parkinsonism	Psychogenic parkinsonism
Huntington's disease	Vascular parkinsonism
Multiple system atrophy	Wilson's disease

trials is that two of these four components must be present to establish a diagnosis of parkinsonism (Mitchell and Rockwood 2001).

There are many diseases and syndromes that have parkinsonism as a prominent symptom complex. Some of these diagnoses are listed in Table 19.1. The spectrum of neuropsychological symptoms are largely determined by the specific disorder causing the parkinsonism. As discussed below, early detection of cognitive deficits can be a clue to the proper diagnosis.

Neuroanatomy and Parkinsonism

The neuropathology of PD and movement disorders is typically associated with dysfunction involving the basal ganglia and/or cerebellum. The basal ganglia are a complex of deep gray matter brain nuclei illustrated in Fig. 19.1. They receive input from a variety of regions of the cerebral cortex and send output back to the cortex (via the *thalamus*) and *brain stem*. The basal ganglia are traditionally associated with the initiation and control of motor movements (eye and body), but also are involved in a variety of cognitive and affective processing as well (see below).

The basal ganglion is often subdivided into the *striatum* and the *globus pallidus* (Fig. 19.2). The striatum is further subdivided into the *caudate nucleus* and the *putamen*. The putamen and globus pallidus are sometimes together referred to as the *lentiform nucleus*. The globus pallidus is divided into the *globus pallidus interna (GPi)* and the *globus pallidus externa (GPe)*. Other structures of the basal ganglia include the *subthalamic nucleus (STN)* and *substantia nigra*, which is divided into the *substantia nigra pars compacta (SNc)* and *substantia nigra pars reticulata (SNr)*. The *nucleus accumbens* (which lies in the anteroventral region of where the head of the caudate nucleus and the putamen fuse), *ventral pallidum*, and *intralaminar nuclei of the thalamus* are also often included in the basal ganglia.

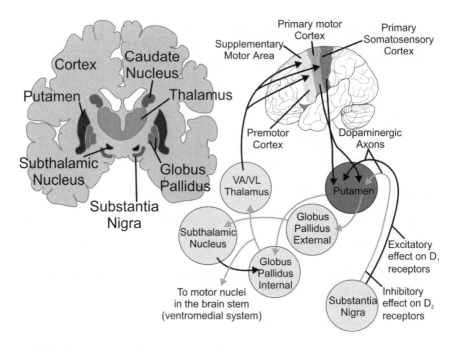

Fig. 19.1 Anatomy (coronal section) of basal ganglia

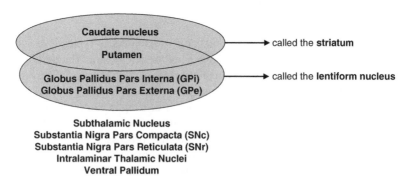

Fig. 19.2 The subcomponents of the basal ganglia

Blood supply of the basal ganglia is mostly from the *lenticulostriate* branches of the *middle cerebral artery (MCA)* (see Chap. 3 for more information about cerebral vasculature), although branches of the internal carotid artery may supply the medial globus pallidus and branches from the anterior cerebral artery can supply the caudate nucleus/lentiform nucleus.

Input, Output, and Intrinsic Connections of the Basal Ganglia

The main inputs to the basal ganglia are projections from the frontal lobes (motor and associative/cognitive) and limbic system (affective/cognitive) to the striatum (caudate and putamen) and the nucleus accumbens (ventral striatum). The inputs are generally excitatory and glutamatergic. The SNc, a midbrain structure pigmented black to the naked eye, also provides input to the striatum via dopaminergic projections.

Output from the basal ganglia is primarily through the GPi and the SNr. Limbic outputs occur from SNr and ventral pallidum.

Direct and Indirect Pathways

Classically, processing through the basal ganglia had been described in terms of a *direct pathway* and *indirect pathway* (see Fig. 19.3). While this framework has provided an important model for the understanding and testing of basal ganglia function, there are exceptions not well explained by the model that has led to the development of new theories. New findings have increased the complexity of the basal ganglia networks and altered how some aspects of the indirect and direct pathways interact. However, because of the intrinsic value this model has for understanding core concepts of basal ganglia function, we provide an overview of the direct and indirect pathways below and also diagram this model in Figures 19.3, 19.4, and 19.5.

The *direct pathway* consists of inhibitory neurons from the striatum to the GPi and SNr, which in turn inhibit the cortex via thalamic nuclei (VA and VL as well as medial dorsal).

The *indirect pathway* consists of striatal neurons projecting to GPe using GABA, which is inhibitory. Then, inhibitory pathways from GPe project to the STN using GABA, and the STN projects to GPi and SNr using glutamate, which is excitatory. GPi and SNr then have inhibitory (GABA) projections to thalamic nuclei (VL and VA), which send excitatory glutamatergic projections to the cortex.

The SNc projections to the striatum involve dopamine and are *excitatory* toward the direct pathway, but *inhibitory* toward the indirect pathway (see Fig. 19.3). Thus, the dopaminergic neurons from the SNc generally *activate the direct pathway* and inhibit *the indirect pathway*. The net effect of the direct pathway is excitation of cerebral cortex, whereas the net effect of the indirect pathway is cortical inhibition.

Rule of thumb: Basal ganglia two major functional neuroanatomic systems

- *Indirect* pathway *Inhibits* action of cortex
- *Direct* pathway *Excites* the cerebral cortex.

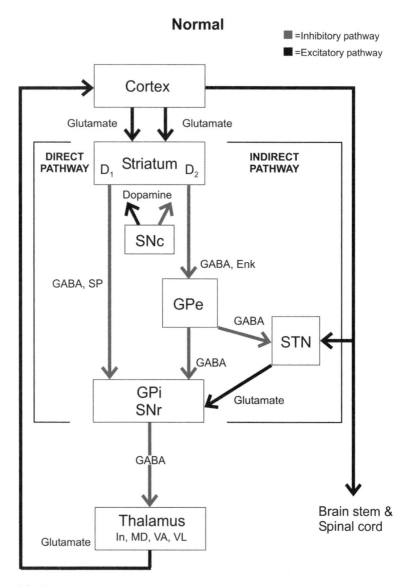

Fig. 19.3 Figure of the basal ganglia circuitry function in healthy individual

In PD, the loss of dopaminergic neurons in the SNc favors the indirect pathway, causing a net inhibition of cortex and hence motor inactivity, a hypokinetic movement disorder (see Fig. 19.4).

Data from Deep brain stimulation (DBS) surgery using a high-frequency electrical stimulation as well as pathological studies have demonstrated much more complex

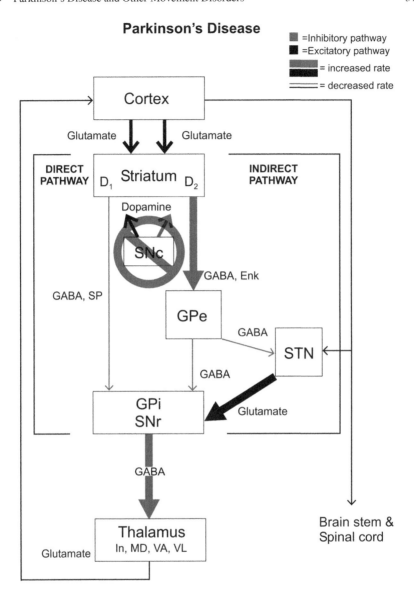

Fig. 19.4 Figure of the basal ganglia circuitry function in a patient with Parkinson's disease. *Note*: D=dopamine recepter (1 & 2), Enk=Enkephalin, GABA=y-aminobutyric acid, GPe=globus pallidus externa, GPi=globus pallidus interna, In=intralaminar nuclei of thalamus, MD=medial dorsal nucleus of thalamus, VA=ventral anterior nucleus of thalamus, VL=ventral lateral nucleus of thalamus, SP=substance P, SNc=Substantia nigra pars compacta, SNr=substantia nigra pars reticulata, STN=subthalamic nucleus

interactions among the previously described direct and indirect pathways, cerebral cortex, and brain stem nuclei. These more complex interactions account for the limited ability of the traditional direct and indirect models to explain or predict the effects of DBS and surgical lesion pathway on of various movement disorders (see below). Another model for understanding the basal ganglia consists of a series of major parallel pathways coursing through the basal ganglia, as described below.

Major Pathways of the Basal Ganglia

The basal ganglia are functionally and structurally connected to the cortex and thalamus by five (5) parallel circuits that are anatomically and functionally segregated, but have projections to shared brain regions to provide for feedback from other circuits. The five circuits are: (1) *motor*, (2) *oculomotor*, (3) *dorsolateral frontal*, (4) *lateral orbitofrontal*, and (5) *medial frontal/anterior cingulate*. Each circuit shares common neuroanatomical structures (e.g., basal ganglia, frontal cortex, thalamus) and neurotransmitters (e.g., dopamine, GABA, glutamate), but utilizes. Each circuit unique neuroanatomic pathways within each anatomic structure, which are maintained throughout the circuit (e.g., the orbital frontal area has projections to the ventral pallidum, while the supplementary motor and primary motor pathways of the frontal lobe project to the lateral caudate and putamen).

Motor pathway is associated with general motor control. The basal ganglion influences function of the lateral motor pathways (corticospinal tracts) and the medial motor systems (reticulospinal and tectospinal tracts), enabling smooth, regulated motor control. Major input is from the cortex via the putamen. Major output is through the GPi and SNr to the VL and VA thalamic nuclei, and subsequently to the sensory and motor cortex.

Oculomotor pathway is involved in the control of eye movements. Major input is from the frontal eye fields and posterior parietal cortices via the caudate nucleus. Output is via GPi and SNr to the VA thalamic nuclei, then to frontal and supplementary eye fields.

Dorsolateral frontal pathway is associated with cognitive executive functions such as organization, mental flexibility, and problem solving. Damage leads to impaired problem solving, perseveration, stimulus-bound behaviors, and poor mental flexibility. Major input is from cortex via the dorsolateral caudate. Major output is to the dorsolateral GPi and then cortex via the intralaminar thalamic nuclei (VA and MD).

Lateral orbitofrontal pathway is involved in processing the affective value of reinforcers (stimuli such as money, taste of food, social benefits) and planning behavior in response to reinforcement or punishment. Damage can lead to behavioral disinhibition (such as public swearing, telling off-color jokes, hypersexuality, excessive gambling, and increased alcohol/drug use) and environmental dependency. Input is from cortex to ventral GPi/nucleus accumbens. Major output is to ventral GPe (ventral pallidum) to cortex via intralaminar thalamic nuclei (VA and MD).

Medial frontal/anterior cingulate pathway is associated with motivation, emotional regulation, and memory functions. An individual's appreciation of the mental state of others has been associated with medial frontal functions. Damage can lead to akinetic states, anterograde amnesia, and lack of motivation and behavioral apathy. Major inputs are projections from limbic structures (hippocampus, amygdala) to ventral striatum/nucleus accumbens. Major output is ventral GPe (ventral pallidum) to cortex via intralaminar thalamic nuclei (MD).

In summary, one can think the motor pathway is involved in motor control, the oculomotor pathway is involved in eye movements, and the dorsolateral, orbitofrontal, and medial frontal/anterior cingulate pathways are involved in cognition and emotions.

Parkinson's Disease

Parkinson's disease (PD) is the most common subtype of parkinsonism, with a prevalence of about 100–200 patients per 100,000 population (Marras and Tanner 2004). The prevalence of PD increases with age, with a peak age of onset around 60 years. Persons who develop symptoms before 40 years of age are often said to have *young-onset PD*.

Diagnostic Criteria

PD is defined pathologically by the loss of dopaminergic cells within the *substantia nigra*, projecting to the *striatum*, and by the presence in surviving nigral neurons of intracellular inclusion bodies called *Lewy bodies*. Lewy bodies are round eosinophilic cytoplasmic inclusions that have a peripheral halo. In Parkinson's disease, Lewy bodies are found in the substantia nigra, locus ceruleus, dorsal vagal nucleus, nucleus basalis of Meynert, hypothalamus, and autonomic ganglia. However, parkinson's disease can be clinically diagnosed based on history and physical examination findings. It is thought the clinical features of PD present after about 70% (range 50–80%) of dopaminergic neurons in the substantia nigra are lost.

To diagnose PD clinically, parkinsonism must be present (see Table 19.2 for signs and symptoms of PD). Most often, a symptom such as resting tremor or loss of dexterity starts unilaterally (usually in an arm). With time, symptoms will begin to affect the other side of the body, but the side manifesting symptoms first often remains more severely affected. Soft voice (hypophonia), lack of facial expression (masked facies), small handwriting (micrographia), and paucity and slowness of all voluntary movement (akinesia or bradykinesia) are classic manifestations of PD. Resting tremor is absent in a minority of patients (Gelb et al. 1999). In PD, postural instability is usually a late development, generally only after a decade or more. Some authors describe two subtypes of Parkinson's disease reflecting the predominant characteristics of the disease: (1) a tremor-predominant, or (2) postural instability/akinesia-predominant type (sometimes referred to as rigidity-predominant type). In making a diagnosis of PD, it is important to look for

Table 19.2 Parkinson's disease cardinal symptoms and classic signs

Cardinal symptoms	Classic signs
Tremor (resting, 4–6 Hz)	Hypophonia (quiet soft voice)
Rigidity (cogwheel or lead-pipe)	Masked facies (reduced facial expression)
Akinesia/Bradykinesia (slow movement)	Micrographia (small handwriting)
Postural Instability	Shuffling gait (small steps and arms do not swing when walking)
	Stooped posture (with no arm swing)

Table 19.3 Features suggestive of an atypical parkinsonism

Atypical features on history or examination	Disease or syndrome that is suggested by the atypical feature
Acute onset	Vascular or drug-induced parkinsonism
Ataxia	MSA
Chorea, dementia and family history	HD
Early or prominent dementia	Vascular parkinsonism, HD, DLBD
Disproportionate gait disturbance	Vascular parkinsonism
Dystonia and liver disease	Wilson's disease
Early falls	PSP or MSA
History of neuroleptic medication	Drug-induced parkinsonism
Prominent orthostasis or dysautonomia	MSA
Unilateral apraxia, reflex myoclonus	CBGD
Vertical eye movement abnormality	PSP

CBGD cortical-basal ganglionic degeneration, *DLBD* diffuse Lewy body disease, *HD* Huntington's disease, *MSA* multiple system atrophy, *PSP* progressive supranuclear palsy

so-called atypical features that might indicate an alternative diagnosis. Some of these features, and diagnoses that they may suggest, are listed in Table 19.3.

Parkinson's disease includes nonmotor features or components in addition to the classical motor manifestations described above. Foremost among these are neuropsychological (cognitive) deficits, symptoms of depression, autonomic disturbances and sleep disturbances. Nonmotor manifestations of PD reflect nervous system pathology outside the substantia nigra.

The severity of PD can be quantified in several ways. The *Modified Hoehn and Yahr Scale* rates only the severity of motor manifestations (parkinsonism). The *Unified Parkinson's Disease Rating Scale (UPDRS)*, on the other hand, assesses nonmotor as well as motor symptoms (Fahn and Elton 1987). It includes questions about cognition and mood, activities of daily living, and complications of therapy, and lists numerous motor items to be scored by the examiner. The *Schwab & England Scale* asks patients to evaluate their independence and ability to perform activities of daily living on a spectrum from 0% (helpless) to 100% (normal).

Generally, evolution of PD is considered to be slow and relentlessly progressive, but is highly variable. The mean time from diagnosis to being chair-bound without medical treatment was about 7–8 years, although some patients exhibit a much more gradual decline with few changes noted over a 10-year time period (e.g., Victor and Ropper 2001). In general, data suggest differences in the progression of symptoms between patients with onset of PD in younger adulthood (at age 40 or younger) versus those with onset of PD in later adulthood (at age 70 or older). Patients with early onset PD tend to exhibit a slower progression of PD symptoms, but are more sensitive to levodopa-induced dyskinesias than are late-onset patients, who exhibit more rapid progression of PD symptoms. Recently, it was found that neuropsychological variables predicted the progression of PD motor symptoms, and particularly progression of cognitive deficits in PD, compared to SPECT (cerebral blood flow) data (Dujardin et al. 2004).

Neuropsychological Symptoms

Neuropsychological deficits are found in a majority of nondemented PD patients, and the prevalence of neuropsychological deficits increases with disease duration (Caballol et al. 2007). Neuropsychological decline can occur early in the course of the disease, particularly for individuals with PD onset later in life, but is not pronounced. Dementia, if it occurs, does not present until later in the course of PD. Neuropsychological deficits in PD are well described, and include: bradykinesia/bradyphrenia (slowed psychomotor speed/information processing speed) and impairments in visuoperceptual/visuoconstructional, attention/executive, memory, and language functions. Visuospatial and visuoconstructional problems often present early in the course of PD and can be quite pronounced, exceeding deficits that could be attributed to tremor alone. Memory deficits are not predominant early in the disease, although reduced retrieval and efficiency in encoding is consistently found. Thus, spontaneous recall is often impaired, but recognition memory is normal or near normal. Language problems include hypophonia and micrographia. Verbal fluency and confrontation naming are not typically impaired early in the course, but become impaired later in the disease course.

Depression and anxiety are common in PD, and many patients (up to 90%) with PD meet diagnostic criteria for a mood disorder (Nuti et al. 2004), with about 40% of the patient sample meeting criteria for depression diagnoses, of which 21% met criteria for major depression and 19% met criteria for dysthymia. Additionally, 40% of patients with PD met diagnostic criteria for Generalized Anxiety Disorder (11%) or Panic Disorder (30%). Pathological studies demonstrate the mood disorder symptoms are associated with the neuropathologic changes that occur in PD

Rule of thumb: Neuropsychological deficits in PD

- Bradykinesia/Bradyphrenia
- Attention/executive deficits,
- Visuoperceptual/visuoconstructional deficits
- Language (hypophonia, micrographia)
- Memory (poor retrieval, intact recognition)
- Depression and anxiety symptoms (80–90%)

(e.g., dopamine depletion), rather than simply a response to chronic illness (Wolters and Braak 2006; Nuti et al. 2004; Levy et al. 1998). Indeed, symptoms of depression are more related to "off" periods of levodopa motor response, and may improve with administration of levodopa. Apathy is common among patients with PD, and is not necessarily secondary to depression (Levy et al. 1998). Apathy exhibited by patients with PD may, however, be exacerbated by symptoms of depression including sadness, social isolation, hopelessness, etc. Apathy can be very troubling to patients' families and is often not adequately addressed by medical treatment. Apathy may be mistaken for "laziness," but is associated with neuropsychological dysfunction in initiating activities.

Dementia in Parkinson's disease (PD-D) has been well described (see Chap. 14, this volume). The lifetime incidence of overt dementia in PD is controversial, but is typically thought to be about 20–30% (Caballol et al. 2007; Emre et al. 2007), although up to 70% of patients with diagnosed Parkinson's disease developed dementia after 10 years of motor symptoms (McKeith and Mosimann 2004). The risk of developing dementia over a year time period is greater for patients with PD exhibiting more deficits in attention/executive (digit span backwards, Wisconsin Card Sorting Test perseverative errors) and memory (poor list learning and recognition), which support evidenced-based neuropsychology practice (Woods and Troster 2003). Common neuropsychological features of PD-D include bradyphrenia and deficits in attention/executive functions, memory (particularly poor retrieval), language (micrographia, hypophonia, poor semantic and phonemic verbal fluency), and impaired visuoconstructional/visuoperceptual functions (Emre et al. 2007).

The clinical, neuropsychological, radiological, and pathological manifestations of PD-D are similar to those of dementia with Lewy bodies (DLBD/DLB) (see next section and also Chap. 14). Indeed, while classically PD has been differentially diagnosed from DLBD/DLB and Alzheimer's dementia, recent studies have indicated PD-D and DLBD/DLB may be the same disease process manifesting differently early in the disease course. Traditionally, DLBD/DLB has been distinguished from PD by onset of dementia within a year of parkinsonian motor symptoms, fluctuating mental status, and visual hallucinations not associated with levodopa/carbidopa medications.

Diffuse Lewy Body Disease/Dementia with Lewy Bodies

Diffuse Lewy Body disease (DLBD), also known as dementia with Lewy Bodies (DLB) often presents with dementia and parkinsonian symptoms including stiffness, akinesia, slow shuffling gait, and resting tremor (see also Chap. 14). Other early features include fluctuating mental status (waxing and waning of mental status during the daytime such that patients appear confused, disoriented, lethargic or drowsy, and staring off into space), visual hallucinations, delusions, and dysautonomia (Broderick and Riley 2008). The name reflects the pathology, with a diffuse distribution of Lewy bodies throughout the brain (McKeith et al. 1996). Patients with Lewy body disease can present with primarily parkinsonism (Parkinson's disease), autonomic (Primary autonomic failure), or cognitive (DLB) manifestations.

The paragraph below reflects a traditional clinical viewpoint in which PD and PD-D is differentially diagnosed from DLBD/DLB and Alzheimer's disease. This has been an important distinction for selection of treatment, both in terms of medications and surgical candidacy. However, an emerging literature suggest PD, PD-D and DLBD/DLB share a common disease process, and the different clinical diagnostic criteria is based on a variable phenotypic presentation of the same disease process. Similar to the previous clinical distinctions that had been made for Multiple System Atrophy (MSA, see below), the clinical distinction of PD, PD-D, and DLBD/DLB may be artificial. Based on this framework, patients with Lewy body disease presenting with primarily parkinsonism have PD/PD-D, with primarily autonomic features have Primary autonomic failure, and those with primarily cognitive deficits have DLBD. While the disease pathology of PD, PD-D, and DLBD/DLB remains to be fully delineated, below we provide an overview of the traditional differential diagnostic framework, since this distinction continues to have relevance in treatment planning. Differential diagnosis between DLBD/DLB, PD, and Alzheimer's disease (AD) can be challenging, particularly for patients with onset of PD in older age. The clinical history is often key to differential diagnosis. While patients with PD may develop dementia, it has traditionally been viewed as occurring late in the disease course. In contrast, patients with DLBD/DLB develop dementia within the first year of having parkinsonian motor symptoms (see also Chap. 14: Dementias, this volume). Indeed, patients diagnosed with DLBD often present first with neuropsychological deficits, and then develop parkinsonian symptoms. There is an emerging evidence-based neuropsychological practice in differential diagnosis between DLBD/DLB and Alzheimer's disease, particularly early in the course of the disease (Calderon et al. 2001). Patients with DLBD/DLB exhibit greater deficits in attention/working memory and visuoperceptual functions compared to Alzheimer's disease. Visual hallucinations and onset of REM sleep behavioral disorder are also common early symptoms of DLBD/DLB. Unlike Parkinson's disease, patients with DLBD/DLB can have visual hallucinations prior to starting anti-Parkinson's disease medications, and the patient can have prominent REM sleep behavioral disorder. Patients diagnosed with DLBD/DLB have exhibited sensitivity to neuroleptic medications (i.e., haloperidol) with marked exacerbation of parkinsonian motor symptoms. They also do not show typical benefit from levodopa and may experience an increase in hallucinations with these medications.

Neuropsychological Symptoms

The neuropsychological deficits in DLBD/DLB have been increasingly well delineated (e.g., McKeith and Mosimann 2004; Collerton et al. 2003), with marked deficits in attention/executive and visuoperceptual/visuoconstructional functions. Impairments in memory are typically mild early in the course of the disease, and progressively worsen at a rate more quickly than classically associated with PD/PD-D. Memory deficits are due to inefficient encoding. Language deficits are not pronounced early in DLB, but impaired fluency and confrontation naming do develop. Phonemic and semantic verbal fluency may be impaired (see also Chap. 14).

Mood symptoms of DLBD/DLB can be pronounced early in the course of the disease, with hallucinations and delusions.

"Parkinson's Plus" Syndromes

"Parkinson's plus" is a blanket term encompassing diseases other than PD that are associated with parkinsonism. The more common "Parkinson's plus" diseases and associated clinical features are described below. These diseases tend to be more rapidly progressive than PD and often lead to earlier disability. Patients tend to respond less briskly to medications like levodopa than patients with PD.

Cortical-Basal Ganglionic Degeneration (CBGD)

The classical syndrome of CBGD (also designated as CBD; Corticobasal Degeneration) is strikingly asymmetric in its parkinsonism. Clinical diagnosis requires a combination of symptoms and signs indicating involvement of both cerebral cortex and basal ganglia. The cardinal cerebral cortical features are apraxia, cortical sensory deficits, and the "alien limb phenomenon/alien hand sign." The principal basal ganglia findings are akinesia, rigidity and dystonia. Additional clinical features may include action and focal reflex myoclonus, corticospinal tract signs, impaired ocular and eyelid motility, dysarthria and dementia (see below and Chap. 18, this volume). These various phenomena may render the more involved hand functionally useless to the patient, due to a combination of dystonia, apraxia, akinesia and myoclonus(Riley et al. 1990). Aphasia may occur with dominant hemisphere involvement of CBGD. In a case series of 15 patients in combination with 13 previously reported CBGD cases, our group found a 43% incidence of dementia and a 21% incidence of aphasia (Riley et al. 1990). Depression is also common (Massman et al. 1996). MRI studies have found perirolandic frontal atrophy that is asymmetric. CBGD is a tauopathy and clinical features have been associated with a frontotemporal dementia (Mathuranath et al. 2000).

Neuropsychological Symptoms

Apraxia appears to be the more clinically prominent feature of CBGD, with other than neuropsychological deficits not as pronounced. However, dementia is a common manifestation later in the disease course (Grimes et al. 1999). In addition to apraxia, the early neuropsychological deficits in CBGD are after lateralized, and include CBGD attention/executive and language dysfunction as well as bradyphrenia (slowed information processing speed). Memory may not be adversely affected, and if affected, may present in a lateralized pattern; memory impairments are generally mild with spontaneous recall worse than recognition memory (see Chap. 14, this volume for more details) (Grafman et al. 1995). Cognitive dysfunction in patients with CBGD differed from subjects diagnosed with mild AD dementia in that the CBGD group did not exhibit significant memory impairment, but did exhibit deficits in attention, processing speed, mental control, and verbal fluency. (Massman et al. 1996). Greater involvement of the language-dominant hemisphere is associated with aphasia symptoms, while greater involvement of non-dominant hemisphere associated with more visuospatial/visuoperceptual deficits.

Multiple System Atrophy (MSA)

Once thought to be separate diseases, olivopontocerebellar atrophy (OPCA), Shy-Drager syndrome, and striatonigral degeneration are but different variations of MSA. Patients can present with primarily parkinsonian (striatonigral degeneration), autonomic (Shy-Drager syndrome) or cerebellar (OPCA) manifestations of MSA. MSA is perhaps the form of atypical parkinsonism that is most often mistaken for PD, although MSA progresses more quickly than PD. The cerebellar features are slow in onset and progression. Autonomic features include bowel, bladder, and sexual dysfunction, as well as orthostatic hypotension (a drop in blood pressure with sitting up or standing up). Orthostatic hypotension is sometimes treated with medications to raise blood pressure.

Neuropsychological Symptoms

Neuropsychological deficits of MSA are commonly described as mild and can reflect deficits in attention/executive, slowed information processing speed, visuoperceptual/visuoconstructional skills, verbal fluency (semantic and phonemic), and memory functions (Bürk et al. 2006; Boeve 2007). However, there is considerable variability, as patients with OPCA, also termed MSA-Cerebellar (MSA-C), tend not to exhibit neuropsychological deficits beyond visuoperceptual/visuoconstructional deficits (Jacobson and Truax 1991), while patients with striatonigral degeneration, also termed MSA–Parkinsonism (MSA-P), tend to have more extensive neuropsychological deficits. A recent comparison between patients with MSA-P and MSA-C found patients with MSA-P exhibited more pronounced neuropsychological deficits compared to patients with MSA-C, particularly on measures of verbal fluency and executive functions, but also visuoperceptual/visuoconstructional skills (Kawai et al. 2008).

Progressive Supranuclear Palsy (PSP)

PSP is a syndrome characterized by predominantly axial parkinsonism, vertical eye movement abnormalities, slurred speech (dysarthria), trouble swallowing (dysphagia), and a prominent gait disorder (gait apraxia and rigidity) with early falls. The prominence of postural instability and unexplained falls in PSP has led to a clinical axiom of the 'toppling' disease. PSP must be differentiated from vascular disease within the brain stem, which can cause similar symptoms (Winikates and Jankovic 1994). The vertical gaze palsy of PSP will affect both upward and downward gaze, although deficient downward gaze is more diagnostically useful than upward gaze, since upward gaze is diminished normally with aging. As PSP progresses, horizontal gaze palsy develops. Other clinical features of PSP include patients appearing to have a wide-eyed stare of surprise. Tremor is not common or predominant. Subtypes of PSP have been proposed. A Richardson's syndrome is distinguished by early onset of supranuclear gaze palsy, postural instability, and neuropsychological deficits. A second type, termed PSP-Parkinsonism, has features more consistent with PD, and patients exhibit some clinical response to levodopa. Two other PSP subtypes have been proposed, a pure akinesia and a primarily cerebellar subtype. MRI studies have found atrophy of the midbrain and pons, particularly the upper midbrain.

Neuropsychological Symptoms

Neuropsychological impairments associated with PSP are commonly described as mild to moderate, with deficits in attention/executive, information processing speed, and memory (spontaneous recall worse than recognition memory) functions (see Chap. 14, this volume for more details) (Grafman et al. 1995). Dementia may *not* occur in some patients, and we have been struck by how much the cognitive function can be preserved in some patients with advanced PSP, while these patients present with a severe nontreatment responsive parkinsonism inclusive of progressive paralysis of eye movements. When dementia does develop, the early and predominant executive dysfunction, slowed information processing speed and vertical gaze palsy differentiate PSP-associated dementia from other dementias (Grafman et al. 1995). In addition, patients with PSP often exhibit the "applause sign," in which the patients are unable to inhibit clapping their hands more than three times in succession (patients clap more than three times). This sign discriminated PSP from FTD with 81.2 hit rate and distinguished PSP from Parkinson's disease (Dubois et al. 2005). However, a follow-up study found the applause sign is also found in patients with CBGD, PSP, and MSA (Wu et al. 2008). Depression and behavioral changes (although not psychosis) are commonly associated with later stages of PSP (Chiu and Psych 1995; Rampello et al. 2005). A pseudobulbar syndrome (emotional expression without associated internalized feeling, i.e., crying with no associated sadness) may also occur (Rampello et al. 2005).

Drug-Induced Parkinsonism

Neuroleptic medications can cause parkinsonism, usually after a period of weeks to months of exposure. These psychiatric medications are used mostly to treat psychosis, such as in schizophrenic patients. The "typical" neuroleptics (which include haloperidol, fluphenazine, and pimozide) are more likely to cause parkinsonism. "Atypical" neuroleptics (such as risperidone and olanzapine) and a newer neuroleptic called aripiprazole also cause parkinsonism, though less often (Sharma and Sorrell 2006). Of these, quetiapine and clozapine are the least likely antipsychotic medications to exacerbate or cause parkinsonism (Kurlan et al. 2007). Hence, they are the antipsychotic medications of choice for patients with PD, although the efficacy of quetiapine for psychosis or agitation in PD may be modest, while clozapine requires frequent blood tests (Kurlan et al. 2007). The treatment of choice for drug-induced parkinsonism (DIP) is discontinuing the responsible medication or switching to one that is less likely to cause parkinsonism. Finally, *antidopaminergic alternative medications* (e.g., prochlorperazine, promethazine, and metoclopramide) can cause parkinsonism.

Neuropsychological Symptoms

Neuropsychological testing may be confounded by the underlying psychopathology that was the indication for the antipsychotic medication in the first place. Apraxia is absent with DIP (Leiguarda et al. 1997). Depending upon underlying etiology for psychosis, patients may present with a variety of neuropsychological dysfunction.

Vascular Parkinsonism

Vascular parkinsonism is a usually symmetric parkinsonism caused by either strokes or more often so-called white matter ischemic disease (WMD). WMD is accumulation of many small confluent stroke like lesions, giving the CT scan (or MRI) the appearance of diffuse increased signal. Vascular parkinsonism is usually manifest by a gait disorder with prominent freezing, leading to the nickname "lower-body parkinsonism." The features of vascular parkinsonism are similar to those of PD. Like PD, the patient may have a slow and shuffling gait and take many small steps to turn around (called en-bloc turns). In addition, patients with vascular disease often present with bradykinesia/bradyphrenia (slowed psychomotor speed and processing speed) and postural instability. Typically, the upper extremities are less affected by parkinsonism features, although not always. Tremor may also be present, but it is more likely to be postural than resting tremor. Importantly, vascular parkinsonism is frequently associated with other features of cerebrovascular disease, including dementia (see below) and focal neurological signs (i.e., Babinski reflex, spasticity, visual field cuts, sensory loss, etc.). Patients with vascular parkinsonism often have comorbid hypertension and/or diabetes, and it is not uncommon for these individuals to have a history of previous strokes/Transient Ischemic Attacks (TIAs). Patients with vascular parkinsonism may have intact sense of smell, which is frequently impaired among patients with PD.

Neuropsychological Symptoms

Multi-infarct dementia is a common accompaniment of vascular Parkinsonism, including deficits in attention/executive, memory, language, and visuoperceptual/visuoconstructional functions (see Chaps. 13 and 14, this volume, for more details of cerebrovascular disease-based impairments) (Román 2003). Briefly, neuropsychological deficits tend to reflect greater impairments in attention/executive, visuoperceptual/visuoconstructional, and language functions. Memory may not be initially impaired, but is often impaired in later stages of disease (Román 2003). The treatment of vascular dementia consists of addressing cerebrovascular risk factors (blood pressure, cholesterol, diabetes, etc.) and symptom treatment when available.

Other Movement Disorders

Essential Tremor

Essential tremor (ET) is the most common cause of tremor in humans, and results in an *action and postural tremor*, as opposed to the resting tremor that is seen in parkinsonism (see Chap. 2 for description of tremor types). Tremor most often affects the arms, but also can affect the head and larynx (voice box). The 8- to 12-Hz tremor typically begins slowly, and often adversely affects daily activities such as writing, eating, and other fine motor tasks. In addition to tremor, patients often exhibit deficits with tandem gait and balance along with non-motor deficits in neuropsychological function and psychiatric/psychological functioning (see below). Prevalence ranges for 4.0–5.6% among people older than 40 years old, and 9% among individuals aged older than 60 years of age. Etiology appears to be complex, inclusive of genetic and environmental factors. Pathophysiology has not been firmly established, but cerebellar dysfunction is clearly involved. Frontal lobe dysfunction is also suspected. Neuroimaging (i.e., SPECT, fMRI, PET) studies identify cerebellar dysfunction and SPECT studies have found bilateral frontal hypometabolism.

Neuropsychological Symptoms

Neuropsychological deficits have not traditionally been associated with ET; however, patients with ET often exhibit mild neuropsychological deficits in attention/executive (i.e., complex auditory and visual attention, behavioral inhibition, set-shifting), immediate memory (short-term recall for a word list), and language (i.e., phonemic verbal fluency and confrontation naming) (Benito-León et al. 2006). Deficits in visuoperceptual functions have been found, but not consistently.

Visuoconstructional skills (taking into account tremor) are generally unaffected. Furthermore, a larger proportion of patients with ET were found to meet diagnostic criteria for dementia (25%) than a comparable age-matched sample (9.2%), suggesting that ET increases risk of dementia (Louis 2009). The pattern of neuropsychological deficits generally reflect cortico-striatal-thalamic-cerebellar dysfunction. When compared to patients with PD without dementia, patients with ET and no dementia exhibited greater impairment on verbal fluency and working memory tasks (Lombardi et al. 2001), while patients with PD exhibited greater impairment in visuospatial/visuoconstructional skills. Finally, patients with ET frequently report symptoms of depression and/or anxiety (Benito-León et al. 2006). Recent data suggest symptoms of depression were present before the onset of tremor, suggesting psychiatric/psychological symptoms may be associated with the ET disease process rather than a psychiatric response to tremor (Louis 2009).

Rule of thumb: Neuropsychological deficits in ET

- Attention/executive deficits (mild),
- Language (phonemic verbal fluency, confrontation naming, dystonic speech (vocal tremor quality))
- Memory (often normal, but there may be mild deficits in immediate recall for list learning tests)
    - Neuropsychological deficits can become more pronounced, with higher rates of dementia found for patients with ET
- Depression and anxiety symptoms typically present

Dystonia

Dystonia is characterized by sustained muscle contractions, usually resulting in abnormal postures. Dystonia can cause coarse clonic (jerky) as well as tonic movements, and can even be paroxysmal (intermittently present) in rare cases. Dystonia is classified as *focal, multifocal, segmental,* or *generalized*, depending on the affected body region(s). For example, torticollis (or cervical dystonia) is a focal dystonia characterized by abnormal muscle contractions in the neck, causing a forced turning of the head. Other dystonias can involve the face, limbs or trunk. Dystonia is also subclassified into *primary* (occurring as a spontaneous or genetic condition) or *secondary* (caused by an identifiable general medical condition or injury) categories.

Neuropsychological Symptoms

Neuropsychological studies in dystonic patients have generally been normal, although semantic word fluency deficits were found in a sample of patients with primary dystonia (Jahanshahi et al. 2003). Problems with the set-shifting were found in another study that aimed to recruit only patients with primary dystonia, but may have included patients with secondary dystonia (Scott et al. 2003).

Tourette Syndrome

Tourette syndrome (TS) is a neurologic condition characterized by motor and phonic tics, which are stereotyped movements and/or sounds that can sometimes be quite complex. Diagnosis of TS requires at least two motor tics and at least one phonic tic (also referred to as a sonic or vocal tic) over a 1-year period before the age of 18 years (American Psychiatric Association 2000; Watkins et al. 2005). The tics generally start at 5–7 years of age, peak in late childhood, and decline in frequency and severity in adolescence and early adulthood, although TS may persist, or rarely worsen, in adulthood. Comorbid attention deficit-hyperactivity disorder (ADHD) is reported in 21–90% of patients with TS, while obsessive-compulsive disorder/obsessive compulsive behaviors (OCD/OCB) have been reported in 11–80% of patients with TS.

Neuropsychological Symptoms

Neuropsychological deficits associated with TS traditionally were characterized as impairments in fine motor coordination, visuoperceptual/visuoconstructional, attention/executive (particularly behavioral disinhibition), memory, and verbal fluency (Watkins et al. 2005). However, early studies of TS included individuals with comorbid ADHD and/or OCD, and more recent studies with patients having no comorbid ADHD or OCD show less neuropsychological dysfunction

Patients with uncomplicated TS generally demonstrate mild deficits in fine motor coordination, visuoperceptual/visuoconstructional skills and less consistently, executive function deficits (Crawford et al. 2005; Como 2001). In one recent study (Crawford et al. 2005), patients with uncomplicated TS scored worse on two measures of inhibition, the Flanker task (Eriksen and Eriksen 1974) and Haylings Test (Burgess and Shallice 1997), but otherwise performed normally on a variety of tests associated with frontal lobe function (e.g., Stroop Color-Word test and Wisconsin Card Sorting test).

Rule of thumb: Tourette's syndrome

- 2 motor and at least one phonic (vocal) tic by 18 years old
- Neuropsychological deficits in:
    - Fine motor coordination
    - Visuoperceptual/visuoconstructional skills
    - Executive dysfunction (types of inhibition)
- Neuropsychological deficits likely worse if comorbid ADHD and/or OCD

Huntington's Disease

Huntington's disease (HD) is a hereditary disorder transmitted in autosomal dominant fashion. In HD, the cytosine-adenine-guanine (CAG) trinucleotide are excessively repeated as a mutation of the HD gene, which results in synthesis of proteins that contain excess glutamine. While the cardinal features of HD are chorea (a series of brief, randomly occurring twitching movements), dementia and psychiatric symptoms, other features of HD include eye movement abnormalities, dystonia, parkinsonism, and gait disturbances.

Neuropsychology Symptoms

Dementia and psychiatric symptomatology are prominent and often early findings in HD (see Chap. 14 this volume for details). Age of onset is often in 30's or 40's, but earlier and later onset have been reported. Briefly, prominent deficits typically occur in attention/executive, psychomotor speed, memory, and visuoconstructional functions (Ward et al. 2006). There is an elevated rate of depression among HD patients, with a high suicide rate. Personality and mood changes can be the first symptom of HD. For example, Leroi et al. (2002) reported 81% of patient with HD met criteria for a personality disorder and/or a mood disorder. The most common symptoms reported were of mood lability, apathy, disinhibition, and paranoia. A total of 42.8% of patients with HD met diagnostic criteria for a mood disorder

Ataxia

Ataxia is a descriptive term meaning the loss of ability to coordinate previously learned motor movements, not attributable to weakness. Ataxia presents with a characteristic dyscocordination of the arms and/or legs. The gait tends to be wide-based and the patient may appear to be on the brink of falling, always shifting his/her position to avoid falling over (see Chap. 2 for illustration of ataxic gait). Speech can be difficult to understand due to being slurred (slurring dysarthria), or speech with variable intonation and volume, termed (scanning dysarthria). Ataxia, like parkinsonism, is a symptom that has many different causes, including medications such as anticonvulsants, alcohol abuse, and MSA, as discussed above.

Genetic ataxia syndromes are subdivided into *autosomal dominant* (*AD*) and *autosomal recessive* (*AR*) etiologies. Autosomal dominant ataxia disorders most commonly consist of the spinocerebellar ataxias (SCAs), which also cause a host of other neurological symptoms. Like HD, most SCAs are CAG repeat disorders, and genetic tests for some SCAs are commercially available. Dentatorubropallidoluysian atrophy (DRPLA) is another AD ataxia. A common autosomal recessive ataxia is Friedreich's ataxia, which is due to GAA repeat on chromosome 9q, and accounts for almost half of all cases of hereditary progressive ataxia. Onset of Friedreich's ataxia is from age 2 or 3 to about age 25 years old, although some patients with onset in late 20's and early 30's have been reported. However, most patients develop symptoms before age 10 years. Initial symptom is ataxia of the legs, most often bilateral, although unilateral onset has been infrequently reported. Ataxia progresses, and most patients have difficulty walking within 5 years of first symptom. Involvement of the upper extremities and speech develop. There is no specific treatment for the genetic causes of ataxia (with the exception of ataxia with vitamin E deficiency). However, physical therapy can be helpful to these patients.

Neuropsychological Symptoms

Neuropsychological deficits have been associated with SCAs, including dementia and prominent mood disorders (e.g., Leroi et al. 2002), but have not been reported among patients with Friedreich's ataxia (Bürk et al. 2003; McMurtray et al. 2006; Evidente et al. 2000). Patients with SCAs 1–3, the most common SCA mutations, often exhibit deficits in memory and executive functions (particularly in SCA 1 patients), but no visuoperceptual deficits (Bürk et al. 2003). Depressive symptoms were present in 60% of SCA 3 patients (McMurtray et al. 2006), and another study found 67.7% of a mixed patient sample, inclusive of patients with degenerative cerebellar disorders (MSA, sporadic spinocerebellar atrophy, and SCA variants), exhibited symptoms sufficient for a diagnosis of a DSM-IV mood disorder. (Leroi et al. 2002). Dementia can also occur in DRPLA and some other SCAs, and psychosis can occur in DRPLA (Evidente et al. 2000).

Myoclonus

Myoclonus is a rapid jerking movement. Some forms of myoclonus are within normal physiologic experience, such as hiccups (myoclonus of the diaphragm) and hypnic jerks (single generalized myoclonic jerks when falling asleep). However, excessive myoclonus may indicate a neurological or toxic-metabolic disorder that requires treatment. For instance, myoclonus can occur in some epilepsy syndromes, and several genetic diseases. Most commonly, myoclonus is caused by a general medical condition such as liver failure or kidney failure or as a side effect of certain medications, including serotonin selective reuptake inhibitors (SSRI's).

Neuropsychological Symptoms

Neuropsychological function is typically completely normal. However, if myoclonus occurs in setting of delirium, diffuse neuropsychological impairments are observed, including altered sensorium. The most common symptomatic treatment for myoclonus is clonazepam, but several other medications can be used.

Stiff-Person Syndrome

Stiff-person (also called stiff-man) syndrome presents in adulthood, and causes intermittent uncontrolled proximal and axial muscle contractions that are present only during wakefulness. The muscle contractions may be precipitated by a variety of stimuli, including movement, noise, or application of heat or cold to the patient. The cramps are often extremely painful. Stiff-person syndrome is thought to be an autoimmune disorder. It is treated long-term with diazepam, clonazepam, or other muscle relaxants. The action of muscle contractions is blocked by curare or nerve blocking agents. Patients with stiff-person syndrome have been incorrectly diagnosed with a psychogenic movement disorder before either their condition has been is accurately recognized.

Neuropsychological Symptoms

Aside from anticipatory anxiety (precipitated by the unpredictability of their episodes of stiffness), patients did not demonstrated neuropsychological deficits (Ameli et al. 2005).

Section II: Medical and Surgical Treatment of the Movement Disorders

In this section, we outline the medical and surgical treatments for the movement disorders. In general, the goal of treatment is to eliminate symptoms and return the patient to previous functional level. However, the treatment of most movement disorders either medically or surgically does not allow for complete resolution of symptoms, although for many return to previous functional status is possible. The medication-based therapies are reviewed first, followed by surgical therapies.

Medication Effects and Neurological and Neuropsychological Side Effects

Parkinson's Disease

Treatment of PD is symptomatic, and can be thought of as balancing the acetylcholine-dopamine systems in the striatum which, because of the dopamine deficiency in PD, is tipped toward acetylcholine in PD patients. It is now recognized that most patients will develop long-term complications of levodopa treatment. As a result, levodopa sometimes is not initiated in the earliest stage of the disease until symptoms become too troublesome. Patients eventually require medical treatment, and levodopa (administered as carbidopa/levodopa) is the most effective PD treatment. As the disease progresses, patients develop a variety of increasingly troublesome symptoms, some in response to medical treatment, including "on-off" fluctuations, "wearing off" phenomena, peak-dose dyskinesia/dystonia, and "off" period dystonia/freezing. Patients eventually develop increasingly shorter and less predictable periods of unmedicated "off" *state* (in which they are at or near their worst motor function) or the medicated "on" *state* (in which they are at or near their best motor function). The "wearing off" phenomenon refers to the increasingly brief "on" state. During "off" states, patients may exhibit akinesia (freezing), tremor, and dystonias as well as parasthesias, GI upset (belching, constipation), tachycardia, and shortness of breath can occur. Visual halucinations and psychoses can occur as a levodopa side effect.

Entacapone (Comtan) and tolcapone (Tasmar) can lengthen the duration of levodopa effect, and can therefore augment the side effects of levodopa. Other PD medications include the dopamine agonists: pramipexole (Mirapex), ropinirole (Requip), the rotigotine transdermal system (Neupro), and apomorphine (Apokyn, Uprima) injections. Selegiline (Eldepryl) and rasagiline (Azilect) are MAO-B inhibitors that can be helpful either in early PD or as adjunct therapy for later stages of PD. Amantadine (Symmetrel) is used primarily to treat dyskinesia. Anticholinergic medications, such as benztropine (Cogentin), diphenhydramine (Benadryl), and trihexyphenidyl (Artane) are especially useful in treating resting tremor. However, anticholinergics should be avoided in elderly or demented patients, since they are the worst offenders among antiparkinsonian drugs in causing sedation, cognitive impairment, and psychiatric changes. Similarly, dopamine agonists can cause cognitive impairment and psychosis in the elderly.

Diffuse Lewy Body Disease/Lewy Body Dementia

Levodopa is less useful and less well tolerated by patients with DLBD/LBD compared to patients with PD. However, one study reported no cognitive or neuropsychiatric adverse effects in a small sample of patients with DLBD/LBD (Molloy et al. 2006). Nootropics (some cognitive enhancing medications) can be used to treat dementia in patients with Parkinsonism. Neuroleptic medications, which treat hallucinations or delusions by blocking dopamine receptors, are not well tolerated by patients with DLBD/LBD due to aggravation of concomitant PD symptoms (Weintraub and Hurtig 2007).

The "Parkinson's Plus" Syndromes

Compared to patients with PD, patients with Parkinson's plus diseases benefit much less from levodopa. In MSA, levodopa and especially dopamine agonists may cause more adverse effects, including exacerbation of symptoms of orthostatic hypotension. Symptoms of orthostasis can be treated with medication, and ataxia can be addressed with physical therapy. Patients with PSP or CBGD typically show no response, good or bad, to medication.

Essential Tremor

The most effective medication for treating symptoms of ET are primidone and propranolol. Topiramate, gabapentin, methazolamide, mirtazapine and clonazepam can also be used. Most of these medications are sedating, and primidone and propranolol are poorly tolerated in some elderly patients.

Dystonia

The first line of therapy for dystonia is botulinum toxin, which is injected directly into affected muscles. Other common medications used to treat dystonias include anticholinergic medications such as trihexyphenidyl and muscle relaxant medications.

Tourette's Syndrome

Treatment of TS is symptomatic. A variety of medications, all of which have a potential to be sedating, can be used to treat tics. These include alpha-2 adrenergic agonist medications (clonidine and guanfacine) tetrabenazine and neuroleptic medications. Depression and OCD are often treated with antidepressant medication. ADHD may be treated with a stimulant medication, which has the potential to exacerbate tics, although clinical studies indicate stimulants are well tolerated by TS patients.

Huntington's Disease

Treatment of HD is symptomatic, as with almost all the disorders discussed in this chapter. The chorea is treated if it is bothersome to the patient. Generally, chorea is first treated using an atypical neuroleptic medication, but typical neuroleptics may be used, particularly to treat more severe chorea. Tetrabenazine is a FDA-approved medication that can be useful in treating chorea, and may have fewer long-term side effects than neuroleptic medications. Tetrabenazine has the potential to worsen depression. Unfortunately, treatment of chorea often does not result in improved quality of life, because of persistent parkisonism and other symptoms of HD. Neuroleptics can cause lethargy or can exacerbate parkinsonism. Behavioral and psychiatric symptoms of HD may respond to treatment with antidepressant or neuroleptic medication.

Common Side Effects of Medications to Treat Movement Disorders

Rather than trying to list all of the possible side effects associated with the many possible medications to treat the movement disorders reviewed in this chapter, this section will briefly review some of the more common medications and associated side effects. Table 19.4 lists common medications involved in the treatment of movement disorders and the frequent physical and cognitive side effects. An important comorbidity of neuroleptic use is neuroleptic malignant syndrome, which is a life-threatening condition associated with muscle rigidity, elevated temperature (hyperthermia), along with confusion and agitation (progressing to somnolence and coma).

Table 19.4 Medications and medication side-effects commonly used to treat movement disorders

Medication class	Medication	Physical side-effects	Neuropsychological side-effects
Alpha-2 adrenergic agonists	Clonidine, guanfacine, etc.	Cardiac rhythm changes Dizziness Dry mouth/eyes Orthostatic hypotension	Sedation/somnolence Depression Vivid dreams
Anti-viral	Amantadine	Edema (particularly legs) Dizziness Insomnia Dyscoordination GI symptoms (nausea, vomiting, diarrhea, constipation) Headache Weakness	Confusion Depression Drowsiness Hallucinations Slurred speech *Note*: Improved neuropsychological function (i.e., nootropic qualities), including delay in dementia onset reported for patients with PD and HD
Anticholinergic medications	Trihexyphenidyl, benztropine, procyclidine, biperiden, ethopropazine, diphenhydramine, orphenadrine	Constipation Dry mouth Narrow angle glaucoma Urinary retention.	Confusion Visual hallucinations Impaired memory

(continued)

Table 19.4 (continued)

Medication class	Medication	Physical side-effects	Neuropsychological side-effects
Anticonvulsant/ Antiepileptics	Gabapentine, primidone, lamotrigine, levetiracetam, oxcarbazepine, topiramate, etc.	Ataxia Decreased appetite Fatigue Drowsiness/ somnolence/ sedation GI symptoms (emesis and nausea) Headache Vision changes (diplopia, nystagmus)	Mood changes (depression, irritability, emotional lability) Cognitive adverse effects (generally mild): • attention/concentration • processing speed • memory • language *Note*: Some newer AEDs (lamotrigine, levetiracetam, gabapentin, etc.) have little adverse cognitive effects.
			Note: Topiramate and zonisamide have greater cognitive adverse effects in some patients, particularly on verbal fluency, memory, and processing speed, but adverse effects are reduced with lower doses and slower titration.
Neurotoxin	Botulinum toxin	Few side effects of focal IM injected dosing	No cognitive adverse effects
COMT[a] inhibitors	Entacapone, tolcapone	GI problems (e.g., nausea, vomiting, constipation, diarrhea) Headache Hyperkinetic movements (e.g., dyskinesias) Hypotension Sedation (generally mild) Sleep disorders Tolcapone can result in increased liver tansaminase enzyme levels and fulminant hepatitis Neuroleptic malignant syndrome has been reported	Hallucinations (related to L-Dopa medication) Mild positive effects on working memory/ short-term memory reported.

(continued)

Table 19.4 (continued)

Medication class	Medication	Physical side-effects	Neuropsychological side-effects
Dopamine agonists	Bromocriptine, pergolide, pramipexole, ropinirole, etc.	GI symptoms (constipation, diarrhea, nausea) Hyperkinetic movement disorders (dyskinesias, choreiform movements, hemiballismus) Insomnia Postural hypotension Somnolence (including rapid and unpredictable onset of extreme tiredness and somnolence at inappropriate times.)	Confusion Hallucinations (often visual) Impulse control behavior problems (compulsive gambling, shopping, and/ or sexual behaviors) has been reported (estimated prevalence 0.5 to 7%). Risk of impulse control problems with medication is more likely among individuals with a history of impulse control problems prior to onset of PD. Delusions (frequently paranoid).
	L-Dopa (Levodopa)	Acute effects: nausea dizziness insomnia Cardiac irregularities Orthostatic hypotension Anorexia Emesis Late effects (particularly with increased L-Dopa dosages): Hyperkinetic movements (dyskinesias, choreiform movements, hemiballismus)	Acute effects: Anxiety Confusion Depression and/or anxiety Late effects: Hallucinations (visual) Delusions Increased psychomotor speed May improve performance on complex executive function measures among patients with severe PD. Improved subjective alertness (Richard et al. 2004; Molloy et al. 2006). Improved mood (Richard et al. 2004)

Table 19.4 (continued)

Medication class	Medication	Physical side-effects	Neuropsychological side-effects
Neuroleptics	Clozapine, Olanzapine, Risperidone, Quetiapine, etc.	Cardiac rhythm changes (arrhythmias, tachycardia) Dry skin/eyes Hyperthermia or hypothermia Urinary retention Movement disorders (parkinsonism, akathisia, dystonia, dyskinesias, tardive dyskinesia) Orthostatic hypotension Seizures Sedation	Acute: Reduced vigilance/ attention (younger patients) Improved orientation and memory (some older patients). Late: Increased rate of cognitive decline for patients with dementia
Antihypertensives/ Beta blockers	Propranolol	Dizziness Fatigue Weakness Weight gain (some older beta-blockers) Insomnia	Depression Mild memory impairment for individuals with dementia

aCOMT catechol-O-methyl transferase is an enzyme that degrades catecholamine neurotransmitters (e.g., dopamine, epinephrine, norepinephrine)

Surgical Treatment: Neurological and Neuropsychological Effects

Patients being considered for neurosurgical treatment of movement disorder typically undergo a comprehensive pre-surgical evaluation to maximize the likelihood of a positive response to the surgical procedure and minimize risks to neurological, neuropsychological, and psychiatric comorbidity. A detailed review of the medical/ neurological and psychiatric evaluation is beyond the scope of this chapter, however, general guidelines for surgical selection is provided below, along with a more detailed review of neuropsychological variables in evaluating surgical candidacy.

General Surgical Candidacy Inclusion/Exclusion Criteria

There have been no universally agreed upon criteria for selecting candidates for surgical procedures to treat movement disorders. Generally, surgical candidacy is dependent upon the type of movement disorder, proposed surgical target, and particular patient characteristics. However, some general inclusion/exclusion criteria are provided below.

General Surgical Inclusion/Exclusion Criteria

The general criteria below reflect our opinion based on review of the literature and experience.

- Diagnosis of the movement disorder is accurate
- Motor symptoms are disabling
- Motor symptoms are refractory to medication treatment (either due to lack of adequate response or that dosage of medication(s) required result in intolerable side effects).
- No comorbid life threatening systemic illness/disease
- No pronounced dementia (although neuropsychological deficits may be present)
- Mood disorder/Psychiatric illness, if present, is not predominate. If present, is being treated
- Patient consent.

In addition, Speelman et al. (2010) also highlight six (6) other factors to consider in patient selection for DBS in dystonia, but is more generally applicable: (1) is the targeted symptom(s) for treatment the predominant source of disability; (2) has other causes of disability been ruled-out, (3) what is likelihood DBS will result in symptom reduction/relief, (4) what is risk of surgical treatment, (5) can a sufficient post-operative recovery plan be developed; and (6) is patient/family expectations for surgery reasonable? We now turn to components of the presurgical evaluation that may be directly assessed with a neuropsychological evaluation.

Presurgical Neuropsychological Evaluation

Neuropsychological evaluation can be a crucial component in assessing a patient's candidacy for surgical treatment (e.g., Smelding et al. 2009). Neuropsychological data can be helpful in reducing post-operative risks to cognitive function (Smeding et al. 2009 but see also Kalbe et al. 2009). While the particular emphasis of pre-surgical neuropsychological evaluations will vary depending upon the type of movement disorder, patient characteristics, and proposed surgical procedure, a triad of general objectives should generally be considered:

Rule of thumb: Pre-surgical neuropsychological evaluation

- Rule-out prominent dementia and quantify cognitive strengths/weakness
- Assess for psychologic risk factors (hypomania, suicidal ideation/attempts)
- May assist to assess patient's decision making capacity
- Extent patient can cooperate in post-surgical follow-up.
- At a minimum, assess attention/executive, verbal memory, verbal fluency (semantic and phonemic), and mood (anxiety, depression)

1. Rule out presence of pronounced dementia. Assessment should quantify extent and severity of neuropsychological impairment [mild to moderate cognitive impairment does not rule DBS for PD (Okun et al. 2004)]
   - Psychological function should also be assessed, including psychosis, manic behaviors, and history of suicidal ideation.
2. Assist in evaluating a patient's decision making capacity and appreciation of the risks/benefits of surgical treatment.
   - Evaluate limitations for the patient to cooperate in post-surgical follow-up care.
3. Establish a baseline for future comparison of neuropsychological domains more likely to be affected by surgical treatment, including attention/executive, verbal fluency (semantic and phonemic), and verbal memory and also mood (anxiety and depression).

Post-operative neuropsychological evaluations indicated to assist in treatment planning, monitor for treatment benefit, and help with placement decisions. For example, the neuropsychological evaluation can identify if, and to what extent, the patient's cognitive function changes over time, develop rehabilitation programming, and determine risks to completing activities of daily living.

Details regarding particular surgical procedures are reviewed below, beginning with ablation procedures followed by a review of DBS. The discussion below includes disease-specific information, including neuropsychological aspects of surgery and selection criteria.

Ablation Techniques

Neurological surgery for the treatment of movement disorders predates the pharmacological approach to these diseases, including PD, ET, dystonia, tardive dyskinesia, and TS. Open surgical procedures to treat movement disorders began in the late nineteenth century with corticotomies in the premotor area to cure choreoathetosis. Stereotactic technique, or 'the touching of tissue with respect to a specific three-dimensional coordinate reference system', was first developed by Horsley and Clarke in 1903 (Horsley and Clarke 1908). Spiegel and colleagues stereotactically targeted the pallidum to treat a variety of movement disorders in the 1940s (Spiegel et al. 1947). The surgical procedures involved a variety of ablation methods to destroy brain tissue using heat, freezing, compression, or neurotoxins. The benefits of neurological surgery are often most appreciated contralateral to the side of surgery, reflecting the decussation of motor and sensory pathways in the central nervous system (see Chap. 3, this volume for review).

Interest in surgical treatment for PD decreased with the introduction of levodopa in 1961. However, by the 1970s, the effects of chronic dopaminergic agonist treatment and progression of the disease became evident (reviewed above), and a renewed interest in movement disorder surgery began. The first resurgence began with ventral intermediate nucleus of the thalamus (VIM) thalamotomies for asymmetrical tremor and posteroventrolateral pallidotomies ablating the globus pallidus interna (GPi) for the side effects of chronic levodopa treatment.

Table 19.5 Surgical benefit and adverse effects of palidotomy and thalamotomy

Ablation procedure	Benefits	Adverse effects
Pallidotomy (i.e., GPi)		

Parkinson's disease	Tremor
	Bradykinesia
	Drug-induced dyskinesias
	"On–Off" dystonias
	"On–Off" motor
	  fluctuations
		Perioperative mortality (death) in
		  0.4–1% of patients
		Contralateral hemiparesis (1–6%)
		Seizures (<1.3%)
		Aphasia
		Ataxia
		Apraxia
		Abulia
		Paresthesias (1–2%) usually
		  involving lips and/or finger tips
		Dysarthria (up to 20% of patients)
		Dysphagia

Thalamotomy (i.e., VIM)		

Parkinson's disease	Tremor (reduction of
	  45–92%
	  from pre-surgical
	  baseline)
	Rigidity (reduction of
	  41–92%
	  from pre-surgical
	  baseline)
	Ten year outcome of
	  bilateral thalamotomy
	  found sustained benefit
	  of reduced tremor by
	  33–73% and rigidity by
	  22–74% compared to
	  pre-surgical baseline
	  (Kelly and Gillingham
	  1980a; Kelly and
	  Gillingham 1980b).
		Bilateral thalamotomy
		• Dysarthria (worsened in up to
		  33% of patients)
		• Dysphagia
		• Aphasia
		• Apraxia
		• Abulia
		• Ataxia
		• Seizures (<1.3%)
		• Contralateral hemiparesis
		  (1–26%)
		• Paresthesias (1–3%) usually
		  involving lips and/or finger tips
		• Perioperative mortality (death)
		  in 0.4–6% of patients

Essential Tremor	Tremor (reduction of
	  75–95%
	  from pre-surgical
	  baseline)
		Same as thalamotomy for
		  Parkinson's disease.

Deep brain stimulation, in which an electrode is permanently implanted at targeted sites allowing for application of continuous electrical stimulation, was introduced in the 1980s by Alim Benabid and colleagues (e.g., Benabid et al. 1998; Benabid et al. 1987). DBS surgery has become the preferred surgical treatment for movement disorders because it: (1) provides a nondestructive and potentially reversible technique, (2) the range of stimulation can be adjusted easily and safely postoperatively to maximize patient response, and (3) the rate of neurological complications is lower for DBS than ablative procedures. Despite the popularity of DBS, some selected patients are still offered ablative surgical treatments. Lesion techniques most often involve radiofrequency heating of tissue with thermocouple probes, or stereotactic radiosurgery with devices such as the Leksell Gamma Knife.

Ablation Surgical Candidacy Inclusion/Exclusion Criteria

Ablation surgeries are rarely offered to patients with diseases resulting in refractory movement disorder symptoms. However, there may be cases in which ablation may be a surgical option when a patient is judged to be a poor candidate for DBS surgery and/or refuses DBS surgery. In these rare cases, selection criteria are similar to those mentioned above for DBS.

General Surgical Inclusion/Exclusion Criteria in Ablation Surgeries

- Patients must not be candidates for DBS and/or refuse DBS surgery.
    - Surgical candidate should demonstrate decision-making capacity and awareness he/she is not a candidate for DBS and/or reasons for refusing DBS treatment.
- No pronounced dementia
- Motor symptoms are medication refractory and result in significant disability and reduced quality of life.
- Mood disorder, if present, is not predominant, and if present, is being treated.

Ablation Surgery for Parkinson's Disease

Surgical treatment of PD has a long history and the interested reader is referred to Tarsy et al. (2003) for review. This history includes ablative surgeries which are rarely performed today. Except in circumstances where either the patient is unwilling or unable to undergo DBS implantation procedures, ablative surgeries are not considered to be treatment options. These surgeries have included pallidotomies and thalamotomie, ablating either targeted areas of the globus pallidus (e.g., GPi) or thalamus (e.g., VIM). These surgeries have fallen out of favor as treatments of choice because of their side effects, introduction of DBS, and data suggesting reduced effectiveness over time. Table 19.5 list the side effects and long-term complications from the ablative surgeries.

Pallidotomy

Pallidotomy (generally targeting GPi) has been a surgical treatment for patients with PD since the 1950s (Tarsy et al. 2003 for review). Initial ablation techniques targeted the anterodorsal pallidum, which resulted in reduction of tremor and rigidity. However, both rigidity and tremor re-occurred in up to 25% of patients in some surgical series. Laitinen and colleagues (1992) after reporting surgerical ablation resulted in reduction of contralateral tremor, rigidity, and akinesia. Dystonia, postural instability, dysarthria, and drug-induced dyskinesias also improved, but benefit to balance and gait were temporary.

Surgical Inclusion/Exclusion Criteria for Pallidotomy in PD

Pallidotomy is rarely offered to patients today. Pallidotomy may be offered in cases in which DBS is judged to be a poor option.

- As specified in general surgical guidelines for ablative surgery AND Patients must obtain clear benefit from dopamine agonists (e.g., levodopa) in reduction of PD motor symptoms
- Medication refractory symptoms of PD may reflect either significant PD motor deficits that are no longer responsive to medication and/or significant medication-induced motor deficits (e.g., "On–Off" fluctuations, dyskinesias, dystonias).

Thalamotomy

Thalamotomy was found to result in a lower rate of recurrence of rigidity and tremor (11%) compared to anterodorsal pallidotomy. While thalamotomy has demonstrated benefit, bilateral thalamotomy has been associated with an increased incidence of adverse neurological and neuropsychological adverse affects (see Table 19.5). Thus, thalamotomy is rarely offered to patients, particularly as bilateral thalatomy is associated with higher incidences of complications involving speech (worsening of dysarthria or aphasia) and/or dysphagia as well as possible worsening of postural instability. Thalamotomy is rarely, if ever, offered, and unilateral thalamotomy may be offered in very unusual circumstances to patients who are unwilling or unable to undergo DBS surgery.

Surgical Inclusion/Exclusion Criteria for Thalamotomy in PD

- As specified in general surgical guidelines for ablative surgery AND Thalamotomy may be offered to patients with PD manifesting as tremor predominant. The resting tremor must be refractory to medication and of sufficient severity to markedly disable a patient's quality of life.
- Patients should obtain benefit from dopamine agonists (e.g., levodopa) in reduction of tremor, although cases of dopaminergic agonist-resistant tremor responding to thalamotomy do occur.

The "Parkinson's Plus" Syndromes

Although patients suffering from Parkinson's plus syndromes can demonstrate improved motor function from neurosurgical interventions, the associated signs and symptoms of Parkinson's plus syndromes (e.g., dementia, autonomic dysfunction, psychiatric disease) do not respond favorably to neurosurgical intervention. Because any benefits from reducing motor dysfunction are overshadowed by their unchanged or even worsened cognitive deficits, surgery is rarely offered in this context.

Essential Tremor

Thalamotomy has been a target for treating the cardinal feature of essential tremor since the 1950s, and between the 1950s and 1970s a number of stereotactic neurosurgeons treating tremor came to favor targeting the VIM nucleus of the thalamus over the VL nucleus (see Tarsy et al. 2003, for review). Deep brain stimulation has largely replaced thalamotomy, but unilateral thalamotomy remains a surgical option among very select patients who cannot or choose not to undergo DBS surgery.

Surgical Inclusion/Exclusion Criteria for Thalamotomy in ET

- As specified in general surgical guidelines for ablative surgery AND Patients should have failed to achieve complete relief of tremor with primidone or propranolol.
- Essential tremor is medication-refractory (lack of adequate response to medication and/or onset of intolerable side effects (sedation)) *and* symptoms adversely affects the patient's quality of life

Deep Brain Stimulation (DBS) Surgery and Chronic High-Frequency Stimulation

Deep brain stimulation (DBS) surgery has become a mainstay in ameliorating medication refractory symptoms of Parkinson's disease (PD), essential tremor (ET), and generalized and focal dystonia (Grimes et al. 1999; Mathuranath et al. 2000; Weaver et al. 2009). Surgical targets for DBS in the basal ganglia include the globus pallidus interna (GPi), subthalamic nuclei (STN), and the ventral intermediate nucleus (VIM) of the thalamus (Grimes et al. 1999; Mathuranath et al. 2000). Chronic high-frequency electrical stimulation of basal ganglia nuclei has been found to decrease the primary motor manifestations of PD, ET, and generalized dystonia. Data regarding the benefit of DBS to reduce the motor and phonic (sonic) tics in Tourette's syndrome has shown early benefit (e.g., Maciunas et al. 2007; Visser-Vandewalle et al. 2003).

Rather than reviewing DBS treatment individually for each movement disorder, a general description of DBS and the resulting motor benefit as well as neurological, neuropsychological, and psychiatric side effects will be reviewed below. This will be followed by unique comments or findings for DBS in particular movement disorders.

The DBS Surgical Procedure

Surgery may involve unilateral or bilateral electrode placement, either in staged procedures weeks or months apart, or increasingly commonly, during the same day. At the onset of the surgical procedure for DBS, the patient undergoes application of a stereotactic headframe. The patient then undergoes volumetric stereotactic imaging. Imaging data are transferred electronically to a computer workstation with stereotactic treatment-planning software in the surgical theater. Using high-resolution MR scans, the surgeon defines coordinate reference points. The trajectory to the target avoids, whenever possible, traversing any cerebral vasculature, sulci or the ventricular ependyma. These targets and trajectories are translated into geometric parameters relating the sterotactic frame and MRI image to the target and the lead is passed through the substance of the brain to the target. Targeting is precise with tolerances of 1–3 microns. The implantable programmable generator (IPG) is typically implanted in the subcutaneous space above the pectoral muscle. This is often completed 2–4 weeks after placement of the DBS electrodes.

During the surgery, the patient is positioned supine upon the operating table, with the basering of the stereotactic headframe secured to the operating table. After opening the dura, microelectrode recording is carried out along the proposed surgical trajectory to the target (some centers use macroelectrode targeting only). Single cell recording makes apparent neuronal cellular electrical activity that enables the surgical team to identify specific deep gray nuclei and the surrounding white matter tracts for precise placement of the DBS electrode. The DBS electrode contains four sequential 1.4 mm leads at its tip, and the spacing between leads is either 1.5 or 0.5 mm apart, depending upon electrode model. Intraoperative stimulation can evaluate for untoward effects and confirm benefit to motor function, particularly for tremor. Programming of the DBS system(s) begins in the outpatient setting 2 weeks following implantation of the IGP(s). Optimization can take several programming sessions.

DBS surgery has shown minimal adverse affects, but do include the following:

- Perioperative mortality (death) in 0.4–1% of patients
- Intracranial bleeding (2.0–2.5%)
- Contralateral hemiparesis (1–6%)
- Seizures (<1.3%)

- Aphasia
- Ataxia
- Apraxia
- Abulia
- Paresthesias (1–2%) usually involving lips and/or finger tips
- Dysarthria (up to 20% of patients)
- Dysphagia

Mechanism of Action for DBS and Chronic High-Frequency Stimulation

Acute surgical effect

Evidence suggests there is a microlesioning effect lasting several days in the DBS surgical procedure. This microlesioning effect is suggested by the brief (hours to days) resolution of PD or ET motor symptoms without the DBS electrodes being attached to a power source.

Chronic high-frequency electrical stimulation

The physiological mechanisms accounting for the clinical benefits observed with chronic high-frequency stimulation remain to be fully understood (e.g., Hauser et al. 1995; Haslinger et al. 2003; Moro et al. 2002). Based on the observation that both DBS and lesions of the STN , GPi, and VIM thalamus are similarly effective in treating PD, dystonia, and ET, respectively; one might assume the therapeutic effect of chronic high frequency electrical stimulation is inhibitory. However, studies using several different modes of investigation now suggest DBS produces a net effect of stimulating output of the target nuclei. Unfortunately, a model based on increased activity of the target nuclei can not easily explain the therapeutic effect of STN DBS in reducing the cardinal motor manifestations of PD.

The mechanisms proposed to explain the therapeutic effects of DBS include: 1) Activation of inhibitory presynaptic axons terminating in the target structure, (2) depolarization blockade, (3) blockage of ion channels, (4) synaptic exhaustion, or (5) jamming (Benazzouz, Piallat, Pollak and Benabid 1995; Benazzouz, Gao, Ni, Piallat, Bouali-Benazzouz and Benabid 2000; Benabid, Benazzous and Pollak, 2002). These models must also account for the spread of electrical current with DBS, such that current decreases as the square of the distance from the active electrode contact (Rank, 1975; Tehovnik, 1996), but is generally thought to reflect a spherical electrical field with a radius of about 3 mm.

Theories 1 through 4 would require stimulation to have an inhibitory effect on target nucleus activity, which is generally not been observed. Rather, it appears DBS causes an alteration of the pattern of neural activity by "jamming" or interrupting abnormal neural signals responsible for many of the symptoms of dystonia

(Windels, Bruet, Poupard, Urbain, Chouvet, Feuerstein and Savasta 2000; Jech, Urgosik, Tintera, Nebuzelsky, Krasensky, Liscak, Roth and Ruzicka 2001; Vitek 2002; Anderson, Postupna and Ruffo 2003).

Hashimoto et al. (2003) showed chronic stimulation of the subthalamic nucleus in parkinsonian monkeys that resulted in a reduction in akinesia and rigidity was associated with an increased mean discharge of neurons in GPi, suggesting *activation* of glutamatergic subthalamic neurons projecting to GPi. There appeared to be a dose-response relationship between STN stimulation and GPi activity: With subtherapeutic stimulation parameters (no clinical benefit), there were nearly equal numbers of neurons with increased, decreased or unchanged activity. During therapeutic stimulation (clinical benefit), however, the proportion of neurons that increased their discharge rate significantly increased (Vitek 2002). Furthermore, the pattern of neural activity was stimulus locked with an increased regularity. As the mean discharge rate increased, parkinsonian symptoms paradoxically improved. Thus, a rate model does not explain the mechanism by which STN DBS improves PD symptoms. Instead, a regularization of the discharge pattern during stimulation supports the role of altered patterns of neuronal activity in the pallido thalamo-cortical circuit in the development of hypo- and hyperkinetic movement disorders.

Support for activation of the output from the site of stimulation has also been demonstrated by studies in normal monkeys (Anderson et al., 2003) and rats (Windels et al. 2000).

A differential effect of voltage (amplitude) and frequency (pulse rate) on neuronal circuitry and motor function is well recognized with DBS (Haslinger et al. 2003; Moro et al. 2002). In VIM DBS, higher voltage was found to result in a linear increase in cerebral blood flow to thalamic areas in close proximity to the microelectrode, while simultaneously increasing blood flow in a nonlinear fashion of neuroanatomically linked cortical areas beyond the area receiving DBS. Alternatively, increasing electrical frequency had a nonlinear effect on cortical blood flow around the microelectrode, while a more linear change in cerebral blood flow occurred in anatomically linked areas outside the immediate DBS stimulation area. Thus, despite advances in our understanding of the electroneurophysiology of high frequency electrical stimulation and advanced models for the neuroanatomical circuitry of the basal ganglia; the exact therapeutic mechanisms of DBS remain unknown. It has been proposed the variability in stimulation parameters among individuals with similarly staged movement disorders with similar targets of DBS stimulation is thought to reflect a variety of factors including individual variability in anatomy, disease pathology, and variations in surgical targeting. Table 19.6 provides a summary of general stimulation parameters for DBS for selected movement disorders and surgical targets.

Parkinson's Disease

DBS of the STN and GPi in PD has been demonstrated to be superior over best medical care at reducing the cardinal motor symptoms of PD and improving quality of life (Weaver et al. 2009; Fraix et al. 2006). While STN and GPi are

Table 19.6 Deep brain stimulation basic settings[a] for chronic high-frequency stimulation

	Amplitude (v)	Pulse width (μs) microseconds	Pulse frequency (Hz)
Parkinson's disease			
STN DBS[b]	2.0–3.0	60–90	130–185
GPi DBS	2.0–4.0	60–90	130–185
Essential tremor			
VIM DBS	2.0–7.0	100–300	80–140
Dystonia			
GPi DBS	2.2–7.0	200–400	90–190

[a]Optimal stimulation parameters for DBS have not been established. The values above reflect general settings, but stimulation parameters can vary widely from individual to individual
[b]Patients with more severe PD and gait disturbances have benefited from higher amplitude and lower frequency (e.g., 60 Hz) compared to younger patients

Rule of thumb: Dopamine-equivalent dose

100 mg standard levodopa = 140 mg sustained-release levodopa = 100 mL liquid levodopa = 10 mg bromocriptine = 1 mg pergolide = 5 mg ropinirole = 1 mg pramipexole = 10 mg selegiline

the most common targets, thalamic DBS was the original surgical target in patients with tremor-predominant PD. The STN has increasingly become a popular surgical target, as STN DBS allows for reductions in levodopa-equivalent dose not observed with GPi DBS. It may provide longer motor benefit, but has been associated with more reports of adverse mood and cognitive effects. The reduction in levodopa-equivalent dose varies, but a reduction of about 50% is common at 12 months post-operation compared to pre-surgical dosages. The reduction of medication is thought to account for the sometimes greater reduction in drug-induced dyskinesias reported for STN DBS compared to GPi DBS over the long term. Recently, STN DBS has demonstrated to be economically superior to medication-only treatment over the long-term (estimated time for economic benefit was 2.2 years of DBS vs medication), in part due to reduced medication costs (Fraix et al. 2006). GPi DBS may lose benefit for several cardinal features of PD after 5 years of chronic stimulation, including bradykinesia, postural instability, and in some cases tremor (Volkmann et al. 2004). Alternatively, GPi DBS has fewer reported adverse mood effects than reported for STN DBS, although many more published studies are available for STN DBS, and this may be a sampling bias (e.g., Okun et al. 2009, Parsons et al. 2006). While the debate continues regarding optimal surgical target sites, DBS has demonstrated a frontline treatment for appropriately selected patients with PD (Weaver et al. 2009).

Neurological (Primary) Outcome of DBS for PD

There is clear evidence-based support for DBS in the treatment of PD. The clinical effect of GPi DBS and STN DBS can be appreciated within seconds to minutes of placement of the DBS leads in the surgical theater. The initial benefit observed immediately following DBS surgery (thought to reflect a microlesioning effect) decreases after several days, and does not return until electrical stimulation is applied. The clinical effect of DBS on motor function is lost within seconds to minutes of stimulator deactivation, but is nearly always regained within seconds to minutes of reinitiating stimulation. Below, we detail the PD symptoms responsive to GPi and STN DBS within first year of surgery. Dysarthria, if present, can also be improved with STN DBS. In general, drug-induced dyskinesias, tremor, rigidity, and akinesia are affected more by DBS than is postural instability. Rates of improvement for postural instability vary widely, but improvement tends to be small.

A commonly used metric to quantify motor benefit of DBS in PD is improvement in UPDRS motor scores. Studies have generally found sustained motor benefit from STN DBS with UPDRS motor scores in the *on* DBS and *off* medication condition improved by 44–71% after 6 months, 56% after 12 months, 47–51% after 2 years, and 26–49% after 5 years compared with pre-operative off medication scores (e.g., Hamani et al. 2005). Similar results have generally been found for GPi DBS, at least for the first 3 years such that the *on* DBS and off medication condition improved by 56% after 12 months, 43% after 3 years, but only 24% after 5 years compared to pre-operative off medication scores (Volkmann et al. 2004). In a prospective comparison study, (Okun et al. 2009) reported no difference between STN DBS (29.9% reduction) and GPi DBS (26.6% reduction) in UPDRS motor scores at 7 months post-operation. However, subtest analysis found the STN DBS group exhibited significantly better rigidity scores compared to the GPi DBS group.

Figures 19.5 and 19.6 illustrate the current thought regarding DBS effects on the frontostriatal circuit in PD following GPi DBS and STN DBS, respectively. GPi

---

Rule of thumb: PD symptoms responsive to STN DBS*

- Tremor (40–81% reduction)
- Rigidity (40–63% reduction)
- Akinesia (40–52% reduction)
- Postural instability (27–50% improvement)
- "On–Off" Motor fluctuations
- "On–Off" dystonias
- Drug induced dyskinesias (41–94% reduction)

---

* *Note*: percentages derived from incomplete review of literature. Used as a guideline of treatment effect only.

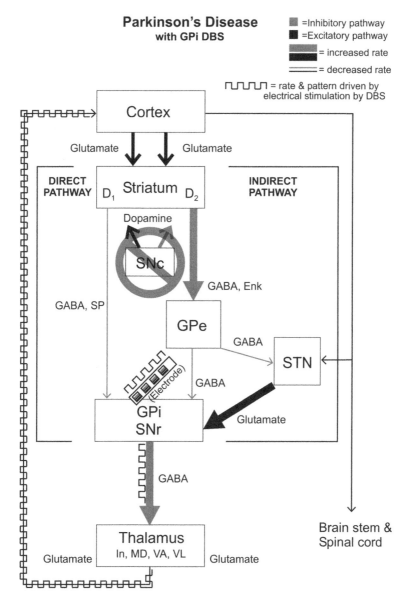

Fig. 19.5 Basal ganglia circuitry function in Parkinson's disease with GPi DBS. Note: D=dopamine recepter (1 & 2), Enk=Enkephalin, GABA=γ-aminobutyric acid, GPe=globus pallidus externa, GPi=globus pallidus interna, In=intralaminar nuclei of thalamus, MD=medial dorsal nucleus of thalamus, VA=ventral anterior nucleus of thalamus, VL=ventral lateral nucleus of thalamus, SP=substance P, SNc=Substantia nigra pars compacta, SNr=substantia nigra pars reticulata, STN=subthalamic nucleus

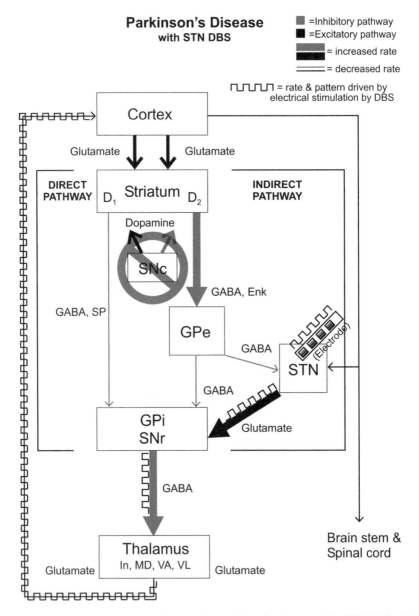

Fig. 19.6 Basal ganglia circuitry function in Parkinson's disease with STN DBS. Note: D=dopamine recepter (1 & 2), Enk=Enkephalin, GABA=γ-aminobutyric acid, GPe=globus pallidus externa, GPi=globus pallidus interna, In=intralaminar nuclei of thalamus, MD=medial dorsal nucleus of thalamus, VA=ventral anterior nucleus of thalamus, VL=ventral lateral nucleus of thalamus, SP=substance P, SNc=Substantia nigra pars compacta, SNr=substantia nigra pars reticulata, STN=subthalamic nucleus

> **Rule of thumb: PD symptoms responsive to GPi DBS***
>
> - Tremor (20–60% reduction)
> - Rigidity (20–60% reduction)
> - Akinesia (20–60% reduction)
> - Postural instability (20–40% improvement)
> - "On–Off" motor fluctuations
> - "On–Off" dystonias
> - Drug-induced dyskinesias (47–89% reduction)
>
> ---
>
> *Note*: percentages derived from incomplete review of literature. Used as a guideline of treatment effect only.

DBS is thought to result in a re-regulation of action by the GPi in PD. STN DBS in PD is thought to lead to re-regulation of action of the STN on the GPe/SNr.

General Surgical inclusion/exclusion criteria for DBS

Identification of patients with PD who are good DBS surgical candidates remains a very challenging and difficult determination. At present, there are no universally agreed upon exclusion criteria, but general selection criteria commonly proposed include:

- Patients must have obtained clear benefit from dopamine agonists (e.g., levodopa) in reduction of PD motor symptoms (minimum of 30% benefit from "off" state is sometimes used).
- No pronounced dementia, particularly dementia with fluctuation in mental status (fluctuating orientation and/or arousal) and/or presence of severe cognitive deficits. Presence of "mild to moderate" cognitive impairment is *not* a contraindication (e.g., Okun et al. 2004).
- Patients must not have history of moderate to severe traumatic brain injury or other comorbid neurodegenerative neurological disease
- Motor symptoms of PD are medication-refractory and result in significant disability.
- Mood symptoms, if present, are not predominate, and if present, are being treated.

The exclusion criteria below are less agreed upon (controversial, and may not preclude DBS surgery), but have been considered as a means to further minimize risk of neuropsychological and/or psychiatric adverse outcomes:

- Patient age at time of surgery less than 70 years old (however, a better criterion to use is the relative health, including neuropsychological function, of the patient rather than an age cut-off).

- Patients with severe mood disorder and/or history of suicide attempts
- Patients with significant premorbid history of gambling, risk-taking behaviors/ impulsivity, and/or hypersexuality.
- Patients with significant language deficits (marked dysarthria or severely impaired verbal fluency likely at increased risk for worse outcome)

The following exclusion criteria may not preclude DBS surgery at some point, but may preclude surgery until the condition is corrected/treated:

- Uncontrolled hypertension or other serious systemic disease
- Current systemic infection (e.g., UTI, pneumonia, etc.)
- Unwilling or unable to cooperate in post-surgical follow-up care, including attending DBS programming
- Abnormal blood clotting (e.g., high-dose Coumadin)

The selection process remains a largely qualitative one, and through 2009 there remains considerable variability in how the general patient selection criteria above are applied across surgical centers. However, a screening questionnaire, the Florida Surgical Questionnaire for PD or FLASQ-PD (Okun et al. 2004) was proposed as a means of providing a more quantitative approach to patient selection. The FLASQ-PD assesses surgical candidacy across 5 domains: (1) extent patients' symptoms meet criteria for the diagnosis of "probable" idiopathic PD, (2) potential contraindications to PD surgery ("red flags"), (3) general patient characteristics, (4) favorable/unfavorable characteristics, and (5) medication trials (response to medications). Higher scores reflect better surgical candidacy, ranging from the best surgical candidate score of 34 with 0 "red flags" to the worst surgical candidate score of 0 and 8 "red flags." A cut-off score of around 25 has been proposed for a good surgical candidate (and/or having any "red flags"), but there remains little validation of this measure. The "red flags" reviewed by (Okun et al. 2004) include many of the general contraindications above (no pronounced dementia, no severe psychosis, motor symptoms are responsive to levodopa, patients are disabled by PD) but also include some additional contraindications including:

1. Snout, grasp, root, or suck reflexes, or Myerson's sign being present
2. Presence of pronounced autonomic dysfunction within the first 1–2 years of onset of parkinsonian motor symptoms (not due to medications or previously chronic medical problem)
3. Ideomotor apraxia/alien hand sign being present
4. Supranuclear gaze palsy
5. History of wide-based gait early in the course of PD symptom presentation

The surgical inclusion/exclusion variables reviewed above reflect data and clinical experience in maximizing response to DBS while minimizing morbidity and mortality (e.g., Okun et al. 2004; Parsons et al. 2006; Weaver et al. 2009). However, predicting individual neuropsychological or psychiatric outcome from DBS for PD remains very challenging (e.g., Kalbe et al. 2009, Parsons et al. 2006; Smeding et al. 2009).

Neuropsychological Outcome following STN or GPi DBS in PD

Increased attention has been given to the post-acute cognitive and emotional effects of DBS surgery and chronic high-frequency electrical stimulation (e.g., Parsons et al. 2006; Woods et al. 2002). Post-operative neuropsychological outcome from DBS surgery and chronic high-frequency stimulation for PD has varied (see Parsons et al. 2006; Weaver et al. 2009; Woods et al. 2002 for reviews), but is generally regarded as cognitively 'safe' (e.g., Funkiewiez et al. 2004; Pillon et al. 2000; Parsons et al. 2006; Weaver et al. 2009). While some authors have observed post-operative declines in attention/executive, memory, and verbal fluency (Gaspari et al. 2006; Gironell et al. 2003; Morrison et al. 2004; Perozzo et al. 2001; Perriol et al. 2006; Saint-Cyr et al. 2000), other studies fail to show declines and some patients exhibit improvement (Gironell et al. 2003; Jahanshahi et al. 2000; Pillon et al. 2000). The pronounced variability in neuropsychological function continues to pose problems for predicting individual outcome, with some individuals exhibiting considerable decline in cognitive functioning, while others with similarly staged PD disease may exhibit little if any significant deterioration in cognitive functioning (e.g., Kalbe et al. 2009; Parsons et al. 2006; Smeding et al. 2009).

The most consistent neuropsychological change in group studies has been a significant decline in generative verbal fluency, with a meta-analysis (Parsons et al. 2006) of STN DBS reporting a moderate effect for semantic verbal fluency (Cohen's $d = 0.73$) and phonemic verbal fluency (Cohen's $d = 0.51$). A recent prospective randomized clinical trial found only a significant decline in phonemic verbal fluency and the Brief Visuospatial Memory Test delayed recall 6 months after STN DBS (Weaver et al. 2009). Decline in measures of verbal memory and attention/executive measures have been inconsistent (Parsons et al. 2006), and overall effect size changes generally small (Cohen's $d < 0.09$), but has been medium in some studies. Effect size reflects a standardized measure of the strength of association between variables or the magnitude of change in a variable over time. Cohen's d values between 0 and 0.3 are considered small, and generally meaningless. Values ranging from above 0.3–0.7 are considered medium. Effect sizes of 0.8 and greater reflect a large effect size, and are considered of particular importance. Table 19.7 summarizes effect size changes in neuropsychological functioning for patients undergoing STN DBS for PD. However, because a particularly challenging aspect of evaluating the effect of DBS on Parkinson's disease is the neurodegenerative process of PD on neuropsychological function, Table 19.8 provides the effect size change in neuropsychological measures among patients with PD who did NOT have surgery, and were treated only with medication. For example, review of Table 19.7 shows that the effect size (Cohen's d) change in verbal fluency for patients undergoing STN DBS ranges from 0.17 (small effect) to 1.02 (large effect), while review of Table 19.8 identifies verbal fluency performance change over time among patients with PD *not* undergoing surgery (reflecting medication controls) ranged from 0.05 to 0.17 (small effect size).

Table 19.7 Effect size change in scores for common neuropsychological measures following bilateral STN DBS for patients with Parkinson's disease

Test or neuropsychological domain	Effect size	Source
Attention and Concentration		
Wechsler Memory Scale – Revised		York et al. (2008)[a]
Digit Span (Total)	0.21[d]	
Attention and Concentration[b]	0.02	Parsons et al. (2006)
Executive Functions		
Wisconsin Card Sorting Test (WCST)		Higginson et al. (2009)
Categories (/6)	0.14[d]	
Perseverative Errors	0.16[d]	
Failure to maintain set	0.00	
Trail Making Test-B	0.32[d]	York et al. (2008)[a]
Executive Functions[b]	0.08[d]	Parsons et al. (2006)
Wisconsin Card Sorting Test (WCST)		Funkiewiez et al. (2004) [1 year/3 year][a]
Categories (/6)	[0.08/0.07][d]	
Total Errors (/128)	[0.04/0.02][d]	
Perseverative Errors	[0.08/n/a][d]	
Failure to maintain set	[0.12/0.12][d]	
Psychomotor Speed		
Trail Making Test-A	0.30[d]	York et al. (2007)[a]
Stroop Word Reading	0.43	
Psychomotor Speed[b]	0.22	Parsons et al. (2006)
Learning and *Memory*		
California Verbal Learning Test		Higginson et al. (2009)
Learning Trials 1–5	0.46[d]	
Long Delay Free Recall	0.17[d]	
Recognition Discriminability	0.30[d]	
Rey Auditory Verbal Learning Test (RAVLT, Rey, 1964)		Contarino et al. (2007) [1 year/5 year][a]
Total for Trials 1–5 (/75)	[0.06/0.22]	
Short delayed recall (/15)		
Long delayed recall (/15)	[0.14/0.41]	
Rey Auditory Verbal Learning Test (RAVLT, Rey, 1964)		York et al. (2008)[a]
Total for Trials 1–5 (/75)	0.28[d]	
Delayed Recall	0.44[d]	
Brief Visual Memory Test-Revised (Benedict, 1997)		
Total Learning	0.10	
Delayed Recall	0.00	
Verbal Functions/Memory[b]	0.21[d]	Parsons et al. (2006)
Grober and Buschke Test[c]		Funkiewiez et al. (2004)
Free recall	[0.03/0.12][d]	[1 year/3 year][a]

(continued)

Table 19.7 (continued)

Test or neuropsychological domain	Effect size	Source
Total recall	[0.08/0.09[d]]	
Delayed free recall	[0.29/0.14][d]	
Delayed total recall	[0.00/0.19][d]	
Recognition	[0.11/0.20][d]	
Language		
Verbal Fluency (semantic, category)	0.50[d]	Higginson et al. (2009)
Verbal Fluency (phonemic, letter)	0.35[d]	
Boston Naming Test	0.07[d]	
Verbal Fluency[b]	0.64[d]	Parsons et al. (2006)
Verbal Fluency (semantic, category)	0.73[d]	
Verbal Fluency (phonemic, letter)	0.51[d]	
Verbal Fluency (phonemic, letter)	[0.51/1.02][d]	Contarino et al. (2007) [1 year/5 year][a]
Verbal Fluency (semantic, category)	[0.48/0.44][d]	Funkiewiez et al. (2004) [1 year/3 year][a]
Verbal Fluency (phonemic, letter)	[0.17/0.23][d]	
Cognitive Screening		
RBANS Index Scores (Randolph, 1998)		Schoenberg et al. (2008)
Total Score	0.18	
Immediate Memory	0.32	
Visuospatial/Constructional	0.32	
Language	0.11	
Attention	0.05	
Delayed Memory	0.23	
RBANS Subtest Scores		
List Learning	0.22	
Story Memory	0.23	
Figure Copy	0.17	
Line Orientation	0.20	
Picture Naming	0.42[d]	
Semantic Fluency	0.49[d]	
Digit Span	0.19[d]	
Coding	0.04[d]	
List Delayed Recall	0.14	
Story Delayed Recall	0.45	
Delayed Figure Recall	0.49	
Dementia Rating Scale (Mattis, 1988)		Funkiewiez et al. (2004) [1 year/3 year][a]
Attention (/37)	[0.10/0.27][d]	
Initiation/Perseveration (/37)	[0.34/0.33][d]	
Construction (/6)	[0.50/0.35][d]	
Conceptualization (/39)	[0.05/0.15][d]	
Memory (/25)	[0.15/0.09][d]	
Total (/144)	[0.15/0.26][d]	

(continued)

Table 19.7 (continued)

Test or neuropsychological domain	Effect size	Source
Mood/Depression		
Beck Depression Inventory	0.34[e]	York et al. (2008)[a]
Beck Depression Inventory	[0.54/0.36][e]	Funkiewiez et al. (2004) [1 year/3 year][a]

RBANS Repeatable Battery of the Assessment of Neuropsychological Status. Eric Rinehardt, PhD, Department of Psychiatry and Neurosciences, University of South Florida, Tampa, FL, USA assisted in the development and formatting of this table

[a]Calculated Cohen's *d* based on mean and SD provided in report

[b]Based on TD Parsons' meta-analysis

[c]From Grober and Buschke (1987)

[d]Indicates cognitive deterioration following STN DBS

[e]Improved mood following STN DBS

The relative significance of any change in function must also be considered in terms of duration in which follow-up was completed (i.e., post-operation at 3 months, 12 months, 2 years, or 5 years) and framed by the neurodegenerative course of Parkinson's disease. Several studies have found initial cognitive declines at 3 months post-operative follow-up (e.g., verbal memory) that resolve and return to baseline levels at the 12 months post-operative follow-up (Pillon et al. 2000). Initially, it was thought STN DBS could be neuroprotective with slowing or reversal of the neurodegeneration process in PD. However, long-term follow-up studies have not found evidence of neuroprotection from DBS, with 5-year follow-up studies observing decline in cognitive function over time (e.g., Contarino et al. 2007; Krack et al. 2003), thought to be reflective of natural course of PD. Finally, PET changes reflecting continued neurodegeneration were observed among a group of patients following STN DBS (Hilker et al. 2005).

Estimating Outcome at an Individual Level

Risk factors for both acute and chronic cognitive decline and behavioral problems have been difficult to identify. However, emerging data suggest patients who are older, exhibit more cognitive or emotional problems and/or have smaller hippocampal volumes at baseline (presurgical assessment) are at greater risk for neuropsychologic morbidity (e.g., Parsons et al. 2006; Saint-Cyr et al. 2000; Smeding et al. 2009). Age has shown to be a risk factor for cognitive morbidity and increased risk of surgical adverse events (Derost et al. 2007; Ory-Magne et al. 2007; Saint-Cyr et al. 2000; Smeding et al. 2009). However, older patients can obtain similar motor benefit (Derost et al. 2007), and there is not a consistent relationship between age and cognitive morbidity (Ory-Magne et al. 2007). Emerging evidence-based neuropsychological data suggest the presence of dementia prior to DBS is generally associated with poor cognitive outcome and reduced quality of life (e.g., Smeding et al. 2009; but see Kalbe et al. 2009). Smeding et al. (2009) found advancing age,

Table 19.8 Effect size change over time on common neuropsychological measures for patients with Parkinson's disease only treated with medication (no surgery)

Test or neuropsychological domain	Effect size	Source
Attention and Concentration		
Wechsler Memory Scale – Revised		Muslimovic et al. (2009)[a]
Digit Span Forward	0.03	
Digit Span Backward	0.07	
Wechsler Memory Scale – Revised		Troster et al. (2007)[b]
Digit Span Forward	0.21[d]	
Digit Span Backward	0.15[d]	
Attention and Processing Speed[c]	0.01	Muslimovic et al. (2007)
Processing Speed		
Trail Making Test-A	0.82[d]	Muslimovic et al. (2009)[a]
Stroop Test (Word Reading)	0.39[d]	
Stroop Test (Color Naming)	0.29[d]	
Executive Functions		
Trail Making Test-B	0.43[d]	Muslimovic et al. (2009)[a]
Stroop Test (Interference)	0.17	
Wisconsin Card Sorting Test		Troster et al. (2007)[b]
Categories (/6)	0.20[d]	
Number of Trials (/128)	0.00	
Perseverative Errors	0.09[d]	
Failure to maintain set	0.34	
Mental Flexibility/Reasoning[c]	0.10[d]	Muslimovic et al. (2009)
Learning and Memory		
Rey Auditory Verbal Learning Test		Muslimovic et al. (2009)[a]
Total for Trials 1–5 (/75)	0.21[d]	
Delayed recall (/15)	0.23[d]	
Delayed recognition	0.34[d]	
Wechsler Memory Scale – III		Muslimovic et al. (2009)[a]
Faces Immediate	0.40	
Faces Delayed	0.07	
California Verbal Learning Test		Troster et al. (2007)[b]
Total Trials 1–5 (/80)	0.14	
List B (/16)	0.04[d]	
Short-Delay free recall (/16)	0.13	
Short-Delay cued recall (/16)	0.18	
Long-Delay free recall (/16)	0.08	
Long-Delay cued recall (/16)	0.15	
Long-Delay discriminability (%)	0.15	
Wechsler Memory Scale – Revised		Troster et al. (2007)[b]
Logical Memory I (/50)	0.12[d]	
Logical Memory II (/50)	0.07	
Memory[c]	0.29[d]	Muslimovic et al. (2007)

(continued)

Table 19.8 (continued)

Test or neuropsychological domain	Effect size	Source
Language		
Boston Naming Test (/60)	0.24[d]	Muslimovic et al. (2009)[a]
Verbal Fluency (semantic, category) Animals	0.09	
Verbal Fluency (semantic, category) Supermarket	0.09	
Verbal Fluency (phonemic, letter) COWAT	0.17[d]	
Verbal Fluency (semantic, category)	0.16[d]	Troster et al. (2007)[b]
Verbal Fluency (phonemic, letter)	0.06	
Verbal Fluency[c]	0.05[d]	Muslimovic et al. (2007)
Boston Naming Test (/60)	0.31[d]	Troster et al. (2007)[b]
Visuospatial Construction		
Visuoconstructive Skills[c]	0.32[d]	Muslimovic et al. (2007)
Cognitive Screening		
Dementia Rating Scale (Mattis, 1988)		Troster et al. (2007)[b]
Attention (/37)	0.30[d]	
Initiation/Perseveration (/37)	0.11	
Construction (/6)	0.50[d]	
Conceptualization (/39)	0.06[d]	
Memory (/25)	0.32[d]	
Total (/144)	0.19[d]	
Global Cognitive Ability[c]	0.40[d]	Muslimovic et al. (2007)
Mood/Depression		
Beck Depression Inventory (/63)	0.37	Troster et al. (2007)[b]

Eric Rinehardt, PhD, Department of Psychiatry and Neurosciences, University of South Florida, Tampa, FL, USA assisted in the development and formatting of this table

[a]Newly diagnosed with PD; Re-test period was 3 years; Calculated Cohen's *d* based on mean and SD provided in report[b]Re-test period was 17 months

[c]Based on D. Muslimovic's meta-analysis

[d]Decline over time

pre-surgical impaired attention, and poor response to L-dopa challenge at baseline to be significant predictors of cognitive outcome and quality of life 12 months after STN DBS. Alternatively, Kalbe et al. (2009) did not find neuropsychological function nor PET metabolism to be predictive of cognitive or metabolic outcome at 6 months post-operation. While all patients demonstrated a decline in right anterior cingulate metabolism following STN DBS, this did not correlate with cognitive outcome. Expectedly, post-operative PET metabolism did correlate with cognitive performance, such that decreased metabolism of the left frontal lobe and dorsal cingulum correlated with decreased verbal fluency and verbal memory. Another potential marker for individual risk is hippocampal volume, and smaller pre-operative hippocampal volume increased the risk of developing dementia an average of 25 months following STN DBS (Aybek et al. 2009). However, there was such overlap in hippocampal volumes between individuals who progressed to dementia after STN DBS and those that did not that no cut-off hippocampal volume could be identified. While individual outcome remains difficult to predict, some general statements can be made regarding reducing cognitive morbidity of DBS in PD.

General risk factors for increased cognitive morbidity following DBS in PD

1. Dementia
   - Pronounced deficits in attention/executive function have initial support as risk factor for poor cognitive outcome
2. Presence of Neuropsychological deficits due to other neurological insult (e.g., history of head injury, herpes encephalitis, etc.)
3. History of hallucinations unrelated to dopamine agonist treatment for PD (e.g., comorbid severe psychiatric disorder)
   - The presence of marked history of gambling, risk-taking behaviors, marked behavioral disinhibition and/or history of active suicidal ideation and/or suicidal attempt(s) are likely risk factors for increased risk of adverse psychiatric comorbidity.

Variables with limited and/or inconsistent support as risk factors for cognitive morbidity

1. Generally poor health status (very old age).
2. Smaller hippocampal volumes

The determination of dementia for a patient with severe PD is very challenging, and the establishment of a cut-off in neuropsychological impairment to determine surgical candidacy can be one of the most challenging aspects of a pre-surgical work-up. It is common for individuals with severe PD to present with neuropsychological deficits in attention/executive, memory, language, and visuoconstructional/visuoperceptual functions (e.g., Lezak et al. 2004). It is also common for these individuals to present with marked limitations in their ability to complete activities of daily living. However, careful clinical evaluation is needed to assess whether poor performances on neuropsychological measures and/or ability to complete activities of daily living is secondary to bradyphrenia and the motor disability associated with PD or dementia. In our opinion, we tend to be quite liberal (not excluding patients who present with some neuropsychological deficits) in the determination of surgical candidacy. We recommend a patient not undergo DBS only for cases in which neuropsychological functioning has been severely compromised, typically reflected by impairment across at least two cognitive domains by scores that fall two or more standard deviations (SD) below demographically matched peers. It is also important to evaluate patient's performance on tasks involving a motor component during "on" periods, as scores on many neuropsychological tests can be adversely affected by slowed psychomotor speed.

Group statistics (effect size) provide general guidance about risk to groups; they are less helpful in predicting outcome of a particular patient who is a candidate for DBS. Much more helpful information to predict individual outcome is evaluation of the proportion of a sample exhibiting a decline that is not due to measurement error and/or the disease process itself (reliable change). Relative risk ratios are also extremely helpful to identify the relative risk of a particular patient having a poor (or better) outcome based on specific risk factors.

Evaluation of the proportion of a study sample that exhibits a decline in function exceeding a specified threshold provides information to delineate the relative magnitude of the sample exhibiting a decline. As an example, similar effect sizes may be reported for two different domains, but for one domain, 100% of patients exhibited a small decline, while in another domain 40% of the sample exhibited a large decline. Clearly, the clinical implications of these two situations is very different. Decline is virtually certain to occur in the first domain (albeit small) while decline in the other domain may or may not occur, but will likely be large if it occurs. Table 19.9 provides the proportion of patients with PD who exhibited a change post-operatively following STN DBS on selected neuropsychological measures. As an example, 18% of patients declined on phonemic verbal fluency, 82% did not change, while no patient exhibited an improvement at 1 year post-operation. At 5 years post-operation, 54% of patients exhibited a decline in phonemic verbal fluency while 46% of patients' scores did not change. More variability in outcome was reported for verbal memory using the Rey Auditory Verbal Memory test (RAVLT; Rey 1964) delayed recall, in which 27% of patients declined, 46% did not change, and 27% exhibited improved performance 1 year after surgery (Contarino et al. 2007). Table 19.10 provides the proportion of patients with PD NOT having surgery (medication only) exhibiting change in performance over time on selected neuropsychological measures. Review of Table 19.10 semantic verbal fluency shows that performance did not decline over time, 97% remained stable, and 3% demonstrated improvement. However, the determination of what threshold a score must change in order to be meaningful has varied in the literature, with some authors reporting change beyond one standard deviation, while others have began to utilize reliable change indices (RCI's; Jacobson and Truax 1991; Temkin et al. 1999).

Reliable Change and Measurement of Change with DBS

The application of Reliable Change Indices (RCIs; Jacobson and Truax 1991; Temkin et al. 1999) has aided in the identification of meaningful change in neuropsychological functioning over time. Reliable Change Indices are developed from individuals with the population of interest (e.g., Parkinson's disease) who receive conservative medical management. The change in neuropsychological function over time would reflect the course of known or suspected neurodegenerative disease, had no (surgical) intervention beyond standard medication treatment been provided. Thus, comparison to a medication management group better allows for identifying change due to surgical intervention itself, rather than the effects of neu-

Table 19.9 Proportion (%) of patients with Parkinson's disease treated with STN DBS exhibiting reliable change[a] on selected neuropsychological measures

Test or neuropsychological domain	Decline	Stable	Improve	Source
Attention and Concentration				
Wechsler Memory Scale – Revised				Contarino et al. (2007) [1 year/5 year][a]
Digit Span Forward	[18/36]	[82/46]	[0/18]	
Digit Span Backward	[0/27]	[73/55]	[27/18]	
Wechsler Memory Scale – Revised				York et al. (2008)[a]
Digit Span (Total)	50	31.8	18.2	
Corsi's Block Span				Contarino et al. (2007)
Forward	[9/27]	[73/55]	[18/18]	[1 year/5 year][a]
Backward	[9/18]	[82/82]	[9/0]	
Executive Functions				
Wisconsin Card Sorting Test (WCST)				Higginson et al. (2009)
Categories (/6)	5.3	89.5	5.3	
Perseverative Errors	0	89.5	10.5	
Failure to maintain set	5.3	89.5	5.3	
Trail Making Test-B	57.1	19.0	23.8	York et al. (2008)[a]
Modified WCST (Jahanshahi et al. 2000)				Contarino et al. (2007) [1 year/5 year][a]
Categories (/6)	[11/22]	[89/67]	[0/11]	
Total Errors (/48)	[22/22]	[45/78]	[33/0]	
Perseverative Errors (/48)	[22/11]	[78/89]	[0/0]	
Wisconsin Card Sorting Test				Funkiewiez et al. (2004)[b]
Categories (/6)	14.9	76.1	9.0	
Total Errors (/128)	9.0	77.6	13.4	
Frontal Score (Benbadis et al.)	21.7	68.2	10.1	
Psychomotor Speed				
Trail Making Test-A	22.7	40.9	36.4	York et al. (2008)[a]
Stroop Word Reading	21.1	73.7	5.3	
Learning and Memory				
California Verbal Learning Test (Dellis et al. 1987)				Higginson et al. (2009)
Learning Trails 1–5	15.8	84.2	0	
Long Delay Free Recall	15.8	84.2	0	
Recognition Discriminability	5.3	94.7	0	
Rey Auditory Verbal Learning Test (Rey, 1964).				Contarino et al. (2007) [1 year/5 year][a]
Total Trials 1–5 (/75)	[18/18][a]	[64/73][a]	[18/9][a]	
List B (/15)	n/a	n/a	n/a	
Short-Delay free recall (/15)	n/a	n/a	n/a	
Long-Delay free recall (/15)	[27/36][a]	[46/55][a]	[27/9][a]	

(continued)

Table 19.9 (continued)

Test or neuropsychological domain	Decline	Stable	Improve	Source
Rey Auditory Verbal Learning Test (Rey, 1964)				York et al. (2008)[a]
Total for Trials 1–5 (/75)	30.4	52.2	17.4	
Immediate Recall	26.1	65.2	8.7	
Delayed Recall	13.0	87.0	0.0	
Brief Visual Memory Test-Revised (Benedict, 1997)				
Total Learning	13.6	68.2	18.2	
Delayed Recall	22.7	63.6	13.6	
Language				
Verbal fluency (semantic, category)	5.6	88.8	5.6	Higginson et al. (2009)
Verbal Fluency (phonemic, letter)	22.2	72.2	5.6	
Boston Naming Test (Kaplan et al., 2001)	0	100	0	
Verbal Fluency (phonemic, letter)	[18/54]	[82/46]	[0/0]	Contarino et al. (2007) [1 year/5 year][a]
Verbal Fluency (semantic, category)	33.3	63.8	2.9	Funkiewiez et al. (2004)[b]
Verbal Fluency (phonemic, letter)	16.0	79.7	4.3	
Cognitive Screening				
Dementia Rating Scale (Mattis, 1988)				Funkiewiez et al. (2004)[b]
Attention (/37)	16.7	75.7	7.6	
Initiation/Perseveration (/37)	19.7	71.2	9.1	
Total (/144)	7.6	90.9	1.5	

Eric Rinehardt, PhD, Department of Psychiatry and Neurosciences, University of South Florida, Tampa, FL, USA assisted in the development and formatting of this table
[a]Change reflects change > +/−1 SD
[b]Change reflects change > +/ −1 SD over 3 years post surgery

rodegenerative disease. While limited at this point, RCIs have become available for several commonly used neuropsychological measures for patients with PD (Troster et al. 2007; see also Rinehardt et al., 2010 for standardized regression-based values (SRBs)), and are summarized in Table 19.11. The RCI values are derived from a test–retest period of about 17 months. For example, a patient's score on the verbal fluency test must decline by more than 7 raw score points (or increase by more than 5 points) to reflect a change in performance that is not likely due to chance, measurement errors, and/or variables related to Parkinson's disease itself.

To account for the apparent variability in outcome from DBS for PD, several variables have been proposed that include: disease variables, methodological limitations of reported studies, and several moderator variables (Parsons et al. 2006). A disease variable that likely accounts for some intra-individual variability in

Table 19.10 Proportion (%) of patients with Parkinson's disease treated with levodopa and/or dopamine agonists exhibiting reliable change from presurgery to post-surgery on selected neuropsychological measures (From Troster et al. 2007)

Test or neuropsychological domain	Decline	Stable	Improve
Attention and Concentration			
Wechsler Memory Scale – Revised			
Digit Span Forward	1.6	95.1	3.3
Digit Span Backward	3.3	95.1	1.6
Executive Functioning			
Wisconsin Card Sorting Test (WCST)			
Categories (/6)	7.4	88.9	3.7
Total Errors (/128)	7.4	83.3	9.3
Perseverative Errors	3.7	92.6	3.7
Failure to maintain set	3.7	92.6	3.7
Learning and Memory			
California Verbal Learning Test (Delis et al. 1987)			
Total Trials 1–5 (/80)	1.6	91.8	6.6
List B (/16)	6.6	90.2	3.3
Short-Delay free recall (/16)	8.2	85.2	6.6
Short-Delay cued recall (/16)	4.9	83.6	11.5
Long-Delay free recall (/16)	8.2	86.9	4.9
Long-Delay cued recall (/16)	1.6	93.4	4.9
Long-Delay discriminability (%)	3.3	93.4	3.3
Wechsler Memory Scale – Revised (Wechsler, 1987)			
Logical Memory I (/50)	5.1	88.1	6.8
Logical Memory II (/50)	5.1	93.2	1.7
Language			
Verbal fluency (semantic, category)	0.0	96.6	3.4
Verbal Fluency (phonemic, letter)	3.4	89.8	6.8
Boston Naming Test (Kaplan et al. 2001)	3.2	96.8	0.0
Cognitive Screening			
Dementia Rating Scale (Mattis, 1988)			
Attention (/37)	3.2	93.5	3.2
Initiation/Perseveration (/37)	3.2	90.3	6.5
Construction (/6)	6.5	93.5	0.0
Conceptualization (/39)	6.5	87.1	6.5
Memory (/25)	6.5	91.9	1.6
Total (/144)	3.2	95.2	1.6
Mood/Depression			
Beck Depression Inventory	7.6	88.7	3.4

Note: $N=62$ older adults with PD; Change reflects RCI methodology determined by base rates; Test-retest about 17 month interval. Eric Rinehardt, PhD, Department of Psychiatry and Neurosciences, University of South Florida, Tampa, FL, USA assisted in the development and formatting of this table

Table 19.11 Reliable Change Indices (RCI's) of common neuropsychological measures for patients with Parkinson's disease treated with medication (From Troster et al. 2007)

Test or neuropsychological domain	90% RCI
Attention and Concentration	
Wechsler Memory Scale – Revised (Wechsler, 1987)	
Digit Span Forward	≤ –3.2, ≥ 2.2
Digit Span Backward	≤ –3.9, ≥ 3.3
Executive Functions	
Wisconsin Card Sorting Test	
Categories (/6)	≤ –3.3, ≥ 2.4
Number of Trials (/128)	≤ –46.0, ≥ 45.5
Perseverative Errors	≤ –24.8, ≥ 21.8
Failure to maintain set	≤ –2.5, ≥ 3.1
Learning and Memory	
California Verbal Learning Test (Delis et al. 1987)	
Total Trials 1–5 (/80)	≤ –10.0, ≥ 13.7
List B (/16)	≤ –2.9, ≥ 2.7
Short-Delay free recall (/16)	≤ 4.0, ≥ 4.9
Short-Delay cued recall (/16)	≤ –2.8, ≥ 4.0
Long-Delay free recall (/16)	≤ –2.9, ≥ 3.5
Long-Delay cued recall (/16)	≤ –3.1, ≥ 4.1
Long-Delay discriminability (%)	≤ –9.9, ≥ 3.0
Wechsler Memory Scale – Revised	
Logical Memory I (/50)	≤ –9.2, ≥ 7.4
Logical Memory II (/50)	≤ –9.3, ≥ 10.3
Language	
Verbal Fluency (semantic, category)	≤ –7.3, ≥ 5.7
Verbal Fluency (phonemic, letter)	≤ –12.7, ≥ 11.1
Boston Naming Test (/60) (Kaplan et al. 2001)	≤ –15.4, ≥ 10.5
Cognitive Screening	
Dementia Rating Scale (Mattis, 1988)	
Attention (/37)	≤ –8.4, ≥ 6.4
Initiation/Perseveration (/37)	≤ –5.2, ≥ 6.1
Construction (/6)	≤ –2.0, ≥ 1.1
Conceptualization (/39)	≤ –7.5, ≥ 7.0
Memory (/25)	≤ –6.3, ≥ 4.2
Total (/144)	≤ –19.8, ≥ 15.2
Mood/Depression	
Beck Depression Inventory (/63)	≤ –6.5, ≥ 10.7

Note: N = 62 older adults with PD; Test–retest about 17 months interval. Eric Rinehardt, PhD, Department of Psychiatry and Neurosciences, University of South Florida, Tampa, FL, USA assisted in the development and formatting of this table

outcome is the inter-individual variability in the neuropathological dysfunction associated with PD (Burton et al. 2006; Jahanshahi et al. 2003). Methodological problems of published data include small sample sizes, poor experimental power, variable patient inclusion/exclusion criteria, and lack of appropriate control groups (Parsons et al. 2006; Voon et al. 2006; Woods et al. 2002). Finally, authors have explored the potential effect of several variables as moderators of cognitive (and motor) outcome of DBS surgery that include patient age, presence of dementia, reductions in dopaminergic medication after surgery, and stimulation parameters (e.g., Francel et al. 2004; Haslinger et al. 2003; Parsons et al. 2006; Trepanier et al. 2000; Troster and Fields 2003; Schoenberg et al. 2008). A recent meta-analysis (Parsons et al. 2006) did not find a significant effect for moderator variables, including stimulation parameters on neuropsychological outcome. However, Francel et al. (2004) and Schoenberg et al. (2008) reported significant correlations between STN DBS stimulation parameters and neuropsychological measures. We believe data are too limited and study variability too great to rule out the differential impact of moderator variables on neuropsychological function. Clearly, changes in DBS stimulation parameters have a marked effect on motor function, and it seems unlikely neuropsychological function cannot be differentially affected by variation in stimulation parameters as well.

Neuropsychological Assessment

Neuropsychological assessment of patients with PD is complicated by several factors. First, most patients with PD who are candidates for surgical treatment will be older adults who present with various comorbid medical conditions that can affect neuropsychological functions. Second, many patients diagnosed with PD will often suffer from unpredictable fluctuations in motor functioning that range from pronounced akinesia and prominent (and painful) dystonias to nearly continuous and uncomfortable dyskinesias. Tremor may also markedly vary during the evaluation. Thus, the duration available to complete the neuropsychological evaluation is often time-limited, with administration of tasks having a strong motor component limited to periods when the patient's motor functioning is at his/her best. Finally, patients may also exhibit a host of related PD symptoms (see Section I), including autonomic problems and psychiatric complications of medication (e.g., visual hallucinations) and/or comorbid depression and/or anxiety. Suicidal ideation is not uncommon. Patients (and their family members) may have high expectations for the treatment benefit from DBS surgery, which can far exceed actual benefit derived from DBS. Risk of suicide should be evaluated, particularly if benefit from DBS does not meet the patient's expectations. The presence of medication-induced pathological gambling, hypersexuality, and other symptoms of hypomania must be assessed, and may increase risk of post-surgical hypomanic symptoms.

Recommended Neuropsychological Evaluation

In addition to providing pre-surgical screening for dementia and psychological complications as well as assessment for a patient's understanding of the relative benefits/risks of surgery, the neuropsychological assessment provides a baseline measure of the patient's pre-surgical functioning against which post-operative evaluations may be compared. Ideally, neuropsychological assessment will quantify general cognitive function (i.e., intellectual function), attention/executive, language (naming, semantic verbal fluency, phonemic verbal fluency), memory, visuoperceptual/visuoconstructional ability, and mood (see Table 19.12). A typical neuropsychological evaluation may total 2 to 4 hours, inclusive of clinical interview and test administration. Assessment of general cognitive ability is often abbreviated or a general index of cognitive functioning used [e.g., Dementia Rating Scale-2 (DRS-2; Jurica et al. 2002) total score].

Rule of thumb: Overview of DBS for Parkinson's disease

- Effective at reducing cardinal symptoms of PD
- Cognitively safe for carefully selected patients
- Psychiatric complications rare, but possible
- Neuropsychologic Evaluation:
  - Rule out prominent dementia
  - Assess for psychologic risk factors
  - May assist to assess patient's decision making/cooperate in follow-up
  - Minimal: attention/executive, verbal memory, verbal fluency and mood

---

Post-surgical follow-ups can be an important component of medical care for patients who have undergone DBS surgery, with a common practice being 3-month post-operative evaluations followed by a 1-year follow-up evaluation. The follow-up time frames noted above are guidelines, and adjustment of the post-surgical follow-up evaluation is often made for patients who require post-surgical rehabilitation and/or experience post-operative complications. Post-surgical neuropsychological battery should, ideally, use the same tests (alternate forms when available), but not all tests (e.g., estimating premorbid intellectual function) need to be repeated.

Essential Tremor

DBS for the treatment of ET has generally targeted the VIM nucleus of the thalamus. VIM DBS has been found to be remarkably effective treatment for reducing debilitating essential tremor in the contralateral limb.

VIM DBS is approved for ET as a unilateral surgical procedure. However, patients can subsequently have both sides implanted if bilateral benefit is important for functional improvement. Some patients may be offered bilateral DBS is necessary for functional improvement and surgical risks are deemed appropriate. The

Table 19.12 Possible neuropsychological battery for patients with PD whom are candidates for DBS

Neuropsychological test/task	Domain(s) assessed
North American Adult Reading Test (NAART) and/or Oklahoma Premorbid Intelligence Estimate – 3 (OPIE-3) and/or Wide Range Achievement Test – 4th Ed. (WRAT-4) Reading subtest	Premorbid General Cognitive Function
Repeatable Battery for the Assessment of Neuropsychological Status (RBANS; Randolph 1998). OR Dementia Rating Scale – 2nd edition (DRS-2; Jurica et al. 2002).	General neuropsychological function (includes screen of attention, memory, language, visuoperceptual/visuoconstructional)
Trail Making Test, parts A and B (Reitan 1958)	Attention/Executive
Stroop Color-Word Test (Golden 1978) or for more impaired patients: Go, No-Go task (Luria 1943)	Attention/Executive
In higher functioning patients, Wisconsin Card Sorting Test-64 (WCST-64, Kongs et al. 2000) or California Card Sorting Test (Delis et al. 1992)	Attention/Executive
Boston Naming Test (Kaplan et al. 2001)	Language
Verbal Fluency [Controlled Oral Word Association Test (phonemic fluency; Benton and Hamsher 1989; Spreen and Strauss 1998) and Category fluency]	Language
Repetition of simple and complex sentence.	Language
Comprehension (simple command, complex command)	Language
Read and Write (e.g., write sentence and read it)	Language
Sensory exam (see Chap. 4)	Sensory
Evaluation for Ideomotor Apraxia (See Chap. 4)	Motor/Motor Planning
Halstead Reitan Finger Tapping Test	Motor
Beck Depression Inventory – 2nd Edition (or Geriatric Depression Scale)	Mood/Psychological
Spielberger State-Trait Anxiety Inventory (or Beck Anxiety Inventory)	Mood/Psychological
SVT's or imbedded measures of task engagement	Task engagement and motivation

average age of patients undergoing VIM DBS for the treatment of ET is in the 50s, but patients aged from the 30s to the 90s have undergone surgery. Like DBS for PD, the surgical benefit of VIM DBS for the treatment of ET occurs within minutes of when the DBS is activated following IPG placement. The microlesion effect is reduced tremor contralateral to the electrode placement, which gradually decreases, resulting in return of the action tremor.

The surgical complication rate for Vim DBS is generally similar to that for GPi or STN DBS. It is more common for patients with ET to have unilateral DBS as compared to patients with PD, because bilateral STN implantation is required in PD in order to obtain the benefit of postoperative medication reduction with its concomitant reduction in medication-induced side effects. The decision to propose bilateral DBS for treatment of ET depends upon the degree of asymmetry of the disease and the patient's resultant functional disability.

ET Symptoms Responsive to VIM DBS

- Action or postural tremor of contralateral limbs
- Tremor involving the axial muscles (jaw and head) may also be ameliorated, although this is typically less significantly achieved as a benefit.

Surgical Inclusion/Exclusion Criteria

Unilateral VIM DBS is more common than bilateral VIM DBS. Surgical inclusion criteria are as follows:

- No pronounced dementia
- Patients should have failed to achieve satisfactory reduction of tremor from either primidone and/or propranolol. This may reflect either significant unilateral tremor that prevents completion of activities of daily living and/or bilateral involvement (one side will be more affected than the other in true ET). Response to medication may still occur, but require doses that produce intolerable side effects (e.g., sedation).
- Mood disorder, if present, is not predominant, and if present, is being treated.

Neuropsychological Assessment

See neuropsychological battery recommended in Table 19.12.

Neuropsychological Outcome following DBS in ET

Neuropsychological outcome from DBS for ET is generally considered good (e.g., Troster et al. 1999). Post-operative neuropsychological outcome from VIM DBS surgery and chronic high-frequency stimulation have limited data (see Troster et al. 1999).

Troster et al. found changes in neuropsychological function for VIM DBS to treat ET were small, with marked improvement in tremor. Like DBS for PD, the most consistent findings have been declines in semantic and phonemic verbal fluency and verbal memory. Table 19.13 provides effect size change for patients with ET having undergone unilateral VIM DBS. As expected, motor function with the dominant hand (target for unilateral VIM DBS) markedly improves (i.e., $d = 1.30$) for Grooved Pegboard test (Matthews and Klove, 1964), measures of cognitive function generally exhibited a small change (either improvement or decline), although changes in phonemic verbal fluency varied from small to large in effect size (i.e., $d = 0.77–0.20$). We are unaware of any published RCI values for patients with ET.

Estimating Outcome at an Individual Level

Risk factors for both acute and chronic cognitive decline and behavioral problems have been difficult to identify. However, data suggest patients with ET who are older and have more cognitive or emotional problems at baseline (pre-surgical assessment) are at greater risk. Increasing age had been considered a risk factor for cognitive morbidity, however, reports of individuals as old as 90 years have benefited from VIM DBS. While individual outcome remains difficult to predict, some general statements can be made regarding reducing cognitive morbidity from VIM DBS for patients with ET.

General risk factors for increased cognitive morbidity following DBS in ET

1. Presence of dementia
2. Neuropsychological deficits due to other neurological insult (e.g., history of head injury, encephalitis, etc.)
3. Presence of psychosis unrelated to medication.

Dystonia

Two randomized trials have established DBS is effective in treating primary generalized dystonias (Kupsch et al., 2006; Vidailhet et al., 2005). Furthermore, considerable data suggest DBS is effective in treating focal dystonias, particularly cervical dystonias (also known as spasmodic torticollis) (see Speelman et al. 2010 for review) generalized dystonias as well as focal dystonias, particularly cervical dystonias (also known as spasmodic torticollis). Both STN and GPi have been targeted.

Table 19.13 Summary of effect size change on common neuropsychological measures for patients with essential tremor following unilateral thalamic DBS

Test or neuropsychological domain	Effect size	Source
Attention and Concentration		
Wechsler Memory Scale – Revised (Wechsler, 1987)		Fields et al. (2003) [3 months/ 12 months][a]
Digit Span Forward	[0.14/0.16]	
Digit Span Backward	[0.20[c]/0.03]	
Wechsler Memory Scale – Revised		Troster et al. (1999)[b]
Digit Span Forward	<0.23	
Digit Span Backward	0.29[c]	
Visual Span Forward	<0.23	
Visual Span Backward	0.61	
Executive Functions		
Wisconsin Card Sorting Test		Fields et al. (2003) [3 months/
Categories (/6)	[0.07[c]/0.11]	12 months][a]
Trials to first category (/128)	[0.02/0.11]	
Perseverative Errors	[0.11/0.06]	
Failure to maintain set	[0.32[c]/0.11]	
Wisconsin Card Sorting Test		Troster et al. (1999)[b]
Categories (/6)	<0.23	
Trials to first category (/128)	0.28	
Perseverative Responses	0.28	
Perseverative Errors	0.28	
Stroop Neuropsychological Screening		
Color-Word Condition	<0.23[c]	
Psychomotor Speed		
Grooved Pegboard		Fields et al. (2003) [3 months/
Dominant Hand	[0.9/0.68]	12 months][a]
Non-dominant Hand	[0.06/0.01]	Troster et al. (1999)[b]
Grooved Pegboard	1.30	
Dominant Hand	<0.23	
Non-dominant Hand		
Learning and Memory		
California Verbal Learning Test		Fields et al. (2003) [3 months/
Total Trials 1–5 (/80)	[0.06/0.46]	12 months][a]
Short-Delay free recall (/16)	[0.18/0.38]	
Long-Delay free recall (/16)	[0.27/.039]	
Recognition hits	[0.66/0.71]	
Wechsler Memory Scale – Revised (Wechsler et al., 1987)		
Logical Memory I (/50)	[0.13/0.28]	
Logical Memory II (/50)	[0.39/0.54]	

(continued)

Table 19.13 (continued)

Test or neuropsychological domain	Effect size	Source
California Verbal Learning Test (Delis et al., 1987)		Troster et al. (1999)[b]
Immediate recall	<0.23[c]	
Short-Delay free recall (/16)	0.30	
Long-Delay free recall (/16)	0.46	
Recognition hits	0.57	
Recognition discriminability%	<0.23[c]	
Wechsler Memory Scale – Revised		
Figural Memory	<0.23	
Logical Memory I (/50)	0.30	
Logical Memory II (/50)	0.69	
Language		
Verbal Fluency (semantic, category)	[0.04/0.05][c]	Fields et al. (2003) [3 months/
Verbal Fluency (phonemic, letter)	[0.20/0.20][c]	12 months][a]
Boston Naming Test (/60)	[0.03[c]/0.28]	
Verbal Fluency (semantic, category)	<0.23[c]	Troster et al. (1999)[b]
Verbal Fluency (phonemic, letter)	0.77[c]	
Boston Naming Test (/60)	<0.23[c]	
Cognitive Screening		
Dementia Rating Scale		Fields et al. (2003) [3 months/
Attention (/37)	[0.21[c]/0.07]	12 months][a]
Initiation/Perseveration (/37)	[0.31/0.30]	
Construction (/6)	[0.72/0.7]	
Conceptualization (/39)	[0.10[c]/0.26]	
Memory (/25)	[0.28/0.14]	
Mattis Dementia Rating Scale		Troster et al. (1999)[b]
Attention (/37)	<0.23	
Initiation/Perseveration (/37)	0.25	
Construction (/6)	0.91	
Conceptualization (/39)	<0.23[c]	
Memory (/25)	0.41	
Total (/144)	0.43	

Note: Eric Rinehardt, PhD, Department of Psychiatry and Neurosciences, University of South Florida, Tampa, FL, USA assisted in the development and formatting of this table
[a]Calculated Cohen's *d* based on mean and SD provided in report
[b]Calculated Cohen's *d* based on t-score provided in report
[c]Indicates cognitive deterioration following unilateral thalamic DBS

GPi DBS is effective for medication-refractory focal and segmental dystonia affecting the cranial and cervical regions. STN DBS has also been reported to be effective for treating generalized and cervical dystonia. However, some patients with GPi DBS exhibited subtle motor disturbances in previously non-dystonic body regions (i.e., arms and legs), which have not been observed for patients with STN DBS used

Rule of thumb: Overview of DBS for essential tremor

- Effective at reducing tremor
- Cognitively safe for carefully selected patients
- Complications generally rare, but possible
- Neuropsychologic Evaluation:
  - Rule out prominent dementia
  - Assess for psychologic risk factors (psychosis not related to meds)
  - May assist to assess patient's decision making/cooperate in follow-up
  - Minimal: attention/executive, verbal memory, verbal fluency, and mood

for cranial and cervical dystonia. Greatest benefit is observed contralateral to the side of DBS, although some ipsilateral benefit is observed for both GPi DBS and STN DBS. DBS is usually not recommended for patients suffering from hemi-facial spasm. Hemifacial spasm is typically treated by botulinum toxin injections, or occasionally by microvascular decompression surgery, in which an arterial loop is often found impinging on the seventh cranial nerve at the nerve root entry zone on the brainstem surface. The impingement is resolved by placement of a Teflon pledget around the nerve. In addition to patients with primary (idiopathic) dystonias obtaining benefit from DBS, patients with secondary (i.e., traumatic, or medication-induced) dystonias also gain benefit from GPi DBS.

Surgical benefit of GPi DBS for dystonia is typically slow, with reduction in muscle dystonia not observed for weeks to months of chronic high-frequency DBS. Unlike DBS for PD or ET, DBS for dystonia will often not result in an immediate therapeutic benefit upon activation of the DBS system. The surgical complication rate in treating dystonia is similar to that for ET (see above).

Dystonic Symptoms Responsive to GPi DBS Include

- Primary Generalized Dystonias
  - Motor dystonia scores improved 21-95% (typically 60-70%)
- Cervical dystonias
  - Motor dystonia scores improved 43-76%
- Secondary Dystonias
  - Motor dystonia improvement less robust than primary or cervical dystonias overall (28-54%).

  BUT Myoclonus-Dystonia response has been excellent (100%) of cases have a dystonia score improvement of 75% or more.
- Muscle dystonias of contralateral limbs are more affected by unilateral GPi DBS, although significant ipsilateral effects are also noted.

- Dystonia involving the axial muscles (jaw, head, or back) may also be ameliorated, although to a lesser extent.
- Pain due to dystonic posturing reduced
- Secondary tremor improved

Surgical Inclusion/Exclusion Criteria

DBS of the GPi or STN can be offered to patients under a humanitarian device exemption as of 2009. Guidelines for surgical inclusion/exclusion criteria are provided below:

- As specified in general surgical inclusion/exclusion criteria above (i.e., correct diagnosis, dystonia is disabling and refractory to medications, no comorbid systemic diseases, etc.). Patients may have obtained some benefit from botulinum toxin
- No gross dementia, but neuropsychological deficits can be present. Patient's status post-moderate to severe traumatic brain injury with structural damage to basal ganglia structures have benefited from GPi DBS (Chang et al. 2002; see Speelman et al. 2010 for review). Pronounced dementia likely risk for worse outcome, but limited data at this time.
- Primary dystonia duration greater than 15 years associated with poorer outcome (Speelman et al. 2010).
- Mood disorder, if present, is not predominant, and if present, is being treated. Speelman et al. (2010) also highlight six (6) other factors to consider in selecting patients with dystonia: (1) is the target symptom the predominant source of disability; (ii) are there other possible sources of disability; (iii) is it possible that DBS will improve the target symptoms; (iv) what is the risk of surgical adverse events; (v) formulation of realistic goals for the rehabilitation of the patient; and (vi) the relation of the patient's own expectation from the surgery for these goals

Neuropsychological Assessment

See neuropsychological battery recommended in Table 19.12.

Neuropsychological Outcome following GPi DBS in Dystonia

Neuropsychological outcome from DBS for cervical dystonia is generally similar to that reported for DBS in PD, and is generally considered cognitively safe (e.g., Halbig et al. 2005; Vidailhet et al. 2007). however, there are less likely to be pronounced neurodegenerative neuropsychological deficits in idiopathic dystonia. Post-operative neuropsychological outcome from DBS surgery and chronic high-frequency stimulation for dystonia have limited data (Halbig et al. 2005; Vidailhet et al. 2007). Initial studies suggest neuropsychological outcome is similar to DBS procedures in general, with no marked decline in general cognitive function. However, significant declines (greater than 2 SD) have been reported for verbal fluency (phonemic and semantic) and, less often, memory scores. Table 19.14 provides effect size change following bilateral GPi DBS for patients with dystonia. Outcome has varied markedly, and overall small decline (Cohen's $d=0.29$) to moderate-sized improvement (Cohen's $d=0.64$) in semantic verbal fluency have been reported.

Table 19.14 Summary of effect size change on common neuropsychological measures for patients with dystonia following bilateral pallidal (GPi) DBS

Test or neuropsychological domain	Effect size	Source
Attention and Concentration		
Wechsler Memory Scale – Revised		Gruber et al. (2009)[a,c]
Digit Span Forward	0.08[b]	
Digit Span Backward	0.09[b]	
Wechsler Memory Scale – Revised		Halbig et al. (2005)[a]
Digit Span Forward	0.06	
Digit Span Backward	0.00	
Executive Functions		
Wisconsin Card Sorting Test		Vidailhet et al. (2007) [1 year/3 years][a]
Categories (/6)	[0.35/0.83]	
Perseverative Errors	[0.17/0.72[b]]	
Failure to Maintain Set	[0.44/0.97]	
Total Errors	[0.38/1.19]	
Wisconsin Card Sorting Test		Pillon et al. (2006)[a]
Categories (/6)	0.35	
Perseverative Errors	0.17	
Failure to Maintain Set	0.44	
Total Errors	0.38	
Trail Making Test-B	0.00	
Stroop Neuropsychological Screening		Halbig et al. (2005)[a]
Color-Word Condition	0.22[b]	
Trail Making Test-B	0.44	
Processing Speed		
Trail Making Test-A	0.28	Pillon et al. (2006)[a]
Trail Making Test-A	0.59	Halbig et al. (2005)[a]

(continued)

Table 19.14 (continued)

Test or neuropsychological domain	Effect size	Source
Learning and Memory		
Rey Auditory Verbal Learning Test		Gruber et al. (2009)[a,e]
Total for Trials 1–5 (/75)	0.46	
List B (/15)	0.85[b]	
Delayed recall (/15)	0.14	
Delayed recognition	0.26[b]	
Grober and Buschke Test		Vidailhet et al. (2007) [1 year/3 years][a]
Free recall	[0.34/0.47]	
Total recall	[0.53/0.59]	
Recognition	[0.41/0.41]	
Delayed free recall	[0.00/0.25]	
Delayed total recall	[0.40/0.46]	
Grober and Buschke Test[d]		Pillon et al. (2006)[a]
Free recall	0.34	
Total recall	0.53	
Recognition	0.42	
Delayed free recall	0.00	
Delayed total recall	0.41	
Rey Auditory Verbal Learning Test		Halbig et al. (2005)[a]
Total for Trials 1–5 (/75)	0.22	
List B (/15)	0.34	
Delayed recall (/15)	0.23	
Delayed recognition	0.19[b]	
Language		
Verbal Fluency (semantic, category)	0.64	Gruber et al. (2009)[a,e]
Verbal Fluency (phonemic, letter)	0.57	
Verbal Fluency (semantic, category)	[0.29[b]/0.02]	Vidailhet et al. (2007) [1 year/3 years][a]
Verbal Fluency (phonemic, letter)	[0.24[b]/0.10]	
Verbal Fluency (semantic, category)	0.29[b]	Pillon et al. (2006)[a]
Verbal Fluency (phonemic, letter)	0.24[b]	
Verbal Fluency (semantic, category)	0.20	Halbig et al. (2005)[a]
Verbal Fluency (phonemic, letter)	0.04	
Cognitive Screening		
Dementia Rating Scale		Gruber et al. (2009)[a,e]
Attention (/37)	0.00	
Initiation/Perseveration (/37)	0.31	

(continued)

Table 19.14 (continued)

Test or neuropsychological domain	Effect size	Source
Construction (/6)	0.00	
Conceptualization (/39)	0.40	
Memory (/25)	0.03	
Total (/144)	0.03[b]	
Mini Mental Status Exam	0.20	Pillon et al. (2006)[a]
Dementia Rating Scale		Halbig et al. (2005)[a]
Attention (/37)	0.31	
Initiation/Perseveration (/37)	0.45[b]	
Construction (/6)	0.00	
Conceptualization (/39)	0.22[b]	
Memory (/25)	0.46	
Total (/144)	0.52	
Mood/Depression		
Montgomery-Asberg Depression Scale	1.33[c]	Gruber et al. (2009)[a,e]
Beck Depression Inventory	[0.41/0.48][c]	Vidailhet et al. (2007) [1 year/3 years][a]
Beck Depression Inventory	0.41[c]	Pillon et al. (2006)[a]
Beck Depression Inventory	0.42[c]	Halbig et al. (2005)[a]

Note: Eric Rinehardt, PhD, Department of Psychiatry and Neurosciences, University of South Florida, Tampa, FL, USA assisted in the development and formatting of this table

[a] Calculated Cohen's *d* based on mean and SD provided in report

[b] Indicates cognitive deterioration following bilateral GPi DBS

[c] Improved mood following STN DBS

[d] From Grober and Buschke (1987)

[e] Study based on tardive dystonia rather than generalized dystonia

Estimating Outcome at an Individual Level

There are very limited data for neuropsychological outcome of DBS for dystonia. At this time, risk factors for neuropsychological decline are based on data derived from other patient populations in which DBS has been applied, particularly ET and PD. Thus, patients with dystonia who are older and have more cognitive or emotional problems at baseline (presurgical assessment) are at greater risk (e.g., Vidailhet et al. 2007). While individual outcome remains difficult to predict, some general statements can be made regarding reducing cognitive morbidity with DBS.

General risk factors for increased cognitive morbidity following DBS in dystonia

1. Pronounced dementia. However, several case reports world-wide have reported patients status-post moderate to severe traumatic brain injuries and later secondary

> **Rule of thumb: Overview of DBS for dystonia**
>
> - Effective treating generalized and focal dystonias
>   - Symptom relief may not be evident for months after DBS.
> - Cognitively safe for carefully selected patients.
> - Complications generally rare, but possible.
> - Neuropsychologic Evaluation:
>   - Document cognitive function.
>   - Patients with traumatic brain injury have shown benefit.
>   - Assess for psychologic risk factors (suicide/homicide ideation, psychosis not related to meds)
>   - May assist to assess patient's decision making/cooperate in follow-up
>   - Minimal: attention/executive, memory, verbal fluency, and mood

dystonia have reported good benefit from GPi DBS without significant cognitive morbidity (e.g., Chang et al. 2002; Speelman et al. 2010; Vidaihet et al. 2007).

2. Psychosis unrelated to medications

Tourette Syndrome

DBS for the treatment of Tourette syndrome (TS) motor symptoms (motor and phonic/sonic) tics refractory to medication has recently gained increasing attention (Visser-Vandewalle et al. 2003; Mink et al. 2006; Maciunas et al. 2007; Shprecher and Kurlan 2009). Surgical sites continue to be explored, but several sites have shown promise including several nuclei of the anterior ventral lateral thalamus. Other potential sites include the anterior limb of the internal capsule and the motor GPi or GPe. Visser-Vandewalle et al. (2003) first reported a clinical reduction to motor and phonic (vocal) tics for three patients with TS following bilateral TL thalamic DBS. In a recent trial, (Maciunas et al. 2007) found bilateral VL thalamic DBS was effective at significantly reducing motor and phonic tics using a randomized, double-blind, cross-over study in patients with medication refractory TS aged 18 and older. Four of the five patients with TS exhibited a significant decline in motor and sonic tics 12 months after DBS surgery. We found no significant benefit from unilateral DBS stimulation in reducing motor or phonic (vocal) tics. Symptoms may continue to show improvement for months with thalamic DBS. In addition to a reduction in motor and phonic (vocal) tics, our experience has shown significant reductions in symptoms of anxiety and depression at 3 months, and even greater improvement at 12 months post-surgery. The reduction in anxiety symptoms reflected significant declines in obsessive and compulsive disorder behaviors for several patients who presented with this co-morbid psychiatric condition.

In our experience, patients who exhibited a clear benefit from thalamic DBS in reducing motor and phonic (vocal) tics, exhibited a transient reduction in tics within minutes of electrode placement (microlesion effect).

Deep brain stimulation in the treatment of adults with refractory TS is a controversial issue (e.g., Mink et al. 2006; Riley et al., 2007). Mink and Colleagues (2006) recommended criteria for patient selection and trial design in evaluating the potential application of DBS for the treatment of TS. The criteria proposed by Mink and colleagues were similar to those employed by (Maciunas et al. 2007) (see below). However, notable differences are a rather arbitrary age cut-off of greater than 25 years old and more limited neuropsychological assessment that was proposed by Mink and colleagues. While early data have supported DBS as a treatment for refractory TS, a review (Shprecher and Kurlan 2009) asserted DBS surgical therapy continued to lack sufficient empirical validation.

The surgical complication rate in treating TS is low, and similar to that for PD, dystonia, or ET (see above).

Tourette Syndrome Symptoms Responsive to Thalamic DBS

- Significant reduction of motor tics varying from a low of 30% to a high of 95%.
- Reduction in vocal (sonic) tics varying from low of 30% to high of 95%.
- Comorbid psychiatric symptoms of obsessive compulsive disorder may also be reduced following thalamic VL DBS.

Surgical Inclusion/Exclusion Criteria

DBS for treatment of TS is not currently approved by the FDA, and can only be offered as an experimental procedure or with a humanitarian exemption. To date, mostly adult patients with refractory TS have been offered DBS, although one adolescent male was reported by Jankovic to have benefitted from GPi DBS. Our (Maciunas et al. 2007) surgical inclusion/exclusion criteria were as follows:

- Patients must have onset of motor and at least one vocal (sonic) tic before age 18.
- Patients must have been tried and failed two dopamine blockers. Response to medication may still occur, but require doses that produce intolerable side effects (e.g., sedation, hallucinations, motor dyskinesias).
- No pronounced neuropsychological impairment, although mild neuropsychological dysfunction was anticipated based on previous work in TS, including:
  - Neuropsychological deficits in fine motor, visuospatial/visuoconstructional and executive functions have been reported in patients with TS (Watkins et al. 2005). The neuropsychological deficits are more likely among patients with TS and comorbid obsessive-compulsive disorder (OCD) and/or attention

deficit-hyperactivity disorder (ADHD) (Watkins et al. 2005). Mild deficits in neuropsychological function did not exclude participants from DBS surgery.

- Motor and, if present, vocal (sonic) tics are refractory to medication.
- The extent, frequency, and/or severity of motor and/or vocal tics are of sufficient severity to limit the individual's quality of life as evidenced by difficulty completing functional activities (eating, bathing, dressing), impairment in ability to attend school/vocational training, and/or unable to work.
- Comorbid psychiatric syndromes of Obsessive-Compulsive Disorder or Attention Deficits-Hyperactivity Disorder (ADHD) are not predominate.

Neuropsychological Evaluation

While Mink et al. (2006) propose a limited neuropsychological battery be included in studies of DBS for the treatment of TS, our data suggest patients may experience considerable variability in neuropsychological outcome following bilateral thalamic DBS (i.e., Visser-Vandewalle et al. 2003; Maciunas et al. 2007). Thus, we argue insufficient data are available to propose limiting neuropsychological studies at this time. Our current neuropsychological protocol is provided in Table 19.15. Of note, we have found the Grooved Pegboard test (Mathews & Klove, 1964) to be too frustrating for patients with severe motor tics. Psychological and personality functioning should include assessment for hypomania symptoms, pathological gambling, and/or hypersexuality, as these behaviors have been reported with patients with TS following DBS. Use of alcohol, nicotine, and caffeine should also be reviewed. Postoperative evaluation at 3 months and at 12 months is ideal.

Neuropsychological Outcome following DBS in TS

Neuropsychological outcome from DBS for TS is, at this time, generally unknown. Data are limited to several case reports and the five patients reported in the prospective clinical trial by Maciunas et al. (2007; Schoenberg et al. 2009; Visser-Vandewalle et al. 2003). Post-operative neuropsychological outcome from bilateral VL thalamic DBS for TS have reported declines in verbal fluency (phonemic and semantic), memory (verbal and visual) and attention. However, some patients have not exhibited any meaningful change in neuropsychological functions (Visser-Vandewalle et al. 2003). Neuropsychological outcome from our study (Maciunas et al. 2007) was variable, and although most of the participants exhibited little change overall, small to medium effect size change declines were found for verbal fluency and memory (Schoenberg et al. 2009). However, one patient exhibited a marked decline in verbal memory. Overall, limited data suggest neuropsychological outcome from bilateral thalamic DBS has no pronounced cognitive morbidity, although at least one patient exhibited an unnoticed but marked decline in memory and verbal fluency.

Table 19.15 Proposed neuropsychological battery for DBS in patients with refractory Tourette's syndrome

Neuropsychological test/task	Domain(s) assessed
North American Adult Reading Test (NAART) and/ or Oklahoma Premorbid Intelligence Estimate – 3rd Edition (OPIE-3) and/or Wide Range Achievement Test – 4th Ed. (WRAT-4) Reading subtest	Premorbid General Cognitive Function
Wechsler Intelligence Scales. Wechsler Adult Intelligence Scale – 3rd Edition (WAIS-III, Wechsler 1997) selected subtests:	Current General Cognitive Function
a. Block Design	Attention/concentration
b. Matrix Reasoning	Visuoperceptual/Visuoconstructional
c. Digit span	Visual Reasoning
d. Similarities	Verbal Reasoning
Rey Auditory Verbal Learning Test (Rey 1964)	Verbal Memory
Rey-Osterrieth Complex Figure Test (Osterrieth 1944)	Non-verbal memory
Boston Naming Test (Goodglass et al. 2000)	Language
Verbal Fluency [phonemic and semantic (category) fluency tests]	Language
Repetition of simple and complex sentence.	Language
Comprehension of simple and complex instruction	Language
Read and Write (write sentence and then read it).	Language
Trails A and B (Reitan 1958)	Attention/Executive
Ruff Figural Fluency Test (Ruff et al. 1987)	Attention/Executive
Stroop Color-Word Test (Golden 1978)	Attention/Executive
Wisconsin Card Sorting Test – 64 (WCST-64; Kongs et al. 2000)	Attention/Executive
Continuous Performance Test-2nd Ed. (CPT-II; Conners, 2000)	Reaction time and Attention/Executive
Finger Tapping Test (Reitan, 1969)	Motor
Yale-Brown Obsessive-Compulsive Scale (Goodman et al. 1989)	Mood/Psychological
Beck Depression Inventory – 2nd Edition (Beck et al. 1996)	Mood/Psychological
Hamilton Rating Scale for Anxiety (Hamilton, 1959)	Mood/Psychological
SVT's or imbedded measures of task engagement	Task engagement and motivation

Estimating Outcome at an Individual Level

At this time, there are insufficient data to establish individual risk factors for cognitive decline.

Chapter Summary

This chapter provided a detailed review of the clinical presentation of movement disorders. Each movement disorder's neurological, neuropsychological, and behavioral features were presented. The next section reviewed therapeutic treatment, first medication and later neurosurgical treatments. The neuropsychological aspects of various medications were reviewed. Finally, considerable attention was provided to the neurosurgical treatments for movement disorders, including ablative therapies followed by DBS. Neuropsychological outcome from DBS was reviewed, both at a group and individual level.

References

Ameli, R., Snow, J., Rakocevic, G., et al. (2005). A neuropsychological assessment of phobias in patients with stiff person syndrome. *Neurology, 64*, 1961–1963.

American Psychiatric Association. (2000). *Diagnostic and statistical manual of mental disorders, DSM-IV-TR* (4th ed.). Washington: American Psychiatric Association.

Anderson, M. E., Postupna, N. et al. (2003). Effects of high-frequency stimulation in the internal globus pallidus on the activity of thalamic neurons in the awake monkey. *J Neurophysiol, 89*, 1150–1160.

Aybek, S., Lazeyras, F., Gronchi-Perrin, A., Burkhard, P. R., Villemure, J. G., & Vingerhoets, J. G. (2009). Hippocampal atrophy predicts conversion to dementia after STN-DBS in Parkinson's disease. *Parkinsonism & Related Disorders, 15*, 521–524.

Beck, A. T., Steer, R. A, & Brown, G. K. (1996) *Manual for the Beck Depression Inventory – 2nd Edition (BDI-II)*. San Antonio, TX: The Psychological Corporation.

Benabid, A. L., Benazzouz, A., Hoffmann, D., Limousin, P., Krack, P., & Pollack, P. (1998). Long-term electrical inhibition of deep brain targets in movement disorders. *Movement Disorders, 13*(suppl. 3), 119–125.

Benedict, R. D. (1997). Brief Visuospatial Memory Test – Revised. In:Psychological Assessment Resources, Lutz, FL.

Benabid, A. L., Benazzouz, A., & Pollack, P. (2002). Mechanisms of deep brain stimulation. *Movement Disorders, 17*(suppl 3), S73–4.

Benabid, A. L., Pollak, P., Louveau, A., Henry, S., & de Rougemont, J. (1987). Combined (thalamotomy and stimulation) stereotactic surgery of the VIM thalamic nucleus for bilateral Parkinson disease. *Applied Neurophysiology, 50*(1–6), 344–346.

Benazzouz, A., D. Gao, M. et al. (2000). Effect of high-frequency stimulation of the subthalamic nucleus on the neuronal activities of the substantia nigra pars reticulata and ventrolateral nucleus of the thalamus in the rat. *Neuroscience, 99*, 289–295.

Benazzouz, A., Piallat, B. et al. (1995). Responses of substantia nigra pars reticulata and globus pallidus complex to high frequency stimulation of the subthalamic nucleus in rats: electrophysiological data. *Neurosci Lett, 189*, 77–80.

Benito-León, J., Louis, E. D., Bermejo-Pareja, F., et al. (2006). Population-based case-control study of cognitive function in essential tremor. *Neurology, 66*, 69–74.

Benton, A. L., Hamsher, K., & de, S. (1989). *Multilingual aphasia examination* . Iowa City, IA: AJA Associates.

Benton, A. L., Hamsher, K., & Sivan, A. B. (1994). *Multilingual aphasia examination.* Iowa City: AJA Associates.

Boeve, B. F. (2007). Parkinson-related dementias. *Neurologic Clinics, 25*, 761–81.

Benedict, R. D. (1997). *Brief Visuospatial Memory Test – Revised. In:Psychological Assessment Resources*, Lutz, FL.

Broderick, M., & Riley, D. E. (2008). Parkinson's Plus Disorders. In S. A. Factor & W. J. Weiner (Eds.), *Parkinson's disease: Diagnosis and clinical management* (2nd ed., pp. 727–739). New York: Demos.

Burgess, P. W., & Shallice, T. (1997). *The Hayling and Brixton tests: Manual.* Bury St Edmonds: Thames Valley Test Company.

Bürk, K., Daum, I., & Rüb, U. (2006). Cognitive function in multiple system atrophy of the cerebellar type. *Movement Disorders, 21*(6), 772–6.

Bürk, K., Globas, C., Bosch, S., et al. (2003). Cognitive deficits in spinocerebellar ataxia type 1, 2, and 3. *Journal of Neurology, 250*, 207–211.

Burton, C., Strauss, E., Hultsch, D., Moll, A., & Hunter, M. (2006). Intraindividual variability as a marker of neurological dysfunction: A comparison of Alzheimer's disease and Parkinson's disease. *Journal of Clinical and Experimental Neuropsychology, 28*, 67–83.

Caballol, N., Martí, M. J., & Tolosa, E. (2007). Cognitive dysfunction and dementia in Parkinson disease. *Movement Disorders, 22*(S17), S358–S366.

Calderon, J., Perry, R. J., Erzinclioglu, S. W., Berrios, G. E., Dening, T. R., & Hodges, J. R. (2001). Perception, attention, and working memory are disproportionately impaired in dementia with Lewy bodies compared with Alzheimer's disease. *Journal of Neurology, Neurosurgery and Psychiatry, 70*, 157–164.

Chang, J.W., Choi, J.Y., Lee, B.W., Kang, U.J., & Chung, S.S. (2002). Unilateral globus pallidus internus stimulation improves delayed onset post-traumatic cervical dystonia with an ipsilateral focal basal ganglia lesion. *Journal of Neurology, Neurosurgery, and Psychiatry, 73*, 588–590.

Chiu, H. F. K., & Psych, M. R. C. (1995). Psychiatric aspects of progressive supranuclear palsy. *General Hospital Psychiatry, 17*, 135–143.

Collerton, D., Burn, D., McKeith, I., & O'Brien, J. (2003). Systematic review and meta-analysis show that dementia with lewy bodies is a visual-perceptual and attentional-executive dementia. *Dementia and Geriatric Cognitive Disorders, 16*, 229–237.

Como, P. G. (2001). Neuropsychological Function in Tourette syndrome. *Advances in Neurology, 85*, 103–111.

Conners, C. K. (2000). *Conners' Continuous Performance Test user's manual.* Toronto, Canada: Multi-Health Systems.

Contarino, M. F., Daniele, A., Sibilia, A. H., Romito, L. M. A., Bentivoglio, A. R., Gainotti, G., et al. (2007). Cognitive outcome 5 years after bilateral chronic stimulation of subthalamic nucleus in patients with Parkinson's disease. *Journal of Neurology, Neurosurgery and Psychiatry, 78*, 248–252.

Crawford, S., Channon, S., & Robertson, M. M. (2005). Tourette's syndrome: Performance on tests of behavioural inhibition, working memory, and gambling. *Journal of Child Psychology and Psychiatry, 46*, 1327–1336.

Delis, D. C., Kramer, J., Kaplan, E., & Ober, B. A. (1987). *California verbal learning test (CVLT) manual.* San Antonio: Psychological Corporation.

Delis, D. C., Squire, L. R., Bihrle, A., & Massman, P. (1992). Componential analysis of problem-solving ability: Performance of patients with frontal lobe damage and amnesic patients on a new sorting test. *Neuropsychologia, 30*, 683–697.

Derost, P. P., Ouchchane, L., Morand, D., et al. (2007). Is DBS-STN appropriate to treat severe Parkinson disease in an elderly population? *Neurology, 68*, 1345–55.

Dubois, B., Slachevsky, A., Pillon, B., Beato, R., Villalponda, J. M., & Litvan, I. (2005). "Applause sign" helps to discriminate PSP from FTD and PD. *Neurology, 64*, 2132–2133.

Dujardin, K., Defbvre, L., Duhamel, A., Lecouffe, P., Rogelet, P., Steinling, M., et al. (2004). Cognitive and SPECT characteristics predict progression of Parkinson's disease in newly diagnosed patients. *Journal of Neurology, 251*, 1432–1459.

Emre, M., Aarsland, D., Brown, R., et al. (2007). Clinical diagnostic criteria for dementia associated with Parkinson's disease. *Movement Disorders, 22*(12), 1689–707.

Eriksen, B. A., & Eriksen, C. W. (1974). Effects of noise letters upon the identification of a target letter in a nonsearch task. *Perception & Psychophysics, 16*, 143–149.

Evidente, V. G. H., Gwinn-Hardy, K. A., Caviness, J. N., et al. (2000). Hereditary ataxias. *Mayo Clinic Proceedings, 75*, 475–490.

Fahn, S., & Elton, R. L. (1987). Members of the UPDRS Development Committee: Unified Parkinson's Disease Rating Scale. In S. Fahn, C. D. Marsden, D. B. Calne, & M. Goldstein (Eds.), *Recent developments in Parkinson's disease* (Vol. 2, pp. 153–163). Florham Park: Macmillan Health Care Information.

Fraix, V., Houeto, J. L., Lagrange, C., Le Pen, C., Krystkowiak, P., Guehl, D., et al. (2006). Clinical and economic results of bilateral subthalamic nucleus stimulation in Parkinson's disease. *Journal of Neurology, Neurosurgery and Psychiatry, 77*, 443–449. on behalf of the SPARK Study Group.

Francel, P., Ryder, K., Wetmore, J., Stevens, A., Bharucha, K., Beatty, W. W., & Scott, J. (2004). Deep brain stimulation for Parkinson's disease: association between stimulation parameters and cognitive performance. *Stereotact Funct Neurosurg., 82*, 191–193.

Funkiewiez, A., Ardouin, C., Caputo, E., Krack, P., Fraix, V., & Klinger, H., et al. (2004). Long term effects of bilateral subthalamic nucleus stimulation on cognitive function, mood, and behaviour in Parkinson's disease. *J Neurol Neurosurg Psychiatry, 75*, 834–839.

Gaspari, D. D., Siri, C., Gioia, M., Antonini, A., Isella, V., Pizzolato, A., Landi, A., Vergani, F., Gaini, S. M., Appollonio, I. M., & Pezzoli G. (2006). Clinical correlates and cognitive underpinnings of verbal fluency impairment after chronic subthalamic stimulation in Parkinson's disease. *Parkinsonism Relat Disord., 12*, 289–295.

Gironell, A., Kulisevsky, J., Rami, L., Fortuny, N., Garcia-Sanchez, C., & Pascual-Sedano, B. (2003). Effects of pallidotomy and bilateral subthalamic stimulation on cognitive function in Parkinson's disease: A controlled comparative study. *Neurology, 250*, 917–923.

Gelb, D. J., Oliver, E., & Gilman, S. (1999). Diagnostic criteria for Parkinson disease. *Archives of Neurology, 56*, 33–39.

Golden, C. J. (1978). Stroop color and word test. In *A manual for clinical & experimental users*. Wood Dale: Stoelting.

Goodman, W. K., Price, L. H., Rasmussen, S. A., Mazure, C., Fleischmann, R. L., Hill, C. L., Heninger, G. R., & Charney DS. (1989). The Yale-Brown Obsessive Compulsive Scale: I. Development, use, and reliability. *Archives of General Psychiatry, 46*, 1006–1011.

Goodglass, H., Kaplan, E., & Barresi, B. (2000). *The Boston diagnostic aphasia examination (BDAE-3)* (3rd ed.). Philadelphia: Lippincott Williams & Wilkins.

Grafman, J., Litvan, I., & Stark, M. (1995). Neuropsychological features of progressive supranuclear palsy. *Brain and Cognition, 28*, 311–320.

Grimes, A., Lang, A. E., & Bergeron, C. B. (1999). Dementia as the most common presentation of cortical-basal ganglionic degeneration. *Neurology, 53*, 1969.

Grober, H., & Buschke, H. (1987). Genuine memory deficits in dementia. *Developmental Neuropsychology, 3*, 13–36.

Gruber, D., Trottenberg, T., Kivi, A., Schoenecker, T., Kopp, U. A., Hoffman, K. T., Schneider, G. H., Kuhn, A. A., Kupsch, A. (2009). Long-term effects of Pallidal deep brain stimulation in tardive dystonia. *Neurology, 73*, 53–58.

Halbig, T. D., Gruber, D., Kopp, U. A., Schneider, G. H., Trottenberg, T., & Kupsch, A. (2005). Pallidal stimulation in dystonia: Effects on cognition, mood, and quality of life. *Journal of Neurology, Neurosurgery and Psychiatry, 76*, 1713–6.

Hamilton, M. (1959). The assessment of anxiety states by rating. *British Journal of Medical Psychology, 32*, 52–55.

Hashimoto, T., C., Elder, M., et al. (2003). Stimulation of the subthalamic nucleus changes the firing pattern of pallidal neurons. *J Neurosci, 23*, 1916–1923.

Haslinger, B., Boecker, H., Buchel, C., Vesper, J., Tronnier, V. M., Pfister, R., Alesch, F., Moringlane, J. R., Krauss, J. K., Conrad, B., Schwaiger, M., & Ceballos-Baumann, A. O. (2003). Differential modulation of subcortical target and cortex during deep brain stimulation. *Neuroimage, 18*, 517–524.

Hauser R. A., Freeman T, B., Olanow C, W., (1995). Surgical therapies for Parkinson's disease; in Kurlan R (ed): *Treatment of Movement Disorders*. (pp 57–93) Philadelphia, PA: Lippincott.

Haslinger, B., Boecker, H., Buchel, C., Vesper, J., Tronnier, V. M., Pfister, R., Alesch, F., Moringlane, JR, Krauss, JK, Conrad, B, Schwaiger, M, Ceballos-Baumann, AO. (2003). Differential modulation of subcortical target and cortex during deep brain stimulation. *Neuroimage, 18*, 517–524.

Hamani, C., Richter, E., Schwalb, J. M., & Lozano, A. M. (2005). Bilateral subthalamic nucleus stimulation for Parkinson's disease: A systematic review of the clinical literature. *Neurosurgery, 56*, 1313–21.

Hellström, P., Edsbagge, M., Archer, T., et al. (2007). The neuropsychology of patients with clinically diagnosed idiopathic normal pressure hydrocephalus. *Neurosurgery, 61*(6), 1219–26.

Higginson, C. I., Wheelock, V. L., Levine, D., King, D. S., Pappas, C. T., & Sigvardt, K. A. (2009). The clinical significance of neuropsychological changes following bilateral subthalamic nucleus deep brain stimulation for Parkinson's disease. *J Clin Exp Neuropsychol, 31*, 65–72.

Hilker, R., Portman, A., Voges, J., Stall, M., Burghaus, L., van Laar, T., et al. (2005). Disease progression continues in patients with advanced Parkinson's disease and effective subthalamic nucleus stimulation. *Journal of Neurology, Neurosurgery & Psychiatry, 76*, 1217–1221.

Horsley, V., & Clarke, R. H. (1908). The structure and function of the cerebellum examined by a new method. *Brain, 31*, 45–124.

Jacobson, N. S., & Truax, P. (1991). Clinical significance: A statistical approach to defining meaningful change in psychotherapy research. *Journal of Consulting and Clinical Psychology, 59*, 12–19.

Jahanshahi, M., Ardouin, C. M., Brown, R. G., et al. (2000). The impact of deep brain stimulation on executive function in Parkinson's disease. *Brain, 123*, 1142–5.

Jahanshahi, M., Rowe, J., & Fuller, R. (2003). Cognitive executive function in dystonia. *Movement Disorders, 18*, 1470–81.

Jech, R., Urgosik, D., et al. (2001). Functional magnetic resonance imaging during deep brain stimulation: a pilot study in four patients with Parkinson's disease. *Mov Disord, 16*, 1126–1132.

Jurica, P. J., Leitten, C. L., & Mattis, S. (2002). *Dementia rating scale-2 (DRS-2). Professional manual*. Odessa: Psychological Assessment Resources.

Kaplan, E., Goodblass, H., & Weintraub, S. (2001). *The Boston Naming Test (2nd Ed.)*. Philadelphia: Lippincott Williams & Wilkins.

Kalbe, E., Voges, J., Weber, T., Haarer, M., Baudrexel, S., Klein, J. C., et al. (2009). Frontal FDG-PET activity correlates with cognitive outcome after SNT-DBS in Parkinson's disease. *Neurology, 72*, 42–49.

Kaplan, E., Goodglass, H,, & Weintraub, S., (2000). *The Boston Naming Test-Revised*. Philadelphia: Lea & Febiger, 2000.

Kawai, Y., Suenaga, M., Takeda, A., Ito, M., Watanabe, H., Tanaka, F., et al. (2008). Cognitive impairments in multiple system atrophy: MSA-C vs. MSA-P. *Neurology, 70*, 1390–1396.

Kelly, P. J., & Gillingham, F. J. (1980a). The long-term results of stereotaxic surgery and L-dopa therapy in patients with Parkinson's disease. A ten year follow-up study. *Journal of Neurosurgery, 53*, 332–337.

Kelly, P. J., & Gillingham, F. J. (1980b). The long-term results of stereotactic surgery and L-dopa in patients with Parkinson's disease. *Journal of Neurosurgery, 53*, 332–337.

Kongs, S. K., Thompson, L. L., Iverson, G. L., & Heaton, R. K. (2000). *Wisconsin card sorting test-64 card version. Professional manual*. Odessa: Psychological Assessment Resources.

Krack, P., Batir, A., Blercom, N. V., Chabardes, S., Fraix, V., Ardouin, C., et al. (2003). Five-year follow-up of bilateral stimulation of the subthalamic nucleus in advanced Parkinson's disease. *The New England Journal of Medicine, 349*, 1925–34.

Kupsch, A., Benecke, R., Müller, J., et al. (2006). Pallidal deep-brain stimulation in primary generalized or segmental dystonia. *New England Journal of Medicine, 355*, 1978–1990.

Kurlan, R., Cummings, J., Raman, R., et al. (2007). Quetiapine for agitation or psychosis in patients with dementia and Parkinsonism. *Neurology, 68*, 1356–1363.

Laitinen, L. V., Bergenheim, A. T., & Hariz, M. I. (1992). Leksell's posteroventral pallidotomy in the treatment of Parkinson's disease. *Journal of Neurosurgery, 77*, 487–488.

Leiguarda, R. C., Pramstaller, P. P., Merello, M., et al. (1997). Apraxia in Parkinson's disease, progressive supranuclear palsy, multiple system atrophy and neuroleptic-induced Parkinsonism. *Brain, 120*, 75–90.

Leroi, I., O'Hearn, E., Marsh, L., Lyketsos, C. G., Rosenblatt, A., Ross, C. A., Brandt, J., & Margolis, R. L. (2002). Psychopathology in patients with degenerative cerebellar diseases: A comparison to Huntington's disease. *American Journal of Psychiatry, 159*, 1306–1314.

Levy, M. L., Cummings, J. L., Fairbanks, L. A., et al. (1998). Apathy is not depression. *The Journal of Neuropsychiatry and Clinical Neurosciences, 10*, 314–319.

Lezak, M. D., Howieson, D. B., & Loring, D. W. (2004). *Neuropsychological assessment* (4th ed.). New York: Oxford University Press.

Lombardi, W. J., Woolston, D. J., Roberts, J. W., & Gross, R. E. (2001). Cognitive deficits in patients with essential tremor. *Neurology, 57*, 785–790.

Louis, E. D. (2009). Essential tremor as a neuropsychiatric disorder. *Journal of the Neurological Sciences*. doi:10.1016/j.jns.2009.08.029.

Maciunas, R. J., Maddux, B. N., Riley, D. E., Whitney, C. M., Schoenberg, M. R., & Ogrocki, P. O., et al. (2007). A prospective randomized double-blind trial of bilateral thalamic deep brain stimulation in adults with Tourette syndrome. *Journal of Neurosurgery, 107*, 1004–14.

Marras, C., & Tanner, C. M. (2004). Epidemiology of Parkinson's disease. In R. L. Watts & W. C. Koller (Eds.), *Movement disorders: Neurologic principles & practice* (2nd ed., pp. 177–195). New York: McGraw-Hill.

Massman, P. J., Kreiter, K. T., Jankovic, J., et al. (1996). Neuropsychological functioning in cortical-basal ganglionic degeneration: Differentiation from Alzheimer's disease. *Neurology, 46*(3), 720–726.

Matthews, C.G. & Klove, H., (1964) In: *Instruction manual for the Adult Neuropsychology Test Batlery*, University of Wisconsin Medical School, Madison, WI.

Mathuranath, P. S., Xuereb, J. H., Bak, T., et al. (2000). Corticobasal ganglionic degeneration and/or frontotemporal dementia? A report of two overlap cases and review of literature. *Journal of Neurology, Neurosurgery and Psychiatry, 68*(3), 304–12.

Mattis, S. (1988). *Dementia rating scale (DRS)*. Lutz, FL: Psychological Assessment Resources.

McKeith, I. G., Galasko, D., Kosaka, K., et al. (1996). Consensus guidelines for the clinical and pathologic diagnosis of dementia with Lewy bodies (DLB): Report of the consortium on DLB international workshop. *Neurology, 47*, 1113–1124.

McKeith, I. G., & Mosimann, U. P. (2004). Dementia with Lewy bodies and Parkinson's disease. *Parkinsonism & Related Disorders, 10*(Suppl 1), S15–8.

McMurtray, A. M., Clark, D. G., Flood, M. K., et al. (2006). Depressive and memory symptoms as presenting features of spinocerebellar ataxia. *The Journal of Neuropsychiatry and Clinical Neurosciences, 18*, 420–422.

Mink, J. W., Walkup, J., Frey, K. A., Como, P., Cath, D., DeLong, M. R., et al. (2006). Tourette Syndrome Association. Inc. Patient selection and assessment recommendations for deep brain stimulation in Tourette syndrome. *Movement Disorders, 21*, 1831–1838.

Mitchell, S. L., & Rockwood, K. (2001). Defining Parkinsonism in the Canadian study of health and aging. *International Psychogeriatrics, 13*(S1), 107–113.

Molloy, S. A., Rowan, E. N., O'Brien, J. T., et al. (2006). Effect of levodopa on cognitive function in Parkinson's disease with and without dementia and dementia with Lewy bodies. *Journal of Neurology, Neurosurgery and Psychiatry, 77*, 1323–1328.

Moreau, C., Defebvre, L., Destee, A., Bleuse, S., Clement, F., Blatt, J. L., et al. (2008). STN-DBS frequency effects on freezing of gait in advanced Parkinson's disease. *Journal of Neurology, Neurosurgery and Psychiatry, 71*, 80–84.

Moro, E., Esselink, R. J. A., Xie, J., Hommel, M., Benabid, A. L., Pollak, P. (2002). The impact of Parkinson's disease of electrical parameter settings in STN stimulation. *Neurology, 59*, 706–713.

Morrison, C. E., Borod, J. C., Perrine, K., Beric, A., Brin, M. F., Rezai, A., Kelly, P., Sterio, D., Germano, I., Weisz, D., Olanow, C. W., (2004). Neuropsychological functioning following bilateral subthalamic nucleus stimulation in Parkinson's disease. *Archives of Clinical Neuropsychology, 19*, 165–181.

Muslimovic, D., Post, B., Speelman, J. D., De Haan, R. J., & Schmand, B. (2009). Cognitive decline in Parkinson's disease: a prospective longitudinal study. *J Int Neuropsychol Soc, 15*(3), 426–437.

Muslimovic, D., Post, B., Speelman, J. D., & Schmand, B. (2005). Cognitive profile of patients with newly diagnosed Parkinson disease. *Neurology, 65*(8), 1239–1245.

Muslimovic, D., Schmand, B., Speelman, J. D., & De Haan, R. J. (2003). Course of cognitive decline in Parkinson's disease: A meta-analysis. *Journal of the International Neuropsychological Society, 13*, 920–932.

Noe, E., Marder, K., Bell, K. L., Jacobs, D. M., Manly, J. J., & Stern, Y. (2003). Comparison of dementia with Lewy bodies to Alzheimer's disease and Parkinson's disease with dementia. *Movement Disorders, 19*, 60–67.

Nuti, A., Ceravolo, R., Piccinni, A., Dell'Agnello, G., Bellini, G., Gambaccini, G., et al. (2004). Psychiatric comorbidity in a population of Parkinson's disease patients. *European Journal of Neurology, 11*, 315–320.

Okun, M. S., Fernandez, H. H., Pedraza, O., Misra, M., Lyons, K. E., Pahwa, R., et al. (2004). Development and initial validation of a screening tool for Parkinson disease surgical candidates. *Neurology, 63*, 161–163.

Okun, M. S., Fernandez, H. H., Wu, S. S., Kirsch-Darrow, L., Bowers, D., Bova, F., et al. (2009). Cognition and mood in Parkinson's disease in subthalamic nucleus versus globus pallidus interna deep brain stimulation: the COMPARE trial. *Annals of Neurology, 65*, 586–595.

Ory-Magne, F., Brefel-Courbon, C., Simonetta-Moreau, M., et al. (2007). Does ageing influence deep brain stimulation outcomes in Parkinson's disease? *Movement Disorders, 22*, 1457–63.

Osterrieth, P. A. (1944). Le test de copie d'une figure complexe. *Archives de Psychologie, 30*, 206–356.

Parsons, T. D., Rogers, S. A., Braaten, A. J., Woods, S. P., & Troster, A. I. (2006). Cognitive sequelae of subthalamic nucleus deep brain stimulation in Parkinson's disease: a meta-analysis. *Lancet Neurol, 5*, 578–588.

Perriol, M., Krystkowiak, P., Defebvre, L., Blond, S., Destee, A., & Dujardin, K., (2006). Stimulation of the subthalamic nucleus in Parkinson's disease: Cognitive and affective changes are not linked to the motor outcome. *Parkinsonism Relat Disorders, 12*, 205–210.

Pillon, B., Ardouin, C., Damier, P., Krack, P., Houeto, J. L., Klinger, H., Bonnet, A. M., Pollak, P., Benabid, A. L., & Agid, Y., (2000). Neuropsychological changes between 'off' and 'on' STN or GPi stimulation in Parkinson's disease. *Neurology, 55*, 411–418.

Randolph, C., (1998). *RBANS: Repeatable Battery for the Assessment of Neuropsychological Status – Manual*. New York, Harcourt Brace & Co.

Rampello, L., Buttà, V., Raffaele, R., et al. (2005). Progressive supranuclear palsy: A systematic review. *Neurobiology of Disease, 20*(2), 179–186.

Rank, J. B., (1975). Which elements are excited in electrical stimulation of mammalian central nervous system: A review. Brain Research, 98, 417–440.

Reitan, R. M. (1958). Validity of the trail making test as an indicator of organic brain damage. *Perceptual and Motor Skills, 8*, 271–276.

Reitan, R. M. (1969). Manual for the administration of Neuropsychological test batteries for adults and children. Indianapalis, IN: Author.

Richard, I. H., Frank, S., McDermott, M. P., et al. (2004). The ups and downs of Parkinson disease: A prospective study of mood and anxiety fluctuations. *Cognitive and Behavioral Neurology, 17*, 201–207.

Riley, D. E., Lang, A. E., Lewis, A., et al. (1990). Cortical-basal ganglionic degeneration. *Neurology, 40*, 1203–12.

Riley, D.E., Whitney, C.M., Maddux, B.N., Schoenberg, M.R., & Maciunas, R.J. (2007). Patient selection and assessment recommendations for deep brain stimulation in Tourette's syndrome. *Movement Disorders, 22*, 1366.

Román, G. C. (2003). Vascular dementia: Distinguishing characteristics, treatment, and prevention. *Journal of the American Geriatrics Society, 51*(5 Suppl Dementia), S296–304.

Ruff, R. M., Light, R. H., & Evans, R. W. (1987). The ruff figural fluency test: A normative study with adults. *Developmental Neuropsychology, 3*, 37–51.

Saint-Cyr, J. A., Trepanier, L. L., Kumar, R., et al. (2000). Neuropsychological consequences of chronic bilateral stimulation of the subthalamic nucleus in Parkinson's disease. *Brain, 123*, 2091–2108.

Schoenberg, M. R., Ogrocki, P., Maddux, R., Gould, D., Whitney, C., Riley, D., & Maciunas, R. J., (2009). Bilateral thalamic DBS for the treatment of refractory Tourette's syndrome. Paper presented at Adult Grand Rounds at the 29th Annual Conference of the National Academy of Neuropsychology, New Orleans, LA, October, 2009. *Archives of Clinical Neuropsychology, 24*, 432.

Schoenberg, M. R., Mash, K. M., Bharucha, K. J., Francel, P. C., & Scott, J. G., (2008). DBS stimulation parameters associated with neuropsychological function in STN DBS for refractory Parkinson's disease. *Stereotactic and Functional Neurosurgery, 86*: 337–344

Scott, R. B., Gregory, R., Wilson, J., et al. (2003). Executive cognitive deficits in primary dystonia. *Movement Disorders, 18*, 539–50.

Sharma, A., & Sorrell, J. H. (2006). Aripiprazole-induced Parkinsonism. *International Clinical Psychopharmacology, 21*(2), 127–129.

Shprecher, D., & Kurlan, R. (2009). The management of tics. *Movement Disorders, 24*, 15–24.

Smeding, H. M. M., Speelman, J. D., Huizenga, H. M., Schuurman, P. R., & Schmand, B. (2009). Predictors of cognitive and psychosocial outcome after STN DBS in Parkinson disease. *Journal of Neurology, Neurosurgery & Psychiatry*. doi:10.1136/jnnp. 2007.140012.

Speelman, J. D., Contarino, M. F., Schuurman, P. R., Tijssen M. A. J., & De Bie, R. M. A. (2010). Deep brain stimulation for dystonia: Patient selection and outcomes. *European Journal of Neurology, 17(s1)*, 102–106.

Spiegel, E. A., Wycis, H. T., Marks, M., et al. (1947). Stereotaxic apparatus for operations on the human brain. *Science, 106*, 349–350.

Spreen, O., & Straus, E. (1998). *A compendium of neuropsychological tests: Administration, norms, and commentary (2nd Ed.).* New York: Oxford University Press.

Tarsy, D., Vitek, J. L., & Lozano, A. M. (2003). *Surgical treatment of Parkinson's disease and other related movement disorders (current clinical neurology).* Totowa: Humana Press Inc.

Tehovnik, E. J, (1996). Electrical stimulation of neural tissue to evoke behavioral responses. *Journal of Neuroscience Methods, 65*, 1–17.

Temkin, N. R., Heaton, R. K., Grant, I., & Dikmen, S. S. (1999). Detecting significant change in neuropsychological test performance: A comparison of four models. *Journal of the International Neuropsychological Society, 5*, 357–369.

Trepanier, L. L., Kumar, R., Lozano, A. M., Lang, A. E., Saint-Cyr, J. A., (2000). Neuropsychological outcome of GPi pallidotomy and GPi or STN deep brain stimulation in Parkinson's disease. *Brain Cognition, 42*, 324–347.

Tröster, A. I., Fields, J. A., (2003). In D. Tarsy, J. L. Vitek, & A. M. Lozano (eds.). *Surgical Treatment of Parkinson's Disease and Other Movement Disorders.* Totowa, NJ: Humana Press. (pp. 213–40).

Troster, A. I., Fields, J, A., Pahwa, R., Wilkinson, S, B., Straits-Troster, K. A., Lyons, K., Kieltyka J., & Koller, W. C., (1999). Neuropsychological and quality of life outcome after thalamic stimulation for essential tremor. *Neurology, 53*, 1774–1780.

Troster, A. I., Woods, S. P., & Morgan, E. E. (2007). Assessing cognitive change in Parkinson's disease: Development of practice effect-corrected reliable change indices. *Archives of Clinical Neuropsychology, 22*, 711–718.

Victor, M., & Ropper, A. H. (2001). *Adams and Victor's principals of neurology* (7th ed.). New York: McGraw-Hill.

Vidailhet, M., Vercueil, L., Houeto, J. L., et al. (2005). Bilateral deep-brain stimulation of the globus pallidus in primary generalized dystonia. *N Engl J Med., 352*, 459–467.

Vidailhet, M., Vercueil, L., Houeto, J. L., Krystkowiak, P., Lagrange, C., Yelnik, J., et al. (2007). Bilateral, pallidal, deep-brain stimulation in primary generalised dystonia: A prospective 3 year follow-up study. *Lancet Neurology, 6*, 223–9.

Visser-Vandewalle, V., Temel, Y., Boon, P., et al. (2003). Chronic bilateral thalamic stimulation: A new therapeutic approach in intractable Tourette syndrome. A report of three cases. *Journal of Neurosurgery, 99*, 1094–1100.

Vitek, J. L. (2002). Mechanisms of deep brain stimulation: excitation or inhibition. *Mov Disord, 17* (s3), S69–72.

Voon, V., Kubu, C., Krack, P., Houeto, J., Troster, A. I., (2006). Deep brain stimulation: Neuropsychological and neuropsychiatric issues. *Movement Disorders, 21*, 305–326.

Volkmann, J., Allert, N., Voges, J., Sturm, V., Schnitzler, A., & Freund, H. J. (2004). Long-term results of bilateral pallidal stimulation in Parkinson's disease. *Annals of Neurology, 55*, 871–875.

Ward, J., Sheppard, J.-M., Shpritz, B., et al. (2006). A four-year prospective study of cognitive functioning in Huntington's disease. *Journal of the International Neuropsychological Society, 12*, 445–54.

Watkins, L. H., Sahakian, B. J., Robertson, M. M., et al. (2005). Executive function in Tourette's syndrome and obsessive-compulsive disorder. *Psychological Medicine, 35*, 571–82.

Weaver, F. M., Follett, K., Stern, M., Hur, K., Harris, C., Marks, W. J., Jr., et al. (2009). For the CSP 468 study group. Bilateral deep brain stimulation vs best medical therapy for patients with advanced Parkinson's disease. *The Journal of the American Medical Association, 301*, 63–73.

Wechsler, D. (1987). *Wechsler memory scale – revised (WMS-R) manual*. San Antonio: The Psychological Corporation.

Wechsler, D. (1997). *Wechsler Memory Scale – 3rd Edition (WMS-III) manual*. San Antonio: The Psychological Corporation.

Weintraub, D., & Hurtig, H. I. (2007). Presentation and management of psychosis in Parkinson's disease and dementia with Lewy bodies. *The American Journal of Psychiatry, 164*(10), 1491–8.

Windels, F., N. Bruet, et al. (2000). "Effects of high frequency stimulation of subthalamic nucleus on extracellular glutamate and GABA in substantia nigra and globus pallidus in the normal rat." *Eur J Neurosciences, 12*, 4141–4146.

Winikates, J., & Jankovic, J. (1994). Vascular progressive supranuclear palsy. *Journal of Neural Transmission, 42*, 189–201.

Wolters, E Ch, & Braak, H. (2006). Parkinson's disease: Premotor clinico-pathological correlations. *Journal of Neural Transmission Supplementum, 70*, 309–19.

Woods, S. P., Fields, J, A., Troster, A. I., (2002). Neuropsychological sequelae of subthalamic nucleus deep brain stimulation in Parkinson's disease: A critical review. *Neuropsychology Review, 12*, 111–126.

Woods, S. P., & Troster, A. I. (2003). Prodromal frontal/executive dysfunction predicts incident dementia in Parkinson's disease. *Journal of the International Neuropsychological Society, 9*, 17–24.

Wu, L. J., Sitburana, O., Davidson, A., & Jankovic, J. (2008). Applause sign in Parkinsonian disorders and Huntington's disease. *Movement Disorders, 15*, 2307–2311.

York, M. K., Dulay, M., Macias, A., Levin, H. S., Grossman, R., & Simpson, R., et al. (2008). Cognitive declines following bilateral subthalamic nucleus deep brain stimulation for the treatment of Parkinson's disease. *J Neurol Neurosurg Psychiatry, 79*(7), 789–795.

Chapter 20
Multiple Sclerosis and Other Demyelinating Disorders

Julie A. Bobholz and Shelley Gremley

Abstract Demyelinating disorders are characterized by the destruction of the myelin sheaths of the nerves following normal myelin development. Types of demyelinating conditions can be generally characterized as immune-mediated diseases, infection-mediated diseases, inherited disorders, and toxic disorders (see (Table 20.1; and Joy and Johnston, 2001, for detailed review). This chapter will begin with a brief description of demyelinating conditions representing these categories. Multiple Sclerosis (MS) is the most common demyelinating condition and will be the primary topic of this chapter.

Key Points and Chapter Summary

- There are many demyelinating disorders which have CNS effects including cognitive decline.
- Demyelinating disorders often have a variable course across individuals ranging from relatively mild and transient symptoms to severe, permanent and even deadly courses. The most common presenting complaints of demyelinating disorders are rapid motor and sensory changes (i.e., paresis, visual loss, acute sensory loss)
- The most common cognitive effect from demyelinating diseases is slowed processing speed and attentional deficits which often produce working memory declines; however, focal and diffuse deficits are not uncommon and include memory impairment, and may include changes in reasoning, personality and judgment.

(continued)

J.A. Bobholz(✉)
Department of Neurology, Medical College of Wisconsin, Milwaukee, WI, USA
and
Alexian Neurosciences Institute, Elk Grove Village, IL, USA
e-mail: jbobholz@mcw.edu

M.R. Schoenberg and J.G. Scott (eds.), *The Little Black Book of Neuropsychology: A Syndrome-Based Approach*, DOI 10.1007/978-0-387-76978-3_20,
© Springer Science+Business Media, LLC 2011

Key Points and Chapter Summary (continued)

- Cognitive deficits in demyelinating disorders are associated with the severity, duration and recurrence of the disorder.
- Emotional sequelae of demyelinating disorders are common and should be addressed and treated expeditiously. Untreated, these factors may compound physical and cognitive disability associated with the demyelinating disorder.

Table 20.1 Types of demyelinating conditions that resemble MS

Immune-mediated diseases
- Acute disseminated encephalomyelitis
- Systemic inflammatory or autoimmune diseases

Infection-mediated diseases
- Progressive multifocal leukoencephalitis
- Human T-cell Lymphotropic Virus Type 1

Inherited disorders
- Dysmyelinating disorders (leukodystrophies)

Toxic disorders
- Toxic optic neuropathy, subacute myelo-optic neuropathy

Acute disseminated encephalomyelitis (ADEM) is an immune-mediated demyelinating disease and can be a consequence of a vaccination or an infection, or without a preceding cause (Joy and Johnston 2001). The most common causes of postinfectious ADEM are upper respiratory tract infections and varicella but it can also occur after viral infections such as mumps, rubella, and influenza A and B. ADEM is characterized pathologically by widespread perivenular inflammation and demyelination. Onset of symptoms is sudden and can include monoplegia (paralysis of a single limb) or hemiplegia (paralysis on one side of the body), headache, delirium, lethargy, coma, seizures, stiff neck, fever, ataxia, optic neuritis, transverse myelitis, vomiting, and weight loss. This disorder occurs more often in children (average age around 5–8 years of age) than adults. The incidence rate is about 0.8 per 100,000 people per year. The average time to recover is 1–6 months, and 50–75% of cases experience complete recovery (Schwarz et al. 2001), although there can be recurrence of the disorder. Patients who recover tend to show good functional recovery from a neurologic standpoint; however, neuropsychological studies show that this apparent transient illness is associated with cognitive and social sequelae (Jacobs et al. 2004).

Rule of thumb: Acute Disseminated encephalomyelitis (ADEM)

- Immune-mediated demyelinating disease that typically involves sudden onset of symptoms and is characterized pathologically as widespread periventricular inflammation and demyelination.

Progressive multifocal leukoencephalitis (PML) is an infection mediated demyelinating disease and is a rare and usually fatal viral disease caused by the JC virus (Joy and Johnston 2001). Most patients die within 4 months of onset. It primarily occurs in people with severe immune deficiency (e.g., transplant patients on immunosuppressive medications, AIDS patients). This disorder is characterized by progressive inflammation of the white matter in the brain at multiple locations. Demyelination is most prominent in the occipital lobes and is a result of direct infection of oligodendrocytes, the cells responsible for creating the myelin sheath. Common symptoms include hemiparesis, aphasia, focal seizures, and visual disturbances.

Rule of thumb: Progressive Multifocal Leukoencephalitis (PML)

- Infection mediated disease that is rare and usually fatal. It is characterized as progressive diffuse inflammation of cerebral white matter.

Another infection-mediated demyelinating disease is Human T-cell Lymphotropic Virus Type 1 (HTLV-1) which is an RNA retrovirus that is sometimes associated with a syndrome called HTLV-1 associated myelopathy/tropical spastic paraparesis. Patients with this disorder have a progressive myelopathy, sensory disturbance, bladder dysfunction, and optic neuritis.

Inherited demyelinating disorders, or leukodystrophies, are characterized by specific gene defects that result in myelin abnormalities (Joy and Johnston 2001). More specifically, there is either inadequate myelin production or excess breakdown of myelin.

Toxic optic neuropathy is defined by visual impairment do to damage to the optic nerve. This disorder is uncommon and is primarily associated with specific medications, occupational exposures, or tobacco and alcohol abuse. It is more common in developing nations afflicted with famine. Subacute myelo-optic neuropathy (SMON) affects the peripheral nerves, spinal cord, and the eyes. SMON typically leads to a disabling paralysis, blindness, and sometimes death.

Rule of thumb: Toxic Optic Neuropathy

- Optic nerve damage that results in visual impairment and is typically associated with medications, chemical exposures, or tobacco/alcohol abuse.

Clinical Features of Multiple Sclerosis

Pathophysiology

Multiple Sclerosis (MS) is an autoimmune condition in which the immune system attacks the central nervous system (CNS), leading to demyelination. Neurons in both the brain and spinal cord can be affected. Demyelination occurs when a subset of lymphocytes, called T cells, get trapped in the brain due to loss of integrity of the blood–brain barrier (during infection or virus) and destroy oligodendrocytes (Joy and Johnston 2001). This eventually leads to thinning or complete loss of myelin, and this demyelinating process can cause changes in motor and sensory functioning, as well as changes in cognition.

Common Symptoms

The most common presenting symptoms of MS include sensory disturbance in limbs, visual loss, and motor disturbance (See Table 20.2 for summary). About 14% of MS begins with a polysymptomatic presentation (Olek 2005). Sensory changes that can occur in MS include numbness in one or more limbs, paresthesia (tingling) in the limbs, and L'hermitte's sign, which involves a sensation like an electric shock in the back and limbs on flexing the neck. Optic neuritis, internuclear ophthalmoplegia, diplopia, and changes in visual acuity can also occur in MS. Common MS-related motor changes include gait disturbance, weakness, balance problems, limb ataxia, slurred speech, decreased coordination, and swallowing difficulty. Spasticity, vertigo, pain, sexual dysfunction, and bladder disturbance are also common symptoms of MS. Paraparesis or hemiparesis can also occur.

Declines in cognitive functioning are a common symptom in MS, with about half of patients experiencing cognitive decline. The functions most frequently affected include abstract conceptualization, recent memory, attention, and information processing speed.

Epidemiology and Prevalence

The onset of MS usually occurs in early adulthood (between 20 and 30 years of age) and is two to three times more common in women. The peak age of onset for

Table 20.2 Most common presenting symptoms of MS (Adapted from Olek 2005)

Symptom	Frequency (%)
Sensory disturbance – limbs	30.7
Visual loss	15.9
Motor disturbance (subacute)	8.9
Diplopia	6.8
Gait disturbance	4.8
Motor (acute)	4.3
Balance problems	2.9
Sensory disturbance – face	2.8

most patients with MS is between 20 and 40 years of age but onset has been has been reported to be as early as 11 months of age and as late as 72 years of age. Onset is also estimated to be approximately 5 years earlier for women (Olek 2005). It is a disease that occurs predominantly in the caucasian population. The prevalence of the disease ranges between 2 and 150 per 100,000 depending on the country or specific population (Rosati 2001). MS is more common among persons of northern European heritage. It is also more common among people who live in northern latitudes during childhood. With this observation, MS is more common in the northern states of the USA. Climate, diet, geomagnetism, toxins, sunlight exposure, and infectious exposure have all been offered as possible reasons for these regional differences.

Disease Course

MS is distinguished by the clinical pattern of disease activity, with current practice typically considering the following categorization of disease activity:

(A) *Relapsing-remitting MS*: The majority of cases of MS begin with a relapsing–remitting course. This course is characterized by clearly defined relapses or unpredictable attacks followed by periods of remission or complete recovery of symptoms. Reported common triggers for relapse include warm weather, infections, and emotional and physical stress.

(B) *Secondary progressive MS*: Secondary progressive course describes around 80% of those with initial relapsing–remitting MS, who then begin to have neurologic decline between their acute attacks without any definite periods of remission. This course represents the most common type of MS.

(C) *Primary progressive MS*: This course type describes approximately 10% of individuals who never had remission after their initial MS symptoms. Decline occurs continuously without clear attacks. The primary progressive subtype tends to affect people who are older at disease onset. Progressive relapsing describes those individuals who, from the onset of their MS, have a steady neurologic decline but also suffer superimposed attacks. This is the least common of all subtypes.

(D) *Progressive relapsing MS*: This disease course is characterized as being progressive since the onset of the disease but with clear acute relapses, and the period between relapses is continued progression of the disease.

Disease course is also described as having two severity outcomes: benign, which is used to describe a course of MS that remains fully functional after 15 years after disease onset, and malignant, which characterizes a rapid progressive course resulting in significant disability or death.

Rule of thumb: Multiple Sclerosis (MS)

- MS can be difficult to diagnosis because the initial symptom(s) are variable, may remit quickly and the course is unpredictable.
- Diagnosis should be considered when individuals present with sensory/ motor symptoms without obvious etiology.
  - Loss of vision/blurred vision
  - Motor weakness
  - Numbness or parasthesias (tingling) of limb(s)
- Symptom onset commonly between 20 and 40 years old.
- Careful history taking is important to appreciate past episodes of sensory/ motor symptoms that may have reflected previous episodes of disease activity.
- Disease course
  - Relapsing–remitting – symptom attacks and remit with return to previous baseline level of function
  - Secondary progressive – decline between symptom attacks without return to previous baseline function
  - Primary progressive – no remission of symptoms after first symptom(s) onset
  - Progressive relapsing – progressive decline since first symptom onset, but have clear episodes of worse symptoms that remit, but function does not return to baseline

Etiology

While no definitive cause of MS has been found, there are many theories regarding the etiology of MS and various risk factors have been identified. A common hypothesis is that a viral infection or retroviral reactivation primes a susceptible immune system for an abnormal reaction later in life. Another theory is that MS is a response to a chronic infection, such as Epstein–Barr virus, spirochetal bacteria infection, Chlamydophila pneumoniae, and Vericella zoster (Joy and Johnston 2001). In addition to these environmental factors, genetics have also been found to help determine risk for developing MS. A 30% concordance rate has been found for identical twins, compared to 3–5% for dizygotic twins. Also, first-degree relatives of MS patients have a 2–5% risk of developing the disease, compared to the average risk in the general population of 0.1% (Vollmer 1999).

Neuropsychological Symptoms of Multiple Sclerosis

Cognitive Deficits

Approximately half of MS patients experience decline in neuropsychological functioning, and cognitive dysfunction is more common in men (Beatty and Aupperle 2002). While it has been found that MS-related cognitive decline tends to increase with disease duration (Amato et al. 2001), studies have shown signs of decline very early in the disease process. Lyon-Caen et al. (1986) found that 85% of patients with MS with less than 2 years disease duration demonstrated some degree of cognitive impairment. Progressive disease course (secondary progressive and primary progressive MS) is associated with more severe cognitive impairment (Huijbregts et al. 2004).

Neuropsychological domains most commonly negatively affected in MS include recent memory, processing speed, and working memory (see Table 20.3 for summary). Deficits in executive functioning, verbal abstraction, and visuospatial perception have also been found (Rao et al. 1991a; Amato et al. 2001; Amato et al. 1995; Ryan et al. 1996). While researchers had initially characterized cognitive dysfunction in MS as predominantly reflective of subcortical dysfunction, studies have clearly demonstrated cognitive difficulties that are not exclusively associated with subcortical dysfunction. Indeed, this growing appreciation of the breath of dysfunction in cognition is coinciding with neuroimaging and immunological research suggesting whole brain involvement in MS.

Memory decline has been reported in approximately 40–60% of MS patients (Rao et al. 1993). Episodic or explicit memory (e.g., remembering what one had

Table 20.3 Neuropsychological functions shown to be impaired in MS

Memory
- Episodic/recent memory
- Working memory

Executive functions
- Abstract reasoning
- Problem solving

Attention/concentration
- Sustained
- Complex

Language functions
- Verbal fluency
- Naming

Speed of information processing

Visuospatial skills

for lunch yesterday) tends to be most affected, while implicit, semantic, and autobiographical memory are typically spared. While debated in the past, memory disruption is likely associated with encoding, storage, and retrieval operations. Some studies have found that MS patients were able to successfully recall information after a delay when they were given more learning trials to ensure that the information was encoded (DeLuca et al. 1994; Demaree et al. 2000). However, another study found that MS patients demonstrated increased brain activation during the recognition trial of a memory task compared to controls, suggesting that retrieval processes are more affected by the disease (Bobholz et al. 2006).

Deficits in processing speed are the most common MS-related cognitive deficit and are thought to be the key component underlying other cognitive deficits in MS. Arnett (2004) found that fewer MS patients performed poorly on a measure of story memory when the stories were presented at a slower rate. Another study found that MS patients performed similar to controls on a working memory task when they were given adequate time to process the test stimuli (Demaree et al. 1999). Deficits in processing speed can be seen in both visual and auditory tests.

Working memory deficits can also be seen in individuals with MS (Rao et al. 1993). Working memory is generally thought to be the ability to hold information in memory for a short period, while manipulating that information. Deficits in working memory are thought to be related to deficits in processing speed since these functions related to one another.

Rather consistently, cross-sectional research has found that nearly half of all MS patients show deficits on neuropsychological testing. Longitudinal research suggested that cognitive dysfunction does have some correlation with disease duration but is also associated with disease course and degree of MR abnormality including lesion burden and atrophy.

Rule of thumb: Common neuropsychological deficits in MS

- Recent memory
- Processing speed
- Working memory

Deficits that may also occur:

- Executive function/verbal abstraction, and
- Visuospatial perception.

Impact of Cognitive Dysfunction in MS

Research has shown that the presence of cognitive dysfunction can have significant impact on daily living. The rates of unemployment are high in MS, with some estimates as high as 70–80% just 5 years after diagnosis. Furthermore, studies have shown that individuals who have cognitive dysfunction are more likely to have problems with employment compared to those without cognitive deficits (Rao et al. 1991a, b; Beatty et al. 1995). Recent studies have also raised concern regarding driving safety in MS patients with cognitive dysfunction. Cognitive dysfunction has been associated with poorer performance on computerized assessment of driving skill and accident rates (Shawaryn et al. 2002; Kotterba et al. 2003; Schultheis et al. 2002).

Correlates with Neuropsychological Deficits

Some general trends have become apparent in the research examining correlates of neuropsychological dysfunction. Disease course tends to be associated with severity of neuropsychological dysfunction, with primary progressive and secondary progressive disease course typically performing more poorly than patients with relapsing–remitting MS. Disease duration is also a relatively strong correlate of neuropsychological dysfunction, with longer periods of disease associated with increasing cognitive deficits (Thorton and Naftail 1997).

While MS more commonly affects women, MS-related cognitive dysfunction tends to occur more frequently in men (Beatty and Aupperle 2002).

Fatigue is thought to be the most common symptom associated with MS, and can significantly impact performance on neuropsychological measures. In fact, MS patients performance on cognitive measures that were repeated worsened following an effortful cognitive task, while controls demonstrated the inverse relationship, such that their performance improved on cognitive measures that were repeated (Krupp and Elkins 2000).

Sleep disturbance is another symptom of MS that can act as a potential correlate of MS-related neuropsychological dysfunction. Research has shown that poor sleep is twice as prevalent in MS patients compared to controls and can be due to a variety of factors, including pain, depression, medication side effects, and nocturnal movement disorders (Lobentanz et al. 2004).

Acute, sub-acute and chronic pain, including Trigeminal neuralgia, tonic spasms, continuous dysesthetic pain, acute radicular pain, and optic neuritis, muscle cramps, headache, and back pain may interfere with test performance. Approximately 55–65% of MS patients experience pain, and cognitive complaints are common among individuals with chronic pain (Roth et al. 2005). Currently, the relationship between pain in MS and cognitive is not well researched, but likely has some impact on performance on cognitive testing and day-to-day functioning. Worth noting is that disease modifying medications typically are not associated with cognitive side effects.

Mood disturbance is another common symptom in MS. There is an estimated lifetime prevalence of 50% of major depression. Brain lesions and psychosocial issues are considered risk factors for mood disturbance, while physical disability does not appear to be closely associated with depression (Goldstein Consensus Group 2005). Mood disturbance has also been found to be associated with cognitive deficits.

Arnett et al. (1999) found that deficits in attention, executive functioning, and processing speed were related to changes in affect and personality, suggesting that mood disturbance may be due to a disruption of frontal-subcortical pathways. Fortunately, mood disturbance associated with MS can be treated. Cognitive Behavioral Therapy (CBT) has been found to have a similar, positive effect to antidepressant medications (Mohr et al. 2001), and both treatments have been found to help improve quality of life (Hart et al. 2005).

Earlier studies examining neuroanatomical variables with standard magnetic resonance imaging (MRI) typically found moderate correlations between cognitive performances on T2 lesion burden. More recent imaging research has demonstrated greater magnitude of correlation between measures of atrophy as measured by third ventricle dilation and cognitive dysfunction. Furthermore, this association appears to be strongly related to thalamic and neocortical atrophy.

Many MS patients remain cognitive intact, despite having positive MR findings. Functional MRI (fMRI) research has shown considerable evidence to suggest that, to some extent, functional reorganization or recruitment of cortical regions occur during cognitive, motor, and visual challenges.

Evidence-Based Neuropsychology: Predicting Outcome

Cognitive dysfunction is a symptom of MS that is typically not a primary feature of the disease used for diagnosis. However, patients often present with cognitive dysfunction as their initial disease symptom and, for some, this can remain their primary symptom throughout their disease. In MS, neuropsychological evidence-based practice/research is in its early stages and has potential to address outcome variables related to disease progression, the impact the disease has on quality of life and day-to-day functions such as employment status, and the effects of treatments (Chelune, 2010). Chelune and Stone (2005a) performed a study that was designed to determine if processing speed was useful in distinguishing patients with relapsing–remitting MS from those with secondary progressive MS. The authors examined performances on three measures of processing speed and found the WAIS-III Processing Speed Index (PSI) was most useful in differentiating the two MS groups. Using contingency table analyses, the authors determined that individuals in their sample were nearly 6 times more likely to have secondary progressive MS, rather than relapsing–remitting MS, if their PSI T-score was 36 or less. Chelune and Stone (2005b) also reported data that showed patients with secondary progressive MS were more likely than patients with relapsing–remitting to perform below the 5th percentile on WAIS-WMS-III factors, with reported odds ratios ranging between 2.7 and 8.3. Further analysis of these data also showed that there was slightly greater risk for men to have lower auditory memory than women (odds ratio of 1:76) but that sex differences were not apparent with the other factors examined. This study also showed an interaction between sex and disease course, as men were found to be 5.2 times more likely than women to have verbal memory deficits if they had secondary progressive MS.

Assessment of Neuropsychological Deficits in MS

The assessment of cognitive functioning varies depending on the reason the MS patient is being referred for neuropsychological evaluation. Often, MS patients are referred for an evaluation in order to establish a baseline before treatment and to monitor disease progression. At other times, an evaluation is helpful in determining the reasons for difficulties at work and/or home, and in determining whether changes in treatment approach are necessary. Many times, a neuropsychological evaluation is needed to determine one's work capacity and/or application for disability. Therefore, the length and depth of the evaluation may differ based on the purpose of the assessment. While some of these referral questions require comprehensive evaluation to best characterize one's cognitive status, patients with MS often fatigue easily and have difficulty tolerating testing sessions that last several hours. Comprehensive test batteries are not always necessary to answer referral questions.

In 2001, an international panel was convened in order to develop an ideal, minimal record of neuropsychological function (Benedict et al. 2002). The panel developed a 90-minute neuropsychological battery called the Minimal Assessment of Cognitive Function in MS (MACFIMS). The MACFIMS is composed of seven tests designed to assess the cognitive domains commonly affected in MS (see Table 20.4). The tests included in this consensus battery are the Paced Auditory Serial Addition Task (working memory/processing speed), Symbol Digit Modalities Test (processing speed), California Verbal Learning Test-II (verbal memory), Brief Visual Memory Test-Revised (visual memory), Judgment of Line Orientation (visuospatial perception), Controlled Oral Word Test (verbal fluency/executive functioning), and Sorting subtest from DKEFS (executive functioning/novel).

In addition to the MACFIMS, there are several other brief neuropsychological batteries that have been developed to assess cognitive functioning in MS. The Brief Repeatable Battery assesses verbal memory, spatial memory, attention, and verbal fluency. The Basso Screening Battery assesses verbal learning, verbal fluency, and auditory attention, and the Screening Evaluation for Cognitive Impairment measures verbal memory, general verbal ability, and attention. Another method for addressing assessment of cognitive dysfunction is the use of the MS Neuropsychological Questionnaire, which is a brief screening questionnaire that can be completed by

Table 20.4 Tests included in the Minimal Assessment of Cognitive Function in MS (MACFIMS) battery (Benedict et al. 2002)

Test	Function
Controlled oral word association test	Language
Judgment of line orientation test	Spatial processing
California verbal learning test, 2nd edition	New learning and memory
Brief visuospatial memory test – revised	New learning and memory
Symbol digit modalities test	Processing speed and working memory
Paced auditory serial addition test	Processing speed and working memory
Delis-Kaplan executive function system – sorting test	Executive function

the MS patient and significant others in the clinic setting. Unlike the batteries of objective measures described above, this measure would assess subjective experience to assist the clinician in management of this symptom. A high rate of cognitive complaints would likely trigger more comprehensive neuropsychological evaluation to better appreciate the concerns and to assist with treatment plans.

There are clinical challenges of assessing cognitive dysfunction in MS that should be considered. While a brief screen of cognitive functions (e.g., Mini Mental State Exam) will likely result in missing or under appreciating the cognitive deficits that can be associated with MS, on the other hand, long comprehensive evaluations can sometimes be difficult for MS patients to tolerate due to issues such as fatigue. The clinician is encouraged to carefully consider the reason for evaluation and to assess accordingly. In cases where the referral question relates to the individual's ability to work or academic functions, a more comprehensive evaluation may be warranted. In contrast, some individuals are referred for evaluation to assess for cognitive problems or monitor course of symptoms. As with motor symptoms or sensory symptoms, neurologists are often requesting neuropsychological evaluations to monitor cognitive symptoms. Often, a relatively briefer evaluation still targeting the areas vulnerable to decline may be considered.

While it is important for the clinician to characterize the nature and severity of cognitive problems, consideration of other issues such as depression, sleep deprivation, pain, and fatigue must be considered when developing treatment recommendations. As with any situation of repeat cognitive testing, clinicians must also consider issues such as test–retest reliability and practice effects.

Treatment Neuropsychological Deficits in MS

As noted above, cognitive dysfunction occurs rather frequently in MS. While neuroanatomical correlates are important in understanding the underlying cause of cognitive difficulties in MS, clinical attention to variables such as mood disturbance, sleep disturbance, fatigue, and pain is also important in considering treatment directions for those MS patients who present with cognitive difficulties.

Studies in the past decade have begun to consider medication treatment options for managing the symptom of cognitive dysfunction in MS. Studies examining the effects of disease modifying medications may help in prevention of cognitive decline (Fischer et al. 2000). However, more recently, efforts to manage the symptom of cognitive dysfunction have focused on donepezil (Krupp et al. 2004), amantadine and pemoline (Geisler, et al. 1996), Prokarin (Gillson et al. 2002) and have found promising results. Porcel and Montalban (2006) offer a review of generally promising research in use of anticholinesterase inhibitors in managing cognitive dysfunction in MS.

Finally, studies have considered treatment options using cognitive rehabilitation and cognitive behavioral therapy for managing cognitive dysfunction in MS.

These studies have focused on strategies aimed at helping patients adapt and cope with cognitive dysfunction. O'Brien and colleagues (2008) have provided a recent review of studies examining cognitive rehabilitation in MS and offer some strong suggestions for future directions.

References

Amato, M., Ponziani, G., Pracucci, G., et al. (1995). Cognitive impairment in early-onset multiple sclerosis: Pattern, predictors, and impact on everyday life in a 4-year followup. *Archives of Neurology, 52*, 168–172.

Amato, M., Ponziani, G., Siracusa, G., et al. (2001). Cognitive dysfunction in early- onset multiple sclerosis: A reappraisal after 10 years. *Archives of Neurology, 58*, 1602–1606.

Arnett, P. (2004). Speed of presentation influences story recall in college students and persons with multiple sclerosis. *Archives of Clinical Neuropsychology, 19*, 507–523.

Arnett, P., Higginson, C., Voss, W., et al. (1999). Depressed mood in multiple sclerosis: Relationship to capacity demanding memory and attentional functioning. *Neuropsychology, 13*, 434–446.

Beatty, W. W., & Aupperle, R. L. (2002). Sex differences in cognitive impairment in multiple sclerosis. *The Clinical Neuropsychologist, 16*, 472–480.

Beatty, W. W., Blanco, C., Wilbanks, S., & Paul, R. (1995). Demographic, clinical and cognitive characteristics of multiple sclerosis patients who continue to work. *Journal of Neurologic Rehabilitation, 9*, 167–173.

Benedict, R., Fischer, J., Archibald, C., et al. (2002). Minimal neuropsychological assessment of MS patients: A consensus approach. *The Clinical Neuropsychologist, 16*, 381–397.

Bobholz, J., Rao, S., Lobeck, L., et al. (2006). fMRI study of episodic memory in relapsing-remitting MS: Correlation with T2 lesion volume. *Neurology, 67*, 1640–1645.

Chelune, G.J. (2010). Evidence-based research and practice in clinical neuropsychology. *The Clinical Neuropsychologist, 24*, 454–467.

Chelune, G. J., & Stone, L. (2005a). Risk of processing speed deficits among patients with relapsing and remitting and secondary progressive multiple sclerosis. *Journal of Clinical and Experimental Neuropsychology, 11*, 52.

Chelune, G. J., & Stone, L. (2005b). Relative risk of cognitive impairment is mediated by disease course and sex in multiple sclerosis. *Journal of Clinical and Experimental Neuropsychology, 11*(SI), 42–43. (S2), 52.

DeLuca, J., Barbieri-Berger, S., & Johnson, S. (1994). The nature of memory impairments in multiple sclerosis: Acquisition versus retrieval. *Journal of Clinical and Experimental Neuropsychology, 16*, 183–189.

Demaree, H., DeLuca, J., Gaudino, E., et al. (1999). Speed of information processing as a key deficit in multiple sclerosis: Implications for rehabilitation. *Journal of Neurology, Neurosurgery and Psychiatry, 67*, 661–663.

Demaree, H., Gaudino, E., DeLuca, J., et al. (2000). Learning impairment is associated with recall ability in multiple sclerosis. *Journal of Clinical and Experimental Neuropsychology, 22*, 865–873.

Fischer, J. S., Priore, R. L., Jacobs, L. D., et al. (2000). Neuropsychological effects of interferon beta-1a in relapsing-remitting multiple sclerosis. Multiple Sclerosis Collaborative Research Group. *Annals of Neurology, 48*(6), 885–892.

Geisler, M. W., Sliwinski, M., Coyle, P. K., et al. (1996). The effects of amantadine and pemoline on cognitive functioning in multiple sclerosis. *Archives of Neurology, 53*(2), 185–188.

Gillson, G., Richard, T. L., Smith, R. B., & Wright, J. V. (2002). A double-blind pilot study of the effect of Prokarin on fatigue in multiple sclerosis. *Multiple Sclerosis, 8*(1), 30–35.

Goldman Consensus Group. (2005). The Goldman consensus statement on depression in multiple sclerosis. *Multiple Sclerosis, 11*, 328–337.

Hart, S., Fonareva, I., Merluzzi, A., et al. (2005). Treatment for depression and its relationship to improvement of quality of life and psychological well-being in multiple sclerosis patients. *Journal of Consulting and Clinical Psychology, 69*, 942–949.

Huijbregts, S., Kalkers, N., de Sonneville, L., et al. (2004). Differences in cognitive impairment of relapsing remitting, secondary, and primary progressive MS. *Neurology, 63*, 335–339.

Jacobs, R. K., Anderson, V. A., Neale, J. L., & Kornberg, A. J. (2004). Neuropsychological outcome after acute disseminated encephalomyelitis: impact of age at illness onset. *Pediatric Neurology, 31*(3), 191–197.

Joy, J. E., & Johnston, R. B. (Eds.). (2001). *Multiple Sclerosis: Current status and strategies for the future*. Washington: National Academy Press.

Kotterba, S., Orth, M., Eren, E., Fangerau, T., & Sindern, E. (2003). Assessment of driving performance in patients with relapsing-remitting multiple sclerosis by a driving simulator. *European Neurology, 50*(3), 160–164.

Krupp, L., & Elkins, L. (2000). Fatigue and declines in cognitive functioning in multiple sclerosis. *Neurology, 55*, 934–939.

Krupp, L. B., Christodoulou, C., Melville, P., et al. (2004). Donepezil improved memory in multiple sclerosis in a randomized clinical trial. *Neurology, 63*, 1579–1585.

Lobentanz, I., Asenbaum, S., Vass, K., et al. (2004). Factors influencing quality of life in multiple sclerosis patients: Disability, depressive mood, fatigue, and sleep quality. *Acta Neurologica Scandinavia, 110*, 6–13.

Lyon-Caen, O., Jouvent, R., Hauser, S., et al. (1986). Cognitive function in recent-onset demyelinating diseases. *Archives of Neurology, 43*, 1138–1141.

Mohr, D., Boudewyn, A., Goodkin, D., et al. (2001). Comparative outcomes for individual cognitive-behavior therapy, supportive-expressive group psychotherapy, and sertraline for the treatment of depression in multiple sclerosis. *Journal of Consulting and Clinical Psychology, 69*, 942–949.

O'Brien, A. R., Chiaravalloti, N., Goverover, Y., & DeLuca, J. (2008). Evidence-based cognitive rehabilitation for persons with Multiple Sclerosis: A review of the literature. *Archives of Physical Medicine and Rehabilitation, 89*, 761–769.

Olek, M. J. (Ed.). (2005). *Multiple Sclerosis: Etiology, diagnosis, and new treatment strategies*. Totowa: Humana Press.

Porcel, J., & Montalban, X. (2006). Anticholinesteraaics in the treatment of cognitive impairment in multiple sclerosis. *Journal of the Neurological Sciences, 245*, 177–181.

Rao, S., Leo, G., Bernardin, L., et al. (1991a). Cognitive dysfunction in multiple sclerosis: Frequency, patterns, and prediction. *Neurology, 41*, 685–691.

Rao, S. M., Leo, G. J., Ellington, L., et al. (1991b). Cognitive dysfunction in multiple sclerosis II: Impact on employment and social functioning. *Neurology, 41*, 692–696.

Rao, S., Grafman, J., & Dijkerman, H. (1993). Memory dysfunction in multiple sclerosis: Its relation to working memory, semantic encoding, and implicit learning. *Neuropsychology, 7*, 364–374.

Rosati, G. (2001). The prevalence of multiple sclerosis in the world: An update. *Journal of the Neurological Science, 22*(2), 117–139.

Roth, R., Geisser, M., Theisen-Goodvich, M., et al. (2005). Cognitive complaints are associated with depression, fatigue, female sex, and pain catastrophizing in patients with chronic pain. *Archives of Physical Medicine and Rehabilitation, 86*, 1147–1154.

Ryan, L., Clark, C., & Klonoff, H. (1996). Patterns of cognitive impairment in relapsing-remitting multiple sclerosis and their relationship to neuropathology on magnetic resonance images. *Neuropsychology, 10*, 176–193.

Schultheis, M. T., Garay, E., Millis, S. R., & DeLuca, J. (2002). Motor vehicle crashes and violations among drivers with multiple sclerosis. *Archives of Physical Medicine and Rehabilitation, 83*(8), 1175–1178.

Schwarz, S., Mohr, A., Knauth, M., Wildemann, B., & Storch-Agenlocher, B. (2001). Acute disseminated encephalomyelitis: A follow-up study of 40 adult patients. *Neurology, 56,* 1313–1318.

Shawaryn, M., Schultheis, M., Garay, E., & DeLuca, J. (2002). Assessing functional status: Exploring the relationship between the multiple sclerosis functional composite and driving. *Archives of Physical Medicine and Rehabilitation, 83,* 1123–1129.

Thorton, A. E., & Naftail, R. (1997). Memory impairment in multiple sclerosis: A quantitative review. *Neuropsychology, 11,* 357–366.

Vollmer, T. L. (1999). Multiple Sclerosis: The disease and its diagnosis. In S. van den Noort & N. J. Holland (Eds.), *Multiple Sclerosis in clinical practice* (pp. 1–22). New York: Demos Medical Publishing, Inc.

Chapter 21
Moderate and Severe Traumatic Brain Injury

Grant L. Iverson and Rael T. Lange

Abstract Traumatic brain injuries arise from open or closed head injuries. Most traumatic brain injuries result from closed head injuries (an example of an open head injury is an object penetrating the skull). Brain injuries occur as the result of acceleration-deceleration forces (linear or angular), blunt trauma, or both. Traumatic brain injuries occur on a broad continuum of severity, from very mild transient injuries to catastrophic injuries resulting in death or severe disability. The continuum of severity of traumatic brain injury is illustrated in Fig. 21.1.

Key Points and Chapter Summary

- Traumatic brain injuries occur on a broad continuum of severity, from very mild transient injuries to catastrophic injuries resulting in death or severe disability.
- The severity of TBI typically is classified using the Glasgow Coma Scale, duration of unconsciousness, and duration of post-traumatic amnesia.
- Most parts of the brain are vulnerable to traumatic injury. However, the anterior portion of the brain is most likely to be affected (i.e., frontal and temporal regions).
- *Traumatic axonal injuries* are often referred to as diffuse axonal injuries, shearing injuries, or *deep white matter injures*. Traumatic axonal injury is the preferred terminology.
- Moderate and severe traumatic brain injuries can result in temporary, prolonged, or permanent neurological or neuropsychiatric problems such as

(continued)

G.L. Iverson (✉)
University of British Columbia, Vancouver, BC, Canada
and
British Columbia Mental Health and Addiction Services, Coquitlam, BC, Canada
e-mail: giverson@interchange.ubc.ca

M.R. Schoenberg and J.G. Scott (eds.), *The Little Black Book of Neuropsychology:*
A Syndrome-Based Approach, DOI 10.1007/978-0-387-76978-3_21,
© Springer Science+Business Media, LLC 2011

Key Points and Chapter Summary (continued)

  (1) motor impairments and movement disorders, (2) balance and dizziness, (3) visual impairments, (4) cranial nerve impairments, (5) headaches,
- (6) sexual dysfunction, (7) fatigue and sleep problems, (8) depression and anxiety disorders, (9) psychotic disorders, (10) personality changes and apathy, and (11) lack of awareness.
- Moderate or severe TBIs frequently result in permanent neurocognitive and neurobehavioral impairments. As a general rule, as injury severity increases, the magnitude of impairment increases.
- The vast majority of recovery from moderate to severe TBI occurs within the first year, although some additional recovery can occur thereafter.
- The short- and long-term effects of moderate and severe TBI present a number of challenges that make adjustment back to everyday life difficult for both patient and family members. Some of the most common issues relate to substance abuse, family and marital integration, return to work, and community integration.

Epidemiology

In the United States, between 1995 and 2001, 1.4 million people per year attended an Emergency Department (ED) following TBI. Of these, 79.6% of patients (1.1 million) were treated and discharged from the ED, 16.8% (235,000) were hospitalized, and 3.6% (50,000) died as a result of their injuries (Langlois et al. 2004). In Canada, it is estimated that there are 120,000 TBIs each year (Brain Association of British Columbia 2002).

Traumatic brain injuries occur across all ages, with the highest rates found in 15–24 year olds and those over the age of 75 (Thurman et al. 2007). In terms of emergency department visits and hospital admissions, reported rates of mild, moderate, and severe TBI vary depending on the nature of the referral institution (e.g., Annegers et al. 1980; Jagger et al. 1984; Klauber et al. 1981; Kraus et al. 1986; MacKenzie et al. 1989; Thurman and Guerrero 1999; Whitman et al. 1984) (Fig. 21.1). For example, some institutions (e.g., Level 1 trauma center) are more likely to receive patients with severe injuries compared to others. However, taken as a whole, the severity distribution of patients admitted to a hospital following TBI in the past 25 years is approximately 80% mild (GCS 13–15), 10% moderate (GCS 9–12), and 10% severe (GCS 3–8) (Kraus and Chu 2005).

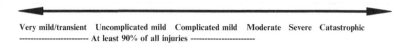

Very mild/transient   Uncomplicated mild   Complicated mild   Moderate   Severe   Catastrophic
------------------------- At least 90% of all injuries -----------------------

Fig. 21.1 Continuum of traumatic brain injury severity

Mild traumatic brain injuries are especially common. Bazarian and colleagues (2005) reported that 56/100,000 people are evaluated in the emergency department each year for an *isolated* mild traumatic brain injury (MTBI). Sosin et al. (1996), based on the National Health Interview Survey in 1991, estimated that 1.5 million

Americans suffer a traumatic brain injury each year (i.e., 618/100,000), with the vast majority being mild in severity. This, of course, is much higher than previous estimates based on hospital admissions because many people who sustain a mild traumatic brain injury are not evaluated in the emergency department or admitted to the hospital (Sosin et al. 1996).

Terminology and Classification Considerations

Traumatic brain injuries are classified as mild, moderate, severe, or catastrophic. There are no universally accepted classification criteria. However, the most common criteria utilize the Glasgow Coma Scale, duration of unconsciousness, and duration of post-traumatic amnesia.

Glasgow Coma Scale

The Glasgow Coma Scale (GCS) is the most widely used rapid screening instrument for evaluating brain injury severity. The GCS is used to evaluate three components of arousal: (1) the stimulus required to induce eye opening, (2) the best motor response, and (3) the best verbal response. Scores on the GCS range from 3 to 15. The GCS is used most often by emergency medical technicians at the scene of an accident and emergency room personnel.

Glasgow Coma Scale (GCS) score range 3–15.
- Eye Opening = 1–4 (Spontaneously = 4, To Speech = 3, To Pain = 2, None = 1)
- Best Verbal Response = 1–5 (Oriented = 5, Confused = 4, Inappropriate = 3, Incomprehensible = 2, None = 1)
- Best Motor Response = 1–6 (Obeying = 6, Localizes Pain = 5, Withdraws (Pain) = 4, Flexion (Pain) = 3, Extension (Pain) = 2, None = 1)

Loss of Consciousness/Coma

The expression *loss of consciousness* (LOC) generally refers to being rendered in what resembles a sleep-like state. A brief loss of consciousness often can be observed in a boxing match when a boxer is "knocked out." Technically, the term *unconsciousness* "is taken to imply lack of awareness of the self or the environment" (Jennett 1996). Therefore, the term does not distinguish between patients in a coma or in a vegetative state. There can be lack of clarity in the use of the term *coma*. Jennett (1996) noted "it is now generally accepted that "coma" should be confined to describing patients whose eyes are continuously closed and who cannot be aroused to a wakeful state" (p.4). Some patients with severe traumatic brain injuries emerge from a coma to a *vegetative state*. The vegetative state involves *wakefulness without awareness* (Jennett 1996). The person cannot speak or communicate through gestures or eye movements. These patients may moan or groan, and move in response to pain, but they show no evidence of meaningful cognitive or emotional functioning. There are differing positions regarding when to use the phrase *persistent vegetative state*, be it after 1 month (American Neurological Association Committee on Ethical Affairs 1993), 3 months (Higashi et al. 1977), or 1 year (Berrol 1986; British Medical Association Medical Ethics Committee 1992).

Rule of thumb: Loss of consciousness and coma

- Loss of consciousness (LOC) is associated with lack of awareness, with the person appearing to be in sleep-like state.
- Coma refers to being in sleep-like state, with eyes continuously closed, and the person cannot be aroused to a state of wakefulness.

Retrograde and Post-Traumatic Amnesia

Individuals who experience TBIs often experience different forms of memory disruption. Some patients are unable to remember events that occur immediately after their injury. They may not be able to keep track of the day of the week or remember if a family member visited them in the hospital. This memory disturbance, called *post-traumatic amnesia*, may last for minutes, hours, days, weeks, or months. It is important to realize that a patient's self-report of PTA can be adversely impacted by several things, including intoxication, pain medication, or the effects of general anesthesia. *Retrograde amnesia* (RTA) is essentially the opposite of post-traumatic amnesia. The duration of retrograde amnesia refers to the loss of memory for events prior to the TBI. The length of RTA is related to the severity of the injury; for example, a person may have no memory for what they did an hour or a week prior to the injury.

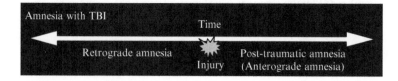

Classification of Severity

By convention, traumatic brain injuries frequently are graded in severity based on the Glasgow Coma Scale (GCS). The severity classification ranges for GCS scores are as follows: Mild = 13–15, Moderate = 9–12, and Severe = 3–8. The classification system based on GCS is widely, but not universally, used in clinical practice and research. There is far less agreement on a classification system based on the

Table 21.1 Common[a] classification system for traumatic brain injury

Classification	Duration of unconsciousness	Glasgow coma scale	Post-traumatic amnesia
Mild	<30 minutes	13–15[b]	<24 hours
Moderate	30 minutes–24 hours	9–12	1–7 days
Severe	>24 hours	3–8	>7 days

[a]This is not a universally agreed upon classification system
[b]Defined as the lowest GCS score obtained 30 min or more post-injury

duration of loss of consciousness and post-traumatic amnesia. A commonly used classification system for mild, moderate, and severe traumatic brain injury is summarized in Table 21.1.

Pathoanatomy and Pathophysiology

Most parts of the brain are vulnerable to traumatic injury. However, the anterior portion of the brain is most likely to be affected (i.e., frontal and temporal regions). There are primary and secondary pathophysiologies that contribute to TBI-associated cognitive and neurobehavioral impairment. Primary damage involves axonal injury, vascular injury, and hemorrhage. Secondary damage can arise from the endogenous evolution of cellular damage or from secondary systemic processes, such as hypotension or hypoxia. The endogenous secondary pathophysiologies include: (1) ischemia, excitotoxicity, energy failure, and cell death cascades (e.g., necrosis and apoptosis), (2) edema, (3) traumatic axonal injury, and (4) inflammation (Kochanek et al. 2007).

Terminology for Injuries to the Head and Brain

Most skull fractures resulting from head injuries are of two types, linear and depressed. *Linear fractures* are usually thin and straight. A dent in the skull is referred to as a *depressed skull fracture*. A *diastatic fracture* is a linear fracture that extends into a suture (the line where two skull bones join).

A *contusion* is a bruise on the brain that is usually associated with swelling and some bleeding. A *coup/contrecoup injury* is a classic lesion pattern resulting from serious falls. If a person falls backward and hits the back of her head, she may have a relatively small contusion at the site of impact ("coup") and a large contusion at the opposite side of the brain (front; "contrecoup"). This is due to the physics of translational forces on the brain (see Fig. 21.2). The areas of the brain most likely to be contused are illustrated in Fig. 21.3.

Hemorrhage represents bleeding in or around the brain. Hemorrhages due to trauma may be *intracerebral (intraparenchymal), intraventricular, subarachnoid, sudural,* and/or *epidural* and represent an independent source of injury to the brain that is unrelated to the mechanics of the trauma itself (whether open or closed head injury). Trauma can result in a combination of hemorrhages within the skull.

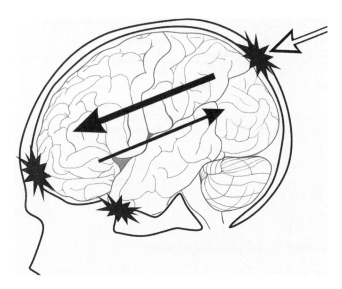

Fig. 21.2 Coup/Contrecoup brain injury

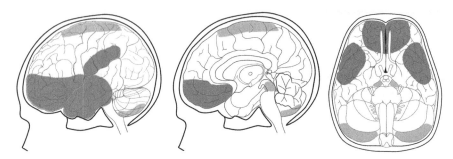

Fig. 21.3 Areas affected by contusions. *Note*: These schematic diagrams of contusion locations in lateral, sagittal midline, and base views show the areas most commonly affected by contusions (*dark gray*) and those that are occasionally affected by contusions (*light gray*). Areas commonly affected by contusions include the orbitofrontal cortex, anterior temporal lobe, and posterior portion of the superior temporal gyrus area, with the adjacent parietal opercular area. Areas that are less commonly affected include the lateral midbrain, inferior cerebellum and adjacent tonsil, and the midline superior cerebral cortex (These drawings were adapted from Morales et al. 2007)

Hemorrhages within the brain are caused by damage to an artery or vein (see also Chap. 13 for discussion of hemorrhagic stroke not due to trauma). Increased symptom onset 2–4 days after the trauma can occur, presenting as a patient who initially shows good functional recovery from the injury, but then deteriorates over a period of several hours with confusion and obtundation.

A *hematoma* is an accumulation of blood in a specific location. Hemorrhages and hematomas *around* the brain may be in three locations: *epidural, subdural,* and *subarachnoid*. Epidural hemorrhages are located between the skull and the dura, and can be life threatening. A blow to the side of the head may damage the middle meningeal artery causing an epidural hematoma. Classically, the clinical presentation involves an initial loss of consciousness associated with a head trauma, followed by recovery of consciousness and a return to broadly normal function (patient appears lucid and walks and talks normally) for a few hours. This is followed by rapid deterioration in function (hours to a day). Epidural hemorrhage due to damage to a vein results in slower progression of symptoms while arterial hemorrhages tend to exhibit faster progression of symptoms and greater likelihood for brain herniation.

Subdural and subarachnoid hematomas are collections of blood located below the dura mater and below the arachnoid mater, respectively (see Chap. 3 for review of anatomy of meninges). Acute subdural hematomas typically are the consequence of head trauma, but sometimes no identifiable head trauma can be identified. Older adults are at increased risk for these hematomas following relatively minor head trauma. Subdural hemorrhage can result in brain compression or herniation. Subdural hemorrhages usually occur over the brain convexity, but can also present along the interhemispheric fissure, the tentorium, or, sometimes, the posterior fossa. When associated with laceration of a bridging vein, there can be an initial traumatic LOC, followed by an interval of return to broadly normal function, followed by deterioration in function over several hours to days. Deterioration in function can be very slow in some cases, particularly among older adults such that the presentation of neuropsychological dysfunction can be mistaken for a dementia. Treatment may involve craniotomy with removal of the blood if the hematoma is large. Smaller hematomas may not require surgical intervention.

A collection of blood within the brain may be referred to as an *intraparenchymal* (within the parenchyma, "brain tissue") hematoma. Intracerebral hemorrhage can result in mass effect. Serial CT studies show that this type of hemorrhage can enlarge over time and/or several smaller hemorrhages may coalesce into a single larger pool of blood. Intraparenchymal hemorrhages can extend to the ventricle (intraventricular hemorrhage extension) and/or subarachnoid space (subarachnoid hemorrhagic extension). Small hemorrhages may resolve (be broken down by the body) resulting in minimal or no obvious encephalomalacia at the site of hemorrhage visible on imaging.

Edema is the term used to describe swelling in the brain. Swelling can be minor, as in the case of a small contusion, or severe, when associated with multiple or severe contusions. Diffuse brain swelling can cause compression or *herniation*. Herniation is more likely when diffuse edema is coupled with a hemorrhage. Herniation is best understood by considering the basic anatomy of the skull. The brain is compartmentalized within the skull. These compartments are formed by structural dividers, such as the falx which separates the left and right hemispheres of the cerebral cortex. The tentorium is like a roof above the lower rear portions of the brain; that is, the brainstem and cerebellum. Major swelling (edema) or a collection of blood (hematoma) can cause the brain to shift (herniate) against these structural dividers or through natural openings in the skull.

Figure 21.4 illustrates several possible areas of brain herniation, involving: (1) the mesial temporal lobe (transtentorial herniation), (2) brainstem and/or mesial temporal lobes (central herniation), (3) cingulate gyrus and related structures, and (4) brain stem and cerebellum through the foramen magnum (tonsillar herniation, a form of central herniation). Transtentorial herniation is sometimes referred to as

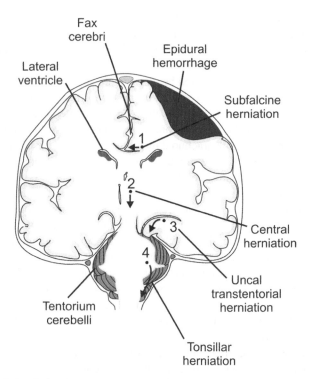

Fig. 21.4 Brain herniations

uncal herniation because the uncus is herniated through the tentorial notch. This is associated with a triad of clinical features: (1) hemiplegia, (2) dilated (blown) pupil, and (3) coma. Hemiplegia (or paresis) contralateral to the side of the mass can occur due to compression of the corticospinal tract. Rarely, due to different physics and tissue displacement, this type of herniation can be associated with ipsilateral motor impairment (Kernohan's phenonmenon). With Kernohan's phenomena, the hemiplegia occurs on the ipsilateral side because, as the midbrain is pushed to the side by the herniating mesial temporal structures (uncus), it is pushed away from the side of the mass (hemorrhage), and the side opposite to where the hemorrhage is becomes compressed against the tentorial notch and results in ipsilateral hemiplegia. Subfalcine herniation is a term to describe large unilateral supratentorial masses that can result in the cingulate gyrus and associated midline structures to herniate under the falx cerebri from the ipsilateral to contralateral side of the brain.

Central herniation describes the downward displacement of the brainstem with herniation through the foramen magnum. Mild central herniation can result in cranial nerve IV dysfunction (abducens nerve palsy) due to "stretching" of the nerve. Greater herniation due to a mass in the supratentorial region (above the posterior fossa) can result in bilateral uncal herniation through the tentorial notch. Very severe mass effects can result in herniation of the brainstem and cerebellum through the foramen magnum (tonsillar herniation), leading to respiratory failure and cardiovascular dysfunction, often resulting in death.

Ventricular Dilation, also referred to *hydrocephalus ex vacuo,* can occur following severe traumatic brain injury. Cerebrospinal fluid is produced in the ventricles and it circulates within and around the brain. A traumatic brain injury can cause damming of the small passages or holes through which the CSF circulates. This results in a condition called *hydrocephalus* which is characterized by *ventricular dilation* (i.e., expansion). Ventricular dilation may also result from the gradual dying off and removal of brain cells (i.e., hydrocephalus ex vacuo). That is, after a traumatic brain injury-damaged cells essentially shrink and then are removed, with the residual space being filled by the ventricles expanding. *Cortical atrophy* (shrinking) and ventricular dilation have been identified in patients with traumatic brain injuries through neuroimaging conducted 6 weeks to 1 year post-injury (Anderson and Bigler 1995; Bigler et al. 1992).

Traumatic axonal injuries are often referred to as diffuse axonal injuries, shearing injuries, or *deep white matter injures.* Traumatic axonal injury is the preferred terminology. Axonal injuries result from severe rotational and/or linear acceleration/deceleration forces on the brain. These injuries typically occur in specific brain regions such as the gray and white matter interfaces of the cerebral cortex, the long fibers of the internal capsule that carry motor information, the crossing fibers that connect the two cerebral hemispheres (corpus callosum; see Fig. 21.5), and the upper brainstem (Gentry et al. 1988a; Orrison et al. 1994). Traumatic axonal injury is described in more detail in the section below.

Rule of thumb: Terminology

- Skull fractures can be linear (straight), depressed ("caved in") or diastatic (linear to suture)
- Hemorrhages can be epidural, subdural, subarachnoid, or interparenchymal
- Edema (swelling) of the parenchyma combined with hemorrhage can result in herniation
- Traumatic axonal injury is a complex process that typically does not result in primary axotomy, but can result in secondary axotomy

---

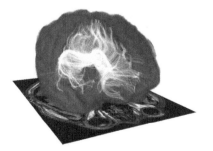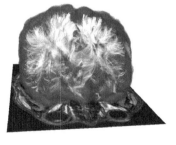

Fig. 21.5 White matter fiber tracks reconstructed from diffusion tensor imaging depicting the corpus callosum (*left*) and the entire white matter fiber population. Images provided courtesy of Dr. Burkhard Mädler (Philips Healthcare, Best, Netherlands).

Traumatic Axonal Injury

In general, unless exposed to very serious forces, axons do not "shear" at the point
of injury (see Fig. 21.6). What was originally conceptualized as "shearing" in
patients with severe to catastrophic brain injuries (Nevin 1967; Peerless and
Rewcastle 1967; Strich 1961) is actually a gradual process where stretched and
badly damaged axons swell and eventually separate (Povlishock et al. 1983). The
pathophysiologic sequence that leads to traumatic injury to neurons is "a process,
not an event" (Gennarelli and Graham 1998, p. 163). However, it is important to
appreciate that axons can stretch and twist without being sheared or torn (Christman
et al. 1994; Povlishock and Becker 1985; Povlishock et al. 1983; Yaghmai and
Povlishock 1992), even after repeated stretch injuries (Slemmer et al. 2002).
In other words, stretch causes a temporary deformation of an axon that gradually
returns to the original orientation and morphology even though internal damage
might have been sustained (Smith et al. 1999).

Axons contain numerous microscopic elements including microtubules and
neurofilaments (see Fig. 21.7). Microtubules are thick cytoskeletal fibers and consist of long polar polymers constructed of protofilaments packed in a long tubular
array. They are oriented longitudinally in relation to the axon and are associated
with fast axonal transport (Schwartz 1991). Neurofilaments are essentially the
"bones" of the axon and are the most abundant intracellular structural element in
axons (Schwartz 1991). Following axonal stretch, small ion species enter the axons.
This initiates metabolic dysfunction and when acceleration/deceleration forces are
sufficiently high, a progressive series of intracellular events will occur that result in
damage to the cytoskeleton and microtubules (Christman et al. 1994; Erb and
Povlishock 1991; Grady et al. 1993; Pettus et al. 1994; Povlishock and Becker
1985; Povlishock et al. 1983; Yaghmai and Povlishock 1992).

Various characteristics of neurons themselves appear to make them more susceptible to injury. Where axons change direction, enter target nuclei, or where they
decussate, they can be more easily damaged (Adams et al. 1977; Grady et al. 1993;
Oppenheimer 1968; Povlishock 1993; Yaghmai and Povlishock 1992). Large caliber

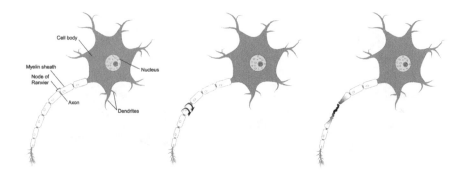

Fig. 21.6 Traumatic axonal injury

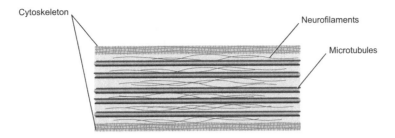

Fig. 21.7 Internal structure of an axon

neurons are injured more often than smaller neurons that surround them (Yaghmai and Povlishock 1992). Injured axons are observed more often where a change in tissue density occurs, such as at the gray/white matter interface near cerebral cortex (Gentry et al. 1988b; Grady et al. 1993; Peerless and Rewcastle 1967; Povlishock 1993). In summary, a single acceleration/deceleration event might result in (1) no apparent change in structure or function, (2) functional or metabolic change, (3) eventual structural change in the axon, or (4) frank separation of the axon into proximal and distal segments. These outcomes are dependent on the force applied to the brain.

Neuroimaging

On neuroimaging, macroscopic abnormalities can be seen within the brain tissue or outside the brain, in what is often referred to as the extra-axial space. Within the brain, injuries include hemorrhagic contusions, non-hemorrhagic contusions, hemorrhagic or non-hemorrhagic shearing injuries, herniations, and cerebral edema. Outside the brain tissue, injuries include epidural hematomas, subdural hematomas, subdural hygromas [collection of cerebrospinal fluid (CSF)], subarachnoid hemorrhage, intraventricular hemorrhage, and hydrocephalus (Barkley et al. 2007). It is possible to sustain a severe brain injury, traumatically-induced coma, and severe and persistent cognitive impairment, yet have a normal day-of-injury CT scan (Gean 1994; Harris and Harris 2000). However, many of these patients experience ventricular dilation and reduced brain volume. This occurs gradually, following diffuse brain injury, as the result of neuronal loss. In its more serious form, it is visible with the naked eye on static CT or MR images. It can be illustrated more elegantly and precisely, however, using quantitative imaging methods.

One of the most common post-acute findings in patients who sustain severe TBIs is white matter atrophy (Bigler 2005; Charness 1993; Huisman et al. 2004; Inglese et al. 2005b; MacKenzie et al. 2002; McAllister et al. 2001; Nakayama et al. 2006). This can be readily identified, using quantitative imaging methods, in the corpus callosum (Adams et al. 1980; Arfanakis et al. 2002; Gorrie et al. 2001; Inglese et al. 2005b; Levin 2003; Levin et al. 1990; Salmond et al. 2006; Sundgren et al. 2004). Those regions of the corpus callosum found to be most vulnerable are the genu and splenium (Huisman et al. 2004; Le et al. 2005; Nakayama et al. 2006; Wilde et al. 2006). Of particular interest are neuroimaging studies using DTI, a sophisticated, high resolution MRI technique that is able to examine the integrity of white matter in the brain at a *micro*structural level. The advantage of DTI compared to conventional MRI techniques is that DTI is superior for detecting white matter changes in the brain. Studies using DTI have consistently found decreases in white matter integrity of the corpus callosum in patients following TBI compared to control subjects (Inglese et al. 2005a; Miles et al. 2008; Nakayama et al. 2006; Wilde et al. 2006).

Neurological and Neuropsychiatric Problems

Moderate and severe traumatic brain injuries can result in temporary, prolonged, or permanent neurological or neuropsychiatric problems. Some of these problems are listed in Table 21.2.

Motor Impairments and Movement Disorders

Motor impairments, such as paresis (weakness) or plegia (paralysis), sometimes occur following severe traumatic brain injury. Some patients experience spasticity (increased muscle tone and exaggerated reflexes), ataxia (loss of muscle coordination), or both. Post-traumatic movement disorders manifest by either slowness or poverty of movement (hypokinesia) or by excessive involuntary movements (hyperkinesia).

The two most common classifications of movement disorders are tremors and dystonias (see Krauss and Jankovic 2007 for a review). Tremors are characterized

Table 21.2 Neurological and neuropsychiatric problems associated with TBI

Balance problems and dizziness

Cranial nerve impairments (e.g., olfactory, ocular/optic, face movement/sensation, and auditory/balance)

Depression and anxiety disorders

Fatigue and sleep disturbance

Headaches

Lack of awareness (e.g., anosognosia, anosodiaphoria, lack of insight/judgment)

Movement disorders (e.g., bradykinesia, tremor, dystonias, myoclonus)

Motor impairments (e.g., hemiparesis, ataxia, apraxia)

Psychotic disorders

Personality changes, apathy, and decreased motivation

Sexual dysfunction

Visual impairments (blurred vision, double vision)

by rhythmic, oscillatory movements. Tremor types include (1) *resting* (or "rest tremor"; seen when the body part is at rest), (2) *postural* (seen when holding a body part out, such as outstretched arms), and (3) *kinetic* (also referred to as an "intention tremor"; seen when moving a body part, such as during the finger-to-nose test). Dystonia is characterized by sustained muscle contractions that cause twisting or repetitive movements, and/or abnormal postures or positions (e.g., athetosis, chorea, and akathisia). Post-traumatic dystonias sometimes co-occur with tremors. Dystonias can affect any part of the body (e.g., arms and legs, trunk, neck, head, or face). They are classified according to bodily distribution (i.e., focal, segmental, multifocal, and generalized).

Balance and Dizziness

It is well established that individuals who sustain traumatic brain injuries (TBI) can experience temporary or permanent deficits in static or dynamic balance (Campbell and Parry 2005; Gagnon et al. 1998; Geurts et al. 1996; Greenwald et al. 2001; Kaufman et al. 2006; McCrea et al. 2003; Rinne et al. 2006). Moreover, dizziness is a common complaint in patients with traumatic brain injuries of all severities. Vertigo (i.e., a spinning sensation) is less common than "dizziness" and typically is caused by a peripheral injury to the vestibular system. It is a mistake to assume uncritically that difficulties with imbalance or dizziness are due to traumatically-induced brain damage. This is because imbalance and dizziness can be related to multiple potential causes. For example, balance is related to the vestibular system, visual system, and the somatosensory and proprioceptive systems. Multiple anatomical structures, peripheral pathways, and central interconnections are involved. Of course, direct damage to the brainstem or cerebellum can be a central cause for balance problems.

Visual Impairments

Visual impairments and ocular abnormalities can arise from orbital fractures; cornea, lens, or retinal injuries; cranial neuropathies; brain stem damage; or damage to subcortical or cortical regions involved with the visual system (see Kapoor and Ciuffreda 2005; Padula et al. 2007). A patient might experience blurred vision, binocular vision problems [e.g., double vision (diplopia), changes in depth perception, or difficulty localizing objects in space], nystagmus, difficulty with visual tracking (i.e., deficit of smooth pursuit), or difficulty reading or rapidly localizing objects in space (i.e., deficit of saccadic movement – quick simultaneous movement of both eyes in the same direction). Although uncommon following TBI, it is possible to have a frank visual field defect.

Cranial Nerve Impairments

The cranial nerves provide motor and sensory innervation to the head and neck and can, of course, be damaged as a result of traumatic injuries to the head or brain. Cranial nerves can be damaged due to skull fractures (e.g., olfactory, optic, facial, and auditory-vestibular), shearing forces (e.g., at the level of the cribriform plate), intracranial hemorrhages or hematomas, or uncal herniation. Damage to a cranial nerve can cause problems with olfaction, vision, hearing, balance, eye movements, facial sensation, facial movement, swallowing, tongue movements, and neck strength.

Headaches

Temporary or chronic headaches can occur following injuries to the neck, head, or both. Post-traumatic headaches are defined as new headaches that emerge within the first week post-injury. Fortunately, post-traumatic headaches typically resolve within 3 months. Headaches are conceptualized as chronic if they last for more than 3 or 6 months. The most common types of headaches following injuries to the neck or head are: (1) muculoskeletal headaches (typically a cap-like discomfort), (2) cervicogenic headaches (typically unilateral sub-occipital head pain with secondary oculo-frontotemporal discomfort), (3) neuritic and neuralgic head pain (e.g., sharp and shooting pain arising from the development of a neuroma in the occipital or parietal region of the scalp), (4) post-traumatic migraine (typically throbbing with associated nausea and sometimes vomiting), and (5) post-traumatic tension headache (typically bilateral vice-like pain in the temporal regions) (Zasler et al. 2007). Headaches can also be associated with depression and psychological distress (Breslau et al. 2003; Mitsikostas and Thomas 1999; Pine et al. 1996; Zwart et al. 2003), and these problems can be mutually reinforcing.

Sexual Dysfunction

Changes in sexuality and sexual functioning are commonly reported by patients or spouses. These changes can involve desire, drive, arousal, and sexual functioning. Human sexuality is influenced by physical, cognitive, emotional, and social factors. Thus, traumatic injuries to the brain can lead to changes in sexuality and functioning through multiple mechanisms. Sandel and colleagues emphasized that sexual dysfunction following TBI can be caused by numerous factors including damage to specific brain regions, neurochemical changes relating to brain damage, endocrinologic abnormalities, medication side effects, secondary medical conditions, physical limitations, cognitive impairments, emotional problems, behavioral problems, and interpersonal difficulties (Sandel et al. 2007).

Fatigue and Sleep Problems

Fatigue and sleep problems are commonly reported following TBI (Fellus and Elovic 2007; Rao et al. 2005; Thaxton and Patel 2007). Fatigue is highly subjective and difficult to assess. It is commonly experienced as tiredness, weakness, or exhaustion. Approximately 16–32% of patients who sustain TBIs (mostly moderate–severe) report significant problems with fatigue 1 year post-injury (Bushnik et al. 2008), 21–68% at 2 years post-injury (Bushnik et al. 2008; Hillier et al. 1997; Olver et al. 1996), and 37–73% at 5 years post-injury (Hillier et al. 1997; Olver et al. 1996). Fatigue can interfere with cognitive functioning and a person's day-to-day activities. Sleep disturbances following traumatic brain injury are typically characterized as (1) insomnia (difficulty initiating or maintaining sleep), (2) hypersomnia (excessive sleep or excessive daytime sleepiness), or (3) disturbed sleep–wake (circadian) cycles. Fatigue and sleep disturbances can be related to traumatic brain damage, co-occurring depression, or both.

Depression and Anxiety Disorders

The estimated prevalence of depression following TBI varies widely, ranging from 11 to 77% (e.g., Jorge et al. 1993; Silver et al. 2001; Varney et al. 1987). Depression is most common in the first year post-injury (Dikmen et al. 2004; Jorge et al. 2004), with rates generally decreasing over time (Ashman et al. 2004; Dikmen et al. 2004). However, chronic depression and late onset depression have been reported 3 years post-injury (14 and 10%, respectively, Hibbard et al. 2004). High rates of depression in TBI populations have also been reported over the course of 8 years (61%; Hibbard et al. 1998) and 30 years (26.7%; Koponen et al. 2002) post-injury. It is not clear whether depression arises as a biological consequence of the TBI and/or as a psychological reaction to deficits and psychosocial problems associated with having a brain injury. Differential diagnoses of post-TBI depression include adjustment disorder with depressed mood, apathy, emotional lability, and post-traumatic stress disorder (Robinson and Jorge 2005).

Compared to depression, the emergence of post-injury anxiety disorders is less common, though still problematic. Anxiety disorders may include generalized anxiety disorder (GAD), panic disorder, obsessive compulsive disorder (OCD), specific phobia, social phobia, and post-traumatic stress disorder (PTSD). The reported prevalence rates of anxiety disorders following TBI are 8–24% for GAD, 2–7% for panic disorder, 1–9% for OCD, less than 25% for specific phobia (especially driving), and 0–42% for PTSD. It is important to note, however, that these prevalence rates include patients with mild TBI, and the prevalence in moderate to severe TBI alone is not known (Warden and Labbate 2005). Exacerbation of pre-injury anxiety problems in people who sustain an MTBI is commonly seen in clinical settings.

A particularly controversial and confusing issue is whether a person who sustains a TBI can develop PTSD when that person has no memory for the traumatic event. Researchers have reported that individuals with marked amnesia around the time of the event are at relatively low risk for developing PTSD (Bombardier et al. 2006; Levin et al. 2001; Sbordone and Liter 1995). Warden and colleagues followed 47 active-duty service members, who sustained moderate traumatic brain injuries, and who had neurogenic amnesia for the event. None of them developed full criteria for PTSD, despite the fact that some individuals appeared to develop a PTSD-like anxiety disorder (Warden and Labbate 2005). Gil and colleagues reported that individuals who sustained a mild TBI and had no memory for the event are less likely to develop PTSD. However, a small percentage of patients with no memory for the event did report PTSD symptomatology (Gil et al. 2005).

Other researchers have reported that PTSD can exist as a co-morbid condition with TBI (Harvey and Bryant 2000; Hickling et al. 1998; Mather et al. 2003; Mayou et al. 2000). It is hypothesized that some injured people can experience some degree of fear conditioning even while in a state of post-traumatic amnesia or confusion. Moreover, they can reconstruct their traumatic experiences over time, with a combination of accurate and possibly inaccurate information, and this might intermingle with the original fear conditioning to perpetuate anxiety symptoms. These reconstructed memories might be re-experienced, fulfilling one of the hallmark criteria for PTSD. Of course, it is also possible for a person to experience traumatic events as they are emerging from post-traumatic amnesia and these might be sufficiently distressing to contribute to later PTSD symptoms.

Psychotic Disorders

Psychotic disorders following TBI are generically referred to as *post-traumatic psychosis*. Post-traumatic psychosis is a term used to describe the onset of symptoms defined by the DSM-IV-TR diagnostic criteria for *psychotic disorder due to a general medical condition* (American Psychiatric Association 2000). It is difficult for a clinician to definitively demonstrate that any case of post-traumatic psychosis is directly caused by TBI. However, there does appear to be a relationship between TBI and psychosis in some patients. Some researchers have reported the prevalence of post-traumatic psychosis tends to be higher in individuals who have sustained a TBI than in the general population (e.g., Achte et al. 1991; Hillbom 1960; Thomsen 1984). Other researchers have reported individuals with psychotic disorders are more likely to have had a prior TBI than the general population (e.g., AbdelMalik et al. 2003; Gureje et al. 1994; Malaspina et al. 2001). Risk factors may include: (1) injuries to the left hemisphere, particularly the temporal and parietal lobes, (2) increased severity of brain injury, (3) closed head injury, as opposed to a penetrating head injury, (4) vulnerability and/or predisposition to psychosis, (e.g., having a first degree relative with a psychotic disorder), (5) presence of pre-morbid neurological pathology, (e.g., prior brain injury, seizures, ADHD), and (6) post-traumatic epilepsy (Corcoran et al. 2005).

Personality Changes, Apathy, and Motivation

Traumatic brain injuries can cause changes in personality and behavior. Personality changes can result from damage to specific regions of the brain. For example, damage to the frontal lobes can result in impulsivity, emotional liability, socially inappropriate behaviors, apathy, decreased spontaneity, lack of interest, or emotional blunting. Damage to the temporal lobes can result in episodic hyper-irritability, aggressive outbursts, or dysphoric mood states (Lucas 1998). However, personality changes can also manifest as a consequence of individuals' reactions to their injury as they experience cognitive and behavioral deficits and major changes in their lifestyle. Depression, anxiety, irritability, restlessness, low frustration tolerance, and apathy are common in this regard (O'Shanick and O'Shanick 2005). Personality changes typically manifest as a consequence of a complex interaction between the direct consequences of the brain injury and secondary reactions to impairment or loss (Lezak et al. 2004).

Lack of Awareness

Up to 45% of persons who sustain moderate to severe TBIs are reported to have reduced awareness of medical, physical, and/or cognitive deficits (Flashman and McAllister 2002). Lack of awareness tends to be function specific, in which some deficits may be accurately assessed by the patient (e.g., hemiplegia), while other deficits are assessed less reliably (e.g., cognitive skills). In general, patients tend to underestimate the severity of their cognitive and behavioral impairments when compared to ratings of family members. In addition, although many patients tend to exhibit some awareness of cognitive and speech deficits, they are less likely to report changes in personality and behavior.

Lack of awareness has been described using the following neurologic and psychodynamic terminology: (1) *Agnosia:* Impaired recognition of previously meaningful stimuli that cannot be attributed to primary sensory defects, attentional disturbances, or a naming disorder; (2) *Anosognosia:* A lack of knowledge, or unawareness of cognitive, linguistic, sensory, and motor deficits following neurological assault; (3) *Anosodiaphoria:* Lack of concern for serious neurological impairments, without denying their existence; (4) *Denial of Insight:* A psychological explanation to account for symptoms of anosognosia. Patients with anosognosia are thought to be motivated to block distressing symptoms from awareness by using a defense mechanism (denial); and (5) *Lack of Insight:* A multidimensional construct that describes a spectrum of concepts, ranging from a psychological defense mechanism to lack of cognitive skills that permit understanding of deficits (Flashman et al. 2005). We believe that in most cases involving severe traumatic brain injury, the underlying cause of the lack of awareness is neurological not psychological.

Functional and Neuropsychological Outcome

All aspects of recovery and outcome are affected by injury severity. Many individuals with severe brain injuries have persistent neuropsychological impairments, functional disability (e.g., difficulty managing day-to-day affairs), and poor return to work rates (Dikmen et al. 1993, 1994). The Glasgow Outcome Scale (Jennett and Bond 1975) was designed to categorize global functional outcome following traumatic brain injury. The five outcome categories are: (1) dead, (2) vegetative state, (3) severe disability (unable to live alone for more than 24 hours), (4) moderate disability (independent at home, able to utilize public transportation, able to work in a supported environment), and (5) good recovery (capable of resuming normal occupational and social functioning, although there might be minor residual physical or mental deficits). Patients who sustain severe traumatic brain injuries are at risk for moderate or severe disability. A substantial percentage, however, have good recovery. As a rule, patients with mild traumatic brain injuries have a good recovery, using this crude scale. Of course, good recovery includes patients with mild cognitive impairment, mild cognitive diminishment, and broadly normal cognitive functioning.

Cognitive impairment following traumatic brain injury is highly individualized and difficult to predict. Nonetheless, it is a truism that when considering groups of patients, those with severe traumatic brain injuries are *likely* to have some degree of persisting impairment and those with mild traumatic brain injuries are *unlikely* to have persisting impairment (Dikmen et al. 1995, 2001; Schretlen and Shapiro 2003). Mild TBIs can be associated with obvious cognitive impairment in the initial days and sometimes weeks post-injury (Bleiberg et al. 2004; Hughes et al. 2004; Lovell et al. 2004; Macciocchi et al. 1996; McCrea et al. 2002, 2003). Due to natural recovery, however, most patients with mild TBI do not experience measurable cognitive impairment beyond a few months post-injury (e.g., Bijur et al. 1990; Dikmen et al. 1995, 2001; Fay et al. 1993; Gentilini et al. 1985; Goldstein et al. 2001; Lahmeyer and Bellur 1987; Ponsford et al. 2000).

As a rule, the vast majority of recovery from moderate to severe TBI occurs within the first year, although some additional recovery can occur during the second year. Substantial improvements after 2 years are not realistic for most patients. However, improvement in functioning can and does occur as the result of learned accommodations and compensations in the years following injury.

Moderate or severe TBIs frequently result in permanent neurocognitive and neurobehavioral impairments. Neurobehavioral changes can include personality changes, problems regulating one's emotions, apathy, disinhibition, and anosognosia (loss of awareness of deficits and limitations). From a neurocognitive perspective, impairments are most notable in attention, concentration, working memory, speed of processing, and memory (Dikmen et al. 1986, 1995, 2001, 2003; Iverson 2005; Lezak et al. 2004; Mearns and Lees-Haley 1993; Spikman et al. 1999; Whyte et al. 2000). However, impairments are certainly not restricted to these domains. As injury severity increases, there is a greater likelihood of global cognitive deficit that may include motor skills, verbal and visual-spatial ability, and reasoning skills (Dikmen et al. 1995).

A linear relationship between injury severity and the magnitude and number of cognitive abilities affected is nicely illustrated by Dikmen and colleagues who compared the neuropsychological test performance of 121 general trauma patients with 436 patients with TBI 1-year post-injury, stratified by time to follow commands. The effect size for each measure has been calculated and is presented in Table 21.3 (with four specific variables illustrated visually in Fig. 21.8). Effect sizes, by convention, are considered as follows: 0.2 = small, 0.5 = medium, and 0.8 = large. As injury severity increases, we can see that the magnitude of impairment increases linearly, but there is also an increased number of impaired abilities across all cognitive domains. Notice that, on average, individuals who are able to

Table 21.3 Effect sizes of neuropsychological performance between general trauma and TBI patients stratified by time to follow commands (Dikmen et al. 1995)

	Time to follow commands					
	<1 hours	1–24 hours	1–6 days	7–13 days	14–28 days	≥29 days
Motor functions						
Finger tapping – DH	.26	.28	.91***	.90**	1.76***	3.14***
Finger tapping – NDH	.15	.18	.98***	.94**	1.67***	2.55***
Name writing – DH	.01	.07	.48	.64*	1.34***	2.74***
Name writing – NDH	.15	.28	.62	.86***	1.39***	2.50***
Attention and flexibility						
Seashore rhythm test	.01	.14	.37	.67	1.38***	2.51***
TMT part A	.09	.12	.39**	.62*	1.42***	2.72***
TMT part B	.11	.15	.16	.37	1.29***	2.22***
Stroop CWT – Part 1	.01	.25	.53	1.04***	1.84***	2.84***
Stroop CWT – Part 2	.06	.26	.41	.90***	1.72***	2.58***
Memory						
WMS-LM	.12	.30	.44	.53	1.00**	1.99***
WMS-VR	.14	.04	.09	.15	.91*	1.94***
SR-RCL	.11	.47	.56*	1.18***	1.86***	3.04***
WMS-LM delayed	.17	.42	.57*	.68*	1.19***	2.07***
WMS-VR delayed	.16	.07	.26	.25	1.19***	2.15***
SR-RCL, 30 min delay	.21	.48	.46	1.29***	1.78***	2.56***
SR-RCL, 4 h delay	.09	.34	.11	.91***	1.24***	2.32***
Verbal						
WAIS VIQ	.10	.22	.32	.61	1.07***	2.11***
Performance skills						
WAIS PIQ	.04	.36	.74***	.76**	1.65***	2.69***
TPT-T	.13	.03	.43***	.62***	1.25***	2.54***
Reasoning						
Category test	.21	.05	.40	.46	1.40***	2.20***
Overall						
Halstead Impairment Index	.01	.22	.71***	.60**	1.67***	2.53***

Cohen's effect sizes were calculated using data presented in Appendix B of Dikmen et al. Abbriviations: *DH* dominant hand, *NDH* non-dominant hand, *TMT* trail making test, *CWT* Color and Word test, *WMS* Wechsler memory scale, *LM* logical memory, *VR* visual reproduction, *SR-RCL* selective reminding test, *WAIS* Wechsler adult intelligence scale, *VIQ* verbal intelligence quotient, *PIQ* performance intelligence quotient, *TPT-T* tactual performance test, Time per block
All p values are reported from Dikmen et al.: *$p < .05$, **$p < .01$, ***$p < .001$

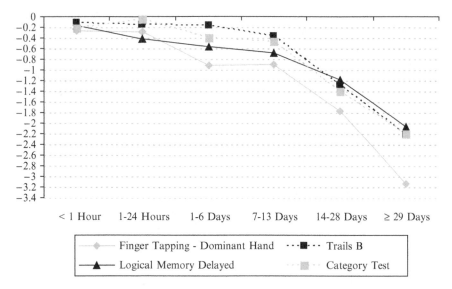

Fig. 21.8 Visual depiction of relation between brain injury severity and neurocognitive outcome at 1 year.

Note: Time to follow commands was used to sort patients into severity groups. Four test scores were selected to illustrate fine motor speed, processing speed and flexibility, delayed verbal memory, and reasoning. The values represent effect sizes compared to trauma control subjects. By convention, Cohen's effect sizes are interpreted as follows: 0.2 = small, 0.5 = medium, and 0.8 = large (From Dikmen et al. (1995))

follow simple commands within the first hour post-injury have nonsignificant, very small cognitive diminishments at 1-year post-injury (compared to trauma controls). In contrast, patients who take longer than 24 hours to follow simple commands are more likely to have widespread and substantial cognitive difficulties, with both the frequency and severity of deficits increasing in relation to injury severity.

Rule of thumb: Functional and Neuropsychological Outcome

- Neuropsychological and functional outcome is related to injury severity
- Acquired long-term deficits are common in moderate and severe brain injuries, but uncommon in mild brain injuries
- Most recovery from moderate to severe TBI occurs within the first year.
  - Additional recovery is possible in next year (2 years post-injury)
  - Substantial recovery of function 3+ years following moderate to severe TBI is not generally present, although accommodations and compensation strategies for deficits can improve functioning in every day tasks.
- Recovery of symptoms from mild TBI generally occurs in the first days to weeks following injury
  - Measurable cognitive deficits are usually not present after several months of injury

Neuropsychological Assessment Issues

The Diagnostic and Statistical Manual of Mental Disorders, 4th Edition (DSM-IV; American Psychiatric Association 1994) offers several categories for diagnosing cognitive problems that are due to a general medical condition, such as a moderate or severe traumatic brain injury. The categories that are the most relevant include cognitive disorder not otherwise specified (NOS) and dementia.

Cognitive disorder NOS is an Axis I DSM-IV diagnosis applied to people who have acquired cognitive impairments from a traumatic brain injury, neurological condition or disease (e.g., stroke or multiple sclerosis), or a general medical condition that affects the brain (e.g., systemic lupus erythematous). Cognitive disorder NOS (CD-NOS) is diagnosed if there is impairment in one, two, or more cognitive domains as the direct result of a general medical condition, but the level of impairment is not sufficient to meet criteria for dementia. CD-NOS is further broken down into two categories, mild neurocognitive disorder and post-concussional disorder (included as research criteria).

To identify a person as having mild neurocognitive disorder, there must be impairment in *at least two domains*, which can include attention or speed of information processing, memory, language, perceptual-motor abilities, and executive functioning. These cognitive impairments must be (1) due to a neurological or general medical condition, (2) considered abnormal or a decline from previous functioning, and (3) cause marked psychological distress or impairment in social, occupational, or other areas of functioning. However, according to the DSM-IV, a person with a traumatic brain injury needs to have impairment in only one domain (i.e., attention or memory) to meet criteria. The reader is encouraged to review the chapter by Iverson and Brooks in this book regarding strategies for improving our ability to accurately identify cognitive impairment.

When assessing patients who have sustained a moderate or severe traumatic brain injury, the clinician is placed in the potentially uncomfortable position of diagnosing the controversial post-concussional disorder. Post-concussional disorder, a specific diagnostic example with research criteria falling under CD-NOS, is distinguished from mild neurocognitive disorder by lesser and more specific criteria for cognitive impairment (e.g., impairment must include *attention or memory*) and a more specific etiology for the identified problems (i.e., traumatic brain injury). In addition, the person must have specific symptoms (e.g., headache and fatigue) that are believed to be due to the traumatic brain injury.

Clinicians can, however, simply diagnose CD-NOS and not post-concussional disorder. Diagnostic accuracy is strengthened, in our view, if the person has impairment in two or more domains and the cognitive impairment interferes with social or occupational functioning. The differential diagnosis between CD-NOS and dementia is based on the severity of impairments. For example, if evaluating a patient who has frank cognitive impairments, significant difficulties with social and occupational functioning, and evidence of a severe traumatic brain injury, the differential diagnosis would be CD-NOS versus dementia due to head trauma. According to the DSM-IV-Text Revision (DSM-IV-TR), CD-NOS is diagnosed if there is "less impairment and less impact on daily activities" (p. 763; American Psychiatric Association 2000) than would be expected for a diagnosis of dementia. Dementia, by definition, is characterized by seriously compromised cognitive functioning and frank impairment in the person's activities of daily living. Dementia is uncommon following a moderate TBI. Dementia can be diagnosed, of course, in a subset of patients with serious residual cognitive and functional impairments arising from a severe traumatic brain injury.

Psychosocial Outcome

The short- and long-term effects of moderate and severe TBI present a number of challenges that make adjustment back to everyday life difficult for both patient and family members. Some of the most common issues relate to substance abuse, family and marital integration, return to work, and community integration.

Substance Abuse

Substance abuse following TBI is common and can interfere with rehabilitation. The prevalence of substance abuse in patients following TBI is typically higher than those without TBI. In a population-based study, Silver and colleagues reported that the prevalence of alcohol and drug abuse disorders was 25 and 11%, respectively, in persons with a history of TBI, compared to 10 and 5% in those without a history of TBI (Silver et al. 2001). Risk factors for substance abuse following TBI include (1) pre-injury history of substance abuse, (2) onset of depression since injury, (3) better physical functioning, (4) male gender, (5) younger age, (6) being uninsured, and (7) not being married (Horner et al. 2005). Combinations of these factors might be related to resumption of, or development of, substance abuse problems following a TBI.

For the majority of people, substance abuse problems following TBI reflect the *resumption* of substance use patterns that existed prior to the injury. Researchers have found high prevalence rates of pre-injury substance abuse problems in TBI rehabilitation populations, with 43–58% having alcohol abuse problems, 29–39% having illicit drug abuse problems, and 48–61% having either or both problems (Bombardier et al. 2003; Corrigan et al. 2001, 2003). The prevalence of pre-injury alcohol and drug abuse problems in a TBI population are much higher than those found in the general population (e.g., 13–29% alcohol abuse problems and 9–22% illicit drug problems; Miller 1991).

Following TBI, patients will typically consume less alcohol or drugs in the acute stages of recovery, similar to other hospitalized patients (Bombardier et al. 2003; Corrigan et al. 1995; Jones 1989; Kreutzer et al. 1996). However, patients tend to return to pre-injury usage levels. Studies examining the rate of return of alcohol consumption post-injury have demonstrated a decline in alcohol consumption in the first year, with incremental increases in consumption at 1, 2, and 3 years post-injury (Bombardier et al. 2003; Corrigan et al. 1998; Kreutzer et al. 1996). Resumption of illicit drug use is much slower than alcohol, with fewer than 25% of previous users reporting any use after 2 years (Kreutzer et al. 1996).

Although the large majority of substance abuse problems following TBI may be related to the resumption of pre-injury usage patterns, some individuals who did not have a history of substance abuse may develop problems following injury (Corrigan 2007). Bombardier and colleagues reported that 14.8% of persons who reported an abstinence or only light consumption of alcohol before injury were reporting consuming moderate or heavy amounts of alcohol at 1-year post-injury (Bombardier et al. 2003). Increases in alcohol use post-injury may be related to self-medication attempts to alleviate pain, depression, and/or anxiety (Corrigan 2007), though this issue has received little research to date and is poorly understood.

Return to Work

Vocational outcome following TBI is important for patients and society as a whole. For many individuals, the inability to return to work results in a number of economic, social, family, and interpersonal problems (Dikmen et al. 1994; Kraus et al. 2005; Wrightson and Gronwall 1981). In addition, the economic burden placed on society is of concern (e.g., long-term sickness benefits and unemployment benefits), particularly because many individuals who sustain a TBI tend to be young and have their whole working lives ahead of them (Ruffolo et al. 1999).

Injury severity is related to successful return to work. Individuals who have sustained moderate or severe TBIs have consistently lower return to work rates when compared to individuals who have sustained a mild TBI (e.g., Asikainen et al. 1996; Dawson et al. 2004; Dikmen et al. 1994; Hawley et al. 2004; Stambrook et al. 1990; Uzzell et al. 1987). For example, Dikmen and colleagues (Dikmen et al. 1994) reported successful return to work rates after 2 years post-injury in 38% of those with severe TBIs, 66% for moderate TBIs, and 80% for mild TBIs. Return to work rates following moderate to severe TBI reported in the literature range from (1) 13–44% within the first 6 months, (2) 26–56% after 1 year, (3) 37–64% after 2 years, and (4) 35–77% after 4–5 years (Dawson et al. 2004; Dikmen et al. 1994; Greenspan et al. 1996; Mazaux et al. 1997; Olver et al. 1996; Ponsford et al. 1995; Ruff et al. 1993; Stambrook et al. 1990).

Evidence-based factors that statistically increase the risk of poor return to work include: (1) being married, male, age greater than 40, or having low education; (2) previous employment in semi- or unskilled manual jobs; (3) starting a new job; (4) low level of social support; (5) greater cognitive, physical, and psychosocial impairment; (6) changes in personality; and (7) a history of substance abuse. There is empirical evidence that neuropsychological variables are one factor related to return to work. Factors that may increase the probability of a *successful return to work* include: (1) using a multidisciplinary team approach during the acute rehabilitation stage, (2) providing a socially inclusive work environment, (3) having health insurance, (4) having social interaction on the job, (5) returning to a job with greater decision-making latitude, (6) providing environmental modifications, and (7) focusing the position on the vocational strengths of the individual (West et al. 2007).

Rule of thumb: Return to work
_____

- Negative predictors of return to work include more severe injuries, age greater than 40, low education, greater physical or cognitive impairment, personality change, and substance abuse.
- Positive predictors of return to work include using a multidisciplinary team approach during the acute rehabilitation stage, providing a socially inclusive work environment, providing environmental modifications, and focusing the position on the strengths of the individual.

Marital and Family Issues

TBIs in family members result in adverse effects for the entire family system (Cavallo and Kay 2005). The impact of TBI on the family varies depending on the relationship between injured and uninjured family members. The greatest burden is usually placed on the *spouse* in which a previously equal partnership is broken and they assume some caregiver or supervision responsibilities. Couples may be faced with increased financial burden, changes of lifestyle, loss of support from the injured spouse, sexuality and intimacy problems, and separation/divorce. When a child is injured, *parents* may be impacted by increased tension in their marital relationship, neglect of their other children, and decreased adult social interaction with friends. *Children* of parents with brain injury may be faced with the loss of nurturance and love from the parent or emergence of behavioral problems due to changes in their family situation. Uninjured *siblings* may feel neglected by their parents and develop behavior problems. Adult children and adult siblings are often torn between the needs of their own lives and the needs of the injured parent or sibling (Cavallo and Kay 2005).

Regardless of the family relationship, there is an obvious increased burden for those family members who have assumed the role of caregiver. Cavallo and Kay (2005) emphasized four important themes that have emerged from studies examining subjective burden on caregivers. Researchers have reported that subjective burden of family members (1) tends to increase, not decrease, over time; (2) is most related to changes in personality, emotions, and behavior, of which the person with brain injury is least aware; (3) is largely the result of neurobehavioral manifestations of TBI and not the neurological severity per se; and (4) tends to be determined by the ability of the family members to adjust to the new situation (Cavallo and Kay 2005).

Community Integration

Community integration following TBI is important for improving quality of life. The most common community integration issues are: (1) family adjustment, (2) social isolation, (3) limited community mobility, and (4) returning to work. Family adjustment and return to work issues have been discussed. Social isolation commonly manifests as a consequence of the person not being able to fulfill or resume a social role following injury. This may be caused by psychosocial or emotional problems (e.g., depression, anxiety, fatigue), or a loss of other skills to develop and maintain personal relationships (e.g., language deficits and personality changes). Limited community mobility is related to transportation problems, such as driving restrictions or inability to independently use public transportation. This might be due to: (1) physical or sensory impairments (e.g., motor incoordination, visual deficits, post-traumatic epilepsy), (2) cognitive deficits (e.g., distractibility, judgment problems), and/or (3) behavioral changes (e.g., impulsivity). Driving can be a very difficult issue for some patients because it is an unattainable, highly desired, personal goal (Kneipp and Rubin 2007).

Rule of thumb: Community Integration

- Community integration is facilitated by good family support, presence of social and peer support, access to transportation (being able to drive), and returning to work.

Conclusions

Traumatic brain injuries are common. It is estimated that there are more than 1.4 million TBIs in the United States each year. These injuries occur on a broad continuum of severity, from very mild to catastrophic. The vast majority (at least 80%) are mild in severity. The severity of injury typically is classified based on combinations of severity criteria derived from the duration of unconsciousness, Glasgow Coma Scale score, duration of post-traumatic amnesia, and, sometimes, the results of neuroimaging.

Moderate and severe TBIs can result in temporary, prolonged, or permanent neurological or neuropsychiatric problems. These problems may include motor impairments, movement disorders, poor balance and dizziness, visual impairments, cranial nerve impairments, headaches, sexual dysfunction, fatigue and sleep problems, depression and anxiety disorders, psychotic disorders, personality changes, apathy, and a lack of awareness.

Many individuals with severe brain injuries have persistent functional disabilities (e.g., managing day-to-day affairs) and poor return to work rates. Problems with returning to work results in a number of economic, social, family, and interpersonal problems for the patients. In addition, there is an increased economic burden on society because many of these individuals are young and have their whole working lives ahead of them.

Without question, moderate and severe TBI can result in permanent neurocognitive impairments. In general, there is a linear relationship between injury severity and the magnitude and number of cognitive abilities affected. Impairments are most notable in attention, concentration, working memory, speed of processing, and memory. As injury severity increases, there is a greater likelihood of widespread cognitive deficits. As a rule, the vast majority of recovery from moderate to severe TBI occurs within the first year, with some additional recovery expected during the second year. Substantial improvements after 2 years are not expected for most patients. However, improvement in functioning can and does occur as the result of learned accommodations and compensations in the years following injury.

It is important to appreciate that the long-term neurological, neuropsychiatric, functional, and neurocognitive deficits and problems associated with moderate to severe TBI are not restricted to the injured person. TBI in a family member results in adverse effects for the entire family system. The greatest burden is typically placed on those family members that assume the role of caregiver. The level of burden placed on the caregiver is significantly influenced by changes in the family system and role responsibilities, financial difficulties, and the level of independence exhibited by the injured person as he or she attempts to integrate back into the community.

Acknowledgments The authors thank Ms. Elena Dupont for providing Figs. 21.2, 21.3, 21.5, and 21.6.

References

AbdelMalik, P., Husted, J., Chow, E. W., & Bassett, A. S. (2003). Childhood head injury and expression of schizophrenia in multiply affected families. *Archives of General Psychiatry, 60*(3), 231–236.

Achte, K., Jarho, L., Kyykka, T., & Vesterinen, E. (1991). Paranoid disorders following war brain damage. Preliminary report. *Psychopathology, 24*(5), 309–315.

Adams, H., Mitchell, D. E., Graham, D. I., & Doyle, D. (1977). Diffuse brain damage of immediate impact type. Its relationship to 'primary brain-stem damage' in head injury. *Brain, 100*(3), 489–502.

Adams, J. H., Graham, D. I., Scott, G., Parker, L. S., & Doyle, D. (1980). Brain damage in fatal non-missile head injury. *Journal of Clinical Pathology, 33*(12), 1132–1145.

American Neurological Association Committee on Ethical Affairs. (1993). Persistent vegetative state: Report of the American Neurological Association Committee on Ethical Affairs. ANA Committee on Ethical Affairs. *Annals of Neurology, 33*(4), 386–390.

American Psychiatric Association. (1994). *Diagnostic and statistical manual of mental disorders* (4th ed.). Washington, DC: American Psychiatric Association.

American Psychiatric Association. (2000). *Diagnostic and statistical manual of mental disorders* (Text Revision 4th ed.). Washington, DC: American Psychiatric Association.

Anderson, C. V., & Bigler, E. D. (1995). Ventricular dilation, cortical atrophy, and neuropsychological outcome following traumatic brain injury. *The Journal of Neuropsychiatry and Clinical Neurosciences, 7*(1), 42–48.

Annegers, J. F., Grabow, J. D., Kurland, L. T., & Laws, E. R., Jr. (1980). The incidence, causes, and secular trends of head trauma in Olmsted County, Minnesota, 1935–1974. *Neurology, 30*(9), 912–919.

Arfanakis, K., Haughton, V. M., Carew, J. D., Rogers, B. P., Dempsey, R. J., & Meyerand, M. E. (2002). Diffusion tensor MR imaging in diffuse axonal injury. *American Journal of Neuroradiology, 23*(5), 794–802.

Ashman, T. A., Spielman, L. A., Hibbard, M. R., Silver, J. M., Chandna, T., & Gordon, W. A. (2004). Psychiatric challenges in the first 6 years after traumatic brain injury: Cross-sequential analyses of Axis I disorders. *Archives of Physical Medicine and Rehabilitation, 85*(4 Suppl 2), S36–S42.

Asikainen, I., Kaste, M., & Sarna, S. (1996). Patients with traumatic brain injury referred to a rehabilitation and re-employment programme: Social and professional outcome for 508 Finnish patients 5 or more years after injury. *Brain Injury, 10*(12), 883–899.

Barkley, J. M., Morales, D., Hayman, L. A., & Diaz-Marchan, P. J. (2007). Static neuroimaging in the evaluation of TBI. In N. D. Zasler, D. I. Katz, & R. D. Zafonte (Eds.), *Brain injury medicine: Principles and practice* (pp. 129–148). New York: Demos.

Bazarian, J. J., McClung, J., Cheng, Y. T., Flesher, W., & Schneider, S. M. (2005). Emergency department management of mild traumatic brain injury in the USA. *Emergency Medicine Journal, 22*(7), 473–477.

Berrol, S. (1986). Evolution and the persistent vegetative state. *The Journal of Head Trauma Rehabilitation, 1*, 7–13.

Bigler, E. D. (2005). *Structural imaging*. London: American Psychiatric Publishing, Inc.

Bigler, E. D., Kurth, S. M., Blatter, D., & Abildskov, T. J. (1992). Degenerative changes in traumatic brain injury: Post-injury magnetic resonance identified ventricular expansion compared to pre-injury levels. *Brain Research Bulletin, 28*(4), 651–653.

Bijur, P. E., Haslum, M., & Golding, J. (1990). Cognitive and behavioral sequelae of mild head injury in children. *Pediatrics, 86*(3), 337–344.

Bleiberg, J., Cernich, A. N., Cameron, K., Sun, W., Peck, K., Ecklund, P. J., et al. (2004). Duration of cognitive impairment after sports concussion. *Neurosurgery, 54*(5), 1073–1078. discussion 1078–1080.

Bombardier, C. H., Temkin, N. R., Machamer, J., & Dikmen, S. S. (2003). The natural history of drinking and alcohol-related problems after traumatic brain injury. *Archives of Physical Medicine and Rehabilitation, 84*(2), 185–191.

Bombardier, C. H., Fann, J. R., Temkin, N., Esselman, P. C., Pelzer, E., Keough, M., et al. (2006). Posttraumatic stress disorder symptoms during the first six months after traumatic brain injury. *The Journal of Neuropsychiatry and Clinical Neurosciences, 18*(4), 501–508.

Brain Association of British Columbia (2002). Retrieved Jan, 2006, from www.lmbia.org/qs/page/1499/0/-1

Breslau, N., Lipton, R. B., Stewart, W. F., Schultz, L. R., & Welch, K. M. (2003). Comorbidity of migraine and depression: Investigating potential etiology and prognosis. *Neurology, 60*(8), 1308–1312.

British Medical Association Medical Ethics Committee. (1992). *Discussion paper of patients in persistent vegetative state*. London: BMA.

Bushnik, T., Englander, J., & Wright, J. (2008). The experience of fatigue in the first 2 years after moderate-to-severe traumatic brain injury: A preliminary report. *The Journal of Head Trauma Rehabilitation, 23*(1), 17–24.

Campbell, M., & Parry, A. (2005). Balance disorder and traumatic brain injury: Preliminary findings of a multi-factorial observational study. *Brain Injury, 19*(13), 1095–1104.

Cavallo, M. M., & Kay, T. (2005). The family system. In J. M. Silver, T. W. McAllister, & S. C. Yudofsky (Eds.), *Textbook of traumatic brain injury* (pp. 533–558). Arlington, VA: American Psychiatric Publishing, Inc.

Charness, M. E. (1993). Brain lesions in alcoholics. *Alcoholism, Clinical and Experimental Research, 17*(1), 2–11.

Christman, C. W., Grady, M. S., Walker, S. A., Holloway, K. L., & Povlishock, J. T. (1994). Ultrastructural studies of diffuse axonal injury in humans. *Journal of Neurotrauma, 11*(2), 173–186.

Corcoran, C., McAllister, T. W., & Malaspina, D. (2005). Psychotic disorders. In J. M. Silver, T. W. McAllister, & S. C. Yudofsky (Eds.), *Textbook of traumatic brain injury* (pp. 213–229). Arlington, VA: American Psychiatric Publishing, Inc.

Corrigan, J. D. (2007). The treatment of substance abuse in persons with TBI. In N. D. Zasler, D. I. Katz, & R. D. Zafonte (Eds.), *Brain injury medicine* (pp. 1105–1115). New York: Demos Medical Publishing, LLC.

Corrigan, J. D., Lamb-Hart, G. L., & Rust, E. (1995). A programme of intervention for substance abuse following traumatic brain injury. *Brain Injury, 9*(3), 221–236.

Corrigan, J. D., Smith-Knapp, K., & Granger, C. V. (1998). Outcomes in the first 5 years after traumatic brain injury. *Archives of Physical Medicine and Rehabilitation, 79*(3), 298–305.

Corrigan, J. D., Bogner, J. A., Mysiw, W. J., Clinchot, D., & Fugate, L. (2001). Life satisfaction after traumatic brain injury. *The Journal of Head Trauma Rehabilitation, 16*(6), 543–555.

Corrigan, J. D., Bogner, J., Lamb-Hart, G., & Sivik-Sears, N. (2003). *Technical report on problematic substance use variables.* The Center for Outcome Measurement in Brain Injury. Retrieved 18 Mar 2008, from http://www.tbims.org/combi/subst

Dawson, D. R., Levine, B., Schwartz, M. L., & Stuss, D. T. (2004). Acute predictors of real-world outcomes following traumatic brain injury: A prospective study. *Brain Injury, 18*(3), 221–238.

Dikmen, S., McLean, A., Jr., Temkin, N. R., & Wyler, A. R. (1986). Neuropsychologic outcome at one-month postinjury. *Archives of Physical Medicine and Rehabilitation, 67*(8), 507–513.

Dikmen, S., Machamer, J., & Temkin, N. (1993). Psychosocial outcome in patients with moderate to severe head injury: 2-year follow-up. *Brain Injury, 7*(2), 113–124.

Dikmen, S., Temkin, N. R., Machamer, J. E., Holubkov, A. L., Fraser, R. T., & Winn, H. R. (1994). Employment following traumatic head injuries. *Archives of Neurology, 51*(2), 177–186.

Dikmen, S., Machamer, J. E., Winn, R., & Temkin, N. R. (1995). Neuropsychological outcome 1-year post head injury. *Neuropsychology, 9*, 80–90.

Dikmen, S., Machamer, J., & Temkin, N. (2001). Mild head injury: Facts and artifacts. *Journal of Clinical and Experimental Neuropsychology, 23*(6), 729–738.

Dikmen, S., Machamer, J. E., Powell, J. M., & Temkin, N. R. (2003). Outcome 3 to 5 years after moderate to severe traumatic brain injury. *Archives of Physical Medicine and Rehabilitation, 84*(10), 1449–1457.

Dikmen, S., Bombardier, C. H., Machamer, J. E., Fann, J. R., & Temkin, N. R. (2004). Natural history of depression in traumatic brain injury. *Archives of Physical Medicine and Rehabilitation, 85*(9), 1457–1464.

Erb, D. E., & Povlishock, J. T. (1991). Neuroplasticity following traumatic brain injury: A study of GABAergic terminal loss and recovery in the cat dorsal lateral vestibular nucleus. *Experimental Brain Research, 83*(2), 253–267.

Fay, G. C., Jaffe, K. M., Polissar, N. L., Liao, S., Martin, K. M., Shurtleff, H. A., et al. (1993). Mild pediatric traumatic brain injury: A cohort study. *Archives of Physical Medicine and Rehabilitation, 74*(9), 895–901.

Fellus, J. L., & Elovic, E. P. (2007). Fatigue: Assessment and treatment. In N. D. Zasler, D. I. Katz, & R. D. Zafonte (Eds.), *Brain injury medicine* (pp. 545–555). New York: Demos Medical Publishing, LLC.

Flashman, L. A., & McAllister, T. W. (2002). Lack of awareness and its impact in traumatic brain injury. *NeuroRehabilitation, 17*(4), 285–296.

Flashman, L. A., Amador, X., & McAllister, T. W. (2005). Awareness of deficits. In J. M. Silver, T. W. McAllister, & S. C. Yudofsky (Eds.), *Textbook of traumatic brain injury* (pp. 353–367). Arlington, VA: American Psychiatric Publishing, Inc.

Gagnon, I., Forget, R., Sullivan, S. J., & Friedman, D. (1998). Motor performance following a mild traumatic brain injury in children: An exploratory study. *Brain Injury, 12*(10), 843–853.

Gean, A. D. (1994). White matter shearing injury and brainstem injury. In A. D. Gean (Ed.), *Imaging of head trauma* (pp. 207–248). New York: Raven Press.

Gennarelli, T. A., & Graham, D. I. (1998). Neuropathology of the head injuries. *Seminars in Clinical Neuropsychiatry, 3*(3), 160–175.

Gentilini, M., Nichelli, P., Schoenhuber, R., Bortolotti, P., Tonelli, L., Falasca, A., et al. (1985). Neuropsychological evaluation of mild head injury. *Journal of Neurology, Neurosurgery and Psychiatry, 48*(2), 137–140.

Gentry, L. R., Godersky, J. C., & Thompson, B. (1988a). MR imaging of head trauma: Review of the distribution and radiopathologic features of traumatic lesions. *American Journal of Roentgenology, 150*(3), 663–672.

Gentry, L. R., Godersky, J. C., Thompson, B., & Dunn, V. D. (1988b). Prospective comparative study of intermediate-field MR and CT in the evaluation of closed head trauma. *American Journal of Roentgenology, 150*(3), 673–682.

Geurts, A. C., Ribbers, G. M., Knoop, J. A., & van Limbeek, J. (1996). Identification of static and dynamic postural instability following traumatic brain injury. *Archives of Physical Medicine and Rehabilitation, 77*(7), 639–644.

Gil, S., Caspi, Y., Ben-Ari, I. Z., Koren, D., & Klein, E. (2005). Does memory of a traumatic event increase the risk for posttraumatic stress disorder in patients with traumatic brain injury? A prospective study. *The American Journal of Psychiatry, 162*(5), 963–969.

Goldstein, F. C., Levin, H. S., Goldman, W. P., Clark, A. N., & Altonen, T. K. (2001). Cognitive and neurobehavioral functioning after mild versus moderate traumatic brain injury in older adults. *Journal of the International Neuropsychological Society, 7*(3), 373–383.

Gorrie, C., Duflou, J., Brown, J., Gibson, T., & Waite, P. M. (2001). Extent and distribution of vascular brain injury in pediatric road fatalities. *Journal of Neurotrauma, 18*(9), 849–860.

Grady, M. S., McLaughlin, M. R., Christman, C. W., Valadka, A. B., Fligner, C. L., & Povlishock, J. T. (1993). The use of antibodies targeted against the neurofilament subunits for the detection of diffuse axonal injury in humans. *Journal of Neuropathology and Experimental Neurology, 52*(2), 143–152.

Greenspan, A. I., Wrigley, J. M., Kresnow, M., Branche-Dorsey, C. M., & Fine, P. R. (1996). Factors influencing failure to return to work due to traumatic brain injury. *Brain Injury, 10*(3), 207–218.

Greenwald, B. D., Cifu, D. X., Marwitz, J. H., Enders, L. J., Brown, A. W., Englander, J. S., et al. (2001). Factors associated with balance deficits on admission to rehabilitation after traumatic brain injury: A multicenter analysis. *The Journal of Head Trauma Rehabilitation, 16*(3), 238–252.

Gureje, O., Bamidele, R., & Raji, O. (1994). Early brain trauma and schizophrenia in Nigerian patients. *The American Journal of Psychiatry, 151*(3), 368–371.

Harris, J. H., & Harris, W. H. (2000). *The radiology of emergency medicine* (4th ed.). Philadelphia: Lippincott, Williams & Wilkins.

Harvey, A. G., & Bryant, R. A. (2000). Two-year prospective evaluation of the relationship between acute stress disorder and posttraumatic stress disorder following mild traumatic brain injury. *The American Journal of Psychiatry, 157*(4), 626–628.

Hawley, C. A., Ward, A. B., Magnay, A. R., & Mychalkiw, W. (2004). Return to school after brain injury. *Archives of Disease in Childhood, 89*(2), 136–142.

Hibbard, M. R., Uysal, S., Kepler, K., Bogdany, J., & Silver, J. (1998). Axis I psychopathology in individuals with traumatic brain injury. *The Journal of Head Trauma Rehabilitation, 13*(4), 24–39.

Hibbard, M. R., Ashman, T. A., Spielman, L. A., Chun, D., Charatz, H. J., & Melvin, S. (2004). Relationship between depression and psychosocial functioning after traumatic brain injury. *Archives of Physical Medicine and Rehabilitation, 85*(4 Suppl 2), S43–S53.

Hickling, E. J., Gillen, R., Blanchard, E. B., Buckley, T., & Taylor, A. (1998). Traumatic brain injury and posttraumatic stress disorder: a preliminary investigation of neuropsychological test results in PTSD secondary to motor vehicle accidents. *Brain Injury, 12*(4), 265–274.

Higashi, K., Sakata, Y., Hatano, M., Abiko, S., Ihara, K., Katayama, S., et al. (1977). Epidemiological studies on patients with a persistent vegetative state. *Journal of Neurology, Neurosurgery and Psychiatry, 40*(9), 876–885.

Hillbom, E. (1960). After-effects of brain-injuries. Research on the symptoms causing invalidism of persons in Finland having sustained brain-injuries during the wars of 1939–1940 and 1941–1944. *Acta Psychiatrica Scandinavica. Supplementum, 35*(142), 1–195.

Hillier, S. L., Sharpe, M. H., & Metzer, J. (1997). Outcomes 5 years post-traumatic brain injury (with further reference to neurophysical impairment and disability). *Brain Injury, 11*(9), 661–675.

Horner, M. D., Ferguson, P. L., Selassie, A. W., Labbate, L. A., Kniele, K., & Corrigan, J. D. (2005). Patterns of alcohol use 1 year after traumatic brain injury: A population-based, epidemiological study. *Journal of the International Neuropsychological Society, 11*(3), 322–330.

Hughes, D. G., Jackson, A., Mason, D. L., Berry, E., Hollis, S., & Yates, D. W. (2004). Abnormalities on magnetic resonance imaging seen acutely following mild traumatic brain injury: Correlation with neuropsychological tests and delayed recovery. *Neuroradiology, 46*(7), 550–558.

Huisman, T. A., Schwamm, L. H., Schaefer, P. W., Koroshetz, W. J., Shetty-Alva, N., Ozsunar, Y., et al. (2004). Diffusion tensor imaging as potential biomarker of white matter injury in diffuse axonal injury. *American Journal of Neuroradiology, 25*(3), 370–376.

Inglese, M., Bomsztyk, E., Gonen, O., Mannon, L. J., Grossman, R. I., & Rusinek, H. (2005a). Dilated perivascular spaces: Hallmarks of mild traumatic brain injury. *American Journal of Neuroradiology, 26*(4), 719–724.

Inglese, M., Makani, S., Johnson, G., Cohen, B. A., Silver, J. A., Gonen, O., et al. (2005b). Diffuse axonal injury in mild traumatic brain injury: A diffusion tensor imaging study. *Journal of Neurosurgery, 103*(2), 298–303.

Iverson, G. L. (2005). Outcome from mild traumatic brain injury. *Current Opinion in Psychiatry, 18*, 301–317.

Jagger, J., Levine, J. I., Jane, J. A., & Rimel, R. W. (1984). Epidemiologic features of head injury in a predominantly rural population. *The Journal of Trauma, 24*(1), 40–44.

Jennett, B. (1996). Clinical and pathological features of vegetative survival. In H. S. Levin, A. L. Benton, J. P. Muizelaar, & H. M. Eisenberg (Eds.), *Catastrophic brain injury*. New York: Oxford University Press.

Jennett, B., & Bond, M. (1975). Assessment of outcome after severe brain damage. *Lancet, 1*(7905), 480–484.

Jones, G. A. (1989). Alcohol abuse and traumatic brain injury. *Alcohol Health and Research World, 13*(2), 104–109.

Jorge, R. E., Robinson, R. G., Starkstein, S. E., & Arndt, S. V. (1993). Depression and anxiety following traumatic brain injury. *The Journal of Neuropsychiatry and Clinical Neurosciences, 5*(4), 369–374.

Jorge, R. E., Robinson, R. G., Moser, D., Tateno, A., Crespo-Facorro, B., & Arndt, S. (2004). Major depression following traumatic brain injury. *Archives of General Psychiatry, 61*(1), 42–50.

Kapoor, N., & Ciuffreda, K. J. (2005). Vision problems. In J. M. Silver, T. W. McAllister, & S. C. Yudofsky (Eds.), *Textbook of traumatic brain injury* (pp. 405–415). Arlington, VA: American Psychiatric Publishing.

Kaufman, K. R., Brey, R. H., Chou, L. S., Rabatin, A., Brown, A. W., & Basford, J. R. (2006). Comparison of subjective and objective measurements of balance disorders following traumatic brain injury. *Medical Engineering & Physics, 28*(3), 234–239.

Klauber, M. R., Barrett-Connor, E., Marshall, L. F., & Bowers, S. A. (1981). The epidemiology of head injury: A prospective study of an entire community-San Diego County, California, 1978. *American Journal of Epidemiology, 113*(5), 500–509.

Kneipp, S., & Rubin, A. (2007). Community re-entry issues and long-term care. In N. D. Zasler, D. I. Katz, & R. D. Zafonte (Eds.), *Brain injury medicine* (pp. 1085–1104). New York: Demos Medical Publishing, LLC.

Kochanek, P. M., Clark, R. S. B., & Jenkins, L. W. (2007). TBI: Pathobiology. In N. D. Zasler, D. I. Katz, & R. D. Zafonte (Eds.), *Brain injury medicine: Principles and practice* (pp. 81–96). New York: Demos.

Koponen, S., Taiminen, T., Portin, R., Himanen, L., Isoniemi, H., Heinonen, H., et al. (2002). Axis I and II psychiatric disorders after traumatic brain injury: A 30-year follow-up study. *The American Journal of Psychiatry, 159*(8), 1315–1321.

Kraus, J. F., & Chu, L. D. (2005). Epidemiology. In J. M. Silver, T. W. McAllister, & S. C. Yudofsky (Eds.), *Textbook of traumatic brain injury* (pp. 3–26). Arlington, VA: American Psychiatric Publishing, Inc.

Kraus, J. F., Fife, D., Ramstein, K., Conroy, C., & Cox, P. (1986). The relationship of family income to the incidence, external causes, and outcomes of serious brain injury, San Diego County, California. *American Journal of Public Health, 76*(11), 1345–1347.

Kraus, J., Schaffer, K., Ayers, K., Stenehjem, J., Shen, H., & Afifi, A. A. (2005). Physical complaints, medical service use, and social and employment changes following mild traumatic brain injury: A 6-month longitudinal study. *The Journal of Head Trauma Rehabilitation, 20*(3), 239–256.

Krauss, J., & Jankovic, J. (2007). Movement disorders after TBI. In N. D. Zasler, D. I. Katz, & R. D. Zafonte (Eds.), *Brain injury medicine* (pp. 469–489). New York, NY: Demos Medical Publishing, LLC.

Kreutzer, J. S., Witol, A. D., & Marwitz, J. H. (1996). Alcohol and drug use among young persons with traumatic brain injury. *Journal of Learning Disabilities, 29*(6), 643–651.

Lahmeyer, H. W., & Bellur, S. N. (1987). Cardiac regulation and depression. *Journal of Psychiatry Research, 21*(1), 1–6.

Langlois, J. A., Rutland-Brown, W., & Thomas, K. E. (2004). *Traumatic brain injury in the United States: Emergency department visits, hospitalizaitons, and deaths*. Atlanta, GA: Centers for Disease Control and Prevention, National Center for Injury Prevention and Control.

Le, T. H., Mukherjee, P., Henry, R. G., Berman, J. I., Ware, M., & Manley, G. T. (2005). Diffusion tensor imaging with three-dimensional fiber tractography of traumatic axonal shearing injury: An imaging correlate for the posterior callosal "disconnection" syndrome: Case report. *Neurosurgery, 56*(1), 189.

Levin, H. S. (2003). Neuroplasticity following non-penetrating traumatic brain injury. *Brain Injury, 17*(8), 665–674.

Levin, H. S., Williams, D. H., Valastro, M., Eisenberg, H. M., Crofford, M. J., & Handel, S. F. (1990). Corpus callosal atrophy following closed head injury: Detection with magnetic resonance imaging. *Journal of Neurosurgery, 73*(1), 77–81.

Levin, H. S., Brown, S. A., Song, J. X., McCauley, S. R., Boake, C., Contant, C. F., et al. (2001). Depression and posttraumatic stress disorder at 3 months after mild to moderate traumatic brain injury. *Journal of Clinical and Experimental Neuropsychology, 23*(6), 754–769.

Lezak, M. D., Howieson, D. B., & Loring, D. W. (2004). *Neuropsychological assessment* (4th ed.). New York: Oxford University Press.

Lovell, M. R., Collins, M. W., Iverson, G. L., Johnston, K. M., & Bradley, J. P. (2004). Grade 1 or "ding" concussions in high school athletes. *The American Journal of Sports Medicine, 32*(1), 47–54.

Lucas, J. A. (1998). Traumatic brain injury and post concussive syndrome. In P. J. Snyder & P. D. Nussbaum (Eds.), *Clinical neuropsychology* (pp. 243–265). Washington, DC: American Psychological Association.

Macciocchi, S. N., Barth, J. T., Alves, W., Rimel, R. W., & Jane, J. A. (1996). Neuropsychological functioning and recovery after mild head injury in collegiate athletes. *Neurosurgery, 39*(3), 510–514.

MacKenzie, E. J., Edelstein, S. L., & Flynn, J. P. (1989). Hospitalized head-injured patients in Maryland: Incidence and severity of injuries. *Maryland Medical Journal, 38*(9), 725–732.

MacKenzie, J. D., Siddiqi, F., Babb, J. S., Bagley, L. J., Mannon, L. J., Sinson, G. P., et al. (2002). Brain atrophy in mild or moderate traumatic brain injury: A longitudinal quantitative analysis. *American Journal of Neuroradiology, 23*(9), 1509–1515.

Malaspina, D., Goetz, R. R., Friedman, J. H., Kaufmann, C. A., Faraone, S. V., Tsuang, M., et al. (2001). Traumatic brain injury and schizophrenia in members of schizophrenia and bipolar disorder pedigrees. *The American Journal of Psychiatry, 158*(3), 440–446.

Mather, F. J., Tate, R. L., & Hannan, T. J. (2003). Post-traumatic stress disorder in children following road traffic accidents: A comparison of those with and without mild traumatic brain injury. *Brain Injury, 17*(12), 1077–1087.

Mayou, R. A., Black, J., & Bryant, B. (2000). Unconsciousness, amnesia and psychiatric symptoms following road traffic accident injury. *The British Journal of Psychiatry, 177*, 540–545.

Mazaux, J. M., Masson, F., Levin, H. S., Alaoui, P., Maurette, P., & Barat, M. (1997). Long-term neuropsychological outcome and loss of social autonomy after traumatic brain injury. *Archives of Physical Medicine and Rehabilitation, 78*(12), 1316–1320.

McAllister, T. W., Sparling, M. B., Flashman, L. A., & Saykin, A. J. (2001). Neuroimaging findings in mild traumatic brain injury. *Journal of Clinical and Experimental Neuropsychology, 23*(6), 775–791.

McCrea, M., Kelly, J. P., Randolph, C., Cisler, R., & Berger, L. (2002). Immediate neurocognitive effects of concussion. *Neurosurgery, 50*(5), 1032–1040.

McCrea, M., Guskiewicz, K. M., Marshall, S. W., Barr, W., Randolph, C., Cantu, R. C., et al. (2003). Acute effects and recovery time following concussion in collegiate football players: The NCAA Concussion Study. *Journal of the American Medical Association, 290*(19), 2556–2563.

Mearns, J., & Lees-Haley, P. R. (1993). Discriminating neuropsychological sequelae of head injury from alcohol-abuse-induced deficits: A review and analysis. *Journal of Clinical Psychology, 49*(5), 714–720.

Miles, L., Grossman, R. I., Johnson, G., Babb, J. S., Diller, L., & Inglese, M. (2008). Short-term DTI predictors of cognitive dysfunction in mild traumatic brain injury. *Brain Injury, 22*(2), 115–122.

Miller, N. S. (1991). *The pharmacology of alcohol and drugs of abuse and addiction.* New York: Springer-Verlag.

Mitsikostas, D. D., & Thomas, A. M. (1999). Comorbidity of headache and depressive disorders. *Cephalalgia, 19*(4), 211–217.

Morales, D., Diaz-Daza, O., Hlatky, R., & Hayman, L. A. (2007). *Brain, Contusion.* Retrieved April 22, 2009, from http://emedicine.medscape.com/article/337782-overview

Nakayama, N., Okumura, A., Shinoda, J., Yasokawa, Y. T., Miwa, K., Yoshimura, S. I., et al. (2006). Evidence for white matter disruption in traumatic brain injury without macroscopic lesions. *Journal of Neurology, Neurosurgery and Psychiatry, 77*(7), 850–855.

Nevin, N. C. (1967). Neuropathological changes in the white matter following head injury. *Journal of Neuropathology and Experimental Neurology, 26*(1), 77–84.

O'Shanick, G. J., & O'Shanick, A. M. (2005). Personality disorders. In J. M. Silver, T. W. McAllister, & S. C. Yudofsky (Eds.), *Textbook of traumatic brain injury* (pp. 245–258). Arlington, VA: American Psychiatric Publishing, Inc.

Olver, J. H., Ponsford, J. L., & Curran, C. A. (1996). Outcome following traumatic brain injury: A comparison between 2 and 5 years after injury. *Brain Injury, 10*(11), 841–848.

Oppenheimer, D. R. (1968). Microscopic lesions in the brain following head injury. *Journal of Neurology, Neurosurgery and Psychiatry, 31*(4), 299–306.

Orrison, W. W., Gentry, L. R., Stimac, G. K., Tarrel, R. M., Espinosa, M. C., & Cobb, L. C. (1994). Blinded comparison of cranial CT and MR in closed head injury evaluation. *American Journal of Neuroradiology, 15*(2), 351–356.

Padula, W., Wu, L., Vicci, V., Thomas, J., Nelson, C., Gottlieb, D., et al. (2007). Evaluating and treating visual dysfunction. In N. D. Zasler, D. I. Katz, & R. D. Zafonte (Eds.), *Brain injury medicine* (pp. 511–528). New York: Demos Medical Publishing, LLC.

Peerless, S. J., & Rewcastle, N. B. (1967). Shear injuries of the brain. *Canadian Medical Association Journal, 96*(10), 577–582.

Pettus, E. H., Christman, C. W., Giebel, M. L., & Povlishock, J. T. (1994). Traumatically induced altered membrane permeability: Its relationship to traumatically induced reactive axonal change. *Journal of Neurotrauma, 11*(5), 507–522.

Pine, D. S., Cohen, P., & Brook, J. (1996). The association between major depression and headache: Results of a longitudinal epidemiologic study in youth. *Journal of Child and Adolescent Psychopharmacology, 6*(3), 153–164.

Ponsford, J. L., Olver, J. H., Curran, C., & Ng, K. (1995). Prediction of employment status 2 years after traumatic brain injury. *Brain Injury, 9*(1), 11–20.

Ponsford, J., Willmott, C., Rothwell, A., Cameron, P., Kelly, A. M., Nelms, R., et al. (2000). Factors influencing outcome following mild traumatic brain injury in adults. *Journal of the International Neuropsychological Society, 6*(5), 568–579.

Povlishock, J. T. (1993). Pathobiology of traumatically induced axonal injury in animals and man. *Annals of Emergency Medicine, 22*(6), 980–986.

Povlishock, J. T., & Becker, D. P. (1985). Fate of reactive axonal swellings induced by head injury. *Laboratory Investigation, 52*(5), 540–552.

Povlishock, J. T., Becker, D. P., Cheng, C. L., & Vaughan, G. W. (1983). Axonal change in minor head injury. *Journal of Neuropathology and Experimental Neurology, 42*(3), 225–242.

Rao, V., Rollings, P., & Spiro, J. (2005). Fatigue and sleep problems. In J. M. Silver, T. W. McAllister, & S. C. Yudofsky (Eds.), *Textbook of traumatic brain injury* (pp. 369–384). Arlington, VA: American Pychiatric Publishing, Inc.

Rinne, M. B., Pasanen, M. E., Vartiainen, M. V., Lehto, T. M., Sarajuuri, J. M., & Alaranta, H. T. (2006). Motor performance in physically well-recovered men with traumatic brain injury. *Journal of Rehabilitation Medicine, 38*(4), 224–229.

Robinson, R. G., & Jorge, R. E. (2005). Mood disorders. In J. M. Silver, T. W. McAllister, & S. C. Yudofsky (Eds.), *Textbook of traumatic brain injury* (pp. 201–212). Arlington, VA: American Psychiatric Publishing.

Ruff, R. M., Marshall, L. F., Crouch, J., Klauber, M. R., Levin, H. S., Barth, J., et al. (1993). Predictors of outcome following severe head trauma: Follow-up data from the Traumatic Coma Data Bank. *Brain Injury, 7*(2), 101–111.

Ruffolo, C. F., Friedland, J. F., Dawson, D. R., Colantonio, A., & Lindsay, P. H. (1999). Mild traumatic brain injury from motor vehicle accidents: Factors associated with return to work. *Archives of Physical Medicine and Rehabilitation, 80*(4), 392–398.

Salmond, C. H., Menon, D. K., Chatfield, D. A., Williams, G. B., Pena, A., Sahakian, B. J., et al. (2006). Diffusion tensor imaging in chronic head injury survivors: Correlations with learning and memory indices. *Neuroimage, 29*(1), 117–124.

Sandel, M. E., Delmonico, R., & Kotch, M. J. (2007). Sexuality, reproduction, and neuroendocrine disorders following TBI. In N. D. Zasler, D. I. Katz, & R. D. Zafonte (Eds.), *Brain injury medicine* (pp. 673–695). New York: Demos Medical Publishing, LLC.

Sbordone, R. J., & Liter, J. C. (1995). Mild traumatic brain injury does not produce post-traumatic stress disorder. *Brain Injury, 9*, 405–412.

Schretlen, D. J., & Shapiro, A. M. (2003). A quantitative review of the effects of traumatic brain injury on cognitive functioning. *International Review of Psychiatry, 15*(4), 341–349.

Schwartz, J. H. (1991). Synthesis and trafficking of neural proteins. In E. R. Kandel, J. H. Schwartz, & T. M. Jessell (Eds.), *Principles of neural science* (3rd ed., pp. 49–65). New York: Elsevier.

Silver, J. M., Kramer, R., Greenwald, S., & Weissman, M. (2001). The association between head injuries and psychiatric disorders: Findings from the New Haven NIMH epidemiologic catchment area study. *Brain Injury, 15*(11), 935–945.

Slemmer, J. E., Matser, E. J., De Zeeuw, C. I., & Weber, J. T. (2002). Repeated mild injury causes cumulative damage to hippocampal cells. *Brain, 125*(Pt 12), 2699–2709.

Smith, D. H., Wolf, J. A., Lusardi, T. A., Lee, V. M., & Meaney, D. F. (1999). High tolerance and delayed elastic response of cultured axons to dynamic stretch injury. *The Journal of Neuroscience, 19*(11), 4263–4269.

Sosin, D. M., Sniezek, J. E., & Thurman, D. J. (1996). Incidence of mild and moderate brain injury in the United States, 1991. *Brain Injury, 10*(1), 47–54.

Spikman, J. M., Timmerman, M. E., van Zomeren, A. H., & Deelman, B. G. (1999). Recovery versus retest effects in attention after closed head injury. *Journal of Clinical and Experimental Neuropsychology, 21*(5), 585–605.

Stambrook, M., Moore, A. D., Peters, L. C., Deviaene, C., & Hawryluk, G. A. (1990). Effects of mild, moderate and severe closed head injury on long-term vocational status. *Brain Injury, 4*(2), 183–190.

Strich, S. J. (1961). Shearing of nerve fibers as a cause of brain damage due to head injury. *Lancet, 2*, 443–438.

Sundgren, P. C., Dong, Q., Gomez-Hassan, D., Mukherji, S. K., Maly, P., & Welsh, R. (2004). Diffusion tensor imaging of the brain: Review of clinical applications. *Neuroradiology, 46*(5), 339–350.

Thaxton, L. L., & Patel, A. R. (2007). Sleep disturbance: Epidemiology, assessment, and treatment. In N. D. Zasler, D. I. Katz, & R. D. Zafonte (Eds.), *Brain injury medicine* (pp. 557–575). New York: Demos Medical Publishing, LLC.

Thomsen, I. V. (1984). Late outcome of very severe blunt head trauma: A 10–15 year second follow-up. *Journal of Neurology, Neurosurgery and Psychiatry, 47*(3), 260–268.

Thurman, D., & Guerrero, J. (1999). Trends in hospitalization associated with traumatic brain injury. *Journal of the American Medical Association, 282*(10), 954–957.

Thurman, D. J., Coronado, V., & Selassie, A. (2007). The epidemiology of TBI: Implications for public health. In N. D. Zasler, D. I. Katz, & R. D. Zafonte (Eds.), *Brain injury medicine* (pp. 45–55). New York: Demos Medical Publishing, LLC.

Uzzell, B. P., Langfitt, T. W., & Dolinskas, C. A. (1987). Influence of injury severity on quality of survival after head injury. *Surgical Neurology, 27*(5), 419–429.

Varney, N., Martzke, J., & Roberts, R. (1987). Major depression in patients with closed head injury. *Neuropsychology, 1*, 7–8.

Warden, D. L., & Labbate, L. A. (2005). Posttraumatic stress disorder and other anxiety disorders. In J. M. Silver, T. W. McAllister, & S. C. Yudofsky (Eds.), *Textbook of traumatic brain injury* (pp. 231–243). Arlington, VA: American Psychiatric Publishing.

West, M., Targett, P., Yasuda, S., & Wehman, P. (2007). Return to work following TBI. In N. D. Zasler, D. I. Katz, & R. D. Zafonte (Eds.), *Brain injury medicine* (pp. 1131–1147). New York: Demos Medical Publishing, LLC.

Whitman, S., Coonley-Hoganson, R., & Desai, B. T. (1984). Comparative head trauma experiences in two socioeconomically different Chicago-area communities: A population study. *American Journal of Epidemiology, 119*(4), 570–580.

Whyte, J., Schuster, K., Polansky, M., Adams, J., & Coslett, H. B. (2000). Frequency and duration of inattentive behavior after traumatic brain injury: Effects of distraction, task, and practice. *Journal of the International Neuropsychological Society, 6*(1), 1–11.

Wilde, E. A., Chu, Z., Bigler, E. D., Hunter, J. V., Fearing, M. A., Hanten, G., et al. (2006). Diffusion tensor imaging in the corpus callosum in children after moderate to severe traumatic brain injury. *Journal of Neurotrauma, 23*(10), 1412–1426.

Wrightson, P., & Gronwall, D. (1981). Time off work and symptoms after minor head injury. *Injury, 12*(6), 445–454.

Yaghmai, A., & Povlishock, J. (1992). Traumatically induced reactive change as visualized through the use of monoclonal antibodies targeted to neurofilament subunits. *Journal of Neuropathology and Experimental Neurology, 51*(2), 158–176.

Zasler, N. D., Horn, L. J., Martelli, M. F., & Nicolson, K. (2007). Post-traumatic pain disorders: Medical assessment and management. In N. D. Zasler, D. I. Katz, & R. D. Zafonte (Eds.), *Brain injury medicine* (pp. 697–721). New York: Demos Medical Publishing, LLC.

Zwart, J. A., Dyb, G., Hagen, K., Odegard, K. J., Dahl, A. A., Bovim, G., et al. (2003). Depression and anxiety disorders associated with headache frequency. The Nord-Trondelag Health Study. *European Journal of Neurology, 10*(2), 147–152.

Chapter 22
Mild Traumatic Brain Injury

Grant L. Iverson and Rael T. Lange

Abstract Mild traumatic brain injuries (MTBI) are heterogeneous. This injury falls on a broad spectrum, from very mild neurometabolic changes in the brain with rapid recovery to permanent problems due to structural brain damage. It is incorrect to assume that MTBIs *cannot* cause permanent brain damage and it is incorrect to assume that MTBIs *typically* cause permanent brain damage. This is a highly individualized injury – most people recover relatively quickly and fully. However, some people have long-term problems. These long-term problems can be caused or maintained by multiple factors. Brain damage, although possible, is probably not the root cause of long-term problems in most patients. Instead, a diverse set of pre-existing and co-occurring conditions and factors likely cause and/or maintain symptoms and problems in most patients (e.g., personality characteristics; pre-existing health and mental health problems; co-morbid chronic pain, depression, anxiety disorders; social psychological factors; and litigation). It is important to carefully consider a multitude of factors that can cause or maintain symptom reporting long after an MTBI before concluding that a person is likely to have permanent damage to the function of his or her brain.

Key Points and Chapter Summary

- It is estimated that there are approximately 1.12 million people who sustain a mild traumatic brain injury in the United States each year. However, this is considered to be an underestimate of the actual prevalence rate.
- Mild traumatic brain injuries (MTBI) are heterogeneous. This injury falls on a broad spectrum of pathophysiology, from very mild neurometabolic

---

(continued)

G.L. Iverson (✉)
University of British Columbia, Vancouver, BC, Canada
and
British Columbia Mental Health and Addiction Services, Vancouver, BC, Canada
e-mail: giverson@interchange.ubc.ca

M.R. Schoenberg and J.G. Scott (eds.), *The Little Black Book of Neuropsychology: A Syndrome-Based Approach*, DOI 10.1007/978-0-387-76978-3_22,
© Springer Science+Business Media, LLC 2011

Key Points and Chapter Summary (continued)

- changes in the brain with rapid recovery to permanent problems due to structural brain damage.
- An important subtype within the MTBI spectrum is an injury character- ized by the presence (complicated MTBI) or absence (uncomplicated MTBI) of abnormalities on day-of-injury computed tomography scans.
- A concussion, by definition, is a mild traumatic brain injury.
- The natural history of MTBI is reasonably well understood. There is a substantial evidence base indicating that neurocognitive deficits typically are not seen in athletes after 1–3 weeks and in trauma patients after 1–3 months in prospective group studies.
- There is reasonably good evidence that early intervention, as simple as edu- cation and reassurance of a likely good outcome, can reduce the number and frequency of post-concussion symptoms and increase return to work rates.
- Depression is fairly common following mild traumatic brain injury. Symptoms of depression can mimic the persistent post-concussion syndrome because many of the symptoms are nearly identical in these conditions.

Epidemiology of MTBI

It is estimated that there are more than 1.4 million people who sustain a traumatic brain injury in the United States (US) each year (Langlois et al. 2004). MTBI is most common, with an estimated 80% of all traumatic brain injuries classified as falling in the mild range (Kraus and Chu 2005). Based on these figures, we can deduce that there are approximately 1.12 million MTBIs per year in the US. However, this is considered to be an underestimate of the actual prevalence rate. Many people who sustain an MTBI seek no medical attention after their injury and are not evaluated in the emergency department or admitted to the hospital (Sosin et al. 1996), and are therefore not captured in studies that rely on hospital based data (McCrea 2008). For example, mild injuries, such as concussions in sport, are very common. In a recent study, 30% of high school football players reported at least one previous concussion; 15% reported that they experienced a concussion during the current football season (McCrea et al. 2004).

Terminology and Diagnostic Criteria

There is no universally agreed upon definition of MTBI, but most commonly used definitions are similar. There are three commonly cited definitions of MTBI developed by (1) the Mild Traumatic Brain Injury Committee of the Head Injury

Interdisciplinary Special Interest Group of the American Congress of Rehabilitation Medicine (ACRM MTBI Committee), (2) Center for Disease (CDC) Control working group (CDC working group), and (3) World Health Organization (WHO) Collaborating Centre Task Force on Mild Traumatic Brain Injury (WHO Collaborating Centre Task Force).

ACRM MTBI Committee Definition

A widely cited definition of MTBI is presented in Table 22.1. This definition was developed by the Mild Traumatic Brain Injury Committee of the Head Injury Interdisciplinary Special Interest Group of the American Congress of Rehabilitation Medicine (1993). Obviously, this definition includes a broad spectrum of injury severity. This definition includes injuries characterized by seconds of confusion to injuries involving 20 minutes of unconsciousness, several hours of post-traumatic amnesia, and a focal contusion visible on day-of-injury computed tomography (CT).

Table 22.1 ACRM (Mild Traumatic Brain Injury Committee 1993) definition of mild traumatic brain injury

A traumatically induced physiological disruption of brain function, as manifested by *at least* one of the following:

1. Any loss of consciousness
2. Any loss of memory for events immediately before or after the accident
3. Any alteration in mental state at the time of the accident (e.g., feeling dazed, disoriented, or confused) and
4. Focal neurological deficit(s) that may or may not be transient

But where the severity of the injury does not exceed the following

- Loss of consciousness of approximately 30 minutes or less
- After 30 minutes, an initial Glasgow Coma Scale (GCS) of 13–15 and
- Posttraumatic amnesia (PTA) not greater than 24 hours

Note: A better conjunction after point #3 should have been "or" as opposed to "and"

CDC Working Group Definition

A Center for Disease Control (CDC) working group proposed a conceptual definition of MTBI (2003). This definition is provided in Table 22.2. The working group noted that this definition does not define subtypes of MTBIs. They emphasized that the presence of an intracranial abnormality was one injury characteristic, as a potential injury subtype, that should routinely be reported when available.

Table 22.2 National Center for Injury Prevention and Control (2003) conceptual definition of MTBI

The conceptual definition of MTBI is an injury to the head as a result of blunt trauma or acceleration or deceleration forces that result in *one or more* of the conditions listed below

Any period of observed or self-reported

- Transient confusion, disorientation, or impaired consciousness
- Dysfunction of memory around the time of injury
- Loss of consciousness lasting less than 30 minutes
- Observed signs of neurological or neuropsychological dysfunction, such as:
  - Seizures acutely following injury to the head
  - Among infants and very young children: irritability, lethargy, or vomiting following head injury
  - Symptoms among older children and adults such as headache, dizziness, irritability, fatigue or poor concentration, when identified soon after injury, can be used to support the diagnosis of mild TBI, but cannot be used to make the diagnosis in the absence of loss of consciousness or altered consciousness. Research may provide additional guidance in this area

More severe brain injuries were excluded from the definition of MTBI and include *one or more* of the following conditions attributable to the injury

- Loss of consciousness lasting longer than 30 minutes
- Post-traumatic amnesia lasting longer than 24 hours
- Penetrating craniocerebral injury

WHO Collaborating Center Task Force Definition

In 2004, a World Health Organization (WHO) Collaborating Center Task Force on Mild Traumatic Brain Injury provided the definition reprinted below. This definition, like all others, is very broad. Nonetheless, it is a reasonable definition for day-to-day clinical practice.

> MTBI is an acute brain injury resulting from mechanical energy to the head from external physical forces. Operational criteria for clinical identification include: (1) 1 or more of the following: confusion or disorientation, loss of consciousness for 30 minutes or less, post-traumatic amnesia for less than 24 hours, and/or other transient neurological abnormalities such as focal signs, seizure, and intracranial lesion not requiring surgery; and (2) Glasgow Coma Scale score of 13–15 after 30 minutes post-injury or later upon presentation for healthcare. These manifestations of MTBI must not be due to drugs, alcohol, medications, caused by other injuries or treatment for other injuries (e.g. systemic injuries, facial injuries or intubation), caused by other problems (e.g. psychological trauma, language barrier or coexisting medical conditions) or caused by penetrating craniocerebral injury (Carroll et al. 2004a, p. 115)

Complicated and Uncomplicated MTBI

We believe an important subtype within the MTBI spectrum is an injury characterized by visible damage on day-of-injury computed tomography (CT) scan. A *complicated* MTBI is diagnosed if the person has a Glasgow Coma Scale (GCS) score of 13–15 but shows some brain abnormality (e.g., edema, hematoma, or contusion) on a CT or magnetic resonance imaging (MRI) scan. Skull fractures were also considered characteristic of complicated injuries (Williams et al. 1990). Williams and colleagues noted that patients with complicated MTBIs are more likely to have worse cognitive functioning acutely compared to uncomplicated MTBI, and their 6-month functional recovery pattern is more similar to persons with moderate brain injuries. Worse outcome associated with complicated MTBIs has been reported by some (Iverson 2006a; Temkin et al. 2003; van der Naalt et al. 1999b; Williams et al. 1990; Wilson et al. 1996), but not all (Hofman et al. 2001; Hughes et al. 2004; McCauley et al. 2001), researchers. The *uncomplicated* MTBI is characterized by having no intracranial abnormality or skull fracture, with all other severity criteria in the mild range. A broad range of injuries fall within the uncomplicated MTBI spectrum, from very mild concussions sustained in sports to more serious injuries sustained in falls or motor vehicle accidents.

Rule of Thumb: Complicated versus Uncomplicated MTBI

- Complicated MTBI is characterized by having a structural abnormality visible on neuroimaging
- Uncomplicated MTBI is characterized by normal neuroimaging

MTBI versus Concussion

A concussion, by definition, is a mild traumatic brain injury. Concussion is the preferred term in sports, both in clinical practice and in research. The term concussion frequently is used in clinical practice in civilian trauma cases, especially for injuries that seem to fall on the milder end of the mild spectrum of injury. An exception would be if an athlete or civilian sustained an injury characterized by prolonged loss of consciousness, prolonged post-traumatic amnesia, or visible damage to his or her brain on CT or MRI. In general, we believe that concussion is the preferred term because it is more readily understood by most patients, it is easier to communicate the favorable prognosis associated with this injury, and it is less likely that the patient will have an adverse psychological reaction to learning about his or her injury. However, iatrogenic psychological reactions can arise from the person becoming somatically and psychologically preoccupied with having an MTBI or a concussion.

In forensic reports, it is common to use the more technical term mild traumatic brain injury, and sometimes the terms are used interchangeably. For patients with injuries on the more severe end of the mild spectrum, such as those with *complicated* mild traumatic brain injuries, we typically do *not* use the term concussion in clinical or forensic practice, or in research.

In clinical and forensic practice, these terms can be used deliberately or unintentionally to convey an opinion that represents the clinician's "world view" or that might appear to be slanted toward the theory of the plaintiff or theory of the defense. For example, it is common for plaintiff-retained experts to write about a remote concussion in the present tense, as if the person "has" a MTBI. It is also common for experts retained by plaintiffs to go to great lengths to establish that a person broke the threshold for the diagnosis of a "mild traumatic brain injury" in the accident and then imply, directly or indirectly, that "a brain injury, is a brain injury, is a brain injury." Clearly, the classification of MTBI is extraordinarily broad, with some injuries being very close to a mild concussion in sports with a 1-day recovery time and other injuries closer to a moderate TBI with some degree of permanent brain damage.

In contrast, experts retained by defendants might be more likely to (1) deny that a concussion ever occurred, or (2) refer to the injury in the past tense. Moreover, experts retained by defendants are more likely to refer to "bad" mild injuries (e.g., complicated MTBIs or mild injuries with severity criteria closer to moderates), or moderate TBIs, as "concussions." This conveys the message that the more serious brain injury should be viewed more like a simple concussion in sports.

It is true, of course, that the vast majority of people who experience an MTBI, especially those on the milder end to the mild continuum, should experience a full recovery. When people report long-term symptoms and problems, there are multiple reasons why this might be the case – only one of which is lingering damage to the structure or function of the brain (see Chap. 24). Therefore, it is important to carefully consider and report the multiple factors that can be related to symptom reporting long after this injury, and not simply assume that if a person reports symptoms they are likely to be caused by the biological effects of the remote injury (see Chap. 24).

Rule of Thumb: What is in the Name: Mild TBI or Concussion?

- Concussions are mild TBIs
- Concussion is the preferred term for sports-related injuries
- Concussions are generally understood to be associated with good recovery

---

Neuropsychological Outcome

The natural history of MTBI is reasonably well understood. Athletes and trauma patients report diverse physical, cognitive, and emotional symptoms in the initial days and weeks post injury. In concussed athletes, the most frequently endorsed symptoms in the initial days post-injury are: headaches, fatigue, feeling slowed down, drowsiness, difficulty concentrating, feeling mentally foggy, and dizziness (Lovell et al. 2006). There is a substantial evidence base indicating that injured athletes and trauma patients perform more poorly on neuropsychological tests in the initial days (Bleiberg et al. 2004; Hughes et al. 2004; Lovell et al. 2004; Macciocchi et al. 1996; McCrea et al. 2003, 2002) and up to the first month following the injury (e.g., Hugenholtz et al. 1988; Levin et al. 1987; Macciocchi et al. 1996; Mathias et al. 2004; Ponsford et al. 2000). Neuropsychological deficits typically are not seen in athletes after 1–3 weeks (Bleiberg et al. 2004; Lovell et al. 2004; Macciocchi et al. 1996; McCrea et al. 2003, 2004; Pellman et al. 2004a) and in trauma patients after 1–3 months (e.g., Gentilini et al. 1985; Lahmeyer and Bellur 1987; Ponsford et al. 2000) in prospective group studies.

Influence of LOC and PTA

Over the years, there has been considerable interest in whether duration of loss of consciousness or post-traumatic amnesia is clearly related to neuropsychological outcome in patients with MTBIs. Researchers studying trauma patients have reported that there is no clear association between *brief* loss of consciousness and short-term neuropsychological outcome (e.g., Iverson et al. 2000; Leininger et al. 1990; Lovell et al. 1999) or vocational outcome (Hanlon et al. 1999). The presence and duration of post-traumatic confusion/amnesia has been associated with worse immediate outcome and slower recovery in athletes (Collins et al. 2003a, b; Lovell et al. 2003; McCrea et al. 2002; Pellman et al. 2004b). Post-traumatic confusion/amnesia in trauma patients also appears to be related to short-term neuropsychological outcome (Iverson et al. 2007). However, by 3 months post-injury this association might disappear (Ponsford et al. 2000). In one study, duration of post-traumatic amnesia was related to 1-year return to work rates, but this effect was mostly due to the inclusion of patients with moderate TBIs and PTA greater than 24 hours (van der Naalt et al. 1999b).

Influence of Intracranial Abnormality

One would naturally assume that patients who sustain a complicated MTBI (i.e., bleeding, bruising, or swelling on their day-of-injury CT) would have worse short-, medium-, and long-term neuropsychological and functional outcome than patients without obvious structural damage. However, the research findings are mixed. Patients with complicated MTBIs tend to perform more poorly on neuropsychological tests in the first 2 months following injury, but only on a small number of tests rather than globally depressed scores (Borgaro et al. 2003; Iverson 2006a; 1999; Kurca et al. 2006; Lange et al. 2005; Williams et al. 1990). When differences do occur between groups, the effect sizes of these differences are lower than expected (i.e., medium to medium–large effect sizes or lower (Borgaro et al. 2003; Hofman et al. 2001; Iverson 2006a; Iverson et al. 1999; Lange et al. 2005; Williams et al. 1990); see Borgaro and colleagues (2003) for an exception). At 6 months post-injury, there are no notable differences in neuropsychological test performance between complicated and uncomplicated mild TBI patients (Hanlon et al. 1999; Hofman et al. 2001). In contrast to neuropsychological functioning, differences in functional outcomes are more apparent. Patients with complicated MTBIs have worse 6–12 months outcome (i.e., Glasgow Outcome Scale) than patients with uncomplicated MTBIs (van der Naalt et al. 1999a; Williams et al. 1990; Wilson et al. 1996) and have similar 3–5 years outcome (i.e., Functional Status Examination) to patients with moderate and severe TBI (Temkin et al. 2003). Interestingly, however, in a well-controlled prospective study, McCauley and colleagues reported that CT abnormalities were not associated with increased risk for post-concussion syndrome at 3 months post-injury (McCauley et al. 2001).

Rule of Thumb: Outcome from Mild TBI: Neuropsychological

- Post-traumatic amnesia is a better predictor of short-term cognitive outcome than duration of loss of consciousness (when LOC is brief)

Meta-Analytic Studies

There are several published meta-analyses (Belanger et al. 2005; Belanger and Vanderploeg 2005; Binder 1997; Schretlen and Shapiro 2003) and reviews (Carroll et al. 2004b; Iverson 2005; Ruff 2005) of the MTBI literature that can be compared to meta-analyses in other areas. This can help put neuropsychological consequences of certain conditions into context. For example, the effects of traumatic brain injuries, of different severities, are compared to the effects of litigation and malingering in Fig. 22.1. In Fig. 22.2, we compare the neuropsychological effects of MTBI to drug abuse. In Fig. 22.3, we compare the neuropsychological effects of MTBI to several psychiatric conditions. These meta-analyses represent the "average" effect of a factor,

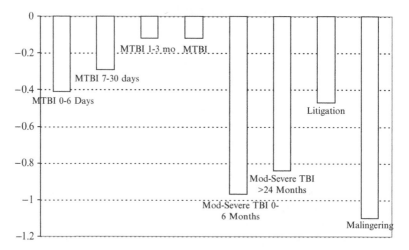

Fig. 22.1 Effects of traumatic brain injuries, litigation, and malingering on neuropsychological functioning. Effect sizes typically are expressed in pooled, weighted standard deviation units. However, across studies, there are some minor variations in the methods of calculation. By convention, effect sizes of .2 are considered small, .5 medium, and .8 large. This is from a statistical, not necessarily clinical, perspective. For this figure, the overall effect on cognitive or neuropsychological functioning is reported. Effect sizes less than .3 should be considered very small and difficult to detect in individual patients because the patient and control groups largely overlap. MTBI 0–6 days, 7–30 days, 1–3 months, moderate-severe TBI 0–6 months, > 24 months, all in Schretlen and Shapiro (2003), 39 studies, *n*=1,716 TBI, *n* = 1,164 controls; MTBI (Binder et al. 1997), 11 studies, *n*=314 MTBI, *n* = 308 controls; Litigation/financial incentives (Binder and Rohling 1996), 17 studies, *n*=2,353 total; Malingering (Vickery et al. 2001), 32 studies published between 1985 and 1998, 41 independent comparisons

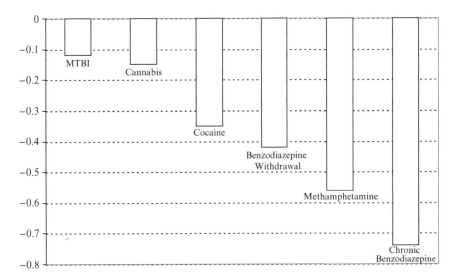

Fig. 22.2 Effects of MTBIs and drug use on neuropsychological functioning. MTBI (Binder et al. 1997), 11 studies, $n=314$ MTBI, $n=308$ controls; Cannabis (Grant et al. 2003), long-term regular use, 11 studies, $n=623$ users, $n=409$ non or minimal users; Cocaine (Jovanovski et al. 2005) dependence/abuse (including some concurrent alcohol abuse), 15 studies, $n=481$ users, $n=586$ healthy normal controls, median (not mean) effect size reported; Benzodiazepine withdrawal (Barker et al. 2004b), 10 studies, long-term follow-up, 44 comparisons; Chronic benzodiazepine use (Barker et al. 2004a), 13 studies, $n=384$, 61 comparisons

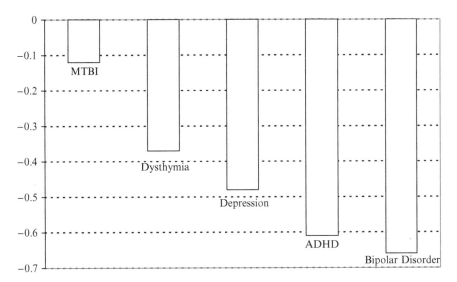

Fig. 22.3 Effects of MTBIs and various psychiatric conditions on neuropsychological function-ing. MTBI (Binder et al. 1997), 11 studies, $n=314$ MTBI, $n=308$ controls; Dysthymia, Depression, and Bipolar Disorder (Christensen et al. 1997), 3 comparisons for dysthymia, 97 comparisons for depression, and 15 comparisons for bipolar disorder; ADHD (Frazier et al. 2004), based on Full Scale IQ, 123 studies

injury, disorder, or condition on cognitive functioning. After a reasonable recovery period (up to several months), *on average*, MTBIs are *not* associated with measurable neuropsychological impairment.

Early Intervention and Return to Work

Clinicians should try to prevent poor outcome in people who have suffered an MTBI. There is reasonably good evidence that early intervention, as simple as education and reassurance of a likely good outcome, can reduce the number and frequency of post-concussion symptoms (Minderhoud et al. 1980) and increase return to work rates (Relander et al. 1972). In most studies, patients participating in early intervention programs consisting of educational materials plus various additional treatments and/or assessments (e.g., neuropsychological testing, meeting with a therapist, reassurance, access to a multidisciplinary team) report fewer post-concussion symptoms at 3 months post-injury (Ponsford et al. 2001, 2002) and at 6 months post-injury (Minderhoud et al. 1980; Mittenberg et al. 1996; Wade et al. 1998) compared to patients who received standard hospital treatment. Educational brochures or sessions typically provide information regarding common symptoms, likely time course of recovery, reassurance of recovery, and suggested coping strategies following MTBI (e.g., Mittenberg et al. 1996; Paniak et al. 2000; Ponsford et al. 2002; Wade et al. 1998).

Early intervention programs are designed to promote uneventful recovery and resumption of normal activities, such as returning to work. Return to work rates following MTBI vary substantially in the literature. Employment rates have ranged from: (1) 25–100% within the first month post-injury (e.g., Dikmen et al. 1994; Haboubi et al. 2001; Stranjalis et al. 2004; Wrightson and Gronwall 1981), (2) 38–83% 6–9 months post-injury (Dikmen et al. 1994; Drake et al. 2000; Friedland and Dawson 2001; Hughes et al. 2004; Kraus et al. 2005; McCullagh et al. 2001), (3) 47–83% 1–2 years post-injury (Dawson et al. 2004; Dikmen et al. 1994; Uzzell et al. 1987; van der Naalt et al. 1999b), and (4) 62–88% 3 or more years post-injury (Asikainen et al. 1996; Dawson et al. 2004; Edna and Cappelen 1987; Stambrook et al. 1990; Vanderploeg et al. 2003). See Iverson et al. (2007) for a review.

The variability in return to work rates is due in large part to methodological differences across studies, such as: (1) differences in definitions of return to work (e.g., return to pre-injury employment versus return to meaningful activity), (2) differences in the inclusion and exclusion of individuals who were unemployed or performing domestic duties before getting injured, and (3) differences in accounting for pre-injury employment status (e.g., return to full-time vs. part-time vs. unemployed).

Rule of Thumb: Return to Work after Mild TBI

- Early intervention programs involving education and reassurance are associated with better outcomes and improved likelihood of return to work

Depression and Mild TBI

Depression is a heterogeneous condition. Depression is fairly common following traumatic brain injury of all severities. Prevalence estimates vary widely (e.g., from 11% to 77%; e.g., Jorge et al. 1993; Silver et al. 2001; Varney et al. 1987). It is likely that depression can arise directly or indirectly from the biological consequences of the traumatic brain injury, it can be a psychological reaction to deficits and problems associated with having a brain injury, or both. It can also arise de novo, incidentally, sometime post injury – such as in response to life stressors. It can also arise as part of a pre-existing chronic relapsing and remitting condition. Rates of depression, in the first 3 months following MTBI, have ranged from 12% to 44% (Goldstein et al. 2001; Horner et al. 2005; Levin et al. 2001, 2005; McCauley et al. 2001; Mooney and Speed 2001; Parker and Rosenblum 1996). It is important to appreciate that people who suffer traumatic brain injuries have higher rates of *pre-injury* psychiatric disorders (Chamelian and Feinstein 2004; Federoff et al. 1992; Hibbard et al. 2004; Jorge et al. 1993), such as depression and substance abuse. This places some patients at risk for post-injury depression.

It is extremely difficult to determine if a person's self-reported symptoms are due to depression, a persistent post-concussion syndrome (see Chap. 24 for additional information), or both because many of the symptoms are nearly identical in these conditions. The problem for clinicians and researchers is that a person with depression is virtually guaranteed to meet diagnostic criteria for a post-concussive disorder (Iverson 2006b), regardless of whether that person (1) has ever injured his brain, or (2) the past injury to his brain is causally related to his current symptoms.

Given the clear overlap between the symptoms of depression and the post-concussion syndrome, some researchers have recommended treatment with antidepressants (e.g., Fann et al. 2000, 2001; McCauley et al. 2001; Zafonte et al. 2002) or cognitive behavior therapy (e.g., Mittenberg et al. 2001, 1996). Those recommending cognitive behavior therapy have set forth a treatment protocol that is based on CBT principles but is tailored toward the post-concussion syndrome and belief systems relating to symptoms and brain damage.

It is important to appreciate that a comprehensive treatment program for depression or post-concussion syndrome should include an exercise component. Exercise has been shown to have positive effects on mood, self-esteem, and it promotes a general sense of well-being. More importantly, exercise can be an effective treatment for mild depression (Dunn et al. 2005; Mead et al. 2008; Penninx et al. 2002). In animal studies, exercise promotes neuroplasticity (Pietropaolo et al. 2008), and exercise done after a period of recovery following MTBI is also associated with neuroplasticity (Griesbach et al. 2007, 2008, 2004).

Rule of Thumb: Depression

- Depression is relatively common after TBIs of all severity
- The cause of depression is difficult to determine in most cases, and is often multifactorial

Mild Traumatic Brain Injury in the Military

Traumatic brain injuries have always been a health problem affecting military personnel. It is well recognized that military personnel are at risk for combat-related and noncombat-related brain injuries. In a survey of active duty soldiers, 23% reported that they had sustained a traumatic brain injury (TBI) after joining the army (Ivins et al. 2003). Paratroopers were much more likely to sustain a TBI than non-paratroopers (Ivins et al. 2003). Noncombat mechanisms of injury include motor vehicle crashes and falls (Ommaya et al. 1996). In past combat situations, helmets offered some protection from shrapnel and fragments, but virtually no protection from bullets (Carey et al. 1982). Modern protective equipment, such as bullet-proof helmets, significantly reduces the risk for penetrating brain injuries (Carey et al. 1998; Peleg et al. 2006). However, penetrating brain injuries still occur in modern combat (Chaudhri et al. 1994).

Post-Deployment Screening Methods

Over the past several years, there has been enormous concern regarding the rates of TBIs among military personnel deployed in the Middle East, most of which are caused by improvised explosive devices (Drazen 2005; Okie 2005; Tanielian and Jaycox 2008). There is considerable scientific interest and practical concern regarding blast-related TBIs (Hoge et al. 2008; Okie 2005; Taber et al. 2006; Warden 2006; Xydakis et al. 2005). There is a need to accurately identify the incidence and prevalence of TBIs, of all severities, in military personnel returning from deployment to Operation Enduring Freedom and Operation Iraqi Freedom. Considerable efforts and resources by the Department of Defense and Veterans Affairs have been directed toward developing and implementing methods for identifying those who sustained a mild brain injury and those who might have residual symptoms.

Post-deployment assessments are used in an attempt to identify the number of military personnel who have experienced a deployment-related mild TBI (Schwab et al. 2007; Tanielian and Jaycox 2008). It is important to appreciate that these are *screening* assessments. The methodology used for screening is typically a methodology that maximizes sensitivity at the expense of specificity. As such, these screening assessments will result in a substantial number of military personnel and veterans being identified as experiencing a deployment-related TBI when, in fact, they did not.

There are a few different versions of the screening tool. Basically, it is a self-report measure asking if the soldier was injured by, or exposed to, a certain event (e.g., fragment, bullet, vehicular accident, fall, or blast). If so, the solider is asked to determine if any of the following occurred: being dazed, confused, or "seeing stars"; not remembering the injury or event; losing consciousness; sustaining a head injury; or having any symptoms of concussion afterward (such as headache, dizziness, irritability). If the soldier or veteran answers affirmatively to this two-question screening process, then the individual is "screened positive." Clearly, in regards to blast-related concussions, a false positive identification is easy when one considers that the soldier or veteran is first asked to think back as to whether he or she was "exposed" to a blast (with or without injury), and then to recall whether he or she felt "dazed" or "confused" after the event. These screening tools will identify uninjured soldiers as having brain injuries in cases where the feeling of being dazed or confused was simply a psychological reaction to combat or a horrific scene.

Over-identification (i.e., false positives) is not necessarily problematic. To maximize the likelihood of identifying true injuries, it is a natural consequence to have high rates of false positives. It is essential, however, to appreciate that *initial screening estimates* of the number of military personnel who have sustained a TBI do *not* represent the *true prevalence* of the injury. Thus, reports estimating that 300,000 military personnel have experienced a deployment-related brain injury (Tanielian and Jaycox 2008), based on a screening methodology, likely represent significantly inflated prevalence estimates. Developing and evaluating more refined and accurate injury surveillance rates is needed.

Proper case identification is the foundation for planning and implementing high quality, evidence-based assessment, treatment, and rehabilitation services for injured active duty military personnel and veterans. This involves (1) accurate injury surveillance, and (2) accurate methods for identifying residual symptoms. Extrapolating from the scientific literature, it is likely that the vast majority of military personnel and veterans who sustain a mild TBI during deployment recovered fully, or nearly fully, from this injury. Some personnel and veterans will continue to report symptoms long after their injuries. It is possible that some or all of these symptoms are due to the residual effects of their mild TBI. However, simply reporting symptoms long after an injury does not mean the symptoms are caused by the past injury. It is likely that in many cases the symptoms are due predominately to other factors such as traumatic stress (e.g., Hoge et al. 2008; Schneiderman et al. 2008), depression, chronic bodily pain, substance abuse, and community-reintegration issues.

> **Rule of Thumb: Post-Deployment Screening**
> - Post-deployment screening for suffering a mild TBI likely results in both false positive errors and false negative errors
> - The occurrence of false positive errors has likely resulted in over-estimating the rate of MTBI in the military

Operational, Health, and Welfare Considerations

Currently, in Iraq and Afghanistan, moderate TBIs, severe TBIs, and penetrating brain injuries can be quickly identified and triaged. Injured personnel can be transported rapidly from forward and far forward positions to a trauma center for treatment, and then to their home country for rehabilitation. Mild TBIs, however, can be very difficult to identify. Moreover, many of those who sustain the mildest form of injury to their brain might simply require rest for a few days before they are fit to return to duty. This is because most of the pathophysiology appears to be reversible.

Blast-related mild TBI is of concern from an operational perspective and a soldier health and welfare perspective. From an *operational perspective*, a soldier might not be fit for duty due to mild cognitive compromise, slowed reaction time, diminished judgment, and modest physical limitations relating to vision and balance. Therefore, it is important to have clinical protocols in place that can provide reliable, valid, and accurate information regarding recovery from injury and fitness for duty. Fortunately, good work in this area has been completed. The Defense and Veterans Brain Injury Center (DVBIC) Working Group on the Acute Management of MTBI in Military Operational Settings published a Clinical Practice Guideline and Recommendations dated December 22, 2006. The guideline involves assessing symptoms and cognition. Similar to the standard of care for athletes who have sustained a concussion (see Chap. 23), it is recommended that military personnel be monitored carefully for resolution of symptoms (at rest) and then be taken through a graded set of physical challenges, with symptom monitoring, before being cleared for return to duty.

From an operational perspective, additional clinical research is needed to refine the assessment methods and algorithms that underlie decision-making regarding fitness for duty. For example, how do you reliably determine whether certain non-specific symptoms are due to concussion versus the physical and mental stains associated with combat? Is full symptom resolution practical or feasible given the working conditions of some soldiers? Which specific light aerobic and heavy exertional protocols are most safe and effective for being used in a sequential manner in the graduated return to duty health assessment?

From a *health and welfare perspective*, there is a need for evidence-based specialized assessment, treatment, and rehabilitation services for active duty personnel and veterans following deployment. The Department of Defense and the Department of Veterans Affairs is faced with providing health care for large numbers of active duty personnel and veterans with complex physical and mental health needs. It can be very difficult to sort out the underlying causes for certain psychological, cognitive, and physical symptoms and problems in combat-exposed and injured military personnel. It is important, however, to carefully assess individuals for a diverse set of possible causes for their problems because differential diagnosis might lead to more effective treatment and rehabilitation services. Some of the most important differential diagnostic considerations are illustrated in Fig. 22.4. Additional information relevant to this is provided in the Chap. 24.

It is essential to note that *longstanding* symptoms and problems in veterans who have sustained one or more MTBIs might be partially or wholly attributable to *co-occurring conditions*. The most important co-occurring conditions are post-traumatic stress disorder, depression, chronic pain, chronic sleep problems, and substance abuse disorders. These conditions are associated with symptoms that are

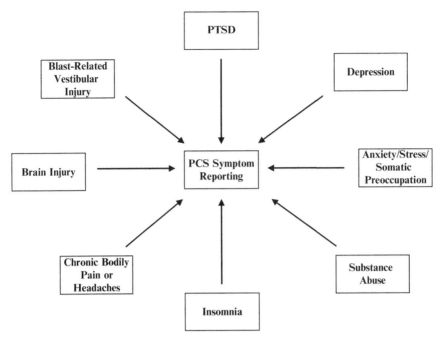

Fig. 22.4 Clinical conditions that influence post-concussion-like symptom reporting acutely, post-acutely, and long after a mild traumatic brain injury in soldiers and veterans

virtually identical to post-concussion symptoms (Gasquoine 2000; Gunstad and Suhr 2004; Iverson and McCracken 1997; Karzmark et al. 1995; McCauley et al. 2001; Smith-Seemiller et al. 2003; Wilde et al. 2004). The symptoms and problems associated with these conditions can co-occur with subtle lingering effects of MTBIs, or mimic the long-term adverse effects of MTBIs. Depression, PTSD, chronic pain, and substance abuse can be associated with diverse psychological problems and cognitive impairment, and they can result in significant disruption in social and occupational functioning. Therefore, it is important to provide accurate differential diagnosis and effective treatment services for veterans with these co-occurring conditions.

Conclusions

There is no universally agreed upon definition of MTBI, but most commonly used definitions are similar. Typically, a mild TBI is characterized by a GCS score of 13–15, duration of LOC less than 30 minutes, and duration of PTA less than 24 hours. A concussion, by definition, is a mild traumatic brain injury. Concussion is the preferred term in sports, both in clinical practice and in research. The term concussion frequently is used in clinical practice in civilian trauma cases, especially for injuries that seem to fall on the milder end of the mild spectrum of injury. An important subtype within the MTBI spectrum is defined by the presence or absence of intracranial abnormality detected on day-of-injury CT (or a later scan). These injuries are termed complicated MTBI (abnormality present) and uncomplicated MTBI (abnormality absent). For patients with *complicated* mild traumatic brain injuries, we typically do *not* use the term concussion in clinical or forensic practice, or in research.

The course of recovery from MTBI is reasonably well understood. Injured athletes and trauma patients perform more poorly on neuropsychological tests in the initial days and up to the first month following the injury. However, neuropsychological deficits typically are not seen in athletes after 1–4 weeks and in trauma patients after 1–3 months. Outcome may be influenced by the presence of day-of-injury intracranial abnormality in which patients with complicated MTBI tend to have worse short-term neuropsychological functioning and functional status compared to uncomplicated MTBI. However, worse long-term outcome in those with complicated MTBIs is related primarily to functional status rather than neuropsychological deficits.

When a person does not recover quickly, healthcare providers are very concerned about the possibility of a persistent post-concussion syndrome, the development of depression, and/or a failure to return to work. It can be extremely difficult to differentiate depression from a post-concussion syndrome. Many of the specific symptoms of depression are similar to the post-concussion syndrome. Clinicians should try to prevent poor outcome in people who have suffered an MTBI. There is reasonably good evidence that early intervention, as simple as education and reassurance of a likely good outcome, can reduce the number and frequency of post-concussion symptoms and increase return to work rates.

It is well recognized that military personnel are at risk for combat-related and noncombat-related brain injuries. Over the past several years, there has been considerable scientific interest and practical concern regarding blast-related traumatic brain injuries. From an *operational perspective*, a soldier might not be fit for duty due to mild cognitive compromise, slowed reaction time, diminished judgment, and modest physical limitations relating to vision and balance. From a *health and welfare perspective*, there is a need for evidence-based specialized assessment, treatment, and rehabilitation services for active duty military personnel and veterans following deployment. Good progress has been made in these areas. Going forward, from a case identification perspective, research is needed to better assist with differentiating military personnel and veterans who were blast exposed from those who were blast exposed *and* who sustained an associated MTBI. Even more difficult is the accurate identification of those individuals with possible residual symptoms from a blast-related MTBI. It is essential to note that *longstanding* symptoms and problems in veterans who have sustained one or more MTBIs might be partially or wholly attributable to *co-occurring conditions*. The most important co-occurring conditions are post-traumatic stress disorder, depression, chronic pain, chronic sleep problems, and substance abuse disorders.

References

Asikainen, I., Kaste, M., & Sarna, S. (1996). Patients with traumatic brain injury referred to a rehabilitation and re-employment programme: social and professional outcome for 508 Finnish patients 5 or more years after injury. *Brain Injury, 10*(12), 883–899.

Barker, M. J., Greenwood, K. M., Jackson, M., & Crowe, S. F. (2004a). Cognitive effects of long-term benzodiazepine use: a meta-analysis. *CNS Drugs, 18*(1), 37–48.

Barker, M. J., Greenwood, K. M., Jackson, M., & Crowe, S. F. (2004b). Persistence of cognitive effects after withdrawal from long-term benzodiazepine use: a meta-analysis. *Archives of Clinical Neuropsychology, 19*(3), 437–454.

Belanger, H. G., Curtiss, G., Demery, J. A., Lebowitz, B. K., & Vanderploeg, R. D. (2005). Factors moderating neuropsychological outcomes following mild traumatic brain injury: a meta-analysis. *Journal of the International Neuropsychological Society, 11*(3), 215–227.

Belanger, H. G., & Vanderploeg, R. D. (2005). The neuropsychological impact of sports-related concussion: a meta-analysis. *Journal of the International Neuropsychological Society, 11*(4), 345–357.

Binder, L. M. (1997). A review of mild head trauma Part II: clinical implications. *Journal of Clinical and Experimental Neuropsychology, 19*(3), 432–457.

Binder, L. M., & Rohling, M. L. (1996). Money matters: a meta-analytic review of the effects of financial incentives on recovery after closed-head injury. *The American Journal of Psychiatry, 153*(1), 7–10.

Binder, L. M., Rohling, M. L., & Larrabee, J. (1997). A review of mild head trauma Part I: meta-analytic review of neuropsychological studies. *Journal of Clinical and Experimental Neuropsychology, 19*(3), 421–431.

Bleiberg, J., Cernich, A. N., Cameron, K., Sun, W., Peck, K., Ecklund, P. J., et al. (2004). Duration of cognitive impairment after sports concussion. *Neurosurgery, 54*(5), 1073–1078. discussion 1078–1080.

Borgaro, S. R., Prigatano, G. P., Kwasnica, C., & Rexer, J. L. (2003). Cognitive and affective sequelae in complicated and uncomplicated mild traumatic brain injury. *Brain Injury, 17*(3), 189–198.

Carey, M. E., Joseph, A. S., Morris, W. J., McDonnell, D. E., Rengachary, S. S., Smythies, C., et al. (1998). Brain wounds and their treatment in VII corps during operation desert storm, February 20 to April 15, 1991. *Military Medicine, 163*(9), 581–586.

Carey, M. E., Sacco, W., & Merkler, J. (1982). An analysis of fatal and non-fatal head wounds incurred during combat in Vietnam by U.S. forces. *Acta Chirurgica Scandinavica. Supplementum, 508*, 351–356.

Carroll, L. J., Cassidy, J. D., Holm, L., Kraus, J., & Coronado, V. G. (2004). Methodological issues and research recommendations for mild traumatic brain injury: the WHO Collaborating Centre Task Force on Mild Traumatic Brain Injury. *Journal of Rehabilitation Medicine, 43*(Suppl), 113–125.

Carroll, L. J., Cassidy, J. D., Peloso, P. M., Borg, J., von Holst, H., Holm, L., et al. (2004). Prognosis for mild traumatic brain injury: results of the WHO collaborating centre task force on mild traumatic brain injury. *Journal of Rehabilitation Medicine, 36*(Supplement 43), 84–105.

Chamelian, L., & Feinstein, A. (2004). Outcome after mild to moderate traumatic brain injury: the role of dizziness. *Archives of Physical Medicine and Rehabilitation, 85*(10), 1662–1666.

Chaudhri, K. A., Choudhury, A. R., al Moutaery, K. R., & Cybulski, G. R. (1994). Penetrating craniocerebral shrapnel injuries during "Operation Desert Storm": early results of a conservative surgical treatment. *Acta Neurochirurgica, 126*(2–4), 120–123.

Christensen, H., Griffiths, K., Mackinnon, A., & Jacomb, P. (1997). A quantitative review of cognitive deficits in depression and Alzheimer-type dementia. *Journal of the International Neuropsychological Society, 3*(6), 631–651.

Collins, M. W., Field, M., Lovell, M. R., Iverson, G., Johnston, K. M., Maroon, J., et al. (2003). Relationship between postconcussion headache and neuropsychological test performance in high school athletes. *The American Journal of Sports Medicine, 31*(2), 168–173.

Collins, M. W., Iverson, G. L., Lovell, M. R., McKeag, D. B., Norwig, J., & Maroon, J. (2003). On-field predictors of neuropsychological and symptom deficit following sports-related concussion. *Clinical Journal of Sport Medicine, 13*(4), 222–229.

Dawson, D. R., Levine, B., Schwartz, M. L., & Stuss, D. T. (2004). Acute predictors of real-world outcomes following traumatic brain injury: a prospective study. *Brain Injury, 18*(3), 221–238.

Dikmen, S., Temkin, N. R., Machamer, J. E., Holubkov, A. L., Fraser, R. T., & Winn, H. R. (1994). Employment following traumatic head injuries. *Archives of Neurology, 51*(2), 177–186.

Drake, A. I., Gray, N., Yoder, S., Pramuka, M., & Llewellyn, M. (2000). Factors predicting return to work following mild traumatic brain injury: a discriminant analysis. *The Journal of Head Trauma Rehabilitation, 15*(5), 1103–1112.

Drazen, J. M. (2005). Using every resource to care for our casualties. *The New England Journal of Medicine, 352*(20), 2121.

Dunn, A. L., Trivedi, M. H., Kampert, J. B., Clark, C. G., & Chambliss, H. O. (2005). Exercise treatment for depression: efficacy and dose response. *American Journal of Preventive Medicine, 28*(1), 1–8.

Edna, T. H., & Cappelen, J. (1987). Return to work and social adjustment after traumatic head injury. *Acta Neurochirurgica, 85*(1–2), 40–43.

Fann, J. R., Uomoto, J. M., & Katon, W. J. (2000). Sertraline in the treatment of major depression following mild traumatic brain injury. *The Journal of Neuropsychiatry and Clinical Neurosciences, 12*(2), 226–232.

Fann, J. R., Uomoto, J. M., & Katon, W. J. (2001). Cognitive improvement with treatment of depression following mild traumatic brain injury. *Psychosomatics, 42*(1), 48–54.

Federoff, J. P., Starkstein, S. E., Forrester, A. W., Geisler, F. H., Jorge, R. E., Arndt, S., et al. (1992). Depression in patients with acute traumatic brain injury. *The American Journal of Psychiatry, 149*, 918–923.

Frazier, T. W., Demaree, H. A., & Youngstrom, E. A. (2004). Meta-analysis of intellectual and neuropsychological test performance in attention-deficit/hyperactivity disorder. *Neuropsychology, 18*(3), 543–555.

Friedland, J. F., & Dawson, D. R. (2001). Function after motor vehicle accidents: a prospective study of mild head injury and posttraumatic stress. *The Journal of Nervous and Mental Disease, 189*(7), 426–434.

Gasquoine, P. G. (2000). Postconcussional symptoms in chronic back pain. *Applied Neuropsychology, 7*(2), 83–89.

Gentilini, M., Nichelli, P., Schoenhuber, R., Bortolotti, P., Tonelli, L., Falasca, A., et al. (1985). Neuropsychological evaluation of mild head injury. *Journal of Neurology, Neurosurgery and Psychiatry, 48*(2), 137–140.

Goldstein, F. C., Levin, H. S., Goldman, W. P., Clark, A. N., & Altonen, T. K. (2001). Cognitive and neurobehavioral functioning after mild versus moderate traumatic brain injury in older adults. *Journal of the International Neuropsychological Society, 7*(3), 373–383.

Grant, I., Gonzalez, R., Carey, C. L., Natarajan, L., & Wolfson, T. (2003). Non-acute (residual) neurocognitive effects of cannabis use: a meta-analytic study. *Journal of the International Neuropsychological Society, 9*(5), 679–689.

Griesbach, G. S., Gomez-Pinilla, F., & Hovda, D. A. (2007). Time window for voluntary exercise-induced increases in hippocampal neuroplasticity molecules after traumatic brain injury is severity dependent. *Journal of Neurotrauma, 24*(7), 1161–1171.

Griesbach, G. S., Hovda, D. A., Gomez-Pinilla, F., & Sutton, R. L. (2008). Voluntary exercise or amphetamine treatment, but not the combination, increases hippocampal brain-derived neurotrophic factor and synapsin I following cortical contusion injury in rats. *Neuroscience, 154*(2), 530–540.

Griesbach, G. S., Hovda, D. A., Molteni, R., Wu, A., & Gomez-Pinilla, F. (2004). Voluntary exercise following traumatic brain injury: brain-derived neurotrophic factor upregulation and recovery of function. *Neuroscience, 125*(1), 129–139.

Gunstad, J., & Suhr, J. A. (2004). Cognitive factors in Postconcussion Syndrome symptom report. *Archives of Clinical Neuropsychology, 19*(3), 391–405.

Haboubi, N. H., Long, J., Koshy, M., & Ward, A. B. (2001). Short-term sequelae of minor head injury (6 years experience of minor head injury clinic). *Disability and Rehabilitation, 23*(14), 635–638.

Hanlon, R. E., Demery, J. A., Martinovich, Z., & Kelly, J. P. (1999). Effects of acute injury characteristics on neurophysical status and vocational outcome following mild traumatic brain injury. *Brain Injury, 13*(11), 873–887.

Hibbard, M. R., Ashman, T. A., Spielman, L. A., Chun, D., Charatz, H. J., & Melvin, S. (2004). Relationship between depression and psychosocial functioning after traumatic brain injury. *Archives of Physical Medicine and Rehabilitation, 85*(4 Suppl 2), S43–53.

Hofman, P. A., Stapert, S. Z., van Kroonenburgh, M. J., Jolles, J., de Kruijk, J., & Wilmink, J. T. (2001). MR imaging, single-photon emission CT, and neurocognitive performance after mild traumatic brain injury. *American Journal of Neuroradiology, 22*(3), 441–449.

Hoge, C. W., McGurk, D., Thomas, J. L., Cox, A. L., Engel, C. C., & Castro, C. A. (2008). Mild traumatic brain injury in U.S. soldiers returning from Iraq. *The New England Journal of Medicine, 358*(5), 453–463.

Horner, M. D., Ferguson, P. L., Selassie, A. W., Labbate, L. A., Kniele, K., & Corrigan, J. D. (2005). Patterns of alcohol use 1 year after traumatic brain injury: a population-based, epidemiological study. *Journal of the International Neuropsychological Society, 11*(3), 322–330.

Hugenholtz, H., Stuss, D. T., Stethem, L. L., & Richard, M. T. (1988). How long does it take to recover from a mild concussion? *Neurosurgery, 22*(5), 853–858.

Hughes, D. G., Jackson, A., Mason, D. L., Berry, E., Hollis, S., & Yates, D. W. (2004). Abnormalities on magnetic resonance imaging seen acutely following mild traumatic brain injury: correlation with neuropsychological tests and delayed recovery. *Neuroradiology, 46*(7), 550–558.

Iverson, G. L. (2005). Outcome from mild traumatic brain injury. *Current Opinion in Psychiatry, 18*, 301–317.

Iverson, G. L. (2006a). Complicated vs uncomplicated mild traumatic brain injury: acute neuropsychological outcome. *Brain Injury, 20*(13–14), 1335–1344.

Iverson, G. L. (2006b). Misdiagnosis of persistent postconcussion syndrome in patients with depression. *Archives of Clinical Neuropsychology, 21*(4), 303–310.

Iverson, G. L., Franzen, M. D., & Lovell, M. R. (1999). Normative comparisons for the controlled oral word association test following acute traumatic brain injury. *The Clinical Neuropsychologist, 13*(4), 437–441.

Iverson, G. L., Lange, R. T., Gaetz, M., & Zasler, N. D. (2007). Mild TBI. In N. D. Zasler, H. T. Katz, & R. D. Zafonte (Eds.), *Brain injury medicine: principles and practice* (pp. 333–371). New York: Demos Medical Publishing.

Iverson, G. L., Lovell, M. R., & Smith, S. S. (2000). Does brief loss of consciousness affect cognitive functioning after mild head injury? *Archives of Clinical Neuropsychology, 15*(7), 643–648.

Iverson, G. L., & McCracken, L. M. (1997). 'Postconcussive' symptoms in persons with chronic pain. *Brain Injury, 11*(11), 783–790.

Ivins, B. J., Schwab, K. A., Warden, D., Harvey, L. T., Hoilien, M. A., Powell, C. O., et al. (2003). Traumatic brain injury in U.S. Army paratroopers: prevalence and character. *The Journal of Trauma, 55*(4), 617–621.

Jorge, R. E., Robinson, R. G., Starkstein, S. E., & Arndt, S. V. (1993). Depression and anxiety following traumatic brain injury. *The Journal of Neuropsychiatry and Clinical Neurosciences, 5*(4), 369–374.

Jovanovski, D., Erb, S., & Zakzanis, K. K. (2005). Neurocognitive deficits in cocaine users: a quantitative review of the evidence. *Journal of Clinical and Experimental Neuropsychology, 27*(2), 189–204.

Karzmark, P., Hall, K., & Englander, J. (1995). Late-onset post-concussion symptoms after mild brain injury: the role of premorbid, injury-related, environmental, and personality factors. *Brain Injury, 9*(1), 21–26.

Kraus, J., Schaffer, K., Ayers, K., Stenehjem, J., Shen, H., & Afifi, A. A. (2005). Physical complaints, medical service use, and social and employment changes following mild traumatic brain injury: a 6-month longitudinal study. *The Journal of Head Trauma Rehabilitation, 20*(3), 239–256.

Kraus, J. F., & Chu, L. D. (2005). Epidemiology. In J. M. Silver, T. W. McAllister, & S. C. Yudofsky (Eds.), *Textbook of traumatic brain injury* (pp. 3–26). Arlington: American Psychiatric Publishing, Inc.

Kurca, E., Sivak, S., & Kucera, P. (2006). Impaired cognitive functions in mild traumatic brain injury patients with normal and pathologic magnetic resonance imaging. *Neuroradiology, 48*(9), 661–669.

Lahmeyer, H. W., & Bellur, S. N. (1987). Cardiac regulation and depression. *Journal of Psychiatry Research, 21*(1), 1–6.

Lange, R. T., Iverson, G. L., Zakrzewski, M. J., Ethel-King, P. E., & Franzen, M. D. (2005). Interpreting the trail making test following traumatic brain injury: comparison of traditional time scores and derived indices. *Journal of Clinical and Experimental Neuropsychology, 27*(7), 897–906.

Langlois, J. A., Rutland-Brown, W., & Thomas, K. E. (2004). *Traumatic brain injury in the United States: emergency department visits, hospitalizaitons, and deaths.* Atlanta: Centers for Disease Control and Prevention, National Center for Injury Prevention and Control.

Leininger, B. E., Gramling, S. E., Farrell, A. D., Kreutzer, J. S., & Peck, E. A., 3rd. (1990). Neuropsychological deficits in symptomatic minor head injury patients after concussion and mild concussion. *Journal of Neurology, Neurosurgery and Psychiatry, 53*(4), 293–296.

Levin, H. S., Brown, S. A., Song, J. X., McCauley, S. R., Boake, C., Contant, C. F., et al. (2001). Depression and posttraumatic stress disorder at three months after mild to moderate traumatic brain injury. *Journal of Clinical and Experimental Neuropsychology, 23*(6), 754–769.

Levin, H. S., Mattis, S., Ruff, R. M., Eisenberg, H. M., Marshall, L. F., Tabaddor, K., et al. (1987). Neurobehavioral outcome following minor head injury: a three-center study. *Journal of Neurosurgery, 66*(2), 234–243.

Levin, H. S., McCauley, S. R., Josic, C. P., Boake, C., Brown, S. A., Goodman, H. S., et al. (2005). Predicting depression following mild traumatic brain injury. *Archives of General Psychiatry, 62*(5), 523–528.

Lovell, M. R., Collins, M. W., Iverson, G. L., Field, M., Maroon, J. C., Cantu, R., et al. (2003). Recovery from mild concussion in high school athletes. *Journal of Neurosurgery, 98*(2), 296–301.

Lovell, M. R., Collins, M. W., Iverson, G. L., Johnston, K. M., & Bradley, J. P. (2004). Grade 1 or "ding" concussions in high school athletes. *The American Journal of Sports Medicine, 32*(1), 47–54.

Lovell, M. R., Iverson, G. L., Collins, M. W., McKeag, D., & Maroon, J. C. (1999). Does loss of consciousness predict neuropsychological decrements after concussion? *Clinical Journal of Sport Medicine, 9*(4), 193–198.

Lovell, M. R., Iverson, G. L., Collins, M. W., Podell, K., Johnston, K. M., Pardini, D., et al. (2006). Measurement of symptoms following sports-related concussion: reliability and normative data for the post-concussion scale. *Applied Neuropsychology, 13*(3), 166–174.

Macciocchi, S. N., Barth, J. T., Alves, W., Rimel, R. W., & Jane, J. A. (1996). Neuropsychological functioning and recovery after mild head injury in collegiate athletes. *Neurosurgery, 39*(3), 510–514.

Mathias, J. L., Beall, J. A., & Bigler, E. D. (2004). Neuropsychological and information processing deficits following mild traumatic brain injury. *Journal of the International Neuropsychological Society, 10*(2), 286–297.

McCauley, S. R., Boake, C., Levin, H. S., Contant, C. F., & Song, J. X. (2001). Postconcussional disorder following mild to moderate traumatic brain injury: anxiety, depression, and social support as risk factors and comorbidities. *Journal of Clinical and Experimental Neuropsychology, 23*(6), 792–808.

McCrea, M., Guskiewicz, K. M., Marshall, S. W., Barr, W., Randolph, C., Cantu, R. C., et al. (2003). Acute effects and recovery time following concussion in collegiate football players: the NCAA Concussion Study. *JAMA, 290*(19), 2556–2563.

McCrea, M., Hammeke, T., Olsen, G., Leo, P., & Guskiewicz, K. (2004). Unreported concussion in high school football players: implications for prevention. *Clinical Journal of Sport Medicine, 14*(1), 13–17.

McCrea, M., Kelly, J. P., Randolph, C., Cisler, R., & Berger, L. (2002). Immediate neurocognitive effects of concussion. *Neurosurgery, 50*(5), 1032–1040.

McCrea, M. A. (2008). *Mild traumatic brain injury and postconcussion syndrome: the new evidence base for diagnosis and treatment*. New York: Oxford University Press.

McCullagh, S., Oucherlony, D., Protzner, A., Blair, N., & Feinstein, A. (2001). Prediction of neuropsychiatric outcome following mild trauma brain injury: an examination of the Glasgow Coma Scale. *Brain Injury, 15*(6), 489–497.

Mead, G. E., Morley, W., Campbell, P., Greig, C. A., McMurdo, M., & Lawlor, D. A. (2008). Exercise for depression. *Cochrane Database Syst Rev*(4), CD004366.

Mild Traumatic Brain Injury Committee, A. C. o. R. M., Head Injury Interdisciplinary Special Interest Group. (1993). Definition of mild traumatic brain injury. *The Journal of Head Trauma Rehabilitation, 8*(3), 86–87.

Minderhoud, J. M., Boelens, M. E., Huizenga, J., & Saan, R. J. (1980). Treatment of minor head injuries. *Clinical Neurology and Neurosurgery, 82*(2), 127–140.

Mittenberg, W., Canyock, E. M., Condit, D., & Patton, C. (2001). Treatment of post-concussion syndrome following mild head injury. *Journal of Clinical and Experimental Neuropsychology, 23*(6), 829–836.

Mittenberg, W., Tremont, G., Zielinski, R. E., Fichera, S., & Rayls, K. R. (1996). Cognitive-behavioral prevention of postconcussion syndrome. *Archives of Clinical Neuropsychology, 11*(2), 139–145.

Mooney, G., & Speed, J. (2001). The association between mild traumatic brain injury and psychiatric conditions. *Brain Injury, 15*(10), 865–877.

National Center for Injury Prevention and Control. (2003). *Report to congress on mild traumatic brain injury in the United States: steps to prevent a serious public health problem*. Atlanta: Centers for Disease Control and Prevention.

Okie, S. (2005). Traumatic brain injury in the war zone. *The New England Journal of Medicine, 352*(20), 2043–2047.

Ommaya, A. K., Ommaya, A. K., Dannenberg, A. L., & Salazar, A. M. (1996). Causation, incidence, and costs of traumatic brain injury in the U.S. military medical system. *The Journal of Trauma, 40*(2), 211–217.

Paniak, C., Toller-Lobe, G., Reynolds, S., Melnyk, A., & Nagy, J. (2000). A randomized trial of two treatments for mild traumatic brain injury: 1 year follow-up. *Brain Injury, 14*(3), 219–226.

Parker, R. S., & Rosenblum, A. (1996). IQ loss and emotional dysfunctions after mild head injury incurred in a motor vehicle accident. *Journal of Clinical Psychology, 52*(1), 32–43.

Peleg, K., Rivkind, A., & Aharonson-Daniel, L. (2006). Does body armor protect from firearm injuries? *Journal of the American College of Surgeons, 202*(4), 643–648.

Pellman, E. J., Lovell, M. R., Viano, D. C., Casson, I. R., & Tucker, A. M. (2004). Concussion in professional football: neuropsychological testing-part 6. *Neurosurgery, 55*(6), 1290–1305.

Pellman, E. J., Viano, D. C., Casson, I. R., Arfken, C., & Powell, J. (2004). Concussion in professional football: Injuries involving 7 or more days out-Part 5. *Neurosurgery, 55*(5), 1100–1119.

Penninx, B. W., Rejeski, W. J., Pandya, J., Miller, M. E., Di Bari, M., Applegate, W. B., et al. (2002). Exercise and depressive symptoms: a comparison of aerobic and resistance exercise effects on emotional and physical function in older persons with high and low depressive symptomatology. *The Journals of Gerontology. Series B: Psychological Sciences and Social Sciences, 57*(2), 124–132.

Pietropaolo, S., Sun, Y., Li, R., Brana, C., Feldon, J., & Yee, B. K. (2008). The impact of voluntary exercise on mental health in rodents: a neuroplasticity perspective. *Behavioural Brain Research, 192*(1), 42–60.

Ponsford, J., Willmott, C., Rothwell, A., Cameron, P., Ayton, G., Nelms, R., et al. (2001). Impact of early intervention on outcome after mild traumatic brain injury in children. *Pediatrics, 108*(6), 1297–1303.

Ponsford, J., Willmott, C., Rothwell, A., Cameron, P., Kelly, A. M., Nelms, R., et al. (2002). Impact of early intervention on outcome following mild head injury in adults. *Journal of Neurology, Neurosurgery and Psychiatry, 73*(3), 330–332.

Ponsford, J., Willmott, C., Rothwell, A., Cameron, P., Kelly, A. M., Nelms, R., et al. (2000). Factors influencing outcome following mild traumatic brain injury in adults. *Journal of the International Neuropsychological Society, 6*(5), 568–579.

Relander, M., Troupp, H., & Af Bjorkesten, G. (1972). Controlled trial of treatment for cerebral concussion. *British Medical Journal, 4*(843), 777–779.

Ruff, R. (2005). Two decades of advances in understanding of mild traumatic brain injury. *The Journal of Head Trauma Rehabilitation, 20*(1), 5–18.

Schneiderman, A. I., Braver, E. R., & Kang, H. K. (2008). Understanding sequelae of injury mechanisms and mild traumatic brain injury incurred during the conflicts in Iraq and Afghanistan: persistent postconcussive symptoms and posttraumatic stress disorder. *American Journal of Epidemiology, 167*(12), 1446–1452.

Schretlen, D. J., & Shapiro, A. M. (2003). A quantitative review of the effects of traumatic brain injury on cognitive functioning. *International Review of Psychiatry, 15*(4), 341–349.

Schwab, K. A., Ivins, B., Cramer, G., Johnson, W., Sluss-Tiller, M., Kiley, K., et al. (2007). Screening for traumatic brain injury in troops returning from deployment in Afghanistan and Iraq: initial investigation of the usefulness of a short screening tool for traumatic brain injury. *The Journal of Head Trauma Rehabilitation, 22*(6), 377–389.

Silver, J. M., Kramer, R., Greenwald, S., & Weissman, M. (2001). The association between head injuries and psychiatric disorders: findings from the New Haven NIMH Epidemiologic Catchment Area Study. *Brain Injury, 15*(11), 935–945.

Smith-Seemiller, L., Fow, N. R., Kant, R., & Franzen, M. D. (2003). Presence of post-concussion syndrome symptoms in patients with chronic pain vs mild traumatic brain injury. *Brain Injury, 17*(3), 199–206.

Sosin, D. M., Sniezek, J. E., & Thurman, D. J. (1996). Incidence of mild and moderate brain injury in the United States, 1991. *Brain Injury, 10*(1), 47–54.

Stambrook, M., Moore, A. D., Peters, L. C., Deviaene, C., & Hawryluk, G. A. (1990). Effects of mild, moderate and severe closed head injury on long-term vocational status. *Brain Injury, 4*(2), 183–190.

Stranjalis, G., Korfias, S., Papapetrou, C., Kouyialis, A., Boviatsis, E., Psachoulia, C., et al. (2004). Elevated serum S-100B protein as a predictor of failure to short-term return to work or activities after mild head injury. *Journal of Neurotrauma, 21*(8), 1070–1075.

Taber, K. H., Warden, D. L., & Hurley, R. A. (2006). Blast-related traumatic brain injury: what is known? *The Journal of Neuropsychiatry and Clinical Neurosciences, 18*(2), 141–145.

Tanielian, T., & Jaycox, L. H. (Eds.). (2008). *Invisible wounds of war: psychological and cognitive injuries, their consequences, and services to assist recovery.* Santa Monica: Rand Corporation.

Temkin, N. R., Machamer, J. E., & Dikmen, S. S. (2003). Correlates of functional status 3–5 years after traumatic brain injury with CT abnormalities. *Journal of Neurotrauma, 20*(3), 229–241.

Uzzell, B. P., Langfitt, T. W., & Dolinskas, C. A. (1987). Influence of injury severity on quality of survival after head injury. *Surgical Neurology, 27*(5), 419–429.

van der Naalt, J., Hew, J. M., van Zomeren, A. H., Sluiter, W. J., & Minderhoud, J. M. (1999). Computed tomography and magnetic resonance imaging in mild to moderate head injury: early and late imaging related to outcome. *Annals of Neurology, 46*(1), 70–78.

van der Naalt, J., van Zomeren, A. H., Sluiter, W. J., & Minderhoud, J. M. (1999). One year outcome in mild to moderate head injury: the predictive value of acute injury characteristics related to complaints and return to work. *Journal of Neurology, Neurosurgery and Psychiatry, 66*(2), 207–213.

Vanderploeg, R. D., Curtiss, G., Duchnick, J. J., & Luis, C. A. (2003). Demographic, medical, and psychiatric factors in work and marital status after mild head injury. *The Journal of Head Trauma Rehabilitation, 18*(2), 148–163.

Varney, N., Martzke, J., & Roberts, R. (1987). Major depression in patients with closed head injury. *Neuropsychology, 1*, 7–8.

Vickery, C. D., Berry, D. T., Inman, T. H., Harris, M. J., & Orey, S. A. (2001). Detection of inadequate effort on neuropsychological testing: a meta-analytic review of selected procedures. *Archives of Clinical Neuropsychology, 16*(1), 45–73.

Wade, D. T., King, N. S., Wenden, F. J., Crawford, S., & Caldwell, F. E. (1998). Routine follow up after head injury: a second randomised controlled trial. *Journal of Neurology, Neurosurgery and Psychiatry, 65*(2), 177–183.

Warden, D. L. (2006). Military TBI during the Iraq and Afghanistan wars. *The Journal of Head Trauma Rehabilitation, 21*(5), 398–402.

Wilde, E. A., Bigler, E. D., Gandhi, P. V., Lowry, C. M., Blatter, D. D., Brooks, J., et al. (2004). Alcohol abuse and traumatic brain injury: quantitative magnetic resonance imaging and neuropsychological outcome. *Journal of Neurotrauma, 21*(2), 137–147.

Williams, D. H., Levin, H. S., & Eisenberg, H. M. (1990). Mild head injury classification. *Neurosurgery, 27*(3), 422–428.

Wilson, J. T. L., Hadley, D. M., Scott, L. C., & Harper, A. (1996). Neuropsychological significance of contusional lesions identified by MRI. In B. P. Uzzell & H. H. Stonnington (Eds.), *Recovery after traumatic brain injury* (pp. 29–50). Mahway: Lawrence Erlbaum Associates.

Wrightson, P., & Gronwall, D. (1981). Time off work and symptoms after minor head injury. *Injury, 12*(6), 445–454.

Xydakis, M. S., Fravell, M. D., Nasser, K. E., & Casler, J. D. (2005). Analysis of battlefield head and neck injuries in Iraq and Afghanistan. *Otolaryngology – Head and Neck Surgery, 133*(4), 497–504.

Zafonte, R. D., Cullen, N., & Lexell, J. (2002). Serotonin agents in the treatment of acquired brain injury. *The Journal of Head Trauma Rehabilitation, 17*(4), 322–334.

Chapter 23
Sport-Related Concussion

Grant L. Iverson

Abstract Concussions in sports typically arise from a hard blow to the head. In soccer, for example, head-to-head impacts carry a high risk for concussion (Withnall et al., Br J Sports Med 39(Suppl 1):i49–i57, 2005). In the National Football League (NFL), an injury reconstruction study revealed that a striking player often lines up his head, neck, and torso to deliver maximum force to the other player in helmet-to-helmet impacts that result in concussive injuries to the player being struck (Viano and Pellman, Neurosurgery 56(2):266–280, 2005). Fortunately, most injuries in sports fall on the milder end of the spectrum of mild traumatic brain injuries (MTBI). Occasionally, however, athletes experience complicated mild, moderate, or severe traumatic brain injuries. In equestrian and auto racing, for example, accidents can result in much more serious injuries to the brain.

Key Points and Chapter Summary

- In sport-related concussion, loss of consciousness is usually not present, post-traumatic amnesia is relatively brief in duration, and full recovery is expected to occur within 2–28 days.
- Most concussions are likely associated with relatively low levels of axonal stretch resulting in temporary changes in neurophysiology. Fortunately, for the vast majority of affected cells, there appears to be a reversible series of neurometabolic events.
- The role of the neuropsychologist is to evaluate and quantify athletes' subjectively experienced symptoms and/or to determine neurocognitive diminishment on objective measures.

(continued)

G.L. Iverson (✉)
University of British Columbia & British Columbia Mental Health
and Addiction Services, Vancouver, BC, Canada
e-mail: giverson@interchange.ubc.ca

M.R. Schoenberg and J.G. Scott (eds.), *The Little Black Book of Neuropsychology:*
A Syndrome-Based Approach, DOI 10.1007/978-0-387-76978-3_23,
© Springer Science+Business Media, LLC 2011

Key Points and Chapter Summary (continued)

- As a rule, the athlete should not return to play the day of injury. Injured athletes should rest until asymptomatic. They should then begin a graded series of exertional activities to make sure that exercise or light contact does not elicit symptoms. Athletes should be medically cleared prior to return to play.
- There is concern that the multiple injured athlete will be at increased risk for (1) future injuries, (2) slower recovery, and (3) long-term changes to the structure or function of his or her brain. In the most serious cases, when athletes have sustained multiple concussions or otherwise are especially susceptible to concussions, the athlete, his or her family, coach, trainer, and physician need to explore the possibility of retirement.

According to the American Academy of Neurology (AAN): "Concussion is a trauma-induced alteration in mental status that may or may not include a loss of consciousness" (American Academy of Neurology 1997, p. 582). Following a Concussion in Sport conference in Vienna, the following definition was published: "Concussion is defined as a complex pathophysiological process affecting the brain, induced by traumatic biomechanical forces" (Aubry et al. 2002, p. 6). The features of this injury are defined below.

1. Concussion may be caused either by a direct blow to the head, face, neck, or elsewhere on the body with an "impulsive" force transmitted to the head.
2. Concussion typically results in the rapid onset of short-lived impairment of neurological function that resolves spontaneously.
3. Concussion may result in neuropathological changes, but the acute clinical symptoms largely reflect a functional disturbance rather than structural injury.
4. Concussion results in a graded set of clinical symptoms that may or may not involve loss of consciousness. Resolution of the clinical and cognitive symptoms typically follows a sequential course.
5. Concussion is typically associated with grossly normal structural neuroimaging studies (Aubry et al. 2002, p. 6).

Neurobiology and Pathophysiology

Most injuries in sports can be characterized as relatively mild concussions. These injuries fall at the mild end of the MTBI severity continuum. Loss of consciousness usually is not present, and post-traumatic amnesia is typically brief. This injury is likely associated with low levels of axonal stretch resulting in temporary changes in neurophysiology. Giza and Hovda (2004) described the complex interwoven cellular and vascular changes that occur following concussion as a multilayered neurometabolic cascade. The primary mechanisms include ionic shifts, abnormal energy metabolism, diminished cerebral blood flow, and impaired neurotransmission (see Figs. 23.1, 23.2, and 23.3). Fortunately, for the vast majority of affected cells, there appears to be a reversible series of neurometabolic events (Giza and Hovda 2001, 2004; Iverson 2005, 2007).

The neurometabolic derangements associated with concussion are studied through animal and in vitro experimental models (Giza and Hovda 2001, 2004). The stretching of axons due to mechanical force results in an indiscriminate release of neurotransmitters and uncontrolled ionic fluxes. Mechanoporation allows calcium (Ca^{2+}) influx and potassium (K) efflux, contributing to rapid and widespread depolarization. Cells respond by activating ion pumps in an attempt to restore the normal membrane potential. This pump activation increases glucose utilization (i.e., accelerated glycolysis). There also appears to be impaired oxidative metabolism. These factors contribute to a state of hypermetabolism, which occurs in tandem with decreased cerebral blood flow, further compounding the hypermetabolism. The sustained influx of Ca^{2+} can result in mitochondrial accumulations of this ion and contribute to metabolic dysfunction and energy failure. The energy production of the cell is compromised further by over-utilization of anaerobic energy pathways and elevated lactate as a by-product. Moreover, intracellular magnesium levels appear to decrease significantly and remain depressed for several days following injury. This is important because magnesium is essential for the generation of adenosine-triphosphate (ATP – energy production). Magnesium is also essential for the initiation of protein synthesis and the maintenance of the cellular membrane potential.

The ultimate fate of the neuron is related to the extent of traumatic axonal injury, summarized elegantly by Buki and Povlishock (2006). High intracellular Ca^{2+} levels, combined with stretch injury, can initiate an irreversible process of destruction of microtubules within axons. The disruption of the microtubular and neurofilament components contributes to axonal swelling and detachment (i.e., secondary axotomy).

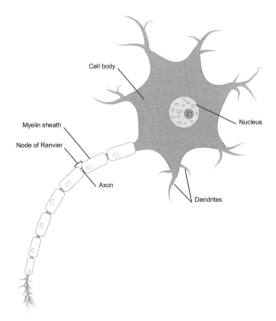

Fig. 23.1 Neuron

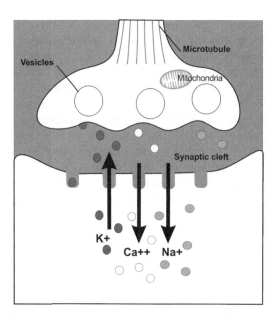

Fig. 23.2 Ionic shifts. This figure illustrates immediate ionic shifts followed by an ensuing energy crisis as the cell attempts to restore homeostasis. K+ Potassium, Ca++ Calcium, Na+ Sodium, and *ATP* Adenosine Triphosphate. ATP plays a vital role in intracellular energy transfer; it assists with transporting chemical injury within cells for metabolism. Metabolism is a general term for chemical reactions within cells which, in this context, help the cell maintain structure and respond to environmental demands. A state of hypermetabolism creates in imbalance between ATP supply and demand (Inspired and adapted from images presented by Professor David Hovda at the National Academy of Neuropsychology, October 22, 2008, New York City)

Some, but not all, cells that experience secondary axotomy will degenerate and die through necrotic or apoptotic mechanisms. In general, however, most injured cells (1) do not undergo secondary axotomy, and (2) appear to recover normal cellular function. In most sport-related concussions, it appears as if the brain undergoes dynamic restoration and the athlete returns, in due course, to normal functioning.

Rule of thumb: Features of complex neurometabolic cascade following concussion

- Influx of calcium
- Efflux of potassium
- Cerebrovascular blood flow subtly decreases
- Neurons enter state of hypermetabolism
- Anaerobic energy production and build-up of intracellular lactate
- Intracellular magnesium levels remain low for days after concussion
- In general, most injured cells (1) do not undergo secondary axotomy, and (2) appear to recover normal cellular function

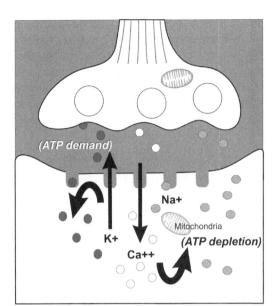

Fig. 23.3 Energy crisis. This figure illustrates immediate ionic shifts followed by an ensuing energy crisis as the cell attempts to restore homeostasis. K^+ Potassium, Ca^{++} Calcium, Na^+ Sodium, and *ATP* Adenosine Triphosphate. ATP plays a vital role in intracellular energy transfer; it assists with transporting chemical injury within cells for metabolism. Metabolism is a general term for chemical reactions within cells which, in this context, help the cell maintain structure and respond to environmental demands. A state of hypermetabolism creates in imbalance between ATP supply and demand (Inspired and adapted from images presented by Professor David Hovda at the National Academy of Neuropsychology, October 22, 2008, New York City)

Recovery Time

Researchers have reported that concussions cause acute adverse changes in subjectively experienced symptoms, balance, and neuropsychological test performance (Barr and McCrea 2001; Collins et al. 1999; Delaney et al. 2001; Erlanger et al. 2003a, 2001; Guskiewicz et al. 2001; Macciocchi et al. 1996; Makdissi et al. 2001; Matser et al. 2001; McCrea et al. 2003, 2002; Peterson et al. 2003; Riemann and Guskiewicz 2000; Warden et al. 2001). When analyzing group data, researchers consistently report that athletes recover within 2 weeks (Bleiberg et al. 2004; Lovell et al. 2004a; Macciocchi et al. 1996; McCrea et al. 2003, 2002; Pellman et al. 2004a). When analyzing individual cases, however, some athletes take longer to recover and their slower recovery can be obscured in group analyses (Iverson et al. 2006b).

Collins et al. (2006) found it took 28 days before 90% of a large cohort of high school foot ball players were believed to have recovered from their concussions. The high school football players took considerably longer to recover than university (McCrea et al. 2003) or professional (Pellman et al. 2006, 2004a, b) football players.

The reasons for this are unclear, but could be related to numerous factors including neurodevelopmental differences in response to concussion-related neuropathophysiology, genetics, and injury resilience. In addition, commonsense would suggest that young athletes who are particularly susceptible to concussions, and slow recovery, might not advance to higher levels of play. Thus, the more rapid recovery time in college and professional athletes could, in part, reflect a selection bias. Not surprisingly, additional research with younger athletes has been encouraged (McCrory et al. 2004).

Rule of thumb: Recovery Time from Concussion

- 2 days to 2 weeks for most college and professional players
- High school players can take longer to recover (a few days to 1 month for most athletes)

Classification Systems

Over the past 25 years, there have been many attempts to grade the severity of sport-related concussions. More than 20 systems have been suggested; however, none have strong empirical basis. Therefore, clinicians and researchers should not assume at this point in time, that any particular system is the "best" system. Two concussion grading systems are presented in Table 23.1.

The American Academy of Neurology (AAN) grading system and management guidelines, published in 1997, evolved out of the Colorado Medical Society Guidelines from 1990. In retrospect, it is clear that these guidelines are limited in at least three important ways. First, Grade 1 concussions cannot actually be identified accurately on the day of injury because many athletes who appear to have this type of injury (e.g., their mental status changes appear to resolve in less than 15 min and they do not appear particularly symptomatic) actually have significant post-concussion symptoms later that day and possibly for several days thereafter. The lingering symptoms can be exacerbated by physical and/or mental activity. Second, there is limited and equivocal research to support the notion that brief loss of consciousness is the hallmark of the "worst" type of concussion. Third, the system does not address the duration of post-concussion symptoms and problems well.

The revised Cantu (2001) system is more elaborate and more carefully considers the duration of post-traumatic amnesia, which is a severity marker that bears some positive correlation with recovery time. Moreover, Cantu's system more carefully considers the duration of post-concussion symptoms. A problem with the system, as worded, is that it is not clear how to grade concussions that have any duration of PTA less than 24 hours *and* 2–7 days of post-concussion symptoms.

In 2004, following the Second Conference on Concussion in Sport held in Prague, a new classification system was proposed. This *"simple–complex"* classification system is binary and based on recovery time. Thus, the athlete is classified

Table 23.1 Example Concussion Grading Scales

Guideline	Qualitative descriptors of concussion severity		
AAN (1997)	**Grade 1**	**Grade 2**	**Grade 3**
	1. Transient confusion	1. Transient confusion	1. Loss of consciousness (brief or prolonged)
	2. No loss of consciousness	2. No loss of consciousness	
	3. Concussion symptoms or mental status changes resolve in less than 15 minutes	3. Concussion symptoms or mental status change lasts longer than 15 minutes	
Cantu (2001)	**Mild concussion**	**Moderate concussion**	**Severe concussion**
	1. No loss of consciousness	1. Loss of consciousness lasts less than 1 minute	1. Loss of consciousness lasts more than 1 minute
	OR	OR	OR
	2. Post-traumatic amnesia[a] or signs/symptoms lasts less than 30 minutes	2. Post-traumatic amnesia[a] last longer than 30 minutes but less than 24 hours	2. Post-traumatic amnesia[a] lasts longer than 24 hours
		OR	OR
		3. Post-concussion signs or symptoms last longer than 30 minutes but less than 24 hours	3. Post-concussion signs or symptoms last longer than 7 days

AAN American Academy of Neurology

[a]Cantu conceptualized PTA as either retrograde or anterograde amnesia.

as having a certain type of concussion, not based on characteristics of the injury, but based on the number of days he or she takes to recover. If the athlete recovers within 10 days the injury is classified as "simple" and if recovery takes more than 10 days it is classified as "complex." The concept of a simple concussion fits reasonably well with the scientific literature to date. Most university and professional athletes appear to recover quickly and fully from a concussion. There is considerable evidence that concussions in sports are self-limiting injuries that are not associated with long-term cognitive or neurobehavioral problems.

Iverson (2007) conducted an exploratory case–control study to determine if injured high school football players ($n = 114$), retrospectively classified as having a simple or a complex concussion, could be differentiated in the first 48 hours post-injury on the basis of symptom reporting or neuropsychological testing. Within 72 hours post-injury, players with complex concussions performed much more poorly on neuropsychological testing, and reported far more symptoms, than those with simple concussions. Athletes with complex concussions who were slow to recover were 18 times more likely to have three unusually low neuropsychological test scores than those with simple concussions. Three interesting findings relating to the new simple–complex classification system emerged. First, complex concussions were much more common than expected in this sample of injured high school football players (52%). Second, those athletes with complex concussions presented differently, clinically, in the acute period (i.e., first 72 hours). They reported far more symptoms and performed much more poorly on computerized neuropsychological testing. This provides commonsense support for the idea that those who are destined to be slower to recover have worse concussions – as measured by level of symptoms and cognitive impairment in the initial days after injury. Third, according to the new system, athletes with past concussions could be automatically classified as complex. However, in this study the athletes with previous concussions did not recover more slowly.

Readers should note that the intent of the Prague article was, I think, to say that complex concussions are defined by recovery time and *may (or may not)* be associated with other factors such as duration of unconsciousness, convulsions, and history of previous concussions (which are, essentially, speculative variables in regards to predicting recovery time). Having these variables unintentionally yoked to the definition of complex concussion might inadvertently encourage the clinician to treat an athlete with those characteristics differently than an athlete without those characteristics. That would, of course, run counter to the recommendations set out in both the Vienna and Prague statements emphasizing that all athletes should be treated individually according to their clinical needs. Recently, at the 3rd International Conference on Concussion in Sport, held in Zurich, it was decided by consensus to drop the simple–complex classification (McCrory et al. 2009).

Multiple Concussions

Under normal circumstances, athletes appear to recover quickly and fully from a concussion. This recovery typically occurs within 2–28 days. Full recovery is assumed if (1) the athlete has no lingering subjectively experienced symptoms, (2) balance testing is normal, and (3) there is no obvious neurocognitive diminishment. Greater concern arises, however, when an athlete experiences multiple concussions. There is concern that the multiple injured athlete will be at increased risk for (1) future injuries, (2) slower recovery, and (3) long-term changes to the structure or function of his or her brain. There is some research evidence that justifies these concerns.

In several studies, it has been reported that athletes who sustain a concussion are at statistically increased risk for sustaining another concussion (Delaney et al. 2000; Gerberich et al. 1983; Guskiewicz et al. 2003; Zemper 2003). The reasons for this are unclear, but could relate to style of play, position, genetics, or lowering a biological susceptibility threshold. It has also been reported that some athletes with prior concussions might recover more slowly (Covassin et al. 2008; Guskiewicz et al. 2003). Researchers have reported that some athletes with multiple concussions (usually three or more) report more symptoms and have worse neuropsychological test performance than athletes with no history of concussion (Collins et al. 1999; Gaetz et al. 2000; Iverson et al. 2004a; Thornton et al. 2007; Wall et al. 2006). This might reflect a long-lasting consequence of multiple injuries (Shuttleworth-Rdwards and Radloff 2008). However, the cross-sectional research designs do not permit confident causal inferences. Moreover, some researchers have not found evidence of lingering effects (Broglio et al. 2006; Collie et al. 2006c; De Beaumont et al. 2007).

There is much reference to the so-called second impact syndrome (Cantu 1998) in the literature and in academic presentations relating to sport concussion. The second impact syndrome, as a true clinical entity, is controversial (McCrory 2001; McCrory and Berkovic 1998). It has been noted in the literature that diffuse cerebral swelling is a very rare and catastrophic consequence of a *single* seemingly mild brain injury – creating a conceptual problem for the assumption that the small number of cases really represent second impact syndrome. Nonetheless, the syndrome is believed to be an extraordinarily rare and catastrophic consequence of a *second* blow to the head while the athlete is still recovering from a concussion (18 cases identified in a literature review; Mori et al. 2006). A catastrophic series of pathophysiological events, including diffuse brain swelling, ensues leading to death or severe disability.

In my view, concern about second impact syndrome has frequently been overstated, and at times it has taken on an alarmist tone, which can actually distract from the bigger issue of preventing more subtle but important magnified pathophysiology attributable to overlapping injuries. For example, there is interesting and emerging evidence in the experimental animal literature that there is a temporal window of vulnerability in which a second injury results in magnified cognitive and behavioral deficits, and greater levels of traumatic axonal injury (Laurer et al. 2001; Longhi et al. 2005; Vagnozzi et al. 2007). Specifically, mice that are re-injured during this "temporal window" have worse behavioral and neurophysiological outcome than mice who are re-injured after the temporal window. Whether one is concerned about second impact syndrome or magnified pathophysiology from overlapping injuries – the end result, from a management perspective, is the same. Athletes should not be returned to contact sports during the *acute recovery stage* from concussion. As a rule, athletes should not be returned to contact sports until they are believed to be *recovered* from their concussion.

Emerging Evidenced-Based Neuropsychology

There is a rapidly emerging specialty area of practice called sports neuropsychology. This area of practice has its roots in the pioneering work of Barth and colleagues with collegiate athletes (Barth et al. 1989). Lovell and colleagues started a similar program with the Pittsburgh Steelers in approximately 1992 (Lovell 1999), and this experience evolved into neuropsychological assessment programs in both the NFL and the National Hockey League (NHL). See Table 23.2 for the test batteries used by the NFL and the NHL (Lovell 2006). Several books are available to assist clinicians in this area (e.g., Echemendia 2006; Lovell et al. 2004), and the National Academy of Neuropsychology published a position paper on the usefulness of neuropsychological evaluation for monitoring recovery from concussions in sports

Table 23.2 Test batteries used in professional sports

NFL neuropsychological test battery	NHL neuropsychological test battery
Orientation Questions	Orientation Questions
Hopkins Verbal Learning Test (HLVT)	Concussion Symptom Inventory
Brief Visuospatial Memory Test-Revised (BVMT-R)	Hopkins Verbal Learning Test (HVLT)
Trail Making Test	Brief Visuospatial Memory Test-Revised
Controlled Oral Word Fluency	Color Trail Making
WAIS-III Symbol Search	Controlled Oral Word Association Test
WAIS-III Digit Symbol	Penn State Cancelation Test
WAIS-III Digit Span	Symbol Digit Modalities
Post-Concussion Symptom Scale	Delayed recall from HVLT
Delayed recall from HVLT	
Delayed recall from BVMT-R	

(Moser et al. 2007). Several published studies provide empirical support the usefulness of neuropsychological assessment in the management of sport-related concussion (Belanger and Vanderploeg 2005; Collie et al. 2006a; Collins et al. 2006; Fazio et al. 2007; Iverson 2007; Iverson et al. 2006b, 2003, 2005; Van Kampen et al. 2006).

Neuropsychologists can get involved at two points in time: preseason and post-injury. Voluntary preseason neuropsychological testing has been adopted by many athletic teams in North America. In this role, the neuropsychologist participates in the baseline testing of entire teams. The preseason test results provide a benchmark for each individual player to help the neuropsychologist and team physician gauge recovery should the player get concussed during the season. As such, the preseason testing is often not considered a "clinical service," and no neuropsychological consult report is generated. Rather, the purpose is to have baseline neuropsychological data for future comparison.

In many settings, however, neuropsychologists become involved only after an athlete has been injured from a concussion. This can occur any time, including within days of injury, several weeks following injury, or in the off-season. The primary role of the neuropsychologist is to determine if the athlete has subjectively experienced symptoms and/or neuropsychological impairments. Assessment procedures typically include an interview with the athlete, post-concussion self-report questionnaires, and administering neuropsychological tests. Following concussion, the neuropsychologist, as a consultant, might set out specific recommendations for return-to-play, advise about any potential for establishing short-term accommodations in school and/or work, and provide data to the player and team on the recovery of neuropsychological function following more serious concussions or persisting injuries. In some cases involving multiple injuries, the neuropsychologist can be helpful if discussions progress to the athlete considering retiring from sports. Neuropsychologists can also become involved in an athlete's care when the player sustains an injury to the head as a result of non-athletic related activities (e.g., accidents, falls, and assaults). In these cases, the role of the neuropsychologist can be similar to when a player is concussed playing sports, but referral questions can differ depending upon the nature and severity of injury the player sustained.

Computerized Neuropsychological Test Batteries

Neuropsychologists can use traditional or computerized neurocognitive testing. It has become increasingly popular to use computerized testing – especially when baseline testing large numbers athletes. There are numerous advantages to using computerized testing in clinical and research settings. These include, but are not limited to: (1) the relatively large amount of information that can be obtained in a brief amount of time, (2) the reduced cost of being able to administer a battery of tests via computer, (3) the ability to have alternate versions and present the test in various languages, and (4) the ability to precisely measure time-sensitive tasks in small units of time (i.e., milliseconds for reaction time). A brief overview of several computerized batteries designed for use in sports neuropsychology is provided below.

Impact (Immediate Post-Concussion Assessment and Cognitive Testing)

ImPACT is a computerized neuropsychological test battery that consists of six individual test modules that measure multiple aspects of cognitive functioning including attention, memory, working memory, visual scanning, reaction time, and processing speed. The test takes 20–25 minutes. Four composite (i.e., summary) scores are tabulated based upon these individual test scores: Verbal Memory, Visual Memory, Reaction Time, and Processing Speed. An Impulse Control composite is generated, too, but this measure has not been included in most studies. In addition to the cognitive measures, ImPACT also contains a Post-Concussion Scale that consists of 22 subjectively experienced symptoms (e.g., headache, dizziness, concentration problems, and fogginess). A total score is derived from this 22-item scale. Normative data are stratified by age, gender, and level of education. Specifically, norms are based on: (1) boys, 13–15, $n = 183$; (2) boys, 16–18, $n = 158$; (3) girls 14–18, $n = 83$; (4) university males, $n = 410$; and (5) university females, $n = 97$. A recent large-scale normative study of high school students in Hawaii ($n = 751$) produced similar results in comparison to the original ImPACT norms (Tsushima et al. 2008). The authors concluded that there was a non-significant trend toward high school students in Hawaii performing somewhat more poorly than students from the mainland. The ImPACT software has built-in reliable change analyses. The sensitivity of the battery to the acute effects of concussion has been examined in a number of studies (e.g., Broglio et al. 2007a; Collins et al. 2003b, 2006; Covassin et al. 2007; Fazio et al. 2007; Iverson 2007; Iverson et al. 2006b, 2002, 2003, 2004a; Lovell et al. 2003; McClincy et al. 2006; Mihalik et al. 2007; Schatz et al. 2006; Van Kampen et al. 2006). In general, ImPACT has more research in sport concussion than all other traditional or computerized batteries.

HeadMinder Concussion Resolution Index

The Concussion Resolution Index is a computerized neurocognitive test battery that takes approximately 25 minutes to complete. The battery consists of six tests designed to measure (1) simple reaction time, (2) complex reaction time, and (3) visual scanning and psychomotor speed. There are two tests in each of these three domains. The scores derived are: (1) simple reaction time index, (2) simple reaction time index errors, (3) complex reaction time index, (4) complex reaction time index errors, and (5) processing speed index. There appear to be three normative samples for this test battery: (1) Junior High and High School, ages 13–17, $n=220$; (2) High School and University, ages 18–25, $n=194$; and (3) Adults, ages 23–59, $n = 126$, as reported by Kaushik and Erlanger(2006). The Concussion Resolution Index software program has built-in analyses for interpreting change. Change can be evaluated based on reliable change or regression methodologies. The reliable change methodology is used by default. The sensitivity of the battery to the effects of concussion has been examined in a number of studies (e.g., Broglio et al. 2007b; Broshek et al. 2005; Erlanger et al. 2003b; Sosnoff et al. 2007).

CogSport

CogSport is a computerized neurocognitive test battery that takes approximately 12–15 minutes to complete (although baseline testing involves two trials, the first for practice). The battery consists of five tests measuring simple reaction time, choice reaction time, sustained attention, working memory, and new learning. All five tests are based on the "playing card metaphor." That is, all tests utilize a computerized deck of playing cards as the stimuli. CogSport also has a built-in post-concussion questionnaire and post-concussion symptom checklist. The primary normative data for CogSport is derived from 300 people between the ages of 16–40 (i.e., 269 males and 31 females). Three normative scores are presented (i.e., speed, variability, and accuracy) for each test. New normative data for children and adolescents, ages 9–10 ($n=63$), 11–12 ($n=48$), 13–14 ($n=28$), 15–16 ($n = 24$), and 17–18 ($n=30$), were presented in a book chapter (Collie et al. 2006b). The sensitivity of the battery to the effects of concussion has been examined in a number of studies (e.g., Collie et al. 2006a; Makdissi et al. 2001).

Automated Neuropsychological Assessment Metrics (ANAM)

The ANAM was developed in the 1980s through a series of US Department of Defense (DOD) projects. It was developed for military use to study the cognitive effects of chemical and environmental stressors. Recently, a sports medicine version of the battery has been proposed. This version consists of seven individual tests:

Simple reaction time, Code Substitution, Running Memory Continuous Performance Test, Mathematical Processing, Spatial Processing, and a delayed recall task for Code Substitution. In general, this battery measures reaction time, processing speed, and working memory. There is a small amount of research supporting its use in sports (e.g., Warden et al. 2001), and research is underway to develop normative data for the sports medicine version of the ANAM (Brown et al. 2007).

Concerns about Computerized Testing

A potential problem with computerized testing is that the baseline might not represent the athlete's true ability. For example, testing might have been done under non-optimal conditions, such as after a vigorous practice. Moreover, some athletes are tested in groups. It is possible that group testing in school computer laboratories contributes to some athletes not taking the testing as seriously as they should.

Another concern expressed by some neuropsychologists is that it can be (1) difficult to know what some of the computerized tests are actually measuring, and (2) how similar or different the computerized tests are to mainstream traditional paper-pencil tests (for which neuropsychologists tend to be more comfortable). There are no easy answers to these concerns. In my view, it is very difficult to determine what *most* neuropsychological tests are truly measuring (i.e., traditional or computerized). Is Trails B, for example, a test of attention, divided attention, processing speed, set shifting, or cognitive flexibility? Do the correlations between Trails B and other measures truly help us determine what the test is measuring? In a mixed clinical sample ($n=56$), for example, Trails B had the following correlations (The Psychological Corporation 2002, p. 164): Verbal Comprehension Index ($-.40$), Perceptual Organization Index ($-.62$), Working Memory Index ($-.65$), Processing Speed Index ($-.55$), and Full Scale IQ ($-.66$). The psychometrics of all neuropsychological tests are complex – we must, in my view, be careful to not equate familiarity and comfort with psychometric confidence. I find it necessary to simply carefully study the task requirements and conceptualize them in behavioral terms.

These batteries have varying degrees of research support for use in concussion management programs. They all have strengths and limitations. Their strengths and limitations, from a purely psychometric perspective, are similar to the strengths and limitations of traditional neuropsychological tests. It is a mistake to view computerized testing, based on the research to date, as being summarily inferior to traditional neuropsychological testing.

Use of Symptom Ratings

There have been numerous studies illustrating that concussions cause a diverse set of symptoms and problems. In one study (Lovell et al. 2006), for example, the most commonly reported symptoms in the initial days post-injury were headaches,

Table 23.3 Normative data for the post-concussion scale total score
(Lovell et al. 2006)

Classification	High School and University Students	
	Males ($n = 1,391$)	Females ($n = 355$)
Low–normal	0	0
Broadly normal	1–5	1–9
Borderline	6–12	10–20
Very high	13–26	21–43
Extremely high	27+	44+

fatigue, feeling slowed down, drowsiness, difficulty concentrating, feeling mentally foggy, and dizziness. These individual symptoms were endorsed by 60–79% of the sample ($n = 260$). The least frequently endorsed symptoms were nervousness, feeling more emotional, sadness, numbness or tingling, and vomiting. These individual symptoms were endorsed by fewer than 25% of the sample.

Symptom ratings are critically important for the documenting the effects of a concussion and monitoring recovery. A commonly used measure is the 22-item Post-Concussion Scale (Lovell 1996, 1999; Lovell and Collins 1998). Variants of this scale have been adopted by the National Football League (Lovell 1996) and National Hockey League (Lovell and Burke 2002; Lovell et al. 2004c), and this scale has been used in numerous published studies (e.g., Collins et al. 2003a; Iverson et al. 2004a, b; Lovell et al. 2003, 2004a). The measure is based on a 7-point Likert scale with 0 and 6 reflecting the anchor points. Athletes report symptoms based on the severity of each symptom that day.

Normative data for the scale are based on 1,391 young males and 355 young females (Lovell et al. 2006). There were no differences within genders when comparing high school students to university students. Thus, the high school and university samples were combined. As seen in Table 23.3, however, females endorse more symptoms on average than males. Thus, normative data are presented separately by gender. It should be noted that borderline scores correspond to "above average" symptom reporting, very high scores occur in 10% or fewer, and extremely high scores occur in 2% or fewer of normative subjects.

Return to Play

It is widely accepted in amateur athletics that athletes who sustain a concussion should not return to the practice or game in which they were injured. The now widely cited recommendation is that athletes should rest until they are asymptomatic. In general, rest means no vigorous physical activity or heavy mental exertion. From a practical perspective, this often means taking a few days off school. When asymptomatic, a return to light aerobic exercise is recommended as described in the two agreement statements following the International Concussion in Sport Conferences in Vienna (Aubry et al. 2002) and Prague (McCrory et al. 2005).

The protocol involves an athlete moving through the following exertional steps in 24-hour periods: (1) light aerobic exercise (e.g., walking or a stationary biking), (2) sport-specific training (e.g., ice skating in hockey or running in soccer), and (3) non-contact training drills (usually heavily exertional). Athletes then progress to contact or full return to play. If the athlete's previously resolved post-concussion symptoms return at any step, the athlete should return to the previous exertion level at which they were last asymptomatic.

Rule of thumb: Return to Play Following Concussion

- Athlete should not return to play the day of injury
- Athlete should rest until asymptomatic
- Athlete should not return to play until asymptomatic with exertion

---

British Columbia Concussion Rehabilitation Program (BC-CRP)

Following the International Symposium on Concussion in Sport that was held in Prague in November of 2004, Gaetz and Iverson began developing the British Columbia Concussion Rehabilitation Program (BC-CRP) (Gaetz and Iverson 2005, 2009; Gaetz et al. 2006). We recognized the need to develop and evaluate a *specific* protocol that followed these agreement recommendations and improved upon the transition between stages 1–3 (complete rest to sport-specific exercise). In addition, this program can be used (through adaptation) as form of active rehabilitation for slow-to-recover athletes and civilians (Iverson et al. 2006a).

The BC-CRP was designed for use with athletes from any sport once they are asymptomatic at rest and before they begin stage two of the Prague 2004 return to play protocol that recommends "Light aerobic activity" (McCrory et al. 2005). The program represents a supervised step 2 (i.e., light aerobic activity). The program uses three steps of graduated difficulty separated by a minimum of 24 hours. The protocol involves both *mental and physical exertion*. First, the athlete completes a symptom rating scale and a standardized balance test. Second, he or she completes a computerized test of sustained attention (i.e., the CPT-II). Immediately thereafter he or she completes a 15-minutes cycle ergometry protocol. There are three levels of difficulty for the cycle ergometry protocol. If the athlete becomes symptomatic during, immediately after, or hours after the cognitive and physical exertion protocol, then the athlete returns to a lower level of physical exertion (Gaetz and Iverson 2005, 2009). The goal of the BC-CRP is to use an active rehabilitation philosophy to help the athlete safely move from being asymptomatic at rest, to being asymptomatic while under a relatively high cognitive and cardiovascular stress load. Thus, the BC-CRP ensures that the athlete becomes increasingly active in a supervised setting with progressive and well-defined benchmarks for recovery.

Active Rehabilitation for Slow to Recover Children and Adolescents

Children who are slow-to-recover from sport-related concussions present unique challenges for health care providers and the school system. It has been recommended that a more conservative approach to concussion management be used with injured children (Lovell and Fazio 2008). The general recommendation that youth athletes avoid exercise until completely asymptomatic at rest works well for most children, most of the time. However, when children are very slow to recover, there is a risk that their symptoms and problems will (1) become chronic, and (2) be caused in whole or part by factors that might not be directly related to the neurobiology of the original concussion. Moreover, from a practical perspective, it is very difficult to ensure that mildly symptomatic children will not engage in physical exertion (e.g., vigorous playing and running).

Gagnon, Galli, Friedman, and Iverson (under review) described an innovative program of active rehabilitation for injured youth athletes that is in place at Montreal Children's Hospital. They presented a consecutive series of cases illustrating that involvement in controlled and closely monitored rehabilitation in the post-acute period promotes recovery. All 10 of the slow-to-recover children and adolescents who participated in the program experienced a relatively rapid recovery and they returned to their normal lifestyles and sport participation. This program is illustrated in Fig. 23.4.

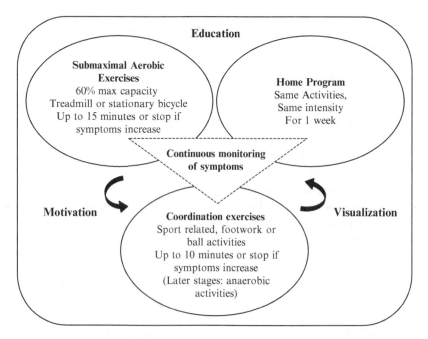

Fig. 23.4 Montreal Children's Hospital Rehabilitation after Concussion Program (Adapted from Gagnon et al. (2009). Copyright © Gagnon et al. (2009))

The active rehabilitation at Montreal Children's Hospital is designed to be used *post-acutely* for the very small percentage of children who have persistent symptoms for many weeks. For this group, significant lifestyle restrictions, including avoiding physical activity, can actually contribute to symptom mainte-nance over time. That is, the longer a child (or adult) has symptoms, the more likely it is that other factors that are separate from or only partially related to the neurobiology of the original injury are causing or maintaining the symptoms. Thus, at some point, active rehabilitation seems indicated. The rationale for active rehabilitation comes from diverse literature. First, exercise has been shown to have positive effects on mood, self-esteem, and it promotes a general sense of well-being (Duman 2005). Second, in adults, exercise can be an effective treat-ment for mild depression (Dunn et al. 2005; Mead et al. 2008; Penninx et al. 2002). Third, exercise promotes neuroplasticity in animal studies (Pietropaolo et al. 2008), and exercise done after a period of recovery in animal studies involving MTBI is also associated with neuroplasticity (Griesbach et al. 2007, 2008, 2004). Finally, active rehabilitation and exercise is used with older adults following stroke. Therefore, a gradual, closely supervised active rehabilitation program for children and adolescents, in the post-acute period (i.e., after 1 month post injury), seems appropriate.

Retirement from Sport Decisions

It can be extraordinarily difficult to determine when a person should retire from contact sports. This is, essentially, a personal choice, and psychologists are encour-aged to respect autonomy and freedom of choice. However, the athlete and his or her family, coach, trainer, and physician need good information upon which they can make informed decisions.

According to Echemendia and Cantu (2003), there are two main changes that should raise concern about when the athlete should retire from contact sports. The first change relates to the *duration* of post-concussive symptoms. Usually, post-concussive symptoms resolve within a few days or weeks. However, a progressively increasing period of symptom duration in athletes who have sus-tained multiple concussions is one warning sign that return to competition may not be advisable. The second change that should raise concern is the *force* required to produce a concussion. Blows that produce concussion almost always strike the head. However, there is anecdotal evidence that some athletes with a history of multiple injuries become more susceptible to a concussion from blows to other parts of the body, especially the chest and back. Apparent changes in the athlete's susceptibility to concussions could be an impetus for discussions about retirement. Unfortunately, the literature used to support a clinician's decision for returning an athlete to sport (or not) remains somewhat inconclusive and has several methodological limitations. Much more work is needed in this area.

Rule of thumb: Retirement Considerations
• Long duration symptoms following concussion (e.g., increasingly long periods to recover from concussion)   • Force required to sustain concussion progressively becomes less (e.g., athlete may note (s)he seems to suffer from concussion symptoms much more easily)   • Results of structural neuroimaging find evidence of brain damage

Conclusions

Concussions in sports are caused from a direct blow to the head, face, or neck, or indirectly, due to an "impulsive" force caused by a blow elsewhere on the body. Most involve hard blows to the head. Most concussions are likely associated with relatively low levels of axonal stretch resulting in temporary changes in neurophysiology. The primary mechanisms include ionic shifts, abnormal energy metabolism, diminished cerebral blood flow, and impaired neurotransmission. Fortunately, for the vast majority of affected cells, there appears to be a reversible series of neurometabolic events.

Concussions in sports typically fall along the milder end of the MTBI severity continuum and appear grossly normal on structural neuroimaging studies. Loss of consciousness is usually not present, post-traumatic amnesia is relatively brief in duration, and full recovery is expected to occur within 2–28 days. Greater concern arises, however, when an athlete experiences multiple concussions. There is concern that the multiply injured athlete will be at increased risk for (1) future injuries, (2) slower recovery, and (3) long-term changes to the structure or function of his or her brain. There is some research evidence that justifies these concerns.

The role of the neuropsychologist is to evaluate and quantify athletes' subjectively experienced symptoms and/or to determine neurocognitive diminishment on objective measures. There is an emerging evidenced-base for neuropsychological assessment in concussion management. Measuring both cognition and symptom ratings is important for documenting the effects of concussion and monitoring recovery. Accordingly, the natural point of insertion for neuropsychological services is at preseason (to establish baseline performance, when possible) or, as is most often the case, post injury.

Neuropsychologists can play an important role in helping athletes function better in school, and determining when it is safe for athletes to return to play. It is recommended that athletes rest until they are asymptomatic. Once asymptomatic, they should be encouraged to engage in light aerobic exercise. This is done in progressive steps of increasing levels of exertion. If previously resolved post-concussion symptoms return, athletes should return to previous exertion levels at which they were asymptomatic. In the most serious cases, when athletes have sustained multiple concussions or otherwise are especially susceptible to concussions, the athlete, his or her family, coach, trainer, and physician need to explore the possibility of retirement.

References

American Academy of Neurology. (1997). Practice parameter: The management of concussion in sports (summary statement). Report of the Quality Standards Subcommittee. *Neurology, 48*(3), 581–585.

Aubry, M., Cantu, R., Dvorak, J., Graf-Baumann, T., Johnston, K., Kelly, J., et al. (2002). Summary and agreement statement of the First International Conference on Concussion in Sport, Vienna 2001. Recommendations for the improvement of safety and health of athletes who may suffer concussive injuries. *British Journal of Sports Medicine, 36*(1), 6–10.

Barr, W. B., & McCrea, M. (2001). Sensitivity and specificity of standardized neurocognitive testing immediately following sports concussion. *Journal of the International Neuropsychological Society, 7*(6), 693–702.

Barth, J. T., Alves, W., Ryan, T., Macciocchi, S., Rimel, R. W., Jane, J. J., et al. (1989). Mild head injury in sports: Neuropsychological sequelae and recovery of function. In H. Levin, J. Eisenberg, & A. Benton (Eds.), *Mild head injury* (pp. 257–275). New York: Oxford University Press.

Belanger, H. G., & Vanderploeg, R. D. (2005). The neuropsychological impact of sports-related concussion: A meta-analysis. *Journal of the International Neuropsychological Society, 11*(4), 345–357.

Bleiberg, J., Cernich, A. N., Cameron, K., Sun, W., Peck, K., Ecklund, P. J., et al. (2004). Duration of cognitive impairment after sports concussion. *Neurosurgery, 54*(5), 1073–1078. discussion 1078–1080.

Broglio, S. P., Ferrara, M. S., Piland, S. G., Anderson, R. B., & Collie, A. (2006). Concussion history is not a predictor of computerised neurocognitive performance. *British Journal of Sports Medicine, 40*(9), 802–805. discussion 802–805.

Broglio, S. P., Macciocchi, S. N., & Ferrara, M. S. (2007a). Neurocognitive performance of concussed athletes when symptom free. *Journal of Athletic Training, 42*(4), 504–508.

Broglio, S. P., Macciocchi, S. N., & Ferrara, M. S. (2007b). Sensitivity of the concussion assessment battery. *Neurosurgery, 60*(6), 1050–1057. discussion 1057–1058.

Broshek, D. K., Kaushik, T., Freeman, J. R., Erlanger, D., Webbe, F., & Barth, J. T. (2005). Sex differences in outcome following sports-related concussion. *Journal of Neurosurgery, 102*(5), 856–863.

Brown, C. N., Guskiewicz, K. M., & Bleiberg, J. (2007). Athlete characteristics and outcome scores for computerized neuropsychological assessment: A preliminary analysis. *Journal of Athletic Training, 42*(4), 515–523.

Buki, A., & Povlishock, J. T. (2006). All roads lead to disconnection? – Traumatic axonal injury revisited. *Acta Neurochirurgica (Wien), 148*(2), 181–193. discussion 184–193.

Cantu, R. C. (1998). Second-impact syndrome. *Clinical Sports Medicine, 17*(1), 37–44.

Cantu, R. C. (2001). Posttraumatic retrograde and anterograde amnesia: Pathophysiology and implications in grading and safe return to play. *Journal of Athletic Training, 36*(3), 244–248.

Collie, A., Makdissi, M., Maruff, P., Bennell, K., & McCrory, P. (2006). Cognition in the days following concussion: Comparison of symptomatic versus asymptomatic athletes. *Journal of Neurology, Neurosurgery and Psychiatry, 77*(2), 241–245.

Collie, A., Maruff, P., Darby, D., Makdissi, M., McCrory, P., & McStephen, M. (2006). CogSport. In R. Echemendia (Ed.), *Sports neuropsychology: Assessment and management of traumatic brain injury* (pp. 240–262). New York: The Guilford.

Collie, A., McCrory, P., & Makdissi, M. (2006). Does history of concussion affect current cognitive status? *British Journal of Sports Medicine, 40*(6), 550–551.

Collins, M. W., Field, M., Lovell, M. R., Iverson, G., Johnston, K. M., Maroon, J., et al. (2003). Relationship between postconcussion headache and neuropsychological test performance in high school athletes. *The American Journal of Sports Medicine, 31*(2), 168–173.

Collins, M. W., Grindel, S. H., Lovell, M. R., Dede, D. E., Moser, D. J., Phalin, B. R., et al. (1999). Relationship between concussion and neuropsychological performance in college football players. *Journal of the American Medical Association, 282*(10), 964–970.

Collins, M. W., Iverson, G. L., Lovell, M. R., McKeag, D. B., Norwig, J., & Maroon, J. (2003). On-field predictors of neuropsychological and symptom deficit following sports-related concussion. *Clinical Journal of Sport Medicine, 13*(4), 222–229.

Collins, M. W., Lovell, M. R., Iverson, G. L., Ide, T., & Maroon, J. (2006). Examining concussion rates and return to play in high school football players wearing newer helmet technology: A three year prospective cohort study. *Neurosurgery, 58*(2), 275–286.

Covassin, T., Schatz, P., & Swanik, C. B. (2007). Sex differences in neuropsychological function and post-concussion symptoms of concussed collegiate athletes. *Neurosurgery, 61*(2), 345–350. discussion 341–350.

Covassin, T., Stearne, D., & Elbin, R. (2008). Concussion history and postconcussion neurocognitive performance and symptoms in collegiate athletes. *Journal of Athletic Training, 43*(2), 119–124.

De Beaumont, L., Brisson, B., Lassonde, M., & Jolicoeur, P. (2007). Long-term electrophysiological changes in athletes with a history of multiple concussions. *Brain Injury, 21*(6), 631–644.

Delaney, J. S., Lacroix, V. J., Gagne, C., & Antoniou, J. (2001). Concussions among university football and soccer players: A pilot study. *Clinical Journal of Sport Medicine, 11*(4), 234–240.

Delaney, J. S., Lacroix, V. J., Leclerc, S., & Johnston, K. M. (2000). Concussions during the 1997 Canadian Football League season. *Clinical Journal of Sport Medicine, 10*(1), 9–14.

Duman, R. S. (2005). Neurotrophic factors and regulation of mood: Role of exercise, diet and metabolism. *Neurobiology of Aging, 26 (Suppl 1)*, 88–93.

Dunn, A. L., Trivedi, M. H., Kampert, J. B., Clark, C. G., & Chambliss, H. O. (2005). Exercise treatment for depression: Efficacy and dose response. *American Journal of Preventive Medicine, 28*(1), 1–8.

Echemendia, R. J. (2006). *Sports neuropsychology: Assessment and management of traumatic brain injury*. New York: The Guilford.

Echemendia, R. J., & Cantu, R. C. (2003). Return to play following sports-related mild traumatic brain injury: The role for neuropsychology. *Applied Neuropsychology, 10*(1), 48–55.

Erlanger, D., Feldman, D., Kutner, K., Kaushik, T., Kroger, H., Festa, J., et al. (2003). Development and validation of a web-based neuropsychological test protocol for sports-related return-to-play decision-making. *Archives of Clinical Neuropsychology, 18*(3), 293–316.

Erlanger, D., Kaushik, T., Cantu, R., Barth, J. T., Broshek, D. K., Freeman, J. R., et al. (2003). Symptom-based assessment of the severity of a concussion. *Journal of Neurosurgery, 98*(3), 477–484.

Erlanger, D., Saliba, E., Barth, J., Almquist, J., Webright, W., & Freeman, J. (2001). Monitoring resolution of postconcussion symptoms in athletes: Preliminary results of a web-based neuropsychological test protocol. *Journal of Athletic Training, 36*(3), 280–287.

Fazio, V. C., Lovell, M. R., Pardini, J. E., & Collins, M. W. (2007). The relation between post concussion symptoms and neurocognitive performance in concussed athletes. *NeuroRehabilitation, 22*(3), 207–216.

Gaetz, M., Goodman, D., & Weinberg, H. (2000). Electrophysiological evidence for the cumulative effects of concussion. *Brain Injury, 14*(12), 1077–1088.

Gaetz, M., & Iverson, G. L. (2005). The British Columbia Concussion Rehabilitation Program (BC-CRP).

Gaetz, M., & Iverson, G. L. (2009). Sex differences in self-reported symptoms following aerobic exercise in non-injured athletes: Implications for concussion management programs. *British Journal of Sports Medicine, 43*, 508–513.

Gaetz, M., Parrott, H., & Iverson, G. L. (2006). The British Columbia Concussion Rehabilitation Program (BC-CRP): Normative and case data. Poster presented at the Brain Injury of the Americas Conference (North American Brain INjury Society – NABIS), Maimi, FL, September 14–16.

Gagnon, I., Galli, C., Friedman, D., Grilli, L., & Iverson, G. L. (2009). Active rehabilitation for children who are slow to recover following sport-related concussion. *Brain Injury, 23*(12), 956–964.

Gerberich, S. G., Priest, J. D., Boen, J. R., Straub, C. P., & Maxwell, R. E. (1983). Concussion incidences and severity in secondary school varsity football players. *American Journal of Public Health, 73*(12), 1370–1375.

Giza, C. C., & Hovda, D. A. (2001). The neurometabolic cascade of concussion. *Journal of Athletic Training, 36*(3), 228–235.

Giza, C. C., & Hovda, D. A. (2004). The pathophysiology of traumatic brain injury. In M. R. Lovell, R. J. Echemendia, J. T. Barth, & M. W. Collins (Eds.), *Traumatic brain injury in sports* (pp. 45–70). Lisse: Swets & Zeitlinger.

Griesbach, G. S., Gomez-Pinilla, F., & Hovda, D. A. (2007). Time window for voluntary exercise-induced increases in hippocampal neuroplasticity molecules after traumatic brain injury is severity dependent. *Journal of Neurotrauma, 24*(7), 1161–1171.

Griesbach, G. S., Hovda, D. A., Gomez-Pinilla, F., & Sutton, R. L. (2008). Voluntary exercise or amphetamine treatment, but not the combination, increases hippocampal brain-derived neurotrophic factor and synapsin I following cortical contusion injury in rats. *Neuroscience, 154*(2), 530–540.

Griesbach, G. S., Hovda, D. A., Molteni, R., Wu, A., & Gomez-Pinilla, F. (2004). Voluntary exercise following traumatic brain injury: Brain-derived neurotrophic factor upregulation and recovery of function. *Neuroscience, 125*(1), 129–139.

Guskiewicz, K. M., McCrea, M., Marshall, S. W., Cantu, R. C., Randolph, C., Barr, W., et al. (2003). Cumulative effects associated with recurrent concussion in collegiate football players: The NCAA Concussion Study. *Journal of the American Medical Association, 290*(19), 2549–2555.

Guskiewicz, K. M., Ross, S. E., & Marshall, S. W. (2001). Postural stability and neuropsychological deficits after concussion in collegiate athletes. *Journal of Athletic Training, 36*(3), 263–273.

Iverson, G. L. (2005). Outcome from mild traumatic brain injury. *Current Opinion in Psychiatry, 18*, 301–317.

Iverson, G. L. (2007). Predicting slow recovery from sport-related concussion: The new simple-complex distinction. *Clinical Journal of Sport Medicine, 17*, 31–37.

Iverson, G. L., Brooks, B. L., Azevedo, A., & Gaetz, M. (2006a). Modifying the British Columbia Concussion Recovery Program for use with injured adults with postconcussion syndrome. Poster presented at the Brain Injury of the Americas Conference (North American Brain Injury Society – NABIS), Maimi, FL, September 14–16.

Iverson, G. L., Brooks, B. L., Collins, M. W., & Lovell, M. R. (2006). Tracking neuropsychological recovery following concussion in sport. *Brain Injury, 20*(3), 245–252.

Iverson, G. L., Gaetz, M., Lovell, M. R., & Collins, M. W. (2002). Relation between fogginess and outcome following concussion. *Archives of Clinical Neuropsychology, 17*, 769–770.

Iverson, G. L., Gaetz, M., Lovell, M. R., & Collins, M. W. (2004a). Cumulative effects of concussion in amateur athletes. *Brain Injury, 18*(5), 433–443.

Iverson, G. L., Gaetz, M., Lovell, M. R., & Collins, M. W. (2004b). Relation between subjective fogginess and neuropsychological testing following concussion. *Journal of the International Neuropsychological Society, 10*, 904–906.

Iverson, G. L., Lovell, M. R., & Collins, M. W. (2003). Interpreting change on ImPACT following sport concussion. *The Clinical Neuropsychologist, 17*(4), 460–467.

Iverson, G. L., Lovell, M. R., & Collins, M. W. (2005). Validity of ImPACT for measuring processing speed following sports-related concussion. *Journal of Clinical and Experimental Neuropsychology, 27*(6), 683–689.

Kaushik, T., & Erlanger, D. M. (2006). The headminder concussion resolution index. In R. Echemendia (Ed.), *Sports neuropsychology: Assessment and management of traumatic brain injury* (pp. 216–239). New York: The Guildford.

Laurer, H. L., Bareyre, F. M., Lee, V. M., Trojanowski, J. Q., Longhi, L., Hoover, R., et al. (2001). Mild head injury increasing the brain's vulnerability to a second concussive impact. *Journal of Neurosurgery, 95*(5), 859–870.

Longhi, L., Saatman, K. E., Fujimoto, S., Raghupathi, R., Meaney, D. F., Davis, J., et al. (2005). Temporal window of vulnerability to repetitive experimental concussive brain injury. *Neurosurgery, 56*(2), 364–374. discussion 364–374.

Lovell, M. R. (1996). Evaluation of the professional athlete. Poster presented at the New Developments in Sports-Related Concussion Conference, Pittsburgh, PA.

Lovell, M. R. (1999). Evaluation of the professional athlete. In J. E. Bailes, M. R. Lovell, & J. C. Maroon (Eds.), *Sports-related concussion*. St. Louis: Quality Medical.

Lovell, M. R. (2006). Neuropsychological assessment of the professional athlete. In R. J. Echemendia (Ed.), *Sports neuropsychology: Assessment and management of traumatic brain injury* (pp. 176–190). New York: The Guilford.

Lovell, M. R., & Burke, C. J. (2002). The NHL concussion program. In R. Cantu (Ed.), *Neurologic athletic head and spine injury* (pp. 32–45). Phildelphia: WB Saunders.

Lovell, M. R., & Collins, M. W. (1998). Neuropsychological assessment of the college football player. *The Journal of Head Trauma Rehabilitation, 13*(2), 9–26.

Lovell, M. R., Collins, M. W., Iverson, G. L., Field, M., Maroon, J. C., Cantu, R., et al. (2003). Recovery from mild concussion in high school athletes. *Journal of Neurosurgery, 98*(2), 296–301.

Lovell, M. R., Collins, M. W., Iverson, G. L., Johnston, K. M., & Bradley, J. P. (2004). Grade 1 or "ding" concussions in high school athletes. *The American Journal of Sports Medicine, 32*(1), 47–54.

Lovell, M. R., Echemendia, R. J., Barth, J. T., & Collins, M. W. (Eds.). (2004). *Traumatic brain injury in sports*. Lisse: Swets & Zeitlinger.

Lovell, M. R., Echemendia, R. J., & Burke, C. J. (2004). Traumatic brain injury in professional hockey. In M. R. Lovell, R. J. Echemendia, J. Barth, & M. W. Collins (Eds.), *Traumatic brain injury in sports: An international neuropsychological perspective* (pp. 221–231). Amsterdam: Swets-Zietlinger.

Lovell, M. R., & Fazio, V. (2008). Concussion management in the child and adolescent athlete. *Current Sports Medicine Reports, 7*(1), 12–15.

Lovell, M. R., Iverson, G. L., Collins, M. W., Podell, K., Johnston, K. M., Pardini, D., et al. (2006). Measurement of symptoms following sports-related concussion: Reliability and normative data for the post-concussion scale. *Applied Neuropsychology, 13*(3), 166–174.

Macciocchi, S. N., Barth, J. T., Alves, W., Rimel, R. W., & Jane, J. A. (1996). Neuropsychological functioning and recovery after mild head injury in collegiate athletes. *Neurosurgery, 39*(3), 510–514.

Makdissi, M., Collie, A., Maruff, P., Darby, D. G., Bush, A., McCrory, P., et al. (2001). Computerised cognitive assessment of concussed Australian Rules footballers. *British Journal of Sports Medicine, 35*(5), 354–360.

Matser, J. T., Kessels, A. G., Lezak, M. D., & Troost, J. (2001). A dose-response relation of headers and concussions with cognitive impairment in professional soccer players. *Journal of Clinical and Experimental Neuropsychology, 23*(6), 770–774.

McClincy, M. P., Lovell, M. R., Pardini, J., Collins, M. W., & Spore, M. K. (2006). Recovery from sports concussion in high school and collegiate athletes. *Brain Injury, 20*(1), 33–39.

McCrea, M., Guskiewicz, K. M., Marshall, S. W., Barr, W., Randolph, C., Cantu, R. C., et al. (2003). Acute effects and recovery time following concussion in collegiate football players: The NCAA Concussion Study. *Journal of the American Medical Association, 290*(19), 2556–2563.

McCrea, M., Kelly, J. P., Randolph, C., Cisler, R., & Berger, L. (2002). Immediate neurocognitive effects of concussion. *Neurosurgery, 50*(5), 1032–1040.

McCrory, P. (2001). Does second impact syndrome exist? *Clinical Journal of Sport Medicine, 11*(3), 144–149.

McCrory, P., & Berkovic, S. F. (1998). Second impact syndrome. *Neurology, 50*(3), 677–683.

McCrory, P., Collie, A., Anderson, V., & Davis, G. (2004). Can we manage sport related concussion in children the same as in adults? *British Journal of Sports Medicine, 38*(5), 516–519.

McCrory, P., Johnston, K., Meeuwisse, W., Aubry, M., Cantu, R., Dvorak, J., et al. (2005). Summary and agreement statement of the 2nd International Conference on Concussion in Sport, Prague 2004. *British Journal of Sports Medicine, 39*(4), 196–204.

McCrory, P., Meeuwisse, W., Johnston, K., Dvorak, J., Aubry, M., Molloy, M., et al. (2009). Consensus Statement on Concussion in Sport: The 3rd International Conference on Concussion in Sport held in Zurich, November 2008. *British Journal of Sports Medicine, 43 (Suppl 1)*, i76–90.

Mead, G. E., Morley, W., Campbell, P., Greig, C. A., McMurdo, M., & Lawlor, D. A. (2008). Exercise for depression. *Cochrane Database of Systematic Reviews* (4), CD004366.

Mihalik, J. P., McCaffrey, M. A., Rivera, E. M., Pardini, J. E., Guskiewicz, K. M., Collins, M. W., et al. (2007). Effectiveness of mouthguards in reducing neurocognitive deficits following sports-related cerebral concussion. *Dental Traumatology, 23*(1), 14–20.

Mori, T., Katayama, Y., & Kawamata, T. (2006). Acute hemispheric swelling associated with thin subdural hematomas: Pathophysiology of repetitive head injury in sports. *Acta Neurochirurgica. Supplementum, 96*, 40–43.

Moser, R. S., Iverson, G. L., Echemendia, R. J., Lovell, M. R., Schatz, P., Webbe, F. M., et al. (2007). Neuropsychological evaluation in the diagnosis and management of sports-related concussion. *Archives of Clinical Neuropsychology, 22*(8), 909–916.

Pellman, E. J., Lovell, M. R., Viano, D. C., & Casson, I. R. (2006). Concussion in professional football: Recovery of NFL and high school athletes assessed by computerized neuropsychological testing-part 12. *Neurosurgery, 58*(2), 263–274. discussion 263–274.

Pellman, E. J., Lovell, M. R., Viano, D. C., Casson, I. R., & Tucker, A. M. (2004). Concussion in professional football: Neuropsychological testing-part 6. *Neurosurgery, 55*(6), 1290–1305.

Pellman, E. J., Viano, D. C., Casson, I. R., Arfken, C., & Powell, J. (2004). Concussion in professional football: Injuries involving 7 or more days out-part 5. *Neurosurgery, 55*(5), 1100–1119.

Penninx, B. W., Rejeski, W. J., Pandya, J., Miller, M. E., Di Bari, M., Applegate, W. B., et al. (2002). Exercise and depressive symptoms: A comparison of aerobic and resistance exercise effects on emotional and physical function in older persons with high and low depressive symptomatology. *The Journals of Gerontology. Series B: Psychological Sciences and Social Sciences, 57*(2), P124–132.

Peterson, C. L., Ferrara, M. S., Mrazik, M., Piland, S., & Elliott, R. (2003). Evaluation of neuropsychological domain scores and postural stability following cerebral concussion in sports. *Clinical Journal of Sport Medicine, 13*(4), 230–237.

Pietropaolo, S., Sun, Y., Li, R., Brana, C., Feldon, J., & Yee, B. K. (2008). The impact of voluntary exercise on mental health in rodents: A neuroplasticity perspective. *Behavioural Brain Research, 192*(1), 42–60.

Riemann, B. L., & Guskiewicz, K. M. (2000). Effects of mild head injury on postural stability as measured through clinical balance testing. *Journal of Athletic Training, 35*(1), 19–25.

Schatz, P., Pardini, J. E., Lovell, M. R., Collins, M. W., & Podell, K. (2006). Sensitivity and specificity of the ImPACT test battery for concussion in athletes. *Archives of Clinical Neuropsychology, 21*(1), 91–99.

Shuttleworth-Rdwards, A. B., & Radloff, S. E. (2008). Compromised visuomotor processing speed in players of Rugby Union from school through to the national adult level. *Archives of Clinical Neuropsychology, 23*(5), 511–520.

Sosnoff, J. J., Broglio, S. P., Hillman, C. H., & Ferrara, M. S. (2007). Concussion does not impact intraindividual response time variability. *Neuropsychology, 21*(6), 796–802.

The Psychological Corporation. (2002). *Updated WAIS-III/WMS-III technical manual*. San Antonio: Author.

Thornton, A. E., Cox, D. N., Whitfield, K., & Fouladi, R. T. (2007). Cumulative concussion exposure in rugby players: Neurocognitive and symptomatic outcomes. *Journal of Clinical and Experimental Neuropsychology, 27*, 1–12.

Tsushima, W. T., Oshiro, R., & Zimbra, D. (2008). Neuropsychological test performance of Hawai'i high school athletes: Hawai'i ImPACT normative data. *Hawaii Medical Journal, 67*(4), 93–95.

Vagnozzi, R., Tavazzi, B., Signoretti, S., Amorini, A. M., Belli, A., Cimatti, M., et al. (2007). Temporal window of metabolic brain vulnerability to concussions: Mitochondrial-related impairment – Part I. *Neurosurgery, 61*(2), 379–388. discussion 379–388.

Van Kampen, D. A., Lovell, M. R., Pardini, J. E., Collins, M. W., & Fu, F. H. (2006). The "value added" of neurocognitive testing after sports-related concussion. *The American Journal of Sports Medicine, 34*(10), 1630–1635.

Viano, D. C., & Pellman, E. J. (2005). Concussion in professional football: Biomechanics of the striking player – Part 8. *Neurosurgery, 56*(2), 266–280. discussion 266–280.

Wall, S. E., Williams, W. H., Cartwright-Hatton, S., Kelly, T. P., Murray, J., Murray, M., et al. (2006). Neuropsychological dysfunction following repeat concussions in jockeys. *Journal of Neurology, Neurosurgery and Psychiatry, 77*(4), 518–520.

Warden, D. L., Bleiberg, J., Cameron, K. L., Ecklund, J., Walter, J., Sparling, M. B., et al. (2001). Persistent prolongation of simple reaction time in sports concussion. *Neurology, 57*(3), 524–526.

Withnall, C., Shewchenko, N., Gittens, R., & Dvorak, J. (2005). Biomechanical investigation of head impacts in football. *British Journal of Sports Medicine, 39 (Suppl 1)*, i49–57.

Zemper, E. D. (2003). Two-year prospective study of relative risk of a second cerebral concussion. *American Journal of Physical Medicine & Rehabilitation, 82*(9), 653–659.

Chapter 24
Post-Concussion Syndrome

Grant L. Iverson and Rael T. Lange

Abstract The post-concussion syndrome (a.k.a., post-concussive disorder and post concussional disorder) has been controversial for decades. Without question, an *acute* post-concussion syndrome can be caused by the neurobiology of a mild traumatic brain injury (MTBI). Without question, a post-concussion syndrome can be worsened by psychological distress, social psychological factors (e.g., the nocebo effect, iatrogenesis, and misattributions), personality characteristics, and co-occurring conditions (e.g., chronic pain and insomnia). If due to the neurobiological effects of an injury to the brain, a post-concussion syndrome should be present in the *first week* post injury. Evaluating someone long after an injury, obtaining a cross-section of symptoms, and then attributing those symptoms to the remote injury can easily result in misdiagnosis.

The widely-cited estimate of 10–20% of patients suffering a long-term post-concussion syndrome is both confusing and incorrect. It is *confusing* because there is often an assumption that if a person reports symptoms long after an MTBI, that the symptoms are causally-related to the biological effects of the injury (by logical inference, the symptoms are related to damage to the structure or function of the brain). However, it is well established that these symptoms could be caused, maintained, or worsened by a large number of factors that are unrelated to traumatically-induced cellular damage. It is *incorrect* because the constellation of symptoms comprising the post-concussion syndrome likely occurs in far fewer than 10–20% of patients with remote MTBIs. The estimates of 10–20% have typically been based on selected, non-representative samples of the entire population of people who sustain an MTBI, and some of the literature has been misinterpreted as showing evidence of a syndrome when it in fact illustrates isolated, non-specific symptom reporting. It is emphasized in this chapter that the post-concussion syndrome is a non-specific cluster of symptoms that can be mimicked by a number of pre-existing

G.L. Iverson (✉)
University of British Columbia, Vancouver, BC, Canada
and
British Columbia Mental Health and Addiction Services, Vancouver, BC, Canada
e-mail: giverson@interchange.ubc.ca

M.R. Schoenberg and J.G. Scott (eds.), *The Little Black Book of Neuropsychology:*
A Syndrome-Based Approach, DOI 10.1007/978-0-387-76978-3_24,
© Springer Science+Business Media, LLC 2011

or comorbid conditions. The biologically-based, traumatically-induced syndrome, theoretically, can also occur in tandem with these conditions.

Key Points and Chapter Summary

- Despite decades of research, the post-concussion syndrome remains controversial.
- The etiology of the *persistent* post-concussion syndrome has never been agreed upon and the validity of this diagnosis as a true syndrome or disorder has been questioned.
- The widely-cited estimate of 10–20% of patients suffering a long-term post-concussion syndrome is likely incorrect.
- The post-concussion syndrome is assumed by many to be a direct and/or indirect consequence of an injury to the head or brain. However, the post-concussion syndrome is a non-specific cluster of symptoms that can be mimicked by a number of pre-existing or co-morbid conditions. A more biologically-based, traumatically-induced syndrome, theoretically, also can occur in tandem with these conditions.
- When considering long-term outcome from mild TBI, it is important to appreciate that a mild injury to the head or brain is not necessary (and often not sufficient) to produce the constellation of symptoms and problems that comprise this syndrome.
- It is imperative for clinicians to systematically evaluate the possible contribution of many differential diagnoses, co-morbidities, and social-psychological factors that may *cause or maintain* self-reported symptoms after MTBI.

Diagnostic Criteria

The International Classification of Diseases, 10th edition (ICD-10), and the Diagnostic and Statistical Manual of Mental Disorders, 4th Edition (DSM-IV) (American Psychiatric Association 1994) include research criteria for the post-concussion syndrome.

International Classification of Diseases, 10th Edition

In 1992, the World Health Organization included research criteria for "Postconcussional Syndrome" in the ICD-10 (World Health Organization 1992). According to these criteria, a person must have a history of "head trauma with a loss of consciousness" preceding the onset of symptoms by *a period of up to 4 weeks* and have at least *three of six* symptom categories listed below.

1. Headaches, dizziness, general malaise, excessive fatigue, or noise intolerance
2. Irritability, emotional lability, depression, or anxiety
3. Subjective complaints of concentration or memory difficulty
4. Insomnia
5. Reduced tolerance to alcohol
6. Preoccupation with these symptoms and fear of permanent brain damage

> "The syndrome occurs following head trauma (usually sufficiently severe to result in loss of consciousness) and includes a number of disparate symptoms such as headache, dizziness (usually lacking the features of true vertigo), fatigue, irritability, difficulty in concentrating and performing mental tasks, impairment of memory, insomnia, and reduced tolerance to stress, emotional excitement, or alcohol. These symptoms may be accompanied by feelings of depression or anxiety, resulting from some loss of self-esteem and fear of permanent brain damage. Such feelings enhance the original symptoms and a vicious circle results. Some patients become hypochondriacal, embark on a search for diagnosis and cure, and may adopt a permanent sick role. The etiology of these symptoms is not always clear, and both organic and psychological factors have been proposed to account for them. The nosological status of this condition is thus somewhat uncertain. There is little doubt, however, that this syndrome is common and distressing to the patient. Diagnostic Guidelines: At least three of the features described above should be present for a definite diagnosis. Careful evaluation with laboratory techniques (electroencephalography, brain stem evoked potentials, brain imaging, oculonystagmography) may yield objective evidence to substantiate the symptoms but results are often negative. The complaints are not necessarily associated with compensation motives" (World Health Organization 1992; section F07.2).

Diagnostic and Statistical Manual of Mental Disorders, Fourth Edition

The DSM-IV has "research criteria" for the "Postconcussional Disorder." According to these criteria, the individual must show *objective evidence* on neuropsychological testing of declines in cognitive functioning, such as attention, concentration, learning, or memory. The person must also report three or more subjective symptoms, present for at least 3 months, from the list below.

1. Becoming fatigued easily
2. Disordered sleep
3. Headache
4. Vertigo or dizziness
5. Irritability or aggression on little or no provocation
6. Anxiety, depression, or affective liability
7. Changes in personality (e.g., social or sexual inappropriateness)
8. Apathy or lack of spontaneity

The DSM-IV includes the additional criteria: "The disturbance causes significant impairment in social or occupational functioning and represents a significant decline from a previous level of functioning." The DSM-IV criteria are much more stringent than the ICD-10 criteria in that they require (1) objective evidence of neurocognitive deficits, and (2) significant impairment in social or occupational functioning. Not surprisingly, when the ICD-10 and DSM-IV criteria are compared in the same set of patients, large diagnostic prevalence differences emerge (Boake et al. 2004; McCauley et al. 2005). Researchers have reported that consecutive patients with mild traumatic brain injuries, seen at a Level I trauma center and followed prospectively, have relatively low rates of diagnosis at 3 months post injury using the DSM-IV criteria (i.e., 11–17%) compared to the ICD-10 criteria (54–64%; Boake et al. 2004; McCauley et al. 2005).

Rule of thumb: Postconcussion syndrome versus Postconcussional disorder

- Postconcussion syndrome is a set of diagnostic criteria in the ICD-10 and requires three of six symptom categories
- Postconcussional disorder is a set of diagnostic criteria outlined in the DSM-IV and requires objective neuropsychological evidence of deficits, three or more subjective symptoms, and impairment in social or occupational functioning
- More people met criteria for ICD-10 Postconcussional syndrome compared to the more stringent DSM-IV Postconcussional disorder

---

Diagnostic Challenges

One of the biggest challenges in applying the ICD-10 and the DSM-IV criteria for the post-concussion syndrome is causally linking the subjective, self-reported symptoms to a remote MTBI. If the syndrome/disorder is clearly documented in the initial weeks post-injury and continues, with only modest improvement over many months, then causation is more clear. However, it is frequently the case that the original severity of injury, acute symptoms in the first week post-injury, and recovery course cannot be determined. In these cases, examining a cross-section of symptoms and problems, months or possibly years after an MTBI, can result in "accurate" syndromal classification but causation might be unrelated to the original injury or be multifactorial.

In fact, the etiology of the *persistent* post-concussion syndrome has never been agreed upon (see Bigler 2008; Evered et al. 2003; Iverson 2005; Ryan and Warden 2003, for reviews). For decades, the validity of this diagnosis as a true syndrome or disorder has been questioned (e.g., Cook 1972; Lees-Haley et al. 2001; Mickeviciene et al. 2002; Mickeviciene et al. 2004; Rutherford et al. 1979; Satz et al. 1999). In prospective studies, the syndrome is rare (e.g., Alves et al. 1993; Rutherford et al. 1979), and concerns regarding the role of financial compensation on symptom reporting have been expressed for many years (Binder and Rohling 1996; Cook 1972; Miller 1961; Paniak et al. 2002; Reynolds et al. 2003). Most researchers suggest that the post-concussion syndrome is the result of the biological effects of the injury, psychological factors, psychosocial factors (broadly defined), chronic pain, or a combination of factors (Bijur et al. 1990; Binder 1986; Brown et al. 1994; Cicerone and Kalmar 1995;

Heilbronner 1993; Larrabee 1997; Lishman 1986; Mittenberg and Strauman 2000; Youngjohn et al. 1995). The bottom-line, however, is that in many cases it can be virtually impossible to determine the etiology of a person's reported symptoms.

Non-Specificity of Symptoms

It is very difficult to disentangle the many factors that can be related to self-reported symptoms in persons who have sustained a remote MTBI. It would be a mistake to assume uncritically that these self-reported symptoms are causally related to a distant MTBI because most individuals with MTBI recover relatively quickly and fully, and because post-concussion symptoms are nonspecific. Researchers have reported that healthy adults and the clinical groups listed below report very similar symptoms. The challenge for the clinician is to determine whether these self-reported, non-specific, symptoms are related or unrelated to the injury.

- Healthy adults (Gouvier et al. 1988; Iverson and Lange 2003; Machulda et al. 1998; Mittenberg et al. 1992; Sawchyn et al. 2000; Trahan et al. 2001; Wong et al. 1994)
- Outpatients seen for psychological treatment (Fox et al. 1995)
- Outpatients with minor medical problems (Lees-Haley and Brown 1993)
- Personal injury litigants (Dunn et al. 1995; Lees-Haley and Brown 1993)
- Post-traumatic stress disorder (Foa et al. 1997)
- Orthopedic injuries (Mickeviciene et al. 2004)
- Chronic pain (Gasquoine 2000; Iverson and McCracken 1997; Radanov et al. 1992; Smith-Seemiller et al. 2003)
- Whiplash (Sullivan et al. 2002)

Differential Diagnoses and Comorbities

When considering a diagnosis of post-concussion syndrome, it is imperative for clinicians to systematically evaluate and eliminate the possible contribution of many differential diagnoses, co-morbidities, and social-psychological factors that may *cause or maintain* self-reported symptoms after MTBI. Common clinical conditions include traumatic cervical injuries due to whiplash-associated disorders; chronic pain, particularly headache and neck pain; depression; and the anxiety spectrum disorders (including post-traumatic stress disorder). Patients with these conditions often report physical, cognitive, and psychological symptoms (e.g., dizziness, fatigue, headaches, poor balance, cognitive diminishment) that are similar to post-concussion-like symptoms. Each of these conditions might co-occur with an MTBI or they might occur independently from a MTBI. If they co-occur, the challenge is trying to determine if the person recovered from the MTBI and the ongoing symptoms and problems reported are more likely to relate to one of the co-morbid conditions.

Factors Relating to the Perception and Reporting of Symptoms

The perception and reporting of symptoms long after an MTBI can be influenced by a diverse range of psychological and social-psychological factors. These factors may include: a person's psychological history, emotional response to injury, coping mechanisms, and psychosocial environment (e.g., work and family).

Personality Characteristics and Disorders

Personality characteristics influence how people respond to illness, injury, or disease. Kay and colleagues (1992) proposed three personality factors that may influence the development and maintenance of symptoms following MTBI, as described below.

- *Differences in individual response style to trauma.* Some individuals tend to over-emphasize cognitive and physical symptoms, whereas others tend to de-emphasize them. A certain symptom might be overwhelming for one person, yet another person may see this same symptom as simply slightly annoying. These differences are not just determined by personality variables, but also by the life circumstances that challenge the person's ability to cope with that symptom.
- *Differences in the emotional significance of an event.* As noted by Kay and colleagues: "for some persons the actual injury, the feelings evoked, and the response – or lack thereof – from others can trigger old, unresolved emotional issues. Often this takes the form of being vulnerable and unprotected, of not being responded to when hurt or sick, or of not being able to gain retribution when one has been wronged. Persons who grew up with significant holes in their emotional nurturing appear more at risk for responding in catastrophic ways to the emotional meaning of the injury" (p. 379–380) (Kay et al. 1992).
- *Vulnerable personality styles.* Five different personality traits have been proposed as being vulnerable to poor outcome following MTBI. These include: (1) over-achievement, (2) dependency, (3) insecurity, (4) grandiosity, and (5) borderline personality characteristics (not disorder). The pre-injury and post-injury prevalence rates of these personality traits in patients with TBI have been found to be higher compared to community-dwelling adults (Evered et al. 2003; Greiffenstein and Baker 2001; Hibbard et al. 2000). Although poorly understood, there is little doubt that personality characteristics influence the development and maintenance of the post-concussion syndrome.

Expectation as Etiology

Expectation as etiology is a term coined by Mittenberg and colleagues (1992) who proposed that for some people the presence of PCS symptoms following MTBI may be due to "the anticipation, widely held by individuals who have had no opportunity to observe or experience post-concussive symptoms, that PCS will occur following mild head injury (p. 202)." Following an injury, a patient may "reattribute benign emotional, physiological, and memory symptoms to their head injury" (p. 203) and disregard or inaccurately recall their pre-injury symptom experience. For example, an individual may attribute an isolated incident of not remembering where he parked the car in a large parking garage post-accident to the injury rather than due to normal forgetfulness or inattention to one's surroundings (Gunstad and Suhr 2001). Other researchers have reported similar, although not identical, results (Ferguson et al. 1999; Gunstad and Suhr 2001). Gunstad and Suhr (2001) emphasized the importance of appreciating a more generalized expectation of negative outcome regardless of the event (e.g., accident, injury, illness, or disease), consistent with the "nocebo effect." The nocebo effect is the causation of sickness by the expectations of sickness and by associated emotional states. That is, the sickness is, essentially, caused by expectation of sickness (Hahn 1997).

"Good Old Days" Bias

The tendency to view oneself as healthier in the past and underestimate past problems is referred to as the "good old days" bias. In some studies, patients with back injuries, general trauma victims, as well as patients who have sustained MTBIs, appear to over-estimate the actual degree of change that has taken place post injury by retrospectively recalling fewer pre-injury symptoms than the base rate of symptoms in healthy adults (Davis 2002; Gunstad and Suhr 2001, 2004; Hilsabeck et al. 1998; Mittenberg et al. 1992). This bias is further complicated involvement in personal injury litigation. Researchers have reported that litigants tend to exhibit a *response bias* in symptom recall compared to non-litigants. That is, personal injury litigants without a history of head trauma, compared to non-litigants, tend to report better past levels of functioning in life in general, self-esteem, concentration, and memory; and fewer symptoms of depression, anxiety, irritability, and fatigue than general medical patients (e.g., Lees-Haley et al. 1996; Lees-Haley et al. 1997). This response bias, combined with an expectation of certain symptoms following MTBI, can have a potent impact on symptom reporting.

Stereotype Threat and Diagnosis Threat

Social psychology researchers have been interested in the concept of *stereotype threat* for many years to help explain performance differences between certain groups (e.g., Aronson et al. 1999; Croizet and Claire 1998; Levy 1996; Leyens et al. 2000; Spencer et al. 1999; Steele 1997; Steele and Aronson 1995; Walsh et al. 1999). The concept proposes that the threat of an inferior and/or negative stereotype can negatively affect an individual's performance on a particular task (Steele and

Aronson 1995; Suhr and Gunstad 2005). For example, Asian-Americans perform better than Caucasians in mathematics, or men perform better than women at using a map to navigate.

Suhr and Gunstad (2002) adopted this concept and applied it to the neuropsychological literature by proposing the concept of *diagnosis threat*. These authors hypothesized that in people with a past MTBI, "calling attention to a personal history of head injury and its potential effects on cognition might lead to worse cognitive performance than that seen in individuals with similar head injury history, but who do not have attention called to either the head injury history or the possible consequences of head injury" (p. 450). In two studies, Suhr and Gunstad 2002, 2005 found that participants who were provided with information highlighting the expected cognitive deficits associated with a mild brain injury (i.e., the diagnosis threat condition) performed worse on measures of intellectual ability, memory, attention/working memory, and psychomotor speed compared to participants in the neutral condition. Quite remarkably, the psychological effect of "diagnosis threat" has a large, adverse effect on neuropsychological test performance (Table 24.1).

Table 24.1 Social psychological factors relating to the post-concussion syndrome

Attributions/misattributions: Arise from the strong human need to "explain" things. In regards to symptoms, a person might misattribute normal or expected emotional, physiological, or memory problems to a remote MTBI when the actual cause is something else.

Diagnosis threat: Applied to MTBI, it is the tendency for individuals to perform worse on neuropsychological testing when attention is called to their history of mild brain injury and the potential negative effects mild brain injuries might have on cognition. That is, people told they are being tested to look for problems relating to a remote MTBI actually perform more poorly than those tested following neutral instructions.

Expectation as etiology: In regards to MTBI, some people might anticipate or expect to have certain symptoms for a long period of time. This might cause them to misattribute future normal, everyday symptoms to the remote injury – or fail to appreciate the relation between more proximal factors (e.g., life stress, poor sleep, and mild depression) and their symptoms.

"Good Old Days" bias: The tendency to view oneself as healthier and higher functioning in the past, and to under-estimate past problems.

Iatrogenesis: A state of ill health or adverse effect caused by medical treatment. For example, diagnosing "brain damage" as an explanation for persistent problems seen long after a concussion can be iatrogenic. Telling her she has brain damage and she will need to cope and compensate, when in fact the probability of permanent brain damage was very low and the probability of an anxiety disorder and sleep disturbance was high, can be iatrogenic. It can also, of course, result in failure to provide the most effective treatment.

Nocebo effect: Causation of sickness by the expectations of sickness and by associated emotional factors. That is, the sickness is, essentially, caused by the *expectation* of sickness.

Assessment Methodology: Interview Versus Questionnaire

When evaluating someone long after an MTBI, two clinicians evaluating the same patient, in close proximity, can easily come to different conclusions. Different symptoms can be documented. Different conditions can be diagnosed. There are many reasons for this, including expertise, "focus" (e.g., neurological versus mental health), context (e.g., brief medical appointment with general physician, psychiatric consultation, or forensic evaluation), and methodology (i.e., how information is gathered). Checklists and questionnaires are widely used to document post-concussion symptoms. They can be a rapid and efficient method for collecting information. One concern, however, is that the use of these measures might lead to the over-endorsement of symptoms and problems.

Iverson et al. (2010) compared spontaneous, interview-based, post-concussion symptom reporting to endorsement of symptoms on a questionnaire in a sample of patients deemed temporarily disabled from work due to an MTBI. The sample consisted of 61 patients consecutively referred for an intake assessment or neuropsychological evaluation over a 27-month period (mean age = 40.3 years, SD = 12.5; mean education = 12.5 years, SD = 1.9; 57% male; 95% Caucasian). All patients were receiving financial compensation through the Worker's Compensation system (mean = 2.3 months post-injury, SD = 1.6, range = 0.8–8.1 months).

The patients were initially asked during a clinical interview to identify the symptoms and problems they had been experiencing over the past couple of weeks. Patients were encouraged to provide a comprehensive list of symptoms and problems during the interview. Patients then completed the British Columbia Postconcussion Symptom Inventory (BC-PSI). The BC-PSI is a 16-item measure designed to assess the presence and severity of post-concussion symptoms. The test was based on ICD-10 criteria for Postconcussional Syndrome.

During the clinical interview, patients spontaneously endorsed an average of 3.3 symptoms (SD = 1.9). However, when given the questionnaire to complete, they endorsed the presence of 9.1 symptoms on average [SD = 3.2; paired samples t test, t (60) = 13.423, $p < .001$]. In addition, 44.4% of the patients reported four or more symptoms during the interview, whereas 91.8% of the patients endorsed four or more symptoms on the questionnaire ($\chi^2 = 45.022$, $p < .001$). It was common for patients to endorse symptoms as *moderate or severe* on the BC-PSI, despite *not* spontaneously reporting those symptoms during the interview.

To our knowledge, only two other studies have compared the influence of interview method on symptom reporting following MTBI. Nolin et al. (2006) compared symptoms endorsed spontaneously versus using an interview-based checklist of symptoms in 108 patients, 12–36 months post-MTBI. Participants reported a significantly greater number of symptoms when responding to a list of symptoms. In addition, there was little similarity in the symptoms reported using each method. Similarly, Gerber and Schraa (1995) compared volunteered versus elicited symptoms in 22 patients in the first 6 months following MTBI. Participants consistently reported a higher number of somatic, cognitive, emotional, and pain related symptoms when elicited using a symptom checklist compared to volunteered recall.

There are multiple reasons why patients report far more symptoms on a questionnaire than during the interview. For example, the questionnaire (1) might remind the patient of a symptom, or (2) encourage the patient to report a symptom that he or she did not think was of interest to the clinician. Moreover, some patients are not very good at articulating their symptoms and problems during an interview, and anxiety or simply feeling rushed or uncomfortable might exacerbate that problem. There are also several reasons, however, to question the validity of questionnaire results. For example, clinicians need to be aware of the possibility of (1) non-specific symptom endorsement (e.g., symptoms due to other causes), (2) symptom exaggeration and over-endorsement (especially in the context of a compensation-related evaluation), (3) symptom expectations influencing symptom endorsement, and (4) the nocebo effect. Moreover, patients periodically do not understand the meaning of a symptom, do not ask for clarification, and simply endorse it. It is also fairly common for patients to report past symptoms as if they are current symptoms (i.e., not properly considering the timeframe of the questionnaire).

Exaggerated Symptoms and Poor Effort on Testing

Patients involved in compensation-related evaluations, long after sustaining an MTBI, have external incentives for providing poor effort during testing or exaggerated symptoms and problems. Without due consideration of these factors, clinicians and researchers may misattribute a poor performance on testing to an underlying deficit when, in fact, the individual has simply failed to give adequate effort. In 2005, the National Academy of Neuropsychology published a position paper on the need for symptom validity assessment in neuropsychological practice (Bush et al. 2005). This position paper solidifies the recommendation for routine effort and validity testing made by clinical researchers for many years (e.g., Doss et al. 1999, p. 17; Green et al. 2001, p. 1,059; Greve et al. 2003, p. 179; Iverson and Binder 2000, p. 853; Iverson and Franzen 1996, p. 38; Mateer 2000, p.54; Millis et al. 1998, p. 172; Sweet 1999, p.278). Specific guidelines for identifying malingering in a neuropsychological evaluation have been available for several years (Slick et al. 1999).

It is important to appreciate poor effort during testing and exaggeration of symptoms are separate behavioral constructs. Poor effort on testing may or may not occur with obvious exaggeration of symptoms and problems, and vice versa (Boone et al. 1995; Larrabee 2003; Rohling et al. 2002; Sumanti et al. 2006; Temple et al. 2003). We prefer using the terms *poor effort* for describing under-performing on neuropsychological tests, and *exaggeration* for describing over-reported symptoms. These terms are simple, descriptive, and communicative. However, under the circumstances where there is equivocal evidence for their presence, the terms "reduced effort" or "variable effort" may be more appropriate (see also Chap. 18 for more details on malingering and factitious disorder).

Clinicians should be encouraged to conceptualize poor effort, exaggeration, and malingering not in simplistic dichotomous terms, but through probabilistic considerations. Effort is a state, not a trait. Effort is a spectrum of behavior, not simply a dichotomous construct. A continuum for conceptualizing effort is as follows: definite poor effort, very likely poor effort, probable poor effort, adequate or good effort, very good effort, and exceptional effort. The accuracy of symptom reporting also falls on a continuum: under-endorsement, accurate reporting, possible exaggeration, probable exaggeration, definite exaggeration. A person's reporting of symptoms and problems can move along this continuum during an evaluation and over time, from evaluation to evaluation. It would be a mistake to conclude that a person provided good effort on the basis of performing normally on a single effort test. Conclusions about level of effort should be based on several sources of converging evidence, not a single test score.

Rule of thumb: Symptom exaggeration or lack of effort

- Symptom exaggeration is not synonymous with lack of effort
  - Symptom exaggeration refers to fabricating or over-reporting symptoms
  - Poor effort describes behavior in which insufficient effort was put forth on testing
- Symptom exaggeration and poor effort are not all or nothing constructs or behaviors; they can vary over time and reflect a continuum of behaviors

---

Post-Concussion Syndrome in Children

Compared to the adult literature, research specifically examining clusters of symptoms following mild TBI in children is limited (Ayr et al. 2009; Mittenberg et al. 1997); literature focusing on behavioral problems is more common (see Satz et al. 1997 for a review) (See also Chap. 25, this volume). Researchers have reported the presence of greater symptoms in children following mild TBI compared to both healthy (Yeates et al. 1999) and orthopaedic controls (Ayr et al. 2009; Farmer et al. 1987; Mittenberg et al. 1997; Ponsford et al. 1999) in the first 3 months following injury. One study found no differences in symptoms in children who sustained an uncomplicated mild TBI, compared to orthopaedic controls, 1 week following injury (Nacajauskaite et al. 2006). On average, symptoms in children tend to largely resolve within 2–3 months (Carroll et al. 2004; Farmer et al. 1987; Kirkwood et al. 2008; Necajauskaite et al. 2005; Ponsford et al. 1999). However, some researchers have reported that a substantial minority (9–17%) continue to have ongoing problems after 3 months (Ayr et al. 2009; Ponsford et al. 1999). In a recent longitudinal study, although parental and child (self) reported somatic symptoms were resolved after 3 months, parental reported cognitive symptoms persisted until 12 months (Taylor et al. 2010). The number of PCS symptoms appears to be related to some injury severity characteristics (Hawley et al. 2002; McKinlay et al. 2002; Mittenberg et al. 1997; Taylor et al. 2010; Yeates et al. 2009), though this is not true for all children (Yeates et al. 2009) or supported by all studies (Ponsford et al. 1999). For example, in one study, acute symptoms were not associated with MRI abnormalities (Taylor et al. 2010).

Many researchers have heavily criticized the literature in this area suggesting a variety of methodological limitations preclude us from understanding the true nature and recovery trajectory in children (Ponsford et al. 1999; Satz et al. 1997; Yeates and Taylor 2005; Yeates et al. 2009). Some of these problems include: (1) imprecise or inconsistent definitions of mild TBI, (2) absence of appropriate comparison groups, (3) reliance on parent reports of symptoms rather than child reports, and (4) lack of longitudinal studies that provide insight into the natural recovery trajectory.

In an effort to rectify some of these methodological shortcomings, Yeates and colleagues (Fay et al. 2010; Taylor et al. 2010; Yeates et al. 2009) conducted a sophisticated prospective longitudinal study that compared the 12-month recovery trajectory of symptoms in 186 children and adolescents who had sustained a mild TBI (uncomplicated and complicated MTBI) and 99 who sustained mild orthopedic injuries (OI). Parental reported post-concussion symptoms were obtained within 3 weeks, and at 1, 3, and 12 months post-injury. Yeates et al. (2009) found that, within 3 weeks post-injury, 24% of the MTBI group reported, on average, 7 to 10 new PCS symptoms (relative to premorbid levels) compared to 6% of orthopedic controls. At 12 months, 9% of the MTBI group reported, on average, four new PCS symptoms compared to 1% of orthopedic controls. These authors identified four distinct recovery trajectories that were characterized as follows: (1) "No PCS" (64% MTBI, 79% OI) – 1.5 new symptoms[1] reported within the first 3 weeks, and 0.5 new symptoms reported at 1, 3 and 12 months post-injury, (2) "Moderate Persistent PCS" (12% MTBI, 15% OI) – four new symptoms reported with 3 weeks post-injury, and at 1, 3 and 12 months, (3) "High Acute/Resolved PCS" (15% MTBI, 5% OI) – seven new symptoms reported within 3 weeks post-injury, followed by a reduction of symptoms at 1 month (three new symptoms), and resolution of the majority of new symptoms by 3 and 12 months (one new symptom), and (4) "High Acute/Persistent PCS" (9% MTBI, 1% OI) – ten new symptoms reported within 3 weeks post-injury, followed by a slight reduction of symptoms at 1 (seven symptoms) and 3 months (six symptoms), followed by a further reduction of symptoms at 12 months (four symptoms).

As in adults, understanding the true nature and recovery trajectory of PCS in children is complicated by the influence of many potential non-injury factors on PCS reporting (e.g., non-specificity of symptoms, comorbidities, social-psychological factors, etc.). It is reasonable to suggest some of the non-injury factors that can affect symptom reporting in adults may have a similar effect on parent- or patient-reported PCS symptoms. Unfortunately, in children, there is little research that have directly evaluated the influence of non-injury factors on symptom reporting (Yeates and Taylor 2005). Some research have suggested PCS symptoms are influenced by a child's cognitive reserve capacity, gender, family socioeconomic status, and age at injury (Fay et al., 2010). Other research examining behavioral problems reported post injury have found behavioral problems may, in part, reflect a confluence of variables, including: (1) premorbid difficulties, (2) the effects of injury more

---

[1]The number of new symptoms reported here reflect the mean of the group. It is reasonable to suggest that many persons in these groups reported a higher or lower number of symptoms. In addition, these data were extracted from Fig. 1 in Yeates et al. 2009. These data are approximate only and have been rounded

generally, (3) specific fears and expectations associated with cerebral trauma, (4) premorbid vulnerability, (5) changes in brain function, and (6) post-injury child and family adjustment (Ganesalingam et al. 2008; Kirkwood et al. 2008; Yeates et al. 2009). As in adults, the differential diagnosis of PCS in children is complex.

Is the Post-Concussion Syndrome Caused by Brain Damage?

The post-concussion syndrome has been extraordinarily controversial for 100 years, because clinicians and researchers have sought simplistic, usually binary, explanations for what causes and maintains the symptoms. Can a person sustain a complicated mild or moderate traumatic brain injury, have permanent measurable neurocognitive deficits that interfere with his life, and experience ongoing subjective symptoms such as cognitive difficulties, low frustration tolerance, fatigue, and balance problems? Of course. Would this person, then, meet criteria for having a post-concussion syndrome? Yes. Would the etiology of the syndrome be damage to the brain? Maybe. As described in this chapter, there are numerous factors that affect how a person perceives and reports post-concussion and post-concussion-like symptoms. In this example, the etiology of the patient's subjectively-experienced symptoms could be depression. Thus, he might not meet criteria for the syndrome – especially if treatment for depression led to resolution of most of the symptoms. In contrast, can a person who is injured, with no obvious concussion or an extremely mild injury, report a constellation of symptoms and problems at 1-year post-accident that appear to be consistent with a post-concussion syndrome? Of course. Is the etiology of the "syndrome" brain damage? No. In this circumstance, numerous factors could be driving the symptom reporting including depression, anxiety, life stress, chronic pain, chronic sleep problems, personality characteristics, misattribution, litigation stress and exaggeration, or even malingering. Thus, we face a fundamental diagnostic accuracy problem – we cannot assume that the widely cited estimates of 5–15% of people having residual symptoms from a mild TBI are accurate. This is because (1) the research methodology in the prospective studies does not allow confident causal inferences, and (2) the diagnostic logic is simply based on remote temporal association. Having symptoms long after an injury does not mean that the injury is the cause of the symptoms. The proximate cause of current symptoms is much more likely, statistically, to be current problems (e.g., depression, anxiety, insomnia, pain, and life stress) than a remote injury. However, having current problems cannot, logically, allow one to completely rule out the possibility that the person has true residual symptoms.

Conclusions

The etiology, pathophysiology, definition, or diagnostic criteria for the post-concussion syndrome have not been universally agreed upon. Obviously, therefore, the syndrome continues to be highly controversial and poorly understood. Following an MTBI, it is clear that most people experience a constellation of symptoms such as headaches, subjective dizziness, fatigue, sleep disturbance, difficulty thinking (e.g., concentration or memory), and/or emotional changes (e.g., irritability). This is well established in the literature. Of course, not everyone experiences all symptoms, or symptoms to the same degree, but a core set of symptoms is commonly experienced.

The post-concussion syndrome is assumed by many to be a direct and/or indirect consequence of an injury to the head or brain. This is very likely to be the case when a person is acutely injured (e.g., the first 2 weeks post-injury). However, when considering long-term outcome, it is important to appreciate that a mild injury to the head or brain is not necessary (and often not sufficient) to produce the constellation of symptoms and problems that comprise this syndrome. The symptoms and problems typically conceptualized as comprising the post-concussion syndrome are non-specific; they can follow a mild injury to the brain or they can arise from other conditions, singly or in combination, such as chronic headaches, chronic bodily pain, depression, or post-traumatic stress disorder. These symptoms are also common in healthy, community-dwelling adults. Symptom reporting can be influenced by psychological distress, social psychological factors (e.g., the nocebo effect, iatrogenesis, and misattributions), and personality characteristics (e.g., pre-injury personality traits). Symptom reporting can also be influence by the methodology in which information is obtained. Patients tend to report far more symptoms when using a questionnaire or symptom checklist compared to spontaneous, interview-based symptom reporting. Of course, patients involved in compensation-related evaluations, long after sustaining an MTBI, have external incentives for providing poor effort during testing or exaggerated symptoms and problems. These factors need to be evaluated carefully.

If the post-concussion syndrome is diagnosed, it should not be assumed, uncritically, that the problems are predominately related to traumatically-induced cellular damage. Traumatically-induced cellular damage, with resulting cognitive and psychological dysfunction, might be a partial causal factor in some patients. However, experienced clinicians who work with this patient population know that the only reasonable perspective is biopsychosocial. The post-concussion syndrome should be considered a diagnosis of exclusion. The clinician should carefully study the history and progression of the symptoms and problems, and systematically attempt to rule out the most obvious differential diagnoses or competing explanations for the symptoms. Once identified, the differential diagnosis should be treated. If no obvious differential diagnosis can be identified and treated, then the clinician should attempt to conceptualize the person's symptoms and problems broadly and descriptively. Then, treatment (psychological and pharmacological) can be implemented that targets the breadth and depth of factors that might be causing and maintaining a person's symptom reporting and problems in daily life.

References

Alves, W., Macciocchi, S. N., & Barth, J. T. (1993). Postconcussive symptoms after uncomplicated mild head injury. *The Journal of Head Trauma Rehabilitation, 8*, 48–59.

American Psychiatric Association. (1994). *Diagnostic and statistical manual of mental disorders* (4th ed.). Washington, DC: American Psychiatric Association.

Aronson, J., Lustina, M. J., & Good, C. (1999). When white men can't do math: Necessary and sufficient factors in stereotype threat. *Journal of Experimental Social Psychology, 35*(1), 29–46.

Ayr, L. K., Yeates, K. O., Taylor, H. G., & Browne, M. (2009). Dimensions of postconcussive symptoms in children with mild traumatic brain injuries. *Journal of the International Neuropsychological Society, 15*(1), 19–30.

Bigler, E. D. (2008). Neuropsychology and clinical neuroscience of persistent post-concussive syndrome. *Journal of the International Neuropsychological Society, 14*(1), 1–22.

Bijur, P. E., Haslum, M., & Golding, J. (1990). Cognitive and behavioral sequelae of mild head injury in children. *Pediatrics, 86*(3), 337–344.

Binder, L. M. (1986). Persisting symptoms after mild head injury: a review of the postconcussive syndrome. *Journal of Clinical and Experimental Neuropsychology, 8*(4), 323–346.

Binder, L. M., & Rohling, M. L. (1996). Money matters: A meta-analytic review of the effects of financial incentives on recovery after closed-head injury. *The American Journal of Psychiatry, 153*(1), 7–10.

Boake, C., McCauley, S. R., Levin, H. S., Contant, C. F., Song, J. X., Brown, S. A., et al. (2004). Limited agreement between criteria-based diagnoses of postconcussional syndrome. *The Journal of Neuropsychiatry and Clinical Neurosciences, 16*(4), 493–499.

Boone, K. B., Savodnik, I., Ghaffarian, S., Lee, A., Freeman, D., & Berman, N. G. (1995). Rey 15-item memorization and Dot counting scores in a "stress" claim worker's compensation population: Relationship to personality (MCMI) scores. *Journal of Clinical Psychology, 51*(3), 457–463.

Brown, S. J., Fann, J. R., & Grant, I. (1994). Postconcussional disorder: Time to acknowledge a common source of neurobehavioral morbidity. *The Journal of Neuropsychiatry and Clinical Neurosciences, 6*(1), 15–22.

Bush, S. S., Ruff, R. M., Troster, A. I., Barth, J. T., Koffler, S. P., Pliskin, N. H., et al. (2005). Symptom validity assessment: Practice issues and medical necessity NAN policy & planning committee. *Archives of Clinical Neuropsychology, 20*(4), 419–426.

Carroll, L. J., Cassidy, J. D., Peloso, P. M., Borg, J., von Holst, H., Holm, L., et al. (2004). Prognosis for mild traumatic brain injury: Results of the WHO Collaborating Centre Task Force on Mild Traumatic Brain Injury. *Journal of Rehabilitation Medicine, 43*(Suppl), 84–105.

Cicerone, K. D., & Kalmar, K. (1995). Persistent postconcussion syndrome: The structure of subjective complaints after mild traumatic brain injury. *The Journal of Head Trauma Rehabilitation, 10*, 1–7.

Cook, J. B. (1972). The post-concussional syndrome and factors influencing recovery after minor head injury admitted to hospital. *Scandinavian Journal of Rehabilitation Medicine, 4*(1), 27–30.

Croizet, J. C., & Claire, T. (1998). Extending the concept of stereotype and threat to social class: The intellectual underperformance of students from low socioeconomic backgrounds. *Personality and Social Psychology Bulletin, 24*(6), 588–594.

Davis, C. H. (2002). Self-perception in mild traumatic brain injury. *American Journal of Physical Medicine & Rehabilitation, 81*(8), 609–621.

Doss, R. C., Chelune, G. J., & Naugle, R. I. (1999). Victoria symptom validity test: Compensation-seeking vs. non-compensation-seeking patients in a general clinical setting. *Journal of Forensic Neuropsychology, 1*(4), 5–20.

Dunn, J. T., Lees-Haley, P. R., Brown, R. S., Williams, C. W., & English, L. T. (1995). Neurotoxic complaint base rates of personal injury claimants: Implications for neuropsychological assessment. *Journal of Clinical Psychology, 51*(4), 577–584.

Evered, L., Ruff, R., Baldo, J., & Isomura, A. (2003). Emotional risk factors and postconcussional disorder. *Assessment, 10*(4), 420–427.

Farmer, M. Y., Singer, H. S., Mellits, E. D., Hall, D., & Charney, E. (1987). Neurobehavioral sequelae of minor head injuries in children. *Pediatric Neuroscience, 13*(6), 304–308.

Fay, T. B., Yeates, K. O., Taylor, H. G., Bangert, B., Dietrich, A., Nuss, K. E., et al. (2010). Cognitive reserve as a moderator of postconcussive symptoms in children with complicated and uncomplicated mild traumatic brain injury. *Journal of International Neuropsychological Society., 16*(1), 94–105.

Ferguson, R. J., Mittenberg, W., Barone, D. F., & Schneider, B. (1999). Postconcussion syndrome following sports-related head injury: Expectation as etiology. *Neuropsychology, 13*(4), 582–589.

Foa, E. B., Cashman, L., Jaycox, L., & Perry, K. (1997). The validation of a self-report measure of posttraumatic stress disorder: The posttraumatic diagnostic scale. *Psychological Assessment, 9*(4), 445–451.

Fox, D. D., Lees-Haley, P. R., Ernest, K., & Dolezal-Wood, S. (1995). Post-concussive symptoms: Base rates and etiology in psychiatric patients. *The Clinical Neuropsychologist, 9*, 89–92.

Ganesalingam, K., Yeates, K. O., Ginn, M. S., Taylor, H. G., Dietrich, A., Nuss, K., et al. (2008). Family burden and parental distress following mild traumatic brain injury in children and its relationship to post-concussive symptoms. *Journal of Pediatric Psychology, 33*(6), 621–629.

Gasquoine, P. G. (2000). Postconcussional symptoms in chronic back pain. *Applied Neuropsychology, 7*(2), 83–89.

Gerber, D. J., & Schraa, J. C. (1995). Mild traumatic brain injury: Searching for the syndrome. *The Journal of Head Trauma Rehabilitation, 10*(4), 28–40.

Gouvier, W. D., Uddo-Crane, M., & Brown, L. M. (1988). Base rates of post-concussional symptoms. *Archives of Clinical Neuropsychology, 3*, 273–278.

Green, P., Rohling, M. L., Lees-Haley, P. R., & Allen, L. M., 3rd. (2001). Effort has a greater effect on test scores than severe brain injury in compensation claimants. *Brain Injury, 15*(12), 1045–1060.

Greiffenstein, F. M., & Baker, J. W. (2001). Comparison of premorbid and postinjury mmpi-2 profiles in late postconcussion claimants. *The Clinical Neuropsychologist, 15*(2), 162–170.

Greve, K. W., Bianchini, K. J., Mathias, C. W., Houston, R. J., & Crouch, J. A. (2003). Detecting malingered performance on the Wechsler Adult Intelligence Scale. Validation of Mittenberg's approach in traumatic brain injury. *Archives of Clinical Neuropsychology, 18*(3), 245–260.

Gunstad, J., & Suhr, J. A. (2001). "Expectation as etiology" versus "the good old days": Postconcussion syndrome symptom reporting in athletes, headache sufferers, and depressed individuals. *Journal of the International Neuropsychological Society, 7*(3), 323–333.

Gunstad, J., & Suhr, J. A. (2004). Cognitive factors in postconcussion syndrome symptom report. *Archives of Clinical Neuropsychology, 19*(3), 391–405.

Hahn, R. A. (1997). The nocebo phenomenon: Concept, evidence, and implications for public health. *Preventive Medicine, 26*(5 Pt 1), 607–611.

Hawley, C. A., Ward, A. B., Magnay, A. R., & Long, J. (2002). Children's brain injury: A postal follow-up of 525 children from one health region in the UK. *Brain Injury, 16*(11), 969–985.

Heilbronner, R. L. (1993). Factors associated with postconcussion syndrome: Neurological, psychological, or legal? *Trial Diplomacy Journal, 16*, 161–167.

Hibbard, M. R., Bogdany, J., Uysal, S., Kepler, K., Silver, J. M., Gordon, W. A., et al. (2000). Axis II psychopathology in individuals with traumatic brain injury. *Brain Injury, 14*(1), 45–61.

Hilsabeck, R. C., Gouvier, W. D., & Bolter, J. F. (1998). Reconstructive memory bias in recall of neuropsychological symptomatology. *Journal of Clinical and Experimental Neuropsychology, 20*(3), 328–338.

Iverson, G. L. (2005). Outcome from mild traumatic brain injury. *Current Opinion in Psychiatry, 18*, 301–317.

Iverson, G. L., & Binder, L. M. (2000). Detecting exaggeration and malingering in neuropsychological assessment. *The Journal of Head Trauma Rehabilitation, 15*(2), 829–858.

Iverson, G. L., & Franzen, M. D. (1996). Using multiple objective memory procedures to detect simulated malingering. *Journal of Clinical and Experimental Neuropsychology, 18*(1), 38–51.

Iverson, G. L., & Lange, R. T. (2003). Examination of "Postconcussion-Like" symptoms in a healthy sample. *Applied Neuropsychology, 10*(3), 137–144.

Iverson, G. L., & McCracken, L. M. (1997). 'Postconcussive' symptoms in persons with chronic pain. *Brain Injury, 11*(11), 783–790.

Iverson, G. L., Brooks, B. L., Ashton, V. L., & Lange, R. T. (2010). Interview versus questionnaire symptom reporting in people with post-concussion syndrome. *Journal of Head Trauma Rehabilitation, 25*(1), 23–30.

Kay, T., Newman, B., Cavallo, M., Ezrachi, O., & Resnick, M. (1992). Toward and neuropsychological model of functional disability after mild traumatic brain injury. *Neuropsychology, 6*(4), 371–384.

Kirkwood, M. W., Yeates, K. O., Taylor, H. G., Randolph, C., McCrea, M., & Anderson, V. A. (2008). Management of pediatric mild traumatic brain injury: A neuropsychological review from injury through recovery. *The Clinical Neuropsychologist, 22*(5), 769–800.

Larrabee, G. J. (1997). Neuropsychological outcome, post concussion symptoms, and forensic considerations in mild closed head trauma. *Seminars in Clinical Neuropsychiatry, 2*(3), 196–206.

Larrabee, G. J. (2003). Exaggerated MMPI-2 symptom report in personal injury litigants with malingered neurocognitive deficit. *Archives of Clinical Neuropsychology, 18*(6), 673–686.

Lees-Haley, P. R., & Brown, R. S. (1993). Neuropsychological complaint base rates of 170 personal injury claimants. *Archives of Clinical Neuropsychology, 8*(3), 203–209.

Lees-Haley, P. R., Williams, C. W., & English, L. T. (1996). Response bias in self-reported history of plaintiffs compared with nonlitigating patients. *Psychological Reports, 79*(3 Pt 1), 811–818.

Lees-Haley, P. R., Williams, C. W., Zasler, N. D., Marguilies, S., English, L. T., & Stevens, K. B. (1997). Response bias in plaintiffs' histories. *Brain Injury, 11*(11), 791–799.

Lees-Haley, P. R., Fox, D. D., & Courtney, J. C. (2001). A comparison of complaints by mild brain injury claimants and other claimants describing subjective experiences immediately following their injury. *Archives of Clinical Neuropsychology, 16*(7), 689–695.

Levy, B. (1996). Improving memory in old age through implicit self-stereotyping. *Journal of Personality and Social Psychology, 71*(6), 1092–1107.

Leyens, J. P., Desert, M., & Croizet, J. C. (2000). Stereotype treat: Are lower status and history of stigmatization preconditions of stereotype threat? *Personality and Social Psychology Bulletin, 26*(10), 1189–1199.

Lishman, W. A. (1986). Physiogenisis and psychogenisis in the 'post-concussional syndrome'. *The British Journal of Psychiatry, 153*, 460–469.

Machulda, M. M., Bergquist, T. F., Ito, V., & Chew, S. (1998). Relationship between stress, coping, and post concussion symptoms in a healthy adult population. *Archives of Clinical Neuropsychology, 13*, 415–424.

Mateer, C. A. (2000). Assessment issues. In S. A. Raskin & C. A. Mateer (Eds.), *Neuropsychological management of mild traumatic brain injury*. New York: Oxford University Press.

McCauley, S. R., Boake, C., Pedroza, C., Brown, S. A., Levin, H. S., Goodman, H. S., et al. (2005). Postconcussional disorder: Are the DSM-IV criteria an improvement over the ICD-10? *The Journal of Nervous and Mental Disease, 193*(8), 540–550.

McKinlay, A., Dalrymple-Alford, J. C., Horwood, L. J., & Fergusson, D. M. (2002). Long term psychosocial outcomes after mild head injury in early childhood. *Journal of Neurology, Neurosurgery and Psychiatry, 73*(3), 281–288.

Mickeviciene, D., Schrader, H., Nestvold, K., Surkiene, D., Kunickas, R., Stovner, L. J., et al. (2002). A controlled historical cohort study on the post-concussion syndrome. *European Journal of Neurology, 9*(6), 581–587.

Mickeviciene, D., Schrader, H., Obelieniene, D., Surkiene, D., Kunickas, R., Stovner, L. J., et al. (2004). A controlled prospective inception cohort study on the post-concussion syndrome outside the medicolegal context. *European Journal of Neurology, 11*(6), 411–419.

Miller, H. (1961). Accident neurosis. *British Medical Journal, 1*, 919–925. 992-998.

Millis, S. R., Ross, S. R., & Ricker, J. H. (1998). Detection of incomplete effort on the Wechsler Adult Intelligence Scale-Revised: A cross-validation. *Journal of Clinical and Experimental Neuropsychology, 20*(2), 167–173.

Mittenberg, W., & Strauman, S. (2000). Diagnosis of mild head injury and the postconcussion syndrome. *The Journal of Head Trauma Rehabilitation, 15*(2), 783–791.

Mittenberg, W., DiGiulio, D. V., Perrin, S., & Bass, A. E. (1992). Symptoms following mild head injury: Expectation as aetiology. *Journal of Neurology, Neurosurgery and Psychiatry, 55*, 200–204.

Mittenberg, W., Wittner, M. S., & Miller, L. J. (1997). Postconcussion syndrome occurs in children. *Neuropsychology, 11*(3), 447–452.

Nacajauskaite, O., Endziniene, M., Jureniene, K., & Schrader, H. (2006). The validity of postconcussion syndrome in children: A controlled historical cohort study. *Brain & Development, 28*(8), 507–514.

Necajauskaite, O., Endziniene, M., & Jureniene, K. (2005). The prevalence, course and clinical features of post-concussion syndrome in children. *Medicina (Kaunas), 41*(6), 457–464.

Nolin, P., Villemure, R., & Heroux, L. (2006). Determining long-term symptoms following mild traumatic brain injury: Method of interview affects self-report. *Brain Injury, 20*(11), 1147–1154.

Paniak, C., Reynolds, S., Toller-Lobe, G., Melnyk, A., Nagy, J., & Schmidt, D. (2002). A longitudinal study of the relationship between financial compensation and symptoms after treated mild traumatic brain injury. *Journal of Clinical and Experimental Neuropsychology, 24*(2), 187–193.

Ponsford, J., Willmott, C., Rothwell, A., Cameron, P., Ayton, G., Nelms, R., et al. (1999). Cognitive and behavioral outcome following mild traumatic head injury in children. *The Journal of Head Trauma Rehabilitation, 14*(4), 360–372.

Radanov, B. P., Dvorak, J., & Valach, L. (1992). Cognitive deficits in patients after soft tissue injury of the cervical spine. *Spine, 17*(2), 127–131.

Reynolds, S., Paniak, C., Toller-Lobe, G., & Nagy, J. (2003). A longitudinal study of compensation-seeking and return to work in a treated mild traumatic brain injury sample. *The Journal of Head Trauma Rehabilitation, 18*(2), 139–147.

Rohling, M. L., Allen, L. M., & Green, P. (2002). Who is exaggerating cognitive impairment and who is not? *CNS Spectrums, 7*(5), 387–395.

Rutherford, W. H., Merrett, J. D., & McDonald, J. R. (1979). Symptoms at one year following concussion from minor head injuries. *Injury, 10*(3), 225–230.

Ryan, L. M., & Warden, D. L. (2003). Post concussion syndrome. *International Review of Psychiatry, 15*(4), 310–316.

Satz, P., Zaucha, K., McCleary, C., Light, R., Asarnow, R., & Becker, D. (1997). Mild head injury in children and adolescents: A review of studies (1970-1995). *Psychological Bulletin, 122*(2), 107–131.

Satz, P. S., Alfano, M. S., Light, R. F., Morgenstern, H. F., Zaucha, K. F., Asarnow, R. F., et al. (1999). Persistent post-concussive syndrome: A proposed methodology and literature review to determine the effects, if any, of mild head and other bodily injury. *Journal of Clinical and Experimental Neuropsychology, 21*(5), 620–628.

Sawchyn, J. M., Brulot, M. M., & Strauss, E. (2000). Note on the use of the postconcussion syndrome checklist. *Archives of Clinical Neuropsychology, 15*, 1–8.

Slick, D., Sherman, E. M., & Iverson, G. L. (1999). Diagnostic criteria for malingered neurocognitive dysfunction: Proposed standards for clinical practice and research. *The Clinical Neuropsychologist, 13*(4), 545–561.

Smith-Seemiller, L., Fow, N. R., Kant, R., & Franzen, M. D. (2003). Presence of post-concussion syndrome symptoms in patients with chronic pain vs mild traumatic brain injury. *Brain Injury, 17*(3), 199–206.

Spencer, S. J., Steele, C. M., & Quinn, D. M. (1999). Stereotype threat and women's math performance. *Journal of Experimental Social Psychology, 35*(1), 4–28.

Steele, C. M. (1997). A threat in the air. How stereotypes shape intellectual identity and performance. *The American Psychologist, 52*(6), 613–629.

Steele, C. M., & Aronson, J. (1995). Stereotype threat and the intellectual test performance of African Americans. *Journal of Personality and Social Psychology, 69*(5), 797–811.

Suhr, J. A., & Gunstad, J. (2002). "Diagnosis Threat": The effect of negative expectations on cognitive performance in head injury. *Journal of Clinical and Experimental Neuropsychology, 24*(4), 448–457.

Suhr, J. A., & Gunstad, J. (2005). Further exploration of the effect of "diagnosis threat" on cognitive performance in individuals with mild head injury. *Journal of the International Neuropsychological Society, 11*(1), 23–29.

Sullivan, M. J., Hall, E., Bartolacci, R., Sullivan, M. E., & Adams, H. (2002). Perceived cognitive deficits, emotional distress and disability following whiplash injury. *Pain Research & Management, 7*(3), 120–126.

Sumanti, M., Boone, K. B., Savodnik, I., & Gorsuch, R. (2006). Noncredible psychiatric and cognitive symptoms in a workers' compensation "stress" claim sample. *The Clinical Neuropsychologist, 20*(4), 754–765.

Sweet, J. J. (1999). Malingering: Differential diagnosis. In J. J. Sweet (Ed.), *Forensic neuropsychology: Fundamentals and practice*. Lisse: Swets & Zeitlinger.

Taylor, A. G., Dietrich, A., Nuss, K. E., Wright, M., Rusin, J., Bangert, B., et al. (2010). Post-concussive symptoms in children with mild traumatic brain injury. *Neuropsychology, 24*(2), 148–159.

Temple, R. O., McBride, A. M., David Horner, M. D., & Taylor, R. M. (2003). Personality characteristics of patients showing suboptimal cognitive effort. *The Clinical Neuropsychologist, 17*(3), 402–409.

Trahan, D. E., Ross, C. E., & Trahan, S. L. (2001). Relationships among postconcussional-type symptoms, depression, and anxiety in neurologically normal young adults and victims of brain injury. *Archives of Clinical Neuropsychology, 16*, 435–445.

Walsh, M., Hickey, C., & Duffy, J. (1999). Influence of item content and stereotype situation on gender differences in mathematical problem solving. *Sex Roles, 41*(3–4), 219–240.

Wong, J. L., Regennitter, R. P., & Barrios, F. (1994). Base rate and simulated symptoms of mild head injury among normals. *Archives of Clinical Neuropsychology, 9*, 411–425.

World Health Organization. (1992). *International statistical classification of diseases and related health problems* – (10th ed.). Geneva, Switzerland: World Health Organization.

Yeates, K. O., & Taylor, H. G. (2005). Neurobehavioural outcomes of mild head injury in children and adolescents. *Pediatric Rehabilitation, 8*(1), 5–16.

Yeates, K. O., Luria, J., Bartkowski, H., Rusin, J., Martin, L., & Bigler, E. D. (1999). Postconcussive symptoms in children with mild closed head injuries. *The Journal of Head Trauma Rehabilitation, 14*(4), 337–350.

Yeates, K. O., Taylor, H. G., Rusin, J., Bangert, B., Dietrich, A., Nuss, K., et al. (2009). Longitudinal trajectories of postconcussive symptoms in children with mild traumatic brain injuries and their relationship to acute clinical status. *Pediatrics, 123*(3), 735–743.

Youngjohn, J. R., Burrows, L., & Erdal, K. (1995). Brain damage or compensation neurosis? The controversial post-concussion syndrome. *The Clinical Neuropsychologist, 9*, 112–123.

Chapter 25
Pediatric Traumatic Brain Injury (TBI): Overview

Cathy Catroppa and Vicki A. Anderson

Abstract The aim of this chapter is to provide an overview of the: (1) prevalence of pediatric TBI; (2) the symptoms associated with pediatric TBI; (3) outcomes and predictors of pediatric TBI; and (4) rehabilitation in this area.

> **Key Points and Chapter Summary**
>
> - The most common type of TBI in children and adolescents is a closed head injury.
> - Pediatric traumatic brain injury (TBI) can result in long-term cognitive and behavioral difficulties, particularly for those sustaining more severe injuries.
> - Neuropsychological testing is important in identifying residual deficits and assisting in designing rehabilitation and educational programs to address deficits.
> - More research is needed to assist in identifying children in need and evaluating intervention effectiveness.

Definition and Prevalence of Pediatric TBI

TBI is a major cause of mortality and disability worldwide, and is associated with a three-fold increase in cognitive, behavioral, social and vocational difficulties (National Paediatric Trauma Registry 1993). While there is difficulty in establishing an accurate

C. Catroppa (✉)
Australian Centre for Child Neuropsychology Studies,
Murdoch Children's Research Institute, Melbourne, Australia
and
Department of Psychology, Royal Children's Hospital,
Flemington Road, Parkville, Melbourne, Victoria, 3052, Australia
and
University of Melbourne, Melbourne, Australia
e-mail: cathy.catroppa@mcri.edu.au

M.R. Schoenberg and J.G. Scott (eds.), *The Little Black Book of Neuropsychology: A Syndrome-Based Approach*, DOI 10.1007/978-0-387-76978-3_25,
© Springer Science+Business Media, LLC 2011

measure of the incidence of pediatric traumatic brain injury (TBI), some rough estimates have been made within particular community settings (Crowe et al. 2009; Goldstein and Levin 1987). Incidence of TBI based on hospital admissions has been reported at between 100 and 300 per 100,000 per year for children and young adults (Cassidy et al. 2004).

The most common type of TBI in children and adolescents is a closed head injury (Davis and Vogel 1995). Specifically, closed head injuries (CHI) lead to brain damage because of the initial compression of the head against an object and also because of the resultant acceleration–deceleration movement of the brain contents inside the skull (see also Chaps. 3 and 21–24, this volume). That is, the brain can move forward, backward and side-to-side (a rotational effect) sequentially and/or simultaneously within the skull. Acceleration and deceleration effects can lead to damage to the brain as it impacts on the bony surface of the skull, both at the site of impact (coup) and opposite to the point of impact (contrecoup). The acceleration and deceleration effects can also stretch and damage nerve axons and blood vessels, contributing to diffuse axonal injury (Fennell and Mickle 1992; Levin and Kraus 1994).

Primary brain injury is due to mechanical damage that occurs at the time of injury as a result of contact between brain matter and the interior skull, and this includes lacerations (tears in brain tissue usually related to depressed skull fractures) and contusions (bruising or microscopic hemorrhages), and these usually occur at the sight of impact or at contrecoup areas. The occurrence of a skull fracture, whether open or closed, can contribute to additional variables affecting the brain, including laceration, hemorrhage, and/or infection of the bone, meninges, brain parenchyma and/or CSF. Internal rotational and velocity forces can also lead to tearing and stretching of axons within white matter (Goldstein and Powers 1994). Following the primary injury, secondary effects, such as hypoxia, hemorrhages, seizures, and edema may also occur. Edema, the rapid diffuse cerebral swelling that is due to increased fluid secondary to trauma, and/or intracranial hemorrhages can exacerbate the damage to brain function related to the primary injury, but can also lead to additional damage to brain parenchyma and further compromise recovery. The brain, cerebrospinal fluid, cerebral blood and extracellular fluid, are all within the skull, and an increase in any one of these areas, (e.g., collection of blood not normally found inside the child's head) will result in raised intracranial pressure (ICP) (Amacher 1988; Chorazy 1985; Fennell and Mickle 1992; Hynd and Willis 1988). Brain damage, related to neuronal apoptosis and/ or degeneration of synapses and/or axons and/or associated neuronal glia result from a complex neurochemical process. The neurochemical processes involve glutamate,

---

Rule of thumb: Pediatric TBI mechanisms of brain damage

- The most common type of TBI in children is a closed head injury.
- Primary brain injury is due to mechanical damage that occurs at the time of injury as a result of contact between brain matter and the interior skull.
- Brain injury may also result from secondary factors such as hypoxia, seizures, edema, ICP and neurochemical changes – it is these factors that medical staff treat in order to minimize/prevent further brain injury.

aspirate, and excitatory amino acids, which are found at elevated levels following TBI, and disrupt cell function (Yeates 1999) (see Chap. 23, this volume for more detail).

Symptoms of TBI

Review of Symptoms of Mild TBI

Mild TBI is most prevalent in the 5–14 age range (Asarnow et al. 1995). Up to half these injuries go unreported, or unrecognised, and are lost to follow-up (Elson and Ward 1994; Evans 1992), making study of "representative" samples difficult. In the weeks post-injury, a number of physical symptoms may occur, including fatigue, headache, drowsiness, irritability, labile mood, dizziness, and nausea and emesis. Research suggests these physical, psychological and cognitive symptoms resolve by 3–6 months post-injury (Alves 1992). However, there is some agreement that there is a group, both children and adults, who continue to experience such symptoms, and go on to develop psychological and cognitive problems including anxiety, irritability and depression, reduced speed of information processing and executive control, and difficulties with memory and attention (Asanow et al. 1991; Klonoff and Lamb 1996; Miller 1996). This has led to the inclusion of a subdivision of mild TBI into; (1) mild TBI, and (2) mild complicated TBI. Mild complicated TBI is distinguished from mild TBI by the presence of subtle structural brain abnormalities and the possibility of neurochemical effects (Roberts et al. 1995; Yeates 1999). Dikman et al. (1995) observed that injuries at the more "severe" extreme of the mild TBI spectrum are more likely to be associated with these persisting post-concussional symptoms, pointing to the heterogeneity within the mild TBI classification (see also Chap. 24 for additional details of post-consussion syndrome). Additional features of mild TBI can include worsening grades (academic performance), social withdraw, and reduced rate of skill development, particularly among children who experience symptoms of mild TBI for longer periods of time, which can limit his/her interaction with their environment, and so may lead to poor skill acquisition and progress in educational and social domains (Anderson et al. 2001a).

Review of Symptoms of Moderate-Severe TBI

Moderate-severe TBI is often associated with loss of consciousness (LOC), post-traumatic amnesia (PTA), and/or focal or diffuse neurological signs. Many symptoms described above associated with mild TBI, such as irritability, headache, fatigue, vision problems, dizziness, etc., occur following moderate to severe TBI. Brain imaging will often identify abnormalities associated with damage to the brain. Consciousness, and the ability to respond appropriately to the environment, depend on the functioning of the centers in the ascending reticular formation and on the level of communication between these centers and the cerebral cortex. Early assessment of the level of consciousness is essential, as it gives an indication of

Table 25.1 Glasgow coma scale (GCS) (Adapted from Teasdale and Jennett 1974)

Category:	Description:	Score:
Eye opening	Spontaneous	4
	To command	3
	To pain	2
	Nil	1
Motor response	Obeys commands	6
	Localizes pain	5
	Normal flexion	4
	Abnormal flexion	3
	Extension	2
	Nil	1
Verbal response	Oriented	5
	Disoriented	4
	Words only	3
	Sounds only	2
	Nil	1
Behavioral response[a]	Smiles, oriented to sound, follows objects	5
	Consolable crying, inappropriate interactions	4
	Inconsistently consolable, moaning	3
	Inconsolable, restless, and irritable	2
	No response	1

[a]Behavioral response replaces verbal response for children of pre-school age and below

how the initial brain injury is impacting brain function (Miller 1991). The Glasgow Coma Scale (GCS); Teasdale and Jennett 1974), is a widely used measure of responsiveness/consciousness. The GCS assesses three aspects of behavior – eye opening, motor responses and verbal responses (see Table 25.1). When using the GCS, the duration of coma (length of time the GCS is less than or equal to eight) is calculated by serial observations (usually 4-hourly), and consists of the time span in which there is no eye opening, an inability to obey commands and the absence of comprehensible speech.

The duration of post-traumatic amnesia (PTA) has also been argued to be a useful measure of the severity of diffuse brain damage (Rutter et al. 1983). After the recovery of consciousness, there may follow a period of time during which recent events are not recalled reliably or accurately. The PTA period refers to a post-injury period of confusion and memory loss, after regaining consciousness, during which the patient is disoriented and unable to register day-to-day information, with older memories relatively resistant to cerebral insult. Therefore, PTA is usually measured up to the point where memory for everyday ongoing events is continuous and reliable. Duration can be measured somewhat reliably as long as PTA lasts for an hour or more (High et al. 1989).

The presence of neurological signs is an indicator of a moderate-severe TBI. Such neurological signs, as reported in research conducted by our research group (Catroppa and Anderson 2003), may include children with differing degrees of hemiparesis-weakness on one side of the body, poor motor control, post-injury

Table 25.2 Symptoms/categorization of childhood TBI (Based/adapted from Begali 1992; Goldstein and Levin 1992; Yeates 1999)

	Mild TBI	Mild-complicated	Moderate TBI	Severe TBI
GCS	13–15	13–15	9–12	8 or less
LOC	<1 hour	<1 hour	1–24 hours	>24 hours
PTA	<24 hours	<24 hours	1–7 days	>7 days
Neurological signs	No	Yes[a]	Yes[a]	Yes[a]
Abnormal imaging	No	Yes[a]	Yes[a]	Yes[a]

[a]May be present

seizures and hearing loss. Additionally, children with a moderate-severe TBI often have abnormalities revealed by imaging techniques. Often, skull fractures (linear and/or depressed) can be seen on an x-ray; however, such fractures are now identified by computed tomography (CT). CT scans are sensitive to the identification of acute intracranial blood products (e.g., subdural and epidural hematomas), and raised intracranial pressure (ICP) (Begali 1987; Miller 1991). Magnetic resonance imaging (MRI) is sensitive to post-acute, acute and chronic effects of brain injury, including very small lesions (as small as several millimetres can be identified), degenerative processes (involving white matter, parenchyma), old blood products, and specific white matter lesions. Advances to the understanding for the gradations in brain injury and distinctions between different forms of diffuse brain damage have increasingly become evident with advances in neuroimaging (Wilson et al. 1988). It bears repeating, however, that neuropsychological studies are the only objective method to measure the effects of TBI on behaviour. Table 25.2 provides a summary of symptoms used to classify (and distinguish between) mild, moderate and severe TBI.

> **Rule of thumb: Indicators of severity of injury**
>
> - Glasgow Coma Scale (GCS).
> - Period of LOC.
> - Length of PTA.
> - Neurological signs.
> - Positive findings on imaging

Differences Between Pediatric TBI and Adult TBI

As seen above, while we are obtaining much information on the consequences of pediatric TBI, long-term outcome remains an active area of research. Indeed, some aspects of recovery from TBI that are generally accepted for adults are less clear in children and adolescents. Like adults, residual physical, cognitive, and psychological/psychiatric problems can occur in children/adolescents. Likewise, problems in educational/vocational and social areas have been reported (Engberg and Teesdale 2004; Hoffien et al. 2001). However, unlike TBI in adults, the developmental level of the child and the child's family and psychosocial support base are of extreme importance with regard to long-term outcome from TBI (Anderson et al. 2001b; Taylor and Alden 1997; Taylor et al. 2002; Taylor et al. 2001). It has been argued that the developing brain is particularly vulnerable to brain trauma (Anderson et al. 2001b; Anderson and Moore 1995), where skills not developed at the time of injury may be at most risk (Dennis 1989). Injuries sustained during childhood are more likely to result in generalized brain pathology, therefore derailing normal developmental processes.

The traditional view in which neurodevelopmental processes and brain plasticity can allow for recovery of cognitive, behavioral, adaptive, and physical functioning among children with TBI has shown to be more true for patients with focal injuries than for patients with diffuse brain injury, particularly for patients with severe diffuse brain injury. While intra- or inter-hemispheric functional neuroanatomical reorganization has shown to account for recovery of previously attained (and/or develop new) cognitive functions following more focal neurological injuries (e.g., Ewing-Cobbs et al. 2003) recovery of function is less pronounced among patients with diffuse brain injuries (Ewing-Cobbs et al. 2003). Like adults, recovery of cognitive functions or skills requires increased recruitment of brain areas, and may result in reduced efficiency.

Clinicians involved in care for children and/or adolescents who are suspected of mild TBI should consider that there can be several important variables that can affect the report of (and outcome from) TBI in children and adolescents that may differ from adults. First, children may be more reticent to report symptoms of mild TBI and/or have trouble expressing these symptoms in a coherent way to parents/clinician. Second, research has suggested that resolution of symptoms following mild TBI in children takes longer than time for adults to be asymptomic. In addition, children whom have suffered a mild TBI are at increased risk for worse academic performance and emotional/behavioral changes that may adversely affect a child's/adolescent's family/friend social support network. Fourth, several demographic variables have been shown to significantly affect recovery from TBI among children, Such factors include age at the time of injury, family support, access to educational accommodation, and appropriate intervention for psychological or psychosocial difficulties post TBI.

Neuropsychological Assessment of Pediatric TBI

What to Do?

Obtain a comprehensive pre-and post-injury history from the family. This gives qualitative information that is difficult to obtain elsewhere and often gives the clinician an insight into the dynamics of the family situation. This information also assists in the choice of assessment battery, frequently giving focus to the areas of difficulty both for the child and family. During this time, the family is also able to ask the clinician questions about TBI, the assessment, recovery issues, and what to expect in the long term. At this time, the child is also able to become acquainted with the clinician, and therefore more comfortable,

Once the assessment is underway, it is important to ensure the child is comfortable in the testing situation and is able to work to the best of their ability. In order to maintain the child's self-esteem, it is beneficial if the child is aware that test items are often easy at first, but then increase in difficulty, with different expectations for different ages (e.g., "some items were developed for kids about your age while others were designed for both younger and older kids."). Children should be aware that it is not expected they be able to answer every question correctly, however, the clinician should encourage the child to perform at his/her best on all items administered. Thus, we advocate the clinician plan the assessment to have breaks (time when no paper and pencil testing is administered, although assessment of gait, coordination, jumping, strength, etc. can be observed and assessed during these breaks) to reduce fatigue, promote motivation, and maintain rapport with the examiner. This is especially true for younger children. As each child is unique, the number and duration of breaks will vary. For some young children, a break of up to 30 minutes is adequate, and they will often have a drink or something to eat. Older children may benefit from several short 10–15 minutes breaks. Alternatively, some children with various neurological, psychiatric, and/or systematic medical diseases may fatigue more quickly or become very anxious, and more frequent breaks of longer duration may be required.

For children with severe impairment, it may be impossible to rely on formal, standardized assessment methods. In such instances, other techniques such as contextual observation (clinic, home, school) and parent and teacher ratings can be used. This can involve the clinician observing the child at home and/or school, and observing how the child interacts and/or behaves in certain settings. The assessment may also be partly based on parental information, where the child's parents are asked to complete questionnaires based on their child's functioning in areas of interest to the clinician (e.g., cognitive or social skills). Furthermore, regular review is important up to 12 months post-injury, and then at key transitional periods, such as school entry or completing primary school and entering secondary school.

Rule of thumb: Assessment in pediatric TBI

- Develop and maintain good rapport (child should be at ease)
- Monitor the child/adolescent for fatigue and/or anxiety/frustration.
- Allow for breaks (suspension of the assessment/testing) during the evaluation
- Test in rooms that minimize distractions, are well lit.

What Not to Do

It is important that when a child is assessed during the acute stage post-TBI that the child is not in PTA. Once the child is no longer in PTA, then a neuropsychological assessment can be arranged. Assessment completed acutely (within days to weeks of the injury) will not, in all likelihood, reflect static (fixed) level of deficits (if any), and change over time, particularly in the first several months from the time of injury, should be expected. Depending upon the severity of the injury, neuropsychological assessment during the acute phase should be tailored to the referral questions and the individual child. Such an assessment is not likely to be lengthy, and may initially be limited to acute bedside assessment. The neuropsychologist should incorporate recommendations above to not test when the child is unable to participate in the assessment (i.e., too distracted, fatigued, irritable). Neuropsychological assessment using psychometric instruments may be postponed if the neuropsychologist believes reliable data could not be obtained. For example, a child with a moderate to severe TBI may be highly distractable post-acutely, and may not be able to sit and attend for a required period of time to administer psychometric-based attention/executive measures.

If a child becomes distressed during the assessment, we advocate the assessment should stop, and to take a break (stop administering psychometric-based tests). As mentioned above, a break of up to 30 minutes is preferable, but at times a longer break may be required. In our experience, most children like to re-unite with their parents during the break, and some may go for a short walk and/or have something to eat or drink. It is important to try and determine the cause of the distress and attempt to make the child comfortable again. Once the child is ready to continue with the assessment, then the session may continue. On rare occasions, if the child is still distressed/anxious after a break, the assessment may be rescheduled for another day. Indeed, it is not uncommon to have more than one office visit initially scheduled for the neuropsychological evaluation to reduce testing demands on the child on any 1 day.

Proposed Neuropsychological Assessment Protocol (Clinical/Research:)

Clinical

The clinician will decide on an assessment battery taking into account: (1) the referral question(s); (2) the child's areas of difficulty as well as the child's age; and, in some situations, (3) questions or concerns of the child's primary caregiver(s). Referral may be from various sources including a neurologist, a neurosurgeon, a general practitioner, a teacher or the parents. The purpose of the referral can often differ depending on the referring party. Common purposes for referral include the identification and description of neuropsychological deficits (and preserved functions) following TBI to assist with diagnosis and rehabilitative efforts (and/or academic programming). Assessments may indicate whether specific skills (e.g., writing, reading, memory, attention) have been 'damaged' due the injury. Such evaluations are useful in guiding interventions in academic and behavioral management treatments. It is not uncommon for the referral question(s) of a physician to differ from questions of a parent, but often it is possible to address questions of both parties with careful consideration of the assessment procedures. Questions about return to normal activities following mild TBI in particular are not uncommon along with questions about school placement, need for special education services, and/or develop speech/cognitive therapy to develop rehabilitation programming. Frequently, in the case of mild TBI, it is our experience that most referrals are generated due to the child/adolescent exhibiting (or complaining of) residual problems or having an unexpected slow recovery from the injury. Difficulties in school are often reported among children and adolescents having residual cognitive deficits from TBI.

When planning the assessment, it is essential the referral question has been addressed (e.g., identify cognitive deficits, assist in developing rehabilitation programming, and/or aide in school re-integration). We generally encourage the clinical assessment to incorporate a measure of general cognitive functioning (i.e., intellectual functioning) along with assessment of attention/executive, memory/learning, language, visuoperceptual/visuoconstructional skills, and an assessment of mood/affect. After evaluation of common neuropsychological domains (and identifying areas of strengths and weakness), the clinician can assess for specific processes or skills which are dysfunctional and contribute to the child's weakness area(s). We also undertake a qualitative assessment of the child's behavior, for example, whether the child is fidgeting, affectively labile, anxious/depressed, apathetic/withdrawn/abulic, etc. Qualitative information provides assessment of brain–behavior relationships not easily measured by currently available psychometric instruments (e.g., orbitofrontal dysfunction), but also guides interpretation of obtained psychometric data based on the degree these variables affected performances on tests. Finally, qualitative information can provide essential information to guide the implementation of treatment programs across a variety of settings.

Research

A neuropsychological assessment protocol for research purposes will be determined by the hypothesis(es) of the study. An example of a research protocol investigating executive functions among adolescents/young adults whom had sustained a head injury between the ages of 7 and 12 years is presented in Table 25.3. When conducting research in our laboratory, feedback is provided to the family and child, and this is often in the form of a neuropsychological report. When required, and with consent from the family, a child may be referred to other clinicians for further assessment or intervention. Again, with consent from the family, the researcher may liaise with the child's school and provide information regarding the child's needs.

Table 25.3 Example of a research based assessment protocol

Assessment protocol:	Publisher:
WISC-III or WAIS-III	Wechsler, D. (1991). *Manual for the Wechsler intelligence scale for children – 3rd Edition (WISC-III)*. San Antonio, TX: The Psychological Corporation.
	Wechsler, D. (1997). *Wechsler adult intelligence scale – third edition manual*. San Antonio: Psychological Corporation.
Rey-Osterrieth complex figure	Rey, A. L'examine psychologique dans les cas d'encephalopathie traumatique (Psychological examination of traumatic encephalopathy). *Archives de Psychologie*.1941; 28:286–290.
Contingency naming test	Taylor, G.H., Schatsneider, C., & Rich, D. (1992). Sequelae of Haemophilus Influenzae meningitis: Implications for the study of brain disease and development. In M.G. Tramontana & S.R. Hooper (Eds.), *Advances in child neuropsychology: Volume 1* (pp.50–108). New York: Springer.
Delis Kaplan executive function system	Delis, D. C., Kaplan, E., & Kramer, J. (2001). *Delis Kaplan executive function system*. San Antonio, TX: The Psychological Corporation.
Questionnaires:	
Behavior rating inventory of executive function	Gioia, G. A., Isquith, P. K., Guy, S. C., & Kenworthy, L. (2000). *Behavior rating inventory of executive function*. Odessa, FL: Psychological Assessment Resources.
Modified Sydney psychosocial reintegration scale	Tate, R. L., Hodgkinson, A., Veerabangsa, A., & Maggiotto, S. (1999). Measuring psychosocial recovery after traumatic brain injury: Psychometric properties of a new scale. *The Journal of Head Trauma Rehabilitation, 14*, 543–557.

Outcome and Recovery from TBI

Mild TBI Outcome

Outcome from mild head injury in children, which comprises up to 90% of all pediatric TBI (Kraus et al. 1986), is not well defined. Some argue mild TBI in children/adolescents is associated with either no detectable sequelae or full recovery (Asarnow et al. 1995; Levin et al. 1987; Papero et al. 1993; Ponsford et al. 1999), while others report significant, ongoing problems (Asarnow et al. 1991; Gronwall et al. 1997). Although there is little empirical support, the cognitive and/or behavioral deficits observed for children within the first few weeks to months of mild TBI is often ascribed to post-concussional syndrome. The more contemporary description of mild-complicated TBI may lead to greater clarity, allowing differentiation of children with greater deficits.

Cognitive aspects of post-concussional syndrome, and mild TBI, when identified in children (and also for adults), include deficits in speed of information processing, memory, and attention/executive control functions (Klonoff and Lamb 1996; Miller 1996; Stablum et al. 1996) (see also Chap. 24 for more details of post concussive syndrome). However, there is little agreement regarding the presence of persisting deficits following mild TBI or the pattern of recovery. Thus, the study of mild TBI in children is made more problematic due to the lack of consensus as to how to operationalize the concept of mild TBI. Within the pediatric TBI literature, mild TBI has been subdivided into mild and mild-complicated TBI (Roberts et al. 1995; Yeates 1999).

Moderate-Severe TBI Outcome

Studies of outcome and recovery from TBI based on pre-school children and school-aged children have identified both acutely, as well as persisting impairments, though the recovery of these skills may differ depending on severity and age at injury (Anderson and Moore 1995). Deficits have been reported at one time point, or longitudinally, in many areas including attentional capacity (Catroppa and Anderson 2005; Catroppa et al. 2007; Fenwick and Anderson 1999; Kaufmann et al. 1993), memory and learning (Anderson and Catroppa 2007; Levin et al. 2004), psychomotor skills (Bawden et al. 1985), linguistic abilities (Brookshire et al. 2000; Catroppa and Anderson 2004), executive functions (Anderson and Catroppa 2005; Gioia and Isquith 2004; Nadebaum et al. 2007); social competence (Muscara et al. 2008), functional skills (Anderson et al. 2005; Catroppa et al. 2008), educational ability (Barnes et al. 1999; Catroppa and Anderson 2007; Hawley 2004), and vocational outcome (Hoofien et al. 2001). Refer to Table 25.4 for a summary of common consequences post-pediatric TBI.

Children that suffer a moderate-severe TBI often exhibit deficits in neuropsychological, behavioral and social areas of functioning. Findings from our laboratory (Anderson et al. 2005, 2006) give an indication of the possible recovery of skills in these areas over time. Figures 25.1, 25.2, and 25.3 show recovery in the areas of intellectual, adaptive, educational skills and memory, for a pediatric group with TBI (injured between the ages of 1–7 years). These data illustrate the vulnerability of children injured at this young age, with the severe TBI injury group generally performing below the level of the control children and those with a mild and also moderate TBI. Figure 25.4 was included to demonstrate the possible impact of age at injury on full-scale intellectual ability (FSIQ), where those with a severe injury perform poorer when compared to children with mild or moderate injuries, regardless of age at injury. However, children sustaining an injury earlier

Table 25.4 Common consequences of childhood traumatic brain injury (From Anderson and Catroppa 2006)

Domain	Specific skills
Neurological impairment	Gross and fine-motor incoordination
	Cranial nerve function/sensory loss
	Speech: e.g., dysarthria, aphasia
	Medical complications: e.g., epilepsy, hydrocephalus
Cognitive impairment	Intellectual impairment
	Attention
	Memory and learning
	Executive function
	Speed of processing
Educational impairment	Reduced progress in content related areas: e.g., reading, mathematics,
	Processing/retention difficulties: e.g., attention, processing speed, memory
	Writing difficulties
	Need for specialist educational placement or support
Emotional/ behavioral	Adjustment difficulties: e.g., reduced self-esteem
	Psychiatric disorders: e.g., depression, anxiety, post-traumatic stress
	Regulatory dysfunction: disinhibition, impulsivity, apathy, reduced insight
Social consequences	Social withdrawal and isolation
	Social anxiety
	In appropriate social skills, reduced social awareness
Lifestyle change	Reduced independence
	Impaired functional communication and mobility
	Increased need for additional assistance
	Reduced recreational options
	Difficulties maintaining pre-injury relationships

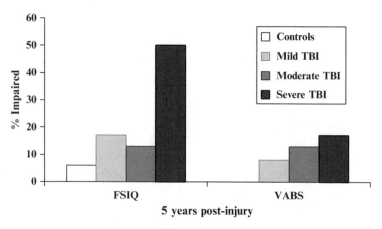

Fig. 25.1 Percentage impaired for full scale intellectual quotient (*FSIQ*) and adaptive functioning (*VABS*) at 5 years post-injury for children injured between 1 and 7 years of age

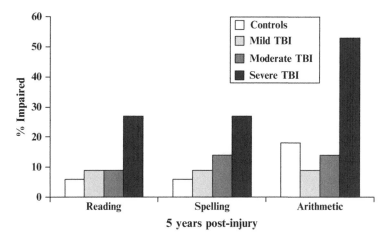

Fig. 25.2 Percentage impaired for educational skills at 5 years post-injury for children injured between 1 and 7 years of age

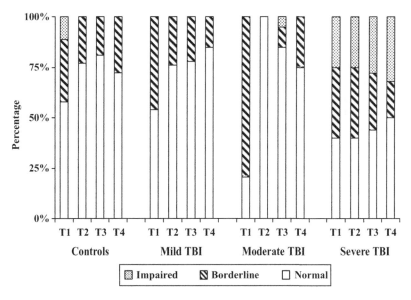

Fig. 25.3 Percentage of children with normal, borderline and impaired memory (acute-18 months post-TBI) for children injured between 1 and 7 years of age: T1=acute, T2=6 month, T3=12 Month, and T4 =18 month

in life tend to exhibit poorer outcome, with younger children whom sustain a severe TBI exhibiting the least recovery (poorest outcome) (Figures adapted from Anderson et al. 2005, 2006).

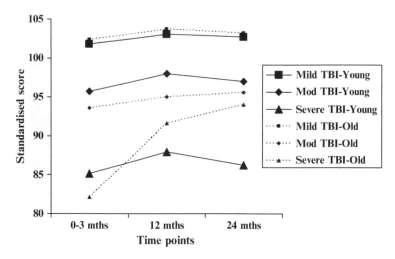

Fig. 25.4 Recovery trajectory for full scale intellectual quotient (FSIQ) for children injured between 1 and 7 years of ages (TBI-young) and between 8 and 12 years of age (TBI-old)

Variables Affecting Outcome and Recovery

Injury severity (as indicated by the GCS, length of PTA, neurological signs – including seizures and epilepsy, abnormalities seen on imaging) has been identified as a reliable predictor of impairment in physical, cognitive and educational domains, with more severe TBI related to greater problems across all age groups (Catroppa and Anderson 1999; Davies et al. 1996; Ewing-Cobbs et al. 2003; Fletcher et al. 1990; Kinsella et al. 1997). However, behavioral outcome may be better predicted by environmental factors, such as socioeconomic status (SES) and family functioning, and these have been argued to contribute significantly to long-term behavioral outcome (Anderson et al. 2001b; Rivara et al. 1994; Yeates et al. 2004). Lower levels of education and SES have been associated with poorer outcome (Coster et al. 1994), while presence of good family cohesion/support to better outcome (Rivara et al. 1994). A combination of severe injury and social disadvantage have been found to be particularly detrimental to recovery following early brain insult (Breslau 1990; Taylor et al. 1995).

Premorbid factors (Anderson et al. 2001b; Schwartz et al. 2003) also contribute to long-term outcome. Ponsford and colleagues (1999), in a longitudinal study of school-aged children sustaining mild TBI, found a clear relationship between pre-injury learning and behavioral problems post-injury. Psychiatric problems may increase post-injury for children where such problems were present pre-injury (Brown et al. 1981; Rutter et al. 1983), with current research interested in areas such as depression and anxiety, and showing that adults that sustained an injury in childhood appear vulnerable to psychiatric problems (Anderson et al. in press). A further potential predictor of poor outcome following child TBI is younger age, or developmental level, at the time of injury (Anderson and Moore 1995).

Furthermore, structural factors may influence the nature of injuries sustained by very young children as they possess a relatively larger head supported by a smaller neck compared to older children and adults, placing them at greater risk for diffuse injuries (Amacher 1988). Thus, damage or disruption may have implications for future skill acquisition, within both cognitive and behavioral domains. From a functional perspective, young children possess few established skills, and so the younger the age at injury, the fewer mature skills available to the child, with the possibility that future skill acquisition may be compromised (Dennis 1989). Table 25.5 provides a summary of predictors of outcome post-TBI.

Table 25.5 Predictors of outcome from childhood brain injury (From Anderson and Catroppa 2006)

Factors found to contribute to outcome from childhood brain injury
Injury factors
Severity (mild, moderate, severe)
Nature (diffuse, focal)
Disability (post-traumatic epilepsy, neurological signs, physical/speech impairment)
Developmental factors
Age at injury
Developmental stage
Pre-injury factors
Pre-injury child function: cognitive ability, personality
Pre-injury family factors: family function, parent mental health
Gender
Environmental factors
Socio-economic status
Access to resources – educational, rehabilitation

Rule of thumb: Variables affecting outcome from TBI

- Severity of injury
- Younger age at injury
- Social disadvantage
- Pre-injury psychological/psychosocial difficulties

Management and Rehabilitation Issues

It is clear that childhood TBI can have long-term adverse affects on neuropsychological, academic, and behavioral functioning. However, professionals report only small numbers of injured children having access to rehabilitation resources (Cronin 2000; Di Scala and Savage 1997). Research indicates children most "at risk" for poor outcome are those who have: (1) more severe injuries at a younger age (Anderson and Moore 1995); (2) a pre-injury history of developmental or behavioral problems (Ponsford et al. 1997); and/or (3) live in poorer functioning and less

Table 25.6 Phases/models of intervention (Adapted from Catroppa and Anderson 2010)

Phase	Intervention
1. During coma	Sensory stimulation
2. Short-term post injury (e.g., 6 hours)	Hypothermia (e.g., Sahuquillo and Vilalta 2007)
3. Post-coma/PTA	Intervention for difficulties in cognition and behavior.
4. Outpatient therapy	Intervention to assist re-entry into home/school/ community:
	Direct approach
	Behavioral compensation
	Environmental modifications and supports
	Behavioral interventions
	Psycho-educational approaches
	Psychological treatments
	Family-based interventions

advantaged families (Rivara et al. 1994). While children with mild-moderate injuries may also benefit from access to intervention and resources, "at risk" children are the most vulnerable, and therefore, most appropriate for rehabilitation efforts. Thus, we argue different models of intervention post-TBI should be considered. Rehabilitation can be divided according to the goal of the intervention, reflecting either (1) Restitution/Restorative or (2) Substitution/Adaptation. Restitution/restorative rehabilitation focuses on restoring function via re-establishment of impaired functions and/or regaining lost skills (Cicerone and Tupper 1990; Sohlberg and Mateer 1989). Substitution/Adaptation focuses on functional adaptation, where intact abilities are utilized to "re-route" skills that have been disrupted. Table 25.6 provides a summary of phases/models of intervention that have been used to develop and implement intervention programs. Currently, intervention programs for children with TBI are scarce, and much work is needed to develop and pilot such rehabilitation programs (Catroppa and Anderson 2010).

Rule of thumb: Rehabilitation approaches

- Restitution/restorative – procedures and interventions designed to restore function of a previously lost skill or behaviour
- Substitution/adaptation – procedures where intact abilities are used to develop adaptations to perform skills that have been disrupted

---

Academic / Vocational Issues

Interventions focused on psychosocial, behavioral and educational/vocational issues may be implemented following acute inpatient treatment utilizing an outpatient setting. For the child, return to school is frequently a major goal of outpatient rehabilitation (Glang et al. 1997). Prior to school return, a number of issues must be considered (Anderson and Catroppa 2006) including the physical incorporation of adaptive equipment, environmental aspects, and instructional adaptations or accommodations that may be necessary. Physical incorporation of adaptive equipment involves consideration of including wheelchairs, special desks, computers, and/or communication devices. Environmental aspects for return to school includes the provision of extra time for assignments, instruction, and/or taking exams, providing a quiet, well-structured classroom, and/or opportunity for the child to receive increased repetition of material and/or opportunities practice skills and revision of assignments, class work, etc. Instructional aspects to consider in returning to school include inclusion of specific educational programming, individual tuition, and social skills retraining. These modifications should be negotiated prior to school return to allow the transition to be as smooth as possible.

For the adolescent or young adult whom has sustained a TBI, the completion of education and entering the workforce is often a time of significant stress. This process may be supported by: (1) providing training for the individual to prepare curriculum vitae/resume; (2) furnishing training to perform adequately in interviews (e.g., behavioral training in social skills, interview skills, relaxation skills, etc.); and (3) consultation with liaison services where counsellors discuss the individual's needs with potential employers, or conduct site visits to determine any environmental modifications which may be required to enhance the individual's performance (e.g., provide referral to vocational counsellors/therapists).

Behavioral/Psychosocial Issues

As noted above, behavioral and psychosocial variables significantly impact outcome from TBI for children and adolescents. We believe providing parent support to families of children whom have sustained a TBI is essential, and the "Signposts for Building Better Behavior" program (Woods et al. 2007), is a modified cognitive behavioral intervention targeting parents of children with TBI. Originally developed by Hudson et al. (2003), this program relies on training parents to implement behavior change strategies at home (Gavidia-Payne and Hudson 2002; Sanders 1999). We expected that parents of children with TBI would benefit from the adapted program (inclusion of a TBI module), and pilot data (Woods et al. 2007) suggests the intervention is of benefit to both parents and children post-TBI, with parent coping strategies improved and child behavior enhanced. We believe there are several benefits of the program: (1) including the family in the intervention process; (2) teaching the family strategies to deal with behavioral issues, and so empowering family members; (3) increasing coping strategies and self-esteem of the family; (4) enhancing a more-so cohesive and adaptive family environment; and (5) improving child behaviors and child well-being.

Intervention, particularly at times of transition, whether with the child, the family, or including external sources (e.g., counsellor) appears to be of benefit. However, as mentioned earlier, the area of intervention in the TBI area is in its infancy, and there is a need for the development, implementation and evaluation of intervention programs for this population (Catroppa and Anderson 2010).

At a minimum, the neuropsychologist working with children whom have suffered a TBI should be aware that pre-injury child and family characteristics, parental and family variables, children's age at injury, presence of diffuse and/or focal injuries, injury severity, and access to social supports may all affect outcome from TBI. We believe providing information to the child's caregivers about these factors, as well as some basic information about common symptoms in the acute and longer-term phases post-injury, and offering support and encouragement during recovery can foster improved outcome from TBI.

Rule of thumb: Factors that may support recovery from TBI

- Increase parental resources/appreciation of recovery processes
- Assure comorbid injury variables (post-traumatic epilepsy, mood disruption, focal neurologic signs) are being treated
- Rehabilitative efforts can be effective
- Consider physical, environmental, and instructional variables for return to school
- Consider vocational counseling/therapy evaluation to plan for work skill development, particularly for adolescents/young adults completing education

---

Conclusions

This chapter has provided a brief summary of a number of areas associated with pediatric TBI, commencing with the prevalence of the injuries to rehabilitation issues. While much is now known regarding outcomes in this population, there is much research required in the intervention area, in order to help these children and their families to achieve a better quality of life.

References

Alves, W. (1992). Natural history of post-concussive signs and symptoms. Physical Medicine and Rehabilitation. *State of the Arts Reviews, 6,* 21–32.

Amacher, A. L. (1988). *Paediatric head injuries: A handbook.* St Louis: Warren H. Green, Inc.

Anderson, V., & Catroppa, C. (2005). Recovery of executive skills following paediatric traumatic brain injury (TBI): A two year follow-up. *Brain Injury, 19*(6), 459–470.

Anderson, V., & Catroppa, C. (2006). Advances in post-acute rehabilitation after childhood acquired brain injury: A focus on cognitive, behavioural and social domains. *American Journal of Physical Medicine & Rehabilitation, 85*(9), 767–787.

Anderson, V., & Catroppa, C. (2007). Memory outcome at 5 years post childhood traumatic brain injury. *Brain Injury, 21*(13–14), 1399–1409.

Anderson, V., & Moore. (1995). Age at injury as a predictor following pediatric head injury: A longitudinal perspective. *Child Neuropsychology, 1*(3), 187–202.

Anderson, V., Catroppa, C., Morse, S., Haritou, F., & Rosenfeld, J. (2001a). Outcome from mild head injury in young children: A prospective study. *Journal of Clinical and Experimental Neuropsychology, 23*(6), 705–717.

Anderson, V., Catroppa, C., Haritou, F., Morse, S., Pentland, L., Rosenfeld, J., & Starga H, R. (2001b). Predictors of acute child and family outcome following traumatic brain injury in children. *Pediatric Neurosurgery, 34*, 138–148.

Anderson, V., Catroppa, C., Morse, S., Haritou, F., & Rosenfeld, J. (2006). *Outcome following TBI sustained at different stages of childhood.* Boston: Meeting of the International Neuropsychological Society (INS).

Anderson, V., Catroppa, C., Morse, S., Haritou, F., & Rosenfeld, J. (2005). *Understanding predictors of functional recovery and outcome five years following early childhood head injury.* Dublin, Ireland: International Neuropsychological Society Meeting (INS).

Asanow, R. F., Satz, P., & Light, R. (1991). Behavior problems and adaptive functioning in children with mild and severe closed head injury. *Journal of Pediatric Psychology, 16*, 543–555.

Asarnow, R. F., Satz, P., Light, R., Zaucha, K., Lewis, R., & McCleary, C. (1995). The UCLA study of mild closed head injury in children and adolescents. In S. H. Broman & M. E. Michel (Eds.), *Traumatic head-injury in children* (pp. 117–146). Oxford University Press: New York.

Barnes, M. A., Dennis, M., & Wilkinson, M. (1999). Reading after closed head injury in childhood. Effects on accuracy, fluency, and comprehension. *Developmental Neuropsychology, 15*(1), 1–24.

Bawden, H. N., Knights, R. M., & Winogron, H. W. (1985). Speeded performance following head injury children. *Journal of Clinical and Experimental Neuropsychology, 7*(1), 39–54.

Begali, V. (1987). *Head injury in children and adolescents.* Brandon: Clinical Psychology Publishing Co., Inc.

Begali, V. (1992). Traumatic head injury: Establishing the parameters. *Head injury in children and adolescents,* Clinical Psychology Publishing Company, Inc.

Breslau, N. (1990). Does brain dysfunction increase children's vulnerability to environmental stress. *Archives of General Psychiatry, 47*, 15–20.

Brookshire, B. L., Chapman, S. B., Song, J., & Levin, H. S. (2000). Cognitive and linguistic correlates of children's discourse after closed head injury: A three year follow-up. *Journal of the International Neuropsychological Society, 6*, 741–751.

Brown, G. C., Chadwick, O., Shaffer, D., Rutter, M., & Traub, M. (1981). A prospective study of children with head injuries: II. Psychiatric sequelae. *Psychological Medicine, 11*, 49–62.

Cassidy, J. D., Carroll, L. J., Peloso, P. M., Borg, J., von Holst, H., Holm, L., et al. (2004). Incidence, risk factors and prevention of mild traumatic brain injury: Results of the WHO collaborating centre task force on mild traumatic brain injury. *Journal of Rehabilitation Medicine, 43*, 28–60.

Catroppa, C., & Anderson, V. (1999). Attentional skills in the acute phase following pediatric traumatic brain injury. *Child Neuropsychology, 5*(4), 251–264.

Catroppa, C., & Anderson, V. (2003). Recovery and predictors of intellectual ability two years following pediatric traumatic brain injury. *Neuropsychological Rehabilitation, 13*(5), 517–536.

Catroppa, C., & Anderson, V. (2004). Recovery and predictors of language skills two years following pediatric traumatic brain injury. *Brain and Language, 88*, 68–78.

Catroppa, C., & Anderson, V. (2005). A prospective study of the recovery of attention from acute to 2 years post pediatric traumatic brain injury. *Journal of the International Neuropsychological Society, 11*, 84–98.

Catroppa, C., & Anderson, V. (2007). Recovery in memory function, and its relationship to academic success, at 24 months following pediatric TBI. *Child Neuropsychology, 13*(3), 240–261.

Catroppa, C., Anderson, V., Morse, S., Haritou, F., & Rosenfeld, J. (2007). Children's attentional skills five years post-TBI. *Journal of Pediatric Psychology, 32*(3), 354–369.

Catroppa, C., Anderson, V., Morse, S., Haritou, F., & Rosenfeld, J. (2008). Outcome and predictors of functional recovery five years following pediatric traumatic brain injury (TBI). *Journal of Pediatric Psychology, 33*(7), 707–718.

Catroppa, C., & Anderson, V. (2010). Cognitive Rehabilitation following padiatric traumatic brain injury. In V. Anderson & K. O. Yeates (Eds.), *New frontiers in pediatric traumatix brain injury*. Cambridge: Cambridge University Press.

Chorazy, A. J. L. (1985). Head injury rehabilitation: Children and adolescents (Introduction). In M. Ylvisaker (Ed.). *Head injury rehabilitation: Children and adolescents*. College Hill Press, Inc.

Cicerone, K., & Tupper, D. (1990). Neuropsychological rehabilitation: Treatment on errors in everyday function. In D. Tupper & K. Cicerone (Eds.), *The neuropsychology of everyday life: Issues in development and rehabilitation* (pp. 271–291). Boston: Kluwer Academic Publishers.

Coster, W. J., Haley, S., & Baryza, M. J. (1994). Functional performance of young children after traumatic brain injury: A 6-month follow-up study. *The American Journal of Occupational Therapy, 48*(3), 211–218.

Cronin, A. F. (2000). Traumatic brain injury in children: Issues in community function. *The American Journal of Occupational Therapy, 55*, 377–384.

Crowe, L., Babl, F., Anderson, V., & Catroppa, C. (2009). The epidemiology of paediatric head injuries: Data from a referral centre in Victoria, Australia. *Journal of Paediatrics and Child Health, 45*, 346–350.

Davis, M. J., & Vogel, L. (1995). Neurological assessment of the child with head trauma. *Journal of Dentistry for Children, 62*(2), 93–96.

Dennis, M. (1989). Language and the young damaged brain. In T. Boll & B. Bryant (Eds.), *Clinical neuoropsychology and brain function: Research, measurement and practice*. Washington DC: American Psychological Association.

Dennis, M., Barnes, M. A., Donnelly, R. E., Wilkinson, M., & Humphreys, R. P. (1996). Appraising and managing knowledge: Metacognitive skills after childhood head injury. *Developmental Neurospychology, 12*(1), 77–103.

Di Scala, C. (1993). National pediatric trauma registry biannual report, phase 2, October.

Di Scala, C., & Savage, R. C. (1997). Children hospitalised for traumatic brain injury: Transition to post-acute care. *Journal of Head Trauma Rehabilitation, 12*, 1–10.

Dikman, S., Machamer, J., Winn, H., & Temkin, N. (1995). Neuropsyhological outcome at 1-year post head injury. *Neuropsychology, 9*, 80–90.

Elson, L., & Ward, C. (1994). Mechanisms and pathophysiology of mild head injury. *Seminars in Neurology, 14*, 8–18.

Engberg, A., & Teesdale, G. (2004). Psychosocial outcome following traumatic brain injury in adults: A long-term population-based follow-up. *Brain Injury, 18*(6), 533–545.

Evans, R. (1992). The postconcussion syndrome and the sequelae of mild head injury. *The Neurology of Trauma, 10*, 815–847.

Ewing-Cobbs, L., Barnes, M. A., & Fletcher, J. M. (2003). Early brain injury in children: Development and reorganization of cognitive function. *Developmental Neuropsychology, 24*, 669–704.

Fennell, E. B., & Mickle, J. P. (1992). Behavioural effects of head trauma in children and adolescents. In M. G. Tramontana & S. R. Hooper (Eds.), *Advances in child neuropsychology – Volume 1*. New York: Springer.

Fenwick, T., & Anderson, V. (1999). Impairments of attention following childhood traumatic brain injury. *Child Neuropsychology, 5*, 213–223.

Fletcher, J.M., Ewing-Cobbs, L., Miner, M. E., Levin, H. S., & Einsberg, H. M. (1990). Behavioral changes after closed head injury in children. *Journal of Consulting and Clinical Psychology, 58*(1), 93–98.

Gavidia-Payne, S. T., & Hudson, A. (2002). Behavioural supports for parents of children with an intellectual disability and problem behaviours: An overview of the literature. *Journal of Intellectual & Developmental Disability, 27*, 31–55.

Gioia, G. A., & Isquith, P. K. (2004). Ecological assessment of executive function in traumatic brain injury. *Developmental Neuropsychology, 25*, 135–158.

Glang, A., Singer, G., & Todis, B. (Eds.). (1997). *Students with acquired brain injury: The school's response*. Baltimore: Paul H. Brookes.

Goldstein, F. C., & Levin, H. S. (1987). Epidemiology of pediatric closed head injury: Incidence, clinical characteristics and risk factors. *Journal of Learning Disabilities, 20*(9), 518–525.

Goldstein, F. C., & Levin, H. S. (1992). Cognitive function after closed head injury: Sequelae and outcome. In Thal, L.J., Moos, W.H., and Gamzu, E.R., *Cognitive Disorders: Pathophysiology and Treatment*, Marcer Dekker, Inc.

Goldstein, B., & Powers, K. S. (1994). Head trauma in children. *Pediatrics in Review, 15*(6), 213–219.

Gronwall, D., Wrightson, P., & McGinn, V. (1997). Effect of mild head injury during the preschool years. *Journal of the International Neuropsychological Society, 3*, 592–597.

Hawley, C. A. (2004). Behaviour and school performance after brain injury. *Brain Injury, 18*(7), 645–659.

High, W. M., Jr., Levin, H. S., & Gary, H. E., Jr. (1989). Recovery of orientation following closed head injury. *Journal of Clinical and Experimental Neuropsychology, 12*(5), 703–714.

Hoofien, D., Gilboa, A., Vakil, E., & Donovick, P. (2001). Traumatic brain injury (TBI) 10-20 years later: A comprehensive outcome study of psychiatric symptomatology, cognitive abilities and psychosocial functioning. *Brain Injury, 15*(3), 189–209.

Hudson, A., Matthews, J., Gavidia-Payne, S., Cameron, C., Mildon, R., & Radler, G. (2003). Evaluation of an intervention system for parents of children with intellectual disability and challenging behaviour. *Journal of Intellectual Disability Research, 47*, 238–249.

Hynd, G. W., & Willis, W. G. (Eds.). (1988). *Intercranial injuries. Paediatric neuropsychology*. New York: Grune and Stratton, Inc.

Kaufmann, P. M., Fletcher, J. M., Levin, H. S., Miner, M. E., & Ewing-Cobbs, L. (1993). Attentional disturbance after pediatric closed head injury. *Journal of Child Neurology, 8*, 348–353.

Kinsella, G. J., Prior, M., Sawyer, M., Ong, B., Murtagh, D., Eisenmajer, R., et al. (1997). Predictors and indicators of academic outcome in children 2 years following traumatic brain injury. *Journal of the International Neuropsychological Society, 3*, 608–616.

Klonoff, P., & Lamb, D. (1996). Mild head injury, significant impairment on neuropsychological test scores, and psychiatric disability. *The Clinical Neuropsychologist, 12*, 31–42.

Kraus, J. F., Fife, D., Cox, P., Ramstein, K., & Conroy, C. (1986). Incidence, severity, and external causes of pediatric brain injury. *American Journal of Epidemiology, 119*, 186–201.

Levin, H., & Kraus, M. F. (1994). The frontal lobes and traumatic brain injury. *The Journal of Neuropsychiatry and Clinical Neurosciences, 6*, 443–454.

Levin, H., Amparo, E., Eisenberg, H., Williams, D., High, W., McCordle, C., et al. (1987). Magnetic resonance imaging and computerised tomography in relation to the neurobehavioural sequelae of mild, and moderate head injuries. *Journal of Neurosurgery, 66*, 706–713.

Levin, H. S., Hanten, G., Zhang, L., Swank, P. R., & Hunter, J. (2004). Changes in working memory after traumatic brain injury in children. *Neuropsychology, 18*, 240–247.

Miller, J. D. (1991). Pathophysiology and measurement of head injury. *Neuropsychology, 5*(4), 235–261.

Miller, L. (1996). Neuropsychology and pathophysiology of mild head injury and the pot-concussion syndrome: Clinical and forensic considerations. *The Journal of Cognitive Rehabilitation, 15*, 8–23.

Muscara, F., Catroppa, C., & Anderson, V. (2008). Social problem solving skills as a mediator between executive function and long-term social outcome following pediatric traumatic brain injury. *Journal of Neuropsychology, 2*, 445–461.

Nadebaum, C., Anderson, V., & Catroppa, C. (2007). Executive function outcomes following traumatic brain injury in young children: A five year follow-up. *Developmental Neuropsychology, 32*(2), 703–728.

Papero, P. H., Prigatano, G. P., Snyder, H. M., & Johnson, D. L. (1993). Children's adaptive behavioural competence after head injury. *Neuropsychological Rehabilitation, 3*(4), 321–340.

Ponsford, J., Willmott, C., Rothwell, A., Cameron, P., Kelly, A., Ayton, G., Curran, C., & Nelms, R. (1997). Cognitive and behavioural outcome following mild traumatic brain injury in children. *Journal of the International Neuropsychological Society, 3,* 225.

Ponsford, J., Willmott, C., Rothwell, A., Cameron, P., Ayton, G., Nelms, R., et al. (1999). Cognitive and behavioural outcome following mild traumatic brain injury in children. *The Journal of Head Trauma Rehabilitation, 14,* 360–372.

Rivara, J. M. B., Jaffe, K. M., Fay, G. C., Polissar, N. L., Fay, G. C., Martin, K. M., et al. (1994). Family functioning and children's academic performance and behaviour problems in the year following traumatic brain injury. *Archives of Physical Medicine and Rehabilitation, 75,* 369–379.

Roberts, M., Manshad, F., Bushnell, D., & Hines, M. (1995). Neurobehavioral dysfunction following mild traumatic brain injury in childhood: A case report with positive findings on positron emission tomography (PET). *Brain Injury, 9,* 427–436.

Rutter, M., Chadwick, O., & Shaffer, D. (1983). Head injury. In M. Rutter (Ed.), *Developmental neuropsychiatry.* New York: Guilford Press.

Sahuquillo, J., & Vilalta, A. (2007). Cooling the injured brain: Does moderate hypothermia influence the pathophysiology of traumatic brain injury. *Current Pharmaceutical Design, 13,* 2310–2322.

Sanders, M. (1999). Triple P Positive Parenting Program: Towards an empirically validated multilevel parenting and family support strategy for the prevention of behavior and emotional problems in children. *Clinical Child and Family Psychology Review, 2,* 71–90.

Schwartz, M., Taylor, H. G., Drotar, D., Yeates, K., Wade, S., & Stancin, T. (2003). Long-term behavior problems following pediatric traumatic brain injury: Prevalence, predictors and correlates. *Journal of Pediatric Psychology, 28,* 251–263.

Sohlberg, M., & Mateer, C. (1989). Training use of compensatory memory books: A three-stage behavioral approach. *Journal of Clinical and Experimental Neuropsychology, 11,* 871–891.

Stablum, F., Mogentale, C., & Umilta, C. (1996). Executive functioning following mild closed head injury. *Cortex, 32,* 261–278.

Taylor, H. G., & Alden, J. (1997). Age-related differences in outcomes following childhood brain insults: An introduction and overview. *Journal of the International Neuropsychological Society, 3,* 555–567.

Taylor, H. G., Drotar, D., Wade, S. L., Yeates, K. O., Stancin, T., & Klein, S. (1995). Recovery from traumatic brain injury in children: The importance of the family. In S. H. Broman & M. E. Michel (Eds.), *Traumatic head injury in children* (pp. 188–218). New York: Oxford University Press.

Taylor, H. G., Yeates, K. O., Wade, S. L., Drotar, D., Stancin, T., & Burant, C. (2001). Bidirectional child-family influences on outcomes of traumatic brain injury in children. *Journal of the International Neuropsychological Society, 7,* 755–767.

Taylor, H. G., Wade, S. L., Stancin, T., Yeates, K. O., Drotar, D., & Minich, N. (2002). A prospective study of short- and long-term outcomes after traumatic brain injury in children: Behavior and achievement. *Neuropsychology, 16,* 15–27.

Teasdale, G., & Jennett, B. (1974). Assessment of coma and impaired consciousness: A practical scale. *Lancet, 2,* 81–83.

Wilson, J. T. L., Wiedmann, K. D., Hadley, D. M., Condon, B., Teasdale, G., & Brooks, D. N. (1988). Early and late magnetic resonance imaging and neuropsychological outcome after head injury. *Journal of Neurology, Neurosurgery and Psychiatry, 51,* 391–396.

Woods, D., Catroppa, C., Anderson, V., Godfrey, C., Matthews, J., Giallo, R., et al. (2007). Treatment acceptability of a family-centred intervention for parents of children with an acquired brain injury (ABI)- Pilot study. In *New frontiers in pediatric traumatic brain injury.* San Diego: Poster.

Yeates, K. (1999). Closed-head injury. In K. O. Yeates, M. D. Ris, & H. G. Taylor (Eds.), *Pediatric neuropsychology: Research, theory and practice* (pp. 192–218). New York: Guilford.

Yeates, K. O., Swift, E., Taylor, H. G., Wade, S. L., Drotar, D., Stancin, T., et al. (2004). Short- and long-term social outcomes following pediatric traumatic brain injury. *Journal of the International Neuropsychological Society, 10,* 412–426.

Chapter 26
Brain Tumors

Kyle E. Ferguson, Grant L. Iverson, and Mike R. Schoenberg

Abstract A brain tumor, or *neoplasm*, is a growth of abnormal cells inside the skull cavity. Most tumors of the Central Nervous System (>90%) originate from glial cells (e.g., astrocytes, oligodendrocytes, microglia, and ependymal cells), and only rarely develop from neurons (1%) (Davis LE, King MK, Schultz JL, Fundamentals of neurologic disease, Demos Medical Publishing, New York, 2005; Kaye AH, Essential neurosurgery, 3rd edn, Blackwell, Oxford, 2005; Victor M, Ropper AH, Adams and Victor's manual of neurology, 7th edn, McGraw-Hill, New York, 2002). Glial cells (glia) provide a number of metabolic, electrical, and mechanical support functions to neurons (Nolte J, The human brain: an introduction to its function anatomy, 5th edn, Mosby, St. Louis, 2002). Although brain tumors often disseminate and seed along the cerebrospinal fluid pathways, they rarely spread outside the central nervous system (Haberland C, Clinical neuropathology, Demos Medical Publishing, New York, 2007). The causes of brain tumors are generally unknown (Schiffer D, Brain tumor pathology: current diagnostic hotspots and pitfalls, Springer, Dordrecht, 2006).

The purpose of this chapter is to provide a brief overview of adult and childhood brain tumors.

The chapter is organized into the following seven sections: (1) Types of Tumors, (2) Epidemiology, (3) Signs and Symptoms, (4) Diagnosis and Neuroimaging, (5), Classification and Survival Rates, (6) Treatment, and (7) Neuropsychological Assessment Issues.

G.L. Iverson (✉)
University of British Columbia & British Columbia Mental Health & Addiction Services,
Vancouver, BC, Canada
e-mail: giverson@interchange.ubc.ca

M.R. Schoenberg and J.G. Scott (eds.), *The Little Black Book of Neuropsychology:*
A Syndrome-Based Approach, DOI 10.1007/978-0-387-76978-3_26,
© Springer Science+Business Media, LLC 2011

Key Points and Chapter Summary

- A brain tumor is a growth of abnormal cells inside the skull cavity. Brain tumors are either benign (noncancerous) or malignant (cancerous).
- There are two types of brain tumors: metastatic and primary. Most metastatic cancers originate in the lungs (50%). Metastatic cancers are twice as common in adults, whereas primary brain tumors are twice as common in children.
- The signs and symptoms of brain tumors vary from asymptomatic to considerable cognitive and behavioral impairment. Seizures are often the presenting symptom that brings a patient with a brain tumor to the attention of physicians. However, the most common symptom of brain tumors is persistent headache in both children and adults.
- Tumors are diagnosed and removed during surgery. Tumors are classified based on their histologic or cellular characteristics, ranging from Grades I through IV.
- There are three standard forms of treatment: (1) surgery, (2) radiation therapy (radiotherapy), and (3) chemotherapy. The treatment goal for lower grades is "curative." In contrast, the treatment goal for higher grades is palliative, to prolong survival and manage symptoms.
- There is no standard battery of neuropsychological tests for brain tumors. Generally, the following neuropsychological domains should be assessed: (1) attention and concentration, (2) language (receptive and expressive), (3) visual-perceptual and spatial skills, (4) learning and memory, (5) executive functioning, and (6) psychological functioning.
- The authors propose using co-normed tests and provide psychometric criteria for Cognitive Disorder NOS using an abbreviated version of the NAB battery.

Types of Tumors

There are two types of brain tumors: *metastatic* and *primary* (National Cancer Institute 2007a). *Metastatic* tumors originate elsewhere in the body and spread to the brain via blood cells and lymph channels. *Metastatic* cancers are twice as common as primary brain tumors in adults. Alternatively, primary brain tumors are twice as common in children (Kebudi et al. 2005).

Adults

The most common brain tumors in adults are metastates from lung cancer (50%), breast cancer (15–20%), and melanomas (10%), respectively (Lassman and DeAngelis 2003; Meyers et al. 2004). As many as 24–40% of adult patients with non-central nervous system tumors will eventually develop metastatic brain cancer (Kebudi et al. 2005; Mehta et al. 2003; Meyers 2002). Prognosis is related to the cancer's primary site. For example, the prognosis for brain metastases from breast cancer is more favorable than metastases from colon cancer (National Cancer Institute 2007b).

Primary brain tumors originate in the brain. Most primary brain tumors in adults develop above the tentorium in the hemispheres (e.g., Davis et al. 2005). Of the primary brain tumors, *Astrocytoma* is the most common (Behin et al. 2003; Mantani and Israel 2001).

Children

Most primary brain tumors in children are found in the posterior fossa (Davis et al. 2005; Mabbott et al. 2008). *Medulloblastoma* is the most common primary brain tumor in children (Crawford et al. 2007; Packer et al. 1999).

Rule of thumb: Terminology

- A brain tumor is a growth of abnormal cells inside the skull cavity
- Brain tumors are either benign (noncancerous) or malignant (cancerous)
- Metastatic tumors originate elsewhere in the body and spread to the brain
- Primary brain tumors originate in the brain

Benign Versus Malignant

Brain tumors have been labeled as either "benign" (noncancerous) or "malignant" (cancerous). The term "benign," is an unfortunate misnomer, as "benign" tumors are not harmless. Benign tumors can undergo malignant transformations and given their location (especially around the brain stem) can become lethal (Behin et al. 2003). Benign tumors do not invade neighboring cells (Torpy et al. 2005). Benign tumors grow slowly by way of expansion (often compressing other areas); are circumscribed; resemble the cell of origin; and tend to be well differentiated (Haberland 2007; Victor and Ropper 2002). Benign tumors include *meningiomas*, *epidermoid tumors*, *dermoid tumors*, *hemangioblastomas*, *colloid cysts*, *pleomorphic xanthoastrocytomas*, *craniopharyngiomas*, and *schwannomas* (which can grow on cranial nerves) (Arthur 2005). Of these, *meningiomas* are the most common, constituting approximately 15% of all adult brain tumors (1/3 of the *gliomas*), reaching peak incidence in middle age, affecting more females than males (Kaye 2005). The gender difference in *meningiomas* is an exception to the rule, because tumors of the CNS are overall more common in males (American Cancer Society 2008; Haberland 2007).

Malignant tumors are anaplastic (cannot be clearly demarcated from normal tissue); they vary in shape, size, and overall pattern; and usually proliferate rapidly (Carriage and Henson 1995; Haberland 2007). The proliferation rate is related to the so-called "aggressiveness" of the tumor (Weber 2007). *Malignant tumors* invade and destroy neighboring cells. The term "malignant," as used here, differs from its common usage with other types of cancer. Because brain tumors rarely metastasize – save *medulloblastoma* and *ependymoma* – "malignant" in this case refers to its aggressive characteristics and prognostic implications (Kaye 2005). *Malignant tumors* are caused by multiple changes in gene expression (predominantly the *p53* gene, located on chromosome 17p), which lead to uncontrolled cell proliferation and cell death (Mantani and Israel 2001; Ruddon 2007; Victor and Ropper 2002). *Oncogenes* and *cancer suppressor genes* are implicated in tumor growth (Haberland 2007). *Malignant* tumors include *anaplastic astrocytoma, glioblastoma multiforme, anaplastic oligodendroglioma, medulloblastomas,* and *pineoblastomas.*

Epidemiology

Rule of thumb: Quick facts

- Malignant brain tumors: 1.4% of all cancers (2% of cancer-related deaths)
- Peak incidence of brain tumors: 74–84 years of age
- Average age of onset (primary brain tumors): 54 years of age
- Gender differences: Greater incidence in boys and men
- GLOBOCAN 2002 worldwide annual incidence of CNS tumors:

    - 3.7 and 2.6 cases per 100,000 for males and females, respectively
    - Total is 7.3 cases per 100,000
    - Higher rates in more developed nations

Note: Information for Quick Facts derived from: (Arthur 2005; 4.0 cases per 100,000; Central Brain Tumor Registry of the United States 2005, 2006) (males: 3.0 cases per 100,000; females: 2.1 cases per 100,000; Central Brain Tumor Registry of the United States 2008)

US incidence rates for 2004 are age-adjusted to the 2000 US population, comprising 19 age groups (e.g., Seattle, New Mexico, Utah, and San Francisco; Ries et al. 2007, Table III-2). The incidence of CNS tumors is 6.5 cases per 100,000 (excluding lymphomas, leukemias, tumors of pituitary and pineal glands, and olfactory tumors within the nasal cavity). The male and female rates are 7.6 and 5.5 cases per 100,000, respectively. Although the incidence of cancer in general is greater in African Americans, incidence rates of CNS tumors are higher in Caucasians (7.2 cases per 100,000) than African Americans (3.9 cases per 100,000; Ries et al. 2007, Table III-2). The mortality rates are 4.5 cases per 100,000 for all races and genders (Ries et al. 2007, Table III-3). The mortality rates for males and females are 5.2 and 3.5 cases per 100,000, respectively. Moreover, mortality rates are higher in Caucasians (4.6 cases per 100,000) than African Americans (2.5 cases per 100,000) (Jemal et al. 2008).

Canadian Cancer Statistics (Steering Committee of the National Cancer Institute of Canada and the Canadian Cancer Society 2005) suggest an overall incidence rate of 8 cases per 100,000; 1,350 of which were males and 1,100 were females. That same year, 1,650 people died from brain cancer; 940 were males and 720 were females.

Bray et al. (2002) examined published estimates from national cancer registries and the World Health Organization mortality data in 38 European countries (Bray et al. 2002, pp. 141–142). The incidence rates for people aged 0–75+ years old was 8.4 male and 5.7 female cases per 100,000, for all 27 countries in the European Union (EU) (e.g., UK, France, and Germany) in 1995. The mortality rates, per 100,000, for that same year for EU countries were: 5.9 male and 3.9 female cases.

China's incidence rate in 2000 was estimated to be 4.4 new cases per 100,000 of brain and nervous system tumors (Yang et al. 2005). The incidence rates of select middle eastern countries are as follows: Based on 1996–2001 data, it was estimated there were 5.2 per 100,000 new cases of CNS tumors in Israel (males: 6.1 cases per 100,000; females: 4.3 per 100,000); 4.0 per 100,000 new cases in Jordan (males: 4.4 cases per 100,000; females: 3.6 cases per 100,000); and 3.7 per 100,000 new cases in Egypt[1] (males: 3.8 cases per 100,000; females: 3.5 cases per 100,000; Inskip and Ron 2006).

Signs and Symptoms

The signs and symptoms of brain tumors vary from essentially asymptomatic to significant cognitive and behavioral impairment. Rapidly growing tumors can cause increased intracranial pressure (Ropper and Brown 2005). Increased intracranial pressure is usually responsible for many signs and symptoms observed in patients (e.g., headache, vomiting, and personality and cognitive changes; American Brain Tumor Association 2005). A rise in intracranial pressure can also lead to "false localizing signs," due to a shift in distal intracranial structures (Wen et al. 2001, p. 219). Significant tumor growth can cause herinations in the temporal (forced through the tentorial opening into the posterior fossa), cerebellar (pressed into the foramen magnum), and subfalcial areas, due to a shift in tissue to compartments where the pressure is lower (Victor and Ropper 2002, p. 260). Additionally, many tumors release unknown substances causing vasogenic edema, which can further increase intracranial pressure (Davis et al. 2005).

The most common symptom of brain tumors is headache for both children and adults. Over 50% of adult patients with brain tumors experience headaches, as early

---

[1] Based on 1999–2001 data.

or late symptoms, whereas headaches occur in 33% of children (Rohkamm 2004; Wilne et al. 2007). Headaches are often described as nonpulsatile and intermittent (Cummings and Trimble 2002), and may resemble migraine or tension headaches. With increased intracranial pressure, a bifrontal or bioccipital headache, regardless of localization, may occur. If lateralized, headache is often ipsilateral to tumor location. Localization signs/symptoms may not be present, and generalized dysfunction is common due to increased intracranial pressure and/or diffuse edema. Partial and/ or generalized seizures are a common symptom, particularly if the tumor is slow growing and affects cortical regions (Behin et al. 2003). Seizures occur in 40–60% of adult patients at some time, and may be the symptom leading to a diagnosis (Wen 1997). Seizures affect 38% of children with brain tumors (Wilne et al. 2007). Lateralized or localizing symptoms can occur. Vomiting, loss of appetite, personality and mood changes, vertigo, fatigue, and cognitive problems may present in adults and children (National Cancer Institute 2007a; Rohkamm 2004; Wilne et al. 2007). Vomiting and vertigo are common symptoms of tumors affecting the posterior fossa. Compression of the brain stem results in motor and/or sensory signs, cranial nerve impairments, and hydrocephalus. Loss of appetite, personality and mood changes can be associated with frontal lobe tumors, particularly when the orbital frontal area is affected. Contralateral motor weakness, expressive language problems, attention and/or memory problems may also occur. Frontal lobe tumors can, however, be asymptomatic. Cognitive symptoms tend to be focal in nature (Meyers 2002). Thus, lesions in the left hemisphere may impair language-mediated functions. In contrast, lesions in the right hemisphere may affect visual-perceptual/ spatial skills. Thalamic tumors also cause cognitive impairment, contralateral sensory loss, hemiparesis, and aphasia, among other symptoms (Wen et al. 2001). Cerebellar and medial temporal lesions cause ataxic symptoms and memory loss, respectively (Victor and Ropper 2002).

Rule of thumb: Signs and symptoms

- Symptoms vary widely among individuals, from asymptomatic to significant cognitive and behavioral impairment
- Headaches are most common for adults and children
- Seizures are also quite common in adults and children
- Cognitive symptoms are often focal in nature (e.g., left hemispheric lesions affect language-mediated functions; right hemispheric lesions affect visual-perceptual/spatial skills)

Paraneoplastic Syndrome

A paraneoplastic syndrome arises from autoimmune reaction to cancers. Autoantibodies are thought to underlie the symptomatic presentation, and several types of autoantibodies have been found. The neurological manifestations can precede cancer diagnosis.

Paraneoplastic syndromes may include more "classical" symptom presentations (e.g., Lambert-Eaton myasthenic syndromes, subacute cerebellar degeneration, and in pediatric patients myclonis/opsoclonus) or those that can be due to cancer or can present as another disease (e.g., amyotrophic lateral sclerosis, polymyositis, and/or polyneuropathy). The five common paraneoplastic syndromes are listed below.

1. Brain and cranial nerves: limbic encephalitis or other dementia, optic neuritis, brain-stem encephalitis, opsoclonus-myoclonus, or subacute cerebellar degeneration.
2. Spinal cord and/or dorsal root ganglia: motor neuron disease, myelitis, myelo-pathies, sensory neuronopathy, subacute motor neuronopathy.
3. Peripheral nerves: autonomic neuropathy, Guillian–Bare syndrome, mononeuri-tis-multiplex and vasculitic neuropathy, subacute sensorimotor peripheral neuropathy.
4. Neuromuscular junction and muscle: Lambert–Eaton myasthenic syndrome, dermatomyositis, myotonia, myasthenia gravis, acute necrotizing myopathy, neuromyopathy.
5. Unknown or combined central and peripheral nervous system: encephalomyelitis, neuromyopathy, stiff-person syndrome.

Diagnosis of paraneoplastic syndrome is a clinical diagnosis of exclusion that can be confirmed by tests for autoantibodies. Onset of symptoms is subacute, inflammatory CSF with increased protein and oligoclonal bands, severe neuro-logic disability, and stereotyped presentation that often affects a specific aspect of the central nervous system. This is thought to reflect the immune response to injury, with a directed autoimmune response to antigens of the tumor and shared nervous system components. The presence of autoantibodies can also assist in the search for underlying cancer. When a paraneoplastic syndrome is present, it suggests a more morbid course than the same tumor without a paraneoplastic syndrome.

Diagnosis and Neuroimaging

Tumors are diagnosed and removed during surgery (National Cancer Institute 2007a). A variety of different conditions – particularly those that cause increased intracranial pressure or produce progressive neurologic symptoms – need to be ruled out when differentially diagnosing brain tumors. These can include subdural hematomas, hydrocephalus, brain abscesses, cerebral infarctions, multiple sclero-sis, and Alzheimer's disease (Wen et al. 2001). Brain biopsy is required to establish histopathologic features, but sometimes to confirm the presence of a brain tumor because some conditions can appear like a brain tumor (e.g., brain abscesses, demy-elinating disease) (Wen et al. 2001). A biopsy may be contraindicated in vital areas, such as the brain stem (e.g., brain stem gliomas). Interested readers are referred to Wen et al. (2001) for a discussion on other diagnostic techniques.

CT and MRI scans are essential in screening for brain tumors and in differential diagnosis (e.g., ruling out hemorrhages and stroke) (Kaye 2005). MR imaging, using gadolinium infusion or not (or "with and without contrast"), is considered the best method of determining the mass' characteristics, which includes location, size, and extent of edema (Behin et al. 2003). Gadolinium pools around cancer cells, making them appear brighter (i.e., contrast-enhanced) (National Cancer Institute 2007a). While not routinely used (due to limited availability and high cost), PET is useful to provide information about blood flow, metabolism, and physiology of brain tumors and surrounding areas (Wen et al. 2001). Functional MRI is useful in cortical mapping during tumor resection, which enables surgeons to avoid damaging eloquent language and motor cortices (Debnam et al. 2007).

Rule of thumb: Diagnosis

- A definitive diagnosis requires a brain biopsy
- A brain biopsy establishes histopathologic features needed to classify or grade brain tumors

---

Classification and Survival Rates

The four-tiered grading system developed by the World Health Organization (WHO) is the most common system of grading brain tumors (Sawrie 2006). According to this system, brain tumors are classified on the basis of their *histologic* or cellular characteristics, ranging from Grades I through IV (Haberland 2007; Louis et al. 2007; see Fig. 26.1).

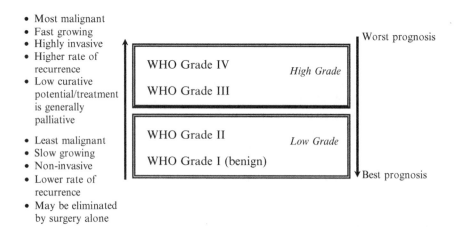

Fig. 26.1 Classification of tumors (Information for this figure was derived from several sources (Behin et al. 2003; El-Zein et al. 2005; Lezak et al. 2004; Reifenberger et al. 2006))

Grade I tumors (e.g., *pilocytic astrocytoma* and *meningioma*) are benign, grow slowly, and have low proliferation potential.

Grade II tumors (e.g., *oligoastrocytoma* and *pineocytomas*) also have low proliferation potential, however, unlike Grade I tumors, often recur and are "infiltrative in nature" (Louis et al. 2007, p. 97). Thus, Grades II and higher suggest malignancy.

Grade III tumors (e.g., *anaplastic astrocytoma* and *anaplastic oligodendroglioma*) are generally malignant, with high proliferation potential, and usually grow again after being removed. Patients with Grade III (and higher) tumors typically receive radiotherapy and/or chemotherapy, in addition to undergoing neurosurgery.

Grade IV tumors (e.g., *glioblastoma multiforme* and *medulloblastoma*) are the most aggressive, and, as such, the most difficult to treat. They also appear very different from normal cells.

Rule of thumb: Grading the tumor

- Grading brain tumors requires histologic sample
- Grade I – low grade tumor, slowly growing, low infiltration potential being encapsulated with clearly defined borders, and tend not to recur
- Grade II – low grade malignant tumor, slowly growing, low infiltration potential being encapsulated but with poorly defined borders, and greater potential for recurrence
- Grade III – high grade malignant tumor, rapid growing, high infiltration potential being poorly encapsulated, and tend to recur
- Grade IV – high grade malignant tumor, rapid growth, high infiltration potential and not encapsulated, identified in multiple areas of brain, and high recurrence potential

---

The WHO grading system is used to predict the "biological behavior" of brain tumors, which is related to survival rates (Louis et al. 2007, p. 106). Carriage and Henson (1995) examined 5,190 cases and found individuals with Grades I or II brain tumors typically had a 50% greater survival rate than individuals with Grade III or IV brain tumors.

Haberland (2007) reported estimated mean survival rates for Grades II to IV. The mean survival rates for Grade II are 5–10 years; 2–3 years for Grade III; and 1–1.5 years for Grade IV. Other variables influencing prognosis include age, the extent of tumor removal, tumor progression, and the location of the tumor (Rohkamm 2004).

Common primary brain tumor types are provided in Table 26.1. The information is organized by type, grade, population affected, and the usual site of the lesion. Benign tumors are indicated with asterisks (*).

Table 26.1 Common brain tumors in adults (Information derived from Central Brain Tumor Registry of the United States 2005, 2006; El-Zein et al. 2005; Kaye 2005; Keles et al. 2006; Kulkarni and McDonald 2006; Louis et al. 2007; Reifenberger et al. 2006; Taylor 2006; van Effenterre and Boch 2006; Victor and Ropper 2002; Weingart et al. 2006; Weller 2006; Westphal 2006; Westphal et al. 2006; Wetjen and Raffel 2006; Wilne et al. 2007)

Brain Tumor Type	Prevalence	WHO grade	Populations affected	Lesion site
Glioblastoma Multiforme	20% of all intracranial tumors (>60% of primary brain tumors)	IV	Mostly >45 years of age (peak age of onset=Sixth or Seventh decade)	Mostly cerebral cortex (although can affect other areas of CNS)
Low-Grade Astrocytoma	25% brain tumors (children); 15% brain tumors (adults)	II	Biphasic age distribution, 2 peak incidences: (1) 6–12 years; (2) 26–46 years	Frontal lobe, followed by temporal and parietal lobes
Anaplastic Astrocytoma	3% of all brain tumors	III	Median age: 51 years	Cerebral cortex (adults)/Brain stem and cerebellum (children)
Oligodendroglioma	5% of all primary brain tumors	II	Mostly affects adults>45 years of age	Frontal lobes
Ependymoma	6–12% of primary brain tumors (children)/1.9% of all intracranial tumors (adults)	I–IV	Young adults and children	Forth ventricle, conus medullaris, and filum terminale
Medulloblastoma	25% (children); rare in adults ≥16 years of age	IV	Mostly children between 5 and 10 years of age, however, can affect all age groups	Cerebellum (mostly in the cerebellar vermis)
Meningioma*	1–3% (children); 15% (male)/30% (female) of all intracranial tumors	I	Mean age=9–13 years	Supratentorial compartment and posterior fossa
Schwannomas*	8% of primary brain tumors	I	30–60 years of age	Cerebellum and Cranial Nerves
Craniopharyngioma*	3–4% of all intracranial tumors; 10% (children)	I	3 age peaks: 7–13 years; 20–25 years; and 60–65 years	Sellar and suprasellar regions

Treatment

There are three standard forms of treatment: (1) surgery, (2) radiation therapy (radiotherapy), and (3) chemotherapy (National Cancer Institute 2007a). The objective of treatment varies with the tumor's grade. For example, the treatment goal for a Grade I tumor is "curative." In contrast, at this time, *glioblastoma multiforme* – a Grade IV tumor – is ultimately fatal, the treatment objective is palliative, to prolong survival and manage symptoms (Davis et al. 2005). A combination of surgery, radiation therapy, and chemotherapy, can prolong "useful" life in persons with *glioblastoma multiforme* by several months (Victor and Ropper 2002, p. 262). In addition to surgery, radiation, and/or chemotherapy, Dexamethasone, a steroid, is often used to reduce swelling and anti-seizure medication (AEDs) may be given to reduce seizures (Torpy et al. 2005). See Wefel et al. (2004) for a discussion on other therapies, including bioimmunotherapy and hormonal therapy.

Surgery

The first treatment of most tumors is usually neurosurgical. This may involve a craniotomy (removal of a section of the skull to gain access) or sometimes bur holes can be used to gain access to the tumor. The goal of surgery is to resect as much of the tumor as possible without causing too much permanent damage (Rohkamm 2004). From surgery, tissue is removed for pathological examination (Mantani and Israel 2001). Surgical armamentarium includes traditional scalpel, laser microsurgery, and ultrasonic aspiration (American Brain Tumor Association 2005). Laser microsurgery is used in conjunction with, or in lieu of, a scalpel. The laser vaporizes tumor cells. Ultrasonic aspiration employs ultrasonic waves, causing vibrations, which break up cancer cells. The loose pieces are then aspirated (vacuumed up).

Surgical resection and debulking are common surgical techniques (American Brain Tumor Association 1993). Resection is the removal of the tumor for curative purposes. Gross total resection is associated with a more favorable prognosis whereas a subtotal resection and/or partial resection (the tumor is not entirely removed) are related to a less favorable prognosis (Nitta and Sato 1995). Debulking entails resecting a portion of the tumor with the primary goal of reducing the tumor's mass. Debulking can improve survival and/or reduce neurologic symptoms by reducing intracranial pressure (Davis et al. 2005).

Radiation Therapy (Radiotherapy)

Many tumors die upon exposure to X- and gamma rays, due to so-called "radiosensitivity" (American Brain Tumor Association 2005). Unilateral and/or bilateral radiation therapy is thus the mainstay treatment for brain tumors (Meyers 2002). Whole-brain radiation therapy (WBRT) is typically employed for brain metastases, irrespective of the number of lesions or location of the tumor (Raizer 2006).

Radiotherapy improves survival over surgery alone, however, side effects of radiation are common (Larson and Wara 1998). These often include anorexia, nausea, and fatigue (Davis et al. 2005). Although delayed damage to multiple neuroanatomic substrates has been documented, no study has yet identified specific regions most sensitive to the effects of radiotherapy (Armstrong et al. 2004). However, generally, radiotherapy affects the white matter tracts and cerebral vasculature, due to axonal demyelination and disruption to vascular endothelial cells, respectively (Wefel et al. 2004).

Radiation therapy is not indicated for children who have undergone complete or nearly complete surgical resection because tumor progression is unlikely (Pollack 1999). Moreover, given the risks to the developing brain, radiotherapy should only be considered when tumors are not well defined and noninfiltrative (Larson and Wara 1998). Although the mechanisms are not fully understood in children, radiation therapy is related to loss of white matter volume or the failure to develop white matter at an appropriate developmental rate (Mulhern et al. 2004). Among other things, compromised white matter integrity is associated with poor intellectual functioning (Mabbott et al. 2008).

Intelligence Quotient (IQ) scores have been chiefly used to measure diminished global cognitive functioning in children who have undergone radiotherapy (Kieffer-Renaux et al. 2005). These adverse effects appear to be dose and, particularly, age dependent, in that very young children (<4 years old) are most susceptible to cognitive deficits (Hoppe-Hirsch et al. 1990; Packer et al. 1989). In light of age effects, when radiotherapy is indicated, chemotherapy is often used to postpone radiation therapy, to allow children's brains to develop as completely as possible (Karajannis et al. 2008). This is especially the case in children under 2 years of age (Albright 1993).

Gamma Knife/Stereotactic Radiosurgery

Stereotactic radiosurgery or gamma knife neurosurgery directs focused gamma radiation (up to 201 ^{60}CO) to a highly circumscribed area, often in a single dose (Sheetz 2009). Gamma-knife neurosurgery has been recommended for targeting smaller tumors (<3 cm in diameter), and, although complications have been documented (e.g., facial numbness and hearing loss), these are rare due to minimal radiation exposure (Kaye 2005). Given its focal delivery, accurate delineation of cancer tissue is critical and usually involves MRI planning (Keles et al. 2007). Better tumor management, improved quality of life, and survival benefits have been documented in select patients using gamma-knife neurosurgery (e.g., those with radio-resistant primary cancers; Jawahar et al. 2002; Sin et al. 2009).

Chemotherapy

Chemotherapy is designed to "poison" cancer cells, and disrupt cell proliferation (American Brain Tumor Association 2005; National Cancer Institute 2007a). Chemotherapy is administered orally or intravenously. Another option is to place a dissoluble wafer (Gliadel wafer) directly on the tumor site (tumor bed) after surgical resection (National Cancer Institute 2007a).

Chemotherapy has immediate and delayed side effects (Klener 1999). Nausea and vomiting are common within 24 hours of treatment. Leukopenia (reduction in white blood cells) and stomatitis (inflammation of the mucous lining in the mouth) can occur within days to weeks. Cardiomyopathy and peripheral neuropathy, with the latter being the most common neurological complication of chemotherapy, can occur within weeks to months of treatment (Kannarkat et al. 2007).

Certain agents used in chemotherapy are known to have neurotoxic effects (e.g., methotrexate and 5-FU cause diffuse white matter changes) (Wefel et al. 2004). Chemotherapy has been shown to cause persistent cognitive deficits (so-called "chemobrain") in approximately 18% of patients undergoing chemotherapy for all cancer types (Meyers 2002; Weiss 2008). Such effects have been observed 2 years after chemotherapy has been discontinued. Chemotherapy may cause deficits of attention, processing speed, verbal memory, visual-spatial functioning, executive functioning, and/or motor functioning (Anderson-Hanley et al. 2003). Additionally, confusion, mental fogginess, fatigue, and significant mood disturbances are subjective complaints of chemotherapy (Taillibert et al. 2007; Weiss 2008). In children, although overall intellectual functioning is often preserved, neurocognitive deficits secondary to treatment remain, including problems with attention and executive functioning (Buizer et al. 2009).

Rule of thumb: Treating brain tumors

- The three standard forms of treatment are (1) surgery, (2) radiation therapy (radiotherapy), and (3) chemotherapy
- The treatment goal for lower grades is "curative"
- The treatment goal for higher grades is palliative, to prolong survival and manage symptoms

Neuropsychological Assessment Issues

Neuropsychological impairment is caused by brain tumors and their treatment (Taphoorn and Klein 2004). There is no standard battery of neuropsychological tests for brain tumors, in part because test selection depends on the clinical and/or research questions (Wefel et al. 2004). Like other clinical populations, some common neuropsychological domains should be assessed including; (1) attention/

concentration, (2) language (receptive and expressive), (3) memory/learning, (4) visual-perceptual/spatial skills, (5) executive functions, and (6) mood/personality variables. In addition, assessing quality of life is often advisable, as brain tumors and their treatments can affect work-related and interpersonal functioning.

Sawrie (2006, p. 425) provide six typical referral questions for patients with brain tumors, which are often representative of the research questions found in the literature. These typical referral/research questions are as follows: (1) Has there been cognitive decline secondary to radiation therapy (Armstrong et al. 2002; 2004; Gregor et al. 1996; Stuschke et al. 1999; Surma-aho et al. 2001; Torres et al. 2003)? (2) Has there been cognitive decline secondary to chemotherapy (Ahles et al. 2002; Castellon et al. 2004; Rohlman et al. 2003)? (3) Has there been cognitive decline secondary to tumor recurrence (Bosma et al. 2007; Glosser et al. 1997)? (4) Does the rehabilitation program or any of its components improve (or affect) cognitive functioning (Kaleita et al. 2004; Langer et al. 2002; Mabbott et al. 2008; Mehta et al. 2003; Meyers et al. 2004)? (5) Can survival rates be predicted using estimates of baseline cognitive functioning (Armstrong et al. 2003; Meyers et al. 2000)? (6) Is cognitive functioning related to quality of life or psychiatric status (Harder et al. 2004; Klein et al. 2001)?

Rationale for Selecting a Test Battery

Although there are no "typical" neuropsychological batteries designed to measure the neuropsychological effects of brain tumors and/or brain tumor treatments, there are a number of recommendations in the literature to guide clinical practice (Sawrie 2006). Tests, for example, should be relatively brief, due to potential fatigue, although comprehensive enough to assess major cognitive domains (i.e., attention, language functioning, visual-spatial and constructional abilities, memory, and executive functioning; Meyers et al. 2004). Sensory and motor tests are also recommended, if there is time (see Lezak et al. 2004, Chaps. 10 and 16 for examples).

Reliable Change Indices

Given that neuropsychological evaluations are sometimes used serially for individuals suffering from brain tumors, we recommend clinicians consider employing measures for which reliable change indices can be calculated (or are known) (see Chelune et al. 1993; Jacobson and Truax 1991; Sawrie et al. 1996 and the chapter by Brooks and colleagues in this book for review of RCI and other psychometric approaches for repeat neuropsychological testing).

Fixed Versus Flexible Batteries

Employing a flexible battery approach is the most common assessment strategy used in Neuropsychology (Lezak et al. 2004). Upon surveying the literature, it also appears to be widely used in assessing neuropsychological functioning in persons with brain tumors. See the chapter by Iverson and Brooks in this book for the advantages of using co-normed tests and the drawbacks of combining tests that have been standardized and normed on different populations.

An alternative is the use of co-normed tests. Iverson and Brooks (2008a, b) evaluated an abbreviated version of the Neuropsychological Assessment Battery (NAB; Stern and White 2003), comprised of 15 of the 24 tests. This abbreviated battery requires approximately 2 hours to administer. A description of the five NAB modules, along with the tests and the 23 primary T scores for this abbreviated battery, are presented below.

Abbreviated NAB Battery for Clinical Practice in Patients with Brain Tumors

The NAB is a comprehensive, modular battery of tests, focusing on multiple areas of cognitive functioning (i.e., attention, language, memory, spatial, and executive functions). The tests in the battery are all new, but most are based on tests commonly used in neuropsychology. All tests were administered to the standardization sample; thus, the normative data applies to every test singly and in combination. The full NAB consists of 24 individual tests. These tests yield 36 demographically corrected (age, education, and sex) T scores, five index scores, and a Total NAB Index score. All of these normative scores were derived from a continuous norming procedure applied to a sample of 1,448 healthy adults between the ages of 18 and 97. A brief measure of intelligence, the Reynolds Intellectual Screening Test (RIST; Reynolds and Kamphaus 2003), was administered to the NAB standardization sample. The RIST is comprised of one verbal and one nonverbal test. Thus, NAB test results can be interpreted in relation to level of intelligence (Iverson et al. 2008). Moreover, base rates of low scores in healthy normals are available (see Iverson et al. 2008).

- NAB Attention Module: Consists of 6 tests, 5 of which contribute to the Attention Index score. This module fully assesses 'attention and speed of information processing. The 5 primary tests are used in the battery. The Numbers and Letters A Efficiency T score are not included in the analyses.
- NAB Language Module: Consists of 6 tests that contribute to the Language Index score. This module clearly measures "language" (e.g., comprehension, word-finding difficulties, and reduced fluency). For the abbreviated NAB, only 2 of the 6 tests are used: Oral Production and Naming. Analyses for this domain are based on 2 T scores.

- NAB Memory Module: The Memory Index is derived from 4 tests assessing verbal and visual learning and memory. For the abbreviated NAB, 3 tests are used: List Learning, Story Learning, and Daily Living Memory.
- NAB Spatial Module: Consists of 4 tests that contribute to the Spatial Index score. This module measures perceptual, spatial, constructional, and spatial-motor abilities. For the abbreviated NAB, only 2 tests are used: Visual Discrimination and Design Construction.
- NAB Executive Functions Module: Measures different aspects of executive functioning. For the abbreviated NAB, 3 of the tests are used: Mazes, Categories, and Word Generation.

Neuropsychological profile analysis involves determining the prevalence of low scores in the domains of attention, language, memory, spatial, and executive functioning. All scores within each domain are considered simultaneously, rather than in isolation. The cutoffs used in our analysis include: <25th %ile; <16th %ile (i.e., <1 SD); <10th %ile; ≤5th %ile; and <2nd %ile (i.e., <2 SDs). Neuropsychological profile analysis is the foundation for the development of new evidence-based psychometric criteria for Cognitive Disorder NOS[2] (Iverson and Brooks 2008b).

Iverson and Brooks (2008a, b) have presented psychometric criteria for Cognitive Disorder NOS using this abbreviated NAB battery. *Possible* impairment is based on having fewer than 20% of healthy adults and *probable* impairment is based on having fewer than 10% of healthy adults obtaining the number of low scores below the given cutoff. In other words, there is a known false positive rate for both possible and probable impairment. Tables were presented illustrating psychometric criteria for possible or probable impairment in each domain.

To use these interpretive tables, there is a three-step procedure: (1) count the number of primary T scores in each domain that fall below the five cutoff scores (i.e., 25th, 16th, 10th, 5th, and 2nd percentiles); (2) refer to the appropriate table that corresponds to the person's level of intelligence[3]; and (3) determine if the number

---

[2]To identify a person as having mild neurocognitive disorder (i.e., a sub-category of the Axis I DSM-IV diagnosis of cognitive disorder not otherwise specified), there must be impairment in *at least two domains*, which can include attention or speed of information processing, language, memory, perceptual-motor abilities, and executive functioning.

[3]We are using the RIST to estimate *current* intellectual abilities. After determining their current RIST score, we combine this information with clinical judgment to estimate premorbid RIST *classification category* (e.g., low average, average, high average, or superior). We usually use the obtained RIST as the best estimate of premorbid RIST classification. However, sometimes we might believe that the obtained RIST under-estimates premorbid ability, and thus we might choose one classification higher. An example would be if a person with significant brain damage obtained a RIST of 109. We might assume that his/her premorbid RIST was more likely to fall in the High Average classification range than in the Average classification range.

of low scores in each cognitive domain is considered *broadly normal, possible impairment,* or *probable impairment.*

We present two case examples of patients who have been treated for brain tumors and have been evaluated using the abbreviated NAB. These case examples illustrate the use of the new psychometric criteria for determining the presence of cognitive impairment. The RIST and NAB test data used for these case examples is presented in Table 26.2. The profile analysis for each subject is presented in Tables 26.3 and 26.4.

Case #1

Age:	47 years
Education:	17 years
Gender:	Male
Ethnicity:	Caucasian
Diagnosis:	Oligodendroglioma
Location:	Right frontal
Resection:	Yes (partial)
Radiation Therapy:	Yes
Chemotherapy:	Yes

His performance on the RIST was high average (RIST Index = 112). His performances in the attention, language, learning and memory, spatial, and executive functioning domains are considered broadly normal. Thus, he does not meet criteria for Cognitive Disorder NOS (i.e., Mild Neurocognitive Disorder).

Case #2

Age:	38 years
Education:	16 years
Gender:	Male
Ethnicity:	Caucasian
Diagnosis:	Glioblastoma Multiforme
Location:	Bifrontal
Resection:	Yes
Radiation Therapy	Yes
Chemotherapy	Yes

His performance on the RIST was average (RIST Index = 103). His performance in the language and spatial domains was broadly normal. He has *possible* impairment in the executive function domain and *probable* impairment on the attention and memory domains. Therefore, he meets criteria for Cognitive Disorder NOS (i.e., Mild Neurocognitive Disorder).

Of course, this abbreviated version of the NAB is simply one option for a battery to use with patients with brain tumors. It is meant to serve as an example. It is limited in that it does not include motor or sensory testing. These tests can be added. There are many other good choices for tests. A core co-normed battery could be created, for example, using WAIS-IV and WMS-IV subtests and then supplementing other tests in other domains of functioning (e.g., Boston Naming

Table 26.2 RIST and NAB test data for the two brain tumor case examples

| | T scores (percentile ranks) | |
Domains/tests	Case 1	Case 2
RIST Index	High Average	Average
Attention & Processing Speed		
Digits Forward	51 (54%)	49 (46%)
Digits Backward	61 (86%)	47 (38%)
Dots	55 (69%)	52 (58%)
Numbers & Letters A Speed	53 (62%)	25 (1%)
Numbers & Letters A Errors	59 (82%)	32 (4%)
Numbers & Letters B Efficiency	54 (66%)	28 (1%)
Numbers & Letters C Efficiency	52 (58%)	42 (21%)
Numbers & Letters D Efficiency	48 (42%)	26 (1%)
Numbers & Letters D Disruption	43 (24%)	46 (34%)
Driving Scenes	52 (58%)	35 (7%)
Language		
Oral Production	63 (90%)	41 (18%)
Naming	52 (58%)	52 (58%)
Learning & Memory		
List Learning A Total Immediate	49 (46%)	37 (10%)
List Learning A Long Delay Recall	58 (79%)	33 (4%)
Story Learning Immediate Recall	55 (69%)	36 (8%)
Story Learning Delayed Recall	55 (69%)	35 (7%)
Daily Living Memory Immediate	47 (38%)	44 (27%)
Daily Living Memory Delayed	58 (79%)	19 (<1%)
Spatial Abilities		
Visual Discrimination	46 (34%)	44 (27%)
Design Construction	58 (79%)	41 (18%)
Executive Functioning		
Mazes	45 (31%)	42 (21%)
Categories	58 (79%)	37 (10%)
Word Generation	67 (96%)	52 (58%)

Table 26.3 Case #1

| | Number of scores below cutoffs | | | | | |
NAB domains	<25th %ile	<16th %ile	<10th %ile	<5th %ile	<2nd %ile	Impairment in domain?
Attention & Processing Speed	1	0	0	0	0	Broadly normal
Language	0	0	0	0	0	Broadly normal
Learning and Memory	0	0	0	0	0	Broadly normal
Spatial	0	0	0	0	0	Broadly normal
Executive Functioning	0	0	0	0	0	Broadly normal

Table 26.4 Case #2

NAB domains	Number of scores below cutoffs					Impairment in domain?
	<25th %ile	<16th %ile	<10th %ile	<5th %ile	<2nd %ile	
Attention & Processing Speed	6	5	5	4	3	Probable
Language	1	0	0	0	0	Broadly normal
Learning and Memory	5	5	4	2	1	Probable
Spatial	1	0	0	0	0	Broadly normal
Executive Functioning	2	1	0	0	0	Possible

Test, Verbal Fluency tests, and other tests of executive functioning). The important point is to cover the primary domains of functioning.

Summary and Conclusions

A brain tumor is a growth of abnormal cells inside the skull cavity and can be either benign or malignant. Benign tumors grow slowly, are circumscribed, and resemble the cell of origin. Malignant tumors grow rapidly, invade and destroy neighboring cells, and vary considerably in shape and overall patterns. There are two major classifications of brain tumors: metastatic and primary. Metastatic brain tumors originate elsewhere in the body and spread to the CNS, whereas primary brain tumors originate in the brain, almost invariably from glial cells (>90%; Davis et al. 2005; Victor and Ropper 2002). Adults are twice as likely to develop a metastatic brain tumor versus a primary brain tumor. As many as 40% of patients with non-central nervous system tumors develop metastatic brain cancer. In contrast, children are twice as likely to suffer from a primary brain tumor versus a metastatic brain tumor. The peak incidence of brain tumors occur between 74 and 84 years of age. Incidence rates of brain tumors are slightly higher in males

Symptoms of brain tumors vary from patient to patient, from asymptomatic to debilitating cognitive, behavioral, and emotional changes. The most frequently reported symptom of brain tumors is headache in children and adults (Rohkamm 2004; Wilne et al. 2007). Many children and adults will also experience seizures at some point during the course of their illnesses, particularly if the tumor is in cortical structures and is slow growing (Wen 1997; Wilne et al. 2007).

Diagnosis of tumors can then be classified histopathologically according to a grading system and is made with a biopsy (National Cancer Institute 2007a). The World Health Organization (WHO) developed a four-tiered grading system, which is the most commonly employed means of classifying brain tumors (Sawrie 2006). Grade I tumors are "benign," grow slowly, and have low proliferation potential. In general, patients with Grade I tumors have the best prognosis. Grades II and III suggest malignancy, are infiltrative in nature, and have a higher proliferation potential than Grade I tumors. Grade IV tumors are the most malignant, most infiltrative, have the highest proliferation potential, and are considered prognostically, the worst.

Most brain tumors are treated surgically, with the goal of excising as much of the tumor as possible. Gross total resection is the goal. Radiation therapy and chemotherapy are also used to destroy cancer cells. After undergoing neurosurgery, many patients receive some form of radiotherapy or chemotherapy, or a combination of the two. Radiotherapy and chemotherapy are successful at destroying cancer cells, but are associated with immediate and delayed cognitive side effects (Taillibert et al. 2007; Wefel et al. 2004; Weiss 2008). Gamma-knife neurosurgery is recommended for targeting smaller tumors. Although they occur in some cases, complications are generally rare, due to limited radiation exposure.

Neuropsychological evaluation services are essential in adult and pediatric oncological settings. Neuropsychological evaluations are used to determine whether there has been cognitive decline secondary to treatment or tumor recurrence; whether a rehabilitation program can improve cognitive functioning; and whether baseline cognitive functioning can predict survival rates (Sawrie 2006). There is no accepted standard neuropsychological battery, and many evaluations employ a flexible battery approach (Lezak et al. 2004). We proposed a 2-hour battery based on the Neuropsychological Assessment Battery (NAB; Stern and White 2003), and provide guidelines for profile analysis of an abbreviated NAB based battery (Iverson and Brooks 2008a, b). This new battery, with corresponding base rate tables, allows a more evidence-based approach for identifying cognitive impairment.

References

Ahles, T. A., Saykin, A. J., Furstenberg, C. T., Cole, B., Mott, L. A., Skalla, K., et al. (2002). Neuropsychologic impact of standard-dose systemic chemotherapy in long-term survivors of breast cancer and lymphoma. *Journal of Clinical Oncology, 20*(2), 485–493.

Albright, A. L. (1993). Pediatric brain tumors. *CA: A Cancer Journal for Clinicians, 43*(5), 272–288.

American Brain Tumor Association (1993). ABTA dictionary for brain tumor patients. From http://neurosurgery.mgh.harvard.edu/abta/diction.htm. Retrieved 10 Jan 2008.

American Brain Tumor Association (2005). A primer of brain tumors (5th ed.). From http://neurosurgery.mgh.harvard.edu/abta/primer.htm. Retrieved 8 Jan 2008.

American Cancer Society. (2008). *Cancer facts & figures 2008*. Atlanta: American Cancer Society.

Anderson-Hanley, C., Sherman, M. L., Riggs, R., Agocha, V. B., & Compas, B. E. (2003). Neuropsychological effects of treatments for adults with cancer: A meta-analysis and review of the literature. *Journal of the International Neuropsychological Society, 9*(7), 967–982.

Armstrong, C. L., Goldstein, B., Shera, D., Ledakis, G. E., & Tallent, E. M. (2003). The predictive value of longitudinal neuropsychologic assessment in the early detection of brain tumor recurrence. *Cancer, 97*(3), 649–656.

Armstrong, C. L., Gyato, K., Awadalla, A. W., Lustig, R., & Tochner, Z. A. (2004). A critical review of the clinical effects of therapeutic irradiation damage to the brain: The roots of controversy. *Neuropsychology Review, 14*(1), 65–86.

Armstrong, C. L., Hunter, J. V., Ledakis, G. E., Cohen, B., Tallent, E. M., Goldstein, B. H., et al. (2002). Late cognitive and radiographic changes related to radiotherapy: Initial prospective findings. *Neurology, 59*(1), 40–48.

Arthur, P. (2005). Brain and spinal tumors. In S. L. Chamberlin & B. Narins (Eds.), *The gale encyclopedia of neurological disorders* (pp. 176–180). Detroit: Thomson Gale.

Behin, A., Hoang-Xuan, K., Carpentier, A. F., & Delattre, J. Y. (2003). Primary brain tumours in adults. *Lancet, 361*(9354), 323–331.

Bosma, I., Vos, M. J., Heimans, J. J., Taphoorn, M. J., Aaronson, N. K., Postma, T. J., et al. (2007). The course of neurocognitive functioning in high-grade glioma patients. *Journal of Neuro-Oncology, 9*(1), 53–62.

Bray, F., Sankila, R., Ferlay, J., & Parkin, D. M. (2002). Estimates of cancer incidence and mortality in Europe in 1995. *European Journal of Cancer, 38*(1), 99–166.

Buizer, A. I., de Sonneville, L. M., & Veerman, A. J. (2009). Effects of chemotherapy on neurocognitive function in children with acute lymphoblastic leukemia: A critical review of the literature. *Pediatric Blood & Cancer, 52*(4), 447–454.

Carriage, M. T., & Henson, D. E. (1995). The histologic grading of cancer. *Cancer, 75,* 406–421.

Castellon, S. A., Ganz, P. A., Bower, J. E., Petersen, L., Abraham, L., & Greendale, G. A. (2004). Neurocognitive performance in breast cancer survivors exposed to adjuvant chemotherapy and tamoxifen. *Journal of Clinical and Experimental Neuropsychology, 26*(7), 955–969.

Central Brain Tumor Registry of the United States (2005, 2006). Primary brain tumors in the United States Statistical Report 1998–2002. From http://www.cbtrus.org/reports//2005-2006/2006report.pdf. Retrieved 9 July 2008.

Central Brain Tumor Registry of the United States (2008). Fact sheet. Retrieved July 13, 2008, from http://www.cbtrus.org/factsheet/factsheet.html

Chelune, G. J., Naugle, R. I., Luders, H., Sedlak, J., & Awad, I. A. (1993). Individual change after epilepsy surgery: Practice effects and base-rate information. *Neuropsychology, 7,* 41–52.

Crawford, J. R., MacDonald, T. J., & Packer, R. J. (2007). Medulloblastoma in childhood: New biological advances. *Lancet Neurology, 6*(12), 1073–1085.

Cummings, J. L., & Trimble, M. R. (2002). *Neuropsychiatry and behavioral neurology* (2nd ed.). Washington: American Psychiatric Publishing.

Davis, L. E., King, M. K., & Schultz, J. L. (2005). *Fundamentals of neurologic disease.* New York: Demos Medical Publishing.

Debnam, J. M., Ketonen, L., Hamberg, L. M., & Hunter, G. J. (2007). Radiology of brain tumors: Structure and physiology. In F. DeMonte, M. R. Gilbert, A. Mahajan, & I. E. McCutcheon's (Eds.), *Tumors of the brain and spine* (pp. 37–51). New York: Springer.

El-Zein, R., Bondy, M., & Wrensch, M. (2005). Epidemiology of brain tumors. In F. Ali-Osman (Ed.), *Brain tumors* (pp. 3–18). Totowa: Humana Press.

Glosser, G., McManus, P., Munzenrider, J., Austin-Seymour, M., Fullerton, B., Adams, J., et al. (1997). Neuropsychological function in adults after high dose fractionated radiation therapy of skull base tumors. *International Journal of Radiation Oncology, Biology, Physics, 38*(2), 231–239.

Gregor, A., Cull, A., Traynor, E., Stewart, M., Lander, F., & Love, S. (1996). Neuropsychometric evaluation of long-term survivors of adult brain tumours: Relationship with tumour and treatment parameters. *Radiotherapy and Oncology, 41*(1), 55–59.

Haberland, C. (2007). *Clinical neuropathology.* New York: Demos Medical Publishing.

Harder, H., Holtel, H., Bromberg, J. E., Poortmans, P., Haaxma-Reiche, H., Kluin-Nelemans, H. C., et al. (2004). Cognitive status and quality of life after treatment for primary CNS lymphoma. *Neurology, 62*(4), 544–547.

Hoppe-Hirsch, E., Renier, D., Lellouch-Tubiana, A., Sainte-Rose, C., Pierre-Kahn, A., & Hirsch, J. F. (1990). Medulloblastoma in childhood: Progressive intellectual deterioration. *Child's Nervous System, 6*(2), 60–65.

Inskip, P. D., & Ron, E. (2006). Brain and other central nervous system cancer. In L. S. Freedman, B. K. Edwards, L. A. G. Ries, & J. L. Young (Eds.), *Cancer incidence in four member countries (Cyprus, Egypt, Israel, and Jordan) of the Middle East Cancer Consortium (MECC) compared with US SEER* (pp. 111–120). Bethesda: National Cancer Institute. NIH Pub. No. 06-5873. From http://seer.cancer.gov/publications/mecc/mecc_brain.pdf. Retrieved 13 July 2008.

Iverson, G. L., & Brooks, B. L. (2008a). Improving accuracy for identifying cognitive impairment. In M. R. Schoenberg & J. G. Scott (Eds.), *The black book of neuropsychology: A syndrome-based approach*. New York: Springer.

Iverson, G. L., & Brooks, B. L. (2008b). New psychometric criteria for DSM-IV cognitive disorder NOS (abstract). *Journal of the International Neuropsychological Society*.

Iverson, G. L., Brooks, B. L., White, T., & Stern, R. A. (2008). Neuropsychological Assessment Battery (NAB): Introduction and advanced interpretation. In A. M. Horton Jr. & D. Wedding (Eds.), *The neuropsychology handbook* (3rd ed., pp. 279–343). New York: Springer.

Jacobson, N. S., & Truax, P. (1991). Clinical significance: A statistical approach to defining meaningful change in psychotherapy research. *Journal of Consulting and Clinical Psychology, 59*(1), 12–19.

Jawahar, A., Willis, B. K., Smith, D. R., Ampil, F., Datta, R., & Nanda, A. (2002). Gamma knife radiosurgery for brain metastases: Do patients benefit from adjuvant external-beam radiotherapy? An 18-month comparative analysis. *Stereotactic and Functional Neurosurgery, 79*(3–4), 262–271.

Jemal, A., Siegel, R., Ward, E., Hao, Y., Xu, J., Murray, T., et al. (2008). Cancer statistics, 2008. *CA: A Cancer Journal for Clinicians, 58*(2), 71–96.

Kaleita, T. A., Wellisch, D. K., Cloughesy, T. F., Ford, J. M., Freeman, D., Belin, T. R., et al. (2004). Prediction of neurocognitive outcome in adult brain tumor patients. *Journal of Neurooncology, 67*(1–2), 245–253.

Kannarkat, G., Lasher, E. E., & Schiff, D. (2007). Neurologic complications of chemotherapy agents. *Current Opinion in Neurology, 20*(6), 719–725.

Karajannis, M., Allen, J. C., & Newcomb, E. W. (2008). Treatment of pediatric brain tumors. *Journal of Cellular Physiology, 217*(3), 584–589.

Kaye, A. H. (2005). *Essential neurosurgery* (3rd ed.). Oxford: Blackwell.

Kebudi, R., Ayan, I., Gorgun, O., Agaoglu, F. Y., Vural, S., & Darendeliler, E. (2005). Brain metastasis in pediatric extracranial solid tumors: Survey and literature review. *Journal of Neurooncology, 71*(1), 43–48.

Keles, G. E., Cha, S., & Berger, M. S. (2007). Magnetic resonance spectroscopy. In G. H. Barnett (Ed.), *High-grade gliomas: Diagnosis and treatment* (pp. 133–140). Totowa: Humana Press.

Keles, G. E., Tihan, T., Burton, E., & Berger, M. (2006). Low-Grade Astrocytoma. In J. C. Tonn, M. Wetphal, J. T. Rutka, & A. Grossman (Eds.), *Neuro-oncology of CNS tumor* (pp. 104–117). New York: Springer.

Kieffer-Renaux, V., Viguier, D., Raquin, M. A., Laurent-Vannier, A., Habrand, J. L., Dellatolas, G., et al. (2005). Therapeutic schedules influence the pattern of intellectual decline after irradiation of posterior fossa tumors. *Pediatric Blood & Cancer, 45*(6), 814–819.

Klein, M., Taphoorn, M. J., Heimans, J. J., van der Ploeg, H. M., Vandertop, W. P., Smit, E. F., et al. (2001). Neurobehavioral status and health-related quality of life in newly diagnosed high-grade glioma patients. *Journal of Clinical Oncology, 19*(20), 4037–4047.

Klener, P. (1999). Chemotherapy side effects and their management. In J. Klastersky, S. Scimpff, & S. Hans-Jarg (Eds.), *Supportive care in cancer a handbook for oncologists* (2nd ed.). New York: Marcel Dekker.

Kulkarni, A. V., & McDonald, P. (2006). Meningiomas. In J. C. Tonn, M. Wetphal, J. T. Rutka, & S. A. Grossman (Eds.), *Neuro-oncology of CNS tumor* (pp. 485–490). New York: Springer.

Langer, T., Martus, P., Ottensmeier, H., Hertzberg, H., Beck, J. D., & Meier, W. (2002). CNS late-effects after ALL therapy in childhood. Part III: Neuropsychological performance in long-term survivors of childhood ALL: Impairments of concentration, attention, and memory. *Medical and Pediatric Oncology, 38*(5), 320–328.

Larson, D. A., & Wara, W. M. (1998). Radiotherapy of primary malignant brain tumors. *Seminars in Surgical Oncology, 14*(1), 34–42.

Lassman, A. B., & DeAngelis, L. M. (2003). Brain metastases. *Neurologic Clinics, 21*(1), 1–23. vii.

Lezak, M. D., Howieson, D. B., & Loring, D. W. (2004). *Neuropsychological assessment* (4th ed.). New York: Oxford University Press.

Louis, D. N., Ohgaki, H., Wiestler, O. D., Cavenee, W. K., Burger, P. C., Jouvet, A., et al. (2007). The 2007 WHO classification of tumours of the central nervous system. *Acta Neuropathologica, 114*(2), 97–109.

Mabbott, D. J., Penkman, L., Witol, A., Strother, D., & Bouffet, E. (2008). Core neurocognitive functions in children treated for posterior fossa tumors. *Neuropsychology, 22*(2), 159–168.

Mantani, A., & Israel, M. A. (2001). Brain tumors. In M. Schwab (Ed.), *Encyclopedic reference of cancer* (pp. 131–134). New York: Springer.

Mehta, M. P., Rodrigus, P., Terhaard, C. H., Rao, A., Suh, J., Roa, W., et al. (2003). Survival and neurologic outcomes in a randomized trial of motexafin gadolinium and whole-brain radiation therapy in brain metastases. *Journal of Clinical Oncology, 21*(13), 2529–2536.

Meyers, C. A. (2002). Cancer patients, cognitive function. In V. S. Ramachandran (Ed.), *Encyclopedia of the human brain* (pp. 587–593). New York: Academic.

Meyers, C. A., Hess, K. R., Yung, W. K., & Levin, V. A. (2000). Cognitive function as a predictor of survival in patients with recurrent malignant glioma. *Journal of Clinical Oncology, 18*(3), 646–650.

Meyers, C. A., Smith, J. A., Bezjak, A., Mehta, M. P., Liebmann, J., Illidge, T., et al. (2004). Neurocognitive function and progression in patients with brain metastases treated with whole-brain radiation and motexafin gadolinium: Results of a randomized phase III trial. *Journal of Clinical Oncology, 22*(1), 157–165.

Mulhern, R. K., Merchant, T. E., Gajjar, A., Reddick, W. E., & Kun, L. E. (2004). Late neurocognitive sequelae in survivors of brain tumours in childhood. *The Lancet Oncology, 5*(7), 399–408.

National Cancer Institute (2007a). Adult brain tumors treatment. From http://www.meb.uni-bonn.de/cancer.gov/CDR0000062697.html. Retrieved 8 Jan 2008.

National Cancer Institute (2007b). Brain cancer. From http://www.nlm.nih.gov/medlineplus/braincancer.html#cat63. Retrieved 20 Nov 2007.

Nitta, T., & Sato, K. (1995). Prognostic implications of the extent of surgical resection in patients with intracranial malignant gliomas. *Cancer, 75*(11), 2727–2731.

Nolte, J. (2002). *The human brain: An introduction to its function anatomy* (5th ed.). St. Louis: Mosby.

Packer, R. J., Cogen, P., Vezina, G., & Rorke, L. B. (1999). Medulloblastoma: Clinical and biologic aspects. *Journal of Neuro-Oncology, 1*(3), 232–250.

Packer, R. J., Sutton, L. N., Atkins, T. E., Radcliffe, J., Bunin, G. R., D'Angio, G., et al. (1989). A prospective study of cognitive function in children receiving whole-brain radiotherapy and chemotherapy: 2-Year results. *Journal of Neurosurgery, 70*(5), 707–713.

Pollack, I. F. (1999). Pediatric brain tumors. *Seminars in Surgical Oncology, 16*(2), 73–90.

Raizer, J. (2006). Radiosurgery and whole-brain radiation therapy for brain metastases: Either or both as the optimal treatment. *The Journal of the American Medical Association, 295*(21), 2535–2536.

Reifenberger, G., Blumcke, I., Pietsch, T., & Paulus, W. (2006). Pathology and classification of tumors of the nervous system. In J. C. Tonn, M. Wetphal, J. T. Rutka, & S. A. Grossman (Eds.), *Neuro-oncology of CNS tumor* (pp. 3–72). New York: Springer.

Reynolds, C. R., & Kamphaus, R. W. (2003). *Reynolds intellectual assessment scales and Reynolds intellectual screening test professional manual*. Lutz: Psychological Assessment Resources.

Ries, L. A. G., Melbert, D., Krapcho, M., Stinchcomb, D. G., Howlader, N., Horner, M. J., et al. (2007). *SEER cancer statistics review, 1975–2005*. Bethesda: National Cancer Institute. From http://seer.cancer.gov/csr/1975_2005/. Retrieved 7 July 2008.

Rohkamm, R. (2004). *Color atlas of neurology*. NY: Thieme Stuttgart.

Rohlman, D. S., Gimenes, L. S., Eckerman, D. A., Kang, S. K., Farahat, F. M., & Anger, W. K. (2003). Development of the behavioral assessment and research system (BARS) to detect and characterize neurotoxicity in humans. *Neurotoxicology, 24*(4–5), 523–531.

Ropper, A. H., & Brown, R. H. (2005). *Adams and Victor's principles of neurology* (8th ed.). New York: McGraw-Hill.

Ruddon, R. W. (2007). *Cancer biology* (4th ed.). Oxford: Oxford University Press.

Sawrie, S. M. (2006). The neuropsychology of adult neuro-onchology. In P. J. Snyder, P. D. Nussenbaum, & D. L. Robins (Eds.), *Clinical neuropsychology* (2nd ed., pp. 415–435). Washington: American Psychological Association.

Sawrie, S. M., Chelune, G. J., Naugle, R. I., & Luders, H. O. (1996). Empirical methods for assessing meaningful neuropsychological change following epilepsy surgery. *Journal of the International Neuropsychological Society, 2*(6), 556–564.

Schiffer, D. (2006). *Brain tumor pathology: Current diagnostic hotspots and pitfalls.* Dordrecht: Springer.

Sheetz, M. (2009). Physical presence during gamma stereotactic radiosurgery. *Health Physics, 96*(2 Suppl), S11–15.

Sin, A. H., Cardenas, R. J., Vannemreddy, P., & Nanda, A. (2009). Gamma Knife stereotactic radiosurgery for intracranial metastases from conventionally radioresistant primary cancers: Outcome analysis of survival and control of brain disease. *Southern Medical Journal, 102*(1), 42–44.

Steering Committee of the National Cancer Institute of Canada and the Canadian Cancer Society (2005). Canadian cancer statistics 2005. From www.cancer.ca/vgn/images/portal/cit_8675111 4/48/28/401594768cw_2005stats_en.pdf. Retrieved 20 Nov 2004.

Stern, R. A., & White, T. (2003). *Neuropsychological assessment battery.* Lutz: Psychological Assessment Resources.

Stuschke, M., Eberhardt, W., Pottgen, C., Stamatis, G., Wilke, H., Stuben, G., et al. (1999). Prophylactic cranial irradiation in locally advanced non-small-cell lung cancer after multimodality treatment: Long-term follow-up and investigations of late neuropsychologic effects. *Journal of Clinical Oncology, 17*(9), 2700–2709.

Surma-aho, O., Niemela, M., Vilkki, J., Kouri, M., Brander, A., Salonen, O., et al. (2001). Adverse long-term effects of brain radiotherapy in adult low-grade glioma patients. *Neurology, 56*(10), 1285–1290.

Taillibert, S., Voillery, D., & Bernard-Marty, C. (2007). Chemobrain: Is systemic chemotherapy neurotoxic? *Current Opinion in Oncology, 19*(6), 623–627.

Taphoorn, M. J., & Klein, M. (2004). Cognitive deficits in adult patients with brain tumours. *Lancet Neurology, 3*(3), 159–168.

Taylor, M. D. (2006). Medulloblastoma. In J. C. Tonn, M. Wetphal, J. T. Rutka, & S. A. Grossman (Eds.), *Neuro-oncology of CNS tumor* (pp. 461–469). New York: Springer.

Torpy, J. M., Lynm, C., & Glass, R. M. (2005). JAMA patient page. Brain tumors. *The Journal of the American Medical Association, 293*(5), 644.

Torres, I. J., Mundt, A. J., Sweeney, P. J., Llanes-Macy, S., Dunaway, L., Castillo, M., et al. (2003). A longitudinal neuropsychological study of partial brain radiation in adults with brain tumors. *Neurology, 60*(7), 1113–1118.

van Effenterre, R., & Boch, A.-L. (2006). Craniopharyngiomas. In J. C. Tonn, M. Wetphal, J. T. Rutka, & S. A. Grossman (Eds.), *Neuro-oncology of CNS tumor* (pp. 505–515). New York: Springer.

Victor, M., & Ropper, A. H. (2002). *Adams and Victor's manual of neurology* (7th ed.). New York: McGraw-Hill.

Weber, J. T. (2007). Experimental models of repetitive brain injuries. *Progress in Brain Research, 161*, 253–261.

Wefel, J. S., Kayl, A. E., & Meyers, C. A. (2004). Neuropsychological dysfunction associated with cancer and cancer therapies: A conceptual review of an emerging target. *British Journal of Cancer, 90*(9), 1691–1696.

Weingart, J. D., McGirt, M. J., & Brem, H. (2006). High-Grade astrocytoma/glioblastoma. In J. C. Tonn, M. Wetphal, J. T. Rutka, & S. A. Grossman (Eds.), *Neuro-oncology of CNS tumor* (pp. 127–138). New York: Springer.

Weiss, B. (2008). Chemobrain: A translational challenge for neurotoxicology. *Neurotoxicology, 29*(5), 891–8. Available online 9 April 2008.

Weller, M. (2006). Oligodendroglioma. In J. C. Tonn, M. Wetphal, J. T. Rutka, & S. A. Grossman (Eds.), *Neuro-oncology of CNS tumor* (pp. 139–144). New York: Springer.

Wen, P. Y. (1997). Diagnosis and management of brain tumors. In P. Black & J. S. Loeffler (Eds.), *Cancer of the nervous system* (pp. 106–127). Cambridge: Blackwell Science.

Wen, P. Y., Teoh, S. K., & Black, P. M. (2001). Clinical, imaging, and laboratory diagnosis of brain tumors. In A. H. Kaye & E. R. Laws (Eds.), *Brain tumors: An encylopedic approach* (2nd ed., pp. 217–248). London: Churchill Livingstone.

Westphal, M. (2006). Ependymomas and ventricular tumors. In J. C. Tonn, M. Wetphal, J. T. Rutka, & S. A. Grossman (Eds.), *Neuro-oncology of CNS tumor* (pp. 145–157). New York: Springer.

Westphal, M., Lamszus, K., & Tonn, J.-C. (2006). Meningiomas and meningeal tumors. In J. C. Tonn, M. Wetphal, J. T. Rutka, & S. A. Grossman (Eds.), *Neuro-oncology of CNS Tumor* (pp. 81–101). New York: Springer.

Wetjen, N., & Raffel, C. (2006). Ependymomas. In J. C. Tonn, M. Wetphal, J. T. Rutka, & S. A. Grossman (Eds.), *Neuro-oncology of CNS Tumor* (pp. 453–460). New York: Springer.

Wilne, S., Collier, J., Kennedy, C., Koller, K., Grundy, R., & Walker, D. (2007). Presentation of childhood CNS tumours: A systematic review and meta-analysis. *The Lancet Oncology, 8*(8), 685–695.

Yang, L., Parkin, D. M., Ferlay, J., Li, L., & Chen, Y. (2005). Estimates of cancer incidence in China for 2000 and projections for 2005. *Cancer Epidemiology, Biomarkers & Prevention, 14*(1), 243–250.

Chapter 27
Neurotoxicity in Neuropsychology

Raymond Singer

Abstract This chapter will provide definitions regarding neurotoxicity, general principles of neurotoxic damage, symptom presentation for common neurotoxic substances, a brief discussion of symptoms/features of the Neurotoxicity Syndrome, and assessment for neurotoxicity.

Key Points and Chapter Summary

- Neurotoxicity is a significant cause of neuropsychological impairment
- Because any nervous system structure or function can be damaged by neurotoxicants, neurotoxicity can be the origin of many common neurologic and psychologic symptoms
- Many types of neurotoxicity are not well recognized among health professionals. The identification of neuropsychological and/or behavioral deficits related to neurotoxic exposure requires awareness and knowledge of neuropsychology and neurotoxicology.
- The chronic symptoms of neurotoxicity include effects on attention/concentration, executive function, learning, information acquisition and consolidation, and emotion. Autonomic functions are also often adversely affected.
- The chronic symptoms of neurotoxicity are similar with many neurotoxicants, and some have proposed the Neurotoxicity Syndrome to describe this constellation of symptoms.
- Neuropsychological assessment is helpful in identifying subtle cognitive and behavioral deficits related to neurotoxic exposure
- The Neurotoxicity Syndrome can be diagnosed with appropriate neuropsychological evaluation procedures.

R. Singer (✉)
National Academy of Neuropsychology, Association for Psychological Science, American Psychological Association, Santa Fe, NM, USA
e-mail: ray.singer@gmail.com

M.R. Schoenberg and J.G. Scott (eds.), *The Little Black Book of Neuropsychology: A Syndrome-Based Approach*, DOI 10.1007/978-0-387-76978-3_27,
© Springer Science+Business Media, LLC 2011

Definitions

Neurotoxicity describes the harmful effects of neurotoxicants (neurotoxic substances and agents) on the nervous system, which can adversely affect cognitive, emotional, behavioral and physical domains. Neurobehavioral toxicity describes the adverse effects of neurotoxicants via neural processes on behavior and neuropsychological function. The symptoms and signs of neurotoxicity may include aspects of neurological, cognitive, behavioral, and affective dysfunction, as neurotoxicants can damage any nervous system structure or function.

Neurotoxicology has had important ramifications for the study of the nervous system and neurological disease. For example, the identification of MPTP (1-methyl-4-phenyl-1,2,3,6-tetrahydropyridine) and its metabolite MPP+ (1-methyl-4-phenylpyridiniuma) as the etiology for a parkinsonian motor disorder due to selective damage to cells in the substantia nigra resulted in advances in our understanding of the neurophysiology of the basal ganglia and Parkinson's disease (Fahn 2002).

As of 1985, more than 850 chemicals had been identified as capable producers of neurobehavioral disorders (Anger and Johnson 1985). The most commonly encountered neurotoxic substances include solvents, metals, pesticides, carbon monoxide, and mold (products of repeated water intrusion). A comprehensive review of the hundreds of agents with toxic effects to humans is beyond the scope of this chapter. Rather, this chapter will provide a review of some commonly encountered toxic substances, and the common neurologic, neuropsychologic, and psychologic effects of exposure. This field of study has become so complex and vast that it is difficult to refer to a comprehensive text. However, the following citations are offered to the interested reader as introductions to the topic (Singer 1990a; Congress and Office of Technology Assessment 1990; Brown 2002; Berent 2005; Kilburn 2004, and Hartman 1995).

Categories of Neurotoxic Agents

Common classes of neurotoxic chemicals include solvents, metals, organophosphates (pesticides), some gases, and the products of repeated indoor water intrusions (mold). Definitions for these classes of neurotoxic substances are reviewed below, followed by more detailed discussion of the recommended neuropsychological evaluation of individuals with known or suspected toxic exposure. In addition, Table 27.1 summarizes the exposure route, common uses, and some of the common acute toxic symptoms of exposure to selected metals, organophosphates, solvents, glycols, and gases.

Organic Solvents (Glues, Cleaning Materials, Varnishes, etc.)

A solvent is a liquid or gas that dissolves a solid, liquid, or gas, resulting in a solution. The most common solvent in everyday life is water. Most other commonly-used

Table 27.1 Major neurotoxic substances and their acute symptoms

Neurotoxic substance class	Exposure route	Common use/exposure	A sample of commonly identified acute symptoms
Metals			
Lead	Inhalation, ingestion	Pre-1960 paint pigmentation; manufacturing production of batteries, lead smelting, brass and copper foundries. Also found in occupations employing lead soldering such as automotive repair and electronics repair	*Inorganic lead*: Systemic pain, joint swelling, constipation, anemia, peripheral neuropathy (historically, foot or wrist drop/weakness) *Organic lead* (found in gasoline in developing countries): Memory impairment, concentration deficits, restlessness, agitation, psychosis and delirium in high concentrations in adults, significant cognitive developmental delays in children
Mercury	Inhalation, ingestion, dermal absorption	Mercury mining, occupations using mercury such as electrical switch manufacturing, chemical production of fungicides, pesticides, and wood preservatives that involve methyl mercury applications: Accidental exposures from multiple broken older thermometers, thermostats and fluorescent lamps	Cerebral encephalopathy, oral hemorrhage, auditory/visual hallucinations, fine motor tremor, insomnia, agitation
Arsenic	Ingestion, inhalation	Industrial applications of pesticides, wood preservatives or agricultural applications; suicide and homicide	Skin rash, gastro-intestinal distress, cardiac arrhythmia, mouth and throat irritation, peripheral neuropathy
Manganese	Inhalation (accumulation is slow)	Manganese mining, manufacturing of batteries, welding rods, fertilizers	Restlessness, agitation, insomnia, anorexia, ataxia, dysarthria, muscle rigidity, parkinsonian symptoms (akinesia, hypertonicity, tremor, ataxia)
Organophosphates (pesticides)			
Malathion/parathion	Inhalation, ingestion, dermal absorption	Primary intoxication occurs in industrial production and agricultural application, but home exposure from improper use or abuse can occur	Weakness, blurred vision, nausea, headache, fatigue, diaphoresis

(continued)

Table 27.1 (continued)

Neurotoxic substance class	Exposure route	Common use/exposure	A sample of commonly identified acute symptoms
Solvents			
Alcohols (includes *Isopropyl alcohol*, *Methyl alcohol* (Methanol), *Ethyl alcohol* (Ethanol))	Primary ingestion, but can be inhalation	*Ethanol*; consumable alcohol *Isopropyl Alcohol*; (rubbing alcohol) Antiseptic, dissolvent, automobile fluids *Methanol*; (wood or cellulose alcohol) engine fuel, aerosol solvent, industrial applications as a solvent and antifreeze	*Ethanol*; CNS depressant, sedation, incoordination, dysarthria *Isopropyl Alcohol*; CNS depressant, much more potent for intoxication than ethanol. Greater neurotoxic effect from breakdown process in the liver to acetone. *Methanol*; Highly toxic-acute blindness. Secondary toxic effect caused by metabolite formation of formaldehyde and subsequently formic acid causing death.
Hydrocarbons (include *Hexene*, *Benzene*, *Toluene*)	Inhalation, ingestion	Commonly used in aerosol applications, cleaning fluids and degreasing agents	Nystagmus, ataxia, incoordination, tremor, cognitive impairment, dysarthria, lethargy, delirium
Halogenated Hydrocarbons (includes *carbon tetrachloride*, *trichlorethane* and *trichloroethylene*)	Inhalation, dermal absorption	Predominately industrial/occupational exposure as dry cleaning solutions, degreasing solutions, and lubrication solvent	Skin rash, peripheral anesthesia if dermal exposure, disorientation, nausea, vomiting if high dose inhalation or if consumed orally
Glycols (includes ethylene glycol, propylene glycol)	Ingestion	Antifreeze, deicers	Transient agitation followed by convulsions, myoclonic jerking, nystagmus, opthalmoplegias
Gases (includes *carbon monoxide* and *carbon dioxide*)	Inhalation	Byproduct of improper combustion or ventilation of fossil fuels	Headache, nausea, dizziness, blurred vision, lethargy, coma

solvents are organic (carbon-containing) chemicals, termed organic solvents. Solvents usually have a low boiling point and evaporate easily, leaving the dissolved substance behind. Common uses for organic solvents are in dry cleaning (e.g., tetrachloroethylene [AKA perchloroethylene; abbreviated as "perc" in the industry and "dry-cleaning fluid" by the public]), as paint thinners (e.g., toluene, turpentine), as nail polish removers and glue solvents (acetone, methyl acetate, ethyl acetate), in spot removers (e.g., hexane, ether), in detergents (citrus terpenes), in perfumes (ethanol), and in chemical syntheses. Many fuels are neurotoxic solvents, including gasoline and diesel.

Metals

In chemistry, a metal is a chemical element whose atoms readily lose electrons to form positive ions (cations), and form metallic bonds between other metal atoms and ionic bonds between nonmetal atoms. A "heavy metal" is a member of an ill-defined subset of elements that exhibit metallic properties. Many different definitions have been proposed – some based on density, some on atomic number or atomic weight, and some on chemical properties or toxicity. An alternative term exists, "toxic metal," for which there also is no consensus of exact definition. Common metals with neurotoxic effects include arsenic, cadmium, lead, manganese, mercury, and thallium.

The toxic effects of lead are reviewed in detail below. Manganese is a known neurotoxicant, capable of producing a parkinsonian syndrome due to extrapyramidal dysfunction. Manganese exposure has been reported to result in neuropsychological and psychological impairments (e.g., Bowler et al. 2006). A primary target of manganese appears to be the dopaminergic neurons in the striatum. Labeled as manganese-induced parkinsonism, the movement disorder has many features similar to idiopathic Parkinson's disease, but there are differences, including reduced response to levodopa treatment. Some research suggested that welders are at increased risk for development of parkinsonism than the general population, with greater prevalence of parkinsonism and onset of symptoms at an earlier age (Racette et al. 2001). However, a recent large study failed to show an increased risk for mortality due to parkinsonism or other neurodegenerative diseases for welders when compared to other peers (Stampfer 2009). Neuropsychological deficits from manganese include impaired psychomotor speed, visuomotor/visuoperceptual skills, verbal fluency (phonemic), working memory/divided attention, and delayed memory. High rates of depression, anxiety, and confusion has also been reported. See Lucchini et al. (2009) for a comprehensive review.

Pesticides

A pesticide is a substance or mixture of substances used to kill a pest. A pesticide may be a chemical substance, biological agent (such as a virus or bacteria), antimicrobial, disinfectant or device used against any pest. Pests include insects, plant pathogens, weeds, mollusks, birds, mammals, fish, nematodes (roundworms) and/or microbes. Although there may be benefits to the use of some pesticides, there are also drawbacks, such as potential toxicity to humans and other animals. Common pesticides include organophosphates, organochlorines, synthetic pyrethroids and toxic metals.

Gases

Some gases are toxic (e.g., Chlorine), while others can be classified as simple asphyxiants. Some toxic gases are corrosive (e.g., Chlorine), in which damage is done directly to tissues and organs (Chlorine damages the lungs). Asphyxia is a condition of severely deficient supply of oxygen to the brain from dysfunctional respiration. Hypoxia describes the condition of reduced oxygen supply to the brain. Since brain cells require almost a constant supply of oxygen to maintain their life, reduced oxygen supply can kill or disable brain cells.

An *asphyxiant* gas is an otherwise nontoxic or minimally-toxic gas which dilutes or displaces oxygen and creates a deficient supply of oxygen to the brain, which can result in hypoxia and ischemia (see Chap. 13, this volume, for details on stroke). Because simple asphyxiant gases are otherwise relatively non-toxic, their dangerous effects may not be noticed until harm is done. An asphyxiant gas (such as carbon monoxide) causes hypoxia by competing with oxygen.

Carbon monoxide, chemical formula CO, is a colorless, odorless, tasteless, yet highly toxic gas. Its molecules consist of one carbon atom covalently bonded to one oxygen atom. Carbon monoxide is produced from the partial oxidation of carbon-containing compounds, notably in internal-combustion engines and gas heaters. Carbon monoxide forms in preference to the more usual carbon dioxide when there is a reduced availability of oxygen present during the combustion process. Carbon monoxide is produced by common household appliances, such as gas space and water heaters. When not properly ventilated, carbon monoxide emitted by these appliances can concentrate to toxic levels

The most common symptoms of CO poisoning are headache, dizziness, weakness, nausea, vomiting, chest pain, and confusion. High levels of CO inhalation can cause loss of consciousness and death. Unless suspected, CO poisoning can be difficult to diagnose because the symptoms mimic other illnesses. People who are sleeping or intoxicated can die from CO poisoning before ever experiencing symptoms.

Carbon monoxide is a leading cause of accidental deaths in America, and has been termed the "Silent Killer." Persons with CO poisoning, as well as their treating doctors, may be unaware of the cause of their symptoms (e.g., headache, nausea, dizziness, or confusion). During 1999–2004, CO poisoning was listed as a contributing cause of death on 16,447 death certificates in the United States. An estimated 11,000 cases of carbon monoxide poisoning among patients presenting to a hospital emergency room could potentially go undetected each year in the United States, if proper screening of all patients for possible CO poisoning is not employed (Suner et al. 2008).

The effect of CO poisoning may not be dose-dependent in some cases, as patients with less severe CO poisoning have exhibited similar cognitive and emotional impairment as those exposed to higher levels of CO. (e.g., Chambers et al. 2008; but their methodology and conclusions have been criticized by Kulig et al. (2009)). Chambers et al. (2008) compared patients identified as having more and less severe CO exposure. Of the 55 patients identified as having less severe CO poisoning, 39% exhibited some cognitive deficits, 21% had depressive symptoms, and 30% of patients reported significant anxiety symptoms 6 weeks after exposure. Of the 201 patients with more severe CO poisoning, 35% had neuropsychological deficits, 16% reported depressive symptoms, and 11% had symptoms of anxiety at 6 weeks after exposure. The prevalence of cognitive dysfunction did not significantly differ between groups at 6 weeks, 6 months, or 12-month follow-up visits. Symptoms of depression and anxiety were commonly reported for both groups.

Mold

Mold neurotoxicity describes the poisonous effects on the human nervous system of mold, mycotoxins and bacteria, which can result from repeated indoor water intrusions. Although not widely known, indoor water intrusions that cause mold infestations also cause growth of various bacterial products that can also be neurotoxic (e.g., Cunningham et al. 2005; Thrasher and Crawley 2009). All the mold and bacterial species from repeated indoor water intrusions that impact human health, as well as the toxic components, have not yet been identified. However, the most common toxic molds include: *Stachybotrys chartarum* (*S. chartarum*), *Aspergillus* spp, *Cladosporium* spp, *Fusarium* spp, and *Penicillium* spp.

Symptoms of chronic mold neurotoxicity that have been reported include difficulty with concentration, learning/memory, sleep, headache, executive dysfunction, personality changes, and other cognitive impairments (see Kilburn 2009; Singer and Gray 2007; Singer 2005a, b).

Notably neurotoxic are the mycotoxins that are emitted by molds, such as trichothecenes, which can be produced by common indoor molds, such as stachybotrys. This substance has been used for biological warfare (Wanamaker and Wiener 1997). Acute effects include anorexia, lassitude, and nausea.

Additional interesting mycotoxins include ergots, generated from *Aspergillus* fumigates, the most common fungal airborne pathogen of humans. *Aspergillus* fumigates are associated with air quality issues in indoor environments, and can produce ergot alkaloids in both culture and in the environment (Panaccione and Coyle 2005). Species of the common indoor mold *Penicillium* can also produce ergot alkaloids. LSD is an ergot mycotoxin, and was first synthesized by Albert Hofmann in 1938 from *ergot*, a grain fungus that grows on rye. Ergot neurotoxicity has occurred in various epidemics in Europe, sometimes associated with non-rational religious movements (Packer 1998). Unexplained delusions or psychosis could be related to ergot mycotoxins under significant indoor moldy conditions.

Definition of Exposure and Symptom Terms for Neurotoxic Agents

Acute exposure is defined as contact with a substance that occurs once or for only a short time (up to 14 days).

Acute effects describe health effects that appear at the time of, or soon after exposure, that persist in a biologic system for only a short time, generally less than a week. The effects can range from symptomless signs, to behavioral changes, to death.

Intermediate duration exposure is defined as contact with a substance that occurs for more than 14 days and less than a year.

Chronic exposure is defined as contact with a substance that occurs over a long time (more than 1 year)

A *chronic health effect* is an adverse health effect persisting for months or years.

The Neurotoxicity Syndrome is a term used or proposed to describe the constellation of chronic symptoms of individuals with neurotoxic exposure. The syndrome reportedly may present from both high-level or repeated low-level exposures. See below for the common symptoms of this condition.

Principals of Identifying and Evaluating Neurotoxic Exposure

Acute and Chronic Symptom Presentation for Two Common Neurotoxic Agents

Acute (short-term) effects of neurotoxic substances certainly vary. Organophosphate poisoning produces hallmark, pathognomonic symptoms, yet the chronic nervous system effects are similar to that of other neurotoxic substances. Lead poisoning also produces commonly recognized acute symptoms, with similar chronic neurotoxic effects as other neurotoxic substances.

Organophosphates (OP's)

Organophosphates are a common ingredient in many pesticides, and are also used as solvents, plasticizers, and extreme pressure lubricants additives. As a pesticide, OPs include compounds that are some of the most toxic chemicals used in agriculture, and as an insecticide are fast acting. An OP tricresyl phosphate (TCP) is used as a gasoline additive.

Acute symptoms

Acute symptoms of OP poisoning will be many, because of the widespread nature and function of the various neurochemical receptors affected by OPs. Acute exposure to high level organophosphates can lead to a variety of acute symptoms affecting multi-organ systems, including (Ecobichon and Joy 1994): cardiovascular, respiratory, gastrointestinal, genitourinary, glandular, and neurological.

Muscarinic effects by organ systems include the following:

- Cardiovascular – Bradycardia, hypotension.
- Respiratory – Rhinorrhea, bronchorrhea, bronchospasm, cough, severe respiratory distress
- Gastrointestinal – Hypersalivation, nausea and vomiting, abdominal pain, diarrhea, fecal incontinence
- Genitourinary – Incontinence
- Ocular – Blurred vision, miosis
- Glands – Increased lacrimation, diaphoresis.

Nicotinic symptoms include muscle fasciculations, cramping, weakness, and diaphragmatic failure.

Autonomic effects include hypertension, tachycardia, mydriasis, and pallor.

CNS effects include anxiety, emotional lability, restlessness, confusion, ataxia, tremors, seizures, and coma.

Rule of thumb: Organophosphate high level exposure acute effects mnemonics SLUDGE and DUMBELS

Salivation	Diaphoresis and diarrhea
Lacrimation	Urination
Urination	Miosis
Diarrhea	Bradycardia, bronchospasm, bronchorrhea
GI upset	Emesis
Emotional	Lacrimation (excess)
	Salivation

Chronic symptoms

In contrast to the above acute symptoms of OP exposure, chronic symptoms of exposure have been reported (Ecobichon and Joy 1994). These symptoms are more similar to chronic symptoms of many neurotoxic substances. Chronic symptoms reported for OP exposure include (Ecobichon and Joy 1994):

1. Impaired vigilance and reduced concentration
2. Slowing of information processing and psychomotor speed
3. Memory deficit
4. Linguistic disturbance
5. Depression
6. Anxiety and irritability

Additionally, there can be idiosyncratic effects with OP exposure, such as persistent psychologic/psychiatric sequelae. Ecobichon and Joy (1994) reported chronic exposure to OPs among agricultural pilots handling pesticides was linked with "neurotic reactions, obsessive-compulsion, phobia, depression, crying spells, fear of being alone, acute anxiety, irritability, and other personality changes" (pp. 226).

Organophosphates may have a proclivity for promoting anxiety disorders. The particular acute effects of OPs could result in damage to various body systems, including heart function. I propose that the effects of OP exposure can be quite anxiety provoking, and in some individuals, create the conditions ideal for the development of future "panic attacks" and related psychologic/psychiatric illnesses.

> **Rule of thumb: Neurobehavioral symptoms reported for some patients chronically following organophosphate neurotoxicity**
>
> 1. Impaired attention, concentration, vigilance and executive function
> 2. Slowing of information processing and psychomotor speed (bradyphrenia and/or bradykinesia)
> 3. Memory deficit (primarily affecting the acquisition and retention of new material)
> 4. Verbal fluency deficit
> 5. Psychiatric symptoms (depression, anxiety, and increased irritability)

Lead

Another example of differing acute effects of neurotoxicity versus similar chronic effects of neurotoxicity can be seen with regard to lead.

Acute effects

Acute symptoms may initially include lethargy, abdominal cramps, anorexia, and irritability, and can progress to vomiting, clumsiness, ataxia, alternating periods of hyperirritability and stupor, and then finally seizures and coma (Lidsky and Schneider 2006).

Chronic effects

The long-term outcome of lead poisoning on central nervous system function seems to be similar to the long-term outcome of organophosphate exposure. Lidsky and Schneider (2006) reviewed epidemiological studies of lead poisoning, and reported that deficits were found on tests that assess fine motor skills, language, memory, and attention/executive functioning, when the results were averaged over the group. However, individual neuropsychological evaluation revealed more idiosyncratic results per child. Lidsky and Schneider studied 21 children with peak blood lead levels at 7–15 mcg per deciliter (a fairly low level of poisoning) with individual neuropsychological assessment, finding that the effects of lead poisoning on each individual child's neuropsychological performance were variable. Not only did the overall pattern of impairments differ from child to child, but even the particulars of deficits within neuropsychological domains showed patient-specific patterns. While there are some general findings at a group level, including deficits in visual memory and fine motor skills, there was considerable individual variability.

The chronic results of lead poisoning are analogous to the chronic effects of OP poisoning described above. There are deficits in psychomotor speed, reduced vigilance, decreased memory, and mood disorders. Children with high-level lead exposure frequently exhibit learning disorders and lower IQ.

Rule of thumb: Lead neurotoxic exposure symptoms

- Deficits in fine motor skills (particularly in children)
- Deficits in attentional/concentration skills
- Deficits in learning and visual memory
- Cognitive inflexibility/executive dysfunction

Summary

The acute symptoms of disparate neurotoxic substances such as OPs, lead, manganese, CO, and mold can differ substantially; the chronic effects, if any, can be revealed by neuropsychological examination which focuses on attention/executive, speed of information processing, and memory functions. Some commonalities in long-term outcome from toxic exposure to various chemicals has led the author of this chapter and others (Russell et al. 1990) to propose a common symptom presentation, termed "The Neurotoxicity Syndrome."

There are at least five neurobehavioral test batteries that have been developed or applied to assess neurotoxicity (i.e., Kilburn 2004; Russell et al. 1990; Ryan et al. 1987; Thorne et al. 1985; Valciukas et al. 1980). The fundamental basis for these tests is the general recognition by neurotoxicity researchers that common symptoms and dysfunctions may result from diverse neurotoxic substances. The five batteries include those used by: Valciukas et al. 1980 (see below), The Walter Reed Performance Assessment Battery (Thorne et al. 1985), The World Health Organization Neurobehavioral Core Battery (Russell et al. 1990), The Pittsburg Occupational Exposure Test Battery (Ryan et al. 1987), and the Kilburn Neuro-Test Battery (Kilburn 2004). We, (Valciukas et al. 1980) developed a battery that could be administered in about 20 min, and included the Wechsler Adult Intelligence Test-Revised (WAIS-R; Wechsler 1981) Digit Symbol and Block Design subtests the Grooved Pegboard Test (Matthews and Klove 1964), and the Embedded Figures Test (Valciukas and Singer 1982).

A comprehensive review of the application of these batteries to questions of neurotoxicity is beyond the scope of this chapter; however, I believe the overall data show that neurotoxic chemical exposure can cause generalized slowing and cognitive inefficiency (Calne et al. 1986; Singer 1990a). In general, neuropsychological measures known to be sensitive to aging effects have been shown to be the most sensitive indicators of neurotoxicity exposure. These include the Digit Symbol test, Digit Span backwards, the Ruff Selective Reminding Test, the Stroop Color-Word Test, and other tests dependent upon cognitive speed and rapid acquisition of material. While the above-named batteries are important research and clinical tools, and have advanced our understanding of neurotoxicity, they do not replace a comprehensive neuropsychological assessment in many applications, particularly the assessment of "The Neurotoxicity Syndrome." Although the term "The Neurotoxicity Syndrome" has not been widely recognized or accepted, it is reviewed below to orient readers to this proposed nomenclature.

The Neurotoxicity Syndrome

The Neurotoxicity Syndrome is a term used or proposed to describe the characteristic constellation of symptoms and signs of neurotoxicity. The World Health Organization International Classification of Diseases-10 (World Health Organization, 1992) refers to neurotoxicity affecting the brain as "toxic encephalopathy," but the authors did not provide a description of symptoms or signs associated with this condition.

The Neurotoxicity Syndrome presents with a constellation of symptoms associated with dysfunction of the central and peripheral nervous system. (Singer 1990a) (see Chap. 3, this volume, for a review of components of nervous system).

Central nervous system dysfunction can result in neuropsychological deficits in memory (i.e., recent learning and information retrieval) and attention/executive functions (planning, inhibiting responses, strategy development, judgment, problem solving and solution implementation, etc.). Mood affects can include increased irritability, anxiety and/or depressive symptoms and/or personality changes. Autonomic dysfunction can result in disruption of sleep (excessive awakenings) along with reduced energy (fatigue) and libido (Singer 1990a).

When a patient presents with symptoms consistent with neurotoxicity, the clinician should take a careful history, because symptoms could be due to or exacerbated by another cause, such as pre-existing medical or psychological conditions, psychosocial stressors (divorce, children, moving, change of jobs, etc.), or other concurrent physiological conditions. In addition, psychological disorders that are independent of neurotoxicity could contribute to or cause the symptom presentation, such as somatization, conversion, factitiousness, or malingering. The doctor needs to conduct a detailed history, paying attention to the patient's premorbid function and skills, and history of occupation, exposure and symptoms. Symptoms appearing de novo or pre-existing symptoms that are exacerbated could be due to neurotoxicity, and need to be interpreted in light of a comprehensive neuropsychological evaluation.

The mere presence of a pre-existing psychiatric or psychological condition does not prevent neurotoxicity. In my experience, the psychological or psychiatric illness that presents in a patient following neurotoxic exposure may be expressed within the context of pre-existing weaknesses, proclivities and habits. For example, if a patient previously had depressive tendencies, neurotoxicity could exacerbate the pre-existing tendency, possibly leading to a relapse of clinical depression (Singer 2008). The same can be said for patients with premorbid histories for symptoms of obsessive–compulsive behaviors (Singer and Gray, 2007), anxiety (Singer 2002a, b), and thought disorders (Singer 2006). [For further references regarding psychologic/psychiatric disorders and neurotoxicity, see Brown (2002) and Ecobichon and Joy (1994)]. On the other hand, an association of events does not mean causality. An increase in psychological/psychiatric symptoms after neurotoxic exposure may or may not be caused by the neurotoxicant exposure, as psychological symptoms can fluctuate and worsen over time independent of neurotoxic exposure.

Some researchers have searched for specific syndromes to be associated with specific neurotoxic substances (Hartman 1995). However, the study of neurotoxicity has included a variety of instruments and protocols, making comparisons difficult. For example, see above for a description of neurotoxicity test batteries. In addition, the search for neurotoxicity syndromes specific to a particular substance seems to be confounded by the acute symptoms of toxicity, which contrasts with the chronic effects. There are specific sets of symptoms associated with acute exposure to substances affecting multi-organ systems, such as organophosphate pesticides or CO poisoning. However, in contrast to the specific acute effects that might be associated with each neurotoxic substance, the chronic effects or outcomes are more consistent across neurotoxicants. This author believes the core symptoms/signs of chronic neurotoxicity affecting the central nervous system appear to be common and for the most part independent of the particular neurotoxic agent, including reduced performance on speeded attention and divided attention tasks. In addition, relatively idiosyncratic chronic symptoms can develop in the individual patient.

Assessment Batteries for Evaluation of Neurotoxic Effects

Several neurotoxicity neuropsychological batteries have been employed in studying neurotoxicity and exploring long-term neurotoxic deficits (see above for review of common neurotoxicity batteries). Below, I review the Neurotoxicity Screening Survey developed by the current author (Singer 1990a).

Neurotoxicity Screening Survey (Singer 1990a)

The Neurotoxicity Screening Survey (NSS; Singer 1990a) is a self-report instrument developed to rapidly measure symptoms of the Neurotoxicity Syndrome. The NSS assesses consistency and frequency of symptoms consistent with the Neurotoxicity Syndrome across ten domains. Items designed to detect distortion of symptom reporting are also included. Initial work with this instrument has found empirical support for the NSS using several small selected samples (Singer 1990a, 1996).

The NSS was applied to a group of participants having previous significant exposure to neurotoxic substances as determined by the clinical judgment of a neuropsychologist/neurotoxicologist (n = 33) and a control group (n = 36) of relatively healthy subjects without significant neurotoxic exposure as determined by the clinical judgment of the same neuropsychologist/neurotoxicologist. Using a cut-off score for the total Neurotoxicity Indicator score that was greater than 1.5 SD from the average score of the control group, a discriminant analysis found 89% of the controls and 86% of the neurotoxicity study groups were correctly classified. The multiple correlation of the NSS factors with group status was 0.90 (adjusted R^2 = 0.74, p <.001). Results found that self-reported symptoms were highly related with participants having had a significant neurotoxic exposure.

The Neurotoxicity Syndrome symptoms can involve four neurobehavioral domains: (1) Cognitive (neuropsychological), (2) Emotional/personality (neuropsychologic/psychiatric), (3) Central and autonomic nervous system, and (4) Peripheral nervous system. Patients reporting symptoms following neurotoxic exposure may not report all of these symptoms, but health providers can ask questions regarding these domains to produce a more comprehensive diagnosis. These symptoms are reviewed below:

Assessment for Neurotoxicity

Neurotoxic Syndrome: Possible Symptoms and Features

Neuropsychological (Cognitive) deficits

- *Attention/Concentration*: Difficulty maintaining focused attention, particularly in distracting environments. Thoughts may drift and seem fuzzy, with increased susceptibility to distraction.
- *Learning/Memory*: Deficits in new learning and memory (acquisition, encoding or consolidation). Memory for remote events and previously acquired semantic knowledge (word meaning; vocabulary skills) acquired before the known or suspected exposure to the toxicant is often spared.
- *Cognitive and psychomotor slowing (bradyphrenia, bradykinesia)*: Although these symptoms have been associated with confusion and reduced information processing speed, this symptom may be described by the patient as "brain fog."
- *Language*: Complaints of increased difficulty finding correct words (word dysfluency, dysnomia) and more effortful speech has been reported.
- *Executive functions*: Difficulty with planning, multi-tasking, organizing, assessing outcomes and changing plans accordingly.

(continued)

Neurotoxic Syndrome: Possible Symptoms and Features (continued)

Emotional and personality changes

- *Irritability*: Increased irritability and/or reduced tolerance for frustration.
- *Depression and anxiety*: Patients may have increased symptoms of depression and/or anxiety. Evaluate premorbid history of depression or anxiety. Evaluate if other psychosocial or medical conditions affect psychological/personality functioning.
- *Social withdrawal*: Complaints of social withdrawal are common.

Central and autonomic nervous system dysfunction (neurologic)

- *Headache*: Patients may experience headache. Check for previous history of headache.
- *Chronic fatigue*: Subjects may report that they are always tired, with reduced ability to lift, carry, climb stairs, walk distances, or stay awake.
- *Cold sensitivity or temperature dysregulation*: In environments where most people feel comfortable, neurotoxicity patients may feel chilled. Alternatively, they may also be excessively hot, and perspire abnormally.
- *Motor dysfunction* (tremor, reduced dexterity, etc.): Parkinsonism has been reported with neurotoxic exposure (e.g., MPTP [1-methyl-4-phenyl-1,2,3,6-tetrahydropyridine], manganese, etc. exposure). A case report of tremor disorder has been associated with solvent exposure (Singer 2001). Neurotoxic exposure has also been reported to be associated with multiple sclerosis symptoms in at least two case reports (Singer 1990b, 1997).
- *Photophobia*: Sensitivity to bright lights.
- *Sleep disturbance*: Sleep may become disrupted and/or intermittent with frequent awakenings. Disruption of sleep, endocrine and hormonal systems can occur with neurotoxicity. Evaluation for sleep apnea (including obstructive, central and complex apnea) may be helpful. Check for premorbid history of sleep problems. Sleep disturbance can adversely affect neuropsychological function and contribute to complaints of chronic fatigue.

Peripheral nervous system and other associated symptoms
Some neurotoxic agents damage peripheral nerves. Nerves with very long axons, such as nerves that serve the feet (and the hands to a lesser extent) are more susceptible to damage from neurotoxic agents. Disruption of the peripheral nervous system may be described by the patient as numbness, tingling, "pin and needles" sensation, or a feeling that the limb "falls asleep." Other symptoms reported include sexual dysfunction and sensory-perceptual disturbances. Sexual dysfunction complaints include erectile dysfunction for men and decreased libido has been reported for both genders. Sensory-perceptual disturbance complaints include decreased vision, blindness, hearing loss, burning sensation, and kinesthetic dysfunction etc. (Singer 1990a; see Lutz 2008 for a discussion of sense organs toxicology).

Acute Exposure

Health care providers in acute settings where patients with neurotoxicity are treated should, when medically indicated, assess for potential acute effects on the nervous system with appropriate neurological and neuropsychological screening measures. Most neurotoxic substances can deleteriously affect central nervous system function (depending upon various circumstances and conditions). Sometimes, in the confusion of the case presentation, especially in an emergency, this type of testing is neglected, and the patient is discharged without detailed assessment, treatment planning, or follow-up care instructions. In some cases, neurological nor neuropsychological functioning may not substantially improve over time, and deterioration of function (cognitive, emotional, social) may ensue for some patients. In these cases, new symptoms such as depression, amotivation and social dysfunction can arise after discharge.

I suggest that following treatment for acute neurotoxic poisoning, patients from acute care facilities be referred for neurological and neuropsychological evaluation. The purpose of the referral includes the evaluation for possible deficits (and identify strengths), assist in monitoring for any change in neuropsychological function over time, and rehabilitation programming, if necessary. The neuropsychologist can assist with rehabilitation efforts for any identified neuropsychological and physical deficits, including accommodations, adaptations, and/or recuperative programming. Additional treatment, including supportive psychological counseling and adherence to protocols for improving health (better diet, avoidance of toxic chemicals, appropriate physical exercise) may also be suggested.

Post Acute Assessment/Evaluation for Neurotoxicity

Below, I review a set of procedures and methods of evaluation for patients having known or suspected neurotoxic poisoning. Depending upon the referral question, the assessment may be focused on neuropsychological (cognitive, emotional/psychological function etc.), psychiatric, pain, sleep problems sensory/motor dysfunction, and/or a combination of these complaints/symptoms. The assessment for neurotoxicity is commonly completed by a physician and/or neuropsychologist. The focus of the assessment may be treatment oriented or forensic (personal injury, criminal justice applications or disability claim). Because of the increased likelihood such evaluations will become part of a forensic case, the health care provider involved in treating or evaluating the patient complaining of, or suspected of, having neurotoxic exposure may want to consider referring the patient to a specialist in neurotoxicology. The assessment usually involves a detailed assessment of symptoms, history, and evaluation of various clinical and laboratory tests.

Symptom Assessment

A structured symptom assessment procedure, such as the above-described Neurotoxicity Screening Survey (Singer 1990a), can be helpful.

Neurological Examination

A neurological exam can be helpful to assess the extent of sensory and motor complaints, as well as ruling-out other potential causes for symptoms that may not be associated with neurotoxicity. It may also assist in evaluating large and/or small fiber neuropathies, headache, focal neurological dysfunction, radiculopathies, and evaluate peripheral nervous system function, including autonomic function, with various laboratory tests (see below). The neurological exam is, however, not conclusive in most cases of neurotoxicity.

Urine Testing for Neurotoxicants

This type of testing can be helpful in evaluating acute exposure cases, but may not be a sensitive indicator when the specimen collection is delayed. Exceptions include metals, which remain in the body longer than many other substances, and which are often the subject of urine testing. Mold mycotoxins can be detected in urine over a longer period of time, indicating exposure. With regard to specific neurotoxic substances, consult a toxicology textbook to determine the appropriate testing.

Blood Assays – Testing for Traces, Metabolites or Other Indications of Exposure

While blood assays can be valuable when assessing acute exposure, in general these tests have been of little value for assessing the effects of a substance months or years after exposure. However, the antimyelin antibody measure, which is often elevated in neurotoxic conditions, can provide helpful corroborative evidence for neurotoxic exposure and chronic effects. As always, the interpretation of an elevation in a blood assay must be made with caution and in terms of unique patient factors.

Neurophysiological Tests

Nerve conduction velocity tests

Nerve conduction velocity tests offer a reliable way to evaluate peripheral nerve function, which can be affected by neurotoxic exposure (Kimura 2001; Singer 1990a). Nerve fibers more susceptible to neurotoxic effects include the median sensory and sural nerves. However, decreases in nerve function can also occur with compression disorders, metabolic disorders such as diabetes, and other conditions, so results are not specific to neurotoxicity (Singer 1990a). Nerve conduction velocity is recommended when there is numbness or other sensory dysfunction in the limbs.

Somatosensory and other evoked potentials

Evoked potentials of sensory, motor, and visual/auditory attention processes (P300) may be helpful. However, findings in this arena are also not specific to neurotoxicity.

EEG

Routine electroencephalography is often used in acute encephalopathy cases, but is less helpful in chronic neurotoxicity cases. For a review of EEG uses in neurotoxicology, see Seppalainen (1989) who reported EEG abnormalities in subjects with various exposures, including high levels of solvent exposure. However, in my clinical experience, clinical EEGs as performed in the US rarely are read as abnormal in many neurotoxicity cases.

Autonomic studies

Autonomic function studies including cardiac function tests may be helpful for documenting autonomic dysfunction. However, findings in this arena also are not specific to neurotoxicity.

Sleep (Polysomnography) studies

Polysomnography studies are helpful to document sleep disorders. Sleep apnea is a common problem resulting from neurotoxicity, although it can also result from other causes of central nervous system decline, or throat obstruction such as obesity or from a tumor. Sleep apnea was found to be 14 times more prevalent among solvent-exposed workers compared with the general population (Edling et al. 1993), and was found in 39% of patients referred for investigation of possible organic solvent encephalopathy (Monstad et al. 1992).

Neuroimaging

Routine CT and MRI brain imaging studies can be helpful to rule out other causes of pathology. Brain atrophy and/or white matter changes can sometimes be found with neurotoxicity. Changes in brain metabolism have been reported in PET and SPECT functional neuroimaging (Haley et al. 2009). For example, a SPECT imaging study of neurotoxic chemically-exposed Gulf War Veterans found abnormal cholinergic response in deep brain structures as detected by 99mTc-HMPAO-SPECT brain scan (Haley et al. 2009).

Neuropsychological Evaluations

Ideal neuropsychological evaluation in the clinical assessment of known or suspected toxic exposure is comprehensive, assessing functions including intelligence, language (receptive and expressive), learning and memory, visuo-spatial function, executive function, attentional processes (sustained attention, attentional control and processing speed), effort and symptom validity (e.g., Bush et al. 2005), as well as mood, emotion and personality (see Lezak et al. 2004 for review). Much briefer evaluations have been used in epidemiological studies of toxic exposure (Valciukas et al. 1980; Valciukas et al. 1985).

Advantages of neuropsychological assessment in toxicology

Neuropsychological testing is the most sensitive and reliable way to assess brain-behavior function (Lezak et al. 2004). The neuropsychological evaluation as a whole can integrate all of the medical, industrial hygiene reports, toxicology literature, as well as the neurobehavioral test results, interviews and other findings into a coherent and consistent pattern for interpretation of results. This procedure is useful for diagnosis, illness monitoring, prognosis and forensic applications.

Disadvantages of neuropsychological assessment in toxicology

A complete neuropsychological evaluation in cases of neurotoxicity, especially when the report will be used in a forensic context, is time-consuming for the client/patient and the neuropsychologist. Because of the duration and the more complex level of analysis, the evaluation is also frequently financially expensive for the client. From a technical standpoint, there is no single test or neuropsychological battery of tests generally accepted as positive only for neurotoxicity, so all of the data must be integrated to find the most likely causes of neuropsychological impairment (if present).

Neuropsychological evaluation must be interpreted in light of pre-existing conditions, as well as the expected neurotoxic effects of the agent to which the patient had suspected exposure. Neuropsychological assessment requires a high degree of expertise in neuropsychology. The interpretation of test results in neurotoxicology cases requires an integration of disparate disciplines, including neuropsychology, neurosciences, psychometrics, clinical psychology, neuroepidemiology, and detailed toxicological analysis of the potential effect of the specific neurotoxic agent on an individual's cognitive, emotional/psychological and behavioral functioning. Usually, the neuropsychologist is not the first healthcare provider to evaluate a patient/client who requires an evaluation for neurotoxicity. The medical record is frequently quite exhaustive. After review of the medical record, for both consultation and treatment purposes, the neuropsychologist may refer the patient/client to additional healthcare practitioners, which may include, the patient's/client's primary care physician/family medicine as well as specialists in internal medicine, neurology, psychiatry, radiology, psychology, etc.

Neuropsychological examination for post-acute neurotoxic exposure

Below, I provide a capsulated summary of a typical neuropsychological examination for known or suspected post-acute neurotoxic exposure (see Singer 2010; Lezak et al. 2004 for detailed description).

Symptoms and exposures. It is important to take a detailed history of symptoms, as well as a detailed account of estimated exposure to neurotoxic agents (duration and exposure levels). Note the presence of symptoms prior to known exposure, which may impact your interpretation of the symptom cause. (Were symptoms exacerbated? Occurred de novo? Or was there a continuation of prior symptoms?)

The examiner is encouraged to assess for symptom distortion (over- or under-reporting) and/or malingering. Some patients may appear to magnify symptoms, reporting an inaccurate number or degree of symptoms. This could be due to many reasons. The neuropsychologist's review of historical data may find discrepancies between the report of symptoms and observed behavior. These discrepancies themselves may be helpful discussion points in the development of treatment planning for the patient. Careful observation is often helpful in the diagnostic process. Observe and document behavior during the interview, evaluation, possibly including observations when the patient enters and leaves the evaluation setting.

Collateral interviews can help an examiner review the consistency of the examinee's symptoms and history with other's observations of the examinee (Sbordonne et al. 2000). Consistency or discrepancy are important factors in determining the reliability (and veracity) of self-reported symptoms. In addition to family observations, interviews of – or statements from – employers, co-workers, supervisors, teachers or other acquaintances may be helpful.

Historical records. Record review should include any records documenting exposure(s) as well as medical, psychiatric, employment (vocational), and educational records. If applicable, military records may be helpful. It is also important to review the patient's social history.

Neuropsychological Assessment. Neuropsychological assessment should be completed following standard procedures and measures (see Lezak et al. 2004 for review). Various measures of symptom validity can be incorporated throughout the evaluation. Table 27.2 provides an overview of the neuropsychological domains and recommended neuropsychological tests for both a detailed neuropsychological assessment (for forensic and some clinical cases) and then for research or clinical screening purposes.

Summary of the Evaluation of Neurotoxic Exposure

Neurotoxic exposure can produce both acute and toxic effects. Acute effects often vary across and among neurotoxic agents, but generally include central and peripheral nervous system symptoms, particularly affecting autonomic function.

Table 27.2 Neuropsychological domains and recommended measures for clinical evaluations as well as measures to be used in research/screening applications

Domain	A comprehensive evaluation may include some of the following instruments:	Screening, abbreviated or research purposes
General cognitive	Wechsler Intelligence Tests (WAIS-V; Wechsler 2008)	Vocabulary subtest, Wechsler Abbreviated Scale of Intelligence (WASI; Wechsler 2001)
Academic achievement	Woodcock-Johnson Psychoeducational Battery (Woodcock, McGrew, and Mather 2001), Wechsler Individual Achievement Test (WIAT -III; Wechsler 2010) Wide Range Achievement Test 4th Ed. (WRAT-IV; Wilkinson and Robertson 2006)	WRAT-IV
Attention/ executive	Delis-Kaplan Executive Functioning Scales (D-KEFS; Delis, Kaplan, and Kramer 2001), Frontal Systems Behavior Scale (FrSBe; Grace and Malloy 2001), Paced Auditory Serial Addition Test (Gronwall 1977), Trail Making Test, Symbol Digit Modalities Test (SDMT; Smith 1982), Stroop Color/Word Test (Golden 1978), Ruff 2 & 7 Selective Attention Test (Ruff and Allen 1996), Visual Search and Attention Test (Trenerry et al. 1990)	Trail Making Test (AITB 1944), SDMT, Stroop Color/Word Test, Ruff 2 & 7 Selective Attention Test, Visual Search and Attention Test.
Memory/ learning	Wechsler Memory Tests (III, IV: Wechsler 1997, 2008), Test of Memory and Learning (TOML-II; Reynolds and Voress 2007), Ruff Selective Reminding-2nd ed., Benton Visual Retention Test (Benton 1974)	Ruff Selective Reminding, Benton Visual Retention Test
Language	Multilingual Aphasia Examination (MAE; Benton and Hamsher 1989), Western Aphasia Battery (WAB; Kertesz 1982), Boston Diagnostic Aphasia Battery (BDAE; Goodglass, Kaplan and Barresi 2000), Controlled Oral Word Association Test (COWAT), Semantic verbal fluency test (Spreen and Strauss 1998)	COWAT, Semantic verbal fluency test, Boston Naming test (Goodglass and Kaplan 2000)
Visuoperceptual/ constructional	WAIS-R Object Assembly subtest, WAIS-R Block Design Subtest	WAIS-R Object Assembly subtest, WAIS-R Block Design subtest
Mood/personality	Beck Anxiety Inventory (BAI), Beck Depression Inventory (BDI; Beck 1996), Revised Neo Personality Inventory (NEO-PI-R; Costa and McCrae 1995), Profile of Mood States (POMS)	BAI, BDI, NEO, Profile of Mood States
Quality of life/ well being	Alcohol Use Disorders Identification Test, Fatigue Severity Scale, General Well Being Schedule, Human Activity Profile, Quick Environmental Exposure and Sensitivity Inventory (Hojo et al. 2003)	Quick Environmental Exposure and Sensitivity Inventory (Hojo et al. 2003)
Motor	Grooved Pegboard Test	Grooved Pegboard Test
Effort/ dissimulation	Boone et al. Dot Counting Test, Test of Memory Malingering, Dot Counting Test, Portland Digit Recognition Test, Recognition testing, Three Word Memory Test, Twenty-one Item Memory Test, Miller Forensic Assessment of Symptoms Test	Boone et al. Dot Counting Test, Portland Digit Recognition Test, Recognition testing, Three Word Memory Test, Twenty-one Item Memory Test

Neurotoxic poisoning can be fatal, and can result in irreversible damage to the nervous system, as well as damage to sensory and other organs, resulting in conditions including blindness, hepatic and renal failure, and pulmonary and cardiac damage. Neurotoxic exposure can lead to long-term deficits in domains including neurological, neuropsychological (including cognitive, executive function, emotion, etc.), psychological/psychiatric, and/or social functioning.

In the broader realm of diagnosing and treating neurotoxic exposure and poisoning, neuropsychological assessment has taken an increasingly important role in determining the extent of cognitive, emotional and behavioral symptoms and complaints, which are manifested in patients (Singer 1990a, 2007, 2010). Clinical findings and reports generated on patients exposed to neurotoxic agents at work, home or elsewhere, are often used in litigation. The examiner may be asked or required to testify regarding their findings (e.g., Singer 2010). Neurotoxicity has also been a factor in death penalty mitigation cases (Singer 2002c), whereby documentation of neurotoxic effects has been introduced in court to help juries determine the extent of punishment to be applied, as well as culpability.

As is the case for many medical and neuropsychological tests, interpretation will depend upon the skill of the examiner (see Chap. 1 and Chap. 29–32 this volume see also Lezak et al. 2004 for review). In addition to core neuropsychological evaluation skills and training, neuropsychologists will be better equipped to diagnose accurately by studying the neuropsychological, epidemiological and toxicological research regarding neurotoxic effects.

References

Anger, W. K., & Johnson, B. (1985). Chemicals affecting behavior. In Neurotoxicity of Industrial and Commercial Chemicals. In J. O. Donoghue (Ed.), *Neurotoxicity of Industrial and Commercial Chemicals* (Vol. 1). Boca Raton: CRC Press.

AITB (1944). *Army Individual Test Battery, Manual of directions and scoring*, War Department, Adjutant General's Office, Washington, DC.

Beck, A. T., and Steer, R. A. (1993). *Beck Anxiety Inventory Manual*. San Antonio, TX: The Psychological Corporation.

Beck, A.T., Steer, R.A., and Brown, G.K. (1996). *Manual for the Beck Depression Inventory-II*. San Antonio, TX: Psychological Corporation

Benton, A. L. (1974). *Revised Visual Retention Test (4th ed.)*. New York: Psychological Corporation.

Benton, A. L., & Hamsher, K. deS. (1989). *Multilingual Aphasia Examination*. Iowa City, IA: AJA Associates.

Berent, S. (2005). *Neurobehavioral toxicology: Neurobehavioral and neuropsychological perspectives, foundations, and methods (Studies on neuropsychology, development, and cognition)*. New York: Taylor & Francis.

Bowler, R. M., Gysens, S., Diamond, E., Nakagawa, S., Drezgic, M., & Roels, H. A. (2006). Manganese exposure: Neuropsychological and neurological symptoms and effects in welders. *Neurotoxicology, 27*, 315–326.

Brown, J. S. (2002). *Environmental and chemical toxins and psychiatric illness*. Washington, DC: American Psychiatric Publishing.

Bush, S. S., Ruff, R. M., Troster, A. I., Barth, J. T., Koffler, S. P., Pliskin, N. H., et al. (2005). For the NAN Policy & Planning Committee. (2005). NAN position paper. Symptom validity assessment: Practice issues andmedical necessity. *Archives of Clinical Neuropsychology, 20*, 419–426.

Calne, D. B., McGeer, E., Eisen, A., & Spencer, P. (1986). Alzheimer's disease, Parkinson's disease, and motoneurone disease: Abiotropic interaction between ageing and environment? *Lancet, 2*, 1067–70.

Chambers, C. A., Hopkins, R. O., Weaver, L. K., & Key, C. (2008). Cognitive and affective outcomes of more severe compared to less severe carbon monoxide poisoning. *Brain Injury, 22*, 387–395.

Costa, P. T., & McCrae, R. R. (1995). *NEO Personality Inventory-Revised manual*. Lutz, FL: Psychological Assessment Resources.

Cunningham, C., Wilcockson, D. C., Campion, S., Lunnon, K., & Perry, V. H. (2005). Central and Systemic Endotoxin Challenges Exacerbate the Local Inflammatory Response and Increase Neuronal Death during Chronic Neurodegeneration. *Journal of Neurosciences, 25*, 9275–9284

U.S. Congress, Office of Technology Assessment (1990, April). *Neurotoxicity: Identifying and controlling poisons of the nervous system* (OTA-BA-436). Washington, DC: U.S. Government Printing Office.

Delis, D. C., Kaplan, E., & Kramer, J. H. (2001). The Delis-Kaplan Executive Function System (K-KEFS). San Antonio, TX: NCS Pearson.

Ecobichon, D. J., & Joy, R. M. (1994). *Pesticides and neurological diseases* (2nd ed.). Boca Raton: CRC Press.

Edling, C., Lindberg, A., & Ulfberg, J. (1993). Occupational exposure to organic solvents as a cause of sleep apnoea. *Br J Ind Med., 50*, 276–279.

Fahn, S. (2002). The case of the frozen addicts: How the solution of an extraordinary medical mystery spawned a revolution in the understanding and treatment of Parkinson's disease. *The New England Journal of Medicine, 335*, 2002.

Golden, C. J. (1978). *Stroop color and Word Test*. Chicago, IL: Stoelting.

Goodglass, H., & Kaplan, E. (2000). *The Boston Naming Test*. Philadelphia: Lippincott Williams & Wilkins.

Goodglass, H., Kaplan, E., & Barresi, B. (2000). *The Boston Diagnostic Aphasia Examination (BDAE-3) (3rd Ed.)*. Philadelphia: Lippincott Williams & Wilkins.

Grace, J., & Malloy, P. F. (2001). *Frontal Systems Behavior Scale (FrSBe)*. Lutz, FL: Psychological Assessment Resources.

Gronwall, D. M. A. (1977). Paced Auditory Serial Addition Task: A measure of recovery from concussion. *Perceptual and Motor Skills*, 44, 367–373.

Haley, R. W., Spence, J. S., Carmack, P. S., Gunst, R. F., Schucany, W. R., Petty, F., et al. (2009). Abnormal brain response to cholinergic challenge in chronic encephalopathy from the 1991 Gulf War. *Psychiatry Research, 171*, 207–20.

Hartman, H. E. (1995). *Neuropsychological toxicology. Identification and assessment of human neurotoxic syndromes* (2nd ed.). New York: Plenum Press.

Hojo, S., Kumano, H., Yoshino, H., Kakuta, K., & Ishikawa, S. (2003). Application of quick environment exposure sensitivity inventory (QEESI©) for Japanese population: study of reliability and validity of the questionnaire. *Toxicology and Industrial Health, 19*, 41–49.

Kertesz, A. (1982). *Western Aphasia Battery*. San Antonio, TX: Psychological Corporation.

Kilburn, K. H. (2004). *Endangered brains: How chemicals threaten our future*. Birmingham: Princeton Scientific Publishers Co.

Kilburn, K. H. (2009). Neurobehavioral and pulmonary impairment in 105 adults with indoor exposure to molds compared to 100 exposed to chemicals. *Toxicology and Industrial Health, 25*(9–10), 681–92.

Kimura, J. (2001). *Electrodiagnosis of diseases of nerve and muscle: Principles and practice* (3rd Ed.). New York: Oxford University Press.

Kulig, K., Cetaruk, E., Palmer, R., & Brent, J. (2009). The methodology in the paper by Chambers et al., raises serious questions about their conclusions. *Brain Injury, 32*, 3–4.

Lezak, M. D., Howieson, D. B., & Loring, D. W. (2004). *Neuropsychological assessment* (4th ed.). New York: Oxford University Press.

Lidsky, T. I., & Schneider, J. S. (2006). Adverse effects of childhood lead poisoning: The clinical neuropsychological perspective. *Environmental Research, 100*, 284–293.

Lucchini, R. G., Martin, C. J., & Doney, B. C. (2009). From manganism to manganese-induced parkinsonism: a conceptual model based on the evolution of exposure. *Neuromol Med Dec, 11*(4), 311–321.

Lutz, W. D. (2008). Toxicology Principles for the Industrial Hygienist. In W. E. Luttrell, W. W. Jederberg, & K. R. Still (Eds.), *Toxicology of sensory organs*. Fairfax: American Industrial Hygiene Association.

Matthews, C.G., & Klove, H. (1964). *Instruction manual for the Adult Neuropsychology Test Battery*. University of Wisconsin Medical School, Madison, WI.

Monstad, P., Mellgren, S. I., & Sulg, I. A. (1992). The clinical significance of sleep apnea in workers exposed to organic solvents: Implications for the diagnosis of organic solvent encephalopathy. *J Neurol., 239*, 195–198.

Packer, S. (1998). Jewish mystical movements and the European ergot epidemics. *Isr J Psychiatry Relat Sci., 35*(3), 227–39.

Panaccione, D. G., & Coyle, C. M. (2005). Abundant respirable ergot alkaloids from the common airborne fungus Aspergillus fumigates. *Appl. Environ. Microbiol, 71*, 3106–3111.

Racette, B. A., McGee-Minnich, L., Moerlein, S. M., Mink, J. W., & Perlmuter, J. S. (2001). Welding related Parkinsonism: Clinical features, treatment, and pathophysiology. *Neurology, 56*, 8–13.

Reynolds, C. R., & Joress, J. K. (2007). *Test of Memory and Learning-2nd ed. (TOML-II)*. Austin, TX: PRO-ED.

Ruff, R. M., & Allen, C. C. (1996). *Ruff 2 & 7 selective attention test, professional manual*. Lutz, FL: Psychological Assessment Resources.

Russell, R. W., Flattau, P.E., & MacPherson-Pope, A. (1990). *Behavioral measures of neurotoxicity: Report of a symposium*, U.S. National Committee for the International Union of Psychological Science, National Research Council, National Research Council (U.S.). Commission on Behavioral and Social Sciences and Education, National Research Council (U.S.). Washington, DC: National Academies Press, p. 48.

Ryan, C. M., Morrow, L. A., Bromet, E. J., & Parkinson, D. K. (1987). Assessment of neuropsychological dysfunction in the workplace: Normative data from the Pittsburgh occupational exposures test battery. *Journal of Clinical and Experimental Neuropsychology, 9*(6), 665–679. doi:10.1080/01688638708405209.

Sbordonne, et al. (2000). The use of significant others to enhance the detection of malingerers from traumatically brain-injured patients. *Archives of Clinical Neuropsychology, 15*, 465–477.

Seppalainen, A. M. (1989). Electrophysiological approaches to occupational neurotoicology. In L. G. Costa & L. Manzo (Eds.), *Occupational neurotoxicology*. Boca Raton: CRC Press.

Singer, R. (1990a). *Neurotoxicity guidebook*. New York: Van Nostrand Reinhold Co.

Singer, R. (1990b). Neurotoxicity can produce "MS-like" symptoms. *Journal of Clinical and Experimental Neuropsychology, 12*, 68.

Singer, R. (1996). Neurobehavioral screening of breast implant women. *Archives of Clinical Neuropsychology, 11*, 5.

Singer, R. (1997). Wood-preserving chemicals, multiple sclerosis, and neuropsychological function. *Archives of Clinical Neuropsychology, 12*, 404.

Singer, R. (2001). Neurotoxicity evaluation of a new solvent. *Archives of Clinical Neuropsychology, 16*, 697.

Singer, R. (2002a). Neurobehavioral evaluation of residual effects of low-level bystander organophosphate pesticide exposure. *Fundamental and Applied Toxicology, Supplement: The Toxicologist, 55*, 311.

Singer, R. (2002b). Panic disorder can be caused by neurotoxicity. *Archives of Clinical Neuropsychology, 17*, 813–814.

Singer, R. (2002c, April 21st). Death penalty mitigation factors: Neurotoxicity. *18th Annual Symposium of the American College of Forensic Psychology*, San Francisco.

Singer, R. (2005a). Forensic evaluation of a mold (repeated water intrusions) neurotoxicity case. *Archives of Clinical Neuropsychology, 20*, 808.

Singer, R. (2005b). Clinical evaluation of suspected mold neurotoxicity. *Proceedings of the Fifth International Conference on Bioaerosols, Fungi, Bacteria, Mycotoxins and Human Health.* Albany, NY: Boyd Printing.

Singer, R. (2006). Forensic neuropsychological autopsy of a suicide following occupational solvent exposure. *Archives of Clinical Neuropsychology, 21*, 606.

Singer, R. (2007). Neuropsychological assessment of toxic exposures. In *The neuropsychology handbook* (3rd ed., Vol. 2). New York: Springer.

Singer, R. (2008). Forensic evaluation of neuropsychological decline following solvent exposure. *Archives of Clinical Neuropsychology, 23*, 746.

Singer, R. (2010). Forensic neurotoxicology. In A. MacNeill Horton and L. C. Hartlage (Eds.). *The Handbook of Forensic Neuropsychology* (2nd ed.). (pp. 541–560) New York: Springer.

Singer, R., & Gray, M. (2007). Neuropsychological evaluation of a practicing physician with mold exposure. *Archives of Clinical Neuropsychology, 22*, 892.

Smith, A. (1982). *Symbol Digit Modalities Test (SDMT) manual (revised).* Los Angeles: Western Psychological Services.

Stampfer, M. (2009). Welding occupations and mortality from Parkinson's disease and other neurodegenerative diseases among United States men, 1985-1999. *Journal of Occupational and Environmental Hygiene, 6*, 267–272.

Spreen, O., & Strauss, E. (1998). *A Compendium of Neuropsychological Tests* (2nd ed.). New York: Oxford University Press.

Suner, S., Partridge, R., Sucov, A., Valente, J., Chee, K., Hughes, A., et al. (2008). Non-invasive pulse CO-oximetry screening in the emergency department identifies occult carbon monoxide toxicity. *Journal of Emergency Medicine, 34*, 441–450.

Thrasher, J. D., & Crawley, S. (2009). The biocontaminants and complexity of damp indoor spaces: more than what meets the eyes. *Toxicol Ind Health, 25*, 583–615.

Thorne, D. R., Genser, S. G., Sing, H. C., & Hegge, F. W. (1985). The Walter Reed performance assessment battery. *Neurobehav Toxicol Teratol, 7*(4), 415–8.

Trenerry, M. R., Crosson, B., DeBoe, J., & Leber, W. R. (1990). *Visual Search and Attention Test.* Lutz, FL: Psychological Assessment Resources.

Valciukas, J., & Singer, R. (1982). The embedded figures test in epidemiological studies of environmental neurotoxic agents. *Environmental Research, 28*, 183–198.

Valciukas, J., Lilis, R., Singer, R., Fischbein, A., Anderson, H. A., & Glickman, L. (1980). Lead exposure and behavioral changes: Comparisons of four occupational groups with different levels of lead absorption. *American Journal of Industrial Medicine, 1*, 421–426.

Valciukas, J., Lilis, R., Singer, R., Glickman, L., & Nicholson, W. J. (1985). Neurobehavioral changes among shipyard painters exposed to solvents. *Archives of Environmental Health, 40*(1), 47–52.

Wanamaker, R. W., & Wiener, S. L. (1997). Tricholthecene mycotoxin. In R. Zajtchuk (Ed.), *Textbook of military medicine* (Medical aspects of chemical and biological warfare). Washington, DC: Office of the Surgeon General, Borden Institute, Walter Reed Army Medical Center, Office of the Surgeon General United States Army. Chapter 34.

Wechsler, D. (1981). *Wechsler Adult Intelligence Scale-Revised.* New York: The Psychological Corporation.

Wechsler, D. (1997a). *Wechsler Adult Intelligence Scale-3rd ed. (WAIS-III).* San Antonio, TX: The Psychological Corporation.

Wechsler, D. (1997b). *Wechsler Memory Scale-3rd ed. (WAIS-III).* San Antonio, TX: The Psychological Corporation.

Wechsler, D. (2001). *Wechsler Abbreviated Scales of Intelligence (WASI).* San Antonio, TX: The Psychological Corporation.

Wechsler, D. (2008). *Wechsler Adult Intelligence Scale-4th ed. (WAIS-IV).* San Antonio, TX: NCS Pearson.

Wechsler, D. (2010). *Wechsler Individual Achievement Test-3rd ed. (WIAT-III).* San Antonio, TX: NCS Pearson.

Wilkinson, G. S., & Robertson, G. J. (2006). *Wide Range Achievement Test-Fourth Edition*. Lutz, FL: Psychological Assessment Resources.

Woodcock, R. W., McGrew, K. W., & Mather, N. (2001). *Woodcock-Johnson III*. Itasca, IL: Riverside Publishing.

World Health Organization (1992). *The International Classification of Mental and Behavioral Disorders: Clinical Descriptions and Diagnostic Guidelines* (10th ed.). Author: Geneva.

Chapter 28
Cognitive Decline in Childhood or Young Adulthood

Mike R. Schoenberg and James G. Scott

Abstract Childhood dementias are rare, occurring at an incidence rate of 5.6/100,000 (.0056% point prevalence) (Yeates et al., Pediatric neuropsychology: research, theory and practice, Guilford, New York, 2000). Many medical disorders can contribute to deterioration in children where a previously acquired skill is lost or negatively compromised. Such diseases would technically be termed a dementia or dementing illness; however, this term is controversial in children. The term's controversy stems from the opposing interactive forces of continued developmental progress in a child and the counter-developmental effect of ongoing or chronic illness. This controversy aside, this chapter discusses illnesses and issues of deterioration in childhood neuropsychological functioning. This is an often neglected issue in Neuropsychology and the interested reader is guided to in-depth descriptions of many of the diseases discussed found in comprehensive texts in pediatric neuropsychology (see Baron et al., Pediatric neuropsychology in the medical setting, Oxford Press, New York, 1995; Lezak et al., Neuropsychological assessment, 4th edn, Oxford University Press, New York, 2004; Yeates et al., 2000; Yeateset al., Pediatric neuropsychology: research, theory and practice, Guilford, New York, 2010. See also Heilman and Valenstein, Clinical neuropsychology, 4th edn, Oxford University Press, New York, 2003).

Key Points and Chapter Summary

- Cognitive decline in children is rare, but can be caused by many disorders
- Suspected cognitive decline or regression in children should be investigated aggressively as many causes can be treated effectively if identified early
- Neuropsychological testing is essential to differentiating between developmental delays, Mental Retardation and frank cognitive decline

---

(continued)

M.R. Schoenberg (✉)
Departments of Psychiatry and Behavioral Sciences and Neurology,
University of South Florida College of Medicine, Tampa, FL, USA
e-mail: mschoenb@health.usf.edu

M.R. Schoenberg and J.G. Scott (eds.), *The Little Black Book of Neuropsychology: A Syndrome-Based Approach*, DOI 10.1007/978-0-387-76978-3_28, © Springer Science+Business Media, LLC 2011

Key Points and Chapter Summary (continued)

- Repeated assessment may be necessary to measure the effectiveness of intervention or document magnitude of any further decline
- Similar to adults, causes can include genetic, infectious, metabolic, structural abnormalities, immune dysfunction and neurotoxic etiologies

Cognitive deterioration (i.e., technically a 'dementia') in childhood is difficult to identify and diagnose. The DSM-IV provides for diagnosis of dementia in children, which is based on the same criteria as in adults (see Chap.14). Briefly, the diagnosis of dementia requires the presence of significant deterioration in memory and at least one other cognitive domain, which results in difficulty in functioning in social, inter-personal, educational, and/or occupational domains. Deterioration in cognitive and motor skills from a neurodegenerative condition or disease is opposed by neurode-velopmental forces, making it challenging to determine if cognitive and/or motor skills have declined. Because of the insidious nature, it is difficult to ascertain a baseline level of development from which to established when (and which) cognitive skills have deteriorated. Thus, the determination of cognitive deterioration can be challenging with children, particularly for those under the age of 6 years old. It is also difficult to determine if young children are suffering from impairments in edu-cational functioning. Therefore, the diagnosis might have to wait until an adequate evaluation can be obtained. In the interim, the DSM-IV has several diagnoses in which it is recognized that cognitive and motor skills can deteriorate in childhood (e.g., Rett's Disorder, Childhood Disintegration Disorder). This chapter reviews some of the more common and distinct syndromes leading to deterioration of cogni-tive functioning in childhood or early adulthood. A detailed review of all of the childhood disorders that can include loss of cognitive or motor functions is beyond the scope of this book, and interested readers are referred to the comprehensive texts of Yeates et al. (2000, 2010) and/or Adams and *Victor's Principals of Neurology* (9th ed., Ropper and Samuels 2009).

Four general patterns of neuropsychological deterioration have been identified in children reflecting the differing affects of the disease/condition and neurodevel-opmental forces (Shapiro and Balthazor 2000).

1. Normal development slows, plateaus, and then declines as the disease progresses. When viewed over short periods (e.g., weeks to months), then it follows a step-like progression, but when viewed over longer periods (e.g., months to years), then loss of function appears more linear.
2. Normal cognitive and motor skill development gradually slows without any actual loss of an obtained developmental milestone or cognitive function. The rate of development is slow, and significantly lags behind healthy peers (and presumed trajectory based on premorbid estimates). As an example, children and adolescents with HIV (AIDS) present with this course.

3. An acute and rapid decline followed by a cessation of any further cognitive or motor development. Examples of diseases reflecting this pattern include some epileptic encephalopathies and some errects associated with brain tumors (i.e., Radiation necrosis). Rett syndrome also results in this pattern of functional deterioration.
4. An acute and rapid decline followed by a very slow, but otherwise normal, development of cognitive and motor skills. Conditions that can result in this pattern include some neurotoxins, traumatic brain injuries, infections, and inflammatory diseases.

Rule of thumb: Cognitive decline in childhood

- Progressive cognitive decline is rare and must be distinguished from developmental delays and Mental Retardation
- May be due to a variety of acquired brain injuries, but we consider this separate from cognitive deficits due to head injury, stroke, epilepsy, brain tumors, or infections.
- Decline should be documented to be gradual over time
- Deficits must pertain to multiple domains of cognitive functioning and psychosocial functioning
- Deficits should be expected to decline with persistence of the etiological factor
- Earlier onset of cognitive decline typically predicts poorer outcomes
- Many etiologies affect cerebral white matter more than gray matter and thus produce focal deficits or general cognitive slowing and inefficiency without frank Aphasias or Amnesia

---

We now turn to review some of the more common conditions that can present with cognitive deterioration in childhood or early adulthood.

Metabolic Diseases

Lysosomal Storage Diseases (LSDS)

Collectively, LSDs are due to deficiencies of various lysosomal enzymes caused by mutations of genes involved in production of enzyme proteins and/or related cofactors. Lysosome enzymes degrade and recycle most biomolecules and are crucial for cellular health. Disruption of lysosome enzymes results in the storage (accumulation) of products in lysosomes leading to cellular dysfunction, enlargement (ballooning), and, eventually, death. Some of the more commonly occurring (but rare nonetheless) lysosomal storage diseases are reviewed below.

Tay-Sachs Disease

Prevalence: 1/300,000, but is 100 times more common in Ashkenazi Jews.

Onset: Typically in early infancy. Due to deficiency of enzyme that breaks down fatty substance in brain that is called GN12 ganglioside. The enzyme is called hexosaminidase A (HEX A). Deficient HEX A results in the fatty substance accumulating in the brain.

Behavioral symptoms/clinical presentation: Red spot in the macula along with motor weakness (hypotonia), irritability, increased startle reflex, reduced responsiveness and voluntary movements within 8–10 months. Progression of disease leads to blindness, myoclonic seizures, and macrocephaly. Mortality typically occurs by 2–4 years old.

Neuropathology: Initially, abnormality of white matter and basal ganglia, followed by enlargement of caudate nucleus and further white matter degeneration. The last changes reflect general cerebral atrophy.

Juvenile Onset Tay-Sachs

Prevalence: Less common than Tay-Sachs type 1. Inefficient hex A enzyme.

Onset: Typically age 2–5 years old, although onset in early adulthood has been reported.

Behavioral symptoms/clinical presentation: Gait ataxia and incoordination, along with speech and language deficits. Additional deficits in cognitive functions (attention/executive, memory, and visuoperceptual skills) can occur along with apraxias. Patients develop spasticity and seizures later in the course of the disease. A 'vegetative' state ensues that can last years. Mortality usually occurs before age 20, but is later in those with adult onset.

Neuropathology: Primarily cerebellar atrophy (particularly of the vermis). Cerebral atrophy is found less consistently.

Niemann-Pick Disease

A group of inherited disorders causing disruption in the individual's ability to metabolize cholesterol (and other lipids). Three subtypes have been reported: Types A, B, and C (type D was found to have gene mutation of type C). Types A and B are caused by an enzyme deficiency resulting in poor metabolism of lipids. Type C is due to a disruption in ability to metabolize cholesterol, with accumulation in lysosomes.

Prevalence: Type A & B is about 1:250,000 (1:40,000 in Ashkenazi Jew population), and Type C is about 1:150,000

Onset: Infancy to early adulthood.

Behavioral symptoms/clinical presentation: Type A symptoms include failure to thrive, jaundice, ascites (fluid in abdomen), respiratory problems, vision loss and ophthalmoplegia (gaze paralysis), ataxia, myoclonis, and mental retardation. Seizure disorders have been reported, but is more commonly associated with Type C (below). Patients with Type A typically present with early severe neurological and physical deficits and mortality occurs by age 4 years old. Patients with Type B, known as the visceral (organ) form, have less severe symptom presentation, with little to no neurological involvement. Patients with Type B have enlarged liver and spleens with respiratory problems with onset of cardiovascular disease as the disease progresses. Mortality of patients with Type B occurs later with survival into teens or early adulthood. Type C symptoms reflect accumulation of cholesterol in the liver and spleen while other lipids accumulate in the brain. Symptom onset usually occurs in young school age children, but may occur within first year of life or not until early adulthood. Symptom presentation may initially be limited to jaundice (enlarged liver and/or spleen) and/or vertical gaze palsy. Seizures may be present, and are often refractory to antiepileptic medications. Onset of dementia occurs gradually. Motor abnormalities can also include dystonia, incoordination, and breathing difficulties. Mortality often occurs by age 40 years.

Neuropathology: Type C includes diffuse atrophy with neurofibrillary tangles throughout the cerebral cortex and cerebellum.

Metachromatic Leukodystrophy (MLD)

An autosomal recessive lysosomal storage disease resulting in demyelination of the CNS. There are three forms of MLD: early (late infantile) onset type (before age 6 years old), juvenile onset (after age 6 but before adulthood), and adult forms (onset in early adulthood).

Prevalence: 1/100,000.

Behavioral symptoms/clinical presentation: Early onset *type* is characterized by predominate motor symptoms early in the course of the disease, followed by cognitive deterioration of memory and visuoperceptual skills. Language skills (receptive and expressive speech and reading) are relatively spared until late. Social and emotional functioning is generally adequate in these children. Children can present with features of nonverbal learning disorder. Nonverbal learning disorder symptoms typically involve three areas; cognitive deficits, academic problems, and social-emotional difficulties. Individuals may have deficits in attention (visual), memory (visual), executive functions (nonverbal reasoning, sequencing, etc.), language (reading comprehension, writing), fine motor skills/psychomotor speed. Arithmetic skills are commonly disrupted and individuals often have a poor appreciation of social cues and appreciating intent with change in prosody in speech.

Juvenile and adult onset type is characterized by more prominent behavioral and cognitive problems, with features of frontal lobe syndromes. Neuropsychological deficits include pronounced attention problems, memory deficits (verbal more impaired than visual/nonverbal memory) and some deficits in executive functions. Language functions were generally intact. Motor deficits can be present, but not predominate.

Neuropathology: Similar for both early and late onset types, with diffuse deymyelination involving CNS, in which frontal lobe involvement is more affected.

Hurler Syndrome [Mucopolysaccharidose (MPS) Disorder (MPS I)]

Autosomal recessive disease with genetic abnormality on chromosome 4. Results in glycosaminoglycans (GAGs) not being degraded properly by lysosomes. Accumulation occurs in virtually all organ systems.

Onset: Late infancy (after first year of life).

Behavioral symptoms/clinical presentation: Early in infancy, children may appear normal and have normal neurodevelopment. Onset of a variety of abnormalities in motor, sensory, physical functioning begins by 1–2 years of life. Patients present with hepatosplenomegaly, corneal clouding, macrocephaly, hearing loss, respiratory insufficiency, heart disease, enlarged tongue, and hip contractures. Hydrocephalus can be present due to blockage (noncommunicating). Cognitive development and obtaining basic milestones can be normal through year 1, but rate of development slows during the second year, and by age 3 years old, loss of previously acquired developmental milestones is apparent. Thus, cognitive function develops normally, slows, plateaus, and then declines. Mortality generally occurs by 10 years of age.

Neuropathology: Ventriculomegaly is common. White matter may have 'swiss cheese' appearance due to accumulation of CAG.

Neuronal Ceroid Lipofuscinosis (NCL) Disorders

NCL are a group of neurodegenerative disorders resulting from excessive accumulation of lipopigments in body tissues. At present, there are eight distinct disorders; we review three of the most common.

Jansky-Bielschowsky Disease (Infantile NCL)

Fatal autosomal recessive disease (gene location 11p15) characterized by loss of cerebral gray matter neurons and accumulation of lipopigments in the neurons and glial cells in the CNS and PNS.

Onset: Late infancy to age 2–3 years of age.

Prevalence: 1:20,000

Behavioral symptoms/clinical presentation: Early development is normal. Beginning around age 1–2 years old, infants typically present with hyperexcitability, muscular hypotonia, and slowing of fine motor development. Microcephaly is also typically noted (called stage 1), but children will initially continue to acquire developmental milestones. Symptoms progress with slowing in acquiring developmental milestones (stage 2). Subsequently, seizure disorder and deterioration of visual, motor, and cognitive functioning occurs over a period of months (stage 3). Seizures typically present 1–3 years of age, and seizure types include myoclonic, complex partial, or absence seizures. Visual loss is being unable to appreciate light. Other symptoms that may present include choreathetosis, dystonias, truncal ataxia, and myoclonic jerks. This is followed by further loss of visual, motor, and cognitive functioning (stage 4). A vegetative state may ensue for several years before death. Mortality generally occurs by age 11 years, but survival to 16 years old has been reported.

Neuropathology: Thalamic T2 hypointensity are first abnormalities typically appreciated, but only after the first 6 months of age (no abnormalities present early). White matter lesions, particularly involving the periventricular white matter surrounding the lateral ventricle are next appreciated. Cerebral and cerebellar atrophy can be found after age 13 months. After age 2 years old, the macula is often discolored a brownish color along with degeneration of the retina and optic nerve.

Batten Disease (Juvenile NCL)

Fatal autosomal recessive disease (gene location 1p32) characterized by loss of cerebral gray matter neurons and accumulation of lipopigments in the neurons and glial cells in the CNS and PNS. It includes myclonic epilepsy

Onset: 4–9 years of age. Mortality generally occurs by late teens or 20s.

Prevalence: 1/21,000

Behavioral symptoms/clinical presentation: Initially symptom is commonly progressive visual loss beginning at age 4–8 years old, such that children are functionally blind by their 20s. Other changes early in course of disease is neuropsychological deficits, behavioral/personality changes, and motor deficits presenting as truncal ataxia and other Parkinsonian symptoms. Seizures typically present at age 10–11 years, but can be subtle and occur predominately at night, particularly when treated with anti-epileptic medication. Seizures are typically primary or secondary generalized seizures along with complex partial seizures. Seizure frequency can be low, with 1–8 seizures per year. Vision loss may be the initial symptom due to retinal pigmentation. Children may appear increasingly clumsy and uncoordinated with shortened and shuffling gait as Parkinsonism worsens. Progression of cognitive deterioration occurs over years and progresses to blindness, global dementia, and gross motor impairments. Neuropsychological deficits include attention, memory, and speech deficits (dysarthria). Motor impairments lead individuals to become wheel chair bound, typically in adolescence or early adulthood.

Neuropathology: No structural abnormalities observed early (until after age 10 years old). Cerebral and/or cerebellar atrophy that progresses is observed after age 10 years old (typically in early adolescence).

Kuf's Disease Aka Parry's Disease (Adult NCL)

Onset: Typically occurs before age 40 years (usually 15–25 years of age).

Incidence: 1/1,000,000

Behavioral symptoms/clinical presentation: Two subtypes described. One presenting with progressive myclonic epilepsy. Another subtype presents with early personality/behavioral changes (e.g., apathy, increased irritability, depressive features, or emotional liability), cognitive decline (dementia), and facial dyskinesias may be initial symptoms. While visual problems may be present, patients have not progressed to blindness. Cognitive deterioration leading to dementia occurs. Disease course progresses slowly (e.g., 10 years).

Neuropathology: Neuroimaging can also be normal. Atrophy of brain stem, cerebellum, and subcortical gray matter (thalamus and striatum) is also observed.

The Aminoacidopathies

A group of 48 inherited aminoacidopathies in which disruption of various aminoacids occur. We review the most clinically visible of these, the phenylketonurias (PKUs).

Phenylketonurias (PKUS)

Autosomal recessive disease (gene location chromosome 12) characterized by a deficiency of a hepatic enzyme phenylalanine hydroxylase leading to failure to metabolize the amino acid phenylalanine to tyrosine. This results in patients excreting phenylpyruvic acid.

Prevalence: Varies among ethnic groups. 1:10,000 for Caucasians. Much lower in Japanese, Ashkenazi Jewish, Finish, and African ethnic groups. Rates in Turkey is reported the highest, 1:2,600.

Onset: Disorder present at birth. Symptom onset typically occurs within first year of life in undetected children. However, there are considerable variations in severity of PKU, with mild and moderately affected individuals. Children with severe form with autosomal mothers are born with mental retardation. Alternatively, some children with milder forms may not exhibit symptoms until early school age or even early adolescence or not at all. Some patients with very mild forms do not require diet changes.

Behavioral symptoms/clinical presentation: Affected children will present with lighter colored skin, eyes, and hair than siblings/parents. Children may have a unique odor due to phenylpyruvic acid in urine. In untreated children, development is typically normal initially, but after several months, progressive decline in motor skills and deterioration in global cognitive function occurs. Infants may exhibit weight loss, frequent vomiting (emesis), diarrhea, and be sensitive to bright light. Motor abnormalities, with myclonis, tremors, and seizures can occur. In older children, symptoms can progress with repetitive behaviors (rocking, head banging) and self-injurious behaviors. Growth is often slowed and seizures develop if disease is not treated. Progression of untreated disease leads to severe cognitive impairment (mental retardation) with seizures.

Neuropsychological symptoms: Adolescents and young adults with early treated PKU have been found to exhibit normal or near normal general cognitive (intellectual) function with deficits in attention/executive function, verbal fluency and word retrieval problems, and memory. Neuropsychological deficits are associated with childhood treatment indicators (e.g., level of phenylalanine).

Neuropathology: Cerebral and/or cerebellar atrophy can be found, but more often among patients with longer disease course. Early onset neuroimaging is often normal.

Acute Disseminated Encephalomyelitis (ADEM)

This is an acute demyelinating disease that typically follows infection, immunization (rare), or, occasionally no known precipitating infection. In developed countries mortality is now generally rare (~2%), but can be as high as 10–20% in undeveloped countries. Recovery is classically described as complete after several months, with no residual deficits after 1 year. However, about a third of patients can exhibit permanent neurological and/or neuropsychological deficits. Adults with ADEM whom survive tend to present with less permanent neurological or neuropsychological deficits.

Prevalence: 3:100,000 for first decade of life. 1:100,000 for second decade of life. In North America, incidence increases during February/March and are less frequent in July/August. Incidence may be decreasing as worldwide use of immunization to pathogens known to be associated with ADEM has increased, resulting in less ADEM.

Onset: ADEM in childhood occurs most often (80%) before 10 years old. Symptoms typically present within days or weeks following exposure to virus/bacteria, and often when other symptoms of infection have resolved or are resolving.

Behavioral symptoms/clinical presentation: Symptoms present acutely, and include confusion, somnolence, seizures, fever, and/or stiffness of the neck. Ataxia, myoclonis, and choreoathetosis have been reported. Classically, ADEM shares a clinical and pathological resemblance to Multiple Sclerosis (MS), but generally has clinical and pathological features which differentiates ADEM from MS. Typically, ADEM in children occurs as a progressive decline in function in school age children, while MS more typically occurs in late adolescence/early adulthood. There is, however, overlap and ADEM and MS may reflect conditions of a clinical continuum. A form affecting only the cerebellum has been reported [particularly with Varicella (Chicken Pox)], presenting with predominate ataxia. The syndrome can rapidly progress over hours to days with headache, confusion, and neck stiffness being more common. Less commonly, patients will experience stupor, decerebrate rigidity, and coma.

Neuropsychological deficits are associated with the extent of underlying neuropathology present, which can none to significant. Children with severe ADEM can present with global cognitive impairment after recovery, with scores on intelligence based tests at or below 70. Less profound neuropsychological impairments can include deficits in attention/concentration, memory, language, visuoperception, executive, and/or motor skills. Learning and memory scores may fall below normal, but recognition memory is usually better and normal or nearly normal. In some cases, residual ataxia and/or hemiparesis are possible.

Neuropathology: Can exhibit variable bilateral white matter lesions. Classically, ADEM will result in bilateral diffuse white matter lesions early in symptom course that than resolve over time, with little residual pathological evidence of ADEM. Chemokines concentrations elevated in CSF of patients with ADEM.

Rassmussen's Encephaolpathy

Rassmussen's syndrome is an autoimmune disorder which causes severe deficits that start unilaterally, but spread bilaterally if not arrested. The mechanism of immune dysfunction in Rasmussen's syndrome is unknown. It typically leads to hemispheric atrophy.

Prevalence: Very rare (less than 1:100,000)

Onset: The onset of the disease is typically in middle childhood (mean onset peaks at age 6 years old), but can be quite variable (Bien et al. 2005). The onset is marked by unilateral seizures, hemipareisis, and lateralized cognitive and motor symptoms. Progression is insidious and often includes increased seizure frequency, hemiplegia, and marked cognitive and less frequently sensory deficits over an 8- to 12-month time period.

Behavioral symptoms/clinical presentation: As noted, the initial symptoms are often seizures of unknown etiology and hemiparesis. These symptoms are progressive and lead to increased seizure frequency, duration and severity as well as associated hemiplegia. Bien et al. (2005) describes three phases, the first of which is the prodromal phase. The prodromal phase is associated with the initial onset of mild infrequent seizures and, often gradually, hemiparesis that develops often in less than a year (median duration was 7.1 months). The second phase, termed acute phase, results in more frequent and severe seizures, evolving from frequent simple seizures to more complex partial seizures. This stage is also marked by greater hemiparesis or frank hemiplegia, cognitive deterioration (see below) and occasional hemianopsia. This stage is noted to last a median of 8 months. The third stage, or residual stage, is characterized by a decrease in seizure frequency, relatively stable neurological deficits, and additional cognitive decline. In this last stage, some patients may recover from hemiplegia, and exhibit a spastic hemiparesis. Diagnosis is made using criteria of unilateral seizures, unilateral focal physical of cognitive symptoms and unilateral hyperintensities in the cortex and underlying white matter and caudate. Treatment with antiepileptic drugs is typically unsuccessful both in mono-therapy and poly-therapy. Clinical monitoring of the disease course may be achieved by assessing extent of hemiparesis. Hemispherectomy has demonstrated the only effective treatment in controlling seizures, but is not without its residual consequences of spastic hemiplegia and homonymous hemianopsia. Outcome from immunotherapy with Corticosteroids, immunoglobulins (IVIG) and plasmapheresis have been mixed with some patients responding well if these therapies are administered early in the course of the disease.

Neuropsychological deficits are typically striking unilateral deficits in the cognitive domains in the effected hemisphere. In addition to the contralateral motor and sensory symptoms, patients with left hemisphere onset typically have language and verbal memory deficits. Language-based deficits may initially be fluency and naming deficits and progress to frank expressive and/or receptive aphasias (see Chaps. 7 and 12). As these symptoms progress, these patients may have a right hemianopsia, apraxias, and language-based reasoning and problem-solving deficits. In contrast, patients with right hemisphere onset typically have visuospatial processing, left neglect and visual (nonverbal) memory deficits in addition to left sided motor impairments. As these symptoms progress, both nonverbal reasoning and expressive and receptive prosody deficits may emerge in addition to a left hemianopsia. Regardless of the side of onset, these patients demonstrate nonfocal or lateralizing neuropsychological deficits in attention and processing speed. If the disease progression is arrested (often following hemispherectomy) and seizure control can be gained, some recovery of lost functions may be possible. However, residual neurologic and neuropsychological deficits remain, and can be severe. Recovery of function (both motor and neuropsychological) is typically better when treated in younger children. Adolescents and younger adults tend to exhibit less recovery of function, although some recovery may occur. For example, the patient may be ambulatory with a spastic gait and gain some gross motor function of arm and hand. Some neuropsychological recovery of function may occur, including development of some language skills in younger patients (particularly patients younger than 6 years old) as well as attention/executive, memory, and visuoconstructional skills.

Compared to baseline, left hemispherectomy patients exhibited a post-surgical decline in expressive speech, but no other domain, including receptive language functions. The patient's academic functioning may be delayed, but some academic skill acquisition often occurs.

Neuropathology: The etiology remains to be well understood. Originally thought to be due to a virus, data suggest it is an autoimmune disease, with involvement of autoantibodies and T-lymphocyte mediated cytotoxicity. Grossly, most of the brain damage occurs over an 8- to 12-month time frame. MRI findings indicate unilateral cerebral atrophy, particularly involving the insular and peri-insular regions, diffuse and patchy subcortical white matter T2 hyperintensities, and often atrophy of the caudate. FDG PET scans show predominate hypometabolism of the frontotemporal regions during the early stages of disease, but involved more posterior cortex later in disease course.

Vitamin B12 Deficiency (Cobalamin Disorders)

Deficiency in vitamin B12 (cobalamin) can be due to a number of autosomal recessive metabolic disorders and environmental causes.

Prevalence: True prevalence is unknown, and varies substantially among populations. Depending upon the assay used and cut-off threshold (e.g., less than 200 pg/mL vs 300 pg/mL), estimates vary from 3% to 16 % of adults in the USA. Prevalence in Europe has been reported to vary from 1.6% to 10%. Rates in developing countries can be higher, and is higher in subpopulations at risk, including the elderly, vegetarians, and those with diabetes. Recommended daily intake of B12 is 2 mcg for adults and adolescents, and 0.7 mcg for children.

Onset: Most common across age groups is due to poor absorption. May be present at birth due to variety of intrinsic factors: Juvenile/congenital pernicious anemia (unable to absorb B12 due to lack of intrinsic factor in gastric secretions), transport protein abnormalities (e.g., Imerslund-Grasbeck syndrome), abnormalities of intracellular B12 metabolism (methylmalonic aciduria, homocystinuria), pancreatic deficiency, Zollinger-Ellison syndrome, disorders of terminal ileum (e.g., Celiac disease, Whipple Disease), etc. Extrinsic factors include: competition for B12 due to tapeworms, medications (e.g., neomycin), deficient B12 intake, etc. Abnormal B12 metabolism noted for infants born to mothers with B12 deficiency. While onset is rare in children/adolescents, it may occur at any time. For infants, symptoms present after store of B12 obtained in utero is exhausted. Symptoms present more rapidly and more intensely in infancy and early childhood than adults, as liver store from in utero development substantially less than the 2- to 5-year store typical for adults. Treatment often results in rapid improvement, although initial worsening immediately after treatment is initiated has been reported. Outcome is variable, but decreased overall cognitive functioning has been observed relative to the normal population.

Behavioral symptoms/clinical presentation: B12 deficiency in infancy presents with failure to thrive, poor feeding, edema, abdominal pain, pallor, irritability, developmental delays, lethargy, respiratory distress, megaloblastic anemia, and pigmentary retinopathy. Rarely, cobalamin metabolic defects can present in later childhood, and present with a decline in cognitive and motor skills and choreoathetoid movements. Among adults, the classic presentation is triad of weakness, sore tongue, and paresthesias, but these symptoms are rarely the chief complaints (or noted) in children. In adolescence/adulthood early symptoms include weakness, fatigue, loss of appetite (anorexia), nausea, constipation, and parasthesias of the toes and fingers. Other symptoms include brittle nails, dry lips, large spleen, and low grade fever. If not treated, parasthesias may extend to limbs along with onset of limb weakness and ataxia. Autonomic nervous system dysfunction (syncope, heart palpitations, constipation, dyspnea, heartburn, etc.) as well as cognitive/neuropsychological deficits may occur. Common neuropsychological deficits include mental retardation along with impaired attention/executive, memory, language, and visuoperceptual functions. Developmental delays are often present. In older children and young adults (and older adults), general cognitive deterioration from previous ability level occurs. Increased irritability, labile mood, anxiety, paranoia, and hallucinations can occur.

Neuropathology: Diffuse cerebral atrophy with widening of sulci (narrowing of gyri) as well as basal ganglia. Other manifestations include pathology in peripheral and optic nerves, posterior column, and lateral corticospinal tract (subacute combined degeneration of spinal cord).

Galactosemia

Prevalence: Incidence rate is 1/62,000 live births. Carrier frequency is 1/125.

Onset: Autosomal recessive disorder of carbohydrate metabolism with symptoms presenting within weeks of birth.

Behavioral symptoms/clinical presentation: First symptoms are typically jaundice and anorexia. Failure to thrive in infancy, cataracts, and hepatomegaly. Without treatment, symptoms worsen to include emesis, diarrhea, lethargy, poor growth, septicemia, hepatomegaly, aminoaciduria, Often identified as failure to thrive infants. Ataxia, tremor, dysarthria, and hypotonia can be present. Along with cognitive deficits, physical development is diminished. Neuropsychological deficits in intellectual functioning, academic problems, language, and visuoperceptual functions. Treatment is lactose free diet. Despite strict adherence, neuropsychological deficits remain and progressive neuropsychological deficits occur. Mild deficits in mean intellectual function have been identified in groups (Mean FSIQ = 85) (Schweitzer et al. 1993).

Neuropathology: Cerebral and cerebellar atrophy with demyelination (multiple white matter lesions).

Hallervorden-Spatz Syndrome

Fatal disorder thought to be related to disorder of iron metabolism, with mutation of the PANK2 gene. Could be autosomal recessive disorder, but some cases appear sporadic.

Prevalence: 1–3:1,000,000

Onset: Highly variable, but commonly symptoms present by late childhood or early adolescent.

Behavioral symptoms/clinical presentation: Progressive onset of movement disorder and in some patient's, cognitive deterioration. Initial symptom may be optic atrophy (retinal pigment found in 20% of patients) followed by movement disorder and/or cognitive deficits. Motor disorder typically involves a progressive dystonia (particularly involving the feet) with gait ataxia, and dysarthria. Choreoathetosis has been reported in 50% patients.

Cognitive deterioration is slow and progressive. Pattern similar to a "subcortical" dementia pattern with early deficits in fine motor deficits, attention/executive dysfunction, memory loss (recognition cues can improve recall). Visuoperceptual/visuospatial deficits and acalculia may be present. Mood/personality changes occur later in the disease and can include stereotyped and compulsive behaviors and irritability.

Neuropathology: Excessive iron deposition in the globus pallidus, pars reticulata of the substantia nigra (SNr) and red nucleus. Neuroimaging frequently reveals "eye of the tiger" sign in which bilateral hyperintensities are found above globus pallidus and substantia nigra.

Rett Syndrome

A progressive dementia originally thought to only affect young females, but a form also found for young males.

Prevalence: 1/15,000–20,000

Onset: Symptoms present typically by 18 months of age.

Behavioral symptoms/clinical presentation: A period of normal development followed by reversal and deterioration of cognitive and motor skills. Patient's present with autistic features, loss of use of purposeful hand movements, seizures, and ataxia. Children can present with a characteristic hand-wringing movements. Spastic paraparesis develops and physical growth is decreased.

Neuropathology: Cessation or severe reduction in axo-dendritic connections in the CNS. Initially no clear abnormality on neuroimaging, except for volumetric reductions of frontal parenchyma, caudate nucleus, and mid brain. Microcephaly develops.

Hydrocephalus

Hydrocephalus refers to an increase volume of cerebrospinal fluid (CSF) in the ventricles leading to increased intracerebral pressure. Hydorcephalus is not a disease entity, but rather a symptom with many causes (over 180 different causes have been identified). Hydrocephalus can be divided into two categories; (1) congenital hydrocephalus, or (2) acquired hydrocephalus. Another division is by presumed etiology, and includes: (1) communicating hydrocephalus and (2) noncommunicating hydrocephalus. Congenital hydrocephalus is present at birth, and is most often due to neural tube defects, including spina bifida, Dandy–Walker syndrome, congenital foraminal stenosis and meningomyelocele. In addition, congenital hydrocephalus can develop following infection such as meningitis or cyst, or in utero trauma such as hemorrhagic stroke or intraventricular bleeding. Other causes may produce hydrocephalus such as space occupying (tumor or arteriovenous malformation). Hydrocephalus is often treated with ventricular-peritoneal (VP) shunt in which CSF is drained into the peritoneum via a shunt inserted into the affected ventricular system (often lateral ventricle).

Prevalence: 1–2 per 1,000 live births secondary to neural tube defects and 0.5 per 1,000 due to other causes.

Onset: May begin as early as in utero through childhood; however, the incidence after infancy is roughly half that during infancy. Progression can be relatively rapid (days) to chronic (months to years).

Behavioral symptoms/clinical presentation: Varies by age and etiology (congenital vs acquired). Onset of symptoms is slower in children than adults, and may be quite subtle. Children with congenital hydrocephalus can be more difficult to identify in some cases, as a change in clinical status after a period of normal development is not present, and an infant with congenital hydrocephalus may not present with pronounced symptoms. Symptoms may be limited, and appear grossly normal, save for a larger than normal head. Other symptoms can include low energy, poor feeding, and/or irritability. Infants with acquired hydrocephalus, even at birth, can also be difficult to readily identify, but there may be more clinical symptoms, particularly if hydrocephalus is secondary to stroke. As the patients become older, onset of acquired hydrocephalus will typically result in more pronounced clinical changes as reviewed below.

- Infants and young children typically present with lethargy, poor feeding, emesis, and irritability. Acquired developmental milestones can be lost. Other features include separation of skull sutures, increased head circumference, bulging fonanelle, frontal "bossing," downward gaze paralysis (so-called "setting sun sign"), and skull shape can become distorted appearing "globular." Seizures may also occur. Head circumference can rapidly increase over days to weeks.
- Children and adolescents/young adults (age 6 years and older) present with headache involving nausea (often with emesis) that is worse in the morning (and

affected by head position), diplopia, gait apraxia, reduced fine motor coordination, papilledema, CN VI palsy, urinary incontinence, lethargy and social withdraw, increased irritability, and decrease academic performance/loss of academic skills.

Early neuropsychological impairments can be mild (or completely missed). In general, children with hydrocephalus present with mild neuropsychological deficits in psychomotor slowing, attention/executive, memory, and visuospatial functions. Deficits can fluctuate over time. Progression of hydrocephalus can lead to global cognitive impairments, in which some individuals may exhibit profound mental retardation. However, children treated early in the course of acquired hydrocephalus can show recovery of neuropsychological function. Paradoxically, individuals with congenital or slowly developing hydrocephalus may show less severe neuropsychological deficits, but exhibit less recovery of cognitive functions with treatment (VP shunting). Recovery of function is also dependent on any comorbid conditions/disease affecting the brain (e.g., previous stroke, traumatic brain injury, space occupying lesions vs congenital defects, infection, etc.). There have been case reports of individuals with marked hydrocephalus exhibiting normal function in everyday life with mild to moderate neuropsychological deficits, despite extreme hydrocephalus (e.g., Feuillet et al. 2007).

Neuropathology: Hydrocephalus can result from three etiologies: (1) obstruction of CSF flow in the ventricles, (2) insufficient absorption of CSF, and (3) excessive secretion of CSF by choroid plexus (see Chap. 3 for review of the CSF pathway). In general, hydrocephalus is categorized as *communicating* or *noncommunicating.*

Communicating hydrocephalus occurs when there is insufficient re-absorption of CSF due to obstruction of arachnoid villi, draining veins, or subarachnoid space. Termed "communicating" because CSF flow is not obstructed between the ventricles. Causes include intraventricular/subarachnoid hemorrhage or infectious process that irritates the leptomeninges, congenital malformations (i.e., Arnold–Chiari malformation), posttraumatic obstruction, or tumors.

Normal pressure hydrocephalus is a particular subtype of communicating hydrocephalus that characteristically associated with the elderly, but has been reported in adults. It is characterized by normal CSF pressure, but imaging demonstrates enlarged ventricles (particularly lateral ventricles). The exact mechanism remains unknown, but theorized as due to dysfunction of the arachnoid granulations located within the superior sagital sinus.

Noncommunicating hydrocephalus occurs when CSF flow is blocked (or diminished) by intraventricular obstruction involving the foremen of Monro, third ventricle, aqueduct, and/or the foramen of Magendie or Luschka. Common etiologies include aqueductal stenosis, congenital malformations (i.e., acquiductal stenosis), or cysts/tumors (extra- or intra-ventricular).The enlarged ventricles observed with structural neuroimaging is often marked, but may not include the entire ventricular system (will not in cases of noncommunicating hydrocephalus).

Psuedotumor Cerebri (Idiopathic Intracranial Hypertension)

Pseudotumor Cerebri or Idiopathic Intracranial Hypertension (IIH) is a progressive disorder marked by increased intracranial pressure without a known cause. Some divide pseudotumor cerebri to primary (idiopathic) and secondary forms. Primary pseudotumor cerebri there is no clear cause, but with a higher prevalence in obese young adult women. Secondary psuedotumor cerebri is not firmly established, but some potential cause(s) is identified, such as venous sinus thrombosis and increased venous sinus pressure as well as some medications such as retinoic acid, antibiotics, steroids and vitamin A.

Prevalence: In children, it is unknown, but "secondary" pseudotumor cerebri has been reported in children younger than 6 years old. Cases of primary (idiopathic) pseudotumor cerebri is very rare in young children, and more common after age 11 years old. Increasing frequency of pseudotumor cerebri is suspected in children. There is no sex discrepancy in prevalence in children. Highest prevalence is in obese women of childbearing age. Overall incidence rate is 0.9 per 100,000. Incidence in women is 1.6 per 100,000 and 7.9–19.3 cases per 100,000 in obese women (aged 15–44). More common in women than men (8:1). Risk increases with female gender, reproductive age group, obesity, menstrual irregularity. Some evidence of increased risk in children having low thyrotrophin levels and being treated with excessive thyroxine replacement therapy.

Behavioral symptoms/clinical presentation: In children, presenting symptoms usually include headache, fatigue, blurred vision, and nausea/vomiting. In adolescents/young adults, associated with headache, vision loss, papilledema, and horizontal diplopia. Most common symptom in children and adults is nonspecific headache, fatigue, blurred vision, and nausea/vomiting. Other symptoms include horizontal diplopia (with some having a false-localizing CN VI nerve palsy), papilledema (transient visual loss, in which vision blacks out or dims in one or both eyes for short periods of time, often after leaning or bending down; loss of visual fields beginning in the nasal inferior quadrants; blurring or visual distortions – metamorphonsia; or sudden vision loss in one eye – due to intraocular hemorrhage), and pulsatile tinnitus (ringing in one or both ears often in association with heart beat). If untreated, symptoms progress to include lethargy, acute cognitive decline, and, rarely, radiculopathy. Papilledema present in 22–96% of cases. Cases of reduced abduction of one or both eyes (eyes looking away from body) reported Optic nerve damage can be persistent even if ICP is controlled. Treatment usually consists of diuretics and weight loss if no occult cause can be found. Shunting is also common in cases that do not respond to diuretics and weight loss.

Neuropathology: Unknown. Research has demonstrated an increased resistance in arachnoid granulations for absorption of CSF. Some data suggest increased intracranial pressure results in narrowing of the transverse dural venus sinus, which exacerbates the pressure elevation by increasing venous pressure in the superior sagittal sinus. Alternatively, arterial inflow has been shown to be elevated in patients with pseudotumor cerebri (21%) while drainage via the superior sagittal sinus was normal (net increase in pressure due to increased arterial inflow).

Sickle Cell Disease

Prevalence: 1:600 newborn African–American children, but is present in many ethnic populations to a lesser degree.

Onset: Systematic testing of newborns in the USA has lead to identification of the gene at birth. SSD is an autosomal recessive pattern of inheritance and thus would be expected to be carried by 25% of children who have a parent with the gene. For individuals with both parents having the trait, 50% would be expected to manifest the disease. The course is often waxing and waning and can be marked by medical complications in multiple systems (i.e., renal, hepatic, pulmonary, cardiac). The course of neuropsychological function can also be quite variable and is determined by the interplay or the effect of CNS involvement as well as the effect of other systems on CNS functioning over time. Sickle cell anemia is present at birth, and symptoms typically present in infants in which sickle cell disease is not identified/treated after 4 months of age. Infants diagnosed with sickle cell anemia will typically have transcranial Doppler ultrasounds of arteries to identify and reduce risk for strokes.

Behavioral symptoms/clinical presentation: Early in the course, undetected newborns may develop colic symptoms or fever. Other symptoms include headache, dizziness, shortness of breath, swelling/pain/coldness in hands/feet, and pale skin. Swelling and pain of the hands and/or feet may be the first symptom of a sickle cell crisis in infants. A sickle cell "crisis" is associated with sudden pain throughout the body, and occurs when red blood cells clump together. The clumps of red blood cells can obstruct small arteries and veins throughout the body, including the brain. The obstruction of small arteries can lead to damage of organs and tissues throughout the body, and either TIA or clear stroke (see Chap. 13, for detailed description). The pain of a sickle cell crisis can vary from person to person from mild to severe, intense pain that typically lasts several hours to several days in duration. Obstruction of arterial blood can damage any organ, and patients may present with TIA/stroke, vision loss/blindness, and damage to lungs, liver, kidney, stomach, and/or heart. Splenic crisis may occur, and result in a blood transfusion. Patients suffering a stroke may present with either or both ischemic and/or hemorrhagic stroke.

Neuropathology: The primary neuropathology includes the cumulative effect of microvascular cerebral lesions and possibly larger strokes. The associated area of infarct predicts the extent and nature of the deficit seen in these children. Studies consistently demonstrate wide-ranging and variable neuropsychological deficits in attention, memory, processing speed, visuospatial skill, and executive (e.g., reasoning/problem solving, sequencing) skills. These are often accompanied by deficits in academic skill development or frank regression.

Lafora Disease (Aka Lafora Progressive Myoclonic Epilepsy)

Lafora is a autosomal recessive genetic disorder marked by inclusion bodies (lafora) in the brain, skin, liver, and muscles. It is one of five inherited progressive myoclonus epilepsy syndromes. It is ultimately a fatal disease, and mortality generally occurs within 2–10 years of symptom onset. Few individuals with Lafora disease live to be 30 years old.

Prevalence: Unknown, and classified as a "rare" disease, affecting less than 200,000 in the entire USA population. Incidence rate is equal for males and females. May be more common among children of Middle Eastern, Southern European, South Asian, and North African decent.

Onset: Typically in adolescents, but may develop in childhood. While frequently after the first decade of life, a few cases of Lafora disease onset have been reported in early childhood (ages 5 and 6 years old).

Behavioral symptoms/clinical presentation: Initial presenting symptom is often a seizure in late childhood or early adolescence (after age 10 years old). If onset in early childhood, first symptoms tend to be learning problems and onset of neuropsychological deficits. In both cases, the initial symptom is quickly followed by onset of other common symptoms including myoclonus (muscle spasms), ataxic gait, rapidly progressive dementia, temporary blindness, visual hallucinations, and/or depression. Patients with Lafora disease develop several seizures types (myoclonic seizures, generalized tonic-clonoic seizures, focal seizures) and the myoclonus is progressive and severe such that the individual may appear to be having nearly continuous myoclonus along with progressive motor ataxia, and dementia. There are broad and marked neuropsychological deficits, but some data suggests a common neuropsychological pattern. Most profound deficits observed in visuoperceptual/visuoperceptual and attention/executive functions. Memory is impaired. Phonemic verbal fluency more impaired than semantic verbal fluency. Verbal abilities can be initially somewhat spared, although verbal intellectual function was impaired compared to controls. There is no known treatment for Lafora disease and treatment is usually symptomatic relief for seizures and myoclonus.

Neuropathology: Most cases of Lafora disease are caused by genetic mutation of EPM2A and EPM2B on chromosome 6, which code for protein laforin and malin. Most patients (75–85%) with Lafora disease have the EPM2A mutation. Most of the remaining cases are thought to be due to mutations of EPM2B. A few cases are due to an as yet unidentified gene. The mutations leads to formation of lafora bodies within cellular cytoplasm. Formation of these bodies leads to build up of polyglucosans within cells and compromise cell function ultimately leading to cell death. Neuroanatomic studies demonstrates greater metabolic dysfunction of the frontal, parietal, basal ganglia and cerebellum regions using proton magnetic resonance spectroscopy (^{1}[H]MRS) (Pichiecchio et al. 2008; Villanueva et al. 2006).

HIV Associated Progressive Encephalopathy (HPE)/HIV-Associated Neurocognitive Disorders

The vast majority of children infected with HIV are born to infected mothers, with exposure either in utero, during delivery, or from breast milk. HIV infections occur in about 10–30% of infants born to women infected with HIV. HIV-associated progressive encephalopathy is a term used to describe a constellation of neurocognitive, motor, and behavioral symptoms in children mirroring the termed HIV-associated neurocognitive disorders (HAND) in adults. As noted above, there are a number of direct and indirect complications with HIV infection and AIDS that can lead to transitory or permanent neuropsychological deficits.

Prevalence: HPE has been reported in 10–67% of children as the first presenting symptom of HIV infection. In untreated children, the prevalence of HPE is 50–67%, but reports of up to 90% of pediatric samples have exhibited some cognitive dysfunction. In children receiving antiretroviral therapy, the prevalence rate is a low 1.6%.

Risk factors: HIV infection in general, especially with lower CD4 counts.

Onset: Most cases present at infancy. Progression when HIV infection is present in infancy is faster than in adults. Some form of symptoms (whether neurocognitive or not) are usually present by 3 years old. The majority (about 80%) will exhibit clinical symptomatology by 6 months of age. Onset and progression varies, but once AIDS symptoms have started, progression is similar to that of adults. Like adults, course is usually progressive, but reduction in symptoms with antiviral therapy and protease inhibitors (i.e., highly active antiviral therapy) among untreated children has been reported.

Behavioral symptoms/clinical presentation: Among infants, the first manifestation of HPE is often is delays in reaching psychomotor developmental milestones and slowing of global functioning. In young children, developing new motor skills and learning rates is slowed. Fine motor skills and motor coordination development slows, and is often impaired. Behavioral abnormalities with social withdraw, apathy, or emotional liability may occur. Learning disorders may be identified. If infection (or symptom onset) occurs in late childhood and/or adolescence, symptoms mirror that of the adults (see Chap. 14). Neuropsychological deficits mirror those of adults with deficits in attention/executive, visuoperceptual/visuospatial, language (verbal fluency and confrontation naming), and memory functions. Recognition memory likely will be better than delayed recall. As disease progress, patients often present with seizures, prominent motor deficits, increasing cognitive deterioration (worsening dementia), mutism, incontinence, and coma.

Neuropathology: Cerebral atrophy largely due prominent lesions of subcortical white matter and subcortical gray matter structures.

Cerebral Autosomal Dominant Arteriopathy with Subcortical Infarcts and Leukoencephalopathy (CADISIL)

Autosomal dominate disorder presenting in early adulthood with headaches (typically migrainous in nature) and recurrent small strokes that culminate in a dementia syndrome.

Prevalence: 1–9:1,000,000

Onset: Variable, but typically early adulthood. Symptoms present by early 60s.

Behavioral symptoms/clinical presentation: Patients may present with initial cognitive deterioration and or transient neurological symptoms such as hemiparesis or sensory losses consistent with TIA's and small strokes. Ischemic strokes tend to predominate in the subcortical white matter and basal ganglia. Neuropsychologial deficits typically exhibit as a progressive "subcortical dementia pattern" in early to middle adulthood. Patients may present with early attention/executive dysfunction, psychomotor slowing, verbal fluency and word finding problems, and memory deficits. Motor deficits are common, with reduced fine motor coordination, which can be asymmetric. In addition, sensory loss, with hemi-inattention and/or the presence of sensory extinction, may also be present.

Neuropathology: MRI/CT studies identify multiple confluent white matter lesions of various sized predominate involving the subcortical white matter and basal ganglia.

Wilson's Disease (Hepatolenticular Degeneration)

Autosomal recessive disorder of copper metabolism mapped to chromosome 13 (13q14.3). Results in the accumulation of copper in the brain, eyes, kidney and liver. Can be fatal if not detected.

Prevalence: 1:30,000.

Onset: Highly variable, ranging from middle childhood to middle adulthood (e.g., 5–50 years old). Typical symptom onset is 10–21 years old. Onset in early childhood (before age 5 years) is very rare.

Behavioral symptoms/clinical presentation: Symptoms involve two prominent types; complications related to hepatic (liver) dysfunction and symptoms due to neurological dysfunction. Hepatic-based symptom onset typically occurs in late childhood early teens (10–14) while neurological-based symptom onset is often later, occurring in late teens early 20s. Classically, Wilson's disease is associated with jaundice, a greenish-brown ring around the cornea (Kayser–Fleischer rings) due to copper accumulation, motor abnormalities, and cognitive/behavioral problems. While Kayser–Fleischer rings are often thought of as diagnostic of Wilson's disease, they are not (Kayser–Fleischer rings not specific to Wilson's disease and not found in all cases). Jaundice with unknown etiology for acute hepatitis and elevated liver enzymes are found in Wilson's disease, and are often first symptoms. Liver cirrhosis is often found among patients with cognitive and behavioral symptoms. Motor symptoms include asymmetric tremor (may be postural, resting, or kinetic), dysarthria, and Parkinsonian symptoms (masked facies, bradykinesia, ataxia, dyskinesias, and rigidity). Asterixis (hand-flapping tremor) and chorea may also be present. Cognitive and psychiatric symptoms are found in neurologically symptomatic individuals (but few deficits have been found in asymptomatic individuals). Neuropsychological deficits involve complex attention/executive functions, memory, and visuoconstructional skills. Fine motor deficits are frequently observed. Dysarthria is not uncommon. Language functions generally remain grossly intact. Mood/personality changes include affective lability, impulsivity, disinhibition, depression, anxiety symptoms, and psychosis in some patients. Up to 50% of patients with Wilson's disease were diagnosed with psychiatric disorders before Wilson's disease was identified.

Neuropathology: Diffuse atrophy may be present, with greater atrophy of the striatum. There are neuronal loss, astrocytic gliosis, and Opalski cells.

References

Angelini, L., Nardocci, N., Rumi, V., Zorzi, C., Strada, L., & Savoiardo, M. (1992). Hallervorden-Spatz disease: Clinical and MRI study of 11 cases diagnosed in life. *Journal of Neurology, 239*, 417–425.

Baron, I. S., Fennell, E. B., & Voeller, K. K. S. (1995). *Pediatric neuropsychology in the medical setting*. New York: Oxford Press.

Bien, C. G., Granata, T., Antozzi, C., Cross, J., et al. (2005). Pathogenesis, diagnosis and treatment of Rasmussen encephalitis. *Brain, 128*, 454–471.

Feuillet, L., Dufour, H., & Pelletier, J. (2007). Brain of a white-collar worker. *The Lancet, 370*(9583), 262.

Heilman, K. M., & Valenstein, E. (2003). *Clinical neuropsychology* (4th ed.). New York: Oxford University Press.

Lezak, M. D., Howieson, D. B., & Loring, D. W. (2004). *Neuropsychological assessment* (4th ed.). New York: Oxford University Press.

Nunn, K., Williams, K., & Ouvrier, R. (2002). The Australian childhood dementia study. *European Child and Adolescent Psychiatry, 11*, 63–70.

Pichiecchio, A., Veggiotti, P., Cardinali, S., Longaretti, F., Poloni, G. U., & Uggetti, C. (2008). Lafora disease: Spectroscopy study correlated with neuropsychological findings. *European Journal of Paediatric Neurology, 12*, 342–347.

Ropper, A. H., & Samuels, M. A. (2009). *Adams and Victor's principals of neurology* (9th ed.). New York: The McGraw-Hill Companies.

Rourke, B. P. (1995). *Syndrome of nonverbal learning disabilities: Neurodevelopmental manifestations*. New York: Guilford.

Schweitzer, S., Shin, Y., Jakobs, C., & Brodehl, J. (1993). Long term outcome in 134 patients with galactocemia. *European Journal of Pediatrics, 152*, 36–43.

Shapiro, E., & Balthazor, M. (2000). Metabolic and neurodegenerative disorders. In K. Yeates, M. Ris, & H. Taylor (Eds.), *Pediatric neuropsychology: Research, theory, and practice* (pp. 171–205). New York: Guilford.

Villanueva, V., Alvarez-Linera, J., Gomez-Garre, P., Gutierrez, J., & Serratosa, J. M. (2006). MRI volummetry and proton MR spectroscopy of the brain in Lafora disease. *Epilepsia, 47*, 788–792.

Yeates, K. O., Ris, M. D., & Taylor, H. G. (2000). *Pediatric neuropsychology: Research, theory and practice*. New York: Guilford Press.

Yeates, K. O., Ris, M. D., Taylor, H. G., & Pennington, B. F. (2010). *Pediatric neuropsychology: Research, theory and practice*. New York: Guilford Press.

Chapter 29
Application of Motivational Interviewing to Neuropsychology Practice: A New Frontier for Evaluations and Rehabilitation

Mariann Suarez

Abstract A mounting number of persons live with a form of cognitive disability (20 million) (US Department of Health and Human Services, Administration for Children and Families, Federal developmental disabilities programs, US Department of Health and Human Services, Administration for Children and Families, Washington, 2000), with approximately 4.1% of the population aged 6 and over (10.7 million) requiring personal assistance to complete one or more activities of daily living. Although specific types of cognitive impairments result from multiple etiologies and vary throughout the life span, these populations share a core commonality: increased risk for difficulty in treatment compliance (HCH Clinicians' Network, Dealing with disability: Cognitive impairments and homelessness, HCH Clinicians' Network, Nashville, 2003). Furthermore, as a consequence of their disability, these patients may inadvertently sabotage their own progress in treatment by the refusal of necessary services due to an inability to understand the goals and benefits of participating in recommended treatments (Backer and Howard, J Primary Prevent 28:375–388, 2007).

In addition to intra-individual issues, the role of the family for pediatric and adult patients is crucial for those with cognitive disabilities (Gan et al., Brain Injury 20(6):587–600, 2006). The deleterious effects of patient's cognitive impairment on individual family members is well documented (Ergh et al., J Head Trauma Rehabilit 17:155–174, 2002; Gillen et al., J Head Trauma Rehabilit 13:31–43, 1998; Hall et al., Arch Phys Med Rehabilit 75:876–884, 1994; Kreutzer et al., Brain Injury 8:197–210, 1994; Minnes et al., Brain Injury 14:737–748, 2000; Perlesz et al., J Head Trauma Rehabilit 15:909–929, 2000; Wade et al., J Head Trauma Rehabilit 17:96–111, 2002), with some studies reporting family members can be more distraught than the impaired patient (Brooks, J Clin Exp Neuropsychol 13:155–188, 1991; Gan and Schuller, Brain Injury 16:311–322 2002). Additionally, these negative effects on the family have shown to continue well past the initial and acute phase of the patient's disability

M. Suarez (✉)
Department of Psychiatry and Newrosciences, University of South Florida
College of Medicine, Tampa, FL, USA
e-mail: msuarez1@health.usf.edu

M.R. Schoenberg and J.G. Scott (eds.), *The Little Black Book of Neuropsychology: A Syndrome-Based Approach*, DOI 10.1007/978-0-387-76978-3_29, © Springer Science+Business Media, LLC 2011

(Gan et al. Brain Injury, 20(6): 587–600, 2006; Davis et al., Brain Injury 17:359–376, 2003; Brooks et al., J Head Trauma Rehabilit 2:1–13, 1987; Rappaport et al., Arch Phys Med Rehabilit 70:885–892, 1989; Thomsen, J Neurol Neurosurg Psychiatry 47:260–268, 1984). Thus, treatment compliance can be compromised not only as a result of the patient's disability but also as a result of the family member's difficulties in adapting to the responsibilities required to support the patient in their rehabilitation and management (Gan et al., Brain Injury 20(6):587–600, 2006).

Key Points and Chapter Summary

- Motivational Interviewing is a technique that is helpful in maximizing compliance among patients and families participating in patient care
- Motivational Interviewing employs cognitive and behavioral reinforcement techniques to gain consensus on behavioral goals and commitment to the changes process by patients and family/caregivers
- Motivational interviewing utilizes behavioral therapy techniques to identify, measure and change behaviors that impede compliance in the context of counseling
- Motivational interviewing techniques have been shown to be effective in many populations who show noncompliance and/or resistance to treatment

---

A New Approach to Noncompliance and Patient Feedback: Emerging Empirical Support

One emerging approach to addressing issues of noncompliance within the field of neuropsychology is Motivational Interviewing. *Motivational interviewing (MI) is a collaborative, person-centered form of guiding to elicit and strengthen motivation for change* (Miller and Rollnick 2009). Originally developed by William R. Miller and Stephen Rollnick in the 1980s as an alternative to mainstream addictions treatment (Miller and Rollnick 1991), MI has blossomed into an empirically supported intervention across multiple domains and settings for adult populations, including compliance, adherence and treatment participation in medical, judicial, mental health, and substance abuse settings (see Rollnick et al. (2007), Arkowitz et al. (2007), Hettema et al. (2005), and Miller and Rollnick (2002) for review), and in the last decade has shown much potential for intervention with pediatric and adolescent populations ages 11 and older (see Suarez and Mullins (2008), for further review).

Although research with MI and patients with cognitive disability is in its infancy, positive results have been found for studies investigating MI as an addition to treatment for adults with traumatic brain injury (Giles and Manchester 2006), and a forensic peer group program adapted for bullying behavior and antisocial attitudes in young men with traumatic brain injury (Manchester et al. 2007). MI has also shown much promise in the provision of feedback during neuropsychological assessment, recently termed the "next generation of client-centered feedback" (e.g., Collaborative Therapeutic Neuropsychological Assessment, Gorske and Smith (2009)). Interestingly, researchers evaluating MI with the cognitively impaired population have incorporated MI as a core element, but not pure intervention. Thus, based on the degree to which the patient's brain function is compromised, the use of MI may require modifications and tailoring, particularly when applied to younger patients and adults with more significant impairments. Applications of MI to caregivers may also bear of some utility, yet, to date, no studies have evaluated the effects of MI with this population. However, based on the multitude of studies evidencing positive effects on compliance, the use of MI with caregivers of patients with cognitive disabilities appears a logical next step in its clinical applicability. The next sections describe MI and the core components of the method, followed by a review of the major principles and skills for use with both pediatric and adult patients with cognitive disabilities and their caregivers.

Rule of thumb: Evidenced-based practice for motivational interviewing

- Emerging evidence base with utility for some patients with cognitive impairment
- May be a helpful tool when working with caregivers to enhance compliance

---

What Is Motivational Interviewing?

Motivational interviewing is a collaborative, person-centered form of guiding to elicit and strengthen motivation for change (Miller and Rollnick in press). From an MI perspective, behavior changes are best sustained if they are driven by internal motivators. The goal for the clinician lays in guiding the patient/caregiver in a discussion about positive behavior change (about the patient or their caretaking of the patient), engaging with them in a collaborative manner, without the use of coercion or uninvited advice (Miller and Rollnick 2002; Rollnick et al. 2007). While incorporating person-centered communication skills to facilitate rapport, the clinician concurrently uses specific goal-oriented strategies to elicit and selectively reinforce change talk language (i.e., self-motivational statements that reflect the caregiver's desire, ability, reason, and need for change) to help increase motivation and commitment to engage in change behaviors (Amrhein 2004; Amrhein et al. 2003). Finally, once the patient/caregiver determines they want to change their behavior, in effect resolving their ambivalence about change and communicating a readiness to take action, the exchange of information, advice and the creation of a behavioral change and treatment plan with the clinician can occur. With this novel approach to neuropsychology encounters, clinicians can gain greater access to the patient/caregiver's motivation and personal goals, as well as a more comprehensive understanding of the factors impacting resistance to follow recommendations and noncompliance with treatment (Miller and Rollnick 2002; Rollnick et al. 2007).

> **Rule of thumb: What is motivational interviewing?**
>
> • Person-centered form of guiding
> • Elicits and strengthens motivation for positive change
> • Decreases resistance during assessment and feedback process
> • Empowers patients/caregivers to be active collaborators in treatment making decisions and planning

Core Concepts and Principles of MI

> **Rule of thumb: Core concepts in MI**
>
> • Consider using MI when motivation is low, resistance is high and/or non-compliance with recommendations exists
> • Provide feedback in a collaborative manner
> • Offer patients/caregivers the opportunity to discuss their interpretation of your feedback
> • Continue to provide feedback and assess relevancy to the caregiver
> • Listen for and elicit change talk statements (desire, ability, reason, need, and commitment statements). Reinforce these statements to increase motivation

Transtheoretical Model of Change

The transtheoretical model of behavior change, developed by Prochaska et al. (1992), although not a core component of motivational interviewing (MI), provides a useful framework for understanding the process of change and tailoring neuropsychological assessment, treatment planning and rehabilitative clinical care to help patients/caregivers make changes (Miller and Rollnick 2002; Rollnick et al. 2007). The model posits behavior change is not a linear, all or nothing phenomenon, but rather an evolving process, with change conceptualized as occurring in six stages. An important component of the model involves relapse, a possible outcome of the action or maintenance stage, wherein the patient/caregiver is unsuccessful in their attempts at making a behavior change (or in the caring for the patient), and thus, resumes their prior and less effective behaviors. At this point, the patient/caregiver is met with a decision to return to the action or contemplation stage. For the clinician using MI, it becomes important to understand the change process, as a major goal for MI involves accepting the patient/caregiver in the stage they are in, while concurrently supporting progress towards more positive behavioral changes that could be of benefit (Table 29.1).

Table 29.1 Transtheoretical model of behavior change

Precontemplation	Not considering the possibility of change
Contemplation	Considering change but feeling ambivalent to making that change
Preparation	Deciding and committing to change
Action	Engaging in the change behavior
Maintenance	Sustaining progress by making change
Termination	Change behavior has become habitual and embedded in the daily repertoire of behaviors

Rule of thumb: Transtheoretical model of change

- Change is not linear, all or nothing behavior, but a an evolving process occurring in six stages
- Understanding process of change useful to tailor feedback and treatment planning discussions

Principles and SPIRIT of MI

A major tenet of MI is that it is not scripted, and should not be viewed as a cookbook or set of strategies to be applied to during every clinical encounter. The SPIRIT of MI refers to the style of interaction with the patient/caregiver. It emphasizes an openness in collaborating about behavior change by being respectful of autonomy, yet evocative in eliciting personal concerns for change. Patients/caregivers are viewed as experts of themselves, and as possessing the abilities (i.e., personal values, motivations, skills) to make a change, with the clinician's role being a guide, rather than telling the patient/caregiver in a direct manner what they "should" do or their "best" course of action. Moreover, patients/caregivers are viewed as responsible for their own choices, and the subsequent consequences of those decisions, whether or not the clinician agrees with the outcome. The four foundational principles central to conveying the SPIRIT of MI includes: (1) roll with resistance; (2) express empathy; (3) develop discrepancy; and (4) support self-efficacy (Table 29.2).

Table 29.2 SPIRIT of MI

Roll with resistance	Avoid arguing as it is counterproductive to the encounter and can increase resistance to engage in change behavior.
Express empathy	Communicate a genuine understanding of feelings and patient's/caregiver's perspective and acceptance of ambivalence by using skilled reflective listening.
Develop discrepancy	Guide the patient/caregiver to consider discrepancies between current behaviors and broader goals and values.
	It is also the patient's/caregiver's responsibility to articulate the incongruence between their actions and goals, and to present the rationale for change.
Support self-efficacy	Support the patient's/caregiver's belief in his/her own ability to make and effect change, acknowledging past successes and reinforcing intentions to change.

MI Skills and Examples of Strategies

Although there are multiple skills and strategies that can be used within MI, several examples are next provided. For an additional list of skills and strategies, see Miller and Rollnick (2002) and Rollnick et al. (2007) (Table 29.3).

Rule of thumb: MI specific skills and strategies

- SPIRIT of MI: REDS

  - Roll with resistance
  - Express empathy
  - Develop discrepancy
  - Support self-efficacy

- OARS

  - Open-ended questions
  - Affirm
  - Reflections
  - Summarize

- Examples of Strategies:

  - Ask permission to discuss feedback and advice
  - Assess importance, confidence and readiness to change
  - Do not argue with resistance
  - Summarize encounter and include motivational statements and commitment to change

---

Table 29.3 Examples of MI skills and strategies

Asking permission	• After reviewing the patient's assessment results, there are some things that concern me here.
Focuses on pointedly addressing areas of concern, while offering the patient/caregiver the freedom to choose to discuss these topics (or not).	Would it be ok for us to discuss this now?
	• Would you be interested in learning more about how the patient's _____ is affecting his/her daily functioning, planning for how you can use this information in caring for him/her, or something else…?
Using open-ended questions	• How have you tried to change…?
Provides the opportunity for the expression of details and allows the patient/caregiver to describe his/her situation, without being directed to respond in a specific manner by the clinician.	• Tell me what concerns you about…

(continued)

Table 29.3 (continued)

Assessing importance and ability Focuses on the perceived reasons, confidence and readiness to engage in change behaviors and allows the patient/caregiver to evaluate their own reasons and ability to make those changes.	• On a scale from 1 to 10, with 1 being the lowest and 10 being the highest, how important is it for you to change …? • Once the patient/caregiver has chosen his/her value, follow with a statement inquiring about a lower number, such as "Why not a 2 instead of a 4?" • The clinician's asking about the lower (rather than higher value) allows for an opportunity not only to understand the extent to which the patient/caregiver currently views the prospect of making changes but also to direct course of the interaction by focusing on topics that are most relevant.
Affirming Conveys the positive aspects of the patient's/caregiver's intent to engage in actual behavior change, as well as to enhance self-efficacy.	• What you are experiencing is not unusual. Many caregivers report… • That is great that you… What is going to be the best way for you to…?
Responding to resistance Respond in a manner that decreases resistance by not arguing with the caregiver's for reasons to change.	• You don't see… as a problem right now and don't agree with this recommendation. What other recommendations that we've discussed might be of more interest for us to focus on during our time today? • This doesn't seem to be a problem as you see it right now.
Looking forward Helps the patient/caregiver to express optimism about making changes by inquiring about how his/her life might be different without the problematic behavior.	• Imagine how you your life would be different if you didn't struggle with… • How might you see yourself in 5 or 10 years if … is still a problem?
Reflective listening Entails using clarifying statements and conveying an understanding of the meaning of responses.	• It seems like you would like to… but don't think it would work. What have you tried? • It sounds like you are feeling… about making a change in … but are concerned about...
Summarizing the encounter Extends reflective listening and provides a synopsis of the content of the reasons, abilities and themes discussed in making a change. Areas of reluctance to change, if appropriate, are also acknowledged. Commitment to change is reflected and summarized. If commitment is strong, elicit/negotiate a change plan.	• So putting it all together, you are concerned about…, and …. • What I hear you saying is… Is there anything else that I've missed?

Summary

Persons with cognitive disabilities present with unique challenges that can directly impact both the patient and family members who provide them with daily support, as well as decrease compliance with recommendations and treatment. Motivational Interviewing is a novel and emerging evidence-based person-centered collaborative guiding method with potential utility for enhancing neuropsychological practice by eliciting and strengthening a patient's and caregiver's motivation for positive change. Core concepts of the MI method involve the understanding of motivation, resistance, using alternate methods for advice and information exchange, and the effects of language on personal change. The transtheoretical model of change provides a framework for conceptualizing a patient's/caregiver's current stage of change and theoretical guide for working to increase motivation to change. The SPIRIT of MI emphasizes openness in collaborating about behavior change and negotiating the course of treatment. The four foundational principles central to conveying the SPIRIT of MI include: (1) roll with resistance; (2) express empathy; (3) develop discrepancy; and (4) support self-efficacy. In each encounter, MI uses specific communication skills and strategies to support the principles, reduce ambivalence, and facilitate change. The primary skills include: (1) open-ended questions; (2) affirmations; (3) reflective listening; and (4) summarizing. Numerous strategies are available in MI, with several examples provided. In sum, the incorporation of MI into neuropsychological practice holds promise for helping patients (particularly those with the ability to understand his/her deficits and/or treatment recommendations), and caregivers to increase motivation and decrease noncompliance to engage in positive behavior change.

References

Amrhein, P. C. (2004). How does motivational interviewing work? What client talk reveals. *Journal of Cognitive Psychotherapy: An International Quarterly, 18*, 323–336.

Amrhein, P. C., Miller, W., Yahne, C., Palmer, M., & Fulcher, L. (2003). Client commitment language during motivational interviewing predicts behavior outcomes. *Journal of Consulting and Clinical Psychology, 71*, 862–878.

Arkowitz, H., Miller, W. R., Rollnick, S., & Westra, H. A. (Eds.). (2007). *Motivational interviewing in the treatment of psychological problems*. New York: Guilford Press.

Backer, T. E., & Howard, E. A. (2007). Cognitive impairments and the prevention of homelessness: Research and practice review. *The Journal of Primary Prevention, 28*, 375–388.

Brooks, D. N. (1991). The head-injured family. *Journal of Clinical and Experimental Neuropsychology, 13*, 155–188.

Brooks, N., Campsie, L., Symington, C., Beattie, A., & McKinlay, W. (1987). The effects of severe head injury on patient and relative within seven years of injury. *The Journal of Head Trauma Rehabilitation, 2*, 1–13.

Davis, J. R., Gemeinhardt, M., Gan, C., Anstey, K., & Gargaro, J. (2003). Crisis and its assessment after brain injury. *Brain Injury, 17*, 359–376.

Ergh, T. C., Rapport, L. J., Coleman, R. D., & Hanks, R. A. (2002). Predictors of caregiver and family functioning following traumatic brain injury: Social support moderates caregiver distress. *The Journal of Head Trauma Rehabilitation, 17*, 155–174.

Gan, C., & Schuller, R. (2002). Family system outcome following acquired brain injury: Clinical and research perspectives. *Brain Injury, 16*, 311–322.

Gan, C., Campbell, K. A., Gemeinhardt, M., & McFadden, G. T. (2006). Predictors of family system functioning after brain injury. *Brain Injury, 20*(6), 587–600.

Giles, G. M., & Manchester, D. (2006). Two approaches to behavior disorder after traumatic brain injury. *The Journal of Head Trauma Rehabilitation, 21*(2), 168–178.

Gillen, R., Tennen, H., Affleck, G., & Steinpreis, R. (1998). Distress, depressive symptoms, and depressive disorder among caregivers of patients with brain injury. *The Journal of Head Trauma Rehabilitation, 13*, 31–43.

Gorske, T. T., & Smith, S. R. (2009). *Collaborative therapeutic neuropsychological assessment.* New York: Springer Publishing Company.

Hall, K. M., Karzmark, P., Stevens, M., Englander, J., O'Hare, P., & Wright, J. (1994). Family stressors in traumatic brain injury: A two year follow-up. *Archives of Physical Medicine and Rehabilitation, 75*, 876–884.

HCH Clinicians' Network. (2003). *Dealing with disability: Cognitive impairments and homelessness.* Nashville: HCH Clinicians' Network.

Hettema, J., Steele, J., & Miller, W. R. (2005). Motivational interviewing. *Annual Review of Clinical Psychology, 1*, 91–111.

Kreutzer, J. S., Gervasio, A. H., & Camplair, P. S. (1994). Primary caregivers' psychological status and family functioning after traumatic brain injury. *Brain Injury, 8*, 197–210.

Manchester, D., Wall, G., Dawson, P., & Jackson, H. (2007). A forensic peer group approach to bullying after traumatic brain injury. *Neuropsychological Rehabilitation, 17*(2), 206–229.

Miller, W. R., & Rollnick, S. (1991). *Motivational interviewing: Preparing people to change.* New York: Guilford Press.

Miller, W. R., & Rollnick, S. (2002). *Motivational interviewing: Preparing people for change* (2nd ed.). New York: Guilford Press.

Miller, W. R., & Rollnick, S. (2009). Ten things that motivational interviewing is not. *Behavioural and Cognitive Psychotherapy, 37*, 129–140.

Minnes, P., Graffi, S., Nolte, M. L., Carlson, P., & Harrick, L. (2000). Coping and stress in Canadian family caregivers of persons with traumatic brain injuries. *Brain Injury, 14*, 737–748.

Perlesz, A., Kinsella, G., & Crowe, S. (2000). Psychological distress and family satisfaction following traumatic brain injury: Injured individuals and their primary, secondary, and tertiary carers. *The Journal of Head Trauma Rehabilitation, 15*, 909–929.

Prochaska, J. O., DiClemente, C. C., & Norcross, J. C. (1992). In search of how people change. Applications to addictive behaviors. *The American Psychologist, 47*, 1102–1104.

Rappaport, M., Herrero-Backe, C., Rappaport, M. L., & Winterfield, K. M. (1989). Head injury outcome up to ten years later. *Archives of Physical Medicine and Rehabilitation, 70*, 885–892.

Rollnick, S., Miller, W. R., & Butler, C. (2007). *Motivational interviewing in health care: Helping patients change behavior.* New York: Guilford Press.

Suarez, M., & Mullins, S. (2008). Motivational interviewing and pediatric health behavior interventions. *Journal of Developmental and Behavioral Pediatrics, 29*, 417–428.

Thomsen, I. V. (1984). Late outcome of very severe blunt head trauma: A 10–15 year second follow-up. *Journal of Neurology, Neurosurgery and Psychiatry, 47*, 260–268.

US Department of Health, Human Services, Administration for Children and Families. (2000). *Federal developmental disabilities programs.* Washington: US Department of Health and Human Services, Administration for Children and Families.

Wade, S. L., Taylor, H. G., Drotar, D., Stancin, T., Yeates, K. O., & Minich, N. M. (2002). A prospective study of long-term caregiver and family adaptation following brain injury in children. *The Journal of Head Trauma Rehabilitation, 17*, 96–111.

Chapter 30
Reliability and Validity in Neuropsychology[1]

Elisabeth M.S. Sherman, Brian L. Brooks, Grant L. Iverson, Daniel J. Slick, and Esther Strauss

Abstract There are now literally hundreds of neuropsychological tests designed for evaluating cognitive abilities in children, adolescents, adults, and older adults. Given this vast library of instruments, how do test users decide which neuropsychological tests to choose? Like most decisions, choosing a test relies on a careful weighing of the relative balance of strengths and weaknesses. Two critical sources of information for making that decision are evidence of a test's reliability and validity. Carefully examining these will help the user make an informed decision as to whether the test is appropriate for a particular purpose, a particular examinee, and a particular setting. This seems like a straightforward task for most neuropsychologists, who have typically covered basic concepts of reliability and validity during undergraduate or graduate training. Yet, a common mistake is to ask an all-or-none question, such as "is this test reliable?" or "has this test been validated?" Reliability and validity often appear deceptively simple, but continue to be complex topics to master.

The goal of this chapter is to facilitate the process of assessing the reliability and validity of tests for clinical use. We will provide an overview of reliability, including different types of reliability, methods for determining reliability, factors that affect reliability, and limits to reliability. We will also cover basic concepts relating to validity, including specific kinds of evidence contributing to validity, ways of evaluating validity, and basic guidelines for interpreting validity. We will do this while keeping the context focused as much as possible on everyday clinical practice.

---

[1]Some elements from this chapter originally appeared in Strauss et al. (2006).

E.M.S. Sherman (✉)
Alberta Children's Hospital, University of Calgary, Calgary, AB, Canada
e-mail: elisabeth.sherman@albertahealthservices.ca

M.R. Schoenberg and J.G. Scott (eds.), *The Little Black Book of Neuropsychology:*
A Syndrome-Based Approach, DOI 10.1007/978-0-387-76978-3_30,
© Springer Science+Business Media, LLC 2011

Key Points and Chapter Summary

- Understanding the concepts of reliability and validity is a prerequisite for skilled use of tests in clinical and research settings.
- Reliability refers to consistency of measurement, and is not an "all or none" property of tests. Rather, reliability refers to test scores, determined through evaluation of different kinds of reliability evidence (e.g., internal, test-retest, alternate form, and interrater).
- Determining the reliability of a test score is an ongoing process based on information gathered in healthy individuals and clinical populations.
- Similarly, validity is not an "all or none" property of a test. Validity is a property of the meaning attached to a test score in the specific context of test usage. That is, test scores have varying degrees of validity, for specific uses, with specific populations.
- In the tripartite model of validity, there are three broad categories of validity evidence to consider: content-related, construct-related, and criterion-related.
- Within these broad categories, there are many ways of estimating the validity of test scores.
- Similar to reliability, determining the validity of a test score is an ongoing process based on evidence gathered in healthy individuals and clinical populations.
- The selection of neuropsychological tests requires a careful and thoughtful process that involves sifting through multiple sources of psychometric evidence.

Reliability in Neuropsychology

Reliability refers to the *consistency of measurement* of a given score. Reliability is not a unitary psychometric construct. Instead, it is determined through evaluation of different kinds of reliability evidence (see Fig. 30.1), applied in different clinical contexts, to diverse groups. Reliability does not pertain simply to test scores. Reliability also relates to the clinical inferences derived from tests (c.f., Franzen 1989, 2000). Types of reliability include the consistency across test items (*internal reliability* or internal consistency), consistency over time (*test–retest reliability* or test stability), consistency across alternate forms (*alternate form reliability*), and consistency across raters (*interrater reliability*). All these different kinds of reliabilities contribute to an overall assessment of a particular test's reliability, which is simply an estimate of the degree to which a test is free from measurement error. By measurement error, we refer to "fluctuation in scores that results from factors related to the measurement process that are irrelevant to what is being measured"; reliability is therefore a property of test *scores*, not of tests (Urbina 2004). Reliability coefficients therefore fall somewhere between perfectly reliable ($r = 1.00$) and completely unreliable ($r = .00$).

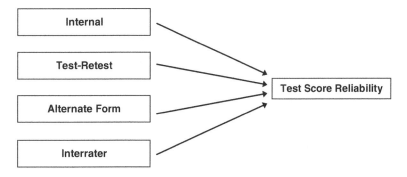

Fig. 30.1 Types of reliability *evidence* to consider for test scores

Rule of thumb: Reliability

- Reliability refers to the consistency of measurement of a given score.
- Reliability is not an "all or none" property.
- Reliability refers to test scores, not to tests.
- Reliability is determined through evaluation of different kinds of reliability evidence.
- There are four types of reliability evidence to consider: Internal, test–retest, alternate form, and interrater reliability.
- Determining the reliability of a test score is an ongoing process based on information gathered in both healthy individuals and clinical populations.

Internal Reliability

Internal reliability, a core concept in classical test theory, reflects the *extent to which the individual items within a test measure the same cognitive domain or construct.* For example, the internal reliability of the WAIS-IV Information subtest is an estimate of the extent to which all of the items on this subtest measure a person's fund of knowledge. It has a high coefficient ($r = .93$) because it has good item cohesiveness and common content. In contrast, low internal consistency generally means that a test is made up of items that do not measure the same construct, or are more heterogeneous than those of tests with high internal consistency. IQ tests are a class of tests that typically are designed to have scores with very high internal reliability (e.g., for the WAIS-IV: $r = .94$ for Vocabulary, $r = .90$ for Matrix Reasoning; Wechsler et al. 2008), whereas instruments designed to sample a variety of content domains over few items will have lower internal reliabilities (e.g., Mini Mental State Exam; MMSE, $r = .31–.96$; Strauss et al. 2006). Internal reliability estimates for the standardization sample and clinical samples for the WAIS-IV are presented in Fig. 30.2.

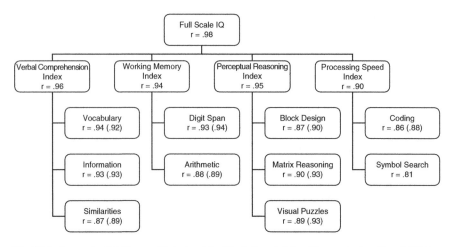

Fig. 30.2 Internal reliability coefficients of the Wechsler adult intelligence scale – Fourth Edition (WAIS-IV). Internal consistency reliability estimates for the total WAIS-IV standardization sample were obtained from p. 42 of the Technical Manual (Wechsler et al. 2008). The reliability estimates in parentheses are averaged for 13 clinical groups; available values were obtained from p. 44 of the Technical Manual. Reliability estimates for the FSIQ or Index scores were not presented for the clinical groups

Internal reliability is usually assessed with an estimate of the average correlation among items within the test. This includes the split-half or Spearman–Brown reliability coefficient, coefficient alpha (Cronbach's alpha), and the Kuder–Richardson reliability coefficient. Descriptions of these different methods are presented in Table 30.1.

Table 30.1 Methods for evaluating internal reliability

Method	Description
Split-half or Spearman–Brown reliability coefficient	• Obtained by correlating two halves of items from the same test
Coefficient alpha (Cronbach's alpha)	• Provides a general estimate of reliability based on all the possible ways of splitting test items.
	• Based on the average intercorrelation between test items and any other set of items, and is used for tests with items that yield more than two response types (e.g., items are scored 0, 1 or 2).
Kuder–Richardson reliability coefficient	• Used for items with dichotomous answers (i.e., yes/no, true/false), or heterogeneous tests where split-half methods must be used (i.e., the mean of all the different split-half coefficients if the test were split into all possible ways).
	• Generally, Kuder–Richardson coefficients will be lower than split-half coefficients when tests are heterogeneous in terms of content (Anastasi and Urbina 1997)

It is important to remember that there is no such thing as a single internal consistency estimate for a given score, let alone a given test. Like other kinds of reliability, internal reliability varies with sample characteristics. This is why the strength of the correlations between items within a test can vary across different age groups and different clinical groups. For example, for the Verbal Comprehension Index subtests of the WISC-IV (Similarities, Vocabulary, and Comprehension), there is a trend towards an overall increase in split-half correlations with increasing age (see Fig. 30.3).

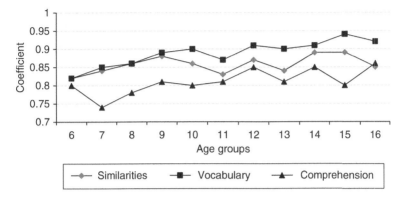

Fig. 30.3 Split-half reliability coefficients for the WISC-IV verbal comprehension index subtests across age groups. This information is adapted from Table 4.1 in the WISC-IV integrated technical and interpretive manual (Wechsler 2004). Each age group has $n = 200$

Greater variability in internal consistency reliability is expected across tests when measuring more variable or less stable cognitive abilities, such as memory and executive functioning. For example, variability in internal consistency reliability across different tests from the Delis-Kaplan Executive Function System (D-KEFS; Delis et al. 2001), by age group, is presented in Fig. 30.4.

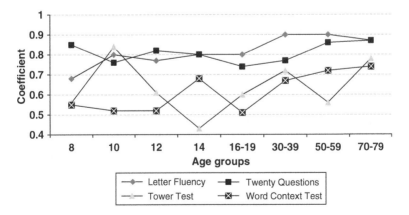

Fig. 30.4 Internal consistency reliability coefficients for selected D-KEFS subtests across age groups. This information is adapted from tables on pp. 22, 34, 37, and 40 of the D-KEFS Technical Manual (Delis et al. 2001)

Internal consistency is reported for most types of cognitive tests and virtually all self-report measures. Examples of reliability estimates for the Ruff Neurobehavioral Inventory (Ruff and Hibbard 2003) for normative and clinical groups are presented in Table 30.2. This example illustrates the basic principle that, all things being equal, a scale with more items such as a composite score (i.e., Cognitive Domain) tends to have higher internal consistency than a scale with few items, such as a subscale score (i.e., Attention & Concentration, Executive Functions, Learning & Memory, or Speech & Language).

Table 30.2 Internal consistency estimates for the Ruff Neurobehavioral Inventory (RNBI)

Scale	Number of items	Standardization sample	Mixed clinical sample
RNBI composite score			
Cognitive domain	24	.90	.93
RNBI subscales			
Attention and concentration	6	.88	.90
Executive functions	6	.79	.80
Learning and memory	6	.81	.87
Speech and language	6	.82	.87

Note: The Ruff Neurobehavioral Inventory (RNBI) standardization sample ($N = 1,024$) reliability estimates are for "postmorbid" ratings. All coefficients were taken from the test manual (Ruff and Hibbard 2003)

Test–Retest Reliability

Test–retest reliability provides an *estimate of the correlation between scores on a test administered twice* over a given time interval. A test score with high test–retest reliability would show little change over time. IQ tests are an example of tests designed a priori to capture stable estimates of an individual's ability levels; these typically have high test–retest correlations. Tests measuring dynamic (i.e., change-able) abilities such as attention or mood may have lower test–retest reliabilities than tests measuring domains that are more trait-like and stable. This is illustrated in Fig. 30.5. In most neuropsychological contexts, the evaluation of both stable and changeable functions are equally important.

The size of test–retest coefficients is influenced by subject characteristics as well as the length of the time interval between test and retest. For example, the test–retest coefficient for Letter Number Sequencing is .48 for 16–29 year olds versus .77 for 55–74 year olds in the normative sample. Other subtests show few differences across age (e.g., Logical Memory 1).

The test–retest interval will depend upon a number of factors, including the particular clinical situation, research question, and availability of relevant re–test data. Across tests, there is no standard time interval for determining test–retest

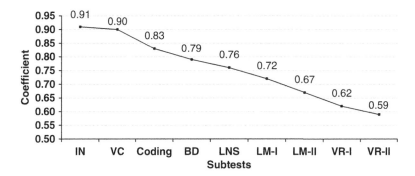

Fig. 30.5 Test–retest correlation coefficients for selected WAIS-IV and WMS-IV subtests. WMS-IV – Wechsler Memory Scale, Fourth Edition (Wechsler et al. 2009). Test–retest coefficients were obtained from p. 48 of the WAIS-IV Technical Manual (Wechsler et al. 2008) and from p. 51 of the WMS-IV Technical Manual (Wechsler et al. 2009). WAIS-IV Subtests: *IN* Information, *VC* vocabulary, *BD* block design, and *LN* letter-number sequencing. WMS-IV Subtests: *LM-I* logical memory-I, *LM-II* logical memory-II, *VR-I* visual reproduction-I, and *VR-II* visual reproduction-II

reliability coefficients. This complicates score comparisons between tests. Retest periods for different tests range from days (e.g., Comprehensive Trail Making Test, Reynolds 2002) to months (e.g., Paced Auditory Serial Addition Test, Sjögren et al. 2000) to years (e.g., Woodcock-Johnson III Tests of Cognitive Abilities, WJIII-COG, McGrew and Woodcock 2001). Many standardized tests provide reliability information for intervals ranging from 2 to 12 weeks, although some tests provide reliability estimates over longer intervals. In particular, the 6-month retest interval for the Neuropsychological Assessment Battery (White and Stern 2003) and the 1-, 3-, and 10-year retest intervals for the WJIII-COG are especially noteworthy.

In most cases, the shorter the time interval between test and retest, the higher the retest reliability coefficient will be. However, the extent to which the time interval affects the test-retest coefficient will depend on the type of ability evaluated (i.e., stable vs more variable) and the type of individual being assessed, because some groups are intrinsically more variable than others. Score fluctuations over time may depend on subject characteristics, including age (e.g., preschoolers vs adults) and neurological status (e.g., brain injured vs healthy). Because this may not necessarily occur in expected patterns across age or demographics, reliability estimates should ideally be provided for both a range of normal individuals and a range of clinical populations.

Alternate Form Reliability

Alternate forms are designed to eliminate the confounding effects of practice when a test must be administered more than once. However, alternate forms can introduce another type of error variance, called content sampling error, in addition to the time

Table 30.3 Factors that increase the reliability of alternate forms

Very high correlations between forms
Very high test–retest reliability for both forms
Equivalence in terms of mean scores from test to retest for both forms
Consistency in score classification within individuals from test to retest

sampling error that accumulates when a test is repeatedly administered over time (see Lineweaver and Chelune 2003). Thus, tests with alternate forms must employ rigorous psychometric standards to avoid introducing new sources of error (see Table 30.3). For example, the Neuropsychological Assessment Battery (Stern and White 2003) was designed to have two parallel alternate forms. A generalizability study was conducted to evaluate the two alternate forms. Of the 36 primary test scores generated from the NAB battery, only 5 fell below the level that would be considered very good reliability (White and Stern 2003). Nevertheless, even though psychometrically-equivalent alternate forms may be designed to eliminate practice effects, prior exposure to similar stimuli and procedures can improve retest scores because of format familiarity and procedural learning despite the use of a different set of items. Thus, it is possible for mean scores to be higher when retesting with an alternate form even though the examinee may not have been previously exposed to the actual content of the test items. See Table 30.3 for factors relevant to constructing good alternate test forms.

Interrater Reliability

Interrater reliability refers to the *degree of consensus between different raters* in scoring items. Test manuals provide specific and detailed instructions on how to administer and score tests according to standard procedures in order to reduce the chances of introducing additional error due to different examiners and scorers. However, some degree of examiner variance remains in individually administered tests, particularly when scores involve a degree of judgment in the scoring procedure. Although many tests are administered and scored in a straightforward manner such that a wrong answer is unequivocally wrong (e.g., Wechsler Digit Symbol), there are other tests that have a subjective component that requires detailed scoring instructions because of the potential for examiner variance (e.g., Wechsler verbal subtests, Rey–Osterrieth Complex Figure, Verbal Fluency). When this is the case, an estimate of the consistency of scores across examiners is needed as additional evidence for the reliability of the test. See Table 30.4 for examples of statistical methods for evaluating interrater reliability.

Table 30.4 Statistical methods for evaluating interrater reliability

Method	Explanation
Percent agreement	This technique is used for nominal data such as classifications or ratings. The number of times each rating is assigned by each rater is divided by the total number of ratings. This method assumes that the data are nominal and it does not adjust for chance agreement between raters.
Kappa	Cohen's kappa is used for comparing two raters; Fleiss' kappa for more than two raters. This technique takes into account the amount of agreement that would be expected to occur by chance. However, the data are treated as nominal.
Pearson's product-moment correlation Spearman's rank correlation	Pearson's coefficient is used for continuous data, Spearman's for ordinal data. Both involve pairwise correlations between the scores of raters. However, because this technique does not take into account the magnitude of the score differences between raters, the scores of two raters could yield a perfect correlation, yet not agree (e.g., Rater 1 = 1, 2, 3, 4; Rater 2 = 7, 8, 9, 10).
Intraclass correlation coefficient (ICC)	The ICC reflects the proportion of variance of an observation due to between-subject variability in the true scores. The ICC will be high when there is little variation between the scores assigned to each item by the raters.
Mean differences and confidence intervals (Bland-Altman plot)	This technique provides information on agreement between raters, and identifies any biases among raters through the derivation of two indices: (1) the mean of the differences between the two raters, and (2) confidence intervals reflecting agreement. If the raters tend to agree, the mean will be near zero. If one rater is usually higher than the other by a consistent amount, the mean will be greater than zero, but the confidence interval will be narrow. If the raters tend to disagree, but without a consistent pattern of one rating higher than the other, the mean will be near zero but the confidence interval will be wide. This information can be graphed using a Bland-Altman plot.

Source: Bland and Altman 1986; Cicchetti and Sparrow 1981; Fastenau et al. 1996; Sattler 2001

Evaluating a Test's Reliability

As we have discussed, tests cannot be described simply as "reliable" or "unreliable." Rather, test scores can be said to possess different kinds and degrees of reliability. The relative importance of one kind of reliability over another will depend on how the test score will be used, with whom, and for what purpose. For instance, a demanding attention test may be highly reliable in normally-functioning adults, but yield unreliable scores in young children or in individuals with severe neurological illness. Importantly, high reliability does not necessarily translate into high validity; some constructs that can be measured with a high degree of precision may be of little use clinically. When faced with deciding between tests with varying reliability, it is usually preferable to choose a test that has slightly lower evidence of reliability if that test has evidence of superior validity (Nunnally and Bernstein 1994).

Given the different kinds of reliabilities, which one matters most when choosing a test? Some have argued that internal reliability is the most important kind of reliability; thus, if alpha is low (regardless of other levels of reliability evidence), a test score should not be considered reliable. Some tests yield scores with relatively lower alpha values yet possess high test–retest reliability. Examples are tests that are made up of heterogeneous items that yield stable scores at retest, such as certain dementia screening instruments. Internal consistency is therefore not necessarily the primary index of reliability, but should be evaluated within the broader context of test–retest and interrater reliability (Cicchetti 1994).

What about test–retest reliability? Does it need to be considered if the test will only be used once and is not likely to be administered again in future? Stability coefficients are essential for evaluating a test's utility because they provide a measure of the degree to which test scores are replicable and stable. For example, a clinician must be reasonably certain that the IQ or memory score obtained now is a good estimate of that person's functioning in future, if that score is to be used for educational planning, or for making a diagnosis regarding a permanent condition such as cognitive disability or dementia. Test scores will have limited clinical utility if they cannot be trusted to give a reasonable estimate of a person's functioning in the future.

Overall, selecting tests – and equally important, selecting test scores – requires that a clinician use an informed and pragmatic (rather than dogmatic) approach to evaluating the reliability of tests for clinical decision making (see Table 30.5). If the goal is to measure a specific, narrowly-defined construct, then high internal reliability might be the most important consideration. High test–retest reliability is usually a requirement of most clinical situations, but may be considered less important if the test is specifically designed to measure state variables that fluctuate. For example, if a depression symptom scale is composed entirely of extremely stable items that are completely resistant to change, it will not be sensitive to treatment-related effects and would be a poor choice for determining whether a patient has benefited from an antidepressant drug regimen. One way around the problem of low test–retest reliability may be to use multiple measures of the specific construct and seek converging evidence to support clinical inferences. In the end, when test

Table 30.5 Examples of interpretations of different patterns of reliability evidence

Reliability			Interpretation of reliability evidence	
Internal	Test–retest	Interrater	Positive interpretation	Negative interpretation
High	High	High	An ideal test for most purposes	None
Low	High	High	Scores reflect a test with heterogeneous item content	Scores are based on items that are measuring something other than the construct the test is designed to measure
High	Low	High	Scores reflect a test measuring a fluctuating ability	Scores are too vulnerable to the effects of normal variability and time

scores have lesser reliability in one domain versus another, such as high internal consistency but low test–retest reliability, there are usually no clear-cut guidelines on how to interpret test scores, or whether the test is appropriate for the specific test usage. It is up to the user to consider all the available evidence and make an informed interpretation of the possible strengths and weaknesses of the test and its scores (see Table 30.5 for examples).

Rule of thumb: Reliability coefficients

- High reliability coefficients are generally preferable, but there are circumstances where lower coefficients may be acceptable
- Low internal consistency may mean that a test is made up of items that do not measure the same construct, or it could mean that the test is designed to measure a broad set of heterogeneous domains (e.g., dementia screening).
- Low test–retest stability may mean that a test is poorly designed and unstable over time, or it could mean that the trait being measured is changeable and dynamic.
- Alternate forms do not eliminate practice effects, and may introduce content sampling error and/or time sampling error.
- It is up to the user to review available evidence on reliability and make an informed interpretation of the strengths and weaknesses of tests

---

Limits to Reliability, Practice Effects, and Effects of Prior Exposure

Although it is possible to have a reliable test score that is not valid for some purpose, it is *not possible to have a valid test score that is highly unreliable*. Despite this statement, it is also conceivable that there are some neuropsychological domains that are very difficult to measure in a highly reliable manner. Thus, even though there is the assumption that questionable reliability is always a function of poor test construction, reliability may depend on the nature of the cognitive process measured and on the nature of the population evaluated. For example, many executive functioning tests scores have relatively modest reliabilities, suggesting that this ability is difficult to assess reliably. Other tests measuring domains such as reaction time or processing speed may yield low coefficients in groups with high response variability, such as preschoolers, elderly individuals, or individuals with brain disorders. Lastly, like validity, reliability is a matter of degree rather than an all-or-none property. Reliability is therefore never actually final. Test scores must be continually re-evaluated from the standpoint of reliability as populations and testing contexts change over time.

One of the most significant influences on test scores re-administered after a period of time is the practice effect. Re-administering a test would be expected to yield better performance at retest, and this is the case in most instances. For example, mean practice effects on the WISC-IV FSIQ range from 4.2 to 8.3 index points (Table 4.4; Wechsler 2004) and on the WAIS-IV FSIQ range from 3.5 to 4.9 index points (Table 4.5; Wechsler et al. 2008). However, not all persons necessarily show a positive practice effect on retest. An examinee may approach tests that he or she had difficulty with previously with heightened anxiety that leads to decreased performance.

The size of a retest reliability coefficient does not indicate the magnitude of practice effects. A test score can have a high stability coefficient, yet have an average retest mean that is several points higher than baseline scores. For example, the WMS-IV Auditory Memory Index has a test–retest reliability estimate of .81, yet has an 11.5 point practice effect over a brief retest interval in healthy adults (Wechsler et al. 2009).

Overall, two main questions must be answered to properly interpret scores in a retest situation: (1) what is the magnitude of the typical expected practice effect, and (2) is the practice effect expected to be consistent across individuals in the group from which the examinee originates? The practical problem for clinicians is that, while most test manuals provide some information on mean practice effects across groups, there is limited information in test manuals for determining the probability of a known practice effect occurring for an individual patient. This is because the majority of practice effects are estimated in healthy subjects, not clinical subjects, and are *averaged* for a group with little information provided regarding the distribution of practice effects across individuals. Therefore, when considering a large group of subjects tested twice, some will likely perform worse, some similarly, some better, and some much better on retest. The *average* practice effect found in a test manual may only apply for an unknown proportion of the sample itself. Reliability coefficients do not provide information on which individuals retain their relative place in the distribution from baseline to retest and which individuals encounter score increases or decreases on retesting. Certain subgroups may benefit more from prior exposure than others (e.g., individuals with above average intelligence; Rapport et al. 1997), or some subgroups may demonstrate more stable scores or consistent practice effects than others. This causes the score distribution to change at retest which will attenuate the correlation. In these cases, the test, retest correlation may vary significantly across subgroups and the correlation for the entire sample will not be the best estimate of reliability for subgroups, overestimating reliability for some and underestimating reliability for others. Despite all these caveats, practice effects, as long as they are relatively systematic and accurately assessed, do not necessarily make a test unusable for clinical practice. Ideally, change scores can be evaluated against a cumulative frequency distribution of test–retest difference scores to determine how frequently a particular test-retest difference occurs in the normative sample (see Brooks et al. 2009). Practically-speaking, for most available tests, the *average* difference score will be the only information available on expected practice effects in healthy people.

Further complicating this situation is the fact that most stability coefficients and practice effects provided in test manuals are based on a single sample of healthy adults retested over a relatively brief interval. This contrasts with the typical clinical scenario of a patient from a specific clinical group tested over longer time intervals. As noted above, test–retest reliability should not be considered an immutable psychometric property of a test, and this is also true of practice effects. Research is needed on the psychometric properties of tests in clinical subjects who are tested over clinically-relevant retest intervals.

Consider the following clinical situation as an example. A 34-year-old man who sustained a moderate traumatic brain injury is assessed with the WMS-III at 1-year post-injury and then again 1 year later. In the test manual, the average practice effect for the WMS-III Logical Memory I subtest in 16–54 year olds tested between 2 and 12 weeks apart is 1.9 scaled score points (Psychological Corporation 2002). If this patient does not show a 1.9 point increase in scores, is this because there was a longer time interval between baseline and retest compared to the normative sample, or was it because the patient had difficulty remembering information and thus did not benefit from re-exposure to the same test items because of his brain injury? These are questions that are not currently well answered by the available data on practice effects for the majority of neuropsychological tests.

It is also essential to note that the actual nature of the test may change with exposure. For instance, tests that rely on a "novelty effect" and/or require deduction of a strategy or problem solving (e.g., Wisconsin Card Sorting Test, Heaton et al. 1993; Tower of London, Culbertson and Zillmer 2005) may not be performed in the same way once the examinee has prior familiarity with the testing paradigm. Practice effects and other effects of prior exposure may plateau after several exposures, and are one reason for including a minimum of test exposures when designing research involving repeated administration of cognitive or psychological tests. Conversely, other tests may simply not be amenable to be administered multiple times in the same patient.

Lastly, it must be kept in mind that factors other than prior exposure may affect test-retest reliability. Variability in scores on the same measure over time can be related to situational variables such as examinee state, examiner state, examiner identity (same vs different at retest), or environmental conditions. With all the different sources of error that can potentially confound measurement at retest, it is quite remarkable that several tests have strong test–retest reliability coefficients.

Validity in Neuropsychology

Test validity may be defined at its most basic level as *the degree to which a test actually measures what it is intended to measure*. Consistent with the construct of reliability, an important point to be made here is that a test cannot be said to have one single level of validity. Rather, it can be said to possess various types and levels of validity across a spectrum of usage and populations. That is, *validity is not a property of a test*, but rather, *validity is a property of the meaning attached to a test score in the specific context of test usage* (c.f., Franzen 1989, 2000). This is a key concept: like reliability, validity relates to test *scores*, not tests (Urbina 2004). As a result, there can be unique factors that can affect validity at the level of individual assessment, such as deviations from standard administration, unusual testing environments, and variable or poor examinee cooperation.

Working knowledge of validity models and the validity characteristics of test scores are a central requirement for responsible and competent test use. From a practical perspective, a working knowledge of validity allows clinicians to chose which tests are appropriate for different uses. For instance, some test scores fail to reach standards for clinical diagnostic purposes of individual patients, but would be perfectly appropriate for research using group data.

Validity Models

Since Cronbach and Meehl (1955), various models of validity have been proposed. The most frequently encountered is the traditional tripartite model (see Fig. 30.6), whereby validity is divided into three core components: content-related, criterion-related, and construct validity (e.g., Anastasi and Urbina 1997; Mitrushina et al. 2005; Nunnally and Bernstein 1994; Sattler 2001). Other validity subtypes, including convergent, divergent, predictive, treatment, clinical, and face validity are subsumed

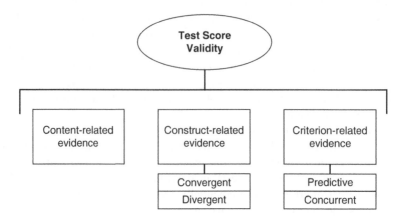

Fig. 30.6 Tripartite model of different types of *evidence* for determining validity of a test score

within these three domains. For example, convergent and divergent validity are most often treated as subsets of construct validity (Sattler 2001), and concurrent and predictive validity as subsets of criterion-validity (e.g., Mitrushina et al. 2005). Concurrent and predictive validity differ in terms of a temporal gradient. Concurrent validity is relevant for tests used to identify existing diagnoses or conditions, whereas predictive validity applies when determining whether a test predicts future outcomes (Urbina 2004).

Although face validity is less studied, the extent to which examinees believe a test measures what it appears to measure can affect motivation, self-disclosure, and effort; consequently, face validity can be seen as a moderator variable affecting concurrent and predictive validity that can be operationalized and measured (Bornstein 1996; Nevo 1985). Face validity matters because it encourages rapport between examiner and examinee, as well as openness and acceptance about test results and their implications (Urbina 2004).

Again, all these labels for distinct categories of validity are ways of providing different types of validity *evidence for test scores*, not different types of validity per se. Lastly, validity is a matter of degree rather than an all-or-none property. Therefore, validity is never actually finalized because test scores must be continually re-evaluated as populations and testing contexts change over time (Nunnally and Bernstein 1994).

Rule of thumb: Validity

- Validity is not an "all or none" property.
- Validity is not a property of tests; it is a property of the meaning attached to a test score in the specific context of test usage.
- There are three broad categories of validity evidence to consider (tripartite model): Content-Related; Construct-Related; and Criterion-Related, but many different ways of determining the validity of test scores.
- Determining validity of a test score is an ongoing process based on information gathered in both healthy individuals and clinical populations.

How to Evaluate the Validity of a Test

There are different kinds and degrees of validity attached to different neuropsychological test scores, and there are numerous features that neuropsychologists can look for when evaluating a test and reviewing test manuals. Not all will have sufficient evidence to satisfy all aspects of validity, but clinicians should have a sufficiently broad knowledge of neuropsychological measures to be able to select one test over another (and one score over another within the same test), based on the quality of the validation evidence available.

Tables 30.6–30.8 present sources of evidence and techniques for critically evaluating the validity of neuropsychological test scores, abstracted from key sources such as Urbina (2004), the American Educational Research Association, American Psychological Association, and National Council on Measurement in Education (1999), Messick (1996), and Yun and Ulrich (2002). Note that there is overlap between the sources of evidence presented in Tables 30.6–30.8. For example, correlations between a specific IQ score and another IQ score can simultaneously provide construct-related and criterion-related evidence of validity.

Content-Related Evidence for Validity

Content-related evidence for validity provides information on whether the test items actually measure the construct they are intended to measure. Content-based

Table 30.6 Questions to ask for evaluating *content-related evidence for validity*

- Is the test based on a theoretical model?
- Is there a literature review with supporting evidence?
- Has the construct being measured been well defined?
- Has the operationalization of the construct (i.e., the translation of theory into test items) been done carefully (e.g., systematic review of the domain from which items are to be sampled)?
- Does the test have a large enough sample of items to be representative of the domain measured?
- Do the items have sufficient range of difficulty for the target population?
- Were items generated with care, using experts in the field or items from previously validated scales?
- Was the final item pool evaluated by experts in the field for accuracy and relevance?
- Will examinees think the test seems valid at face value?

Table 30.7 Questions to ask for evaluating *construct-related evidence for validity*

- Were hypotheses generated to measure the construct?
- Is the construct reliably measured as demonstrated by high reliability coefficients?
- Does it correlate highly with other test scores measuring the same construct?
- Does it have low correlations with test scores measuring different constructs?
- Do factor analytic studies support the construct measured by the test score as it is operationalized in the test?
- Are factor analytic and correlational findings consistent with the theoretical background for the construct measured?

Table 30.8 Questions to ask for evaluating the *criterion-related evidence for validity*

- Is the test score sensitive to expected developmental, demographic, or other differences in the sample?
- Do group difference studies support the test score?
- Is the test score sensitive to treatment effects (e.g., responsiveness)?
- Do classification accuracy statistics (e.g., positive and negative predictive power) support the use of the test score?
- Are there meta-analytic studies on the test score's usage in the population of interest?

sources of information for determining this might include whether test items were generated based on a theoretical model for the construct in question and whether that theoretical model reflects current empirical research on the construct. Additionally, it is important to determine whether the construct has been adequately operationalized in the test's items, and whether the test developers adequately defined the specific construct to be measured by the test. One way in which this is accomplished occurs when a test developer conducts a systematic review of the literature before generating test items, and by employing experts in the field to generate items and/or review item content, ideally after consensus. The goal is to refine the item pool while also balancing the need for a sufficiently broad set of items capable of capturing a range of function across the target group, and retaining good face validity.

Table 30.6 lists some basic questions to aid in determining whether a test has sufficient evidence for content-related validity. Few tests will satisfy each condition in Table 30.6, but a good test should have sufficient evidence satisfying a number of points in the table.

Construct-Related Evidence for Validity

Construct-related evidence for validity overlaps with content-related evidence for validity, as both pertain to what is being measured by the test itself (as opposed to what the test might predict, or have utility for clinically). Table 30.7 shows specific examples of ways in which the construct validity evidence for a test can be evaluated. As with content-related evidence, the presence of a theoretical model or theoretical background supported by empirical evidence is important in test item content, test structure, and test format, but equally important is whether that construct was reliably measured. Examination of reliability evidence therefore becomes crucial for determining construct validity. At the same time, a test that measures a specific construct well should overlap with other tests measuring a similar construct, and show some differentiation in terms of tests measuring different constructs. Methods such as the multitrait/multimethod matrix, factor analysis, and structural equation modeling are ways in which the construct validity of tests is evaluated. These methods answer specific questions such as, is there sufficient empirical evidence for grouping test items hierarchically into specific levels, such as subscales, index scores for specific domains, and global composites?

One common method for presenting validity evidence is through intercorrelations among tests that are believed to measure similar and dissimilar constructs. Realistically, many tests do not yield clear-cut correlation matrices with high correlations to similar tests and low correlations to dissimilar tests. Whenever large numbers of correlations among measures are presented, there tends to be expected and unexpected relationships between variables, and dissociable relations between tests may not occur in a clear-cut manner. Some of the overlapping variance to consider may be due to global factors such as underlying innate intelligence, or to the fact that most neuropsychological tests require multiple basic abilities.

Criterion-Related Evidence for Validity

Content and construct validity are aimed at increasing our understanding of the psychological construct being measured and how a person's performance fits within that frame of reference. A further question asks "what are the criteria that are related to the test score?". In its most basic sense, criterion-related evidence for validity refers to the sensitivity and utility of the test (see Table 30.8). For clinical neuropsychologists, this is the most important aspect of validity. The clinical sensitivity of tests can be assessed by examining whether scores follow an expected developmental curve across age, or show expected gender differences, or else are sensitive to expected demographic differences across examinees such as ethnicity, language, or socioeconomic status. Paradoxically, when a test yields different scores across demographic groups, it may have inherent bias or error, but a test that shows no ability to detect known differences may be insensitive to real individual differences across examinees. Also crucial is whether the test is capable of detecting changes in performance after treatment or intervention (responsiveness), and whether it is sensitive to the expected natural course of neurological, medical, or psychiatric conditions (e.g., fluctuating, declining, or stable). Classification accuracy statistics relating to test scores are also used to determine the validity of test scores. Although a detailed discussion is beyond the scope of this chapter, this relates to the adequacy of statistics such as positive and negative predictive power in predicting the presence or absence of specific diagnoses or conditions based on test scores. Ideally, well-validated test scores have also been tested through meta-analytic studies to determine effect sizes describing the sensitivity of different neuropsychological tests in different contexts and with different groups. However, studies of this kind are few and far between in the field of neuropsychology.

Conclusions

The goal of this chapter was to help clinicians and researchers in assessing the reliability and validity of tests for clinical use. We discussed different types of reliability, factors that affect reliability, and limits to reliability. Reliability refers to the consistency of measurement of a given score. It is not an "all or none" property of a test. Rather, reliability refers to test scores, determined through evaluation of different kinds of reliability evidence (e.g., internal, test–retest, alternate form, and interrater). Determining the reliability of a test score is an ongoing process based on information gathered in both healthy individuals and clinical populations.

Similarly, validity is not an "all or none" property of a test. Validity is a property of the meaning attached to a test score in the specific context of test usage. That is, test scores have varying degrees of validity, for specific uses, with specific populations. There are three broad categories of validity evidence to consider (tripartite model): content-related, construct-related; and criterion-related. Within these broad categories, there are many ways of estimating the validity of test scores. Similar to reliability, determining the validity of a test score is an ongoing process based on information gathered in both healthy individuals and clinical populations.

The selection of neuropsychological measures requires a careful and thoughtful process that involves sifting through multiple sources of psychometric evidence. The process depends heavily on test publishers' ability to include comprehensive information in test manuals that clinicians need for selecting and administering tests, but it is equally critical for clinicians to review test manuals carefully and scrutinize the information that is being presented. In the end, evaluating the reliability and validity of neuropsychological tests is a gradual process involving numerous studies over extended periods of time. Perhaps one of the most important components of reliability and validity is the *clinical inferences derived from tests* (see Franzen 1989, 2000; Strauss et al. 2006). Our field has come a long way but there is still much progress to make in this domain.

References

American Educational Research Association, American Psychological Association, & National Council on Measurement in Education. (1999). *Standards for educational and psychological testing*. Washington, DC: American Psychological Association.

Anastasi, A., & Urbina, S. (1997). Psychological testing (7th edition) Upper Saddle River, New Jersey, Prentice-Hall.

Bland, J. M., & Altman, D. G. (1986). Statistical methods for assessing agreement between two methods of clinical measurement. *Lancet, i*, 307–310.

Bornstein, R. F. (1996). Face validity in psychological assessment: Implications for a unified model of validity. *American Psychologist, 51*(9), 983–984.

Brooks, B. L., Iverson, G. L., & White, T. (2009). *Advanced interpretation of the Neuropsychological Assessment Battery (NAB) with older adults: Base rate analyses, discrepancy scores, and interpreting change*. Unpublished manuscript.

Cicchetti, D. V. (1994). Guidelines, criteria, and rules of thumb for evaluating normed and standardized assessment instruments in psychology. *Psychological Assessment, 6*(4), 284–290.

Cicchetti, D. V., & Sparrow, S. S. (1981). Developing criteria for establishing interrater reliability of specific items: Applications to assessment of adaptive behavior. *American Journal of Mental Deficiency, 86*, 127–137.

Cronbach, L. J., & Meehl, P. E. (1955). Construct validity in psychological tests. *Psychological Bulletin, 52*(4), 281–302.

Culbertson, W. C., & Zillmer, E. A. (2005). *Tower of London – Drexel University* (2nd ed.). North Tonawanda: MHS.

Delis, D. C., Kaplan, E., & Kramer, J. H. (2001). *Delis Kaplan executive function system technical manual*. San Antonio: The Psychological Corporation.

Fastenau, P. S., Bennett, J. M., & Denburg, N. L. (1996). Application of psychometric standards to scoring system evaluation: Is "new" necessarily "improved"? *Journal of Clinical and Experimental Neuropsychology, 18*(3), 462–472.

Franzen, M. D. (1989). *Reliability and validity in neuropsychological assessment*. New York: Plenum Press.

Franzen, M. D. (2000). *Reliability and validity in neurological assessment* (2nd ed.). New York: Kluwer Academic/Plenum Press.

Heaton, R. K., Chelune, G. J., Talley, J. L., Kay, G. G., & Curtis, G. (1993). *Wisconsin card sorting task (WCST) manual, revised and expanded*. Odessa: Psychological Assessment Resources.

Lineweaver, T. T., & Chelune, G. J. (2003). Use of the WAIS-III and WMS-III in the context of serial assessments: Interpreting reliable and meaningful change. In D. S. Tulsky, D. H. Saklofske, G. J. Chelune, R. K. Heaton, R. Ivnik, R. Bornstein, A. Prifitera, & M. F. Ledbetter (Eds.), *Clinical interpretation of the WAIS-III and WMS-III* (pp. 303–337). New York: Academic press.

McGrew, K. S., & Woodcock, R. W. (2001). *Woodcock-Johnson III technical manual*. Itasca: Riverside Publishing.

Messick, S. (1996). Validity of psychological assessment: Validation of inferences from persons' responses and performances as scientific inquiry into score meaning. *American Psychologist, 50*(9), 741–749.

Mitrushina, M. N., Boone, K. B., Razani, J., & D'Elia, L. F. (2005). *Handbook of normative data for neuropsychological assessment* (2nd ed.). New York: Oxford University Press.

Nevo, B. (1985). Face validity revisited. *Journal of Educational Measurement, 22*, 287–293.

Nunnally, J. C., & Bernstein, I. H. (1994). *Psychometric theory* (3rd ed.). New York: McGraw-Hill, Inc.

Psychological Corporation. (2002). *WAIS-III/WMS-III technical manual*. San Antonio: Psychological Corporation.

Rapport, L. J., Brines, D. B., & Axelrod, B. N. (1997). Full scale IQ as a mediator of practice effects: The rich get richer. *Clinical Neuropsychologist, 11*(4), 375–380.

Reynolds, C. R. (2002). *Comprehensive trail making test*. Austin: PRO-ED.

Ruff, R. M., & Hibbard, K. M. (2003). *Ruff neurobehavioral inventory*. Lutz: Psychological Assessment Resources, Inc.

Sattler, J. M. (2001). *Assessment of children: Cognitive applications* (4th ed.). San Diego: Jerome M. Sattler Publisher, Inc.

Sjögren, P., Thomsen, A., & Olsen, A. (2000). Impaired neuropsychological performance in chronic nonmalignant pain patients receiving long-term oral opioid therapy. *Journal of Pain and Symptom Management, 19*(2), 100–108.

Stern, R. A., & White, T. (2003). *Neuropsychological assessment battery (NAB)*. Lutz: Psychological Assessment Resources.

Strauss, E., Sherman, E. M. S., & Spreen, O. (2006). *A compendium of neuropsychological tests* (3rd ed.). New York: Oxford University Press.

Urbina, S. (2004). *Essentials of psychological testing*. Hoboken: John Wiley & Sons.

Wechsler, D. (2004). *Wechsler intelligence scale for children* (Integrated technical and interpretive manual 4th ed.). San Antonio: The Psychological Corporation.

Wechsler, D., Coalson, D. L., & Raiford, S. E. (2008). *Wechsler adult intelligence scale* (Technical and interpretive manual 4th ed.). San Antonio: NCS Pearson, Inc.

Wechsler, D., Holdnack, J. A., & Drozdick, L. W. (2009). *Wechsler memory scale* (Technical and interpretive manual 4th ed.). San Antonio: NCS Pearson, Inc.

White, T., & Stern, R. A. (2003). *Neuropsychological assessment battery (NAB): Psychometric and technical manual*. Lutz: Psychological Assessment Resources.

Yun, J., & Ulrich, D. A. (2002). Estimating measurement validity: A tutorial. *Adapted physical activity quarterly, 19*, 32–47.

Chapter 31
Psychometric Foundations for the Interpretation of Neuropsychological Test Results[*]

Brian L. Brooks, Elisabeth M.S. Sherman, Grant L. Iverson, Daniel J. Slick, and Esther Strauss

Abstract The purpose of this chapter is to illustrate how an understanding of the psychometric properties of tests, normative samples, and test scores are an essential foundation for meaningful and accurate clinical interpretations and reduces the likelihood of misinterpreting test results. Our goal is to present this information in an easy-to-understand format that facilitates clinicians' knowledge of basic psychometrics in the context of test score interpretation. Clinical examples using commonly used tests will be provided throughout to illustrate the relevance and utility of these concepts in clinical practice.

With regard to sample distributions, we will review concepts relating to non-normality and the influence of score distribution characteristics on derived scores. Floor and ceiling effects, equivalence of normative data sets, and truncated distributions will be discussed with regard to test items and test norms. When comparing scores between tests, we will review the role of test measurement error. We will also discuss normal variability and briefly comment on the prevalence of low test scores in healthy people, and how to use this information for supplementing clinical judgment. Finally, we will provide an overview of various methods for interpreting change in test performance over time.

Key Points and Chapter Summary

- Interpreting and communicating test performance depends on having an appropriate (comparative) sample and a common "language" of descriptors.
- Sample characteristics, such as non-normal distributions, skew, or truncated samples, will impact interpretation of test performance.

(continued)

---

*The current chapter is based upon the chapter, "Psychometrics in neuropsychological assessment," from Strauss et al. (2006) and co-written with Daniel J. Slick.

B.L. Brooks (✉)
Alberta Children's Hospital, University of Calgary, Calgary, AB, Canada
e-mail: brian.brooks@albertahealthservices.ca

M.R. Schoenberg and J.G. Scott (eds.), *The Little Black Book of Neuropsychology: A Syndrome-Based Approach*, DOI 10.1007/978-0-387-76978-3_31,
© Springer Science+Business Media, LLC 2011

Key Points and Chapter Summary (continued)

- Comparison of performance across tests is affected by normative sample differences, measurement error, score magnitude and rank in the distribution, extreme scores, ceiling and floor effects, and extrapolation/interpolation of derived scores.
- It is normal for healthy people have some variability across tests and to have some low scores on a battery of neuropsychological tests. This normal variability must be considered in the interpretation of isolated low test scores.
- Interpreting test scores over time requires sophisticated psychometric models to minimize clinical bias and error and supplement clinical judgment.

Interpreting and Communicating Test Performance in Clinical Practice

A person's raw score on a neuropsychological test has little meaning without (1) a comparison to a normative sample and (2) a method for interpreting and communicating the meaning of that comparison. For example, if Mr. Doe, a 62-year-old male, obtains a raw score of 26 on a test of speeded information processing, this fact does not hold much meaning by itself. However, if a sample of 200 men between the ages of 60 and 65 years obtain a mean score of 25 on the same test, with a standard deviation (SD) of 5.0 points,[1] then two things become readily apparent. First, Mr. Doe's performance is within +1SD of the mean for his age group. Second, it is unlikely that Mr. Doe has a clinically-significant problem with information processing speed as measured by this test. In short, the performance of a normative sample allows clinicians to determine the relative standing of an individual's performance. Overall, the notion of relative standing is a key concept in neuropsychology, and serves as the basis for all test score interpretations. Almost all scores used by neuropsychologists provide information on relative standing, whether these consist of z scores (mean = 0, SD = 1), scaled scores (mean = 10, SD = 3), T scores (mean = 50, SD = 10), index scores (mean = 100, SD = 15), or percentiles.

Having a methodology for comparing performance on a test to a representative sample is an important step in understanding a person's ability on a test of a cognitive ability. However, the result of a person's performance on the test needs to be communicated to other neuropsychologists, to other professionals, to the patient, and to others involved in the patient's care. Without a system for interpreting and communicating the results, again, the patient's performance on the test remains meaningless.

A psychometric approach, based on the theoretical normal distribution, has been used for the interpretation of intelligence test results for decades. The modern version of this psychometric approach is based on the Wechsler classification system and is illustrated in Table 31.1. This classification scheme is based on fairly precise estimates of where a person falls in the distribution of scores obtained by

---

[1] This example assumes that the scores are normally distributed. This example also assumes that higher raw scores reflect better performance.

healthy persons with no cognitive, psychiatric, or neurological problems. Another classification and interpretation system, based on a system popularized by Heaton and colleagues (Heaton et al. 1993, 1991, 2004) and used for the Neuropsychological Assessment Battery (NAB; Stern and White 2003a), is also presented in Table 31.1. Considering the above example with Mr. Doe's performance on the speeded information coding test (i.e., his performance is equal to a z score of +0.2, a T score of 52, and is at the 58th percentile), the clinician is able to interpret and communicate that this performance is "average" compared to 60–65 year olds according to both the Wechsler and Heaton-NAB classification systems. (*Note*: We do not advocate one classification system over the other, but we do suggest that clinicians use the same system throughout a report. Reporting scores using different classification systems, within the same report, can be conceptually confusing for readers.)

Table 31.1 Commonly used classification ranges, along with their corresponding standard scores and percentile ranks

Wechsler classification ranges[a]	Scaled score range $M = 10, SD = 3$	IQ/index score range $M = 100, SD = 15$	T score range $M = 50, SD = 10$	Percentile ranks
Very superior	16+	130 +	70 +	98 +
Superior	14–15	120–129	64–69	91–97
High average	13	110–119	57–63	75–90
Average	8–12[b]	90–109	44–56	25–74
Low average	7	80–89	37–43	9–24
Unusually low (Borderline)[c]	5–6[d]	70–79	30–36	2–8
Extremely low	≤ 4[e]	<70	<30	<2

Heaton-NAB classification ranges[f]	Index score range $M = 100, SD = 15$	T score range $M = 50, SD = 10$	Percentile ranks
Very superior	130–155	70–81	98+
Superior	115–129	60–69	84–97
Above average	107–114	55–59	68–82
Average	92–106	45–54	30–67
Below average	85–91	40–44	16–27
Mildly impaired	77–84	35–39	6–15
Mildly-to-moderately impaired	70–76	30–34	2–5
Moderately impaired	62–69	25–29	0.6–1.9
Moderately-to-severely impaired	55–61	20–24	0.13–0.5
Severely impaired	45–54	19	<.12

M mean, *SD* standard deviation

[a] Note that this is similar to the Wechsler system of classification

[b] A scaled score of 12 is at the 75th percentile, but is described as being "average" in this classification system

[c] The Wechsler system refers to scores between the 2nd and 8th percentiles as "borderline"

[d] A scaled score of 6 is at the 9th percentile, but is classified as being "unusually low" (borderline)

[e] A scaled score of 4 is at the 2nd percentile, but is considered "extremely low"

[f] Note that this is similar to the Heaton system of classification. Classifications for interpreting scores according to the Wechsler system were derived from Tables 2.2 and 2.3 in the WAIS-III Technical Manual (Wechsler 1997a). Classifications for interpreting Index and T scores according to the NAB-Heaton method were derived from Tables 6.8 and 6.9, respectively, from the NAB Administration, Scoring, and Interpretation Manual (Stern and White 2003b)

> **Rule of thumb: Interpreting and communicating test performance in Neuropsychology**
>
> Interpreting and communicating test performance depends on having an appropriate comparative sample and a common "language" of descriptors (i.e., classification system). Regardless of the classification system that is used, it is recommended clinicians be consistent throughout a report.

Sample Characteristics and Test Score Interpretation

The Adequacy of the Normative Sample

Neuropsychological tests typically provide numerous test scores that are derived from a comparison of a person's performance to the performance of a representative normative sample, including z scores, T scores, scaled scores, index scores, IQ scores, and percentiles (for a discussion on the derivation of each of these score types, see Sattler 2001; Strauss et al. 2006; Urbina 2004). All these scores are derived from *samples*. Importantly, these scores are not population values, and any limitations of generalizability due to normative sample composition or testing circumstances must be taken into consideration when standardized scores are interpreted. Some tests, for example, may have normative samples that are (1) limited in heterogeneity, (2) samples of convenience, (3) small in size, and (4) outdated. An obvious example would be the practice of computing z scores for the Auditory Consonant Trigrams test based on a sample of 30 adults from Eastern Canada who completed the test in the 1980s. This is the first consideration when using norms: does the test have an adequate normative sample and what are the limitations of this sample?

The Boston Naming Test (BNT) is a good example of a test in widespread use that, historically, has had problems with inadequate normative data. For example, the original normative data for adults were based on 178 adults (Kaplan et al. 1978). Although this is a respectable number overall, the age range covered by the norms is large. Thus, the actual cell sizes when broken down by age are as low as 11 individuals in some age groups. Moreover, it turned out to be inappropriate to apply the original normative information to adults 60 years and older (i.e., the highest age group was 50–59 years, $n = 22$). Van Gorp et al. (1986) extended normative data for older adults up to 95 years of age, although the sample was small in size ($n = 78$) and was high functioning (i.e., mean Verbal IQ scores were in the high average to superior ranges). The Tombaugh and Hubley (1997) norms consisted of only 219 people between 25 and 88 years of age (cell sizes for age ranged from $n = 18$ to 33; cell sizes for age × education ranged from $n = 26$ to 78), although once again the sample was relatively well educated. Further improvements on the BNT normative data have been published, and include the Mayo's Older American Normative Studies (i.e., $n = 663$, ages 57–97; Ivnik et al. 1996) and the Mayo's Older African American Normative Studies (i.e., n = 309 ages 56–94; Lucas et al. 2005) and the Expanded Halstead-Reitan Neuropsychological Battery norms (i.e., n = 1,000; Heaton et al. 2004).

Although there have been some improvements in the adequacy of the BNT normative data, having numerous (and different) comparative groups creates a problem for the clinician. Do meaningful interpretive differences exist, depending on which normative data is used? Figure 31.1 illustrates the differences in obtained percentiles that occur based on the use of different comparative normative samples. Consider the interpretation of a raw score of 51 for a 72-year-old African American woman with 10 years of education using the MOANS and MOAANS normative samples. According to the MOANS norms, this would be at the 37th percentile (scaled score = 9). However, according to the MOAANS norms, this would be at the 75th percentile (scaled score = 12). This difference in normative scores can create substantial interpretive differences, particularly as the performance declines below clinically-meaningful cutoff scores. These differences can be at least partially accounted for by the nearly all Caucasian (i.e., 99.1%) and relatively well-educated (i.e., 83.6% had at least high school, 50.3% had at least some post-secondary education, and 26.0% had at least a bachelor's degree) MOANS sample for the BNT normative data. Importantly, as seen for the BNT scores of 43 and 40, normative systems that are not adjusted for ethnicity will yield scores that are "impaired" whereas ethnicity-adjusted systems will yield scores that are average.

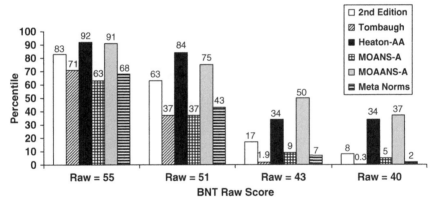

Fig. 31.1 Comparison of normative systems for the Boston Naming Test: 72-year-old African American woman with 10 years of education (percentile ranks).

Note: Percentile ranks are presented. If a percentile rank included a range (e.g., 10–25 percentile), then the highest value in the range is presented in the figure. 2nd edition – BNT-second edition, which includes normative data obtained from Kaplan et al. (2001). Tombaugh – Tombaugh and Hubley (1997) sample, which was relatively well-educated and had small sample sizes. To calculate the percentiles presented for the Tombaugh and Hubley (1997) norms, z scores were calculated using the age-adjusted mean (M = 52.5) and standard deviation (SD = 4.6) from Table 31.1 in the manuscript (despite the raw scores *not* being normally distributed). Heaton-AA – African American normative data from the Expanded Norms for the Halstead-Reitan Neuropsychological Battery (Heaton et al. 2004). MOANS-A – Age-adjusted normative data from the Mayo's Older Americans Normative Studies (Ivnik et al. 1996). MOAANS-A – Age-adjusted normative data from the Mayo's Older African Americans Normative Studies (Lucas et al. 2005). Normative data for MOANS-A and MOAANS-A were derived from pp. 906–907 of Strauss et al. (2006). Meta Norms – Meta-normative data from Mitrushina et al. (2005) on p. 725

Another example of how normative data can affect clinical interpretation relates to the California Verbal Learning Test (CVLT; Delis et al. 1987). In the manual for the second edition (CVLT-II; Delis et al. 2000), a comparison study between the CVLT and CVLT-II was presented. Healthy adults ($n = 62$) took both versions in counter-balanced order. The raw scores derived from the two tests were remarkably similar. Examples are as follows: Trials 1–5 Recall was 58.76 (SD = 8.94; CVLT) and 58.47 (SD = 9.98; CVLT-II) and Long Delay Free Recall was 12.94 (SD = 2.73; CVLT) and 13.26 (SD = 2.86; CVLT-II). Although the raw scores are similar, the *normative scores* are different (see Fig. 31.2). Why? Because the original CVLT norms were based on a research sample that was well educated (mean education level = 13.8 years, SD = 2.7) and less representative of healthy adults in the community than the CVLT-II.

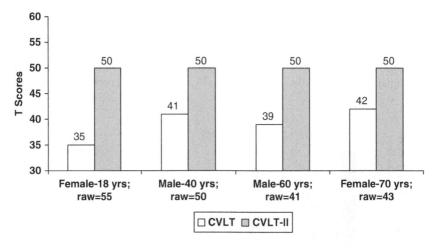

Fig. 31.2 CVLT versus CVLT-II trials 1–5 total score: Normative comparisons (T-scores). Age-adjusted T scores for the CVLT and CVLT-II were derived from Table 6.8 (p. 80) of the CVLT-II manual (Delis et al. 2000)

The clinical implications for CVLT interpretation, based on normative differences, are striking. In the past, many examinees with average or low average scores (based on performance on the CVLT-II) would have been labeled as "impaired" when using the original CVLT. When this happens over many cases in one's clinical practice, it is natural to assume that the test is "highly sensitive" to actual impairment. This is particularly true if other memory tests show no such pattern of impairment, and thus appear comparatively less sensitive. The problem is that more than 30% of people with average scores were being falsely classified as "below average" or "impaired" based on the original CVLT norms. Well-informed clinicians were aware that there were problems with the original CVLT norms, and it was appropriate to use these norms with examinees who matched the normative sample (i.e., had higher education).

However, clinicians who were not aware of the specific characteristics of this normative dataset were at risk of overestimating memory deficits in healthy people. The newer normative dataset for the CVLT-II clearly addresses this problem and therefore provides a more broadly usable normative dataset than its predecessor.

Clearly, the quality and representativeness of normative data can have a dramatic effect on the clinical interpretation of test scores. For example, it is well understood that education is related to test performance. Moreover, ethnicity is related to test performance (perhaps as a surrogate for factors such as quality of education). However, many neuropsychological tests do not have education- or ethnicity-adjusted normative data; or, if it is available, it is not commonly used. The effects of education and ethnicity, on WTAR-demographics predicted Full Scale IQ, are illustrated in Fig. 31.3. As seen in this figure, estimated Full Scale IQ is positively associated with years of education and varies by ethnicity. The direction of difference between ethnic groups is consistent across all levels of education and is quite large, exceeding one standard deviation for some comparisons.

What are the clinical and interpretive implications of Fig. 31.3? First, Full Scale IQ scores are related to education and ethnicity. Second, as discussed in more detail later in this chapter (i.e., it is not illustrated in Fig. 31.3), Full Scale IQ is positively correlated with other cognitive test scores. Therefore, those individuals with below average IQ are expected to have far more low neuropsychological test scores than those with above average IQ. Finally, many normative sets used in clinical practice are adjusted for age only. Therefore, variables such as education, IQ, and ethnicity are left uncontrolled and must be subject to clinical judgment, as opposed to being considered psychometrically.

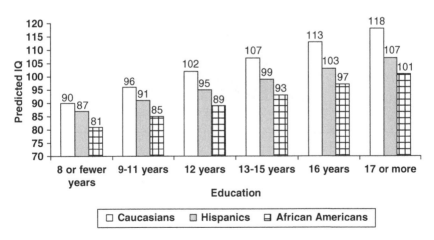

Fig. 31.3 Effects of education and ethnicity on demographics-predicted WAIS-III Full Scale IQ in men. Demographics-predicted WAIS-III FSIQ scores were derived from p. 114 of the Wechsler Adult Reading Test Manual (The Psychological Corporation 2001)

The Shape of the Distribution: Non-normality and Skew

The normal curve is the basis of most commonly used (parametric) statistical and psychometric models in neuropsychology. When a new test is constructed, non-normality can be "corrected" by examining the distribution of scores on the proto-type test, adjusting its properties, and re-sampling until a normal distribution is reached. More commonly, normality is achieved by various "smoothing" proce-dures. This facilitates clinical interpretation, for reasons that we will discuss below.

A true normal distribution is perfectly symmetrical about the mean and has a skew of zero. Positive skew indicates a frequency distribution where more scores fall below the mean compared to above the mean. Negative skew refers to distribu-tions where more scores fall above the mean compared to below the mean. Perfect symmetry and zero skew might be more theoretical than practical (see Fig. 31.4 for a theoretical normal distribution, as well as "classic" examples of skewed distribu-tions). Many actual distributions of test scores deviate somewhat from the theoretical distribution that we have come to expect. What happens when scores for the normative sample for a test are not normally distributed?

Rule of thumb: Distribution descriptors

- Direction of the tail that tells the tale
- Tail "pointing" to the right (positive) is a positively skewed distribution
- Tail "pointing" to the left (negative) is a negatively skewed distribution

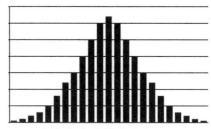

Theoretical normal distribution

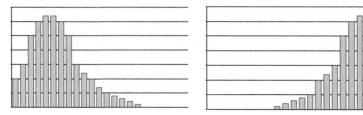

Positively skewed distribution   Negatively skewed distribution

Fig. 31.4 Theoretical examples of normal, positively skewed, and negatively skewed distribu-tions. The visual examples of positively and negatively skewed distributions represent "classic" examples of skew

First, when distributions are skewed, the mean and median are not identical (i.e., the mean will not be at the midpoint in rank) and z scores will not accurately translate into sample percentile rank values. The error in mapping of z scores to sample percentile rank increases as skew increases. Self-report questionnaires typically have positively skewed distributions in healthy people because they are assessing problem behaviors that are typically found at a higher frequency or severity in clinical populations. For example, the Behavior Rating Inventory of Executive Function (Gioia et al. 2000) assesses the severity of executive dysfunction; consequently, most of the children in the normative sample had few elevated scores, and hence the normative distribution has a negative skew (high scores indicate more problems and thus the normative group reports relatively few symptoms). However, the degree of skew differs slightly across BRIEF subscales, which means that T scores (which are linear transformations of the z scores) are not directly comparable across subscales. Percentiles derived directly from a skewed raw score distribution are therefore a more accurate way to compare these subscales to each other. In other words, as a general rule percentile ranks obtained from the natural distribution of raw scores, regardless of skew, are more comparable than transformed scores.

Second, tests with a normal distribution of scores in samples from the general population may show significant skew or other divergence from normality when given to a population that differs considerably from the average individual. For example, the performances of Elderly Hispanic persons on an English Vocabulary test might result in scores clustering at the low end of the distribution. These scores are unlikely to reflect actual impairment or decline. Thus, the distribution of scores on a test's normative sample should be evaluated for congruence with the individual being assessed to determine whether there are factors that might skew score distributions (e.g., in this example, English fluency and possible cultural differences).

In some circumstances, a normal distribution of scores simply does not exist. For instance, the ability being measured may not be normally distributed in the population. An example of this might be a test of orientation, where almost all healthy individuals score almost perfectly (i.e., a highly positively skewed distribution where most persons perform perfectly). Alternatively, one may want only to identify and/or discriminate between patients who have known cognitive impairment (i.e., identify differences between groups at one end of the normal distribution only). Thus, the measure might be designed specifically to sample a range of abilities in patients with impairments. If one is not interested in the rest of the distribution, items that would provide discrimination in that region can be omitted to save administration time.

In general, the degree to which a sample distribution approximates the underlying population distribution increases as sample size increases, and becomes less accurate as sample size decreases. This has important implications for norms comprised of small samples. Thus, a larger sample will on average produce a more normal distribution, but only if the underlying characteristic (i.e. height) in the population distribution from which the samples is obtained is normal (i.e., a large n does not "correct" for nonnormality of an underlying population distribution). Small samples may yield a nonnormal distribution due to random sampling effects, even though the population from which the sample is drawn has a normal distribution. As a result, clinicians should be cautious when interpreting tests with normative samples less than 50 per age group.

The Range of the Distribution: Truncated Distributions

Significant skew often indicates the presence of a truncated distribution. This may occur when the range of scores is restricted on one side of the distribution but not the other. An example would be a simple effort test, such as the Test of Memory Malingering (TOMM; Tombaugh 1996), where a large proportion of healthy children and adults obtain perfect or near-perfect scores (e.g., 49 or 50/50). Truncated distributions are also present for certain neuropsychological tests, such as those involving tests that healthy people accomplish almost perfectly (e.g., orientation, recognition memory). Some tests do not include a high enough ceiling to allow for discrimination between higher functioning individuals and to detect cognitive deficits in some cases. This can translate into a truncated distribution for such a population. A good example of this is the Failure to Maintain Set (FMS) score on the Wisconsin Card Sorting Test (WCST; Heaton et al. 1993). In the normative sample of 30- to 39-year-old persons, observed raw scores ranged from 0 to 21, but the majority of persons (84%) obtained scores of 0 or 1 and less than 1% obtained scores greater than 3 (see Tables D20–D25 in the WCST Manual). What happens when an individual obtains a low score on a test with a truncated distribution? The clinician might calculate an extreme z or T score with a percentile rank that would not actually exist in the normative sample because the assumption of normality has not been met. Care is therefore required so as not to over-interpret abnormally low score differences based on truncated distributions.

Truncated distributions also occur when specific subgroups are purposefully (or unintentionally) excluded from inclusion in the normative sample. Purposeful exclusion of subgroups occurs when exclusion criteria are used in creating normative samples. This might include omitting persons with cognitive impairments, learning difficulties, or medical conditions to create normative samples composed exclusively of healthy subjects. One of the problems with this approach is that the general population includes a certain proportion of persons falling in the low end of the distribution. Excluding these individuals, therefore, creates norms that are missing the left tail of the distribution or have a left tail that is not heavy enough (as opposed to full-range normative sampling). When these distributions are then used for standardized testing, because low-functioning individuals have been excluded from the norms, the resulting low end of the distribution (or lowest percentiles) are now occupied by persons who would have populated higher percentiles in the full distribution. This can potentially lead to (1) identification of normal individuals as low functioning, (2) difficulties estimating the severity of impaired performance, and (3) potentially, an increase in the number of persons identified as impaired with subsequent test re-norming (e.g., if the test itself is used to consecutively exclude the lowest percentile members each time new norms are created; McFadden 1996).

The PPVT-4 (Dunn and Dunn 2007) is an example of a test with a full-range normative sample, whereas the child sample for the WCST excludes children with a variety of conditions potentially affecting cognition (Strauss et al. 2006). The WISC-IV is an example of a test that screened the sample for conditions, but then re-inserted a specific proportion of special needs children into the sample (5.7%) so that it would reflect the full range of abilities in the general population (Wechsler 2003).

The normative sample for the Test of Verbal Comprehension and Fluency (Reynolds and Horton 2006) also includes people of all ages with known problems, such as learning problems or ADHD. Knowing the inclusion and exclusion criteria that were used in creating normative samples allows better comparison between scores obtained from different measures.

Rule of thumb: Psychometric issues affecting interpretation

Sample characteristics, such as non-normal distributions, skew, or truncated samples, can impact interpretation of test performance.

Comparing Scores Between Tests

Standardizing test scores facilitates comparison of scores across measures. This is most useful, of course, when (1) the raw score distributions for tests that are being compared are approximately normal in the population, and (2) the scores being compared are derived from similar samples, or more ideally, from the same sample (i.e., co-norming). Thus, a score at the 50th percentile on a test normed on a small sample of well-educated Caucasians from Ottawa, Ontario, in the 1980s might not have the same meaning as an "equivalent" score on a test normed on a large, ethnically-diverse sample obtained from Los Angeles, California in 2004.

Measurement Error

When comparing test scores, it is important to consider the reliability of the two measures and their intercorrelation before determining if a reliable or clinically meaningful difference exists (see Crawford and Garthwaite 2002). In some cases, relatively large discrepancies between scores may not actually reflect reliable differences. Moreover, a statistically significant or reliable difference between test scores might occur frequently in a given population, and thus not necessarily be clinically meaningful (e.g., Crawford et al. 2007). For example, large differences between attention (normal range) and IQ (superior range) may occur in some gifted individuals, but this would not necessarily constitute evidence of cognitive dysfunction. Rather, it could be a normal pattern of scores for some gifted individuals.

Score Magnitude and Rank in the Score Distribution

The level of the two scores being compared should also be considered. That is, an absolute difference between two standard scores may be common or uncommon, depending on the level of the scores (e.g., T score of 30 vs 40 as compared to 60 vs 70). One should also keep in mind that, when test scores are not normally distributed, standardized scores may not accurately reflect actual population rank. In these circumstances, differences between standard scores may be misleading.

The relationship between normative scores (e.g., z scores or T scores) and percentiles is not linear. That is, a constant difference between z scores will be associated with a variable difference in percentile scores, as a function of the distance of the two scores from the mean. This is because there are proportionally more scores closer to the mean than farther from the mean (i.e., otherwise, the distribution would be rectangular, or non-normal).

The non-linear relation between z scores and percentiles has important interpretive implications. For example, a one-point difference between two z scores may be interpreted differently, depending on where the two scores fall on the normal curve. The difference between a z score of 0 and a z score of +1 is 34 percentile points, because 34% of scores fall between these two z scores (i.e., the scores being compared are at the 50th and 84th percentile). However, the difference between a z score of +2 and a z score of +3 is less than 3 percentile points, because only 2.2% of the distribution falls between these two points (i.e., the scores being compared are at the 97.7th and 99.9th percentile).

The interpretation of percentile scores with an equivalent "difference" between two percentile rankings might have very different clinical implications if the scores occur at the tail end of the curve versus near the middle of the distribution. For example, an improvement in a standard score from the 5th percentile to the 30th percentile (25 percentile points), compared to an improvement from the 37th to the 62nd percentile (25 percentile points), (1) requires a greater improvement in performance from a *standard score* perspective (i.e., going from the 5th to the 30th percentile is an index score improvement from 76 to 92, which is more than one standard deviation; going from the 37th to the 62nd percentile is an index score improvement from 95 to 105, which is two-thirds of a standard deviation) and (2) might be much more clinically and functionally meaningful (i.e., going from the 5th percentile to the 30th percentile is going from an unusually low score to an average score; scores at the 37th and the 62nd percentile are both in the average range).

Ceiling/Floor Effects and Score Comparisons

Floor and ceiling effects may be defined as the presence of truncated tails in the context of limitations in range of item difficulty. For example, a test may be said to have a *high floor* when a large proportion of the examinees obtain raw scores at or near the lowest possible score. This may indicate that the test lacks a sufficient number and range of easier items. Conversely, a test may be said to have a *low ceiling* when the opposite pattern is present. Floor and ceiling effects may significantly limit the usefulness of a measure. For example, a measure with a high floor may not be suitable for use with low functioning examinees, particularly if one wishes to delineate level of impairment. Misinterpreting results obtained from tests with low ceilings is common. For example, on the TOMM, a clinician might interpret a score of 50/50 as showing "very good" or "excellent" effort – when in fact that score is easily obtained by the majority of people. Thus, it likely better reflects no evidence of non-compliance with the assessment, or "adequate," "normal," or even "minimal" effort. A similar situation occurs with the Boston Naming Test where a score of 60/60 should be considered as reflecting average, not excellent, naming ability.

If a clinician is not well informed of the distribution of test scores, floor and ceiling effects can potentially lead to misinterpretations when comparing across tests. For instance, on the *Wechsler Memory Scale* – Third Edition (WMS-III; Wechsler 1997b), the distribution varies by (1) subtest, and (2) age. An example from WMS-III that serves to illustrate the presence of ceiling effects is presented in Fig. 31.5. A clinician who is not aware of these normative distribution characteristics might inadvertently conclude that a very high functioning examinee who scores in the superior range on the delayed portion of Logical Memory (LMII) performs less well, or has a "relative weakness," on the delayed portion of Verbal Paired Associates (VPAII; note that the maximum possible normative score for VPAII in 20–24 year olds is 12, which is at the 75th percentile).

Another example of a truncated distribution is illustrated in Fig. 31.6. The Boston Diagnostic Aphasia Exam Complex Ideation test (Goodglass and Kaplan 1983) measures language comprehension and short-term memory. The total score ranges from 0 to 12. A perfect score of 12 is achieved by a large percentage of healthy adults, and performance varies considerably based on level of education. This truncation represents a "ceiling effect" in that the test does not measure a broad range of performance in high functioning adults. As seen in Fig. 31.6, a perfect raw score of 12 on this test results in a *T* score of 60 (84th percentile) for a young woman with 9–11 years of education, and 53 (62nd percentile) for young women with university degrees (note: normative data are derived from Heaton et al. 2004). Thus, truncation (ceiling effect in this example) is important to consider,

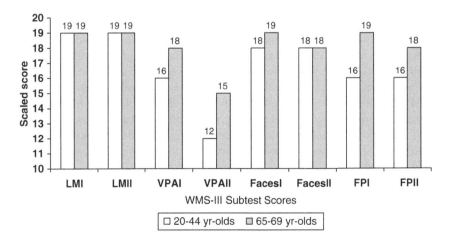

Fig. 31.5 Maximum (ceiling) scaled scores on the WMS-III in two selected age groups.
Note: This information was derived from the normative tables presented in the WMS-III Administration Manual (Wechsler, 1997b)

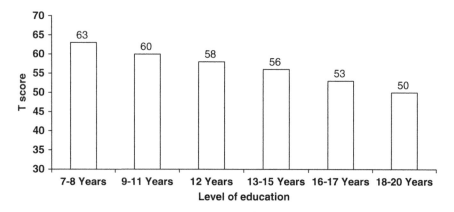

Fig. 31.6 Education-stratified normative scores (*T* scores) corresponding to a perfect raw score (12/12) on the Boston Diagnostic Aphasia Exam Complex Ideation Test: 25-year-old Caucasian female. The BDAE T scores were obtained from the Expanded Halstead-Reitan Battery Normative Manual (Heaton et al. 2004)

especially in high functioning adults, so that the clinician does not inadvertently consider (1) an "average" score in a highly educated adult a "relative weakness" when, in fact, it is a perfect raw score, and (2) a more educated person to have underperformed compared to a less educated person.

Extrapolation/Interpolation of Derived Scores

There are times when norms fall short in terms of range or cell size. This includes missing data in some cells, inconsistent age coverage, or inadequate demographic composition of some cells compared to the population. In these cases, data are often extrapolated or interpolated using the existing score distribution and techniques such as multiple regression. For example, Heaton and colleagues have published sets of norms that use multiple regression to correct for demographic characteristics and compensate for few subjects in some cells (Heaton et al. 1991; 2004). Although multiple regression is robust to slight violations of assumptions, estimation errors may occur when using normative data that violates the assumptions of homoscedasticity (uniform variance across the range of scores) and the distribution of residuals that are necessary for multiple regression are non-normal (Fastenau and Adams 1996).

Age extrapolations beyond the bounds of the actual ages of the individuals in the samples are occasionally seen in published datasets, based on projected developmental curves (e.g., ages 18–19, 25–34, and 45–54 years in the WMS-R normative database; WIAT-II, ages 4 and 5). These norms should be used with caution due to the lack of actual data points in these age ranges (e.g., Mittenberg et al. 1992).

Extrapolation methods, such as those that employ regression techniques, depend on the shape of the distribution of scores. Thus, including only a subset of the distribution of age scores in the regression (e.g., by omitting very young or very old individuals) may change the projected developmental slope of certain tests dramatically. Tests that appear to have linear relationships, when considered only in adulthood, may actually have highly nonlinear relationships when the entire age range is considered. One example is vocabulary, which tends to increase exponentially during the preschool years, shows a slower rate of progress during early adulthood, remains relatively stable with continued gradual increase, and then shows a minor decrease with advancing age. If only a subset of the age range (e.g., adults) is used to estimate performance at the tail ends of the distribution (e.g., preschoolers and elderly), the estimation will not fit the shape of the actual distribution.

Rule of thumb: Comparison of test scores across tests

Comparison of performance across tests is affected by:

- Measurement error
- Score magnitude and rank in the distribution
- Extreme scores
- Ceiling and floor effects
- Extrapolation/interpolation of derived scores.

Normal Variability across Test Batteries and the Prevalence of Low Scores

It is important for clinicians to carefully consider how they interpret an isolated low score or a small number of low scores obtained on a battery of neuropsychological measures. This is because healthy people have variable performance on a battery of tests and the likelihood of obtaining low scores increases (1) as the number of tests increases, (2) as the cutoff for defining a low score becomes more liberal (i.e., the 16th percentile compared to the 5th percentile), and (3) with lower levels of baseline cognitive functioning (i.e., as determined by fewer years of education and/or lower intelligence). The prevalence of low scores on a neuropsychological battery is knowable when considering all test scores *simultaneously* in a co-normed sample. The fact that healthy people obtain some low scores is not a feature of any particular battery. Researchers have reported that obtaining some low scores is expected on the Expanded Halstead-Reitan Neuropsychological Battery (E-HRNB; Heaton et al. 2004), the combined Wechsler Adult Intelligence Scale-III/Wechsler Memory Scale-III battery (WAIS-III/WMS-III; Iverson et al. 2008), the Neuropsychological Assessment Battery (NAB; Brooks et al. 2007; Iverson et al. 2008), the WMS-III in older adults (Brooks et al. 2008), the Children's Memory Scale (CMS; Brooks et al. 2009), in Schretlen's ABC study (Schretlen et al. 2008), de Rotrou's study (de Rotrou et al. 2005), and Palmer's study (Palmer et al. 1998). A simple computer program can also be used to determine the base rates of low scores for a co-normed battery when the test intercorrelations are known and score distributions are assumed to be normal (Crawford et al. 2007).

Although it is important for clinicians to understand that low scores are common, it can be challenging to use this information in everyday clinical practice. The goal is to have interpretive tables that allow clinicians to simply and rapidly look up the prevalence of low scores on a battery of tests using various cutoff scores. For example, consider the following clinical vignette involving a patient with temporal lobe epilepsy. In addition to considering the test performance in relation to functional neuroanatomy, the application of base rate and psychometric information for this battery adds to the clinician's repertoire of interpretive tools.

Joey Smith is a 10-year-old, right-handed boy who presents with intractable epilepsy since he was 3 years old. His epilepsy involves partial complex seizures and frequent episodes of secondary generalization. Joey's current antiepileptic medications include Epival and Lamictal. Based on neurological and radiological investigations, the epileptogenic focus is suspected to be in his left mesial temporal lobe. Joey underwent a neuropsychological evaluation as part of his pre-surgical evaluation, which included the Children's Memory Scale (CMS; Cohen1997). Joey's overall intellectual abilities were low average. His performance on the CMS is presented in Table 31.2. As can be seen in the table, his verbal immediate, verbal delayed, and delayed recognition index scores were below the first percentile, whereas his visual memory abilities were low average. The differences between his verbal and visual indexes are found in fewer than 5% of healthy children (i.e., 4.9% prevalence for the 35-point difference between the visual and verbal immediate indexes; 4.1% prevalence for the 38-point difference between the visual and verbal delayed indexes). When considering the prevalence of low index scores on the CMS[2] (i.e., the base rates information was obtained from a 2009 conference presentation by Brooks and colleagues, with some CMS base-rate information being published in Brooks, Iverson, Sherman, and Holdnack, 2009), having 3 or more index scores below the second percentile was not found in healthy children and adolescents from the CMS standardization sample with below average intelligence. That is, there was a 0.0% prevalence of this many low scores in the standardization sample. Overall, the clinician can have increased confidence that the performance on memory tests makes sense from a neuroanatomical and a psychometric perspective.

---

[2]It is important to note that the General Memory Index was not included in the base rate analyses because it is a summary score for the verbal immediate, verbal delayed, visual immediate, and visual delayed index scores. The Attention/Concentration Index was also not included.

Table 31.2 Performance on the learning and memory indexes from Children's Memory Scale in a 10 year-old with intractable left temporal lobe epilepsy

Children's Memory Scale (CMS) indexes	Index score	Percentile rank	Classification
Learning	91	27th	Average
Visual immediate	85	16th	Low average
Visual delayed	88	21st	Low average
Verbal immediate	50	<1st	Extremely low
Verbal delayed	50	<1st	Extremely low
Delayed recognition	50	<1st	Extremely low
General memory	52	<1st	Extremely low

Classifications are based on a Wechsler system, as presented in Table 31.1

Knowing the prevalence of low scores in healthy children, adolescents, adults, and older adults is critical as part of a clinician's repertoire for interpretation of test performance (see Binder et al. 2009). Further information regarding using the prevalence of low scores on a battery of tests to improve diagnostic accuracy of cognitive impairment is presented in the chapter 32 by Iverson and Brooks in this book.

Assessing Change over Time

Serial assessment in neuropsychology is used to monitor cognition over time and to make inferences regarding improvement or decline in functioning. The fundamental question, of course, is to what degree do changes in test scores reflect "real" changes in function as opposed to measurement error? To what degree do real changes in test scores reflect clinically significant changes in function as opposed to clinically

Rule of thumb: Variability is normal

- Healthy individuals exhibit considerable variability in test performance, and some low scores should be expected given a battery of neuropsychological tests.
- The number of low scores found in healthy people increases with the number of tests being administered and interpreted, fewer years of education, lower levels of intelligence at baseline, and in ethnic minorities.
- Variables that increase or decrease expected variability in neuropsychological performances must be considered when interpreting performance.

trivial changes? To what degree do changes in test scores conform to expectations, given the application of treatments or the occurrence of other events or processes occurring between test and retest, such as brain injury, dementia, or brain surgery?

A number of statistical/psychometric methods have been developed for assessing changes observed over repeated administrations of neuropsychological tests and these differ considerably with respect to mathematical models and assumptions regarding the nature of test data. As with most areas of psychometrics, the problems and processes involved in decomposing observed scores (i.e., change scores) into measurement error and "true" scores are often complex. Moreover, it is important to remember that a statistically meaningful change does not necessarily translate into a clinically meaningful change. A brief overview of the issues and methods are presented below. However, a thorough discussion is beyond this chapter and interested readers are referred to several other sources (Chelune 2003; Crawford and Garthwaite 2007; Dikmen et al. 1999) for more in-depth reviews and discussions of these issues.

Reference Group Change Score Distributions

If a clinical or normative sample is administered a test twice, the distribution of observed change scores can be quantified. When such information is available, individual examinee change scores can be transformed into standardized change scores, thus providing information on the degree of unusualness of any observed change in score. Unfortunately, it is rarely possible for clinicians to use this method of evaluating change due to major limitations in most data available in test manuals. Retest samples tend to be relatively small for many tests, thus limiting generalizability. This is particularly important when change scores may vary with demographic variables (e.g., age and level of education) and/or initial test score level (e.g., normal vs abnormal), because retest samples typically are restricted with respect to both. Second, retest samples are often obtained within a short period of time after initial testing, typically less than 2 months, whereas in clinical practice typical test–retest intervals are often much longer. Therefore, any effects of extended test–retest intervals on change score distributions are not reflected in most change score data presented in test manuals. Lastly, change score information is typically presented in the form of summary statistics (e.g., mean and SD) that have limited utility if change scores are not normally distributed (in which case percentile tables would be much preferable). As a result of these limitations, clinicians often must turn to other methods for analyzing change scores.

Reliable Change

Jacobson and Truax (1991; see also Jacobson et al. 1999) proposed a psychometric method for determining if changes in test scores over time are reliable (i.e., not an artefact of imperfect test reliability). This method involves calculation of a *Reliable Change Index* (RCI). The RCI is an indicator of the probability that an observed difference between two scores from the same examinee on the same test can be attributed to measurement error (i.e., to imperfect reliability). When there is a low probability the observed change is due to measurement error, one may infer that it reflects other factors, such as progression of illness, treatment effects, motivational defects, and/or prior exposure to the test.

The RCI is calculated using the *Standard Error of the Difference* (SE_{diff}), an index of measurement error derived from classical test theory. It is the standard deviation of expected test–retest difference scores about a mean of zero given an assumption that no actual change has occurred. The original formula by Jacobson and Truax (1991) used the internal consistency reliability coefficient at a single point in time for calculating the SE_{diff}, whereas more recent versions have used the test–retest reliability coefficients from time 1 and time 2. Moreover, the original formula used the standard deviation from a single point in time, whereas authors using modified formulas have used the standard deviation from both test and retest. The formulas for the SE_{diff} are:

Using internal consistency reliability (Jacobson and Truax 1991):

$SEM = SD\sqrt{1-\alpha}$ → Standard deviation multiplied by the square root of 1 minus the internal consistency reliability coefficient (Cronbach's α).

$SE_{diff} = \sqrt{2\cdot(SEM)^2}$ → Square root of the product of two times the squared SEM.

Using test–retest reliability:

$SEM_1 = SD_1\sqrt{1-r_{12}}$ → Standard deviation from time 1, multiplied by the square root of 1 minus the test–retest reliability coefficient.

$SEM_2 = SD_2\sqrt{1-r_{12}}$ → Standard deviation from time 2, multiplied by the square root of 1 minus the test–retest coefficient.

$SE_{diff} = \sqrt{(SEM_1)^2 + (SEM_2)^2}$ → Square root of the sum of the square of SEM_1 and the square of SEM_2.

The reliable change methodology has the potential to allow the clinician to reduce the adverse impact of measurement error on test interpretation. To represent clinically significant improvement, the change score must be statistically reliable. Thus, the reliable change methodology is used to *supplement* clinical judgment. For neurocognitive assessments, reliable change is used to determine if there has been improvement or deterioration in functioning that exceeds the probable range of measurement error. For example, when the SE_{diff} is multiplied by 1.64, the clinician knows that scores *outside that range* would be found in fewer than 5% of subjects in each tail of the distribution (i.e., 90% confidence interval). Table 31.3 presents examples of reliable change values, based on the test–retest information, for use with the NAB. A change in performance on the NAB Attention Index of 14 points would be considered reliable at a 90% confidence interval.

There are, however, some drawbacks to the reliable change methodology. First, the reliable change formula implicitly assumes that no practice effects have occurred. When practice effects are present (and they frequently are present), "reliable" improvements may partially or wholly reflect effects of prior test exposure rather than a change in underlying functional level. Second, the reliable change

Table 31.3 Examples of reliable change values for the NAB Indexes in 18–59 year olds

NAB indexes	SD_1	SD_2	r_{12}	SEM_1	SEM_2	SE_{diff}	RCI 80% confidence interval	RCI 90% confidence interval
Attention	16.6	16.0	0.88	5.75	5.54	7.99	10.2	13.1
Language	14.0	14.3	0.55	9.39	9.59	13.42	17.2	22.0
Memory	14.9	15.2	0.74	7.60	7.75	10.85	13.9	17.8
Spatial	16.7	16.3	0.66	9.74	9.50	13.61	17.4	22.3
Executive functions	16.2	18.2	0.68	9.16	10.30	13.78	17.6	22.6
Total index	15.1	17.0	0.80	6.75	7.60	10.17	13.0	16.7

The formula used for calculating the SE_{diff} was: $SE_{diff} = \sqrt{SEM_1^2 + SEM_2^2}$, where $SEM_1 = SD_1\sqrt{1 - r_{12}}$ and $SEM_2 = SD_2\sqrt{1 - r_{12}}$. Standard deviations (SD) and test–retest correlations were obtained from Table 5.15 in the NAB Psychometric and Technical Manual (White and Stern 2003)

information is typically derived from retest performance in healthy participants but is often applied to retest performance in patients. Third, the time between test and retest, which is used to derive the reliable change information, is often substantially shorter (e.g., 1–2 months for most tests) than the actual retest duration in clinical practice (e.g., 1 year retest is often used for traumatic brain injury reassessment; see the Chap. 30 for further discussion on retest data).

Reliable change estimates are not presented in the vast majority of test manuals. Thus, they must be calculated by clinicians or researchers. We have calculated reliable change estimates for the WAIS-IV, WMS-IV, and selected D-KEFS subtests and presented them in Tables 31.4–31.6. We have also computed the average practice effects. By examining these tables, clinicians can gain a better understanding of the probable range of measurement error, in healthy adults, over relatively brief retest intervals. For example, on the WMS-IV, Index scores on the adult battery need to change by 11.2–12.7 points to be considered reliably higher or lower at the 80% confidence interval. These confidence intervals can be adjusted, if desired, by adding or subtracting the average practice effects.

Reliable Change Adjusted for Practice Effects

Chelune (2003) suggested a modification to the calculation of the RCI in which the mean change score for a reference group [i.e., mean change score = (mean score at time 2) – (mean score at time 1)] is subtracted from the observed change score of an individual examinee and the result used as an Adjusted Change Score for purposes of calculating reliable change adjusted for practice effects. Table 31.7 presents data that involves change scores for the NAB using this methodology. For example, if we subtract the practice effect of 6.5 index points from 10.2 (i.e., this is the 80% confidence interval for a reliable decline; that is, 1.28 × SE_{diff}), then a decline greater than 3.7 index points (i.e., 10.2–6.5) would be

Table 31.4 Reliable change on the WAIS-IV

WAIS-IV IQ, indexes, and subtests	Age: 16–29 years				Age: 30–54 years				Age: 55–69 years				Age: 70–90 years			
	SE_{diff}	80% CI	90% CI	Average practice effect	SE_{diff}	80% CI	90% CI	Average practice effect	SE_{diff}	80% CI	90% CI	Average practice effect	SE_{diff}	80% CI	90% CI	Average practice effect
FSIQ	5.0	6.4	8.2	4.4	4.3	5.5	7.1	4.4	4.2	5.4	6.9	4.9	4.6	5.9	7.6	3.5
VCI	4.8	6.1	7.9	2.2	4.3	5.6	7.1	2.7	5.1	6.5	8.3	3.3	4.6	5.9	7.6	2.1
PRI	8.0	10.2	13.1	4.6	7.7	9.8	12.6	4.5	7.2	9.2	11.8	3.6	7.9	10.2	13.0	3.2
WMI	8.8	11.2	14.4	2.7	8.6	11.0	14.1	1.9	6.2	8.0	10.2	4.3	6.6	8.5	10.9	3.2
PSI	7.9	10.1	12.9	4.8	9.8	12.6	16.1	5.3	6.6	8.5	10.8	5.0	7.8	9.9	12.7	2.7
Block design	1.8	2.3	3.0	1.2	1.9	2.4	3.1	1.0	2.0	2.6	3.3	0.6	1.7	2.1	2.7	0.4
Similarities	1.9	2.4	3.1	0.4	1.4	1.8	2.3	0.6	1.5	2.0	2.5	0.7	1.6	2.0	2.6	0.5
Digit span	2.2	2.8	3.6	0.6	1.9	2.5	3.2	0.5	1.4	1.8	2.3	0.8	1.6	2.1	2.7	0.7
Matrix reasoning	2.4	3.1	3.9	0.2	1.9	2.4	3.1	0.1	2.4	3.0	3.9	0.8	2.1	2.6	3.4	0.3
Vocabulary	1.3	1.7	2.2	0.2	1.4	1.7	2.2	0.1	1.5	1.9	2.5	0.2	1.2	1.5	1.9	0.0
Arithmetic	1.6	2.1	2.7	0.5	2.0	2.5	3.2	0.3	1.8	2.3	2.9	0.8	1.8	2.3	2.9	0.4
Symbol search	1.9	2.4	3.1	1.2	2.3	2.9	3.8	1.1	1.9	2.5	3.2	1.1	1.7	2.2	2.8	0.2
Visual puzzles	2.0	2.6	3.3	1.1	2.4	3.0	3.9	1.1	2.2	2.8	3.6	0.4	2.6	3.3	4.2	1.0
Information	1.3	1.7	2.2	0.7	1.5	1.9	2.5	0.8	1.3	1.7	2.1	0.9	1.2	1.5	2.0	0.6
Coding	1.6	2.1	2.7	0.5	1.6	2.1	2.7	0.9	1.5	2.0	2.5	0.6	1.6	2.1	2.6	0.6
Letter-number sequencing	2.1	2.6	3.4	0.7	1.8	2.2	2.9	0.5	2.2	2.8	3.6	0.1	–	–	–	–
Figure weights	2.2	2.8	3.6	1.0	2.0	2.6	3.3	1.0	2.1	2.7	3.5	0.6	–	–	–	–
Comprehension	1.6	2.1	2.7	0.0	1.3	1.7	2.2	0.2	1.6	2.1	2.7	0.0	1.6	2.1	2.7	0.4
Cancelation	2.0	2.5	3.2	1.1	2.3	2.9	3.7	0.5	1.9	2.4	3.1	0.2	–	–	–	–
Picture completion	2.1	2.7	3.5	2.4	2.5	3.2	4.1	2.3	2.1	2.7	3.5	1.8	2.0	2.6	3.3	1.2

$N = 228$. Mean test interval was 22 days (range = 8–82 days). SE_{diff} = Standard error of difference. The formula used for calculating the SE_{diff} was: $SE_{diff} = \sqrt{SEM_1^2 + SEM_2^2}$, where and $SEM_2 = SD_2\sqrt{1 - r_{12}}$. The correlations used were the uncorrected "average stability coefficients." *CI* confidence interval. The standard deviations and correlations used to calculate these reliable change estimates are presented on pp. 49–52 in the WAIS-IV Technical and Interpretive Manual (Wechsler et al. 2008). Average practice effects are calculated by subtracting the age-adjusted mean score at time 2 – mean score at time 1

Table 31.5 Reliable change on the WMS-IV

WMS-IV indexes and subteFsts	Age: 16–69 years (adult battery)				Age: 65–90 years (older adult battery)			
	SE_{diff}	80% CI	90% CI	Average practice effect	SE_{diff}	80% CI	90% CI	Average practice effect
Auditory memory index	8.8	11.2	14.4	11.5	8.2	10.5	13.5	10.6
Visual memory index	9.9	12.7	16.3	12.1	10.3	13.1	16.8	11.0
Visual working memory index	9.0	11.5	14.8	4.3	–	–	–	–
Immediate memory index	9.4	12.0	15.4	12.4	7.9	10.2	13.0	12.4
Delayed memory index	9.4	12.0	15.4	13.7	8.7	11.1	14.3	11.0
Logical memory I	2.1	2.6	3.4	1.9	2.1	2.7	3.5	2.0
Logical memory II	2.3	3.0	3.8	2.3	2.1	2.7	3.4	2.1
Verbal paired associates I	2.3	2.9	3.7	2.3	2.0	2.5	3.2	1.7
Verbal paired associates II	2.0	2.5	3.2	1.0	1.8	2.3	3.0	1.1
Designs I	2.3	3.0	3.8	1.1	–	–	–	–
Designs II	2.2	2.8	3.6	1.7	–	–	–	–
Visual reproduction I	2.4	3.1	4.0	1.9	2.0	2.6	3.3	1.8
Visual reproduction II	2.6	3.4	4.3	2.8	2.5	3.2	4.1	1.8
Spatial addition	2.1	2.7	3.4	0.8	–	–	–	–
Symbol span	2.3	2.9	3.7	0.6	2.3	2.9	3.7	0.6

Adult battery, $n = 144$–173. Older adult battery, $n = 69$–71. Mean test interval was 23 days (range = 14–84 days). SE_{diff} = Standard error of difference. The formula used for calculating the SE_{diff} was: $SE_{diff} = \sqrt{SEM_1^2 + SEM_2^2}$, where $SEM_1 = SD1\sqrt{1 - r_{12}}$ and $SEM_2 = SD2\sqrt{1 - r_{12}}$. The correlations used were the uncorrected "average stability coefficients." CI confidence interval. The standard deviations and correlations used to calculate these reliable change estimates are presented on p. 51 in the WMS-IV Technical and Interpretive Manual (Wechsler et al. 2009). Average practice effects are calculated by subtracting the age-adjusted mean score at time 2 – mean score at time 1

Table 31.6 Reliable change on selected D-KEFS subtests

Selected D-KEFS subtests	Ages: 8–19 years				Ages: 20–49 years				Ages: 50–89 years			
	SE_{diff}	80% CI	90% CI	Average practice effect	SE_{diff}	80% CI	90% CI	Average practice effect	SE_{diff}	80% CI	90% CI	Average practice effect
Visual scanning	2.3	3.0	3.8	2.0	2.6	3.4	4.3	0.7	2.3	3.0	3.8	0.4
Number sequencing	1.7	2.1	2.7	1.0	2.6	3.4	4.3	1.3	2.9	3.7	4.8	1.8
Letter sequencing	2.7	3.5	4.5	1.7	2.9	3.7	4.8	0.9	2.4	3.1	4.0	0.9
Number-letter sequencing	3.8	4.8	6.2	1.1	2.7	3.4	4.4	1.3	3.0	3.8	4.9	0.3
Motor speed	1.6	2.0	2.6	0.4	2.5	3.1	4.0	0.7	2.0	2.6	3.4	0.0
Letter fluency	2.2	2.8	3.6	0.8	2.3	3.0	3.8	0.6	1.8	2.3	3.0	0.3
Category fluency	2.1	2.7	3.5	1.0	2.1	2.7	3.4	0.5	2.2	2.8	3.6	0.1
Category switching-correct	2.2	2.8	3.6	1.3	3.7	4.7	6.0	-1.2	3.6	4.6	5.9	0.1
Category switching-accuracy	2.9	3.7	4.7	0.7	4.3	5.5	7.0	-1.1	3.7	4.7	6.1	0.7
CW: Color naming	1.7	2.2	2.8	1.1	1.5	2.0	2.5	1.0	3.0	3.9	5.0	0.5
CW: Word reading	2.2	2.8	3.6	0.0	2.6	3.3	4.3	0.6	2.7	3.4	4.4	0.5
CW: Inhibition	1.3	1.7	2.1	1.5	1.8	2.4	3.0	1.2	3.3	4.2	5.4	0.5
CW: Inhibition/switching	2.0	2.5	3.2	1.8	2.2	2.8	3.6	1.1	2.9	3.7	4.7	0.5

Sample sizes were as follows: ages 18–19, $n = 26$–28; ages 20–49, $n = 35$; and ages 50–89, $n = 36$–38. Mean test interval was 25 days (range = 9–74 days).

$SEdiff$ Standard error of difference. The formula used for calculating the SE_{diff} was: $SE_{diff} = \sqrt{SEM_1^2 + SEM_2^2}$, where $SEM_1 = SD_1\sqrt{1 - r_{12}}$ and $SEM_2 = SD_2\sqrt{1 - r_{12}}$. CI confidence interval, CW Color-Word Interference subtest. The standard deviations and correlations used to calculate these reliable change estimates are presented on pp. 21, 23, and 29 in the D-KEFS Technical Manual (Delis et al. 2001). Average practice effect is calculated by subtracting the mean age-adjusted score at time 2 – mean score at time 1

Table 31.7 Example of reliable change corrected for practice effects: NAB Attention Index in 18–59 year olds

| | Time 1 | | Time 2 | | Practice effect | | | Confidence intervals | | | |
| | | | | | | | | Reliable decline | | Reliable improvement | |
NAB index	Mean$_1$	SD$_1$	Mean$_2$	SD$_2$	Mean$_2$ – Mean$_1$	r_{12}	SE$_{diff}$	80%	90%	80%	90%
Attention	96.2	16.6	102.7	16	6.5		0.88	7.99	3.7	6.6	16.7	19.6

The formula used for calculating the SE$_{diff}$ was: $SE_{diff} = \sqrt{SEM_1^2 + SEM_2^2}$, where $SEM_1 = SD_1\sqrt{1-r_{12}}$ and $SEM_2 = SD_2\sqrt{1-r_{12}}$. The practice effect was either subtracted from (reliable decline) or added to (reliable improvement) the confidence interval for the SE$_{diff}$. Means, standard deviations (SD), and test-retest correlations were obtained from Table 5.15 in the NAB Psychometric and Technical Manual (White and Stern 2003)

considered reliable at the 80% confidence interval. Likewise, if we add the practice effect of 6.5 points to 10.2 (80% confidence interval for a reliable improvement), then an increase greater than 16.7 index points (10.2 + 6.5) would be considered reliable (80% confidence interval). When considering the previous example of a 14-point change on the NAB Attention Index, a decline of this amount would be reliable at the 90% confidence interval if it is adjusted for practice effects. However, if the 14-point change was an improvement on the Attention Index, then this would not be considered reliable at either the 80% or 90% confidence intervals adjusted for practice effects.

Reliable change corrected for practice effects seems more appropriate for tests where large practice effects are expected. However, it is problematic in a number of ways, first and foremost of which is the use of a constant (group mean) term for the practice effect, which does not take into account the range of practice effects that are actually present in a sample of people tested twice. For example, there is evidence that more able people typically gain more on retesting than less able people (Rapport et al. 1997). Second, the calculation of practice effects is typically based on relatively short retest durations (e.g., 1–2 months). Therefore, practice effects might be overestimated because of the brief retest interval. Third, average practice effects (typically calculated over brief retest intervals) are computed from healthy subjects in normative samples. Practice effects in clinical groups might be different. Fourth, neither standard nor adjusted RCIs account for regression toward the mean (i.e., estimated measurement error is not proportional to extremity of observed change). Finally, the use of practice effects when calculating change scores has been recommended *only* when 75% or more of the sample showed at least some improvement on the test score (Iverson and Green 2001).

Regression Methods

The reliable change methodology may provide useful information regarding the likelihood of a meaningful change in test performance, but it can have limited validity when various variables are systematically associated with changes in scores over time.

These variables include: test–retest interval; scores from other tests; examinee characteristics such as baseline ability level (Time 1 score), gender, education, age, and acculturation; and neurological or medical conditions. In addition, although this methodology factors in test reliability, this is operationalized as a constant error term that does not account for regression to the mean (although some reliable change methods used in clinical psychology have been adjusted for regression to the mean). One method for evaluating change that does allow clinicians to account for additional predictors and also controls for regression to the mean is the use of linear regression models (Crawford and Howell 1998; Hermann et al. 1991).

With linear regression models, *predicted* retest scores are derived and these are compared with *observed* retest scores for purposes of determining if deviations are "significant." This is accomplished by dividing the difference between obtained retest scores and regression-predicted retest scores by the *Standard Error for Individual Predicted Scores* (SE). Because score differences are divided by a standard error measure, the resulting value is considered to be standardized. The resulting standardized score is in fact a *t* statistic that can be translated into a probability value using an appropriate program or table. As with other standardized scores (e.g., *z* scores), standardized regression-based change scores from different measures can be directly compared, regardless of the original test score metric. Regression models can also be used when one wishes to consider change scores from multiple tests simultaneously (see McCleary et al. 1996).

It is important to understand the limitations of regression methods. Regression equations based on smaller sample sizes can lead to large error terms so that meaningful predicted-obtained differences may be missed. However, attenuation of reliability in small samples *is also not factored into reliable change calculations*, which might be based on spuriously low or high test–retest correlations obtained from small samples. Regression equations from large studies, or that have been cross-validated, are therefore preferred. In order to maximize utility, sample characteristics should match populations seen clinically and predictor variables should be carefully chosen to match data that will likely be available to clinicians. Test users should generally avoid interpolation; that is, they should avoid applying a regression equation to an examinee's data (predictor variables and test–retest scores) when the data values fall outside the ranges for corresponding variables comprising the regression equation. For example, if a regression equation is developed for predicting IQ at retest from a sample with initial IQ scores ranging from 85 to 125, it should not be applied to an examinee whose initial IQ is 65. Finally, regression-based change scores should only be derived and used when necessary assumptions concerning residuals are met (see Pedhazur 1997, p. 33–34).

Rule of thumb:

Interpreting change in test performance over time requires sophisticated psychometric models to minimize clinical bias and error associated with clinical judgment

Summary and Conclusions

The purpose of this chapter was to provide an overview of the basic psychometric properties that are necessary for proper neuropsychological test interpretation. Moreover, our goal was to provide this information in a manner that would be easily understood by clinicians. To achieve this goal, we illustrated various psychometric concepts using tests that are commonly used by clinicians in everyday practice.

It was not our intention to suggest that certain cognitive measures, which were used as examples, have better or worse psychometric properties or normative samples than other measures that were not presented. It was also not our intention to suggest that clinicians should not use the tests that were used to illustrate some of the psychometric concepts in this chapter.

It was our intention, however, to draw attention to *all* psychological and neuropsychological tests and to have clinicians carefully consider the psychometric foundations presented in this chapter when interpreting test performance. The highlighted problems with psychometric properties, which can lead to inaccurate interpretation of test performance in some situations, are a reality of many tests in psychology and neuropsychology. However, having these issues addressed has often resulted in test developers and publishers becoming more aware of the problems and striving to address, correct, and/or eliminate these problems on subsequent versions of the tests or on newly developed tests (e.g., WMS to WMS-R: adding measures of visual memory, including longer retention intervals, and including various summary scores; WMS-R to WMS-III: not using interpolated normative data, extending the age range, and providing scaled scores for subtests; WMS-III to WMS-IV: addressing floor effects or range restriction, providing a battery for older adults that is shorter in administration time, and improved methods for excluding controls who might have subtle memory problems).

Based on our review, we offer a number of suggestions for best practice when interpreting test performance. These are presented in Table 31.8. We suggest that clinicians carefully consider the normative data for tests that they administer and interpret, the psychometric properties of the tests, and other psychometrically-based strategies that are designed to improve our interpretation of these tests. The composition of normative samples, in some cases, can have a major effect on test interpretation (e.g., see Fig. 31.2).

There were five main themes discussed in this chapter. First, we believe that interpreting and communicating test performance is facilitated by having a common "language" of descriptors (i.e., classification system). Regardless of the classification system that is used (see Table 31.1), it is recommended that clinicians be consistent throughout a report (see also Chap. 1). Second, sample characteristics, such as non-normal distributions and truncated samples, can impact interpretation of test performance. Third, comparison of performance across tests is affected by

Table 31.8 Points to consider in the interpretation of test scores

• Are the norms adequate (i.e., sufficient sample size; representative of the larger population)?
• Is this individual from a group with a non-normal distribution?
• Is this individual likely from the ends/tails of the normal distribution?
• Does this test have floor effects?
• Does this test have ceiling effects?
• Was score extrapolation/interpolation used in the creation of derived scores?
• When considering scores on two or more tests, are the normative samples equivalent in terms of demographics?
• Does either test have a normative sample with a truncated distribution? (i.e., what were the screening methods used in the recruitment for the normative samples?)
• When comparing two tests, are they equally reliable?
• Does one of the tests have a small normative sample size?
• Is one of the scores an extreme score (i.e., is the magnitude of score size the same)?
• What is the likelihood that having a low score, when interpreting multiple test scores, is considered "broadly normal" compared to healthy people with similar intelligence?
• What is the likelihood that a change over time represents a real change or an artefact?
• What classification system will be used to communicate the results?
• Has the same classification system been used for interpretation of all tests?

measurement error and ceiling and floor effects (see Fig. 31.6). Fourth, it is normal for healthy people to have variability and some low scores across a battery of neuropsychological tests. The number of low scores found in healthy people increases with the number of tests being administered, fewer years of education, lower levels of premorbid intelligence, and in ethnic minorities (see Figs. 31.1 and 31.3). These principles should be considered when interpreting performance. Finally, interpreting change in test performance over time requires sophisticated psychometric models. Toward this end, we provided tables for interpreting change on the NAB Index scores, WAIS-IV, WMS-IV, and selected subtest from the D-KEFS.

Rule of thumb: General guidelines for interpreting neuropsychological data

- A common "language" of descriptors is needed to describe performance (the same descriptors should be used throughout a report)
- Sample characteristics can impact test interpretation
- Measurement error, ceiling effects, and floor effects can impact comparisons of performance across different tests
- It is normal for healthy people to have variability and some low scores when given a battery of tests
- Interpreting test performance over time should include psychometric methods for determining "real" change

References

Binder, L.M., Iverson, G.L., & Brooks, B.L. (2009). To err is human: 'Abnormal' neuropsychological scores and variability are common in healthy adults. *Archives of Clinical Neuropsychology, 24*, 31–46.

Brooks, B. L., Iverson, G. L., Holdnack, J. A., & Feldman, H. H. (2008). The potential for misclassification of mild cognitive impairment: A study of memory scores on the Wechsler Memory Scale-III in healthy older adults. *Journal of the International Neuropsychological Society, 14*(3), 463–478.

Brooks, B. L., Iverson, G. L., Sherman, E. M. S., & Holdnack, J. A. (2009). Healthy children and adolescents obtain some low scores across a battery of memory measures: Base rate analyses on the Children's Memory Scale (CMS). *Journal of the International Neuropsychological Society, 15*(4), 613–617.

Brooks, B. L., Iverson, G. L., & White, T. (2007). Substantial risk of "Accidental MCI" in healthy older adults: Base rates of low memory scores in neuropsychological assessment. *Journal of the International Neuropsychological Society, 13*(3), 490–500.

Chelune, G. J. (2003). Assessing reliable neuropsychological change. In R. D. Franklin (Ed.), *Prediction in forensic and neuropsychology: Sound statistical practices* (pp. 65–88). Mahwah: Lawrence Erlbaum Associates.

Cohen, M. J. (1997). *Children's memory scale (CMS) manual*. San Antonio: The Psychological Corporation.

Crawford, J. R., & Garthwaite, P. H. (2002). Investigation of the single case in neuropsychology: confidence limits on the abnormality of test scores and test score differences. *Neuropsychologia, 40*(8), 1196–1208.

Crawford, J. R., & Garthwaite, P. H. (2007). Using regression equations built from summary data in the neuropsychological assessment of the individual case. *Neuropsychology, 21*(5), 611–620.

Crawford, J. R., Garthwaite, P. H., & Gault, C. B. (2007). Estimating the percentage of the population with abnormally low scores (or abnormally large score differences) on standardized neuropsychological test batteries: a generic method with applications. *Neuropsychology, 21*(4), 419–430.

Crawford, J. R., & Howell, D. C. (1998). Regression equations in clinical neuropsychology: an evaluation of statistical methods for comparing predicted and obtained scores. *Journal of Clinical and Experimental Neuropsychology, 20*(5), 755–762.

de Rotrou, J., Wenisch, E., Chausson, C., Dray, F., Faucounau, V., & Rigaud, A. S. (2005). Accidental MCI in healthy subjects: a prospective longitudinal study. *European Journal of Neurology, 12*(11), 879–885.

Delis, D. C., Kaplan, E., & Kramer, J. H. (2001). *Delis Kaplan executive function system technical manual*. San Antonio: The Psychological Corporation.

Delis, D. C., Kramer, J. H., Kaplan, E., & Ober, B. A. (1987). *California verbal learning test*. San Antonio: The Psychological Corporation.

Delis, D. C., Kramer, J. H., Kaplan, E., & Ober, B. A. (2000). *The California verbal learning test manual* (2nd ed.). San Antonio: The Psychological Corporation.

Dikmen, S. S., Heaton, R. K., Grant, I., & Temkin, N. R. (1999). Test-retest reliability and practice effects of expanded Halstead-Reitan Neuropsychological Test Battery. *Journal of the International Neuropsychological Society, 5*(4), 346–356.

Dunn, L. M., & Dunn, D. M. (2007). *Peabody picture vocabulary test* (4th ed.). Minneapolis: Pearson Assessments.

Fastenau, P. S., & Adams, K. M. (1996). Heaton, Grant, and Matthew's comprehensive norms: An overzealous attempt. *Journal of Clinical and Experimental Neuropsychology, 18*(3), 444–448.

Gioia, G. A., Isquith, P. K., Guy, S. C., & Kenworthy, L. (2000). *Behavior rating inventory of executive function*. Lutz: Psychological Assessment Resources, Inc.

Goodglass, H., & Kaplan, E. (1983). *Boston diagnostic aphasia examination*. Philadelphia: Williams & Wilkins.

Heaton, R. K., Chelune, G. J., Talley, J. L., Kay, G. G., & Curtiss, G. (1993). *Wisconsin card sorting test manual*. Odessa: Psychological Assessment Resources.

Heaton, R. K., Grant, I., & Matthews, C. G. (1991). *Comprehensive norms for an extended Halstead-Reitan Battery: Demographic corrections, research findings, and clinical applications*. Odessa: Psychological Assessment Resources, Inc.

Heaton, R. K., Miller, S. W., Taylor, M. J., & Grant, I. (2004). *Revised comprehensive norms for an expanded Halstead-Reitan Battery: Demographically adjusted neuropsychological norms for African American and Caucasian adults professional manual*. Lutz: Psychological Assessment Resources.

Hermann, B. P., Wyler, A. R. V. R., LeBailey, R. K., Whitman, S., Somes, G., & Ward, J. (1991). Predictors of neuropsychological change following anterior temporal lobectomy: Role of regression toward the mean. *Journal of Epilepsy, 4*, 139–148.

Iverson, G. L., Brooks, B. L., & Holdnack, J. A. (2008). Misdiagnosis of cognitive impairment in forensic neuropsychology. In R. L. Heilbronner (Ed.), *Neuropsychology in the courtroom: Expert analysis of reports and testimony* (pp. 243–266). New York: Guilford Press.

Iverson, G. L., Brooks, B. L., White, T., & Stern, R. A. (2008). Neuropsychological Assessment Battery (NAB): Introduction and advanced interpretation. In A. M. Horton Jr. & D. Wedding (Eds.), *The neuropsychology handbook* (3rd ed., pp. 279–343). New York: Springer Publishing Inc.

Iverson, G. L., & Green, P. (2001). Measuring improvement or decline on the WAIS-R in inpatient psychiatry. *Psychological Reports, 89*(2), 457–462.

Ivnik, R. J., Makec, J. F., Smith, G. E., Tangolos, E. G., & Peterson, R. C. (1996). Neuropsychological tests' norms above age 55: COWAT, BNT, MAE Token, WRAT-R Reading, AMNART, STROOP, TMT, and JLO. *The Clinical Neuropsychologist, 10*, 262–278.

Jacobson, N. S., Roberts, L. J., Berns, S. B., & McGlinchey, J. B. (1999). Methods for defining and determining the clinical significance of treatment effects: description, application, and alternatives. *Journal of Consulting and Clinical Psychology, 67*(3), 300–307.

Jacobson, N. S., & Truax, P. (1991). Clinical significance: A statistical approach to defining meaningful change in psychotherapy research. *Journal of Consulting and Clinical Psychology, 59*(1), 12–19.

Kaplan, E. F., Goodglass, H., & Weintraub, S. (1978). *The Boston naming test*. Boston: E. Kaplan & H. Goodglass.

Kaplan, E. F., Goodglass, H., & Weintraub, S. (2001). *The Boston naming test* (2nd ed.). Philadelphia: Lippincott Williams & Wilkins.

Lucas, J. A., Ivnik, R. J., Smith, G. E., Ferman, T. J., Willis, F. B., Petersen, R. C., et al. (2005). Mayo's older African Americans normative studies: Norms for Boston naming test, Controlled Oral Word Association, Category Fluency, Animal Naming, Token Test, Wrat-3 Reading, Trail Making Test, Stroop Test, and Judgment of Line Orientation. *The Clinical Neuropsychologist, 19*(2), 243–269.

McCleary, R., Dick, M. B., Buckwalter, G., Henderson, V., & Shankle, W. R. (1996). Full-information models for multiple psychometric tests: Annualized rates of change in normal aging and dementia. *Alzheimer's Disease and Associated Disorders, 10*(4), 216–223.

McFadden, T. U. (1996). Creating language impairments in typically achieving children: The pitfalls of "normal" normative sampling. *Language, Speech, and Hearing Services in Schools, 27*, 3–9.

Mitrushina, M. N., Boone, K. B., Razani, J., & D'Elia, L. F. (2005). *Handbook of normative data for neuropsychological assessment*. New York: Oxford University Press.

Mittenberg, W., Burton, D. B., Darrow, E., & Thompson, G. B. (1992). Normative data for the Wechsler Memory Scale-Revised: 25- to 34-year-olds. *Psychological Assessment, 4*(3), 363–368.

Palmer, B. W., Boone, K. B., Lesser, I. M., & Wohl, M. A. (1998). Base rates of "impaired" neuropsychological test performance among healthy older adults. *Archives of Clinical Neuropsychology, 13*(6), 503–511.

Pedhazur, E. (1997). *Multiple regression in behavioral research*. New York: Harcourt Brace.

Rapport, L. J., Brines, D. B., Theisen, M. E., & Axelrod, B. N. (1997). Full scale IQ as a mediator of practice effects: The rich get richer. *The Clinical Neuropsychologist, 11*(4), 375–380.

Reynolds, C. R., & Horton, A. M., Jr. (2006). *Test of verbal conceptualization and fluency, examiner's manual*. Austin: Pro-Ed Publishing.

Sattler, J. M. (2001). *Assessment of children: Cognitive applications* (4th ed.). San Diego: Jerome M. Sattler Publisher, Inc.

Schretlen, D. J., Testa, S. M., Winicki, J. M., Pearlson, G. D., & Gordon, B. (2008). Frequency and bases of abnormal performance by healthy adults on neuropsychological testing. *Journal of the International Neuropsychological Society, 14*(3), 436–445.

Stern, R. A., & White, T. (2003a). *Neuropsychological assessment battery*. Lutz: Psychological Assessment Resources.

Stern, R. A., & White, T. (2003b). *Neuropsychological assessment battery: Administration, scoring, and interpretation manual*. Lutz: Psychological Assessment Resources.

Strauss, E., Sherman, E. M. S., & Spreen, O. (2006). *A compendium of neuropsychological tests: Administration, norms, and commentary* (3rd ed.). New York: Oxford University Press.

The Psychological Corporation. (2001). *Wechsler test of adult reading manual*. San Antonio: Psychological Corporation.

Tombaugh, T. N. (1996). *Test of memory malingering*. North Tonawanda: Multi-Health Systems.

Tombaugh, T. N., & Hubley, A. M. (1997). The 60-item Boston Naming Test: norms for cognitively intact adults aged 25 to 88 years. *Journal of Clinical and Experimental Neuropsychology, 19*(6), 922–932.

Urbina, S. (2004). *Essentials of psychological testing*. Hoboken: John Wiley & Sons.

Van Gorp, W. G., Satz, P., Kiersch, M. E., & Henry, R. (1986). Normative data on the Boston naming test for a group of normal older adults. *Journal of Clinical and Experimental Neuropsychology, 8*, 702–705.

Wechsler, D. (1997a). *Wechsler adult intelligence scale* (3rd ed.). San Antonio: The Psychological Corporation.

Wechsler, D. (1997b). *Wechsler memory scale* (3rd ed.). San Antonio: The Psychological Corporation.

Wechsler, D. (2003). *Wechsler intelligence scale for children* (4th ed.). San Antonio: The Psychological Corporation.

Wechsler, D., Coalson, D. L., & Raiford, S. E. (2008). *Wechsler adult intelligence scale* (Technical and interpretive manual 4th ed.). San Antonio: NCS Pearson, Inc.

Wechsler, D., Holdnack, J. A., & Drozdick, L. W. (2009). *Wechsler memory scale* (Technical and interpretive manual 4th ed.). San Antonio: NCS Pearson, Inc.

White, T., & Stern, R. A. (2003). *Neuropsychological assessment battery: Psychometric and technical manual*. Lutz: Psychological Assessment Resources.

Chapter 32
Improving Accuracy for Identifying Cognitive Impairment

Grant L. Iverson and Brian L. Brooks

Abstract Deficit measurement is the sine qua non of neuropsychology. The risk, of course, is that we can be so focused on deficit measurement – and so focused on describing the nature and severity of a person's cognitive impairment – that we can underappreciate human diversity and overattribute low or unexpected test scores to brain injury or disease. The North American psychometric tradition has long since attempted to minimize possible misattribution of low test scores through a reliance on the normal curve. However, clinicians know that overly formulaic reliance on the normal curve can result in false positive and false negative attributions of cognitive diminishment. Moreover, the normal curve relates to a single test score in relation to a theoretical normal population. Neuropsychologists never rely on single tests. Instead, we administer numerous tests and we interpret performance in combination, not in isolation. Thus, the principles of normative test score interpretation, applied to *single* test scores, are inherently limited when interpreting performance across a *battery* of tests.

Cognitive impairment can arise from a single cause or it can have a multifactorial etiology. There are a large number of medical, psychiatric, and neurological diseases, disorders, and conditions that can have an adverse affect on cognition. Clearly, the accurate identification and quantification of cognitive impairment is important in clinical practice, research, and in clinical trials. However, comprehensive, psychometrically-sophisticated guidelines for identifying and quantifying cognitive impairment, across a battery of tests, are not clearly outlined in the neuropsychological literature. The primary exception to this is the work of Reitan and Wolfson for the Halstead Reitan Neuropsychological Battery (Reitan RM, Wolfson D, The Halstead-Reitan neuropsychological test battery: Theory and clinical interpretation, Neuropsychology Press, Tucson, AZ, 1985; Reitan RM, Wolfson D, The Halstead-Reitan neuropsychological test battery: Theory and clinical interpretation, 2nd edn, Neuropsychology Press, Tucson, AZ, 1993) and Golden and colleagues for the Luria–Nebraska Neuropsychological Battery (Golden C, Purish A, Hammeke T,

G.L. Iverson (✉)
British Columbia Mental Health & Addictions, University of British Columbia,
Vancouver, Canada
e-mail: giverson@interchange.ubc.ca

M.R. Schoenberg and J.G. Scott (eds.), *The Little Black Book of Neuropsychology:*
A Syndrome-Based Approach, DOI 10.1007/978-0-387-76978-3_32,
© Springer Science+Business Media, LLC 2011

Manual for the Luria-Nebraska Neuropsychological Battery, Western Psychological Services, Los Angeles, 1985; Golden CJ, Freshwater SM, Vayalakkara J, The Luria-Nebraska neuropsychological battery, in Groth-Marnat G (ed), Neuropsychological assessment in clinical practice: A guide to test interpretation and integration, Wiley, New York, 2000, pp 263-289; Moses JA Jr, Golden CJ, Ariel R, Gustavson JL, Interpretation of the Luria-Nebraska neuropsychological battery (Vol 1), Grune and Stratton, New York, 1983). Considerable psychometric work has been done regarding how to interpret combinations of scores derived from these batteries.

The purpose of this chapter is to provide clinicians with psychometrically sophisticated information that is designed to improve their accuracy for identifying cognitive problems in daily practice. This chapter begins by presenting information on current definitions of cognitive impairment (*Conceptualizing Cognitive Impairment*). In the second section, we describe some of the various classification systems for conceptualizing cognitive impairment (*Classifying Cognitive Impairment*). Fundamental psychometric principles, derived from analyses on co-normed batteries of tests, are illustrated in the third section (*Evaluating Cognitive Impairment: Five Psychometric Principles to Consider*). In the final section, we present new psychometric criteria for identifying cognitive impairment across a battery of neuropsychological measures that adhere to the five psychometric rules (*Identifying Cognitive Impairment: New Psychometric Criteria for Cognitive Disorder NOS*).

Key Points and Chapter Summary

- Cognitive diminishment or impairment can result from a variety of medical, psychiatric, and/or neurological conditions.
- There are very few empirically-established psychometrically-based guidelines for what constitutes mild impairment in cognition.
- Failing to consider fundamental psychometric principles applied to interpreting multiple test scores can readily result in false positive or false negative diagnoses of cognitive impairment.
- Five psychometric principles for interpreting scores: (1) Low scores are relatively common across all test batteries; (2) Low scores depend on where you set your cutoff score; (3) Low scores vary by number of tests administered; (4) Low scores vary by demographic characteristics of the examinee; and (5) Low scores vary by level of intelligence.
- New empirically-based, psychometrically-derived criteria for identifying DSM-IV-TR Cognitive Disorder NOS are presented in this chapter.

Conceptualizing Cognitive Impairment

There is no universally agreed upon *definition* of cognitive impairment. Establishing a level of cognitive impairment sometimes requires multiple sources of information, including input from family members, review of medical records, review of collateral records (e.g., school or employment), interviews with the patient, observations of the patient's behavior, psychological test results, and neuropsychological test results. Iverson and colleagues have suggested five categories of cognitive impairment that illustrate a continuum of severity (Iverson et al. 2008a; b). These categories are presented below in Fig. 32.1. These categories reflect levels of cognitive impairment in a face valid manner. However, the specific criteria for each level have not been codified or agreed upon.

Neuropsychology, unfortunately, remains far from having uniform psychometric criteria for interpreting the severity of cognitive impairment using neurocognitive tests, nor do we have specific behavioral criteria for quantifying impairment or diminishment in everyday functioning. Research is needed to develop and empirically test criteria for cognitive impairment and impairment in social or occupational functioning. For now, the diagnosis of cognitive impairment, and level of cognitive impairment, is primarily based upon clinical judgment.

Mild Cognitive Diminishment

Mild diminishment in cognitive functioning may or may not be identifiable using neuropsychological tests. This diminishment can, but does not always, have a mild adverse impact on a person's social and/or occupational functioning. This diminishment may or may not be noticeable by others.

Mild Cognitive Impairment

Mild cognitive impairment should be identifiable using neuropsychological tests. This impairment has a mild (sometimes moderate) adverse impact on a person's social and/or occupational functioning.

Moderate Cognitive Impairment

Moderate cognitive impairment has a substantial impact on everyday functioning. This impairment would be noticeable to others in regards to the person's social and/or occupational functioning.

Severe Cognitive Impairment

Severe cognitive impairment has a substantial adverse impact on everyday functioning. The person is incapable of competitive employment, should not be driving a motor vehicle, and would likely have difficulty with activities of daily living.

Profound Cognitive Impairment

The cognitive impairment would render the person incapable of living outside of a nursing home or an institution. If the person lived at home, he or he likely would require 24-hour supervision.

Fig. 32.1 Suggested categories of cognitive impairment along a severity continuum

Classifying Cognitive Impairment

In addition to a lack of consensus on defining cognitive impairment, there are no widely accepted, empirically-validated *psychometric criteria* for identifying the cognitive disorders. The Diagnostic and Statistical Manual of Mental Disorders, Fourth Edition (DSM-IV; American Psychiatric Association 1994) and the ICD-10 Classification of Mental and Behavioral Disorders (World Health Organization 1992) offer several categories for diagnosing cognitive problems that are due to a general medical conditions. In clinical situations when the cognitive impairment is obvious, widespread, and associated with poor daily functioning (i.e., severe or profound cognitive impairment), the most relevant DSM-IV and ICD-10 categories would be the dementias. However, in clinical situations when the cognitive problems and impact on daily functioning following a medical or neurological disease, disorder, or condition are less serious and do not meet DSM-IV or ICD-10 criteria for dementia (i.e., mild cognitive impairment, and perhaps moderate cognitive impairment), then alternative diagnostic classifications are typically considered.

One area of research and clinical practice that has had numerous suggestions for how to define cognitive impairment has been identifying memory impairment in older adults. This has been related to an enormous research effort to identify Alzheimer's disease at a very early stage (i.e., prodromal). One term (along with accompanying criteria) that has gained considerable, but not universal, popularity with clinicians and researchers is mild cognitive impairment (MCI). In particular, this typically refers to amnestic MCI (aMCI).[1] Petersen and colleagues (Petersen et al. 1994, 1999) defined aMCI as being characterized by (1) a subjective memory complaint, (2) an unusually low score on an objective memory measure (based on age only or age and education adjusted normative data), (3) normal general cognitive functioning, (4) normal activities of daily living, and (5) not meeting criteria for dementia. More recent versions of the criteria for aMCI have de-emphasized or dropped the need for a subjective memory complaint. The psychometric criterion for an unusually low score has generally been set at 1.5 SDs below the normative mean for healthy older adults. Of course, this cutoff remains somewhat arbitrary and often researchers might select a psychometric criterion for impairment that ranges anywhere from 1 to 2 SDs below the mean. Even the authors of the recent consensus-based research criteria for probable Alzheimer's disease (Dubois et al. 2007) "have not defined a magnitude of deficit or the comparative norms that should be utilized [for identifying memory impairment]" (p. 742).

The clinical implications for assessing memory functioning in older adults without a solid psychometric foundation are striking. If one assumes that the cutoff score for memory impairment is the 5th percentile, then one accepts a priori that

---

[1]MCI has been divided into several classifications depending on the type of cognitive impairment. Amnestic MCI (aMCI) is the most commonly studied subtype and refers to impairment with memory.

there will be a 5% false positive rate (i.e., 5% of healthy older adults would be falsely diagnosed with MCI). However, that false positive rate applies to a single test score in relation to a theoretical population of healthy older adults. Because a single test score is rarely relied upon, this theoretical false positive rate is not accurate. Clinicians typically administer several tests which yield multiple test scores. Thus, the false positive rate for having *at least one* low score will be considerably greater than 5%. Moreover, the number of low scores varies by level of intelligence. Those older adults with below average intelligence will have more low scores than those with above average intelligence (Brooks et al. 2008; 2007). These points are illustrated in Fig. 32.2. Notice that, for healthy older adults of average intelligence, 22–38% will have one or more scores ≤5th percentile across a battery of memory tests. As seen in this figure, the number of low ("abnormal") memory scores in healthy older adults varies considerably by level of intelligence. This will be addressed in more detail later in this chapter.

Rule of thumb: Classifying cognitive impairment

• There are no universally-accepted psychometrically-established criteria for cognitive impairment
• Diagnoses using DSM-IV-TR or ICD-10 do not contain information about "how to" identify cognitive impairment
• MCI provides a criterion for memory impairment but is subject to false positives when several memory tests are administered and interpreted

---

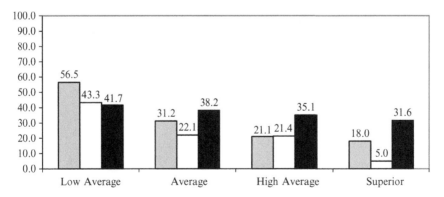

Fig. 32.2 Percent healthy older adults with one or more low memory scores according to the MCI criterion for memory impairment (≤5th percentile). Note: The NAB memory module consists of four tests that yield 10 demographically-adjusted scores. The WMS-III battery consists of four tests that yield 8 age-adjusted (WMS-III age) or demographically-adjusted (WMS-III demo) scores

DSM-IV Cognitive Disorder NOS
(Mild Neurocognitive Disorder)

Cognitive disorder NOS (CD-NOS) is an Axis I DSM-IV diagnosis that can be applied to people who have acquired cognitive impairments from an injury, illness, or disease. Unfortunately, there are no specific empirically-derived, evidence-based criteria for this disorder. CD-NOS can be broken down into two categories, *mild neurocognitive disorder* and *postconcussional disorder*. Our focus in this chapter is mild neurocognitive disorder. To identify mild neurocognitive disorder, there must be impairment in *at least two domains*, which can include attention or speed of information processing, language, learning and memory, perceptual-motor abilities, and/or executive functioning (see Fig. 32.3). These cognitive impairments must be due to a neurological or general medical condition, be considered abnormal or a decline from previous functioning, and cause marked psychological distress or impairment in social, occupational, or other areas of functioning.

Although the criteria for cognitive disorder NOS have been available to clinicians and researchers since the publication of the DSM-IV in 1994, there has yet to be psychometrically-derived, empirically-validated, published criteria, with known sensitivity and specificity, for identifying impairment in these five cognitive domains. There has been some research leading to published guidelines for identifying mild neurocognitive disorder in patients with Human Immunodeficiency Virus (HIV). By consensus, new research criteria for HIV-associated neurocognitive disorders (HAND) were published in October of 2007 (Antinori et al. 2007). These research criteria are similar but not directly applicable to the DSM-IV criteria for mild neurocognitive disorder. Moreover, they were designed for a specific clinical population. These criteria require the person to have *one or more* test scores, in *two or more* cognitive domains, below *1 standard deviation* from the mean on age, sex, and education adjusted normative data. The seven domains of functioning include: attention/working memory; speed of information processing; verbal/language; memory (learning; recall); abstraction/executive; sensory-perceptual; and motor skills (Antinori et al. 2007).

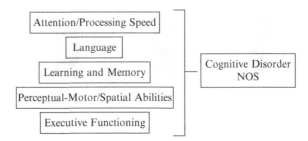

Fig. 32.3 Domains relating to cognitive disorder NOS. Impairment in 2 or more domains is required for diagnosis

Clinicians and researchers should note that specific methodological issues can adversely affect diagnostic accuracy of these new consensus-based criteria. We have conducted extensive psychometric analyses on two large databases of healthy adults and found that (1) the more tests that are given, the more likely a person is to have one or more scores fall below 1 SD from the mean, (2) the prevalence of low scores varies by demographics, and (3) the prevalence of low scores varies by level of intelligence. The criteria for HAND do not establish the number of tests to be administered, and require that a person's performance by considered in regards to his or her age, education, and sex (but not intelligence). Thus, diagnostic accuracy can vary based on the number of tests a clinician or researcher chooses to administer. Regarding intelligence, this will result in a substantial number of *false positives* for people with below average intelligence and an increased rate of *false negatives* for people with above average intelligence. The next section elaborates on these fundamental psychometric principles.

Evaluating Cognitive Impairment: Five Psychometric Principles to Consider

Neuropsychologists typically administer numerous tests that can yield dozens of scores. As part of the interpretive procedure, the neuropsychologist must use his or her clinical judgment to consider all of the test scores simultaneously and make sense of the patient's performance. Although a low score might be suggestive of an acquired impairment, it is important to consider that having inter-subtest variability and obtaining a low score might be "normal" for that person. Obtaining low scores might be attributable to measurement error (broadly defined), normative sample characteristics (i.e., having healthy people, rather than clinical groups, at the lower end of the distribution), longstanding weaknesses in certain areas, fluctuations in motivation and effort, psychological interference, and other situational factors such as inattentiveness, fatigue, or minor illness (Binder et al. under review).

This section introduces and discusses five psychometric principles to consider when evaluating a person for cognitive impairment. Although an understanding of these psychometric principles is invaluable for any clinician, it is important for clinicians to utilize these principles when simultaneously interpreting test scores across a battery of neuropsychological tests.

Principle 1: Low Scores Are Common across All Test Batteries

Any battery of tests, whether fixed or flexible, will have a certain number of low scores when administered to healthy people (Axelrod and Wall 2007; Binder et al. under review; Brooks et al. 2008, 2007; Crawford et al. 2007; Heaton et al. 1991;

2004; Ingraham and Aiken 1996; Iverson et al. 2008b, c; Palmer et al. 1998; Schretlen et al. 2008). This is because there is a substantial amount of intraindividual variability in the cognitive abilities of healthy people. Figures 32.4 and 32.5 illustrate the first principle that low scores are common across all test batteries. These figures present the prevalence of low scores, using one standard deviation (SD) and ≤5th percentile as the cutoff scores, in healthy adults on the Neuropsychological Assessment Battery (NAB; Stern and White 2003), the Expanded Halstead-Reitan Neuropsychological Battery (E-HRNB; Heaton et al. 2004), and the combination of the Wechsler Adult Intelligence Scale – III (WAIS-III; Wechsler 1997a) and Wechsler Memory Scale – III (WMS-III; Wechsler 1997b). As seen in Fig. 32.4, the majority of healthy adults have two or more scores below 1SD on all three batteries. Moreover, a substantial percentage have two or more scores ≤5th percentile on all three batteries (Fig. 32.5).

Rule of thumb: Evaluating cognitive impairment – Principle 1

• Low scores are relatively common in healthy individuals

Principle 2: Low Scores Depend on Where You Set Your Cutoff Score

There is no universal agreement on the definition of a low score. Some neuropsychologists have fixed and consistent definitions of low scores (e.g., 1 SD below the

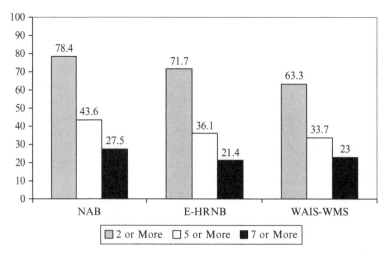

Fig. 32.4 Base rates of low scores across different test batteries: Cutoff < 1 SD. *SD* standard deviation, *NAB* Neuropsychological Assessment Battery; *E-HRNB* Expanded Halstead-Reitan Neuropsychological Battery, *WAIS-WMS* Wechsler Adult Intelligence Scale – III and Wechsler Memory Scale – III. The number of scores considered were as follows: NAB = 36, E-HRNB = 25, WAIS-WMS = 20. Bars represent percent of healthy adults from standardization samples who had (1) 2 or more, (2) 5 or more, or (3) 7 or more scores below 1SD (i.e., *T* < 40 or SS < 7)

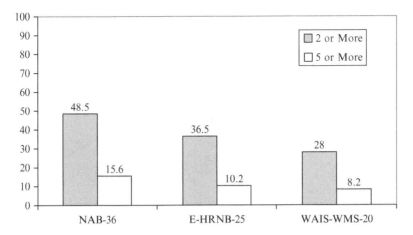

Fig. 32.5 Base rates of low scores across batteries with different numbers of scores being interpreted: Cutoff ≤5th percentile. *SD* standard deviation. NAB-36 = all 36 scores from the full Neuropsychological Assessment Battery; E-HRNB-25 = 25 scores from the Expanded Halstead-Reitan Neuropsychological Battery; and WAIS-WMS-20=all 20 primary scores from the Wechsler Adults Intelligence Scale – III and Wechsler Memory Scale – III. Bars represent percent of healthy adults from standardization samples who had (1) 2 or more or (2) 5 or more scores at or below 5th percentile (i.e., *T* = 34 or SS = 5)

mean, 5th percentile, or 2 SDs below the mean), whereas other neuropsychologists might vary their definition based on the characteristics of the examinee. For example, for a highly educated person, or a person with a superior level of intelligence, the neuropsychologist might choose to interpret some average scores as "low" and some low average scores as "mildly impaired." Both approaches have strengths and weaknesses, psychometrically. The key is to carefully define the psychometric strengths and limitations of the specific approach taken for interpreting neuropsychological tests.

The balance between sensitivity and specificity is related to the cutoff score used. Higher cutoff scores are more likely to correctly identify those who have cognitive problems (improved sensitivity), but they are also more likely to include those who do not have cognitive problems (reduced specificity). This is true when interpreting a single score or multiple scores from a battery. Using data from the NAB and the WAIS-III/WMS-III as examples, Fig. 32.6 and 32.7 illustrate the percentage of healthy people who obtain low scores below four cutoff scores: 1 SD (16th percentile), 10th percentile, 5th percentile, and 2 SDs (2nd percentile). As the cutoff score gets progressively lower, the number of healthy people who would be incorrectly identified (i.e., specificity/false positives) as having cognitive problems declines. For example, having five or more low scores on the NAB would be found in 43.6% of healthy people when using 1SD as the cutoff score but only 5.2% when using 2SD as the cutoff score. Having five or more low scores on the WAIS-III/WMS-III would be found in 33.7% of healthy people when using 1SD as the cutoff score but only 1.9% when using 2SD as the cutoff score.

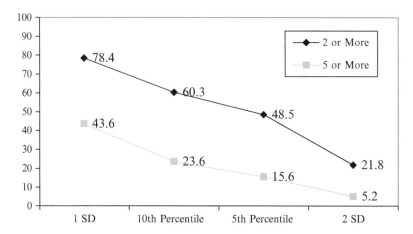

Fig. 32.6 Prevalence of low scores on the NAB across different cutoffs. *SD* standard deviation, *NAB* Neuropsychological Assessment Battery. The 36 primary *T* scores were considered. Each data point represents the percent of healthy adults from the NAB standardization sample who had (1) 2 or more or (2) 5 or more scores below 1 SD (i.e., *T* < 40), below the 10th percentile (i.e., *T* < 37), at or below the 5th percentile (i.e., *T* = 34), or below 2 SDs (i.e., *T* < 30)

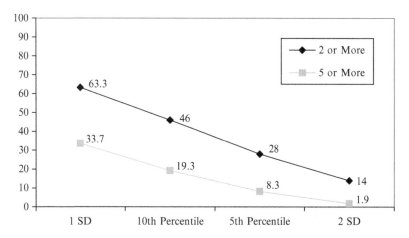

Fig. 32.7 Prevalence of low scores on the WAIS-III/WMS-III across different cutoffs. *SD* standard deviation. WAIS-WMS-20 = all 20 primary scores from the Wechsler Adults Intelligence Scale – III and Wechsler Memory Scale – III. Each data point represents the percent of healthy adults from the WAIS-III/WMS-III standardization sample who had (1) 2 or more or (2) 5 or more scores below 1 SD (i.e., SS < 7), below the 10th percentile (i.e., SS < 6), at or below the 5th percentile (i.e., SS < 5), or below 2 SDs (i.e., SS < 4)

Rule of thumb: Evaluating cognitive impairment – Principle 2

- Different cutoffs can be used to define a low score
- Cutoff scores represent a balance between sensitivity and specificity

Principle 3: Low Scores Depend on the Number of Tests Administered

Comprehensive neuropsychological evaluations often consist of numerous tests that yield several scores. As an example, the NAB is a 3-h battery that consists of 24 tests, which yield 36 primary scores, five index scores, a summary score, and more than 50 secondary scores. As the number of tests administered and interpreted increases, the likelihood of having low scores also increases. Figures 32.8 and 32.9 illustrate this principle using four batteries of varying lengths (i.e., 36 scores from the NAB, 25 scores from the E-HRNB, 20 scores from the WAIS-III/WMS-III, and 16 scores from an abbreviated version of the NAB). It should be noted that regardless of which cutoff score is used, the expected number of low scores increases with lengthier test batteries.

Rule of thumb: Evaluating cognitive impairment – Principle 3
- The more tests that are administered, and scores interpreted, the more likely it is to find low scores in healthy adults

---

Principle 4: Low Scores Vary by Demographic Characteristics of the Examinee

It is well established that many cognitive abilities vary by demographic characteristics. The impact of age on neuropsychological test performance is well appreciated.

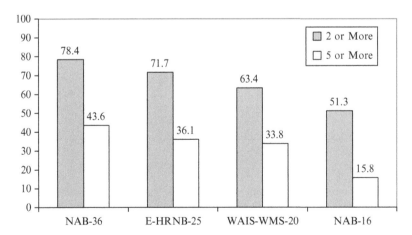

Fig. 32.8 Base rates of low scores across batteries with different numbers of scores being interpreted: Cutoff <1 SD. *SD* standard deviation. NAB-36 = all 36 scores from the full Neuropsychological Assessment Battery; E-HRNB-25 = 25 scores from the Expanded Halstead-Reitan Neuropsychological Battery; WAIS-WMS-20 = all 20 primary scores from the Wechsler Adults Intelligence Scale – III and Wechsler Memory Scale – III; NAB-16 = 16 primary scores from an abbreviated version of the Neuropsychological Assessment Battery. Bars represent percent of healthy adults from standardization samples who had (1) 2 or more or (2) 5 or more scores below 1 SD (i.e., *T* < 40 or SS < 7)

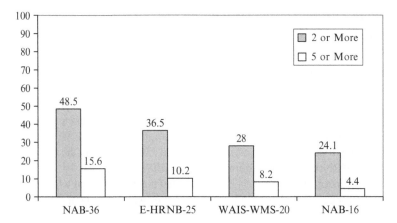

Fig. 32.9 Base rates of low scores across batteries with different numbers of scores being interpreted: Cutoff ≤5th percentile. *SD* standard deviation. NAB-36 = all 36 scores from the full Neuropsychological Assessment Battery; E-HRNB-25 = 25 scores from the Expanded Halstead-Reitan Neuropsychological Battery; WAIS-WMS-20 = all 20 primary scores from the Wechsler Adults Intelligence Scale – III and Wechsler Memory Scale – III; NAB-16 = 16 primary scores from an abbreviated version of the Neuropsychological Assessment Battery. Bars represent percent of healthy adults from standardization samples who had (1) 2 or more or (2) 5 or more scores at or below 5th percentile (i.e., $T = 34$ or SS = 5)

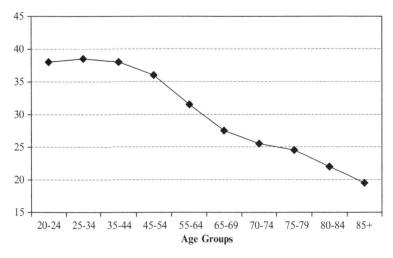

Fig. 32.10 Delayed memory for stories (WRAML-2) by age group. The raw scores corresponding to an age corrected scaled score of 10 are portrayed for each age group (The data was obtained from Sheslow and Adams 2003)

For example, performance on tests of memory and processing speed is lower in older adults versus younger adults. As seen in Fig. 32.10, delayed memory for stories (raw score performance) is fairly consistent between the ages of 20 and 55, but then declines in older adults. Thus, virtually all cognitive tests are normed by age.

For some tests, there are sex differences. The literature on sex differences suggests that women perform better on tasks of verbal learning and memory, verbal fluency, and processing speed (Beatty et al. 2003; Donders et al. 2001; Herlitz et al. 1997; Norman et al. 2000). Motor dexterity has also been shown to be a strength for women compared to men (Schmidt et al. 2000). In contrast, men tend to perform better on motor speed (Schmidt et al. 2000), some visual-spatial and visual-constructional tasks (Beatty et al. 2003; Collaer and Nelson 2002; Voyer et al. 1995), and arithmetic reasoning and computations (Geary et al. 2000). As a result of known differences in cognitive abilities, many normative scores for traditional, paper–pencil, neuropsychological measures (e.g., Wechsler Adult Intelligence Scale-III and Wechsler Memory Scale-III demographic norms, Neuropsychological Assessment Battery, Expanded Halstead-Reitan Neuropsychological Battery, and California Verbal Learning Test-II) are corrected for gender.

Education is an important variable to consider when interpreting cognitive test results (Heaton et al. 2004; Heaton et al. 2003; Ivnik et al. 1996; Morgan et al. 2007; Rosselli and Ardila 2003; Ryan et al. 2005). It has long been recognized that education is correlated with cognitive test performance. For example, predicted WAIS-III Full Scale IQ scores in Caucasian men, stratified by level of education, are as follows: ≤8 years = 90, 9–11 years = 96, 12 years = 102, 13–15 years = 107, 16 years = 113; and ≥17 years = 118 (The Psychological Corporation 2001, p. 114). The effects of education and sex on cognitive functioning are illustrated in Fig. 32.11. Normative scores on each test for 35 year olds, adjusted for sex and education, are presented. Higher scores mean *better performance* relative to the normative sample. For example, the Arithmetic subtest of the WAIS-III measures a person's ability to do mental arithmetic. A raw score on this test of 13 was used for all normative comparisons. First, notice the striking effect of education. A raw score of 13 corresponds to a *T* score of 53 for men with 9 years of education

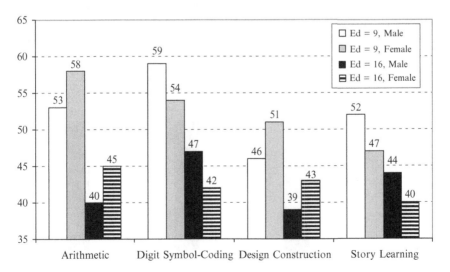

Fig. 32.11 Influence of sex and education on cognitive functioning (normative *T* scores). Normative scores were calculated for 35 year olds based on the following raw scores: WAIS-III Arithmetic = 13, WAIS-III Digit Symbol Coding = 75, NAB Design Construction = 14, and NAB Story Learning Immediate Recall = 61. Education levels of 9 and 16 years were used

(i.e., the 62nd percentile) and 40 for men with 16 years of education (i.e., 16th percentile). Men outperform women on the Arithmetic test; thus, the normative *T* scores for women are higher than the normative *T* scores for men (i.e., a raw score of 13 for women results in a *better* normative score than it does for men). In contrast, women outperform men on Digit Symbol-Coding, a measure of visual-motor processing speed, and immediate memory for stories (thus, the same raw score results in a higher normative *T* score for men versus women). Men outperformed women on the Design Construction test, a measure of visual-spatial ability.

Reading ability, as a correlate of both education and intelligence, is also related to neuropsychological test performance. Reading is believed to be relatively resistant to the effects of brain injury and disease (Bright et al. 2002; Maddrey et al. 1996; Strauss et al. 2006); thus, reading test performance has been used to estimate pre-injury or pre-disease cognitive functioning (Bright et al. 2002; Green et al. 2008; Griffin et al. 2002; Paolo et al. 1996). The relation between reading test scores and cognitive functioning is presented in Fig. 32.12.

Researchers working with diverse groups of people, in different settings and in different countries, have repeatedly demonstrated that ethnic groups frequently perform differently on cognitive testing (Ardila 1995; Brickman et al. 2006; Manly and Echemendia 2007; O'Bryant et al. 2004). For example, Patton and colleagues (2003) compared 50 healthy older African American adults to 50 Caucasians matched on age, education, and gender on the Repeatable Battery for the Assessment of Neuropsychological Status (RBANS; Randolph 1998). The RBANS is a neuropsychological screening battery designed to measure attention/processing speed, expressive language, visual-spatial and constructional abilities, and immediate and delayed memory. The performances of the two groups on the RBANS Index scores are provided in Fig. 32.13. Note that effect sizes ranged from *d* = .52 (Immediate Memory) to *d* = .91 (Total Score).

The practical implication of this study is that ethnic differences are present on neuropsychological tests, both verbal and nonverbal, in people from the same culture who speak the same language. If an elderly African–American was being

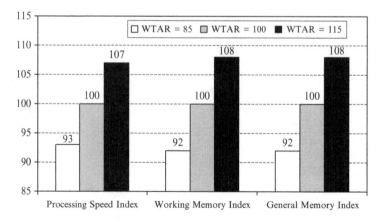

Fig. 32.12 Relation between reading test scores and cognitive functioning in healthy adults. Predicted WAIS-III Processing Speed and WMS-III Working Memory and General Memory Index scores by level of WTAR score

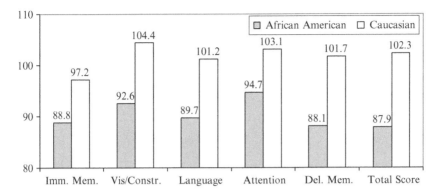

Fig. 32.13 Comparison of healthy African Americans to healthy Caucasians on a neuropsychological screening battery. *Imm. Mem.* Immediate Memory Index, *Vis/Constr.* Visuospatial/Constructional Index, *Del. Mem.* Delayed Memory Index. Values are Index scores with a mean = 100 and standard deviation = 15 (Derived from Patton et al. 2003)

evaluated for cognitive impairment secondary to Alzheimer's disease the psychologist might erroneously conclude that the patient was showing frank evidence of memory impairment if his or her scores were compared to Caucasian normative data instead of African–American normative data.

The relation between demographic variables and cognitive test performance has clear and compelling implications for research and clinical practice. If the goal of testing is to identify the presence of cognitive impairment, especially a decline attributable to a neurological injury or disease, then diagnostic accuracy will be improved if relevant demographic characteristics are considered in the interpretation of test performance.

Rule of thumb: Evaluating cognitive impairment – Principle 4

- Demographic variables (e.g., education and ethnicity) are related to the number of low scores when age-adjusted normative data are used

Principle 5: Low Scores Vary by Level of Intelligence

Perhaps the most often overlooked, yet very important, principle when interpreting multiple scores from a battery of tests is that the number of low scores is related to level of intellectual functioning (Horton 1999; Steinberg et al. 2005a, b; Tremont et al. 1998; Warner et al. 1987). People with below average intellectual abilities are expected to have more low scores than people with above average intelligence. Therefore, it is important to interpret test performance within the context of a person's intellectual abilities. Figures 32.14 and 32.15 illustrate the fourth principle using performance on the NAB and the WAIS-III/WMS-III that is stratified by level of intelligence (Figs. 32.16 and 32.17). As can be seen, the percentage of healthy people with low scores is greater for those with lesser intelligence.

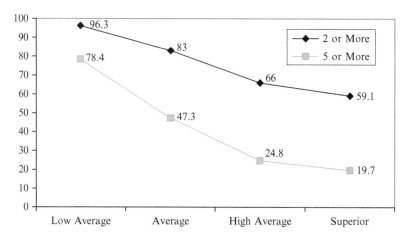

Fig. 32.14 Prevalence of low NAB scores stratified by intelligence (RIST): Cutoff <1 SD. *SD* standard deviation, *NAB* Neuropsychological Assessment Battery. The 36 primary *T* scores were considered. Data points represent the percent of healthy adults from the NAB standardization sample who had (1) 2 or more or (2) 5 or more scores below 1 SD (i.e., *T* < 4 0). Data are presented for different classifications of intellectual abilities based on RIST Index (i.e., low average, RIST = 80–89; average, RIST = 90–109; high average, RIST = 110–119; and superior, RIST ≥ 120)

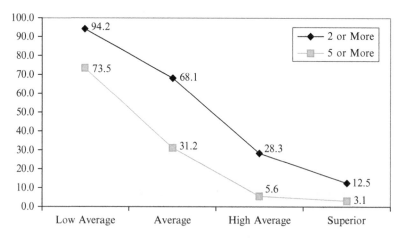

Fig. 32.15 Prevalence of low WAIS-III/WMS-III scores stratified by estimated intelligence (WTAR-Demographics Predicted FSIQ): Cutoff <1 SD. *SD* standard deviation, *WAIS-III* Wechsler Adult Intelligence Scale – Third Edition, *WMS-III* Wechsler Memory Scale – Third Edition. The 20 primary scaled scores from the WAIS-III/WMS-III were considered. Data points represent the percent of healthy adults from the WAIS-III/WMS-III standardization sample who had (1) 2 or more or (2) 5 or more scores at or below the 5th percentile (i.e., SS ≤ 5). Data are presented for different classifications of intellectual abilities based on WTAR-demographics predicted full scale IQ (WTAR-FSIQ; i.e., low average, WTAR-FSIQ = 80–89; average, WTAR-FSIQ = 90–109; high average, WTAR-FSIQ = 110–119; and superior, WTAR-FSIQ ≥ 120)

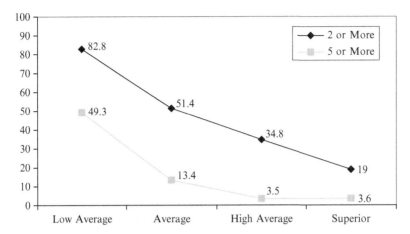

Fig. 32.16 Prevalence of low NAB scores stratified by intelligence (RIST): ≤5th percentile. *SD* standard deviation, *NAB* Neuropsychological Assessment Battery. The 36 primary *T* scores were considered. Data points represent the percent of healthy adults from the NAB standardization sample who had (1) 2 or more or (2) 5 or more scores at or below the 5th percentile (i.e., *T* < 34). Data are presented for different classifications of intellectual abilities based on RIST Index (i.e., low average, RIST = 80–89; average, RIST = 90–109; high average, RIST = 110–119; and superior, RIST ≥ 120)

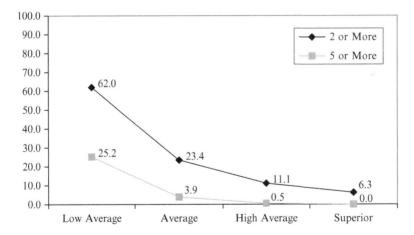

Fig. 32.17 Prevalence of low WAIS-III/WMS-III scores stratified by estimated intelligence (WTAR-Demographics Predicted FSIQ): Cutoff ≤5th percentile. *SD* standard deviation, *WAIS-III* Wechsler Adult Intelligence Scale – Third Edition, *WMS-III* Wechsler Memory Scale – Third Edition. The 20 primary scaled scores from the WAIS-III/WMS-III were considered. Data points represent the percent of healthy adults from the WAIS-III/WMS-III standardization sample who had (1) 2 or more or (2) 5 or more scores at or below the 5th percentile (i.e., SS ≤ 5). Data are presented for different classifications of intellectual abilities based on WTAR-demographics predicted full scale IQ (WTAR-FSIQ; i.e., low average, WTAR-FSIQ = 80–89; average, WTAR-FSIQ = 90–109; high average, WTAR-FSIQ = 110–119; and superior, WTAR-FSIQ ≥ 120)

Rule of thumb: Evaluating cognitive impairment – Principle 5

- Low scores occur at different rates depending upon the intellectual ability of the individual
- Individuals with lower intellectual ability tend to have more low scores

Identifying Cognitive Impairment: New Psychometric Criteria for Cognitive Disorder NOS

The clinical implications of these five fundamental psychometric principles are obvious. Failing to consider the prevalence of low scores, demographic variables, and intelligence carefully and judiciously can result in misdiagnosis or missed diagnosis. For the past 3 years, we have been working on psychometric analyses relating to the base rates of low scores across batteries of neuropsychological tests (Iverson et al. 2008b, c). This work led to the development of new psychometric criteria for the DSM-IV Axis I diagnosis Cognitive Disorder NOS (Iverson and Brooks in press) using the Neuropsychological Assessment Battery (NAB; Stern and White 2003). We have attempted to carefully consider the core psychometric principles discussed in this chapter in the development of these psychometric criteria for CD NOS using the NAB. First, the battery is fixed in number of tests and number of scores that are interpreted (i.e., additional tests can be given, but the fixed number represents the "core" that pertains to the CD NOS psychometric criteria). Second, the battery covers all the domains of functioning for mild neurocognitive disorder. Third, all tests are co-normed, meaning they were all given to a large normative sample. Fourth, all test scores are presented on a common metric (i.e., T scores), and all scores are adjusted for demographic variables (i.e., sex, age, and education). Fifth, criteria for impairment are established for different cut-off scores (e.g., 1 SD, 10th percentile, and 2 SDs below the mean). Sixth, criteria for impairment in each domain were set with known false positive rates. Finally, the criteria for impairment were stratified by level of intelligence because the entire NAB standardization sample was also administered the Reynolds Intellectual Screening Test (RIST; Reynolds and Kamphaus 2003), a brief measure of intellectual abilities.

An *abbreviated version of the NAB*, comprised of 15 of the 24 tests, was used to develop the new psychometric criteria. This abbreviated battery requires approximately 2 h to administer. A brief description of the five NAB modules, along with the tests and the 23 primary T scores selected for the development of the CD NOS criteria, is presented in Table 32.1 (see White and Stern 2003 for additional information about the specific tests).

Development of the criteria involved determining the prevalence of low scores in each domain. All scores within each domain were considered simultaneously, rather than in isolation. The cutoffs used in this study included: <25th percentile; <16th percentile (i.e., <1 SD); <10th percentile; ≤5th percentile; and <2nd percentile (i.e., <2 SDs). For each domain, the number of scores below various cutoffs

Table 32.1 NAB modules and tests used for development of psychometric criteria for CD NOS

- NAB Attention Module: This module fully assesses "attention and speed of information processing" as described for the DSM-IV mild neurocognitive disorder (e.g., concentration and rapidity of assimilating or analyzing information). All five primary tests are used in the abbreviated battery, but the analyses do not include Numbers & Letter A Speed and Errors).
- NAB Language Module: For the abbreviated NAB, only Oral Production and Naming are used.
- NAB Memory Module: This module measures verbal and visual learning and memory. This clearly covers the memory domain for mild neurocognitive disorder (i.e., "learning or recalling new information"). For the abbreviated NAB, analyses are based on 6 T scores (List Learning A Immediate Recall for 3 Trials; List Learning A Long Delayed Recall; Story Learning Immediate Recall; Story Learning Delayed Recall; Daily Living Memory Immediate Recall; Daily Living Memory Delayed Recall).
- NAB Spatial Module: This module measures perceptual, spatial, constructional, and spatial-motor abilities. This is partially related to the DSM-IV category called "perceptual motor abilities" (e.g., "integrating visual, tactile, or auditory information with motor activities"). For the abbreviated NAB, the Visual Discrimination and Design Construction tests are used.
- NAB Executive Functions Module: Measures different aspects of executive functioning (e.g., planning, abstracting, conceptualizing, judgment, and word generativity). This module reasonably covers the "executive functions" domain for mild neurocognitive disorder. For the abbreviated NAB, the Mazes, Categories, and Word Generation tests are used.

suggesting the presence of cognitive impairment was determined from frequency distributions. *Possible* impairment is based on having fewer than 20% of healthy adults and *probable* impairment is based on having fewer than 10% of healthy adults obtaining the number of low scores below the given cutoff. In other words, there is a known false positive rate for both possible and probable impairment.

Table 32.2 presents the psychometric criteria, stratified by level of intelligence, for determining possible or probable impairment in each of the five domains from the abbreviated NAB. To use these interpretive tables, there is a three-step procedure: (1) count the number of primary *T* scores in each domain that fall below the five cutoff scores (i.e., 25th, 16th, 10th, 5th, and 2nd percentiles); (2) refer to the appropriate table that corresponds to the person's level of intelligence[2]; and (3) determine if the number of low scores in each cognitive domain is considered *broadly normal*, *possible impairment*, or *probable impairment*.

These proposed guidelines, *which were established with a false positive rate of less than 20% for possible cognitive impairment and less than 10% for probable cognitive impairment*, are stratified by level of intellectual abilities. However, it is important to note that the false positive rates are established for each domain *in isolation, not for all domains simultaneously*. We have not determined the criteria, yet, for determining how often a person has two or more "impaired" domains. This work is underway.

---

[2] We are using the RIST to estimate *current* intellectual abilities. After determining their current RIST score, we combine this information with clinical judgment to estimate premorbid RIST *classification category* (e.g., low average, average, high average, or superior). We usually use the obtained RIST as the best estimate of premorbid RIST classification. However, sometimes we might believe that the obtained RIST under-estimates premorbid ability, and thus we might choose one classification higher. An example would be if a person with obvious brain damage obtained a RIST of 109. We might assume that his/her premorbid RIST was more likely to fall in the High Average classification range than in the Average classification range.

Table 32.2 Criteria for possible and probable cognitive impairment by domain

Low average intelligence (RIST = 80–89)	
Attention and speed	*Psychometric criteria*
Possible impairment	7 scores < 25th%; 5 scores < 1 SD; 4 scores < 10th%; 3 scores ≤ 5th%
Probable impairment	8 scores < 25th%; 6 scores < 1 SD; 5 scores < 10th%; 2 scores < 2nd%
Language	
Possible impairment	2 scores < 25th%; 1 score < 2 SD
Probable impairment	2 scores < 1 SD
Learning and memory	
Possible impairment	6 scores < 25th%; 5 scores < 1 SD; 4 score < 10th%; 3 scores ≤ 5th%
Probable impairment	6 scores < 1 SD; 5 scores < 10th%; 4 scores ≤ 5th%; 2 scores < 2nd%
Perceptual and spatial	
Possible impairment	2 scores < 1 SD; 1 score < 2nd%
Probable impairment	2 scores < 10th%
Executive functioning	
Possible impairment	3 scores < 25th%; 2 scores < 10th%; 1 score < 2nd%
Probable impairment	3 scores < 1 SD; ; 2 scores ≤ 5th%
Average intelligence (RIST = 90–109)	
Attention and speed	*Psychometric criteria*
Possible impairment	5 scores < 25th%; 3 scores < 1 SD; 2 scores < 10th%; 1 score < 2nd %
Probable impairment	6 scores < 25th%; 4 scores < 1 SD; 3 scores < 10th%; 2 scores < 2nd%
Language	
Possible impairment	1 score < 10th%
Probable impairment	2 scores < 25th%; 1 score < 2 SD
Learning and memory	
Possible Impairment	3–4 scores < 25th%; 2 scores < 1 SD; 1 score < 10th%
Probable Impairment	5 scores < 25th%; 3 scores < 1 SD; 2 scores < 10th%
Perceptual and spatial	
Possible impairment	1 score < 10th%
Probable impairment	2 scores < 25th%
Executive functioning	
Possible impairment	2 scores < 25th%; 1 score < 10th%
Probable impairment	3 scores < 25th%; 2 scores < 1 SD
High average intelligence (RIST = 110–119)	
Attention and speed	*Psychometric criteria*
Possible impairment	4 scores < 25th%; 2–3 scores < 1 SD; 2 scores < 10th%; 1 score ≤ 5th%
Probable impairment	5 scores < 25th%; 4 scores < 1 SD; 3 scores < 10th%; 2 scores ≤ 5th%; 1 score < 2nd%
Language	
Possible impairment	1 score < 1SD
Probable impairment	2 scores < 25th%
Learning and memory	
Possible impairment	3 scores < 25th%; 1 score < 10th%
Probable impairment	4 scores < 25th%; 2 scores < 1 SD

(continued)

Table 32.2 (continued)

Perceptual and spatial	
Possible impairment	1 score < 1 SD
Probable impairment	2 scores < 25th%; 1 score < 10th%
Executive functioning	
Possible impairment	1 score < 1 SD
Probable impairment	2 scores < 25th%; 1 score < 10th%
Superior/very superior intelligence (RIST ≥ 120)	
Attention and speed	*Psychometric criteria*
Possible impairment	4 scores < 25th%; 3 scores < 1 SD;
Probable impairment	6 scores < 25th%; 4 scores < 1 SD; 2 scores < 10th%; 1 score < 2nd%
Language	
Possible impairment	1 score < 1 SD
Probable impairment	2 scores < 25th%; 1 score < 10th%
Learning and memory	
Possible impairment	2 scores < 25th%; 1 scores < 1 SD
Probable impairment	3 scores < 25th%; 2 scores < 1 SD; 1 score ≤ 5th%
Perceptual and spatial	
Possible impairment	1 score < 25th%
Probable impairment	1 score < 1 SD
Executive functioning	
Possible impairment	1 score < 1 SD
Probable impairment	2 scores < 25th%; 1 score < 10th%

Note: Analyses based on subjects between 18 and 79 years of age (*n* = 1,269). Produced by special permission of the Publisher, Psychological Assessment Resources, Inc., 16204 North Florida Avenue, Lutz, Florida 33549, from the standardization data presented in the Neuropsychological Assessment Battery Psychometric and Technical Manual by Travis White, Ph.D. and Robert A. Stern, Ph.D. Copyright 2001, 2003 by PAR, Inc. Further reproduction is prohibited without permission from PAR, Inc. There are slight variations due to rounding

The criteria in Table 32.2 can be used to identify widespread diminishment or frank impairment. For example, for adults of average intelligence, having 5 or more scores below average (i.e., below the 25th percentile) in the Attention and Psychomotor Speed domain reflects widespread low performance ("possible impairment"), whereas having 2 scores below the 2nd percentile (i.e., 2 SDs below the mean) reflects circumscribed frank impairment ("probable impairment"). Of course, some patients will show widespread below average performance punctuated by some extremely low scores.

Rule of thumb: Psychometric criteria for diagnosing cognitive disorder NOS

- Possible cut-off scores include 25th%, 1 SD, 10th%, 5th%, 2nd%
- Number of scores falling below cut-off criteria vary by level of intelligence
- Tables provide base rates of low test scores, in each domain, stratified by intelligence

Case Examples: Patients Treated for Brain Tumors

The new psychometric criteria presented in Table 32.2 allow us to determine whether performance across several measures from a cognitive domain are diminished while still maintaining desired false positive rates. In the tables below, we present case examples of two patients who have been treated for brain tumors and have been evaluated using the abbreviated Neuropsychological Assessment Battery (NAB). These case examples illustrate the use of the psychometric tables for determining the presence of cognitive impairment that would be consistent with cognitive disorder NOS (i.e., Mild Neurocognitive Disorder). The patients' performances on the individual tests comprising the abbreviated NAB are presented in Table 32.3.

Table 32.3 RIST and NAB test data for two brain tumor case examples

	T scores (percentile ranks)	
Domains/tests	Case example 1	Case example 2
RIST index (classification)	High average	Average
Attention and processing speed		
Digits forward	46 (34%)	40 (16%)
Digits backward	52 (58%)	55 (69%)
Dots	58 (79%)	47 (38%)
Numbers and letters A speed	52 (58%)	48 (42%)
Numbers and letters A errors	39 (14%)	27 (1%)
Numbers and letters B efficiency	41 (18%)	32 (4%)
Numbers and letters C efficiency	60 (84%)	35 (7%)
Numbers and letters D efficiency	63 (90%)	36 (8%)
Numbers and letters D disruption	60 (84%)	36 (8%)
Driving scenes	53 (62%)	30 (2%)
Language		
Oral production	48 (42%)	46 (34%)
Naming	55 (69%)	52 (58%)
Learning and memory		
List learning A total immediate	42 (21%)	40 (16%)
List learning A long delay recall	41 (18%)	32 (4%)
Story learning immediate r	59 (82%)	38 (12%)
Story learning delayed recall	57 (76%)	28 (1%)
Daily living memory immediate	42 (21%)	39 (14%)
Daily living memory delayed	45 (31%)	45 (31%)
Perceptual and spatial abilities		
Visual discrimination	61 (86%)	44 (27%)
Design construction	54 (66%)	46 (34%)
Executive functioning		
Mazes	52 (58%)	47 (38%)
Categories	51 (54%)	29 (2%)
Word generation	59 (82%)	40 (16%)

Note: Values represent demographically-adjusted T scores (percentiles) from the abbreviated NAB

Case Example #1 was a 59-year-old Caucasian woman with 13 years of education. She was diagnosed with metastatic brain tumors (from her cervix), located in her left front-temporal region and her left occipital region. She underwent radiation therapy 14 months before this evaluation. She subsequently underwent chemotherapy for the next 7 months. Her performance on the RIST was high average (RIST Index = 116). Therefore, her performance on each domain is compared to the criteria in Table 32.2. Her performances in the attention, language, spatial, and executive functioning domains are considered broadly normal. She has *probable* impairment on the learning and memory module. Thus, she appears to have diminished learning and memory skills. However, she does not appear to meet the psychometric criteria for Cognitive Disorder NOS.

Case Example #2 was a 43-year-old Caucasian man with 14 years of education. He underwent a total resection of a Grade II oligodendroglioma in his right frontal lobe, followed by partial brain radiation therapy and chemotherapy. His surgery was 6.5 years before this evaluation. His performance on the RIST was average (RIST Index = 101). His performance in the language and spatial domains is considered broadly normal. He has *possible* impairment in the executive functioning domain and *probable* impairment in the attention and memory domains. Based on his performance on testing, he meets the psychometric criteria for Cognitive Disorder NOS.

Conclusions

The purpose of this chapter was to provide information for clinicians and researchers that should ultimately improve the accuracy of how we define, conceptualize, and measure cognitive impairment in neuropsychology. Five key psychometric principles that should be considered when interpreting a battery of tests are presented in this chapter. These principles include: (1) Low scores are relatively common across all test batteries; (2) Low scores depend on where you set your cutoff score; (3) Low scores vary by number of tests administered; (4) Low scores vary by demographic characteristics of the examinee; and (5) Low scores vary by level of intelligence.

There are clear implications for these principles in day-to-day clinical practice. If a neuropsychologist administers a 3- to 4-h battery of tests, sets the cutoff for impairment at 1SD below the mean (i.e., $T < 40$), then 30–50% of healthy adults will have *five* or *more* low scores. If a more conservative cutoff for impairment on the battery is set at ≤5th percentile, then 30–50% of healthy adults will have *two* or *more* low scores.

Not surprisingly, the probability of obtaining a low score depends on where you set your cutoff. For example, when considering 36 T scores from the NAB, 44% of healthy adults obtain five or more scores below 1SD and only 5% of healthy adults obtain five or more scores below 2 SD. Similarly, when considering 20 subtest scores from the WAIS-III/WMS-III, 34% have five or more scores below 1SD and only 2% have five or more scores below 2 SD.

The average neuropsychological evaluation might include 20–40 tests that yield 40–60 scores. The more tests that are given, the more likely it is to obtain low scores. For example, if 36 primary T scores are considered across the NAB, then 44% of healthy adults will have five or more scores below 1SD ($T = 39$ or less). If 16 primary T scores from the NAB are considered, then 16% of healthy adults will have five or more scores below 1SD.

The failure to consider the demographic characteristics of a patient or research subject can increase the likelihood of a false positive or a false negative diagnosis of cognitive impairment. For example, if test scores are only adjusted for age, then (1) there will be sex differences on some tests, (2) those with less education will perform more poorly than those with more education on some tests, and (3) ethnic minorities will perform more poorly than majority culture Caucasians on some tests.

Considering cognitive test performance within the context of intellectual ability can improve a clinician or researcher's ability to accurately identify cognitive impairment. When considering 20 subtest scores from the WAIS-III/WMS-III, 31% of healthy adults of *average* intelligence will have *five or more* low scores (scaled score of 7 or lower) compared to only 5.6% of healthy adults with *high average* intelligence. Therefore, considering pre-injury or pre-disease level of intellectual ability should reduce false negative diagnoses of cognitive impairment in those with higher levels of intelligence and reduce false positive diagnoses in those with lower levels of intelligence.

It is important for clinicians and researchers to (1) have an understanding of these principles and (2) to implement these principles in clinical practice, research programs, and clinical trials. It is necessary to apply these principles when developing criteria for cognitive impairment. Failure to appreciate, consider, and apply these principles to cognitive assessment will result in decreased diagnostic accuracy. For example, if trying to identify early evidence of cognitive impairment associated with prodromal Alzheimer's Disease, failure to consider these principles can result in (1) failure to identify true cognitive diminishment in a Caucasian man of high average intelligence (i.e., a false negative), and (2) misdiagnosing a Hispanic woman with 10 years of education as cognitively impaired when she is not (i.e., a false positive).

We have developed new psychometric criteria for determining the presence of cognitive impairment (Iverson and Brooks in press). To our knowledge, this represents the first psychometrically-derived and testable guidelines for identifying plausible psychometric criteria for CD-NOS that (1) take into consideration the five psychometric principles, (2) are consistent with the recommendations for cognitive disorder NOS, and (3) are based on fixed number of tests (i.e., an abbreviated version of the NAB). The procedure outlined in this chapter should result in fewer false positive and false negative diagnoses. Of course, additional research is needed to test these criteria in clinical populations with known cognitive impairment.

The guiding principles and research set out in this chapter have important implications for (1) day-to-day clinical practice, (2) the design of research and clinical trials involving cognition, and (3) the development of new nosology for cognitive impairment. It is our hope that the next edition of the Diagnostic and Statistical Manual of Mental Disorders – Fifth Edition (DSM-V) will provide more guidance for the accurate identification of cognitive impairment in patients with medical, psychiatric, or neurological conditions.

References

American Psychiatric Association. (1994). *Diagnostic and statistical manual of mental disorders* (4th ed.). Washington, DC: American Psychiatric Association.

Antinori, A., Arendt, G., Becker, J. T., Brew, B. J., Byrd, D. A., Cherner, M., et al. (2007). Updated research nosology for HIV-associated neurocognitive disorders. *Neurology, 69*(18), 1789–1799.

Ardila, A. (1995). Directions of research in cross-cultural neuropsychology. *Journal of Clinical and Experimental Neuropsychology, 17*(1), 143–150.

Axelrod, B. N., & Wall, J. R. (2007). Expectancy of impaired neuropsychological test scores in a non-clinical sample. *International Journal of Neuroscience, 117*(11), 1591–1602.

Beatty, W. W., Mold, J. W., & Gontkovsky, S. T. (2003). RBANS performance: influences of sex and education. *Journal of Clinical and Experimental Neuropsychology, 25*(8), 1065–1069.

Binder, L. M., Iverson, G. L., & Brooks, B. L. (2009). To err is human: "Abnormal" neuropsychological scores and variability are common in healthy adults. *Archives of Clinical Neuropsychology, 24*, 31–46.

Brickman, A. M., Cabo, R., & Manly, J. J. (2006). Ethical issues in cross-cultural neuropsychology. *Applied Neuropsychology, 13*(2), 91–100.

Bright, P., Jaldow, E., & Kopelman, M. D. (2002). The National Adult Reading test as a measure of premorbid intelligence: a comparison with estimates derived from demographic variables. *Journal of the International Neuropsychological Society, 8*(6), 847–854.

Brooks, B. L., Iverson, G. L., Holdnack, J. A., & Feldman, H. H. (2008). The potential for mis-classification of mild cognitive impairment: A study of memory scores on the Wechsler Memory Scale-III in healthy older adults. *Journal of the International Neuropsychological Society, 14*(3), 463–478.

Brooks, B. L., Iverson, G. L., & White, T. (2007). Substantial risk of "Accidental MCI" in healthy older adults: Base rates of low memory scores in neuropsychological assessment. *Journal of the International Neuropsychological Society, 13*(3), 490–500.

Collaer, M. L., & Nelson, J. D. (2002). Large visuospatial sex difference in line judgment: possible role of attentional factors. *Brain and Cognition, 49*(1), 1–12.

Crawford, J. R., Garthwaite, P. H., & Gault, C. B. (2007). Estimating the percentage of the population with abnormally low scores (or abnormally large score differences) on standardized neuropsychological test batteries: a generic method with applications. *Neuropsychology, 21*(4), 419–430.

Donders, J., Zhu, J., & Tulsky, D. (2001). Factor index score patterns in the WAIS-III standardization sample. *Assessment, 8*(2), 193–203.

Dubois, B., Feldman, H. H., Jacova, C., DeKosky, S. T., Barberger-Gateau, P., Cummings, J., et al. (2007). Research criteria for the diagnosis of Alzheimer's disease: Revising the NINCDS-ADRDA criteria – a position paper. *Lancet Neurology, 6*, 734–746.

Geary, D. C., Saults, S. J., Liu, F., & Hoard, M. K. (2000). Sex differences in spatial cognition, computational fluency, and arithmetical reasoning. *Journal of Experimental and Child Psychology, 77*(4), 337–353.

Golden, C., Purish, A., & Hammeke, T. (1985). *Manual for the Luria-Nebraska neuropsychological battery*. Los Angeles: Western Psychological Services.

Golden, C. J., Freshwater, S. M., & Vayalakkara, J. (2000). The Luria-Nebraska neuropsychological battery. In G. Groth-Marnat (Ed.), *Neuropsychological assessment in clinical practice: A guide to test interpretation and integration* (pp. 263–289). New York: Wiley.

Green, R. E., Melo, B., Christensen, B., Ngo, L. A., Monette, G., & Bradbury, C. (2008). Measuring premorbid IQ in traumatic brain injury: An examination of the validity of the

Wechsler Test of Adult Reading (WTAR). *Journal of Clinical and Experimental Neuropsychology, 30*(2), 163–172.

Griffin, S. L., Mindt, M. R., Rankin, E. J., Ritchie, A. J., & Scott, J. G. (2002). Estimating premorbid intelligence: Comparison of traditional and contemporary methods across the intelligence continuum. *Archives of Clinical Neuropsychology, 17*(5), 497–507.

Heaton, R. K., Grant, I., & Matthews, C. G. (1991). *Comprehensive norms for an extended Halstead-Reitan battery: Demographic corrections, research findings, and clinical applications.* Odessa: Psychological Assessment Resources, Inc.

Heaton, R. K., Miller, S. W., Taylor, M. J., & Grant, I. (2004). *Revised comprehensive norms for an expanded Halstead-Reitan battery: Demographically adjusted neuropsychological norms for African American and Caucasian adults professional manual.* Lutz: Psychological Assessment Resources.

Heaton, R. K., Taylor, M. J., & Manly, J. (2003). Demographic effects and use of demographically corrected norms with the WAIS-III and WMS-III. In D. S. Tulsky, D. H. Saklofske, G. J. Chelune, R. K. Heaton, R. J. Ivnik, R. Bornstein, A. Prifitera, & M. Ledbetter (Eds.), *Clinical interpretation of the WAIS-III and WMS-III* (pp. 183–210). San Diego: Academic.

Herlitz, A., Nilsson, L. G., & Backman, L. (1997). Gender differences in episodic memory. *Memory & Cognition, 25*(6), 801–811.

Horton, A. M., Jr. (1999). Above-average intelligence and neuropsychological test score performance. *International Journal of Neuroscience, 99*(1–4), 221–231.

Ingraham, L. J., & Aiken, C. B. (1996). An empirical approach to determining criteria for abnormality in test batteries with multiple measures. *Neuropsychology, 10*, 120–124.

Iverson, G. L., & Brooks, B. L. (in press). New psychometric criteria for DSM-IV cognitive disorder NOS. *Journal of the International Neuropsychological Society.*

Iverson, G. L., Brooks, B. L., & Ashton, V. L. (2008). Cognitive impairment: Foundations for clinical and forensic practice. In M. P. Duckworth, T. Iezzi, & W. O'Donohue (Eds.), *Motor vehicle collisions: Medical, psychosocial, and legal consequences* (pp. 243–309). Amsterdam: Academic.

Iverson, G. L., Brooks, B. L., & Holdnack, J. A. (2008). Misdiagnosis of cognitive impairment in forensic neuropsychology. In R. L. Heilbronner (Ed.), *Neuropsychology in the courtroom: Expert analysis of reports and testimony* (pp. 243–266). New York: Guilford Press.

Iverson, G. L., Brooks, B. L., White, T., & Stern, R. A. (2008). Neuropsychological Assessment Battery (NAB): Introduction and advanced interpretation. In A. M. Horton Jr. & D. Wedding (Eds.), *The neuropsychology handbook* (3rd ed., pp. 279–343). New York: Springer Publishing Inc.

Ivnik, R. J., Makec, J. F., Smith, G. E., Tangolos, E. G., & Peterson, R. C. (1996). Neuropsychological tests' norms above age 55: COWAT, BNT, MAE Token, WRAT-R Reading, AMNART, STROOP, TMT, and JLO. *The Clinical Neuropsychologist, 10*, 262–278.

Maddrey, A. M., Cullum, C. M., Weiner, M. F., & Filley, C. M. (1996). Premorbid intelligence estimation and level of dementia in Alzheimer's disease. *Journal of the International Neuropsychological Society, 2*(6), 551–555.

Manly, J. J., & Echemendia, R. J. (2007). Race-specific norms: using the model of hypertension to understand issues of race, culture, and education in neuropsychology. *Archives of Clinical Neuropsychology, 22*(3), 319–325.

Morgan, E. E., Woods, S. P., Scott, J. C., Childers, M., Beck, J. M., Ellis, R. J., et al. (2007). Predictive Validity of Demographically Adjusted Normative Standards for the HIV Dementia Scale. *Journal of Clinical and Experimental Neuropsychology, 20*, 1–8.

Moses, J. A., Jr., Golden, C. J., Ariel, R., & Gustavson, J. L. (1983). *Interpretation of the Luria-Nebraska neuropsychological battery* (Vol. 1). New York: Grune and Stratton.

Norman, M. A., Evans, J. D., Miller, W. S., & Heaton, R. K. (2000). Demographically corrected norms for the California Verbal Learning Test. *Journal of Clinical and Experimental Neuropsychology, 22*(1), 80–94.

O'Bryant, S. E., O'Jile, J. R., & McCaffrey, R. J. (2004). Reporting of demographic variables in neuropsychological research: trends in the current literature. *The Clinical Neuropsychologist, 18*(2), 229–233.

Palmer, B. W., Boone, K. B., Lesser, I. M., & Wohl, M. A. (1998). Base rates of "impaired" neuropsychological test performance among healthy older adults. *Archives of Clinical Neuropsychology, 13*(6), 503–511.

Paolo, A. M., Ryan, J. J., Troster, A. I., & Hilmer, C. D. (1996). Utility of the Barona demographic equations to estimate premorbid intelligence: Information from the WAIS-R standardization sample. *Journal of Clinical Psychology, 52*(3), 335–343.

Patton, D. E., Duff, K., Schoenberg, M. R., Mold, J., Scott, J. G., & Adams, R. L. (2003). Performance of cognitively normal African Americans on the RBANS in community dwelling older adults. *The Clinical Neuropsychologist, 17*(4), 515–530.

Petersen, R. C., Smith, G. E., Ivnik, R. J., Kokmen, E., & Tangalos, E. G. (1994). Memory function in very early Alzheimer's disease. *Neurology, 44*(5), 867–872.

Petersen, R. C., Smith, G. E., Waring, S. C., Ivnik, R. J., Tangalos, E. G., & Kokmen, E. (1999). Mild cognitive impairment: clinical characterization and outcome. *Archives of Neurology, 56*(3), 303–308.

Randolph, C. (1998). *Repeatable battery for the assessment of neuropsychological status manual.* San Antonio: The Psychological Corporation.

Reitan, R. M., & Wolfson, D. (1985). *The Halstead-Reitan neuropsychological test battery: Theory and clinical interpretation.* Tucson: Neuropsychology Press.

Reitan, R. M., & Wolfson, D. (1993). *The Halstead-Reitan neuropsychological test battery: Theory and clinical interpretation* (2nd ed.). Tucson: Neuropsychology Press.

Reynolds, C. R., & Kamphaus, R. W. (2003). *Reynolds intellectual assessment scales and Reynolds intellectual screening test professional manual.* Lutz: Psychological Assessment Resources.

Rosselli, M., & Ardila, A. (2003). The impact of culture and education on non-verbal neuropsychological measurements: a critical review. *Brain and Cognition, 52*(3), 326–333.

Ryan, E. L., Baird, R., Mindt, M. R., Byrd, D., Monzones, J., & Bank, S. M. (2005). Neuropsychological impairment in racial/ethnic minorities with HIV infection and low literacy levels: effects of education and reading level in participant characterization. *Journal of the International Neuropsychological Society, 11*(7), 889–898.

Schmidt, S. L., Oliveira, R. M., Rocha, F. R., & Abreu-Villaca, Y. (2000). Influences of handedness and gender on the grooved pegboard test. *Brain and Cognition, 44*(3), 445–454.

Schretlen, D. J., Testa, S. M., Winicki, J. M., Pearlson, G. D., & Gordon, B. (2008). Frequency and bases of abnormal performance by healthy adults on neuropsychological testing. *Journal of the International Neuropsychological Society, 14*(3), 436–445.

Sheslow, D., & Adams, W. (2003). *Wide range assessment of memory and learning* (Administration and technical manual 2nd ed.). Wilmington: Wide Range, Inc.

Steinberg, B. A., Bieliauskas, L. A., Smith, G. E., & Ivnik, R. J. (2005a). Mayo's Older Americans Normative Studies: Age- and IQ-Adjusted Norms for the Trail-Making Test, the Stroop Test, and MAE Controlled Oral Word Association Test. *The Clinical Neuropsychologist, 19*(3–4), 329–377.

Steinberg, B. A., Bieliauskas, L. A., Smith, G. E., Ivnik, R. J., & Malec, J. F. (2005b). Mayo's Older Americans Normative Studies: Age- and IQ-Adjusted Norms for the Auditory Verbal Learning Test and the Visual Spatial Learning Test. *The Clinical Neuropsychologist, 19*(3–4), 464–523.

Stern, R. A., & White, T. (2003). *Neuropsychological assessment battery.* Lutz: Psychological Assessment Resources.

Strauss, E., Sherman, E. M. S., & Spreen, O. (2006). *A compendium of neuropsychological tests: Administration, norms, and commentary* (3rd ed.). New York: Oxford University Press.

The Psychological Corporation. (2001). *Wechsler test of adult reading manual.* San Antonio: Psychological Corporation.

Tremont, G., Hoffman, R. G., Scott, J. G., & Adams, R. L. (1998). Effect of intellectual level on neuropsychological test performance: A response to Dodrill (1997). *The Clinical Neuropsychologist, 12*, 560–567.

Voyer, D., Voyer, S., & Bryden, M. P. (1995). Magnitude of sex differences in spatial abilities: a meta-analysis and consideration of critical variables. *Psychological Bulletin, 117*(2), 250–270.

Warner, M. H., Ernst, J., Townes, B. D., Peel, J., & Preston, M. (1987). Relationships between IQ and neuropsychological measures in neuropsychiatric populations: within-laboratory and cross-cultural replications using WAIS and WAIS-R. *Journal of Clinical and Experimental Neuropsychology, 9*(5), 545–562.

Wechsler, D. (1997a). *Wechsler adult intelligence scale* (3rd ed.). San Antonio: Psychological Corporation.

Wechsler, D. (1997b). *Wechsler memory scale* (3rd ed.). San Antonio: The Psychological Corporation.

White, T., & Stern, R. A. (2003). *Neuropsychological assessment battery: Psychometric and technical manual*. Lutz: Psychological Assessment Resources.

World Health Organization. (1992). *International statistical classification of diseases and related health problems* (10th ed.). Geneva, Switzerland: World Health Organization.

Index

A

AAN. *See* American Academy of Neurology
Absence seizures, 410, 432
ACRM. *See* American Congress of
    Rehabilitation Medicine
Acromatopsia, 207
Activities of daily living (ADLs), 3, 4, 13, 18
Acute disseminated encephalomyelitis
    (ADEM), 648, 847–848
ADD/ADHD. *See* Attention deficit
    disorder and attention deficit
    with hyperactivity disorder
Adrenal corticotropic hormone (ACTH), 74
Agnosia, 206–209
AEDs. *See* Antiepileptic drugs
Akinesia, 568
Alice in Wonderland /Todd's syndrome,
    206, 207
Alzheimer's disease, 358–359, 926
Amaurosis fugax, 419
American Academy of Neurology (AAN),
    722, 726
American Congress of Rehabilitation
    Medicine (ACRM), 699
Amygdala, 75
Amygadalohippocampectomy, 452–453
ANAM. *See* Automated Neuropsychological
    Assessment Metrics
Anterior temporal lobectomy (ATL), 452–453
  epilepsy surgery
    factoids for, 478–479
    post-surgical neuropsychological
      outcome, 477–478
Anterograde amnesia, 184
Antiepileptic drugs (AEDs), 521, 526
  cognitive and behavioral effects of, 450
Anti-seizure medication, 797
Anxiety disorders, 484–485
  traumatic brain injuries, 677–678

Aphasia syndromes
  alexia, agraphia, and aphemia, 279–281
  aprosodies, 282–283
  assessment
    comprehension, 285
    fluency, 284–285
    naming, 285
    reading and writing, 286
    repetition, 285
  Broca's aphasia, 271–272
  considerations
    cultural, 286
    geriatric, 288
    pediatric, 286–288
    psychiatric, 288–289
  cortical deafness, 281–282
  fluent aphasias
    anomic aphasia, 278–279
    conduction aphasia, 277–278
    transcortical sensory aphasia, 275–276
    Wernicke's aphasia, 274–275
  global aphasia, 269–270
  mixed transcortical aphasia, 270–271
  nonfluent aphasias, 268
  nonverbal auditory agnosia, 281–282
  transcortical motor aphasia, 272–273
  verbal auditory agnosia, 281–282
Aphemia, 172
Apperceptive visual agnosia, 209
Apraxia, 211–212
Aprosodies, 282–284
Arousal
  assessment, 144–146
  delirium, 142–143
  problems, 140–141
  stuporous conditions, 141–142
Arteriovenous malformation, 315
Associative visual agnosia, 209
Astereognosia, 116

M.R. Schoenberg and J.G. Scott (eds.), *The Little Black Book of Neuropsychology:*
A Syndrome-Based Approach, DOI 10.1007/978-0-387-76978-3,
© Springer Science+Business Media, LLC 2011

Ataxia, 587–588
    neuropsychological symptoms, 588
ATL. *See* Anterior temporal lobectomy
Atonic seizures, 432
Atopognosia, 116
Attentional capacity
    anatomy, 150–151
    assessment, 154–155
    auditory attention span, 156
    deficits, 150
    problems
        impulsivity and hyperactivity,
            151–153
        primary attention problems, 153
        vigilance, 153
        without hyperactivity, 152
    vigilance, 157–158
Attention deficit disorder and attention deficit
        with hyperactivity disorder (ADD/
        ADHD), 153
Auditory attention span, 156
Auditory dorsal pathway, 118
Auditory hallucinations, 260
Automated Neuropsychological Assessment
        Metrics (ANAM), 732–733

B
Balint's syndrome, 206–208
Basal ganglia, 76–77
    anatomy, 570
    blood supply, 570–571
    circuitry function
        deep brain stimulation, 572–574
        direct pathway, 571
        healthy individual, 572
        high frequency stimulation, 572
        indirect pathway, 571
        Parkinson's disease, 573
    dorsolateral frontal pathway, 574
    inputs, 571
    lateral orbitofrontal pathway, 574
    medial frontal/anterior cingulate pathway,
        574–575
    motor pathway, 574
    oculomotor pathway, 574
    outputs, 571
    subcomponents, 569–570
Basilar migraine, 414
Batten disease, 845–846
BC-CRP. *See* British Columbia Concussion
        Rehabilitation Program
BC-PSI. *See* British Columbia Postconcussion
        Symptom Inventory

Behavior Rating Inventory of Executive
        Function (BRIEF), 901
Benign childhood epilepsy with centrotempo-
        ral spikes (BECTS), 438–439
Benign paroxysmal positional vertigo
        (BPPV), 413
Benign rolandic epilepsy, 438–439
Benign *vs.* malignant tumor, 789–790
Body mass index (BMI), 529
Boston Naming Test (BNT), 896
BPPV. *See* Benign paroxysmal positional
        vertigo
Bradykinesia, 568
Brain herniation, 669–670
Brainstem syndromes
    leukoariosis, 339–340
    PICA, 333
Brain tumor
    adults, 796
    benign *vs.* malignant, 789–790
    classification, 794–796
    diagnosis and neuroimaging, 793–794
    epidemiology, 790–791
    grading system, 795
    neuropsychological assessment
        causes, 799
        clinical practice, 801–805
        fixed *vs.* flexible batteries, 801
        reliable change, 800
        test battery selection, 800
    neuropsychological evaluation, 806
    peak incidence, 805
    signs and symptoms
        intracranial pressure, 791
        paraneoplastic syndrome, 792–793
        seizures, 792
    treatment
        Chemotherapy, 799
        gamma knife/stereotactic radiosurgery,
            798
        radiation therapy, 797–798
        surgery, 797
    types
        metastatic, 788–789
        primary, 789
BRIEF. *See* Behavior Rating Inventory of
        Executive Function
British Columbia Concussion Rehabilitation
        Program (BC-CRP), 735
British Columbia Postconcussion Symptom
        Inventory (BC-PSI), 753
Broader psychopathology, 485–486
Broca's aphasia, 164, 167–169
Brodmann's area, 101–103

C
CAE. *See* Childhood absence epilepsy
California Verbal Learning Test (CVLT), 898
CAM. *See* Confusion assessment method
Canadian Cancer Statistics, 791
Capgras syndrome, 230–231
CBGD. *See* Cortical basal ganglionic
        degeneration
Center for Disease Control (CDC), 699–700
Central nervous system
    cerebellum, 65
    cerebral peduncle, 68
    diencephalon, 69
    forebrain /procencephalon, 69
    hindbrain/ rhombencephalon, 66–67
    hypothalamus, 73
    midbrain/mesencephalon, 68
    pituitary gland, 73–74
    pons, 67
    pretectum, 69
    tegmentum, 68
    thalamus, 69–73
Cerebellum, 67
Cerebral cortex
    Brodmann's area, 103–105
    heteromodal, 105
    limbic, 105
    paralimbic, 105
    primary sensory-motor, 105
    unimodal, 105
Cerebral peduncle, 68
Cerebro-spinal fluid (CSF), 78–81
Cerebrovascular disease and stroke
    afterstroke conditions
        ACA distribution stroke, 344–346
        left hemisphere, 349–350
        MCA distribution stroke, 343–344
        neuropsychological evaluation, 341–343
        PCA distribution strokes, 346–347
        right hemisphere, 348–349
        subcortical strokes, 347–348
    assessment and rehabilitation, 352–354
    brainstem syndromes
        leukoariosis, 339–340
        PICA, 333
    cerebral artery syndromes, 317–326
    cerebral vasculature
        anterior circulation, 305–307
        circle of Willis, 308
    clinical symptoms
        arteriovenous malformation, 315
        ICH, 312–315
        ischemic strokes, 309–311
        SAH, 315–317

hemorrhagic strokes
    ICH, 299–300
    IVH, 304
    SAH, 300–303
ischemic stroke/ infarction, 295–297
lacunae syndromes, 327–330
midbrain and brain stem, 334–337
pathophysiology, 294–295
subtypes and categorization, 295
thalamic vascular syndromes,
        331–332
TIAs, 297–298
Chemotherapy, 799
Childhood absence epilepsy (CAE), 439–440
CIND. *See* Cognitive impairment
        no dementia
Clonic seizures, 432
Closed head injurys (CHI), 766
Cobalamin disorders, 850–851
Cognitive decline
    Batten disease, 845–846
    deterioration, 840
    galactosemia, 851
    general patterns, 840–841
    Hallervorden-Spatz syndrome, 852
    hepatolenticular degeneration (*see*
            Wilson's disease)
    HIV associated progressive encephalopathy,
            858
    Hurler syndrome (*see* Mucopolysaccharidose
            (MPS) disorder)
    hydrocephalus
        behavioral symptoms, 853
        cerebrospinal fluid, 853
        neuropathology, 854
    juvenile onset Tay-Sachs, 842
    metachromatic leukodystrophy, 843–844
    Niemann-Pick disease, 842–843
    Rett syndrome, 852
    sickle cell disease, 856
    Tay-Sachs disease, 842
Cognitive impairment
    classification
        clinical implications, 926–927
        psychometric criteria, 926
        test score, 927
    clinical practice, 945
    cutoff score
        definition, 930
        NAB, 931, 932
        sensitivity and specificity, 932
        WAIS-III/WMS-III, 931, 932
    demographic characteristics
        delayed memory, 934

Cognitive impairment (*cont.*)
    diagnostic accuracy, 937
    education and sex, 935
    impacts, 933
    RBANS index scores, 936
    test scores *vs.* cognitive functioning, 936
    guiding principles, 946–947
    identification
        criteria, 941–943
        NAB module, 940, 941
        psychometric analyses, 940
    intellectual ability, 946
    intelligence, level
        NAB scores, 937–939
        test performance, 937
        WAIS-III/WMS-III scores, 937–939
    neuropsychological evaluation,
        945–946935–936
    patient treatment
        radiation therapy, 945
        RIST and NAB test data, 944
    severity continuum, 925
    test
        administration, 933, 934
        battery, 929–931
Cognitive impairment no dementia (CIND),
    388, 390–391
Coma, 665–666
Community integration, traumatic brain
    injuries, 687
Complex partial seizures, 410, 431
Computed tomography (CT), 769
Concussion resolution index, 732
Conduction aphasia, 164, 171
Confusion assessment method (CAM), 144
Contusion, 667
Corpus callosotomy, 453
Cortical atrophy, 671
Cortical basal ganglionic degeneration
    (CBGD), 370–372, 377–378,
    580–581
Cortical functional neuroanatomy
    auditory dorsal pathway, 118
    auditory processing, 117
    dorsolateral prefrontal (dysexecutive
        syndrome), 113
    fasciculi, 122
    frontal lobe pathways, 118–119
    insular cortex (lobe), 114–115
    memory/mesial temporal pathway, 118
    mesial frontal/anterior cingulate, 114
    motor cortex, 113
    occipital lobe, 115–116
    orbitofrontal/inferior ventral frontal, 113–114
    parietal lobe, 116
    polymodal/heteromodal processing/STS
        visual processing pathway, 118
    prefrontal cortex, 113
    premotor cortex, 113
    sensory pathways, 117
    temporal lobe, 117
    visual processing, 117–118
Coup/Contrecoup injury, 667
CSF. *See* Cerebro-spinal fluid
CT. *See* Computed tomography
CVLT. *See* California Verbal Learning Test

D

Deep brain stimulation (DBS)
    chronic high frequency stimulation, 601–602
    mechanism of action, 603–604
    neurological (primary) outcome, 606–609
    neuropsychological battery, 625
    Parkinson's disease, 604–605
    reliable change and measurement, 618,
        620, 622–624
    risk factors, 617
    STN or GPi DBS, 611–614
    surgical procedure, 602–603
    VIM DBS, 626–627
Deep brain stimulator implantation, 454–455
Delirium, 142–143, 409
Delis-Kaplan executive function system
    (D-KEFS), 877
Dementia with Lewy bodies (DLB), 361,
    368–370
Demographic characteristics
    delayed memory, 934
    diagnostic accuracy, 937
    education and sex, 935
    impacts, 933
    RBANS index scores, 936, 937
    test scores *vs.* cognitive functioning, 936
Depression, 482–486
    traumatic brain injuries, 677–678
Diagnostic and Statistical Manual of Mental
    Disorders, Fourth Edition
    (DSM-IV), 747–748
Diastatic fracture, 667
Diet and behavioral therapies, 456
Diffuse Lewy body disease/dementia with
    Lewy bodies (DLBD/DLB)
    medication effects, 590
    neuropsychological symptoms, 579–580
Diffusion-weighted magnetic resonance
    imaging (DWI MRI), 297, 318
Dizziness and vertigo

basilar migraine, 414
BPPV, 413
Meniere disease, 414
presyncope, 414
vertebrobasilar TIAs, 413
vestibular neuronitis/labyrinthitis, 414
DLB. *See* Dementia with Lewy bodies
D-KEFS. *See* Delis-Kaplan executive function
        system
Dorsal simultanagnosia, 211
Dorsolateral frontal lobe epilepsy, 446–447
Dorsolateral prefrontal/ dysexecutive
        syndrome
Drug-induced Parkinsonism (DIP), 582–583
DSM-IV. *See* Diagnostic and Statistical
        Manual of Mental Disorders, Fourth
        Edition
DWI MRI. *See* Diffusion-weighted magnetic
        resonance imaging
Dysarthria, 172
Dysfunctional symptoms, frontal lobe
    anatomy, 234, 236
    autonoetic awareness, 230
    Capgras syndrome, 230–231
    environmental dependency, 229
    frontal abulia syndrome, 239
    frontal disinhibition syndrome, 239
    glabbelar reflex, 231
    grasp reflex, 231
    medial frontal syndrome, 238
    neuropsychiatric syndromes, 230
    orbitofrontal syndrome, 235–237
    palmomental reflex, 231
    paratonia, 230
    reduplicative paramnesia, 230
    root reflex, 231
    snout reflex, 231
    suck reflex, 232
    tangentiality /circumloquaciousness, 229
Dystonia
    GPi DBS, 630–635
    medication effects, 591
    neuropsychological symptoms, 585–586

E
Electroencephalogram (EEG), 830
Emotional functioning, 492–493
Emotions and mood
    multiaxial diagnostic system
        axis I, 250–251
        axis II, 252
        axis III, 252–254
        axis IV, 254

        axis V, 254–255
    neurologic illness
        auditory hallucinations, 260
        cognitive deficits, 257
        dorso-lateral-frontal lobe syndrome,
            256
        dysphoria, 258
        emotional and behavioral symptoms,
            258–259
        euphoria, 258
        olfactory and gustatory hallucinations,
            260–264
        somatosensory hallucinations, 260
        visual hallucinations, 260
Epidural hemorrhage, 669
Epilepsy
    classification of, 437
    diagnosing, 427
    diagnostic tools in, 426–427
    encephalopathies, 437
    incidence of, 429–430
    neuropsychological assessment guide
        "executive function," 490
        general cognitive assessment, 489–490
        psychological/emotional functioning,
            492–493
    neuropsychological comorbidity
        cognitive and behavioral dysfunction,
            459
        potentially progressive disorder,
            460–462
        prognosis for patients, 457–459
        seizure onset, 459–460
    neuropsychological tests, 493–501
    potentially progressive disorder,
        460–462
    presumed etiologies, 437
    prevalence of, 429–430
    psychiatric issues
        anxiety disorders, 484–485
        broader psychopathology, 485–486
        depression, 482–484
    quality of life, 486–487
    role of neuropsychologist, 424–425
    syndromes
        frontal lobe epilepsy, 446–448
        idiopathic, 438–440
        juvenile myoclonic epilepsy, 440–441
        Landau–Kleffner syndrome, 443–444
        Lennox–Gastaut syndrome, 442–443
        occipital lobe epilepsy, 448–449
        parietal lobe epilepsy, 448
        temporal lobe epilepsy, 444–446
        West's syndrome, 442

Epilepsy surgery
    cognitive outcome from ATL
        factoids for, 478–479
        post-surgical neuropsychological
            outcome, 477–478
        memory impairment, 475–476
    seizure freedom prediction
        neurological and demographic
            variables, 473
        risk factors for surgery failure, 473–474
        seizure-free rates, 471
        seizure remission, 471–473
    seizure onset, 474
    Wada's procedure, language dominance
        contralateral side of surgery, 480–481
        ipsilateral side of surgery, 480
Epileptic seizures (ES), 524, 543
Episodic neurologic symptoms
    abnormal movements
        acute dystonic reactions, 415–416
        HFS, 416
        simple partial motor seizures, 415
        tics, 416
    aphasia, 419
    consciousness and convulsions, loss
        confusional states, 408–409
        delirium, 409
        dissociative fugue, 411
        hypoglycemia, 407
        narcolepsy, 407
        nonepileptic myoclonus, 407–408
        panic attacks, 411
        parasomnias, 411–412
        PNES, 406–407
        seizures, 406, 410
        syncope, 407
        TIAs, 408
        transient global amnesia, 410–411
    dizziness and vertigo
        basilar migraine, 414
        BPPV, 413
        Meniere disease, 414
        presyncope, 414
        vertebrobasilar TIAs, 413
        vestibular neuronitis/labyrinthitis, 414
    hallucinations, 421
    headaches and facial pain
        cluster headaches, 418
        migraine, 417
        paroxysmal hemicrania, 418
        trigeminal neuralgia, 418
    limb pain, 419
    sensory symptoms, 421
    visual loss

        giant cell arteritis, 420
        migraine, 419–420
        optic neuritis, 420
        pseudotumor cerebri, 420
        transient monocular blindness/
            amaurosis fugax, 419
    weakness
        LEMS, 412
        metabolic myopathies, 413
        migraine auras, 417
        myasthenia gravis, 412
        periodic paralysis, 412–413
        spinal cord/ plexus damage/impinge-
            ment, 417
        TIAs, 416–417
        Todd's paralysis, 417
Essential tremor (ET)
    deep brain stimulation
        chronic high frequency stimulation,
            601–602
        mechanism of action, 603–604
        reliable change and measurement, 618,
            620, 622–624
        risk factors, 617
        STN and GPi, 604–614
        surgical procedure, 602–603
        VIM DBS, 626–627
    medication effects, 591
    neuropsychological symptoms, 584–585
Evidence-based neuropsychological practice
    (EBNP), 3–4
Evidences
    construct-related, 888, 889
    content-related, 888–889
    criterion-related, 888, 890
Expressive aprosody, 163, 174

F
Factoids, 478–479
Familial epilepsies, 437
Febrile seizures, 433–434
FFA. See Fusiform face area
FLE. See Frontal lobe epilepsy
Fluent aphasias
    anomic aphasia, 278–279
    conduction aphasia, 277–278
    transcortical sensory aphasia, 275–276
    Wernicke's aphasia, 274–275
Fluent speech
    anomic aphasia, 171
    conduction aphasia, 171
    transcortical sensory aphasia, 170
    Wernicke's aphasia, 170

fMRI. *See* Functional magnetic resonance imaging
Focal epilepsy, neurocognitive profiles, 462–463
Focal seizures
  complex partial seizures, 431–432
  secondarily generalized seizures, 432
  simple partial seizures, 431
Forebrain /procencephalon, 69
Foundational principles, 870
Frontal disinhibition syndrome, 239
Frontal lobe
  anatomy
    functional organizations, 220
    orbitofrontal region, 221
    prefrontal cortex, 221
  dysfunction
    anatomy, 234, 236
    autonoetic awareness, 230
    Capgras syndrome, 230–231
    environmental dependency, 229
    frontal abulia syndrome, 239
    frontal disinhibition syndrome, 239
    Glabbelar reflex, 231
    Grasp reflex, 231
    medial frontal syndrome, 238
    neuropsychiatric syndromes, 230
    orbitofrontal syndrome, 235–237
    palmomental reflex, 231
    paratonia, 230
    reduplicative paramnesia, 230
    root reflex, 231
    snout reflex, 231
    suck reflex, 232
    tangentiality/circumloquaciousness, 229
  frontal eye fields, 226
  general assessment issues, 240
  motor and sequencing skills
    abstract reasoning, 244–247
    attention assessment, 243
    impulsivity/disinhibition, 243–244
  prefrontal cortex, 226–227
  primary motor cortex
    Broca's area, 225–226
    facial, 222–224
Frontal lobe epilepsy (FLE)
  dorsolateral, 446–447
  neuropsychological findings, 468–469
  opercular, 447
  orbitofrontal, cingulate, and mesial frontal, 447
Frontotemporal dementias (FTD), 360, 370–374
Full scale intellectual quotient (FSIQ), 776, 778
Functional adequacy model, 475–476

Functional magnetic resonance imaging (fMRI), 656
Functional reserve hypothesis, 475
Fusiform face area (FFA), 204

G
GAGs. *See* Glycosaminoglycans
Galveston Orientation and Amnesia Test (GOAT), 142, 143
Gamma-knife radiation, 455
Gamma knife/Stereotactic radiosurgery, 798
GCS. *See* Glasgow coma scale
Generalized epilepsy syndromes, 462
Generalized seizures
  absence seizures, 432
  atonic seizures, 432
  clonic seizures, 432
  myoclonic seizures, 433
  primary generalized tonic-clonic seizures, 433
  tonic seizures, 432–433
Giant cell arteritis, 420
Glabbelar reflex, 231
Glasgow coma scale (GCS), 144, 146, 665, 768
Glial cells, 73–74
Global aphasia, 163, 269
Globus pallidus interna (GPi)
  basal ganglia circuitry function, 607
  neuropsychological outcome, 611–614
  Parkinson's disease, 604–605
Glycosaminoglycans (GAGs), 844
Graphesthesia, 48, 51
Grasp reflex, 229–230

H
Hallervorden-Spatz syndrome, 852
HAND. *See* HIV-associated neurocognitive disorders
HD. *See* Huntington's disease
Headaches, traumatic brain injuries, 676
Hematoma, 668–669
Hemispherectomy, 453
Hemorrhage, 667–668
Hemorrhagic strokes
  ICH, 299–300
  IVH, 304
  SAH, 300–303
Heteromodal cortex, 103
Hindbrain/ rhombencephalon, 66–67
Hippocampus, 75
HIV-associated neurocognitive disorders (HAND), 362, 380–381, 858, 928, 929

HPA. *See* Hypothalamus-pituitary-adrenal
Human immunodeficiency virus (HIV), 928
Human T-cell lymphotropic virus type 1
        (HTLV-1), 649
Huntington's disease (HD), 374–375
    medication effects, 591–595
    neuropsychological symptoms, 587
Hydrocephalus
    behavioral symptoms, 853
    cerebrospinal fluid, 854
    neuropathology, 854
Hypearousal, 140–141
Hypoglycemia, 407
Hypothalamus-pituitary-adrenal (HPA), 75
    amygdala, 76
    basal ganglia, 76–77
    epithalamus, 75
    glial cells, 73–74
    hippocampus, 75
    neocortex, 78
    PVN, 74
    telencephalon and third ventricle, 76

I
ICA. *See* Internal carotid arteries
ICH. *See* Intracerebral/Intraparenchymal
        hemorrhage
IDEA. *See* Individual with Disabilities
        Education Act
Idiopathic epilepsies, 437
Idiopathic intracranial hypertension (IIH). *See*
        Psuedotumor cerebri
Idiopathic syndromes
    benign childhood epilepsy with centrotem-
        poral spikes, 438–439
    childhood absence epilepsy, 439–440
Immediate Post-Concussion Assessment and
        Cognitive Testing (ImPACT), 731
Incidence rate
    China, 791
    US, 790–791
Indeterminate spells (IS), 544
Individual Education Program (IEP), 9, 36
Individual with Disabilities Education Act
        (IDEA), 9, 36
Inpatient medical chart
    abdomen, 46
    back, 46
    blood count and coagulation, 54–55
    cardiovascular, 45
    cerebral spinal fluid, 57
    chemistry descriptors, 55–56
    cranial nerves, 47

    extremities, 46
    family and social, 43–44
    gait and balance, 50–51
    genitourinary, 46
    laboratory evaluations, 51
    lungs/chest, 45
    mental status, 46–47
    motor examination, 47–50
    neck, 45
    neurological, 46
    past medical history, 40
    present illness, 40
    rectal, 46
    review, 44
    sensory, 51
    vital signs, 44–45
Internal carotid arteries (ICA), 85, 86
Internal reliability
    D-KEFS subtests, 877
    evaluation methods, 876, 878
    split-half correlation, 877
    standardization, 875–876
International Classification of Diseases, 10th
        edition (ICD-10), 746–747
International League Against Epilepsy, 428
Interrater reliability, 880–881
Intracerebral/Intraparenchymal hemorrhage
        (ICH), 299–300

J
Jansky-Bielschowsky disease, 844–845
Juvenile myoclonic epilepsy (JME),
        440–441

K
Ketogenic diet, 456
Ketosis, 456
Kuf's, Aka Parry's disease, 846

L
Lacunae syndromes, 327–329
Lafora disease, 857
Lambert-Eaton myasthenic syndrome
        (LEMS), 412
Landau–Kleffner syndrome, 443–444
Language problems and assessment
    alexia with agraphia, 172
    alexia without agraphia, 172
    anatomical correlation
        Brodmann's area, 161–162
        lesions, 163

perisylvian area, 161
prosodic functions, 163
aphemia, 172
aspects, 156–157
bedside assessment, 174–175
cortical deafness, 172
dysarthria, 172
expressive language and aprosodies,
        165–166
fluent speech
    anomic aphasia, 167
    conduction aphasia, 171
    transcortical sensory aphasia, 170
    Wernicke's aphasia, 170
nonfluent speech
    Broca's aphasia, 164
    global aphasia, 168
    mixed transcortical aphasia, 164
    transcortical motor aphasia, 169
nonverbal auditory agnosia, 173
prosodic speech, 173–174
psychometric based assessment, 175–176
pure word deafness, 173
receptive language and aprosodies, 161–163
right hemisphere, 173
LEMS. *See* Lambert-Eaton myasthenic
        syndrome
Lennox–Gastaut syndrome, 442–443
Limbic cortex, 104
Linear fractures, 667
Locked-in syndrome, 142
Long-term memory, 181–182
Loss of consciousness (LOC), 703
Lysosomal storage diseases (LSDS)
    Hurler syndrome
            (*see* Mucopolysaccharidose disorder)
    juvenile onset Tay-Sachs, 842
    metachromatic leukodystrophy, 843–844
    Niemann-Pick disease, 842–843
    Tay-Sachs disease, 842

M
Magnetic resonance imaging (MRI), 769
Malingering and factitious disorder
    definition/terminology, 554
    etiology, 555
    prevalence
        neurocognitive dysfunction, 555
        rate, 555
    vs. somatoform disorder
        determination, 559
        diagnosis, 556
        hypochondriasis, 560

neuroimaging, 558
response bias/effort, 556–558
MCA. *See* Middle superior artery
MCI. *See* Mild cognitive impairment
Medical chart deconstruction
    assessment and consultation, 40
    inpatient chart
        abdomen, 46
        back, 46
        blood count and coagulation, 54–55
        cardiovascular, 45
        cerebral spinal fluid, 57
        chemistry descriptors, 55–56
        cranial nerves, 47
        extremities, 46
        family and social, 43–44
        gait and balance, 50–51
        genitourinary, 46
        laboratory evaluations, 51
        lungs/chest, 45
        mental status, 46–47
        motor examination, 47–50
        neck, 45
        neurological, 46
        past medical history, 40
        present illness, 40
        rectal, 46
        review, 44
        sensory, 51
        vital signs, 44–45
    outpatient chart, 51
Medication effects, movement disorders
    DLBD/LBD, 590
    dystonia, 591
    essential tremor, 591
    Huntington's disease, 591–595
    Parkinson's disease, 589–590
    Parkinson's plus diseases, 591
    side-effects, 595
Memory and learning
    assessment, 193
    bedside/acute assessment, 194
    comprehensive/outpatient laboratory
            assessment, 199
    diencephalon, 190–191
    frontal lobes and forebrain, 191
    impairment terms
        anterograde amnesia, 184
        patterns, 185
        recall, 185–186
        retrograde amnesia, 185
    intermediate/bedside assessment,
            194–199
    laterality, 191–192

Memory and learning (*cont.*)
    model
        long-term memory, 181–182
        sensory storage, 181
        short-term memory, 181
    neuropsychological assessment
        anatomy, 189–190
        evaluation, 186–188
        learning curve patterns, 188
    storage and retrieval, 192–193
    temporal lobe, 190
    types
        declarative/explicit, 183–184
        nondeclarative/implicit, 184
Memory impairment
    evidence-based neuropsychology, 475
    FLE and TLE, 468
Meniere disease, 414
Mesial temporal lobe seizure onset (MTLE),
        445–446
Mesial temporal sclerosis (MTS), 473
Metachromatic leukodystrophy (MLD),
        843–844
Midbrain/mesencephalon, 68
Middle superior artery (MCA), 270, 273,
        275, 277
Middle temporal (MT) area, 204
Migraine, 419–420
Mild cognitive impairment (MCI), 1, 3,
        19, 927
Mild cognitive impairment and dementia
    aging and cognitive impairment, 388
    Alzheimer's disease, 358–359, 365–367
    assessment, 397–399
    CBGD, 371–372
    childhood / young adulthood, 391–392
    CIND, 390–391
    dementia with lewy bodies, 361
    DLB, 368–370
    etiologies, 364
    evidence-based neuropsychology, 396–397
    frontotemporal dementias, 360
    FTD, 370–374
    HAND, 362–364, 380–381
    HD, 374
    MSA, 378–379
    NPH, 381–382
    PD-D, 375–376
    prevalence, 364–365
    progressive supranuclear palsy, 361–362
    pseudodementia, 392–394
    PSP/Steele–Richardson–Olszewski
        syndrome, 376–377
    vascular dementia, 359–360, 367–368

Mild traumatic brain injury (MTBI). *See also*
        Post-concussion syndrome
    depression, 707
    early intervention programs, 706
    epidemiology, 698
    intracranial abnormality, 703
    LOC and PTA, 703
    meta-analytic studies, 704–706
    military, health problems
        operational, health, and welfare
            considerations, 709–711
        post-deployment screening methods,
            708–709
    terminology and diagnostic criteria
        ACRM MTBI Committee, 699
        CDC working group, 699–700
        complicated and uncomplicated,
            700–701
        vs. Concussion, 701–702
        WHO Collaborating Center Task Force,
            700
Minimal Assessment of Cognitive Function
        in MS (MACFIMS), 657
Mixed transcortical aphasia, 170
MLD. *See* Metachromatic leukodystrophy
Montreal Children's Hospital Rehabilitation,
        736
Motivational interviewing (MI)
    cognitive disabilities, 870
    concepts and principles, 866
    definition, 865
    noncompliance and patient feedback,
        864–865
    principles and SPIRIT, 867
    skills and strategies, 868–869
    transtheoretical model, 866–867
Motor system
    neurological-based assessment, 133–134
    neuropsychological-based assessment, 134
Movement disorders
    ataxia, 587–588
    dystonia
        GPi DBS, 630–631
        neuropsychological symptoms, 585–586
    essential tremor
        neuropsychological symptoms, 584–585
        surgical treatment, 601–609
    Huntington's disease, 587
    myoclonus, 588
    stiff-person syndrome, 589
    surgical treatment
        ablation techniques, 597–599
        presurgical neuropsychological
            evaluation, 596–597

Tourette syndrome
neuropsychological symptoms, 586
surgical inclusion/exclusion criteria,
636–639
thalamic DBS, 636
MRI. *See* Magnetic resonance imaging
MSA. *See* Multiple system atrophy
MTBI. *See* Mild traumatic brain injury
MTLE. *See* Mesial temporal lobe seizure onset
MTS. *See* Mesial temporal sclerosis
Mucopolysaccharidose (MPS) disorder, 844
Multiaxial diagnostic system
axis I, 250–251
axis II, 252
axis III, 252–254
axis IV, 254
axis V, 254–255
Multiple sclerosis (MS)
acute disseminated encephalomyelitis, 648
cognitive deficits, 653–654
cognitive dysfunction impact, 654–655
epidemiology and prevalence, 650–651
etiology, 652
neuropsychological deficits
assessment, 657–658
evidence-based neuropsychology, 656
mood disturbance, 655–656
treatment, 658–659
pathophysiology, 649–650
primary progressive, 651
progressive multifocal leukoencephalitis, 649
progressive relapsing, 651
relapsing-remitting, 651
secondary progressive, 651
sensory changes, 650
types, 648
Multiple system atrophy (MSA), 378–379, 581
Myoclonic seizures, 433
Myoclonus, neuropsychological symptoms, 588

N

NAB. *See* Neuropsychological assessment
battery
National Health Interview Survey, 664
Nerve conduction velocity test, 829–830
Nervous system functions
cerebellar and praxis examination,
134–135
higher order, 135–136
motor testing, 133–134
pre–requisite function, 130–132
sensory, 132–133
NES. *See* Nonepileptic seizures

Neuroanatomy primer
asymmetry
cerebral, 122–123
functional, 124
left hemisphere, 123
right hemisphere, 124–125
visual processing regions, 124
central nervous system
cerebellum, 67
cerebral peduncle, 68
diencephalon, 69
forebrain/procencephalon, 69
hindbrain/rhombencephalon, 67
hypothalamus, 73
midbrain/mesencephalon, 68
pituitary gland, 73, 74
pons, 67
pretectum, 69
tegmentum, 68
thalamus, 69–73
cerebral cortex
Brodmann's area, 103–104
heteromodal cortex, 105
limbic cortex, 105
paralimbic cortex, 105
primary sensory-motor cortex, 105
unimodal cortex, 105
cerebro-spinal fluid, 78, 80–81
cerebrovascular system
ICA, 86, 88
venus system, 88–94
cortical functional neuroanatomy
auditory dorsal pathway, 118
auditory processing, 117
dorsolateral prefrontal/dysexecutive
syndrome, 113
fasciculi, 120, 122
frontal lobe pathways, 112–113,
118–119
insular cortex (lobe), 114–115
memory/mesial temporal pathway, 118
mesial frontal/anterior cingulate, 114
motor cortex, 113
occipital lobe, 115–116
orbitofrontal /inferior ventral frontal,
113–114
parietal lobe, 116
polymodal/heteromodal processing/sts
visual processing pathway, 118
prefrontal cortex, 113
premotor cortex, 113
sensory pathways, 117
temporal lobe, 117
visual processing, 117–118

Neuroanatomy primer (*cont.*)
  hypothalamus-pituitary-adrenal (HPA), 75
    amygdala, 76
    basal ganglia, 76–77
    epithalamus, 75
    glial cells, 92–93
    hippocampus, 76
    neocortex, 78
    PVN, 74–75
    telencephalon and third ventricle, 76
  major sensory (afferent) pathways,
    106–108
  motor (efferent) descending system
    pathways, 109–112
  neurophysiology and neurochemical
    activity
    classification, 95
    IPSPs and EPSPs, 94
  organization, 63, 64
  peripheral nervous system (PNS)
    autonomic nervous system, 84, 85
    catecholamine neurotransmitters,
     97–100
    components, 83–85
    small molecule neurotransmitters, 96–97
  spinal cord, 81–83
  structural and functional components
    fasciculi, 121
    heteromodal/multimodal cortex, 120
    semantic memory, 120, 123
Neurocognitive disorder
  domains, 928
  psychometric analyses, 929
Neuroimaging, 830
Neurologic illness
  auditory hallucinations, 260
  cognitive deficits, 257
  dorso-lateral-frontal lobe syndrome, 257
  dysphoria, 258
  emotional and behavioral symptoms, 258
  euphoria, 258
  olfactory and gustatory hallucinations,
    260–264
  somatosensory hallucinations, 260
  visual hallucinations, 259–260
Neuronal ceroid lipofuscinosis (NCL) disorder
  adult (*see* Kuf's, Aka Parry's disease)
  infantile (*see* Jansky-Bielschowsky
    disease)
  juvenile (*see* Batten disease)
Neuropsychological assessment
  anatomy, 189–190
  evaluation, 186–188
  learning curve patterns, 188

Neuropsychological assessment battery (NAB)
  attention module, 801
  cognitive disorder, 803
  executive functions module, 802
  language module, 801
  memory module, 802
  profile analysis, 803–805
  spatial module, 802
  test data, 803, 804
Neuropsychological evaluation
  advantages and disadvantages, 831
  answers, 6
  basics, 128–129
  capacities, 12–13
  decision-making capacity and competence, 12
  description, 18–21
  diagnosis, 8–9
  domains, 832, 833
  EBNP, 3–4
  factors, 129–130
  function, 4
  health improvement, 9–10
  historical record, 832
  medico-legal considerations, 11–12
  nervous system functions
    cerebellar and praxis examination,
     134–135
    higher order, 135–136
    motor testing, 133–134
    pre–requisite function, 130–132
    sensory, 132–133
  optimization, 14
  premorbid cognitive ability, 16–17
  referral
    making, 21–22
    providers, 16
    questions, 18
  report, 11, 22–26
  structure and organization, 4–5
  time, 130
  timelines, 6–7
Neurotoxicity
  acute symptoms, 814–816
  aging effects, 824
  autonomic studies, 830
  batteries, evaluation, 825
  blood assay, 829
  clinical findings, 834
  EEG, 830
  exposure and symptom terms, 820
  gases
    asphyxiant, 818
    CO poisoning, 819
    silent killer, 818

metals, 817
mold, 819
neurobehavioral test battery, 823
neuroimaging, 830
neurological examination, 829
organic solvent, 814, 815
organophosphates (OP's)
    acute symptom, 820–821
    chronic symptom, 821–822
pesticides, 817–818
post acute assessment, 828
premorbid history, 825
psychiatric illness, 824–825
psychological disorders, 824
screening survey, 825–826
sleep studies (*see* polysomnography
    studies)
symptoms and features, 826–827
toxic encephalopathy, 824
urine test, 829
Neurotoxicity Screening Survey (NSS), 825–826
Niemann-Pick disease, 842–843
Noncompliance and patient feedback
applications, 865
cognitive disability, 864
Nonepileptic seizures (NES)
assessment strategies, PNES, 541–542
behavioral semiology, 524, 525
children and adolescent, PNES, 541
co-occurrence (CO), 544
definition, 523
diagnosis, 523–526
etiology
    demographic correlation, 528, 529
    psychiatric history, 531–533
    social history, 530–531
gold standard, 543
indeterminate spells, 524, 544
neuropsychological testing
    neurocognitive function, 535
    SVT failure, 536
paroxysmal events, 526
PNES, prevalence, 528
somatic syndromes, 537–538
treatment
    AEDs, 541
    psychiatric comorbidity, 539
    responsibility, 540
    USA health care system, 539–540
variability, 526
video-EEG (vEEG), 523
Nonfluent aphasias, 268–273
Nonfluent speech
Broca's aphasia, 168

Global aphasia, 168
mixed transcortical aphasia, 169
transcortical motor aphasia, 169
Non-normality and skew. *See* Shape,
    distribution
Nonverbal auditory agnosia, 281–282
Normal variability
change over time, assessment
    mathematical model, 910
    real, 909
clinical vignette, 908
learning and memory index, 909
neuropsychological battery, 907
practice effect, 912–916
regression method
    standard error, 917
    test performance, 916
reliable change
    calculation, 911
    D-KEFS subtest, 912–915
    indicator, 910
    WAIS-IV, 912, 913
    WMS-IV, 912, 914
score distribution, 910
NSS. *See* Neurotoxicity Screening Survey

O
Occipital lobe, 115
Occipital lobe epilepsy (OLE), 448–449
Ocular apraxia, 208
Olfactory and gustatory hallucinations,
    260–264
Opercular frontal lobe epilepsy, 447
Optic ataxia, 206, 207
Optic neuritis, 420
Orbitofrontal syndrome, 235–237
Organophosphates (OP's)
acute symptom, 815–817
chronic symptom
    acute effects, 820–821
    chronic effects, 822
    lead, 822

P
PAI. *See* Personality Assessment Inventory
Pallidotomy, 599–600
Paralimbic cortex, 105
Paraneoplastic syndrome, 792–793
Parasomnias, 411
Paratonia, 230
Paraventricular nucleus (PVN), 74
Parietal lobe, 116

Parietal lobe epilepsy (PLE), 444
Parkinsonism
    drug-induced Parkinsonism, 582–583
    etiologies, 569
    features, 576
    vascular, 583, 584
Parkinson's disease (PD)
    apathy, 578
    atypical features, 576
    cardinal symptoms and classic signs, 576
    DLBD/DLB, 578–579
    history and physical examination, 575
    medication effects, 589–590
    neuroanatomy (see Basal ganglia)
    nonmotor features, 576
    pallidotomy, 599–600
    thalamotomy, 598, 600, 601
    visuospatial and visuoconstructional
        problems, 577
Parkinson's disease with dementia (PD-D),
    375–376
Parkinson's plus syndromes
    cortical-basal ganglionic degeneration,
        580–581
    medication effects, 591
    multiple system atrophy, 581
    progressive supranuclear palsy, 581–582
    surgical treatment, 601
Paroxysmal hemicrania, 418
PCEs. See Posterior cortical epilepsies
PD. See Parkinson's disease
PD-D. See Parkinson's disease with dementia
Pediatric traumatic brain injury
    vs. adult TBI, 769–770
    definition and prevalence, 765
    management and rehabilitation issues
        academic/vocational, 780–782
        behavioral/psychosocial, 781–782
        phases/models of intervention, 780
    mild symptoms, 767, 769–770
    moderate-severe symptoms
        categorization of childhood, 769
        common consequences, 775
        CT scans, 769
        educational skills, 775
        full scale intellectual quotient, 776, 778
        Glasgow coma scale, 768
        magnetic resonance imaging, 769
        post-traumatic amnesia, 768
    neuropsychological assessment
        child's self-esteem, 771
        clinical, 772–773
        parental information, 771
        qualitative information, 769–770
        research, 773–774

predictors of outcome, 779
premorbid factors, 778
socioeconomic status, 778
Peripheral nervous system (PNS)
    autonomic nervous system, 85
    catecholamine neurotransmitters, 97–100
    small molecule neurotransmitters, 96–97
Perisylvian area, 161
Personality Assessment Inventory (PAI), 534
Phenylketonurias (PKUS), 846–847
Physiological nonepileptic seizures (PhyNES),
    544
PICA. See Posterior Inferior Cerebellar
    arteries
PLE. See Parietal lobe epilepsy
PNES. See Psychogenic nonepileptic seizures
PNS. See Peripheral nervous system
Polysomnography studies, 822
Post-concussion syndrome
    brain damage, 757
    children, 755–757
    comorbities, 749
    diagnosis threat, 751–752
    DSM-IV, 746–748
    emotional significance, event, 750
    exaggeration, 754–755
    expectation as etiology, 750–751
    "good old days" bias, 751
    ICD-10, 746–748
    individual response, trauma, 750
    interview vs. questionnaire, 752–754
    lack of effort, 754–755
    non-specificity, 749
    stereotype threat, 751–752
    vulnerable personality styles, 750
Post-deployment screening methods,
    708–709
Posterior cortical epilepsies (PCEs), 469
Posterior inferior cerebellar arteries (PICA), 307
Post-ictal aphasia, 436
Post-ictal mood disorders, 436
Post-ictal psychosis, 436
Post-traumatic amnesia (PTA), 665, 700, 768
Post-traumatic epilepsy (PTE), 430
Post-traumatic seizure (PTS), 430–431
Post-traumatic stress disorder (PTSD), 535
Potentially progressive disorder, 460–462
Prefrontal cortex, 113
Premorbid cognitive ability, 16–17
Premotor cortex, 113
Presurgical epilepsy patients, 469–471
Pretectum, 69
Primary generalized tonic-clonic seizures, 433
Primary sensory-motor cortex, 103
Probably symptomatic partial epilepsies, 444

Progressive multifocal leukoencephalitis
    (PML), 649
Progressive myoclonus epilepsies, 437
Progressive supranuclear palsy (PSP),
    376–377, 581–582
Prosodic speech, 173–174
Prosopagnosia, 211
Pseudodementia, 392–394
Pseudotumor cerebri, 420, 855, 856
Psychiatric issues, in epilepsy
    anxiety disorders, 485–486
    broader psychopathology, 485–486
    depression, 484–502
Psychogenic nonepileptic seizures (PNES),
    406–407
    children and adolescents, 541
    epilepsy co-occurrence, 528
    etiology
        demographic correlation, 528–532
        psychiatric history, 533
        social history, 531
    medical history, 530
    neuropsychological assessment strategies,
        541–542
    subtypes, 537–538
Psychological testing
    configural patterns, 533
    depressed neurotics, 534
    neurocognitive function, 535
    patient profile, 534
    SVT failure, 536
Psychometric properties
    ceiling/floor effects, 904–906
    clinical practice
        classification system, 894–895
        neuropsychological test, 894
        performance, 894
    extrapolation/interpolation, 906–907
    interpretation, test scores, 911, 913
    measurement error, 903
    normal variability
        change over time, assessment,
            909–910
        clinical vignette, 908
        learning and memory index, 908
        neuropsychological battery, 908
        practice effect, 912, 918
        regression method, 916–917
        reliable change, 911–916
        score distribution, 910
    normative sample, adequacy
        BNT, 896
        clinical implications, 898
        comparison, 894–895
        CVLT vs. CVLT-II trials, 898

education and ethnicity, effects, 899
    IQ, 899
range, distribution (see Truncated
    distribution)
score magnitude and rank, 903–904
shape, distribution
    classic examples, 900
    normal curve, 900
    population, 902
Psychopathology, broader, 485–486
PTA. See Post-traumatic amnesia
PTE. See Post-traumatic epilepsy
PTS. See Post-traumatic seizure
PVN. See Paraventricular nucleus

Q
Quality of life (QOL), in epilepsy, 482–483

R
Radiation therapy, 797–798
RAM. See Rapid alternating movements
Rapid alternating movements (RAM), 50
Rassmussen's encephaolpathy
    behavioral symptoms, 848–850
    neuropathology, 850
    prevalence, onset, 848
RCI's. See Reliable change indices
Receptive aprosody, 173
Reflex epilepsies, 437
Refractory epilepsy, 450–451
    anterior temporal lobectomy, 452–453
    corpus callosotomy, 453
    deep brain stimulator implantation, 454–455
    hemispherectomy, 453
    multiple subpial transection, 453–454
    stereotaxic gamma-knife radiation
        treatment, 455
    vagus nerve stimulator implantation, 454
Reliability and validity
    alternate form, 879–880
    construct-related evidence, 889
    content-related evidence, 888–889
    criterion-related evidence, 890
    evaluation, 887–888
    internal reliability
        consistency, 876–878
        D-KEFS subtests, 877
        evaluation methods, 876
        Ruff Neurobehavioral Inventory
            (RNBI), 878
        Split-half reliability coefficients, 877
        WAIS-IV Information subtest, 875–876
    interrater reliability, 880–881

Reliability and validity (*cont.*)
   limitations
      novelty effect, 885
      practice effect, 884
      test score, 883
   neuropsychological measures, 891
   neuropsychology, 874–875
   split-half correlation, 877
   standardization, 875–876
   test–retest
      coefficients, 878–879
      correlation, 878
      score fluctuation, 879
   validity model, 886–887
Reliable change indices (RCI's), 493, 500,
      618, 622, 910–912
Retrograde amnesia, 666
Reynolds intellectual screening test (RIST), 801
Root reflex, 231
Ruff Neurobehavioral Inventory (RNBI), 878

S
SAH. *See* Subarachnoid hemorrhage
Secondarily generalized seizures, 432
Seizures
   classification
      focal seizures, 431–432
      generalized seizures, 432–434
   diagnosing, 427–429
   elective neurosurgical treatment, 451
   incidence of, 429–430
   medication treatment, 449–450
   post-ictal behaviors, 436
   prevalence of, 429–430
   semiology, 434–436
   symptoms of, 428–429
   treatment
      antiepileptic drugs, 449–450
      diet and behavioral therapies, 456
      presurgical evaluation, 456
      pre-surgical neuropsychological
         evaluation, 457
      refractory epilepsies, 450–455
Sensory pathways, 117
Sexual dysfunction, traumatic brain injuries, 676
Shape, distribution
   classic examples, 900
   normal curve, 900
   population, 901
Short-term memory, 181
Simple partial seizures, 431
Simultanagnosia, 211
Skull fractures, 667

Snout reflex, 231
Somatoform disorder
   definition/terminology
      diagnostic criteria, 552
      process, 551
      putative subtypes, 551–552
   etiology, 553–554
   malingering and factitious disorder
      definition/terminology, 554
      etiology, 555
      prevalence, 554–555
   prevalence, 553
   treatment, 560–561
Somatosensory hallucinations, 263
Sport-related concussion
   active rehabilitation, 736–737
   British Columbia Concussion
      Rehabilitation Program, 735
   classification systems
      American Academy of Neurology,
         726
      grading scales, 727
      simple–complex, 726–728
   evidenced-based neuropsychology
      automated neuropsychological
         assessment metrics, 732–733
      CogSport, 732
      computerized neuropsychological test
         batteries, 731
      HeadMinder Concussion Resolution
         Index, 732
      immediate post-concussion assessment
         and cognitive testing, 731
      NHL and NFL, 730
      symptom ratings, 733–734
   exertional steps, 735
   multiple, 728–729
   neurobiology and pathophysiology
      energy crisis, 725
      ionic shifts, 725
      mechanoporation, 723
   recovery time, 725–726
   retirement, 737–738
Steele-Richardson-Olszewski syndrome,
      376–377
Stereotaxic gamma-knife radiation treatment,
      455
Stiff-person syndrome, neuropsychological
      symptoms, 589
Subarachnoid hemorrhage (SAH), 300–303
Subcortical strokes, 347–348
Subdural and subarachnoid hematomas, 669
Substance abuse, traumatic brain injuries,
      684–685

Subthalamic nucleus (STN)
  basal ganglia circuitry function, 608
  neuropsychological outcome, 611–614
  Parkinson's disease, 604–605
Suck reflex, 232
Superior temporal sulcus (STS), 205
Symptomatic epilepsies, 442
Symptom validity test (SVT), 537

T
Tegmentum, 68
Temporal lobe, 117
Temporal lobe epilepsy (TLE)
  language deficits and seizure lateralization,
    464–466
  pathology associated with, 445
  post-operative findings, 467–468
  preoperative findings, 463–464
  risk factors for, 445
  taxonomic description, 466–467
  types of, 445–446
Test of memory malingering (TOMM), 902
Thalamic vascular syndromes, 331–332
Thalamotomy, 598, 600, 601
Thalamus, 69–73
Tonic seizures, 432–433
Tourette syndrome (TS)
  deep brain stimulation
    neuropsychological outcome, 637
    surgical inclusion/exclusion criteria,
      632–635
    thalamic, 636
  medication effects, 591
  neuropsychological symptoms, 586
Transcortical motor aphasia, 169, 272–273
Transcortical sensory aphasia, 275–276
Transient global amnesia, 410–411
Transient monocular blindness, 419
Transtheoretical model, 866–867
Traumatic brain injury (TBI), 1, 3, 7
  classification of, 666–667
  coma, 665–666
  epidemiology of, 664–665
  functional and neuropsychological
    outcome, 680–682
  Glasgow coma scale, 665
  loss of consciousness, 665–666
  neurological and neuropsychiatric problems
    anxiety disorders, 677–678
    balance and dizziness, 675
    cranial nerve impairments, 676
    depression, 677–678
    fatigue and sleep problems, 677

    headaches, 676
    lack of awareness, 679
    motor impairments and movement
      disorders, 674–675
    personality changes, apathy, and
      motivation, 679
    psychotic disorders, 678
    sexual dysfunction, 694
    visual impairments, 675
  neuropsychological assessment issues,
    683–684
  pathoanatomy and pathophysiology
    contusion, 667, 668
    coup/contrecoup injury, 667
    edema, 669–670
    hematomas, 668–669
    hemorrhage, 667–668
    neuroimaging, 673–674
    traumatic axonal injury, 671–673
    ventricular dilation, 671
  post-traumatic amnesia, 684
  psychosocial outcome
    community integration, 687
    marital and family issues, 686
    return to work, 685–686
    substance abuse, 684–685
  retrograde amnesia, 666
Tricresyl phosphate (TCP), 820
Truncated distribution, 902–903

U
Unified Parkinson's disease rating scale
  (UPDRS), 576
Unimodal cortex, 105

V
Vagus nerve stimulation (VNS), 454
Vagus nerve stimulator implantation, 454
Validity
  construct-related evidence, 888, 889
  content-related evidence, 888–889
  criterion-related evidence, 888, 890
  models, 886–887
  neuropsychology, 886
Vascular Parkinsonism, 583–584
Ventral intermediate nucleus (VIM),
  626–627
Ventral simultanagnosia, 211
Ventricular dilation, 671
Verbal auditory agnosia, 281–282
Verbal memory tests, 491
Visual hallucinations, 259–260

Visual loss
  giant cell arteritis, 420
  migraine, 419–420
  optic neuritis, 420
  pseudotumor cerebri, 420
  transient monocular blindness/amaurosis
      fugax, 419
Visual object agnosia, 209
Visuoperceptual/Visuoconstructional skills, 492
Visuospatial/visuoconstructional skills and
      motor praxis
  agnosia, 208–211
  anatomy, 202–204
  apraxia, 211–212
  assessment
    evaluation, 217
    hemisphere functions, 214
    laboratory, 217–218
    occulo-motor movement, 212–213
    recognition, 217
    screening, 214
  Balint's syndrome, 206–208

cortical blindness/"blind sight," 206
deficits, 205–206
visual processing "streams," 204–205
visuoperceptual distortions, 206
Vitamin B12 deficiency. See Cobalamin
    disorders
VNS. See Vagus nerve stimulation

W

Wada's procedure, epilepsy surgery
    contralateral side of surgery, 480–481
    ipsilateral side of surgery, 480
Wechsler adult intelligence scale (WAIS), 930
Wechsler memory scale (WMS), 930
Wernicke's aphasia, 170, 274–276
West's syndrome, 442
WHO Collaborating Center Task Force, 700
Whole-brain radiation therapy (WBRT), 798
Wilson's disease, 859–860
Wisconsin card sorting test (WCST), 902
World Health Organization (WHO), 794

CPSIA information can be obtained at www.ICGtesting.com
Printed in the USA
LVOW01*1047190114

370035LV00001B/1/P